Orthopaedic Basic Science

Foundations of Clinical Practice

FOURTH EDITION

Acknowledgments

Contributors

Matthew J. Allen, VetMB, PhD
Associate Professor, Small Animal Surgery
Department of Veterinary Clinical Sciences
The Ohio State University
Columbus, Ohio

Peter C. Amadio, MD
Lloyd A. and Barbara A. Amundson Professor of Orthopedic Surgery
Department of Orthopedic Surgery
Mayo Clinic
Rochester, Minnesota

Howard S. An, MD
The Morton International Endowed Chair
Professor of Orthopaedic Surgery
Director of Spine Surgery
Department of Orthopaedic Surgery
Rush University Medical Center
Chicago, Illinois

Mohit Bhandari, MD, MSc
Professor and Academic Chair
Department of Orthopaedic Surgery
McMaster University
Hamilton, Ontario, Canada

Suneel B. Bhat, MD, MPhil
Department of Orthopaedics
The Rothman Institute
Thomas Jefferson University Hospital
Philadelphia, Pennsylvania

Julius Bishop, MD
Assistant Professor
Department of Orthopaedic Surgery
Stanford University School of Medicine
Palo Alto, California

Kevin J. Bozic, MD, MBA
Associate Professor and Vice Chair
Department of Orthopaedic Surgery
University of California, San Francisco
San Francisco, California

Susan V. Bukata, MD
Associate Professor of Orthopaedics
Department of Orthopaedics
University of California, Los Angeles
Los Angeles, California

Jason P. Caffrey, BS
Graduate Student
Department of Bioengineering
University of California, San Diego
La Jolla, California

James D. Capozzi, MD
Chairman
Department of Orthopaedics
Winthrop University Hospital
Mineola, New York

James Cashman, MD
Arthroplasty Fellow
Department of Orthopaedics
Rothman Institute
Philadelphia, Pennsylvania

Di Chen, MD, PhD
Professor
Department of Orthopaedics
University of Rochester
Rochester, New York

Constance R. Chu, MD
Albert B. Ferguson Professor of Orthopaedic Surgery
Professor of Bioengineering
Vice Chair for Translational Research
Director, Cartilage Restoration Center
Department of Orthopaedic Surgery
University of Pittsburgh
Pittsburgh, Pennsylvania

Susan Chubinskaya, PhD
Professor, Associate Provost
Department of Biochemistry
Rush University Medical Center
Chicago, Illinois

P. Christopher Cook, MD, FRCSC
Associate Professor, Orthopaedics and Pediatrics
Department of Orthopaedics
University of Rochester
Rochester, New York

Charles L. Cox, MD, MPH
Assistant Professor
Department of Orthopaedic Surgery and Rehabilitation
Vanderbilt University Medical Center
Nashville, Tennessee

Tamim Diab, PhD
Research Scientist
Parker H. Petit Institute for Bioengineering and Bioscience
Georgia Institute of Technology
Atlanta, Georgia

Edward Diao, MD
Professor Emeritus
Department of Orthopaedic Surgery and Neurosurgery
University of California, San Francisco
San Francisco, California

M. Hicham Drissi, PhD
Director of Research
Department of Orthopaedics
University of Connecticut Health Center
Farmington, Connecticut

Reza Firoozabadi, MD
Assistant Professor, Traumatology
Department of Orthopaedic Surgery
Harborview Medical Center
University of Washington
Seattle, Washington

Hemanth Reddy Gadikota, MS
Research Scientist
Department of Orthopaedics
Massachusetts General Hospital
Boston, Massachusetts

Richard H. Gelberman, MD
Fred C. Reynolds Professor and Chairman
Department of Orthopaedic Surgery
Washington University School of Medicine
St. Louis, Missouri

Burhan Gharaibeh, PhD
Assistant Professor
Department of Orthopaedic Surgery
Stem Cell Research Center
University of Pittsburgh
Pittsburgh, Pennsylvania

Stuart B. Goodman, MD, PhD
Professor
Department of Orthopaedic Surgery
Stanford University School of Medicine
Redwood City, California

Hana Goto, BSc, MSc
Research Assistant
Department of Orthopaedic Surgery
Columbia University Medical Center
New York, New York

Chancellor F. Gray, MD
Instructor
Department of Orthopaedic Surgery
Hospital of the University of Pennsylvania
Philadelphia, Pennsylvania

Farshid Guilak, PhD
Laszlo Ormondy Professor
Department of Orthopaedic Surgery
Duke University Medical Center
Durham, North Carolina

Robert E. Guldberg, PhD
Director
Parker H. Petit Institute for Bioengineering and Bioscience
Professor
George W. Woodruff School of Mechanical Engineering
Georgia Institute of Technology
Atlanta, Georgia

Ali Hosseini, PhD
Research Fellow
Department of Orthopaedic Surgery
Massachusetts General Hospital/Harvard Medical School
Boston, Massachusetts

Johnny Huard, PhD
Professor
Department of Orthopaedic Surgery
Stem Cell Research Center
University of Pittsburgh
Pittsburgh, Pennsylvania

Wesley M. Jackson, PhD
Senior Researcher
Department of Surgery
Uniformed Services University
Bethesda, Maryland

Jeffrey N. Katz, MD, MSc
Professor of Medicine and Orthopedics
Department of Orthopedic Surgery
Brigham and Women's Hospital
Harvard Medical School
Boston, Massachusetts

Mary Ann Keenan, MD
Professor
Department of Orthopaedic Surgery
University of Pennsylvania
Philadelphia, Pennsylvania

Oran Kennedy, PhD
Assistant Professor
Biomedical Engineering
The City College of New York
New York, New York

Han-Soo Kim, MD, PhD
Professor
Department of Orthopaedic Surgery
Seoul National University
Seoul, Korea

Mininder S. Kocher, MD, MPH
Associate Director
Division of Sports Medicine
Department of Orthopaedics
Children's Hospital Boston
Boston, Massachusetts

Francis Y. Lee, MD
Chief of Musculoskeletal Tumor Service
Professor with Tenure and Vice Chair of Research
Department of Orthopaedic Surgery
Columbia University Medical Center
New York, New York

Seth S. Leopold, MD
Professor
Department of Orthopaedic and Sports Medicine
University of Washington School of Medicine
Seattle, Washington

Guoan Li, PhD
Director
Bioengineering Laboratory
Department of Orthopaedic Surgery
Massachusetts General Hospital
Harvard Medical School
Boston, Massachusetts

Jing-Sheng Li, MS
Department of Orthopaedic Surgery
Massachusetts General Hospital
Boston, Massachusetts

Elena Losina, PhD, MSc
Associate Professor of Medicine and Orthopedics
Department of Orthopedic Surgery
Brigham and Women's Hospital
Boston, Massachusetts

Lichun Lu, PhD
Associate Professor of Biomedical Engineering and Orthopedics
Department of Orthopedics
Mayo Clinic
Rochester, Minnesota

Robert J. Majeska, PhD
Professor
Department of Biomedical Engineering
The City College of New York
New York, New York

Anne-Marie Malfait, MD, PhD
Assistant Professor
Department of Biochemistry and Rheumatology
Rush University Medical Center
Chicago, Illinois

Kenneth A. Mann, PhD
Research Professor
Department of Orthopedic Surgery
SUNY Upstate Medical University
Syracuse, New York

Richard C. Mather III, MD
Assistant Professor
Division of Sports Medicine
Department of Orthopaedic Surgery
Duke University School of Medicine
Durham, North Carolina

Robert L. Mauck, PhD
Associate Professor
Department of Orthopaedic Surgery and Bioengineering
University of Pennsylvania
Philadelphia, Pennsylvania

Samir Mehta, MD
Chief, Orthopaedic Trauma and Fracture Service
Assistant Professor
Department of Orthopaedic Surgery
Hospital of the University of Pennsylvania
Philadelphia, Pennsylvania

Kofi A. Mensah, MD, PhD
Resident Physician
Department of Orthopaedic Surgery
Hospital for Special Surgery
New York, New York

Saam Morshed, MD, PhD, MPH
Assistant Professor
Orthopaedic Trauma Institute
University of California, San Francisco/San Francisco General Hospital
San Francisco, California

Issac L. Moss, MD, MASc, FRCSC
Assistant Professor
Department of Orthopaedic Surgery
University of Connecticut Health Center
Farmington, Connecticut

Saqib Nizami, BS
Research Associate
Center for Orthopaedic Research
Columbia University
New York, New York

Regis J. O'Keefe, MD, PhD
Professor and Chair
Associate Dean for Clinical Affairs
Department of Orthopaedics
University of Rochester Medical Center
Rochester, New York

Maurizio Pacifici, PhD
Director of Research
Division of Orthopaedic Surgery
The Children's Hospital of Philadelphia
Philadelphia, Pennsylvania

Javad Parvizi, MD, FRCS
Vice Chairman of Orthopaedic Surgery
Department of Orthopaedic Surgery
Rothman Institute
Philadelphia, Pennsylvania

Vincent D. Pellegrini Jr, MD
James L. Kernan Professor and Chair
Department of Orthopaedics
University of Maryland School of Medicine
Baltimore, Maryland

William Reichmann, MA
Biostatistician
Orthopedic and Arthritis Center for Outcomes Research
Brigham and Women's Hospital
Boston, Massachusetts

Katherine E. Reuther, BS
Graduate Student
Department of Bioengineering
University of Pennsylvania
Philadelphia, Pennsylvania

Rosamond Rhodes, PhD
Director, Bioethics Education
Professor, Medical Education
Mount Sinai School of Medicine
New York, New York

Robert L. Sah, MD, ScD
Professor
Department of Bioengineering
University of California, San Diego
La Jolla, California

James O. Sanders, MD
Professor of Orthopaedics and Pediatrics
Department of Orthopaedics and Rehabilitation
University of Rochester
Rochester, New York

Johannah Sanchez-Adams, PhD
Postdoctoral Associate
Department of Orthopaedic Surgery
Duke University
Durham, North Carolina

Mitchell B. Schaffler, PhD
CUNY and Wallace H. Coulter Distinguished Professor of Biomedical Engineering
Director, New York Center for Biomedical Engineering
Department of Biomedical Engineering
Grove School of Engineering
The City College of New York
New York, New York

Andrew H. Schmidt, MD
Professor
Department of Orthopaedic Surgery
University of Minnesota
Minneapolis, Minnesota

Sung Wook Seo, MD, PhD
Assistant Professor
Department of Orthopaedic Surgery
Sungkyunkwan University
Seoul, Korea

David Shearer, MD, MPH
Resident
Department of Orthopaedic Surgery
University of California, San Francisco
San Francisco, California

Louis J. Soslowsky, PhD
Professor and Center Director
Department of Orthopaedic Surgery
University of Pennsylvania
Philadelphia, Pennsylvania

Kurt P. Spindler, MD
Professor and Vice Chairman
Department of Orthopaedic Surgery and Rehabilitation
Vanderbilt University Medical Center
Nashville, Tennessee

Steven D. Stovitz, MD, MS
Associate Professor
Department of Family Medicine and Community Health
University of Minnesota
Minneapolis, Minnesota

Stavros Thomopoulos, PhD
Associate Professor
Department of Orthopaedic Surgery
Washington University
St. Louis, Missouri

Rocky S. Tuan, PhD
Director
Center for Cellular and Molecular Engineering
Department of Orthopaedic Surgery
University of Pittsburgh
Pittsburgh, Pennsylvania

Charles M. Turkelson, PhD
Senior Research Director
Center for Medical Technology Policy
Baltimore, Maryland

Wakenda Tyler, MD, MPH
Assistant Professor
Department of Orthopaedics
University of Rochester Medical Center
Rochester, New York

Kristy Weber, MD
Professor of Orthopaedic Surgery
Johns Hopkins School of Medicine
Baltimore, Maryland

Jennifer J. Westendorf, PhD
Professor of Biochemistry/Molecular Biology and Orthopedics
Department of Orthopedics
Mayo Clinic
Rochester, Minnesota

Nick J. Willett, PhD
Postdoctoral Fellow
George W. Woodruff School of Mechanical Engineering
Georgia Institute of Technology
Atlanta, Georgia

Markus A. Wimmer, PhD
Associate Professor
Department of Orthopaedic Surgery
Rush University Medical Center
Chicago, Illinois

Adam Wright, MD
Resident
Department of Orthopaedic Surgery
University of Pittsburgh
Pittsburgh, Pennsylvania

Michael J. Yaszemski, MD, PhD
Professor of Biomedical Engineering and Orthopedics
John and Posy Krehbiel Professor of Orthopedics Honoring
  Bernard F. Morrey, MD
Department of Orthopedics
Mayo Clinic
Rochester, Minnesota

Chunfeng Zhao, MD
Associate Professor of Orthopedics and Biomedical Engineering
Department of Orthopedic Surgery
Mayo Clinic
Rochester, Minnesota

Michael J. Zuscik, PhD
Associate Professor
Department of Orthopaedics
Center for Musculoskeletal Research
University of Rochester Medical Center
Rochester, Minnesota

Peer Reviewers

Derek Amanatullah, MD, PhD
Chief Resident
Department of Orthopaedic Surgery
University of California, Davis
Sacramento, California

Theodore A. Blaine, MD
Chief of Shoulder and Elbow Surgery
Department of Orthopaedics
Yale University
New Haven, Connecticut

W. Timothy Brox, MD
Program Director
Department of Orthopaedic Surgery
UCSF Fresno
Fresno, California

Brett D. Crist, MD
Associate Professor
Department of Orthopaedic Surgery
University of Missouri
Columbia, Missouri

Thomas A. DeCoster, MD
Professor Emeritus
Department of Orthopaedics and Rehabilitation
The University of New Mexico
Albuquerque, New Mexico

Christopher Evans, PhD
Müller Professor of Orthopaedic Surgery
Center for Advanced Orthopaedic Studies
Beth Israel Deaconess Medical Center
Boston, Massachusetts

Frank J. Frassica, MD
Professor of Orthopaedics and Oncology
Department of Orthopaedics
Johns Hopkins University
Baltimore, Maryland

Leesa M. Galatz, MD
Associate Professor
Department of Orthopaedic Surgery
Washington University School of Medicine
St. Louis, Missouri

Marc T. Galloway, MD
Cincinnati Sports Medicine
Montgomery, Ohio

Kevin L. Garvin, MD
Professor and Chair
Department of Orthopaedic Surgery and Rehabilitation
University of Nebraska Medical Center
Omaha, Nebraska

Shepard Hurwitz, MD
Executive Director
American Board of Orthopaedic Surgery
Chapel Hill, North Carolina

Young-Jo Kim, MD, PhD
Staff Surgeon
Department of Orthopaedic Surgery
Boston's Children's Hospital
Boston, Massachusetts

John S. Kirkpatrick, MD
Professor and Chair
Department of Orthopaedic Surgery
University of Florida College of Medicine, Jacksonville
Jacksonville, Florida

Joseph M. Lane, MD
Chief, Metabolic Bone Disease Service
Department of Orthopaedics
Hospital for Special Surgery
New York, New York

Francis Y. Lee, MD
Chief of Musculoskeletal Tumor Service
Professor with Tenure and Vice Chair of Research
Department of Orthopaedic Surgery
Columbia University Medical Center
New York, New York

Sheldon Suton Lin, MD
Associate Professor
Department of Orthopedic Surgery
University of Medicine and Dentistry of New Jersey
Newark, New Jersey

Ronald W. Lindsey, MD
Professor and Department Chairman
Holder of the John Sealy Distinguished Centennial Chair in
* Rehabilitation Sciences*
Department of Orthopaedic Surgery and Rehabilitation
The University of Texas Medical Branch
Galveston, Texas

Patricio Melean, MD
Orthopedic Surgeon
Shoulder Surgery and Upper Extremity Arthroscopy Unit
Hospital del Trabajador
Santiago, Chile

Anne N. Normand, MD
Orthopaedic Surgeon/Orthopaedic Oncologist
Department of Orthopaedic Surgery
Essentia Health – East
Duluth, Minnesota

James W. Ogilvie, MD
Consultant
Department of Genetic Research
Taueret Laboratories
Salt Lake City, Utah

Javad Parvizi, MD, FRCS
Vice Chairman of Orthopaedic Surgery
Department of Orthopaedic Surgery
Rothman Institute
Philadelphia, Pennsylvania

Jeffrey P. Rouleau, PhD
Senior Manager
Department of Strategy and Scientific Operations
Medtronic, Inc.
Minneapolis, Minnesota

Edward Schwarz, PhD
Professor
Department of Orthopaedics
University of Rochester
Rochester, New York

Kern Singh, MD
Assistant Professor
Department of Orthopaedic Surgery
Rush University Medical Center
Chicago, Illinois

David H. Sohn, JD, MD
Assistant Professor
Department of Orthopaedic Surgery
University of Toledo Medical Center
Toledo, Ohio

Nelson F. SooHoo, MD
Associate Professor
Department of Orthopaedic Surgery
UCLA School of Medicine
Los Angeles, California

Table of Contents

Section 3: Basic Principles and Treatment of Musculoskeletal Disease
Section Editor: Constance R. Chu, MD

Section 4: Clinical Science
Section Editor: Thomas A. Einhorn, MD

Preface

A thorough understanding of the science of the musculoskeletal system is the foundation for outstanding diagnostic skills, clinical judgment, and patient care. Surgery requires more than technical skills and knowledge of anatomy. Excellence in surgical performance requires a broad understanding of tissue structure and function, biomechanics, materials science, pharmacology, immunology, and physiology. The fourth edition of *Orthopaedic Basic Science: Foundations of Clinical Practice* is designed to provide an organized and efficient overview of the scientific principles that enable excellence in the care and management of orthopaedic diseases.

The text was produced to serve as a reference for the practicing orthopaedic surgeon. This edition has four interrelated sections. Section 1, Basic Principles of Orthopaedic Surgery, has content that includes cell and molecular biology, genetics, biomechanics, materials science, immunology, and clinical science. Major principles are presented using examples relevant to orthopaedic practice. Section 2, Physiology of Musculoskeletal Tissues, further extends basic scientific principles toward a more detailed understanding of the normal form and function of the musculoskeletal system. Chapters address growth and development and the physiology of the various tissues of the musculoskeletal system, such as muscle, bone, articular cartilage, tendon and ligament, and nerve. Because of its importance in orthopaedic care, one chapter is dedicated to the clotting system and thromboembolism. Section 3 is Basic Principles and Treatment of Musculoskeletal Disease. Although we are unable to provide a comprehensive review of orthopaedic conditions, this section provides broad insight into the pathophysiology of musculoskeletal diseases. Each of the chapters focuses on a particular musculoskeletal tissue. Particular attention is directed toward an understanding of the regenerative potential of the various tissues and the process of aging. Section 4, Clinical Science, is a new contribution to the fourth edition. The chapters cover the principles of evidence-based medicine, clinical trial design, cost-effectiveness research, healthcare guidelines, bias in research, decision analysis, biostatistics, and ethics in research. In aggregate, these chapters provide a concise overview of clinical research that will enable the practicing orthopaedic surgeon to more critically review findings and care recommendations presented in the orthopaedic literature.

The development of the fourth edition involved the collaborative effort of the American Academy of Orthopaedic Surgeons and the Orthopaedic Research Society. It required the concerted effort of a large number of individuals all dedicated to improving the lives of patients with musculoskeletal disease. The editors and authors wish to express their sincere appreciation to those members of the staff of the American Academy of Orthopaedic Surgeons, without whose tireless efforts this text would not have been possible: Hans Koelsch, PhD, Director of the Publications Department; Lisa Claxton Moore, Managing Editor; Deborah Williams, Senior Editor; Mary Steermann Bishop, Senior Manager, Production and Archives; Courtney Astle, Editorial Production Manager; Suzanne O'Reilly, Graphic Designer; and Karen Danca, Permissions Coordinator. All of these individuals worked with determination and incredible commitment to bring this information to you in such a complete, accurate, and attractive format. Finally, we would like to extend our appreciation for the patience and support of Dr. Evan Flatow, Chair of the AAOS Publications Committee, and the other members of the committee.

Regis J. O'Keefe, MD, PhD
Joshua J. Jacobs, MD
Constance R. Chu, MD
Thomas A. Einhorn, MD

Section I

Basic Principles of Orthopaedic Surgery

Section Editor

Regis J. O'Keefe, MD, PhD

Chapter 1

Molecular and Cell Biology in Orthopaedics

Francis Y. Lee, MD   M. Hicham Drissi, PhD

Michael J. Zuscik, PhD   Di Chen, MD, PhD

Saqib Nizami, BS   Hana Goto, BSc, MSc

Introduction

Although modern medicine has traditionally branched out into numerous medical subspecialties, there has been a recent surge in scientific interdisciplinary translational research since 2000. History in medicine highlights the importance of interdisciplinary research. Significant innovations have been made in the field of orthopaedic surgery because of parallel advances in physics, engineering, material science, chemistry, and biologic science. Breakthrough developments such as CT and MRI, artificial joints, polymethyl methacrylate, fiberglass, arthroscopy, antibiotics, and recombinant proteins have drastically changed orthopaedic practice. Behind these advancements were numerous collaborative efforts between clinicians and basic scientists. These collaborations have yielded a myriad of achievements such as the discovery of insulin,[1] bone morphogenetic protein (BMP) as a bone generation agent,[2] and the first prototype of MRI, which was used to differentiate normal versus tumor cells through nuclear magnetic resonance.[3] Some of these advances have changed the face of orthopaedic diagnostics and treatment.

More recently, the discovery of induced pluripotent stem (iPS) cells opened a new avenue in medical science. iPS cells

Dr. Drissi or an immediate family member serves as a paid consultant to or is an employee of Merck and has received research or institutional support from Merck. Dr. Chen or an immediate family member has received research or institutional support from Amgen. None of the following authors nor any immediate family member has received anything of value from or owns stock in a commercial company or institution related directly or indirectly to the subject of this chapter: Dr Lee, Dr. Zuscik, Mr. Nizami, and Ms. Goto.

were formed by introducing *Oct4*, *Sox2*, *Klf4*, and *cMyc* genes into fibroblasts.[4]

Due to an intricate melding of orthopaedic and basic science knowledge, a plethora of new drugs based on cellular and molecular mechanisms have been introduced over the past 10 years. Orthopaedic surgeons are becoming more aware of personalized medicine, customized medicine, targeted therapy, disease-modifying drugs, compounds, small molecules, growth factors, gene therapy, platelet-rich plasma (PRP), hyaluronic acid, and stem cells. Advancement of orthopaedic care and therapeutic avenues is largely dependent on an integrated education, comprising research techniques applied with clinical knowledge. Patients and the public will expect orthopaedic surgeons to be familiar with the new wave of scientific advances. This chapter will provide information on clinically relevant translational science, research utility, and therapeutic applications.

Clinically Relevant Growth Factors and Cytokines

Musculoskeletal tissues continuously adapt to genetic queues and external environments. Bone mass is tightly regulated by many bone-active cytokines, physical loading, drugs, and genetic mutations (**Figure 1**). Likewise, chondrocytes in the growth plate, articular cartilage, and fracture callus respond to growth factors and cytokines. Growth factors are cytokines and messengers that enable musculoskeletal cells to communicate with local environments and remote organs. For example, osteocytes respond to parathyroid hormone (PTH) or mechanical loading by secreting proteins such as receptor activator of nuclear factor–κB ligand (RANKL) and sclerostin to regulate osteoblastic bone formation and osteoclastic bone resorption (**Figure 2**). Updating knowledge on functions of growth

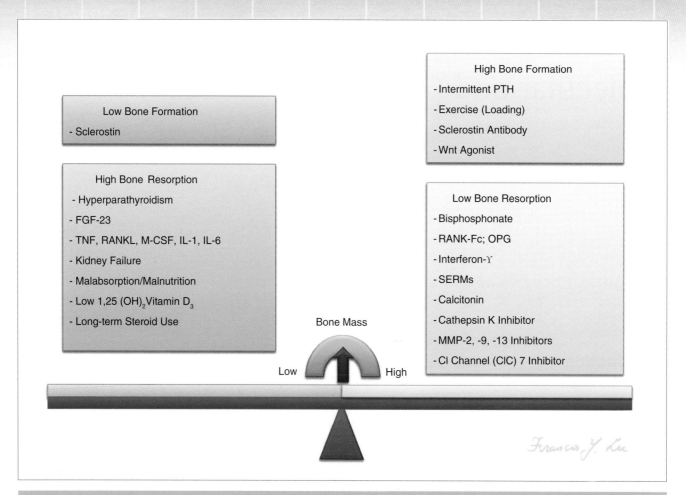

High Bone Formation
- Intermittent PTH
- Exercise (Loading)
- Sclerostin Antibody
- Wnt Agonist

Low Bone Formation
- Sclerostin

High Bone Resorption
- Hyperparathyroidism
- FGF-23
- TNF, RANKL, M-CSF, IL-1, IL-6
- Kidney Failure
- Malabsorption/Malnutrition
- Low 1,25 $(OH)_2$ Vitamin D_3
- Long-term Steroid Use

Low Bone Resorption
- Bisphosphonate
- RANK-Fc; OPG
- Interferon-γ
- SERMs
- Calcitonin
- Cathepsin K Inhibitor
- MMP-2, -9, -13 Inhibitors
- Cl Channel (ClC) 7 Inhibitor

Bone Mass

Low   High

Francis Y. Lee

Figure 1 Biologic factors and pharmacologic drugs affecting bone mass. FGF = fibroblast growth factor; TNF = tumor necrosis factor; M-CSF = macrophage colony-stimulating factor, IL = interleukin; OPG = osteoprotegerin; SERMs = selective estrogen receptor modulators; MMP = matrix metalloproteinase. (Courtesy of Francis Y. Lee, MD, New York, NY.)

factors and cytokines is important to understand emerging drugs for the treatment of osteoporosis or arthritis.

Growth Factors and Hormones (Proteins Affecting Musculoskeletal Cell Function)

Growth factors are proteins that have diverse effects on cellular differentiation, proliferation, and function. These processes are important for development and repair of musculoskeletal disorders. All musculoskeletal tissues produce and respond to growth factors. These proteins activate cell surface receptors either on the same cell (autocrine stimulation) or on nearby cells (paracrine stimulation). Growth factors such as BMPs are used to treat orthopaedic conditions. Conversely, growth factors such as vascular endothelial growth factor (VEGF) are therapeutic targets of cancers.

Bone Morphogenetic Proteins

BMPs are a subfamily of the transforming growth factor–β (TGF-β) superfamily of growth factors.[5] These dimeric dis-

ulfide proteins are involved in the regulation of tooth development, limb development, dorsal patterning of the spinal cord, and bone formation.[6] BMPs are the first known growth factors that induce bone and cartilage formation.[6,7] BMP-1 is a metalloprotease that functions as a C-propeptidase for types I, II, and III collagen. BMP-2 is a growth factor that strongly induces chondrogenic differentiation of mesenchymal cells.[7] BMPs -5, -6, and -7 are closely related and are effective osteoinductive agents. BMP-6 and BMP-7 are located in hypertrophic cartilage and promote the endochondral calcification pathway. BMP expression is also critical for the induction of programmed cell death (apoptosis) in the interdigital web spaces during embryonic development.[6]

Three BMP receptors have been identified that are similar to the TGF-β receptors.[6] There are two type I receptors, A and B, and one type II receptor. Similar to TGF-β, activation of BMP receptors leads to nuclear transport of Smad transcription factors for gene expression.[8] Abnormal function of a BMP type I receptor is associated with fibrodysplasia ossificans progressiva, which is characterized by excessive ectopic bone formation in the soft tissues.

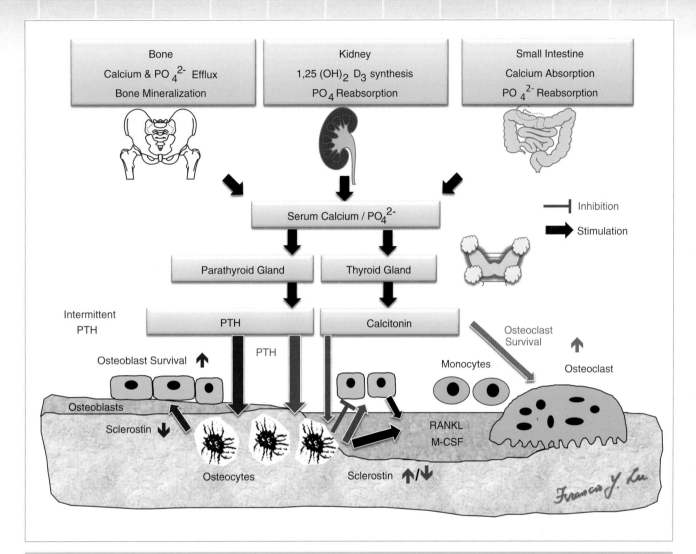

Figure 2 Modern concept of bone homeostasis. Cells use hormones, growth factors, and cytokines to orchestrate communications between cells and regulate intracellular signaling pathways. Osteocytes orchestrate bone homeostasis and other organs by secreting sclerostin, RANKL, and fibroblast growth factor–23. Chief cells of the parathyroid gland and follicular cells of the thyroid gland sense serum calcium and phosphorus concentrations regulated by the kidney, bone, and intestine. PTH acts on osteoblasts and osteocytes, induces secretion of sclerostin and RANKL by osteocytes, and stimulates RANKL secretion by osteoblasts. Sclerostin inhibits osteoblastic bone formation, RANKL promotes osteoclast formation and bone resorption. Calcitonin inhibits sclerostin formation and inhibits osteoclast apoptosis. Intermittent PTH prolongs osteoblast survival and decreases serum sclerostin. These networks of feedback mechanisms maintain bone mass. (Courtesy of Francis Y. Lee, MD, New York, NY.)

Transforming Growth Factor–β

TGF-β comprises a family of structurally related dimeric growth factors[9] and is also classified as a cytokine. TGF-β is produced by many different types of cells including osteoblasts, chondrocytes, and cancer cells. TGF-β signaling has many diverse implications in pathogenesis and therapeutics. TGF-β stimulates proliferation of cells of mesenchymal origin except for normal epithelial cells.[9] Activation of TGF-β is achieved by acidic conditions, heat, or enzymatic cleavage. Binding of this factor to the heteromeric TGF-β receptor initiates signaling cascades leading to the activation of transcription factors collectively known as Smads.[8]

TGF-β signaling has been implicated in metastatic bone cancers, carpal tunnel syndrome, and arthritis. In bone, TGF-β is stored in bone matrix in a latent form. During bone resorption by osteoclasts, TGF-β is released from the bone matrix, and the acidic pH activates the protein. In metastatic breast cancer, breast cancer cells stimulate osteoclastic bone resorption, and released TGF-β promotes cancer cell growth, increases angiogenesis, and inhibits host immune cells. TGF-β stimulates proteoglycan synthesis in chondrocytes and osteoblast proliferation as well as matrix synthesis.[9,10] In Marfan syndrome, excessive TGF signaling was demonstrated in the pathogenesis of aortic dilatation.

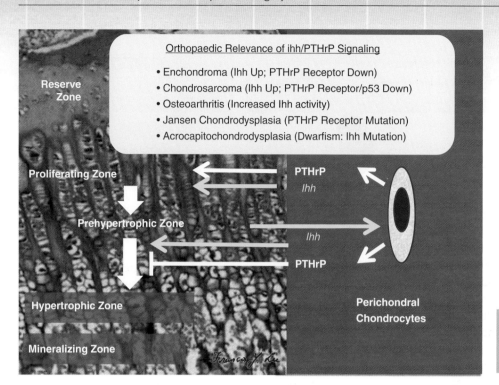

Orthopaedic Relevance of ihh/PTHrP Signaling

• Enchondroma (Ihh Up; PTHrP Receptor Down)
• Chondrosarcoma (Ihh Up; PTHrP Receptor/p53 Down)
• Osteoarthritis (Increased Ihh activity)
• Jansen Chondrodysplasia (PTHrP Receptor Mutation)
• Acrocapitochondrodysplasia (Dwarfism: Ihh Mutation)

Figure 3 Ihh/PTHrP signaling in growth plate chondrocytes.

TGF-targeting antisense peptides or drugs (angiotensin II type I receptor blockers) prevented the progression of such fibrillin-1 deficiency-related Marfan phenotypes. PRP, which gained popularity for the treatment of tendon or arthritis-related disorders, also contains TGF-β.

Parathyroid Hormone and Parathyroid Hormone-Related Peptide

PTH (PTH1-84) consists of 84 amino acids. PTH regulates serum calcium concentration by acting on bone, kidney, and intestine. In bone, osteoblasts have PTH receptors and promote osteoclast formation by producing RANKL in response to PTH. In kidney, PTH stimulates calcium reabsorption and 1,25-dihydroxyvitamin D_3, which then promotes calcium reabsorption in the small intestine. PTH1-34 is a shorter version of PTH1-84 and can activate PTH signaling by binding PTH receptors. In contrast, PTH has anabolic effects on bone (higher bone turnover with more bone formation than resorption) when it is given subcutaneously once a day. Daily injection of PTH1-34 is approved for treatment of osteoporosis by the Food and Drug Administration (FDA). Parathyroid hormone-related protein (PTHrP) is a group of proteins whose structure is similar to that of PTH. PTHrP consists of 139 to 173 amino acids but the first six amino acids in the N-terminal region are identical to PTH. PTHrP and PTH share a common receptor known as the PTH/PHThrP receptor. Therefore, PTHrP has functions similar to PTH.[11,12] It was initially identified in hypercalcemia of malignant tumors, which overproduced this growth factor. PTHrP is a locally acting growth factor or hormone that regulates endochondral bone formation,

growth plate development, and oncogenesis. Activation of the PTH/PTHrP receptor results in induction of signaling proteins, including protein kinase A, phospholipase C, and protein kinase C.[12] These protein activations lead to altered gene transcription. PTHrP stimulates the proliferation of chondrocytes and the suppression of genes involved in chondrocyte maturation.[13]

Indian Hedgehog

Indian hedgehog (Ihh) is a critical factor for chondrocyte and osteoblast differentiation during prenatal bone formation.[14] This growth factor is also important for the maintenance of the growth plate and postnatal skeletal growth.[11] Ihh is present in the prehypertrophic chondrocytes, and promotes chondrocyte proliferation and further differentiation into hypertrophic chondrocytes. Ihh protein secreted from prehypertrophic chondrocytes is dissipated through the cartilage matrix and interacts with perichondral cells that subsequently produce PTHrP. PTHrP provides a negative feedback signal to prehypertrophic chondrocytes undergoing hypertrophic differentiation and maintain a pool of proliferating chondrocytes in the growth plate during skeletal immaturity[14] (**Figure 3**). Mice studies showed the importance of Ihh signaling in endochondral bone formation.[15] Mutation of the Ihh gene is associated with brachydactyly. Normal articular cartilage does not have active Ihh signaling. Osteophytes, a classic sign of osteoarthritis, are formed during pathologic endochondral ossification of quiescent articular chondrocytes. Ihh may be used as a diagnostic marker of osteoarthritis, and Ihh blockers may also be potential targeted therapy for osteoarthritis in the future.

Multiple osteochondromatosis (Ollier disease) has been associated with an increase in Ihh signaling and enhanced cell proliferation by mutations of PTH type I receptor and subsequent loss of Ihh/PTHrP negative feedback.

Insulin-like Growth Factors

Insulin-like growth factors (IGFs; also known as somatomedin C) are anabolic hormone-like proteins whose structure is similar to that of insulin. IGFs regulate a variety of processes in the skeletal muscles, including growth, differentiation, and homeostasis of adult tissues, and include IGF-1 and IGF-2.[16] In a normoxic microenvironment, activation of IGF receptors leads to myoblast differentiation. However, in a hypoxic microenvironment, myoblast differentiation is inhibited and cellular proliferation is stimulated by the activation of the IGF receptors. In addition to these IGF receptors, there is another group of proteins that interact with IGF. These proteins are collectively known as IGF binding proteins and they regulate the activity and availability of this growth factor.[16] IGF-1 deficiency is associated with dwarfism because of the ineffective relaying of signals between growth hormone and growth plates. Aberrant activation of IGF signaling is seen in osteosarcomas.

Fibroblast Growth Factors

Fibroblast growth factors (FGFs) are a group of growth factors found in the matrix of the cartilage and also in the bone tissues.[17] Of the 23 members of this family, FGF-1 and FGF-2 are the most common growth factors present in these tissues.[17] In conjunction with heparin or heparan sulfate, FGFs activate FGF receptors, leading to the activation of signaling cascades and genes involved in cellular processes.[17] These cellular processes include migration, proliferation, apoptosis, angiogenesis, and wound healing. FGF receptor types 1 and 2 (FGFR1 and FGFR2) mutation is associated with craniosynostosis. FGFR3 signaling normally suppresses chondrocyte proliferation. Gain-of-function mutation of FGFR3 causes constitutively active FGFR3 signaling that in turn causes suppression of normal endochondral ossification in achondroplasia. FGF-23 was identified as a causative factor in tumor-induced osteomalacia. FGF-23 inhibits phosphate reabsorption in the proximal renal tubule and also inhibits 1α-hydroxylase, resulting in decreased 1,25-dihydroxyvitamin D_3 levels.

Vascular Endothelial Growth Factor

VEGF is another growth factor that stimulates angiogenesis, which is an important step in not only endochondral bone formation but also bone regeneration.[18] VEGF is produced by the endothelial cells and the bone marrow stromal cells. It is also produced by osteoblasts when there is a bone injury and a bone repair process is necessary.[18] Cancers are associated with autonomous and increased angiogenesis. VEGF-targeting agents are undergoing clinical trials.

Low-Density Lipoprotein Receptor–Related Protein–5 and Wnts

Skeletal radiographs of patients with genetic diseases led to the discovery of many important signaling pathways that have great therapeutic implications. Osteoporosis-pseudoglioma syndrome is associated with loss of bone mass and is caused by loss-of-function mutation of low-density lipoprotein receptor–related protein–5 (LRP5). LRP5 gain-of-function mutation is associated with autosomal recessive osteopetrosis. Further mechanistic studies revealed that LRP5 is linked to Wnt signaling. LRP5 is a coreceptor of the Wnt signaling pathways. The Wnt proteins are a family of highly conserved secreted glycoproteins that act as short-range ligands for receptor-mediated signaling pathways, including those that regulate processes throughout embryonic development and tissue homeostasis.[19] Bone mass–enhancing drugs may be designed by enhancing Wnt signaling pathways. Therefore, it becomes important to understand Wnt signaling pathways. The critical and best characterized form of Wnt signaling is the canonical Wnt pathway,[20] which functions by regulating the amount of the transcriptional coactivator β-catenin and controls key developmental gene expression programs (**Figure 4**). In the absence of Wnt, β-catenin is translated and subsequently marked for degradation by the action of the destruction complex, which is composed of the scaffolding protein Axin1/Axin2, the tumor suppressor adenomatous polyposis coli gene product, casein kinase 1, and glycogen synthase kinase 3.[21] This protein complex promotes the phosphorylation of β-catenin, which leads to its ubiquitination by β-TrCP, an E3 ubiquitin ligase subunit, and to its degradation by 26S proteasome. The Wnt/β-catenin pathway is activated when a Wnt ligand binds to the seven-pass transmembrane Frizzled (Fzd) receptor and its coreceptor, LRP5, or its closely related family member, LRP6.[20] The formation of a Wnt-Fzd-LRP6 complex, together with the recruitment of the scaffolding protein Disheveled (Dvl), results in LRP5/6 phosphorylation and activation and the recruitment of the destruction complex. These events lead to inhibition of the destruction complex, thereby blocking the degradation of β-catenin. β-catenin then accumulates in the nucleus, binds to lymphoid enhancer–binding factor and T cell factor proteins, and activates Wnt-targeted gene expression. Wnt proteins produced by the bone marrow cells and hematopoietic stem cells promote the proliferation and self-renewal of these stem cells. Wnt signaling positively regulates bone mass by promoting the differentiation of mesenchymal stem cells into osteoblasts.[22] In addition, Wnt inhibits osteoclastogenesis by increasing osteoprotegerin (OPG) expression in osteoblasts.[23] OPG is a decoy receptor for RANKL and can inhibit the differentiation of osteoclast precursors. Wnt signaling is inhibited by sclerostin secreted by osteocytes. These dynamic interactions centering on Wnt signaling are logical therapeutic targets to treat osteoporosis by enhancing Wnt signaling or inhibiting sclerostin.

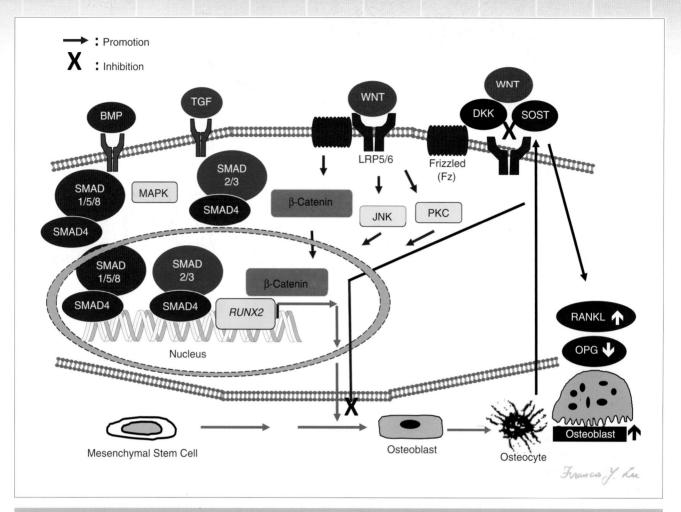

Figure 4 Regulation of bone mass by Wnt signaling. Examples of cell signaling pathways and therapeutic implications. Cytokines, growth factors, kinases, and transcription factors are communicating proteins among organs and cells for skeletal growth and adaptation. Transcription factor activates target gene promoters that regulate synthesis of mRNA and subsequent protein synthesis. Proteins determine phenotypes and function. BMP/TGF signaling via β-catenin and Wnt signaling promotes osteoblastic differentiation. Bone mass is tightly regulated by osteocytes. SOST and DKK from osteocytes negatively regulate osteoblast differentiation by inhibiting Wnt signaling. SOST increases osteoclast formation by increasing RANKL and by decreasing OPG. Wnt agonist or SOST inhibitors increase bone mass and such agents are on clinical trials as of 2013. RANKL blockers such as RANK:Fc (denosumab) are approved by the FDA for the treatment of select osteoporosis and metastatic bone cancers. SOST = Sclerostin; Wnt (Wingless + Integration 1); DKK = *dickkopf* protein; PKC & JNK = kinases; SMAD = SMA gene in C. Elegans + Mothers Against Decapentaplegic in Drosophila. (Courtesy of Francis Y. Lee, MD, New York, NY.)

Cytokines

The cytokines are a diverse group of proteins that modulate immune response and cellular communication. These proteins act on cell membrane receptors, leading to changes in cellular behavior and function. Although cytokines are essential for cellular response to occur, dysregulation of these proteins has been implicated in diseases such as inflammatory arthritis and hypercalcemia due to an increased osteoclastic bone resorption. This section describes the major cytokines and their roles in the musculoskeletal system.

Tumor Necrosis Factor

Tumor necrosis factor (TNF) is a proinflammatory cytokine that stimulates inflammation in response to viral infections and cancer.[24] This cytokine has been shown to regulate osteoclast differentiation and bone resorption. As a result, there is a marked increase in activity in inflammatory joint diseases and osteolytic disorders. TNF works synergistically with another cytokine (RANKL) to stimulate osteoclastogenesis. Furthermore, TNF was shown to stimulate RANKL independent osteoclast differentiation in the presence of macrophage colony-stimulating factor (M-CSF) cytokine. TNF-signaling targeting is currently used to modify inflammatory arthritis.

1: Basic Principles of Orthopaedic Surgery

Interleukins

Like TNF, interleukin-1 (IL-1) is also a proinflammatory cytokine that stimulates inflammation.[24] It plays a major role in innate immune response and causes the expression of proinflammatory genes in macrophages, monocytes, endothelial cells, and epithelial cells.[24] In addition, IL-1 promotes gene expression in chondrocytes and induces bone resorption.[25] This cytokine was shown to enhance TNF-induced osteoclastogenesis in bone marrow stromal cells and the formation of multinucleated osteoclasts.[26,27] IL-1 has been implicated in pathologic conditions such as osteoporosis and inflammatory joint diseases.[28] IL-6 is a proinflammatory cytokine produced during inflammation and is important for B cell maturation. IL-6 is produced by osteoblastic cells, bone marrow stromal cells, and synovial cells that have been stimulated with IL-1 and TNF.[29] The role of IL-6 in bone resorption remains controversial. In vitro studies of osteoclasts revealed that IL-6 activates osteoclasts indirectly by stimulating the expression of factors that induce osteoclast activity. However, this cytokine was also shown to reduce RANKL-induced osteoclast formation and bone resorption in both mouse and human cell lines.[27] Nevertheless, this cytokine is known to mediate bone pathology in several diseases, such as Paget disease and giant cell tumors of the bone.[27] IL-6 receptor blocking antibody is currently being tried for the treatment of rheumatoid arthritis. IL-7 is a cytokine important for the development of memory T cells after an infection.[30] IL-7 plays a role in bone homeostasis, but its exact role in the bone tissues remains uncertain. Several studies have reported IL-7 involvement in osteoclastogenic activity, whereas other studies have shown the role of this cytokine in bone formation and inhibition of osteoclastogenesis.[27] IL-10 is a cytokine that opposes proinflammatory cytokine activities (IL-6, IL-1, and TNF-α).[24] This anti-inflammatory cytokine is produced by numerous immune cells, including T cells, B lymphocytes, and mast cells.[31] Although IL-10 inhibits the production of cytokines involved in inflammation and allergy, it stimulates humoral and cytotoxic immune responses.[24] IL-10 has been shown to attenuate localized inflammation, such as in the case of rheumatoid arthritis and infections of the bone.[27] The IL-17 family of cytokines has numerous immune regulatory functions. Its major notable function is in inducing and mediating proinflammatory responses. The production of various cytokines and chemokines is influenced by IL-17, including IL-6, granulocyte M-CSF, IL-1β, TGF-β, and TNF-α as well as IL-8 and monocyte chemoattractant protein–1. IL-17 interacts with a wide range of cell types such as fibroblasts, endothelial cells, keratinocytes, and macrophages. However, its function is crucial for CD4+ (T helper or Th17) cells, which play a role in many autoimmune diseases, such as rheumatoid arthritis. IL-17 inhibitors are currently being tested as treatment for rheumatoid arthritis, among other diseases.

Transforming Growth Factor–β

As mentioned previously, TGF-β is a growth factor and a cytokine[31] stored in the tissues of the cartilage and bone.[27] As a cytokine, TGF-β acts as a chemoattractant and regulator of IL-1 and other cytokines. Furthermore, it has a role in the stimulation of Th17 cells based on IL-17 expression. TGF-β has been shown to regulate the proliferation and differentiation of osteoprogenitors. In addition, TGF-β is activated by the acidic pH of the resorption pits. The active cytokine induces the migration of bone MSCs to the bone remodeling sites, resulting in the change of bone processes from bone resorption to bone formation.[32]

Interferon-γ

Interferon-γ (IFN-γ) is a type II IFN produced by T cells and natural killer cells.[24] This cytokine is responsible for cell-mediated immunity.[31] Furthermore, IFN-γ has been shown to regulate osteoclast function and formation in human and mouse studies. This cytokine inhibits osteoclastogenesis in vitro, but in vivo experiments revealed an opposite effect.[27]

Receptor Activator of Nuclear Factor–κB Ligand

RANKL belongs to the TNF superfamily of proteins.[27] RANKL, which is produced by osteoblasts, acts as a potent inducer of osteoclast formation and activity[33] and is necessary and required for osteoclast precursor cell differentiation into mature osteoclasts both in vitro and in vivo. Thus, mice lacking RANKL expression develop a severe form of osteopetrosis due to the failure of osteoclast formation.[27] RANKL binds to its specific receptor RANK on the surface of monocyte/macrophage cell populations to trigger a series of signaling pathways essential for the expression of genes required for osteoclast precursor cell fusion and osteoclast function.[27] RANKL has been a successful drug target for osteoporosis as decreased RANKL expression results in inhibited bone loss in osteoporotic patients. The use of anti-RANKL therapy for giant cell tumor of bone is under way.

Macrophage Colony-Stimulating Factor

M-CSF was initially identified as a modulator of macrophage formation;[33,34] it was soon shown to be necessary for proper osteoclast formation. The essential role of M-CSF in osteoclast formation was demonstrated in mice that possessed a spontaneous mutation resulting in a severe osteopetrotic phenotype (op/op mice).[27] These mice were found to be osteopetrotic due to the absence of M-CSF production. This lack of production caused a defect in macrophage/monocyte formation, which resulted in absence of osteoclasts. It is important to know that in addition to its osteoclastogenic potential, partly through enhancing RANK expression, M-CSF also regulates macrophage survival and osteoclast formation.[27]

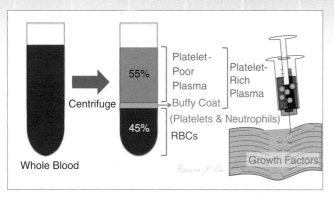

Figure 5 Platelet-rich plasma. (Courtesy of Francis Y. Lee, MD, New York, NY.)

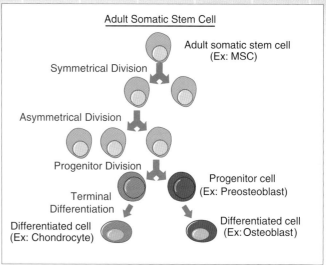

Figure 6 Process of adult somatic stem cell creation.

Osteoprotegerin

OPG, also known as TNFRSF-11B, is a RANKL decoy receptor[33] that belongs to the TNF family of secreted receptors and has the capacity to block osteoclast formation.[27] OPG-overexpressed mice exhibit an osteopetrotic phenotype, whereas OPG knockout mice are severely osteoporotic.[27] OPG, which is secreted by osteoblasts, can also bind to the TNF-like ligand TNF-related apoptosis-inducing ligand.[27]

Platelet-Rich Plasma

PRP is the platelet-enriched fluid portion of whole blood that is separated from red blood cells (RBCs). Plasma consists of approximately 55% whole blood. Plasma contains water (approximately 93%), electrolytes, proteins, and hormones. Cellular components (RBCs, neutrophils, and platelets) are approximately 45% volume fraction of whole blood. Among these, neutrophils and platelets form a buffy coat layer when the whole blood is centrifuged (**Figure 5**). PRP is a mixture of plasma and platelets in the buffy coat, and has a collection of numerous autologous growth factors and cytokines. Platelets contain growth factors and cytokines such as platelet-derived growth factor (PDGF), TGF, IGF, VEGF, and IL-8. PRP has been used in an attempt to promote healing of tendon, ligament, muscle, and cartilage injuries. The ultimate therapeutic efficacy is still uncertain, and evidence supporting the use of PRP requires additional translational research and well-controlled clinical trials.

Stem Cells

Stem cell technologies are being developed with the goal to cure challenging medical conditions such as spinal cord injuries, advanced arthritis, ophthalmologic disorders, and other neurologic disorders. Orthopaedic surgeons are the pioneers in the use of stem cell technology in the delivery of fresh autologous bone marrow for the treatment of bone cysts and nonunions.

Adult Somatic Stem Cells

Adult somatic stem cells are undifferentiated cells in the body that are capable of self-renewal and multipotency.[35] They can divide indefinitely without differentiating and are also capable of generating cells from various cell types (**Figure 6**). This is accomplished through two types of cell division. Symmetrical division allows the somatic stem cells to self-renew and create more somatic stem cells. Asymmetrical division produces a stem cell and a progenitor cell, which eventually differentiates into a particular cell. Progenitor cells are also capable of undergoing multiple divisions without differentiating. There are mesenchymal stem cells (MSCs), hematopoietic stem cells, and neural stem cells. MSCs are adult somatic stem cells that can differentiate into chondrocytes, osteoblasts, fibroblasts, tenocytes, and adipocytes.[35] MSCs can be cultured and differentiated in vitro to provide osteoprogenitor cells, autologous chondrocyte grafts, and other regenerative applications. MSCs are discussed later in this chapter.

Embryonic Stem Cells

Embryonic stem (ES) cells are pluripotent, capable of self-renewal, and harvested from the inner cell mass (ICM) of a blastocyst[36] (**Figure 7**). Pluripotency is the ability to differentiate into any of the three germ layers: mesoderm, endoderm, or ectoderm. This plasticity is unlike adult stem cells, which generally are only multipotent within the lineage. Under the right conditions, ES cells can replicate and stay undifferentiated, thereby propagating more stem cells. Because of these characteristics, ES cells provide a rich ability to study a wide range of diseases as well as the potential for tissue regeneration. However, ES cells might suffer from a graft-versus-host response. This can be mitigated through the use of techniques such as therapeutic cloning to generate the blastocyst and ICM.

iPS Cells

iPS cells are an artificially derived form of pluripotent stem cells (**Figure 8**). Differentiated adult cells are taken from a host to be induced into stem cells by viral transfection of stem cell–associated genes such as *Sox2*, *Oct3/4*, *c-Myc*, and *Klf4* as well as other possible genes to enhance induction ability. iPS cells were successfully reprogrammed by these genes to an ES cell–like state through various functions.[4] *Sox2* (SRY-box2: sex-determining region Y box-2) is an essential factor in self-renewal in undifferentiated ES cells. The SOX family of transcription factors is important in the regulation of embryonic development and cell fate determination. *Oct3/4* encodes for a transcription factor that is vitally important in promoting the self-renewal of undifferentiated cells. In *Oct3/4* knockdown experiments, it has been shown that cells start to differentiate in the absence of *Oct3/4*. *c-Myc* is a proto-oncogene that encodes for a transcription factor that is responsible for regulating the expression of 15% of all genes, many of which are involved in cell proliferation. In iPS cells, *c-Myc* is used for these cell proliferative effects, but aberrant behavior or mutations in the gene can lead to an increased risk of cancer. Scientists are trying to optimize iPS cells by reducing tumor formation or

by replacing with other genes. *Klf4* (Kruppel-like factor 4) plays roles in cell proliferation, differentiation, and survival by working in concert with other transcription factors as a transcriptional activator or repressor. *Nanog* is a transcription factor that promotes pluripotency in ES cells (not shown in **Figure 8**).

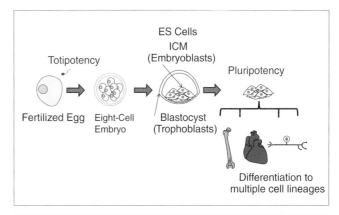

Figure 7 Process of embryonic stem cell creation.

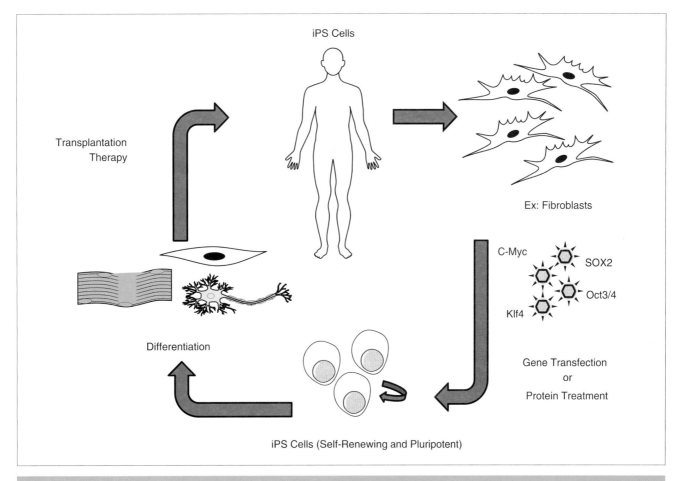

Figure 8 Process of protein-induced pluripotent stem cell creation.

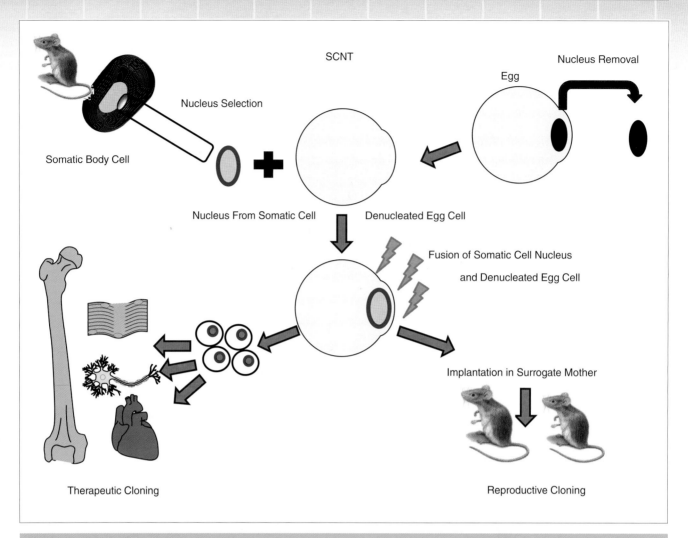

Figure 9 Process of SCNT. This procedure allows for the creation of totipotent cells that can be used in therapeutic cloning, and it can also provide the first step of reproductive cloning.

Although the extent of the similarity between ES cells and iPS cells is still being investigated, there are some parallels that have already been observed. Doubling time, embryoid body formation, teratoma formation, and chromatin methylation patterns have all been observed to be comparable between iPS cells and ES cells. Furthermore, iPS cells are also viable for chimera formation while showing adequate potency and differentiability, much like natural ES cells.

Protein-Induced Pluripotent Stem Cells

Protein-induced pluripotent stem (pIPS) cells have been generated without the use of genetic alteration through viral vector transfection. A poly-arginine tag is fused to the C terminus of the recombinant proteins, which imparts cell permeability.[37] The proteins are then introduced to a culture of mouse embryonic fibroblasts and cultured to produce the pIPS cells.

Somatic Cell Nuclear Transfer

Somatic cell nuclear transfer (SCNT) is used for the creation of totipotent cells that can be used in therapeutic cloning (**Figure 9**). It can also provide the first step of reproductive cloning. The nucleus from a desired somatic cell type is extracted intact and placed into a denucleated egg cell.[38] After administration of an electrical shock, the denucleated ovum and somatic cell nucleus fuse, at which point the host egg cell reprograms the nucleus and starts to divide. After multiple mitotic divisions in cell culture, the single cell forms a blastocyst with the DNA of the transplanted nucleus. The cells can continue to be cultured in vitro for therapeutic cloning purposes or the early-stage embryo can be implanted into a surrogate mother for reproductive cloning.

SCNT garnered massive attention for being the method by which Dolly the sheep was cloned.[39] Despite this success, SCNT as a viable cloning technique is restricted by its

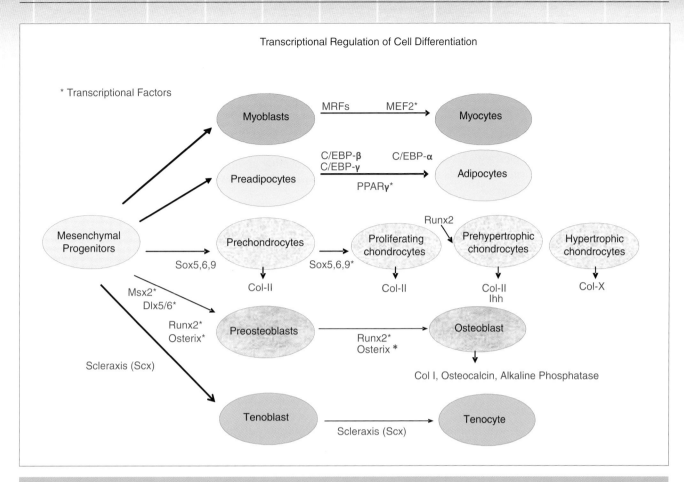

Figure 10 Key transcription factors during MSC differentiation.

1: Basic Principles of Orthopaedic Surgery

resource-intensive nature, high loss of embryos, low number of viable embryos, and uncertainty regarding the specific biochemical reactions that enable reprogramming of the somatic cell nucleus and activation of the egg cell.

SCNT can be used for therapeutic cloning applications such as disease research and cell transplantation therapy. In one envisioned use, cells from a diseased tissue could be cloned to further investigate how a particular disease manifests through gene activity. SCNT can also be used to grow cells for transplantation into a patient who is free from the fear of immune rejection, because the cells originated from the host.

Musculoskeletal Developmental Biology

Transcription Factors (Proteins Affecting Musculoskeletal Cell Differentiation, Function, and Phenotypes)

In order for correct biologic functioning to take place in a cell, gene expression must be tightly regulated. One of the ways in which a cell regulates gene expression is by means of DNA-binding proteins known as transcription factors,

which control the transcription of a gene by binding to the regulatory elements found on the DNA. More than 1,000 transcription factors have been classified into families based on the structural characteristics of their DNA binding domains. Within this group of proteins, several transcription factors have been shown to be essential in the cells of the musculoskeletal system (bone, cartilage, tendon, and muscle). These transcription factors are discussed in the next paragraphs and depicted in **Figure 10**.

Runt-Related Transcription Factor 2

Runt-related transcription factor 2 (Runx2) is a member of the Runt family, and the protein is known to be a key transcription factor for osteoblast differentiation.[35] This transcription factor directs the differentiation of mesenchymal cells to the osteoblast lineage, leading to the formation of immature osteoblasts.[40,41] Runx2 controls the expression of major osteoblast genes, including the genes that encode for osteopotonin, osteocalcin, and type I collagen α-1 chain.[40] In addition, Runx2 plays an important role in the later stages of chondrocyte differentiation[42] as well as the cell cycle.[40]

Osterix

Osterix (Osx) is a zinc finger transcription factor that is expressed exclusively by osteoblasts and acts downstream of Runx2 during osteoblast differentiation.[43] Osx is required for the differentiation of preosteoclasts to mature osteoblasts. The molecular mechanisms underlying the action of Osx are poorly understood. However, it has been shown that Osx inhibits Wnt signaling during bone formation and forms a transcriptional complex with NFATc1.[43] Similar to Runx2, this transcription factor also binds to the promoter of a gene encoding type I collagen.[43]

Twist1

Twist1 belongs to a small family of basic helix-loop-helix transcription factors, which include Dermo1/Twist2, Paraxis, Scleraxis, and most recently identified Hand1 and Hand2. Mutations in *Twist1* (7p21.1) were identified in patients with Saethre-Chotzen syndrome, a genetic condition characterized by premature fusion of skull bones.[44] In addition to its implication in craniosynostosis in both humans and mice, Twist1 also plays a key role in mediating cell patterning during limb morphogenesis and development through cooperative and antagonistic effects on sonic hedgehog and FGF signaling.[44] *Twist1* null mice die during midgestation (E11.5) from vascular and neuronal defects, and these animals exhibit growth retardation of the forelimb buds. The reasoning behind this observation is that Twist1 acts as a potent inhibitor of osteoblast differentiation, possibly through its repressive effects on Runx2 expression and activity.[45] Furthermore, emerging evidence is pointing to a possible role of Twist1 in the etiology of osteoarthritis.

Muscle Segment Homeobox

Muscle segment homeobox 2 (Msx2) is a transcription factor involved in osteoblast differentiation. This transcription factor was shown to be pivotal for cranial bone formation in mice studies.[46] However, the exact function of this transcription factor in osteoblast differentiation remains controversial.

Distal-less Homeobox

Distal-less homeobox (Dlx) 5 and 6 transcription factors are expressed in a similar pattern during the early stages of osteoblast differentiation. Dlx5 was shown to accelerate osteoblast differentiation and induce the expression of *Col1a1* gene, which encodes for type I collagen.[47]

Sex-Determining Region Y Box-9

Sex determining region Y box-9 (SOX-9) is a transcription factor that promotes chondrocytic differentiation by enhancing expression of essential elements of chondrocytic phenotypes such as type II collagen. SOX-9 genetic mutation is associated with campomellic dysplasia that is manifested by shortening and bowing of long bones, cleft palate, clubbing, laryngotracheomalacia, and scoliosis.

c-Fos

c-Fos, a member of the activator protein-1 (AP-1) family of transcription factors, is a key regulator of osteoclast differentiation and bone remodeling. This transcription factor partners with another transcription factor, c-Jun, to form the dimeric transcription complex known as AP-1.[34] AP-1 attaches to the promoter of *NFATc2* and causes the expression of NFATc2 transcription factor. NFATc2 associates with AP-1, forming another transcription factor complex, which leads to the activation of osteoclastogenic genes.[34]

Nascent Polypeptide-Associated Complex and Coactivator α

Nascent polypeptide-associated complex and coactivator α (aNAC) is a transcription factor that is activated by the phosphorylation activity of integrin-linked kinase.[48] aNAC is present in differentiated osteoblasts and acts in combination with AP-1 to potentiate osteocalcin gene transcription. aNAC acts as a stabilizer of the AP-1 transcription factor complex by assisting this transcription factor complex to have a stronger association with the promoter of this gene.[48] The activation of this transcription factor leads to osteoblastic gene transcription.

Myogenic Regulatory Factor

Myogenic regulatory factor (MRF) is a basic helix-loop-helix transcription factor group that has four members: MYOD, MYF5, MYOG (myogenin), and MRF4.[49] MRFs regulate the expression of genes involved in skeletal myogenesis, including *MYOG*. MRF proteins associate with a specific sequence found in the promoter of a gene. This sequence is known as the E box.[49] Activation of these transcription factors leads to genetic changes and an increase in the expression level of myogenin throughout the process of differentiation.[49]

Myocyte Enhancer Factor 2

Myocyte enhancer factor 2 (MEF2) is a family of transcription factors involved in organogenesis. In particular, MEF2 plays a pivotal role in mammalian skeletal myogenesis and it regulates this process by interacting with other transcription factors to control the expression of target genes.[50] One of the gene targets of MEF2 is *MYOG*, which suggests that MEF2 and MRF proteins synergistically activate this gene.[49]

Nuclear Factor of Activated T Cells c1

Nuclear factor of activated T cells c1 (NFATc1) is a crucial transcription factor for RANKL-mediated osteoclastogenesis.[5] This transcription factor, which is a member of the NFAT family, is activated and translocated into the nucleus upon dephosphorylation by calcineurin.[51] NFATc1 is induced by autoregulation of its own promoter.[34] In conjunction with other transcription factors, NFATc1 regulates osteoclast-specific genes, such as tartrate-resistant acid phosphatase (TRAP), cathepsin K, and β3-integrin genes.[34]

Nuclear Factor Kappa-Light-Chain-Enhancer of Activated B Cells

Nuclear factor kappa-light-chain-enhancer of activated B cells (NF-κB) is a group of transcription factors implicated in many biologic processes, such as the immune response and osteoclast differentiation. There are five proteins in this family: cRel, RelA, RelB, p50, and p52. NF-κB is activated by RANKL in the early stages of osteoclast formation and is important in the differentiation and survival for this cell.[34] Activation of this transcription factor is achieved by two different pathways: the classic pathway and the alternative pathway.[34] In the classic pathway, inhibitor of κB (IκB) kinase (IKK) complex degrades IκB, leading to the activation of NF-κB (p50/RelA). In the alternative pathway, NF-κB–inducing kinase (NIK) and IKKα mediate the processing of p100 to generate p52. This leads to the activation of NF-κB (p52/RelB).

Peroxisome Proliferator-Activated Receptor γ

Peroxisome proliferator-activated receptor γ (PPARγ) is not only an important factor for glucose metabolism, but it is also an important factor for adipogenesis in the bone marrow.[52] Activation of this transcription factor leads to the differentiation of MSCs toward the adipogenic lineage.[40] This is supported by the observation that PPARγ activation due to the drug thiazolidinedione leads to the suppression of osteoblastogenic transcription factors such as Runx2 and Osx.[52] However, the exact function of PPARγ in osteoclastogenesis is yet to be clarified.

C/EBP

In addition to PPARγ, the CCAAT-enhancer-binding proteins, or C/EBP transcription factor family, are known to regulate the differentiation of mesenchymal progenitor cells into adipocytes.[53] Of the six members of the basic region-leucine zipper transcription factor family, C/EBPα, C/EBPβ, and C/EBPγ were shown to be expressed in mesenchymal cell differentiation to adipocytes.[53] C/EBPβ and C/EBPγ are expressed early in the adipogenic process, whereas C/EBPα is expressed later. C/EBPα maintains the expression of PPARγ and other adipocyte proteins in the terminal stages of the adipogenic differentiation process.[53]

Scleraxis

Scleraxis (Scx) is a basic helix-loop-helix transcription factor that regulates chondrogenesis. This regulator is commonly used as a marker for tendon and ligament progenitors. It regulates the transcription of aggrecan and collagen genes by binding to the DNA regions known as the E boxes.[54] Scx associates with other transcription factors, such as E47 and Sox-9, to regulate *Col2a1*.[54]

Expression of Cellular Phenotype

The genotype of an organism or a cell refers to the genes present in its genome. However, in any somatic cell, only a fraction of the genes are expressed and that expression profile is usually regulated by specific interactions with the matrix and various factors. The phenotype of a cell is defined by the array of genes that are expressed and their relative levels of expression. When the phenotype of a cell is characterized, the focus tends to be on the genes that are expressed, which are unique or relatively unique to that cell type, due to the fact that there are thousands of genes that all cells express in common. Differentiation of cells refers to acquisition of a specific profile of gene expression that sets the cell apart from other types of cells, and determines its structure and function. In general, cell proliferation and differentiation tend to be inversely regulated. Proliferation of normal cells is prevented by cell-cell contacts, a phenomenon known as contact inhibition.[55] When cells are plated at low densities in culture, there is no contact inhibition and they tend to enter the cell cycle and proliferate. When confluency is attained, contact inhibition triggers mechanisms that inhibit the cell cycle, and cells tend to differentiate, expressing specific characteristics of the tissue from which they were derived. This paradigm has been well established in several skeletally relevant tissues, including in the culture of osteoblasts. Osteoblasts express proteins characteristic of differentiation at confluency such as alkaline phosphatase, osteocalcin, and osteopontin, and ultimately produce a mineralized osteoid matrix.[56] A more detailed description of the behavior of these cells can be found in the next paragraphs.

The cells of most skeletal tissues, including muscle, tendon, ligament, connective tissue, bone, and cartilage, are derived from multipotent cells called MSCs.[57] MSCs give rise to all the skeletal elements during development, and remain present in low numbers in sites such as periosteum and bone marrow throughout life. It is these cells that can differentiate into bone, cartilage, and fibrous tissue following a fracture and generate a reparative callus. MSCs can be isolated from bone marrow, and under the correct culture conditions can be induced to differentiate into osteoblasts, chondrocytes, lipoblasts, myoblasts, fibroblasts, and tenoblasts (**Figure 9**). Most likely they can also be induced to form tenocytes or fibrochondrocytes, although this has not yet been demonstrated specifically. The number of MSCs declines with age, as does their responsiveness to growth factors; hence, the ability to regenerate various mesenchymal tissues declines as a function of aging.[58] The use of MSCs for regenerating bone and repairing osteochondral defects is well under way and feasibility has been demonstrated in several animal models. Several putative markers specific for MSCs, such as STRO1, have been reported,[59] but further work needs to be done to fully characterize these markers.

Osteoblast Phenotype

Several phenotypic parameters are considered features of osteoblasts. Osteoblasts produce and secrete structural proteins such as collagen, and regulatory proteins including growth factors.[60] The study of osteoblasts has been facilitated by the development of methods for isolating them from intact bone tissue, usually by collagenase digestions of rodent calvarial or long bone specimens or human trabecular bone specimens. Osteoblastic cells are derived from tumors or immortalization by viral transformations. Commonly used cell lines include ROS 17.28 (rat), UMR106 (rat), SAOS2 (human), MG63 (human), and MC3T3 (murine).[61] The most abundant extracellular matrix, which is produced by osteoblasts, is called osteoid,[62] and when this matrix is mineralized with crystalline hydroxyapatite, the matrix becomes a bone. The major matrix protein synthesized by osteoblastic cells, which comprises more than 90% of the organic matrix of bone, is type I collagen. Type I collagen is synthesized and secreted as a triple helix with two α1 and one α2 chains (genes designated as COLIA1 and COLIA2).[63] The amino-terminal and carboxy-terminal propeptides are cleaved extracellularly, and the collagen molecules spontaneously self-assemble into collagen microfibrils and fibrils with a quarter-staggered arrangement of the individual molecules. C-propeptide is cleaved by the proteolytic activity of BMP-1, a member of the BMP family that lacks osteoinductive capacity but has some homology to the other members.[6] The C-propeptide and N-propeptide fragments can be detected in serum; these fragments are indicative of bone formation rates.[63] Bone matrix also contains small amounts of type III and type V collagens. The collagen fibrils are laid down parallel to the surface of the osteoblast and spontaneously nucleate hydroxyapatite crystals that initially form preferentially in the "hole zones" between the quarter-staggered collagen molecules.[64] With a periodicity related to the bone formation rate, the orientation of the fibrils changes 90° to the preceding layer, resulting in a plywood-like layered structure that maximizes the tensile strength of the material.[64]

The carboxyglutamic acid–containing glycoprotein osteocalcin, along with two other glycoproteins, osteopontin and osteonectin, are the next most abundant extracellular matrix protein constituents produced by osteoblasts.[65] Osteonectin may function to enhance the binding of hydroxyapatite crystals to the collagen matrix as mineralization proceeds.[66] Osteocalcin is thought to play a role in recruitment of osteoclasts to bone surfaces for bone resorption, but the function of osteopontin remains unclear. Bone matrix also contains a sialoprotein and small amounts of several other glycoproteins and phosphoproteins of uncertain function.[65] The extracellular matrix structural proteins are one set of phenotypic parameters that define the osteoblast. During osteoblast differentiation, there are several shifts in protein synthesis: from a mixture of type III and type I collagen to predominantly type I collagen; from low to high levels of alkaline phosphatase; from versican to fibronectin expression; and from expression of an attachment protein called thrombospondin to expression of the bone glycoproteins osteonectin, osteocalcin, osteopontin, and sialoprotein.[62]

Bone matrix also contains several regulatory proteins deposited by osteoblasts. These include growth factors such as

TGF-β, IGF-I and IGF-II, FGFs, PDGF, and BMPs.[62] Although present quantitatively in minute amounts, these proteins are extremely important in regulating bone remodeling and in conferring osteoinductive capacity on bone, thus enabling bone grafting and transplantation.

Osteoblasts express the PTH/PTHrP receptor and exhibit intracellular signaling responses to PTH or PTHrP.[11] Osteoblasts also express the vitamin D receptor and consequently vitamin D responsiveness.[67] Some transcription factors such as Runx2 and the transcriptional coactivator αNAC have been identified. Glucocorticoids have complex effects on bone, stimulating differentiation of preosteoblasts in culture through a BMP-6–mediated pathway, while inhibiting bone cell proliferation and decreasing bone formation, resorption, and net mass when given systemically in vivo.[68]

Osteocyte Phenotype

Osteocytes are fully differentiated osteoblasts that become encased in the secreted matrix.[62] Osteocytes have numerous long cell processes that extend throughout the bone matrix and are in contact with the cell processes of other osteocytes.[62] Because osteocytes are completely embedded in bone, their culture and study have been difficult, but new functions are being revealed (**Figure 2**). There are several osteocyte-specific phenotypic markers. Dentin matrix protein–1 (DMP-1) is important in osteocyte maturation and phosphate maturation. Genetic deletion of DMP-1 results in immature osteocytes, increased FGF-23 secretion, osteomalacia, and rickets.[69] Sclerostin (encoded by a SOST gene) is predominantly secreted by osteocytes and is a negative regulator of osteoblastic bone formation. Sclerostin secretion is increased by PTH and decreased by calcitonin, thereby acting as a major regulator of bone homeostasis.[70]

The channels in the matrix through which these numerous connecting cell processes extend are called canaliculi. It has been demonstrated that osteocytes express cell-cell channels (gap junctions) called connexins, through which small molecules such as second messengers can pass.[71] This implies that the network of osteocytes is in communication with one another. When the bone is loaded, osteocytes sense oscillating fluid flow in the canaliculi. Osteocytes also perceive tensile strains during normal activities. Sclerostin is downregulated on physiologic mechanical loading and, as a result of loss of inhibition, osteoblastic bone formation increases. It is also known that bone exhibits piezoelectric properties under mechanical loading due to its anisotropic nature; it develops surface electrical charges that are asymmetrically distributed when mechanically loaded. One putative function of osteocyte-osteocyte communication within the larger organization of bone as a tissue may be in sensing and modulating signals that control osteoblastic and osteoclastic activity, enabling the observed ability of bone to increase its mass in areas that are loaded and decrease mass in response to unloading. Recent studies showed that osteocytes are very important in the regulation of bone mass. Conditional knockout of RANKL in osteocytes showed osteopetrosis, suggesting that osteocytes are the predominant source of RANKL in comparison with osteoblasts.[72,73] Osteocytes also express osteocalcin and fibronectin, although the role of these proteins in osteocyte function is unknown.[71]

Chondrocyte Phenotype

Chondrocytes are derived from similar undifferentiated mesenchymal precursor cells to those that give rise to osteoblasts.[12] As chondrocytes differentiate, they also express a pattern of specific genes that define their function. Similar to osteoblasts, chondrocytes are characterized by their production of an abundant extracellular matrix. Chondrocytes undergo differentiation along two major distinct pathways: one in which the cells undergo maturation, hypertrophy, and matrix calcification (the endochondral calcification pathway), and one in which the cells are relatively quiescent, carrying out load-bearing and structural functions. Induction of chondrocyte differentiation from MSC precursors occurs during embryogenesis and also in injury and repair processes such as in the case of fracture callus.[12] The nonendochondral calcification pathway can be activated in quiescent chondrocytes by the onset of maturation and calcification in the deep layers of the articular cartilage during cartilage degeneration.[74] Growth plate chondrocytes generate bone growth through proliferation and hypertrophy during maturation through the endochondral calcification pathway[74] (**Figure 3**).

Chondrocytes can be grown and studied in culture. Isolation of these cells can be achieved by the digestion of the cartilage tissues with collagenase or combinations of collagenase, hyaluronidase, and trypsin. Chondrocytes in monolayer culture tend to dedifferentiate, and lose their expression of type II collagen and other phenotypic markers such as proteoglycan synthesis. Instead, they take on a more fibroblastic phenotype and express type I collagen. When cultured in a suspension culture or in a three-dimensional gel made of collagen, agar, or alginate, the cells will maintain their chondrocytic phenotype, emphasizing the importance of cell-matrix interactions in controlling gene expression.

The predominant matrix protein in cartilage is type II collagen, which is composed of a single chain forming a triple helix.[75] Like type I collagen, it is secreted as triple helical proprotein, which is cleaved extracellularly by proteinases (gene designated as *COLIIA1*).[74] The other major organic component of the matrix is proteoglycan, which includes several proteins containing covalently bound glycosaminoglycan side chains.[62] The major proteoglycan is aggrecan, which consists of a protein core that associates with chondroitin sulfate and keratan sulfate side chains. The proteoglycans confer many of the unique mechanical properties of cartilage, including its ability to absorb repetitive compressive mechanical loads without damage. Aggrecan molecules form noncovalently bound aggregates with hyaluronic acid and a link glycoprotein. In addition, cartilage contains small proteoglycans, such as decorin and biglycan. In addition to

type II collagen and aggrecan, there are a series of minor collagens that also contribute to the chondrocytic phenotype. These include type VI, IX, X, and XI collagens.[75] Type VI collagen is a pericellular matrix protein, whereas type IX is a collagen molecule with a proteoglycan moiety. Type IX collagen molecules coat the outer surface of type II collagen fibrils and interact with the matrix proteoglycan via proteoglycan moieties. This is thought to serve as an interconnection between the collagen and proteoglycan matrix. Type XI collagen is localized within the type II fibrils and may regulate the diameters of fibrils.

Several chondrocyte phenotypic markers are specific to the differentiation pathway of the chondrocyte. For instance, type X collagen is only expressed by hypertrophic chondrocytes, and is a specific marker for this phenotype. In addition, these cells express high levels of alkaline phosphatase, in contrast to the minimal expression observed in chondrocytes that are not committed to maturation. Chondrocytes committed to the endochondral calcification pathway also express several growth factors, including BMP-6 and BMP-7, which promote maturation.[74] Differential expression of these genes in articular and growth plate chondrocytes demonstrates the critical role of regulatory gene products that may operate as determinants of chondrocytic phenotypes.

Osteoclast Phenotype

Osteoclast is a cell responsible for carrying out bone resorption.[76] These cells are extremely specialized, with an array of proteins used for accomplishing the complex task of resorbing calcified matrix. Osteoclasts are derived from monocytic precursors and share some of the characteristics of monocytes and macrophages. Monocytes and macrophages form osteoclasts in response to RANKL and M-CSF, two essential pro-osteoclastogenic cytokines[34] (**Figure 11** and **Figure 12**). Other pro-osteoclastogenic cytokines are IL-1, granulocyte M-CSF, M-CSF, IL-6, RANKL, and prostaglandin E_2.[27] Antiosteoclastogenic cytokines are IFN-β, IFN-γ, and IL-4, and these suppress RANKL-induced osteoclastogenesis.[27] Osteoclasts are multinucleated, and arise through syncytial fusion of several precursor cells under the influence of specific growth factors in the bone marrow. Functional osteoclasts have been isolated from animal and human models using several techniques. In the past, one of the earliest methods of obtaining a sufficient number of osteoclasts from the marrow cavity of long bones was to raise egg-laying chickens on low-calcium diets. Soon after, cells with osteoclast-like characteristics were isolated from human giant cell tumors. Functional osteoclasts currently can be generated from the marrow of long bones of neonatal rats or mice by culturing wafers of cortical bone in the presence of vitamin D and PTH. Although this method leads to a polymorphous cell population, the method readily facilitated the study of osteoclasts in vitro.

Osteoclasts attach to bone surfaces through a specific cell attachment receptor called an integrin. The osteoclast inte-

1: Basic Principles of Orthopaedic Surgery

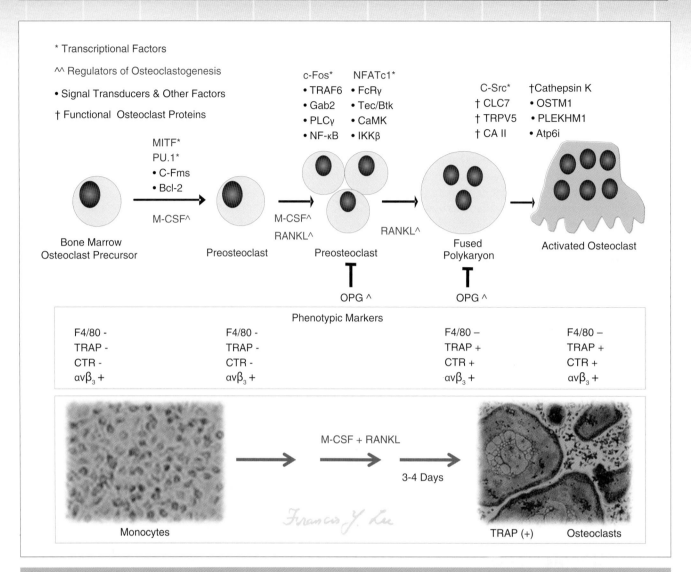

Figure 11 Monocytes and macrophages form osteoclasts in response to RANKL and M-CSF, which are two essential pro-osteoclastogenic cytokines. (Courtesy of Francis Y. Lee, MD, New York, NY.)

grin is known as $\alpha_v\beta_3$, or the vitronectin receptor.[33] Several bone matrix proteins, including collagen, fibronectin, and osteopontin, contain the attachment arginine-glycine-aspartate (RGD) sequences.[76] After attachment to a bone surface, the integrins activate focal adhesion kinases, including c-src, which is a regulatory kinase that contributes to the induction of osteoclast polarization. This involves formation of an extensive series of microscopic invaginations of the plasma membrane surface against the bone matrix surface. These series of invaginations are called the ruffled border, which serves to markedly increase the surface area of membrane next to the bone. A plasma membrane proton pump moves to the ruffled border and pumps protons from the cytosol into the space between the osteoclast and the bone. This acidifies the bone surface, resulting in dissolution of the hydroxyapatite mineral phase of the bone.[76]

Lysosomes move to the ruffled border and discharge their contents of lysosomal enzymes into the resorption re-

gion. These enzymes include acid-activated hydrolases such as cathepsin, which degrades the collagen in the matrix. Furthermore, osteoclasts express an isoform of carbonic anhydrase (CAII), which generates intracellular protons for the acidification process. Osteoclasts also express matrix metalloproteinase (gelatinase B, or MMP) and a specific phosphatase (TRAP), but the functions of these enzymes remain unclear.[76] TRAP and other glycosylated lysosomal enzymes are deposited on the resorption surface and remain there even after the osteoclast has moved away. Many of these enzymes contain glycosylations, which permit these enzymes to bind to receptors such as the IFGII/Mannose-6-phosphate receptor.[76] This receptor is expressed by osteoblasts, and when stimulated, it causes anabolic effects and matrix synthesis. Theoretically, the residue of glycosylated enzymes on the resorption surface may function to target osteoblasts to this location and initiate bone formation, thus representing part of the site-directing coupling mechanism

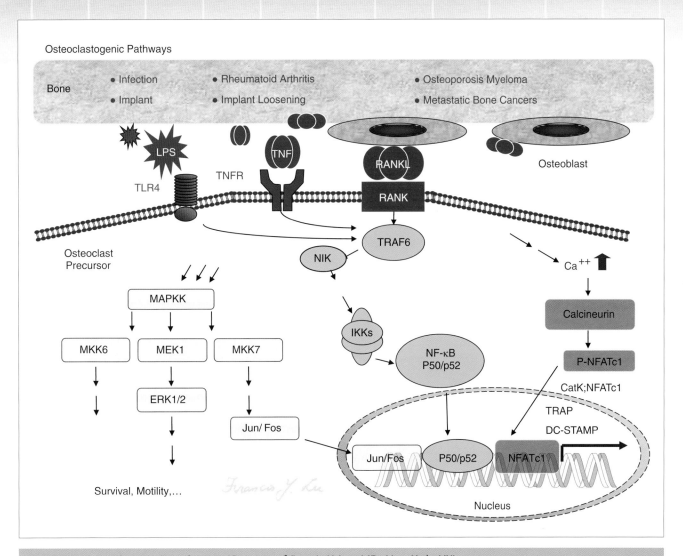

Figure 12 Osteoclastogenic pathways. (Courtesy of Francis Y. Lee, MD, New York, NY.)

between bone formation and resorption. Osteoclasts contain a calcium receptor that may be involved in the movement induction of pseudopodia of the motile osteoclasts, which creep along the bone surface as they excavate the matrix. When the pseudopodia lift up from the bone surface and move to reattach, the high concentration of inorganic ions (calcium and phosphate) that has accumulated from bone matrix resorption becomes discharged into the extracellular space. Some of the matrix and mineral may be removed by endocytosis and transport across the osteoclast, but this is controversial. Osteoclasts have a finite lifetime and are active in bone resorption for an estimated 10 to 14 days, after which they undergo apoptosis.[75]

Several key hormones and local factors control osteoclast function. Systemically, PTH stimulates bone resorption.[11] However, only osteoblasts and not osteoclasts express the PTH receptor. Therefore, the stimulation of resorption by PTH is mediated through indirect signaling from osteoblasts to osteoclasts.[11] One of these signals may be IL-6, a stimulator of osteoclast formation and resorption. Similar

to IL-1, TNF-α is an extremely potent stimulator of osteoclast progenitor proliferation, fusion, and activation of osteoclastic bone resorption. TNF-α, IL-1, and IL-6 are produced by many inflammatory processes and are collectively known as proinflammatory cytokines.[24] These factors are critical to many important clinical disorders and have been implicated in pathologic bone resorption in metastatic and primary bone tumors, infection, prosthetic loosening, nonunion of fractures, osteoporosis, and periarticular bone loss in inflammatory arthropathies (**Figure 12**).

Fibroblastic Phenotype

The hallmarks of the fibroblastic phenotype are synthesis of type I and III collagen and a spindle cell shape.[62] There are relatively few specific markers for the fibroblastic phenotype, and it appears in some ways that there is a default differentiation pathway of the production of fibroblasts from MSCs. Fibroblastic cells express fibronectin and can differentiate along some specialized pathways in generation of ligaments and tendons. Ligaments and tendons contain primarily type I collagen, with a minuscule amount of type XII collagen, which coats the type I fibrils. Type XII collagen is analogous to type IX collagen in cartilage in that it contains a proteoglycan-like moiety thought to interact with the proteoglycans within the matrix.[75] Tendon and ligament contain only small amounts of proteoglycans, biglycan, and decorin, rather than aggrecan.[75] During compression, tendons develop a fibrocartilaginous phenotype due to the expression of aggrecan. This phenotype is observed in areas where tendons are under chronic compressive force, such as in the posterior tibial tendon. Other important components of tendons and ligaments are tenascin and elastin. Recently, two new BMPs have been identified (BMP-12 and BMP-13) by molecular cloning techniques. These two proteins are homologous to previously identified murine growth and differentiation factors (gdf7 and gdf6, respectively). When implanted ectopically, instead of bone production as with the other BMPs, these molecules induced the formation of an organized fibrous tissue that resembled a tissue of a tendon or a ligament. This tissue also expressed tenascin, small proteoglycans, and elastin. Thus, tenascin, proteoglycans, elastins, and BMPs all may have a potential role in regulating tendon and ligament morphogenesis.[77] Expression of these proteins was observed during the formation of the joint capsule, at tendinous attachments to bone, and at ligament sites. In addition, a recent study has shown BMP-12 implantation stimulates patellar tendon healing in an animal model. Growth factors such as basic FGF, PDGF, and TGF-ß have also been demonstrated to enhance the healing of ligaments and tendons in animal models.[75]

Tendon and ligament fibroblast-like cells also respond to mechanical stress, and these cells control the reorganization of the matrix during healing, both to decrease the excessive amount of type III collagen expressed early in healing in favor of increased expression of type I, and to allow realignment of the fibrils with the direction of mechanical force, which increases the strength of the structure. The realignment is thought to occur through matrix remodeling, but little is known about this process. The increased strength and rate of tendon or ligament healing is enhanced by the application of moderate mechanical tensile force. (Excessive force will not enhance healing and it will lead to laxity.) In addition, as the healing process progresses, there is an increased amount of collagen cross-linking and increased diameter of the fibril; both factors again enhance the mechanical structure of the healing tissue.

Functional Matrix Biology: Cell-Matrix Interactions

The matrix is a key factor influencing gene expression in skeletal tissues, and it allows the cells to receive signals from the environment. This is particularly important in the musculoskeletal system due to the load-bearing functions of the tissues, which require responsiveness and adaptability to mechanical forces. Matrix proteins interact with cell surface receptors in a manner similar to growth factors, and this array of stimuli is transduced by intracellular signaling pathways that integrate them to cause activation of genes, which control the cell cycle, and the expression of proteins, which define differentiated functions of target cells.[62]

Some interactions of cells with surrounding matrix are mediated through the cytoskeleton. Cytoskeletal proteins are essential for numerous cellular functions, including mitosis, cell motility, intracellular movement, and organization of organelles. The cytoskeleton is composed of three major types of filaments made by reversible polymerization of specific proteins: actin filaments (actin polymer), microtubules (tubulin polymer), and intermediate filaments (polymers of vimentin or lamin).[62] Cell surface movements are controlled by interactions of the actin molecules with myosins in the cytoplasm, enabling contractility and cell movement. Actin fiber formation is regulated by the Rho family of G proteins. Actin filaments are flexible, whereas microtubules are more rigid structures. Microtubules polymerize and depolymerize continuously in the cell and mediate organelle transport and subcellular organization. Microtubules are critically involved in organizing the events of cell division, and radiate outward through the cell from origin sites within the centrosome, a structure adjacent to the nucleus. Proteins called kinesins and dyneins are cytoplasmic adenosine triphosphate-dependent motors that move in opposite directions along microtubules, carrying bound proteins or vesicles.[78] The cytoplasmic intermediate filaments are thought to function within the cell to resist deformation to external mechanical stress, and have greater strength than actin and tubulin. Numerous cytoplasmic proteins associate with the cytoskeletal proteins and control their structure, contractility, and stability.

One common mechanism linking cells to matrix is the integrin family of cell surface receptors that interact with specific matrix proteins. Integrins consist of transmembrane heterodimeric signaling molecules that reside on the cell surface and interact with matrix proteins containing a specific sequence of amino acids (RGD). Many extracellular matrix proteins, including collagens, contain RGD sequences enabling interaction with integrin receptors. The receptor dimers consist of α and β subunits that associate in specific combinations in different cell types.[79] All mesenchymal cells express specific subsets of integrin receptors on the cell surface. More than 20 heterodimers have been identified between 9 types of β subunits and 14 types of α subunits. In addition to the numerous isoforms of the two integrin subunits, some isoforms have several alternatively spliced forms of the protein, further increasing the diversity of this receptor family. The different heterodimers possess differing and sometimes overlapping specificity for particular matrix RGD-containing proteins. Integrin receptors have relatively lower affinities for their ligands than growth factor and hormone receptors, and are 10 to 100 times more abundant on cell surfaces. The β subunit contains a binding domain that interacts with the cytoskeletal proteins talin and α-actinin.[79] This ligand binding causes formation of linkages to the actin cytoskeleton. These areas of focal receptor/cytoskeletal contact can activate kinases, such as the focal adhesion kinase or the tyrosine kinase product of the *src* gene. This in turn leads to a signal cascade, which can result in changes in gene expression. Because cells are attached to their matrix by the integrins, perturbations of the mechanical environment couple to effects on the cytoskeleton and associated kinases, providing one mechanism whereby cells can respond with changes in gene expression to changes in mechanical loading.

Another class of adhesion molecules is known as the hyaluronan receptor family, which recognizes carbohydrates related to hyaluronate. This is also known as the CD44 receptor group and consists of several isoforms.[80] CD44 has been implicated in the attachment of tumor cells to matrix in target tissues during metastasis. Like other cell surface receptors, CD44 can activate intracellular processes. Some types of cell surface receptors, such as cadherins, receptors with some homology to immunoglobulins, and cell-cell adhesion molecules (CAMs), mediate cell-cell contact events rather than cell-matrix interactions. Activation of cadherins results in binding of these receptors to cytoplasmic proteins called catenins, which interact with the actin cytoskeleton analogous to the manner in which talin and α-actinin link integrin activation to actin. Cadherins and CAMs are homophilic receptors (binding to a like receptor on a different cell to mediate signaling events).[81] Alterations in cadherin expression can change chondrocyte differentiation pathways in embryogenesis, indicating the dependence of gene expression on cell-cell interactions as well as cell-matrix interactions.[81]

Most cells possess stretch-activated ion channels in the plasma membrane, which provide another means of cellular response to mechanical stimuli. These channels control influx of K^+ or Ca^{2+}, the two cations that the cell actively maintains at low intracellular levels through the actions of plasma membrane–based energy-dependent pumps. When the matrix adjacent to an attached cell is mechanically deformed, transient elevations of cations can occur through the action of the stretch-activated channels. These cations can influence other signaling pathways within the cell, thus enabling mechanical input to influence the cell's transcriptional machinery. Stretch-activated channels have been demonstrated in fibroblasts, osteoblasts, and chondrocytes. A family of matrix cell–binding proteins called annexins has features of both a matrix receptor and an ion channel. Annexins are ubiquitous extracellular proteins that associate with the plasma membrane under certain conditions.[82] Annexins II, V, and VI bind to collagen and to the plasma membrane, providing another mechanism for cell-matrix attachment. In addition, some annexins function as calcium channels in the plasma membrane. In chondrocytes, annexins V and VI may function as calcium channels that are activated by binding of type II and type X collagen.[82] The phospholipid composition of the plasma membrane influences annexin association with the membrane, with acidic phospholipids enhancing the membrane binding. Annexin V binding is enhanced by changes in the phospholipids of the plasma membrane that occur as part of the cascade of events in apoptosis, and binding of this annexin has been used as a marker for this process.[82] Annexins provide another connection between the matrix and intracellular signaling pathways.

Bone remodeling provides an excellent prototypical example of matrix control of cell behavior and communication as well as integration of multiple signal inputs by cell-matrix interactions. Osteoblasts secrete the matrix of bone, incorporating growth factors that can be released and activated upon matrix resorption (loss of tissue).[62] Osteoblasts provide the initial signals for bone resorption by osteoclasts, responding to stimuli such as PTH, with production of collagenase, which clears the area for osteoclast attachment as well as production of cytokines that stimulate osteoclast formation and activation. The osteoclast begins resorbing the bone, organizing its functional apparatus in response to integrin signals upon contact with the bone matrix.[79] The osteoclast releases and activates growth factors from the bone matrix as it resorbs the bone tissues that in turn stimulate nearby osteoblast progenitors to differentiate. In addition, the osteoclast deposits signals on the resorption surface before moving on or undergoing apoptosis. These signals attract osteoblasts and stimulate matrix deposition at the previously resorbed surface, replacing the bone matrix. This functional cooperation of osteoblasts and osteoclasts, coupled by the matrix, is under modulation of systemic hormonal controls such as PTH and vitamin D, which regulate systemic calcium metabolism. However, the remodeling process is also under local control through mechanical signal transduction through the bone matrix to the osteoblasts and/or osteoclasts, allowing the bone to remodel according to local mechanical stress. Finally, pathologic processes such as inflammation or tumors can produce local cytokines that alter the balance between formation and resorption, leading to pathologic loss of bone matrix.

Immunology
Innate and Adaptive Immunity

Defense against foreign pathogens is mediated by the early innate immunity response and the late adaptive immunity response. Innate immunity, which provides the early defense line, is stimulated by a certain structure shared by a group of microbes. It responds rapidly to infection and responds in the same way to repeated infections. (Physical barriers include epidermis, dermis, and mucosa; cellular barriers include phagocytotic cells and natural killer cells; chemical barriers include antimicrobial substances, blood proteins [complement system], and cytokines.)

Adaptive immunity memorizes the specific antigens of foreign pathogens. It is able to recognize diverse and specific antigens. The successive exposure to antigens increases the magnitude of immune reaction. There are two types of

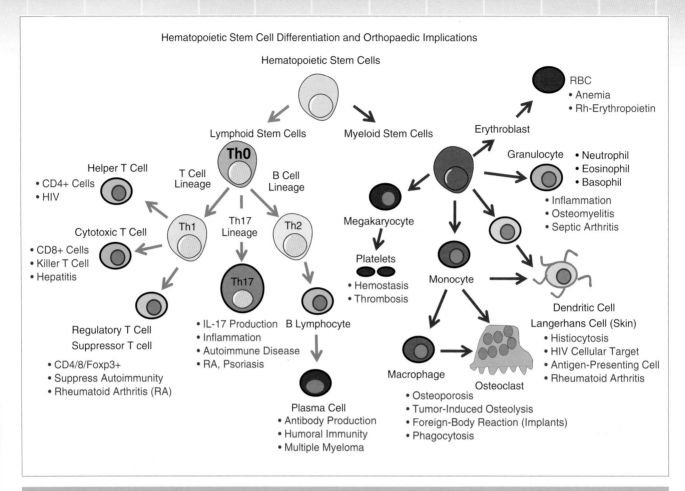

Hematopoietic Stem Cell Differentiation and Orthopaedic Implications

Figure 13 Hematopoietic stem cell differentiation and orthopaedic implications.

adaptive immune responses: humoral immunity and cell-mediated immunity. Humoral immunity is mediated by antibodies produced by B lymphocytes.[31] Cell-mediated immunity is mediated by T lymphocytes.[24] T cells can activate macrophages to kill phagocytosed antigen or directly destroy infected cells. For example, an individual who has had chickenpox will be have immunity against chickenpox for many years.

Types of Immune Cells

Although the immune system is composed of a wide range of cell types, all cells of this system are derived from a specific type of stem cells known as hematopoietic stem cells.[31] This stem cell is further differentiated into two kinds of progenitor cells: the myeloid progenitor cell and the lymphoid progenitor cell (**Figure 13**).

Myeloid Progenitor Cells

Myeloid progenitor cells give rise to various cells that play a prominent role in providing immediate protection against invading pathogens.[83] In addition, myeloid-derived cells mediate allergy and hypersensitivity reactions. In addition to erythrocytes, myeloid progenitor cells give rise to granu-

locytes and phagocytes. There are three types of granulocytes, known as eosinophils, basophils, and neutrophils.[83] Eosinophils are commonly recognized by their retention of large granules and provide defense against parasitic infections. Upon activation, these cells release toxic contents of the granules that target the invading pathogens. In addition to eosinophils, basophils assist in protecting the host from parasitic infections by releasing large amounts of cytokines. Furthermore, basophils display high numbers of immunoglobulin E antibody receptors on the cell surface.[83] Binding of immunoglobulin E antibody to these receptors leads to degranulation of basophils, resulting in the release of heparin and histamine. Heparin and histamine are not only important for causing immune response, but these inflammatory mediators are the key components of allergic reactions. Unlike basophils and eosinophils, neutrophils are considered both granulocytes and phagocytes. This type of immune cell internalizes bacterial pathogens, which become exposed to the toxic reactive oxygen species-filled granules in the cytoplasm of neutrophils. Another phagocytic cell is known as a macrophage. This cell is a renowned immune cell that is derived from monocytes, which circulate in the blood.[83] Motile macrophages phagocytose bacterial patho-

Table 1

Commonly Used DMARDs for the Treatment of Rheumatoid Arthritis

Drug	Drug Type	Target	Mechanism
Abatacept	Recombinant fusion protein	Major histocompatibility complex receptors	Binds to major hisotcompatibility complex receptors on antigen-presenting cells to block T cell activation
Adalimumab	Recombinant monoclonal antibody	TNF-α	Binds to TNF-α and inhibits the interactions of this cytokine to p55 and p75 receptors
Anakinra	Receptor antagonist	IL-1 receptors	Binds to IL-1 receptors to block IL-1 proinflammatory signaling pathway
Canakinumab	Monoclonal IgG antibody	IL-1β	Binds to IL-1β with high affinity to inhibit IL-1β and receptor association
Etanercept	Recombinant fusion protein	TNF-α	Competes with TNF-α receptor for the binding of TNF-α
Infliximab	Recombinant chimeric human-murine monoclonal antibody	TNF-α	Binds to TNF-α. The drug has higher affinity to TNF-α than the receptor, so TNF-α could dissociate from its receptor.
Methotrexate	Folate antagonist	Dihydrofolate reductase	Inhibits dihydrofolate reductase activity, leading to adenosine-dependent inhibition of inflammation
Sulphasalazine	Combination of sulphapyridine and 5-salicylic acid	Unknown	Modulates B cell response and angiogenesis
Tocilizumab	Humanized monoclonal antibody	IL-6 receptors	Binds to IL-6 receptors to inhibit the association between the receptor and IL-6

gens and present the processed components of the pathogen (antigen) to T cells, leading to the activation of the adaptive immunity.

Lymphoid Progenitor Cells

With the exception of natural killer cells, cells derived from the lymphoid progenitor provide long-lasting antigen-specific immunity. This type of progenitor cell gives rise to B cells, T cells, and natural killer cells.[83] As stated earlier, B cells play a large role in the humoral immune response, whereas T cells are primarily responsible for cell-mediated immune response. Upon activation, B cells differentiate into plasma cells and memory B cells. Plasma cells secrete antibodies during the course of infection, whereas memory B cells remain within the host after the infection for quicker immune response in the case of a secondary infection of the same pathogen.[31] In addition, two types of T cells known as the Th cells and cytotoxic T cells have been found. Th cells direct the immune response by releasing cytokines, whereas

cytotoxic T cells induce the death of the pathogen-infected cells by releasing toxic granules.[83] Like cytotoxic T cells, natural killer cells release toxic granules to facilitate the disposal of the invading pathogen. However, the difference between these two killer cells is that only cytotoxic T cells recognize specific antigens.

Pharmaceutical Modification of Immune Response (Disease-Modifying Drugs)
Rheumatoid Arthritis

Rheumatoid arthritis, an autoimmune disease that leads to inflammation of joints, is treated by the use of multiple drugs and drug regimens.[84] Biologic disease-modifying antirheumatic drugs (DMARDs), which target specific components of the inflammation processes, have been used to treat this debilitating disease.[85] With the discovery and research of these novel drugs, the list of DMARDs is currently growing. This section describes the commonly used DMARDs. A complete summary of these drugs is presented in Table 1.

Methotrexate is considered one of the traditional DMARDs and has been used to treat multiple diseases ever since its discovery in the 1940s.[26] Although this drug was initially used to treat cancer, methotrexate was shown to have anti-inflammatory effects against rheumatoid arthritis when given in low doses.[26] This drug specifically targets a metabolic enzyme called dihydrofolate reductase, which is involved in purine metabolism. Inhibition of this enzyme leads to adenosine release, which has anti-inflammatory effects. Another traditional DMARD is sulphasalazine.[84] Although this sulfa drug was shown to inhibit rheumatoid arthritis disease progression, the exact mechanism of this drug remains unclear.

TNF-α is a major cytokine in the cascade of cytokines. It stimulates the production of various inflammatory mediators and recruits immune and inflammatory cells. Three anti-TNFs have been approved for the treatment of rheumatoid arthritis. Infliximab and adalimumab are monoclonal anti–TNF-α antibodies with high affinity to TNF-α. These drugs prevent the cytokine from binding to its receptors.[85] Etanercept is a fusion protein that binds to TNF-α and prevents it from interacting with its receptors.[85] TNF-α inhibitors reportedly reduced the erosive damage and the disability in patients with rheumatoid arthritis.

In addition to TNF-α inhibitors, IL-1 inhibitors have also been discovered and are available on the market for the treatment of rheumatoid arthritis. Anakinra is an analog of IL-1β and thus it competitively binds to the IL-1 cell surface receptor and blocks the downstream IL-1 response.[84] Although anakinra has been shown to be not as effective as TNF-α inhibitors, this drug has been used to treat patients with systemic juvenile idiopathic arthritis as well as those with rheumatoid arthritis who do not respond very well to TNF-α inhibitors. In addition, canakinumab, a drug that was approved by the FDA in 2009 for the treatment of inflammatory disorders, is currently being evaluated for the treatment of rheumatoid arthritis. Canakinumab is another monoclonal antibody that specifically targets IL-1β.[86]

Drugs that suppress IL-6 activity have also been tested and used for the treatment of rheumatoid arthritis. IL-6 has been shown to have immune stimulatory activity. Similar to anakinra, tocilizumab is also a humanized monoclonal antibody. The difference between these two drugs is that the former targets IL-1 receptor, whereas the latter targets IL-6 receptor.[87] Tocilizumab, which was approved by the FDA in 2010, has been shown to dramatically inhibit the disease progression in patients with rheumatoid arthritis.[84] Furthermore, when this drug was administered together with methotrexate, patients with rheumatoid arthritis experienced significant improvement because of the reduction of bone resorption and cartilage turnover.[84]

Another drug with anti-inflammatory activity that targets a receptor is abatacept.[88] This recombinant protein drug has a binding affinity to major histocompatability complex receptors found on the antigen-presenting cell.[88] Binding of abatacept to major histocompatability complex receptors leads to incomplete formation of costimulatory signals between the T cells and antigen-presenting cell.[88] This incompletion leads to inhibition of T cell activation.

Osteoclast Inhibitors

There have been therapeutic interventions to control excessive osteoclastogenesis. RANKL is one of the important factors for osteoclastogenesis. DNA vaccination against RANKL has been attempted on an experimental basis in animals.[89] Furthermore, a synthetic RANK-Fc has been tried clinically for treatment of osteoporosis and bone cancers.[90]

OPG is a secreted member of the TNF receptor family that binds to RANKL. Binding of OPG to RANKL prevents RANKL from associating with RANK, which is a receptor on the osteoclastic linage cell for osteoclast differentiation. Direct OPG injection and modulation of OPG expression in bone cells are considered as possible therapeutic approaches.[33] The use of OPG has been tried once in humans. However, the development of OPG antibody in patients receiving this agent was raised as a concern. Currently, OPG is not used for clinical trials. Other inhibitors of osteoclast such as cathepsin K inhibitors, $\alpha_v\beta_3$ integrin receptor blockers, and osteoclast-selective H1-ATPase inhibitor could potentially be used to block bone resorption.

Molecular Biology for Translational Orthopaedic Research

Cell biology is the study of the structure and function of cells.[79] Examination of different functions, sizes, shapes, and ultrastructures of growth plate chondrocytes is one example of orthopaedic cell biology. Cell biology has advanced since the invention of light microscopy, tissue staining, electron microscopy, and culture techniques, and is once again under the spotlight because of ongoing controversies and the rapidly developing field of stem cell biology. The use of stem cells is attractive in orthopaedic surgery because stem cells can be used to restore or treat damaged bones, ligaments, nerves, muscles and cartilages. Therefore, the basic concepts of stem cells will be discussed in this section.

In physics, a molecule is an extremely minute particle consisting of an electrically neutral group of at least two atoms held together by chemical bonds. In biology and medicine, molecules have a broad meaning on a larger scale and are basic units of cellular structures and functions. Structural molecules are basic building blocks of cellular organelles. Functional molecules are the smallest peptides or fragments of DNA that have distinct functions in a cell, tissue, organ, or individual. For example, proteins are polypeptides, which are templated by RNA according to the genetic information in DNA and synthesized in ribosomes. The smallest functional unit of protein, such as PTHrP, is regarded as a molecule. Molecular biology examines the structure and function of molecules in living cells, tissues, organs, systems, individuals, and populations. The same molecule can have different functions depending on its three-dimensional structures, biochemical environments, and cell types. Studies on BMP molecules are good examples of orthopaedic molecular biology. BMPs exhibit many different functions in the bone, cartilage, tendon, stomach, and brain. Orthopaedic molecular biology research is meant to enhance musculoskeletal health by optimizing the function of orthopaedically important molecules in musculoskeletal disorders. Molecular biology fields have benefited from adoption of high-speed and high-efficiency computer technologies. As a result, new fields such as high-throughput screening, microarray, genomics, proteomics, and nanomedicine have emerged over the past 10 years. These new fields have orthopaedic implications. For example, many scientists are in the process of developing nanostructure-based scaffolds loaded with specific growth factors (molecules) and cells (MSCs) for tissue regeneration.

Orthopaedic surgeons often treat patients with other medical conditions, such as congenital or acquired disorders, cancers caused by genetic mutations, or tumors caused by abnormal gene functions. Therefore, basic understanding of cell and molecular biology, along with the terms molecular targeted therapy, disease-modifying drugs, compounds, small molecules, gene therapy, and stem cells, is essential not only for understanding pathophysiology, but for optimizing treatment.

Basic Cellular Structures and Function

The basic cell structures and other terms pertinent to cell biology are summarized in **Tables 2** through **5**. Some of these structures are discussed in more detail in the following paragraphs.

The Nucleus

The nucleus is a prominent membrane-bound organelle found in all eukaryotic cells.[79] The nucleus contains the genetic blueprint for the organism. DNA molecules, along with accompanying proteins such as histones, form complexes called chromosomes. The genetic information or genome is coded within the genes located on the chromosomes in this structure.[79] Through a vast signaling network, the nucleus is the site of gene and, subsequently, protein expression. The nucleus features its own double membrane, referred to as a nuclear envelope.[91] The outside of the membrane is continuous with the rough endoplasmic reticulum and both are studded with ribosomes. Nuclear pores are channels embedded into the largely impermeable nuclear membrane and they allow the free movement of small molecules and ions.[91] Passage of larger molecules such as proteins is regulated and mediated by carrier proteins. The separation that the nuclear envelope provides to the nucleus from the cytosol allows for posttranscriptional modifications that are not possible in prokaryotes. This enables a large amount of control over gene expression at the transcriptional level. Other nuclear structures include linear DNA organized into structures known as chromosomes.[79]

Under normal conditions, the chromosomes are found in a condensed state known as chromatin. While the cell is undergoing division, they can be observed as the well-defined chromosomes that are seen in karyotypes. Karyotyping is the study of the number and appearance of chromosomes in the nucleus.[79] Within the nucleus, there is a suborganelle structure known as nucleolus, which contains proteins and nucleic acids. This structure is the site of assembly and transcription of ribosomal RNA. The nucleus has a variety of other structures that are present in normal conditions. Some of these structures form functional domains in the nucleus; they include Cajal bodies, Gemini of coiled bodies, polymorphic interphase karyosomal association, promyelocytic leukemia bodies, paraspeckles, and splicing speckles.[92]

Ribonucleic Acid

RNA, along with DNA and proteins, makes up some of the most essential factors for life in an organism.[80] RNA and DNA share some similarity in composition with a few important exceptions: RNA uses ribose as its sugar component, whereas DNA uses deoxyribose, which is a ribose with one fewer oxygen molecule. Three of the four constitutive nucleotides of DNA (adenine, cytosine, and guanine) are present in RNA; however, uracil is substituted for thymine in RNA molecules. Furthermore, although DNA is double stranded and locked in a helical pattern, RNA is single stranded and is able to form complex three-dimensional structures.

There are several subtypes to RNA, which make up the protein synthesis machinery. Messenger RNA (mRNA) encodes the sequence of amino acids in specific peptides. mRNA is transcribed from DNA initially as heterogeneous nuclear RNA (hnRNA or premessenger RNA) and is altered by small nuclear RNA (snRNA) to form mRNA, which is a conduit for the genetic information held in DNA to be interpreted by the cellular protein synthesis mechanisms. Further along the protein synthesis chain, transfer RNA (tRNA) plays a part in building polypeptide chains at the ribosome during the translation of mRNA.[93] It transports specific amino acids by binding to them on its 3' end and then attaching the amino acid to the growing polypeptide chain at the ribosome. It accomplishes this through its three-base anticodon region, which binds to the corresponding three-base region on the mRNA undergoing ribosomal translation.[93] tRNA is aided by ribosomal RNA (rRNA) in decoding mRNA into its corresponding amino acids.[94] rRNA has been shown to have an effective antibiotic focus, with the use of drugs such as rRNA-targeting streptomycin.[95]

Several short RNA varieties exist to alter protein expression based on the cellular environment and requirements. These functions convey high research relevance for studying disease states. Two such types are small interfering RNA (siRNA) and microRNA (miRNA). miRNAs are short RNA molecules of 22 nucleotides in length. miRNAs suppress mRNA by a process called posttranscriptional regulation or gene silencing.[96] miRNAs are also involved in cell processes

Table 2

Definitions and Functions of Cell Structures

Structure	Definition	Clinical Relevance
Nucleus	A double-membrane–enclosed organelle found in eukaryotic cells. It contains chromosomes and various nuclear proteins, which communicate with the surrounding cytosol by transportation through numerous nuclear pores.	Genetic disorders Karyotyping Flow cytometry Mitosis in cancer
Nucleolus	A prominent structure in the nucleus responsible for the production of ribosomes.	Rothmund-Thompson syndrome Bloom syndrome Treacher Collins syndrome
Cytosol/ cytoplasm	Cytosol is an intracellular "soup" where most of the cellular metabolism occurs, including signal transduction pathways and glycolysis. It is also the location where synthesis of proteins, such as intracellular receptors and transcription factors, occurs. Cytoplasm is a collective term for cytosol and the organelles present in cytosol.	Signal transduction Metabolism Synthesis of proteins Degradation
Centrosome/ microtubule organizing center (MTOC)	MTOC is an area where microtubules are produced in a cell. Microtubules form the flagella/cilia of eukaryotic cells and are involved in chromosome separation during mitosis/meiosis.	Cystic kidney disease Mitosis and cancer Drug target (taxane)
Golgi body	A single membrane-bound structure in which enzymatic or hormonal contents are produced, packaged, and released into membrane-bound vesicles from the periphery of this organelle.	Alzheimer disease
Lysosome	An organelle that contains acid hydrolases. These enzymes are responsible for intracellular digestion of aged organelles, cellular waste, and phagocytosed pathogens, including viruses and bacteria.	Lysosomal storage disorders Mucopolysaccharidosis Gaucher disease
Cell membrane	A double layer of phospholipids (lipid bilayer) that encloses cells and acts as a protective barrier from the external environment.	Duchenne muscular dystrophy Long QT syndrome Hemolytic uremic anemia
Peroxisome	A membrane-bound packet of oxidative enzymes that are involved in metabolic pathways such as oxidation of fatty acids, as well as production of cholesterol, bile acids, and plasmalogens.	Brain storage diseases Adrenoleukodystrophy Infantile refsum disease Cerebrohepatorenal syndrome
Mitochondria	Double-membrane organelle that provides energy for the cell to move, divide, and produce secretory products by the production of adenosine triphosphate, a source for power. This organelle is also involved in cell death and amino acid synthesis.	Myopathy Diabetes and deafness Ataxia and epilepsy Optic neuropathy
Smooth/rough endoplasmic reticulum (SER/RER)	SER, which appears as a smooth membrane on the electron microscopy, synthesizes lipid and steroid hormones. In addition, SER degrades lipid-soluble toxins in the liver cells and controls calcium release in the muscle cells. RER has numerous ribosomes on its surface.	Liver endoplasmic reticulum storage disease

Table 2

Definitions and Function of Cell Structures (continued)

Structure	Definition	Clinical Relevance
Ribosome	A machinery unit that makes peptides/proteins by reading the sequence of mRNA and assembling tRNA-bound amino acids	Macrocytic anemia Cartilage hair hypoplasia
Cytoskeleton	A network of microtubules, actin filaments (microfilaments), and intermediate fibers. Its function includes the maintenance of cell shape, the internal movement of cell organelles, cell motility, and muscle fiber contraction.	Cardiomyopathy Deafness Congenital myopathy Osteoclast motility Phagocytosis

Table 3

Terminology Related to DNA

Term	Definition	Clinical Relevance
DNA	A double-stranded polymer formed from multiple pairs of dioxyribonucleotides, which are connected by hydrogen bonds. Dioxyribonucleotides consist of deoxyribose, a phosphate group, and one of the four nucleobases (adenine, guanine, cytosine, or thymine). DNA contains biologic information vital for replication and regulation of gene expression. The nucleotide sequence of DNA determines the specific biologic information.	Diagnosis of diseases DNA vaccines
Chromosome	A nuclear structure that contains linear strands of DNA. Humans have 46 chromosomes (23 pairs).	Abnormalities in number/structure lead to diseases (for example, DiGeorge syndrome)
Gene promoter	Regulatory portion of DNA that controls initiation of transcription adjacent to the transcription start site of a gene.	Mutations lead to certain diseases (for example, Alzheimer disease)
Chromatin	Genetic material composed of DNA and proteins. It is located within the nucleus of the cell and becomes condensed to form chromosomes.	Chromatin remodeling diseases
Gene	A specific DNA segment that contains all the information required for synthesis of a protein, including both coding and noncoding sequences.	Mutations of genes have been linked to certain diseases (for example, cancer, Cockayne syndrome)
Genome	The complete genetic information of an organism.	Genome-wide screening (microarray)
Mitochondrial DNA (mtDNA)	Circular DNA that is found in the mitochondria. mtDNA encodes proteins, which are essential for the function of the organelle. Mammalian mtDNAs are 16 kb in length, contain no introns, and have very little noncoding DNA.	Mutations leading to diseases (for example, thyroid disease, cataracts, diabetes)
DNA polymerase	An enzyme that synthesizes new strands of DNA by polymerizing dioxyribonucleotides.	Mutations in the polymerase can cause diseases (eg, cancer)
Exon	Portion of a gene that encodes for mRNA.	
Intron	Portion of a gene that does not encode for mRNA.	
Gene enhancer	Short regions of a gene that enhance the level of transcription.	Mutations lead to certain diseases (for example, Hirschsprung disease)

1: Basic Principles of Orthopaedic Surgery

Table 3

Terminology Related to DNA (continued)

Term	Definition	Clinical Relevance
Recombinant DNA	DNA that is artificially made by recombining DNA segments, which are usually not found together from splicing.	
Transgene	Gene that is artificially placed into a single-celled embryo. An organism that develops from this embryo will have the gene present in all of its cells.	Genetic disease model
Single nucleotide polymorphism (SNP)	Difference in DNA sequence due to a single nucleotide change. SNPs are found among members of the same biologic species.	Personalized medicine SNP genotyping
Central dogma of molecular biology	A framework that shows how information is passed sequentially in a cell. It is commonly depicted as: DNA→RNA→Protein	
Epigenetics	Study of how environmental factors affect gene expression without changing the DNA sequence itself.	Medical epigenetics for cancer research
Genomics	Study of genomes as well as gene functions.	Genome-wide screening (microarray) Gene imprinting

such as proliferation and differentiation and are sometimes abnormally expressed in cancer, making them important possible therapeutic targets. siRNA is a double-stranded synthetic RNA molecule responsible for knockdown or silencing of target mRNAs.[96] siRNA is used for loss-of-function experiments of genes of interest or therapeutic purpose.

Endoplasmic Reticulum

Endoplasmic reticulum is a network of folded membranes that performs many functions, including protein translocation, lipid synthesis, and regulation of intracellular Ca^{+2} concentrations. These membranes extend from the plasma membrane to the nucleus. In a typical eukaryotic cell, endoplasmic reticulum is classified into three different categories: nuclear endoplasmic reticulum, smooth endoplasmic reticulum, and rough endoplasmic reticulum.[97] Nuclear endoplasmic reticulum is composed of two layers of membrane and wraps around the nuclear envelope.[97] Rough endoplasmic reticulum has ribosomes associated with it, whereas the smooth endoplasmic reticulum lacks these organelles. Smooth endoplasmic reticulum, which is only abundant in selected cell types such as liver cells, muscle cells, and neurons, plays an important role in detoxification of substances, regulation of intracellular calcium, and transportation of molecules to the Golgi apparatus.[98] Unlike the smooth endoplasmic reticulum, the rough endoplasmic reticulum is present in all eukaryotic cells and is involved in processing of the proteins produced by the ribosomes.[98] Because endoplasmic reticulum has multiple roles in the cellular processes, an understanding of its structure and function is important. As mentioned previously, endoplasmic reticu-

lum is known to be a major site for Ca^{+2} storage and plays a role in regulating intracellular Ca^{+2} levels. This is significant because Ca^{+2} is used as a secondary messenger within the cells and the lack of Ca^{+2} regulation could lead to diseases and disorders such as heart and bone diseases.[51,99]

Golgi Apparatus

The Golgi apparatus, an organelle found in most eukaryotic cells, is responsible for directing molecules to their intracellular or extracellular locations. The Golgi apparatus is a collection of flattened membrane-enclosed cisternae commonly located in close proximity to the endoplasmic reticulum and the nucleus.[100] The complex is organized into three compartments: cis-Golgi, medial Golgi, and trans-Golgi.[101] Proteins from the endoplasmic reticulum are retrieved on the cis side of the organelle and transported to their final destinations from the trans-Golgi.[101] In addition, this organelle is a major site for carbohydrate synthesis, which is essential for the addition of oligosaccharide side chains to the proteins derived from the endoplasmic reticulum.[100,102] One of the functions of the Golgi apparatus is proper glycosylation of proteins.[103] Impairment of this function could not only cause inherited diseases, but also epidemic diseases, such as cancer and diabetes.[104] For instance, GnT-V, an enzyme found in the Golgi apparatus, was shown to be highly expressed in metastatic cancer cells.[101]

Lysosome

The lysosome is an organelle that contains acid hydrolases, which are enzymes that degrade aged organelles and cellular waste.[105] In addition to waste disposal, this organelle is

Table 4

Terminology Related to RNA

Term	Definition	Clinical Relevance
RNA	A polymer composed of ribonucleotide monomers that are covalently linked. Ribonucleotide has a ribose, a phosphate group, and a nucleobase (adenine, guanine, cytosine, or uracil). RNA is essential for protein synthesis, biologic reactions, and cellular communication.	Detection of mRNA in pathogens, arthritis, and cancers. rRNA can be used for the detection of bacterial pathogens. siRNAs are currently investigated for the treatment of cancers and viral infections. siRNAs are very useful for the functional genetic study by examining the effect of target gene knockdown. Rifamycin targets RNA polymerase.
Messenger RNA (mRNA)	RNA molecule that depicts the specific amino acid sequence of a protein. It is transcribed from DNA and used for protein synthesis.	
MicroRNA (miRNA)	Small RNA segments (22 nts), which regulate the expression of mRNA molecules. miRNA interacts with mRNA to inhibit the translation of the mRNA.	
Small interfering RNA (siRNA)	Short double-stranded RNA, which interferes with the expression of a specific gene.	
Ribosomal RNA (rRNA)	RNA that is a part of the ribosome and is involved in protein synthesis.	
Small nuclear RNA (snRNA)	Small RNA found in the nucleus. It binds to proteins to form small nuclear ribonucleoprotein particles (snRNPs), which produce functional molecules. Functional molecules are involved in a variety of processes, such as RNA splicing, transcription factor regulation, and maintenance of the telomeres.	
Small nucleolar RNA (snoRNA)	Small RNA molecules involved in methylation or pseudouridylation of rRNAs and other RNA genes.	
Transfer RNA (tRNA)	RNA molecule that carries amino acids to the ribosome for the transfer of these amino acids to the elongating mRNA.	
X-inactive specific transcript RNA	A large RNA molecule that inactivates one of the two X chromosomes in females.	
RNA polymerase I (Pol I)	An enzyme that transcribes the rRNA.	
RNA polymerase II (Pol II or RNAP II)	An enzyme that transcribes protein-encoding genes into mRNA.	
RNA polymerase III (Pol III)	An enzyme that transcribes all the tRNA genes.	
Gene silencing, gene knockdown	Epigenetic process of preventing genes from being expressed. Gene silencing could be performed before transcription of a gene (for example, transposon silencing) or after transcription (for example, RNA interference).	

1: Basic Principles of Orthopaedic Surgery

Table 5

Terminology Related to Gene Expression and Protein Synthesis

Term	Definition	Orthopaedic Implications
Gene expression	Transcription: DNA → mRNA	
Transcription	A reading process of DNA information by RNA polymerase to make specific complementary mRNA.	Correct sequential transcription is essential for protein synthesis and cellular processes.
Splicing	Removal of intronic sequences from newly transcribed RNA, resulting in the production of mRNA.	Splicing variations could result in functional changes of genes and may cause diseases.
Transcription factor	Protein that can initiate transcription by binding to the regulatory elements of the DNA.	Examples: RUNX-2 (Cbfa-1) and Osx for osteoblastic differentiation SOX-9 for cartilage differentiation PPAR for adipose tissue differentiation.
Protein expression	Translation: mRNA → proteins	
Translation	A process of protein synthesis by decoding mRNA sequence to produce amino acid chains. This process is mediated by tRNA and the ribosome machinery. tRNA interprets the code on the mRNA and delivers an amino acid to the elongating peptide chain.	Correct translation of RNA is essential for cell survival. Antibiotics such as tetracycline inhibit tRNA from binding to the ribsosome.
Posttranslational modification	Enzymatic processing of a newly formed peptide. Peptides could be processed in numerous ways, such as disulfide-bridge formation, acetylation, glycosylation, and phosphorylation.	Posttranslational modifications of certain proteins are important for their activities (for example, noncollagenous proteins must undergo proper posttranslational modifications in order for bone mineralization to occur).
Proteomics	A study of all proteins expressed from the genome (proteome).	

important for digestion of phagocytosed pathogens including viruses and bacteria. Components that need to be removed, could be degraded by this organelle through endocytosis, phagocytosis, or autophagy. To carry out this degradative function, lysosome contains a variety of hydrolytic enzymes as well as a proton pump (ATPase), which maintains the organelle's acidic lumen (pH 4.6–5).[105] More than 50 hydrolases have been identified in lysosomes and these include phosphatases, nucleases, proteases, lipases, and glycosidases. In addition, some cell types have specialized lysosomal organelles, which not only possess digestive activities but also the ability to store newly synthesized secretory proteins.[106] Malfunction of lysosomes or lysosomal enzymes have been shown to cause a series of diseases known collectively as lysosomal storage disorders. There are more than 40 known diseases, including Pompe disease and Gaucher disease.[107] In addition, this organelle has been studied extensively due to its potential role in other diseases and cel-

lular processes. For instance, alterations in lysosomal enzyme expression have been observed in cancer cells, whereas several microbial pathogens, such as *Shigella* and *Listeria*, have been noted to avoid contact with lysosomes for their survival inside the host's cell. Furthermore, osteoclasts, which are responsible for bone resorption, are known to break down the bone by the release of lysosomal hydrolases.[106]

Mitochondrion

A mitochondrion, also known as the "powerhouse of the cell," is a rod-shaped organelle that is responsible for most ATP production. In addition to producing energy, this organelle is involved in several other functions, including apoptosis and amino acid production. This organelle is composed of an outer membrane, intermembrane space, inner membrane, cistae membranes, intracristal space, and matrix.[108] Although mitochondria contain DNA in the matrix, most mitochondrial proteins are encoded in the nucleus.[108] ATP is produced by respiration, which involves the citric acid cycle and the electron transport chain. This organelle is also involved in other cellular processes such as apoptosis and production of many molecules such as amino acids, vitamin cofactors, and fatty acids.[109]

Mitochondrial function and dysfunction have been implicated in a wide range of diseases, including neurologic disorders, cardiovascular diseases, myopathies, and diabetes.[110,111] An example of one of these diseases is Barth syndrome, which is a genetic disorder characterized by cardioskeletal myopathy and neutropenia. This disease has been shown to be caused by a mutation that affects the structure of the mitochondria.[112] In addition to the dysfunction of this organelle, mitochondria are known to generate a large number of reactive oxygen species due to respiration. Although this organelle has enzymes to counteract these free radicals, damages to plasma membrane and DNA from these sources may be possible.[111]

Cytoskeleton

Cytoskeleton is an internal network of actin polymers present in all eukaryotic cells.[78] This organelle is not only important for structural support and cell motility, but it also plays a crucial role in cell signaling, mitosis, and the cell cycle. In eukaryotic cells, cytoskeleton is made up of three types of actin polymers: microtubules, microfilaments (also known as actin filaments), and intermediate filaments.[78] Microtubules, which consist of α and β subunits, polymerize and depolymerize from the centrosome and play a role in intracellular transport as well as mitosis.[78] Microfilaments are composed of actin subunits and allow cell motility to occur, whereas intermediate filaments give support for cell structure. Because actin and microtubule systems help regulate many signaling pathways in multiple cell types, scientists are interested in finding the role of these systems in the formation and progression of diseases.[113] In addition, research into the cytoskeleton is important for understanding the change and the behavior of cells. For instance, the cytoskeleton has been shown to be essential for the function of osteoclast, which causes degradation of bone tissue (resorption).[114] For osteoclasts to undergo resorption, these cells reorganize their cytoskeleton for bone attachment.

DNA, RNA, and Proteins: The Central Dogma

In 1958, Francis Crick depicted the relationship among the three major macromolecules in the central dogma of molecular biology.[115] This proposal illustrated the transformation of genetic material into proteins, which are vital components for biologic, structural, and enzymatic processes to occur. The processes required for the formation of a functional protein from DNA is described in this section (**Figure 14**).

Transcription (DNA to RNA)

Transcription is an important process of transferring genetic information into a form of mRNA. RNA polymerase II transcribes DNA from the 3' to the 5' direction to produce pre-mRNA.[60] At the end of transcription, poly (A) tail is added to the 3' end of pre-mRNA in a process known as polyadenylation.[79,116]

For cells to have control over gene transcription, DNA has regulatory regions, which include the gene promoter and gene enhancer. Gene promoter is a DNA segment where transcription factors bind to control the expression of a gene. A promoter of a gene is located adjacent to the gene it controls. One of the most common promoter sequences of a eukaryotic DNA is known as the TATA box. Furthermore, the promoter is the site where RNA polymerase II binds to initiate transcription. Another regulatory region of the DNA is known as the gene enhancer. This DNA segment enhances the rate of transcription of a gene, which could be located upstream or downstream of this enhancer.

After the formation of pre-mRNA, mRNA is produced by a process known as splicing.[117] This essential process removes the introns from the pre-mRNA and joins the exons together. More recently, scientists found multiple ways in which exons are assembled together to form a variety of mRNA molecules.[117] This mechanism is known as alternative splicing, and the discovery of this process led to an understanding of how a single gene could lead to multiple unique mRNA molecules.

Translation (RNA to Protein)

mRNA must be decoded to form a protein in a process known as translation.[118] mRNA, which is released into the cytosol of the cell, is bound by a ribosome. This ribosome reads the codons (trinucleotide sequence) of the mRNA, starting from the start codon. Each codon encodes for an amino acid. The tRNA, which has an amino acid–binding site and anticodon site, delivers the correct amino acid to the ribosome, forming a peptide chain.[60] Translation is terminated when the ribosome reads the stop codon and the peptide is released.[60]

Posttranslational Modification

Shortly after translation, newly made peptides are processed by an event known as posttranslational modification. There are a variety of different ways a peptide could be processed, including attachment of functional groups (for example, acetylation), change in the structure of the peptide (for example, proteolytic cleavage), and change in the chemical nature of the peptide (for example, citrullination).[118] These modifications are important for the appropriate functioning of these proteins.

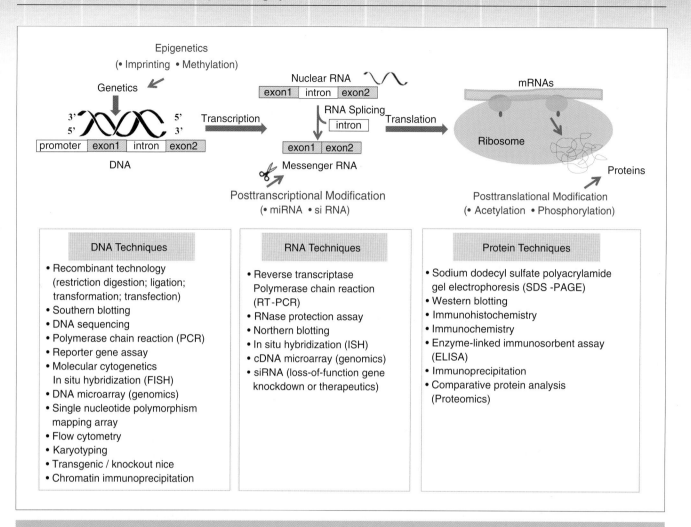

Figure 14 Molecular techniques used for orthopaedic diagnosis and research.

Epigenetics: Beyond the Central Dogma of Molecular Biology

Although DNA was shown to provide important heritable information, as research advances, scientists found heritable changes that affect gene expression, but not the DNA sequence itself. The study of these inherited characteristics is known as epigenetics. The mechanisms of epigenetics involve repression of gene expression without the physical change of the DNA sequence.[119] Epigenetics focuses on remodeling of chromatin—the complex of DNA and the histone proteins around which it is wrapped. The basic concept is the addition of some molecules to the DNA to alter its folding around the histones, thus opening up new parts to the DNA sequence for transcription. Three gene-silencing systems have been identified: DNA methylation, histone modification, and RNA-associated silencing. DNA methylation and histone modification are mechanisms that silence a gene before transcription, whereas RNA-associated silencing is a mechanism of posttranscriptional silencing. DNA methylation, which is one of the well-known silencing mechanisms, occurs with the methylation of cytosine resi-

dues in the DNA by an enzyme known as DNA methyltransferase.[120] In histone modification, histones, which are nuclear proteins associated with DNA, are subjected to numerous modifications. These proteins could be acetylated, methylated, phosphorylated, or ubiquitinated—referring to different additions to the chromatin structure that influence how the DNA sequences are read. Modifications of histones lead to inactivation of the DNA regions, which are associated with these proteins.[121] In RNA-associated silencing, small RNA molecules are used to inhibit gene expression. Some examples of RNA-associated silencing are miRNA, siRNA, and X-inactive specific transcript RNA.[122]

Epigenetics was shown to be linked to many hereditary diseases and numerous cellular mechanisms. Although this field is fairly new, some researchers have found the effects of epigenetics in orthopaedic diseases.[119] An example of the role of epigenetics in orthopaedic diseases is in the case of osteoarthritis.[123] This disease is characterized by pain in the joints due to the loss of cartilage. Recently, scientists have found that one of the causes of this disease is abnormal DNA methylation of metalloproteinase promoter sequences.[124] Furthermore, epigenetics was shown to regulate

Table 6

Commonly Used Molecular Biology Techniques for Diagnosis and Research Related to DNA or mRNA

Technique	Definition	Orthopaedic Implications
Molecular cytogenetics	Techniques that combine molecular biology and cytogenetics for the analysis of a specific DNA in a cell's genome. These techniques include fluorescence in situ hybridization (FISH) and comparative genomic hybridization (CGH).	These cytogenetic techniques have been used for detection of bone tumors as well as orthopaedic research.
In situ hybridization	A technique that involves the use of short, labeled complementary DNA or RNA strand (a probe) for localization and detection of a specific nucleic acid segment in a tissue.	Detection of oncogenes (mRNA) or mutated genes in pathologic specimens is performed by FISH technique.
Flow cytometry	A technique used to sort, analyze, or count biologic components, usually cells, by passing these components through a detection device.	Flow cytometry has been used in orthopaedic research, such as in the assessment of bone tumor malignancy.
Reporter gene assay	A method that uses a signal-producing gene for studying gene expression and localization in cells. A signal-producing gene could be green fluorescence protein, luciferase, or LacZ gene.	Reporter gene assays are commonly used in research for assessing the expression of a specific gene in a cell or tissue.
Polymerase chain reaction (PCR)	A method of amplifying a specific DNA sequence of interest to a detectable level by the use of DNA template, nucleotides, primers, and thermostable DNA polymerase. Double-stranded DNA is denatured into a single strand by increasing the temperature to 92°C to 94°C. Subsequently, the primers anneal (hybridize) to the template at an annealing temperature and at an optimal temperature, and the polymerase elongates the primers forming a double-stranded DNA. These steps are repeated numerous times in a thermal cycle to amplify the specific DNA sequence.	PCR is used for the diagnosis of infection when culturing is not feasible (eg, tuberculosis or HIV). In addition, PCR is used for phenotypic analysis of cancer cells, as well as for the identification of upregulation/downregulation of genes.
Reverse transcription-polymerase chain reaction (RT-PCR)	A sensitive technique that uses both reverse transcription and PCR techniques. RT-PCR is used for detection and quantification of mRNA from a sample. More recently, products of RT-PCR are detected on a real-time basis by a technique known as real-time RT-PCR or quantitative real-time PCR (Q-PCR).	RT-PCR and Q-PCR are used for both diagnosis and research purposes. These techniques are used for testing for the presence of viruses or cancer cells from the patient samples. The technique is also used for the analysis of gene expression levels in research.
Northern blotting	A technique used to identify and quantitate specific RNA molecules. RNA is subjected to agarose gel electrophoresis, which separates RNA by size. Probes, which hybridize specifically to these RNA molecules, are used for detection purposes.	Northern blotting has been used for the detection of mRNA expression in human cells, tissues, and research specimens.

Table 6

Commonly Used Molecular Biology Techniques for Diagnosis and Research Related to DNA or mRNA (continued)

Technique	Definition	Orthopaedic Implications
cDNA microarray	Multiplex chip that is used to interpret genomic information by comparison of control and experimental samples. This microarray requires the isolation of RNA from the samples and the conversion of these molecules into cDNAs, which are labeled with fluorescent probes. These cDNAs are hybridized on the chip and fluorescence is analyzed.	cDNA microarrays are used for comparing gene expression of normal and tumor cells. In addition, cDNA microarrays are tools used in orthopaedic research, such as in the case of examining gene expression profile of macrophages that have been exposed to biomaterials.
DNA sequencing	Methods developed for the detection of DNA sequences. A common method of sequencing is known as the Sanger method of dideoxy chain termination, which uses the fact that dideoxynucleotides do not possess 3'OH groups next to the nucleotides. In this method, four different reactions with each containing a different dideoxynucleotide (ddATP, ddCTP, ddGTP, or ddTTP) are arranged. In each of the four reactions, the DNA polymerase synthesizes DNA from the template by the addition of nucleotides to the primer. Incorporation of the dideoxynucleotide terminates this DNA elongation, resulting in fragments with different lengths. Each of the reactions is placed in different lanes on a gel and the sequences are read by analyzing the position of the bands on the gel.	DNA sequencing is an important tool not only in orthopaedic research, but also in other research fields. This technique is essential for understanding genes, mutations, and polymorphisms.
Southern blotting	A technique of running DNA fragments on agarose gels to identify a specific DNA sequence. After restriction digestion, negatively charged DNA fragments are separated by the gel apparatus, which has a negative and positive charge. These fragments are attracted to the positive-charged pole, causing them to migrate through the gel. The lengths of the DNA fragments could be identified by the comparison of these fragments to the molecular weight standard. The intensity of the band represents the amount of DNA fragments present in the gel.	Southern blotting has been used in orthopaedic research, such as in the analysis of genes of bone specimens.
Recombinant technology	A series of procedures used for the production of a desired protein. Recombinant protein is produced by the introduction of a genetic sequence that encodes for the specific protein into a genome of an organism.	This technology has been used for the production of numerous proteins, such as rhBMP-2, rhBMP-7, erythropoietin, RANKL blocker, TNF blocker, and IL-6 blocker. It is also used for functional studies of genes.
Manipulation of DNA (cutting, pasting, copy)	A series of procedures involving the use of DNA or RNA for the production of a desired DNA, RNA, or amino acid.	

Table 6

Commonly Used Molecular Biology Techniques for Diagnosis and Research Related to DNA or mRNA (continued)

Technique	Definition	Orthopaedic Implications
Restriction digestion (cutting DNA)	A technique that involves the use of restriction enzymes that cut double-stranded DNA at a specific location on the DNA sequence.	Restriction digestion is a widely used molecular technique for removing DNA fragments from other fragments.
Ligation (paste a DNA fragment)	A technique involving the use of an enzyme called ligase, which makes covalent phosphate bonds between nucleotides.	Ligation is a technique used in research for inserting DNA into another DNA fragment.
Transformation	Insertion of recombinant DNA (a plasmid) into a bacterial cell, resulting in genetic modification of that cell.	Transformation is a common technique used in research for isolating a plasmid, which encodes for a gene of interest. It is also a process used for the amplification of a plasmid.
Transfection	A nonviral method of introducing exogenous nucleic acids into a eukaryotic cell for integration of these nucleic acids into the chromosomal DNA of the cell. Insertion of nucleic acids could be performed by several methods, including electroporation and the use of calcium phosphate.	Transfection is an important process used in research for introducing DNA into cell lines.

gene expression in bone cells, such as in the case of osteogenic differentiation.[123]

Molecular Techniques Used for Orthopaedic Diagnosis and Research

In the past century, scientists developed and improved numerous scientific methods and techniques, which have been implicated not only in research, but also for diagnostic purposes. As previously stated, the combined use of computer technology and molecular biology significantly optimized the current understanding of molecular biology. This new information and technology led to the analysis of full DNA sequence of an organism (genome) and created a new field of study known as genomics. Similarly, the amalgamation of technology and biology led scientists to a new scientific field of proteins known as proteomics, the study of all proteins of a single organism (proteome). The combined understandings of genomics, epigenetics, and proteomics as well as the development of new techniques have led to an increased knowledge of cell biology and disease development in humans. The continuing increased knowledge in these fields could lead to the development of personalized medicine. For instance, single nucleotide polymorphisms (SNPs) are unique changes in a single nucleotide of DNA. Several studies have found that certain SNPs increase the tendency of humans to get a disease. These and similar studies would contribute to the understanding of diseases, leading to per-

sonalized medicine. This section summarizes the common techniques applied to current orthopaedic research and diagnostics of diseases (**Figure 14**, **Tables 6** and **7**).

DNA Techniques

Over many years, scientists developed various techniques that use the structure and the molecular characteristics of DNA to improve the understanding of this macromolecule and its effects on the outcome of human health.

After the discovery of DNA structure in 1953, recombinant technology was introduced in 1972.[125] This technology involves the manipulation of DNA to form a recombinant DNA. Recombinant DNA is an artificially prepared DNA produced by molecular techniques such as restriction digestion and ligation.[126] Recombinant proteins, made from such technology, are now almost ubiquitous in research and therapeutic applications. DNA is cut by a procedure known as restriction digestion and is reattached in a process known as ligation. The DNA of interest is frequently ligated into a circular bacterial DNA known as a plasmid.[127] This plasmid is inserted into a competent bacterial cell in a process called transformation.[125] The transformed bacterial cell expresses the genes of the inserted plasmid and the cell grows, leading to the amplification of the plasmid. Similarly, exogenous DNA could also be inserted into a eukaryotic cell in a process called transfection.[79] From the success of expressing exogenous genes in a bacterium and a eukaryotic cell, scientists were able to use this technology in whole organisms to

1: Basic Principles of Orthopaedic Surgery

1: Basic Principles of Orthopaedic Surgery

Table 7

Commonly Used Molecular Biology Techniques for Diagnosis and Research Related to Proteins

Technique	Definition	Orthopaedic Implications
Immunohistochemistry/ immunocytochemistry	A method for detection and localization of a target protein in a cell or tissue. The method involves the use of an antibody specific for the protein of interest. Some of the common target proteins are tumor markers and cytokines.	The technique is used for the diagnosis of musculo-skeletal and hematopoietic tumors.
Enzyme-linked immunosor-bent assay (ELISA)	A biochemical method for detection and quantifica-tion of a specific soluble protein.	ELISA is used for the sero-logic quantifications of enzymes and proteins such as in the case of alkaline phosphatase and amylase.
Bicinchoninic acid assay (BCA assay)	A biochemical test that uses colormetric techniques to determine the total amount of protein present in a solution.	The assay is used in ortho-paedic research for exam-ining the protein concen-tration of a test sample.
Tartrate-resistant acid phos-phatase assay (TRAP assay)	A staining technique for the identification of TRAP enzyme, which is a common marker of osteoclast identity.	TRAP assay is used for quantification and identi-fication of osteoclasts in research.
Sodium dodecyl sulfate polyacrylamide gel electro-phoresis (SDS-PAGE)	A technique that separates proteins according to mo-lecular weight, confirmation, and charge.	SDS-PAGE is an important technique used in research for protein isolation and analysis.
Coomassie Blue staining	A method of visualizing protein bands on SDS-PAGE gels by using dyes (Coomassie Blue) that bind to proteins nonspecifically.	This staining technique is used in research to quickly observe proteins in SDS-PAGE gels.
Western blotting	A technique commonly used after SDS-PAGE to iden-tify a specific protein of interest by using an antibody. This antibody binds to the protein of interest for rec-ognition.	Comparative analysis of protein expression in con-trol and pathologic tissues/experimental groups.
Immunoprecipitation	A method of precipitating a protein out of a solution by the use of a specific antibody that recognizes that protein of interest.	Immunoprecipitation is used in orthopaedic re-search to isolate proteins.
Chromatin immunoprecipi-tation (ChIP) assay ChIP sequencing	A type of immunoprecipitation assay used to examine the interactions and localizations of proteins to DNA in a cell.	ChIP is used in research for the analysis of proteins that are associated with specific regions of DNA. These proteins could be transcription factors.
Comparative proteomic analysis	A method that applies the use of a computer and a peptide sequencing machine for a comprehensive and rapid analysis of entire proteins in both the con-trol and pathologic (experimental) tissues or cells.	The technique is used for the detection of abnormal proteins in pathologic tis-sues.

produce transgenic animals, which are currently used as genetic disease models in research.[126] These genetically modified organisms are made by inserting a transgene into an embryo, which develops into an organism. As the embryo develops into an organism, the transgene will be present and expressed in each cell of the organism.

In addition to the recombinant technology, a method known as Southern blotting was discovered in 1975. In this method, DNA fragments are separated on a gel electrophoresis for the detection of specific DNA sequences. Currently, Southern blotting has been replaced by a new technique known as microarray, which is discussed in further detail in the following paragraphs.

These fundamental procedures have been used for understanding genes and their effect on cell behavior and cell differentiation, such as in the case of osteoclast differentiation. In addition, recombinant technology has been implicated in gene therapy, which involves the transfer of genes to a person for therapeutic purposes.[128] For example, a clinical trial that involves the use of gene therapy, was performed to treat rheumatoid arthritis in 2005.[128]

DNA sequencing is an important tool used in orthopaedic research and for diagnostic purposes. Sequencing of DNA has led to understanding of genetic mutations and how these affect health in humans. For instance, DNA sequencing of patients with fibrodysplasia ossificans progressiva, a rare genetic bone disease, led to the identification of missense mutation in a gene encoding for a BMP type I receptor.[129] In addition to the understanding of gene mutation and its effects on human health, DNA sequencing has been used for the identification of SNP, a single nucleotide change found among the members of the same species.[130]

Less than a decade after the discovery of the two DNA sequencing methods, a new laboratory technique known as polymerase chain reaction (PCR) was developed. In this technique, DNA is amplified by a thermostable DNA polymerase, which uses a DNA template and primers for initiating DNA synthesis.[131] These enzymes and the DNA of interest are placed in a machine to undergo changes in the temperature for optimal DNA separation, enzyme annealing, and DNA elongation to form double-stranded DNA. PCR has been extensively used for research and diagnostic purposes. An example of the use of PCR in diagnosis is in the case of identifying microbial infections from an orthopaedic surgery.

After the advancement of microscopes and computers, new methods related to DNA developed. Some of these common techniques include reporter gene assay, molecular cytogenetics, complementary DNA (cDNA) microarray, and flow cytometry. Reporter gene assay is a method used to indirectly measure the rates of transcription of a specific gene using a signal-producing gene, such as luciferase and *LacZ* gene.[132] Molecular cytogenetics is a series of techniques used to analyze a specific DNA sequence in a cell's genome. One of the well-known techniques in molecular cytogenetics is in situ hybridization. In this technique, a short DNA or RNA probe is used for the detection and localization of a specific nucleic acid segment (DNA or mRNA) within the histologic section.[133-135] In addition to these techniques, cDNA microarray, which was developed in the 1980s, has been used for research purposes as well as clinical cancer screenings. cDNA microarray uses a multiplex chip that consists of microscopic spots with DNA oligonucleotides and probes.[128] cDNA, which is made from reverse transcription of RNA, binds to the oligonucleotide present on the chip. This hybridization is detected with a computer. Microarrays are important tools for comparison of gene expression between different samples. Flow cytometry is often used for the detection and quantification of microscopic particles, such as DNA and cells, by the use of a detection device.[136] All of these methods are important in understanding of genes and their roles in orthopaedic diseases.

Chromatin immunoprecipitation sequencing (ChIP-Seq) technology can be used to determine novel regulatory sequences, which are targeted by a given transcription factor.[137] The power of this technology is that it helps identify areas of protein-DNA interactions within the whole genome.[138] In this assay, chromatin is sheared and immunoprecipitated using a specific antibody that targets a given transcription factor (as stated previously). Subsequently, adapters of known sequences are ligated to the ends of ChIPed DNA fragments. These adapters serve as primers for performing DNA sequencing of all immunoprecipitated fragments. ChIPed and adapter-modified chromatin libraries are used in massively parallel DNA sequencing, using approximately two million 25-nt sequencing reads per sample.[138] DNA binding sites for the transcription factor of interest are identified using the ChIP-Seq peak-calling program and data are then mapped to the species-specific genome to identify target regions to which the transcription factor binding was significantly enriched.[139] These data provide a high-resolution map of all binding sites within the genome with 27- to 50-oligomer resolution. Sequence reads mapped to more than one site within the genome are usually excluded because these likely represent repetitive DNA sequences. Potential targets that are identified by this method are commonly confirmed by real-time reverse transcription–polymerase chain reaction (RT-PCR) as downstream targets of a given transcription factor or in response to a signal that enhances this factor's activity.

RNA Techniques

Similar to DNA techniques, RNA laboratory techniques have been developed for diagnostic and research purposes. Other common laboratory RNA techniques are RT-PCR[131] and Northern blotting.[79] RT-PCR is a variant of PCR, but instead of using DNA as a template, mRNA is reversibly transcribed into cDNA. In the same reaction, PCR techniques are applied to the newly made cDNA. RT-PCR is used for the detection and quantification of mRNA in a test sample. Likewise, Northern blotting is used for the quantification of RNA molecules in a given sample, but in a different method. In Northern blotting, gel electrophoresis is used to run the RNA molecules according to their size. Probes are used to detect specific RNA sequences on the gel. Both RT-PCR and Northern blotting are used mainly for orthopaedic research. ISH is used to detect mRNA expression on pathology slides.[135] RT-PCR has been used for diagnosis of infections related to orthopaedic surgeries.

Protein Techniques

Numerous protein techniques, which have contributed to the knowledge of proteins and the effect of cellular functions on human health, have been produced and applied to research and diagnostics. One of the most frequently used protein techniques is sodium dodecyl sulfate polyacrylamide gel electrophoresis (SDS-PAGE). In this technique, proteins are placed in a gel, which separates these molecules by molecular weight, conformation, or charge.[79] After SDS-PAGE, the protein gels are commonly subjected to other techniques, such as Coomassie Blue staining and Western blotting. Coomassie Blue staining stains all of the proteins present in the polyacrylamide gel nonspecifically.[79] It is often used for quick visualization of the protein on the gel. Western blotting is a technique in which proteins are transferred on a membrane and probed by antibodies.[79] These antibodies are specific for the proteins; thus, the protein of interest could be identified and analyzed in terms of its size. These protein techniques are fundamental to most biologic research fields, including orthopaedic research where proteins associated with bone diseases can be investigated.

In addition to these techniques, some biochemical methods for identification of proteins in cells have been used extensively in research, such as enzyme-linked immunosorbent assay (ELISA), bicinchoninic acid (BCA) assay, and TRAP assay. ELISA is a common laboratory technique based on an antigen-antibody reaction that is used for the detection and quantification of a protein from a sample.[140] Unlike ELISA, which is specific, BCA assay is a colorimetric test used for the quantification of the total protein present in the sample.[141] TRAP assay is used in orthopaedic research for the identification of an enzyme known as TRAP. TRAP is a marker of osteoclast activity, which is commonly found in bone tissues.[142]

As research advances, new protein techniques such as immunoprecipitation, immunohistochemistry/immunocytochemistry, and comparative protein analysis have been developed. Immunoprecipitation is a method of removing a protein of interest out of a solution by the use of a specific antibody, which targets the protein. One of the common immunoprecipitation techniques is ChIP assay. In this technique, proteins, which interact with DNA of a cell, are purified for analysis.[143] ChIP assay allows scientists to conduct analysis of nuclear proteins and the DNA regions associated with these proteins. Immunohistochemistry and immunocytochemistry involve the use of a specific antibody, which has a probe. This antibody is used for detecting and locating a specific protein of interest in a sample. Immunohisto-

chemistry is used for tissue samples, whereas immunocytochemistry is used for cells with extracellular matrix removed.[144] In an effort to analyze and compare all of the proteins in samples at once, comparative protein analysis uses a computer and a peptide sequencing machine for comparison of protein profiles from different tissues. In addition, immunohistochemistry has been implicated in the diagnosis of certain cancers, such as in the case of musculoskeletal tumors, whereas comparative proteomic analysis has been used for the detection of abnormal proteins in pathologic tissue samples.[144]

Summary

The complex nature of bone biology and pathology affords many avenues of research. As the understanding regarding the interplay of the many factors involved in normal and abnormal bone function increases, orthopaedic surgeons will have greater knowledge to pursue and will use new, safer, and more effective therapies. Important developments such as CT, MRI, artificial joints, stem cells, and BMPs have all furthered the field of orthopaedic surgery. It is incumbent upon clinicians to stay abreast of these and possible novel treatment modalities to provide the utmost level of care. New discoveries such as the role of osteocytes in managing bone functions, sclerostin-inhibiting osteoblastic bone formation, and scleraxis-regulating chondrogenesis have shed new light on how bone and cartilage are made and maintained. This knowledge has enabled clinical therapeutic applications such as PRPs to promote tendon, ligament, muscle, and cartilage healing; RANK-Fc (denosumab) for the treatment of osteoporosis; and BMPs to promote bone growth. Additionally, myriad new treatments are developed usch as sclerostin inhibitors, which are undergoing clinical trials. Knowledge of research techniques as well as current and possible molecular treatments will be invaluable for discovering and evaluating new avenues for treatment.

References

1. Rosenfeld L: Insulin: Discovery and controversy. *Clin Chem* 2002;48(12):2270-2288.

2. Reddi AH: Marshall R. Urist: A renaissance scientist and orthopaedic surgeon. *J Bone Joint Surg Am* 2003;85(suppl 3):3-7.

3. Damadian R: Tumor detection by nuclear magnetic resonance. *Science* 1971;171(3976):1151-1153.

4. Takahashi K, Yamanaka S: Induction of pluripotent stem cells from mouse embryonic and adult fibroblast cultures by defined factors. *Cell* 2006;126(4):663-676.

5. Teitelbaum SL, Ross FP: Genetic regulation of osteoclast development and function. *Nat Rev Genet* 2003;4(8):638-649.

6. Hoffmann A, Gross G: BMP signaling pathways in cartilage and bone formation. *Crit Rev Eukaryot Gene Expr* 2001;11(1-3):23-45.

7. Rawadi G, Vayssière B, Dunn F, Baron R, Roman-Roman S: BMP-2 controls alkaline phosphatase expression and osteoblast mineralization by a Wnt autocrine loop. *J Bone Miner Res* 2003;18(10):1842-1853.

8. Yang X, Chen L, Xu X, Li C, Huang C, Deng CX: TGF-beta/Smad3 signals repress chondrocyte hypertrophic differentiation and are required for maintaining articular cartilage. *J Cell Biol* 2001;153(1):35-46.

9. Dennler S, Goumans M-J, ten Dijke P: Transforming growth factor beta signal transduction. *J Leukoc Biol* 2002;71(5):731-740.

10. Zhou S, Eid K, Glowacki J: Cooperation between TGF-beta and Wnt pathways during chondrocyte and adipocyte differentiation of human marrow stromal cells. *J Bone Miner Res* 2004;19(3):463-470.

11. Kronenberg HM: PTHrP and skeletal development. *Ann N Y Acad Sci* 2006;1068:1-13.

12. Schipani E, Provot S: PTHrP, PTH, and the PTH/PTHrP receptor in endochondral bone development. *Birth Defects Res C Embryo Today* 2003;69(4):352-362.

13. Ionescu AM, Schwarz EM, Vinson C, et al: PTHrP modulates chondrocyte differentiation through AP-1 and CREB signaling. *J Biol Chem* 2001;276(15):11639-11647.

14. Maeda Y, Nakamura E, Nguyen MT, et al: Indian Hedgehog produced by postnatal chondrocytes is essential for maintaining a growth plate and trabecular bone. *Proc Natl Acad Sci U S A* 2007;104(15):6382-6387.

15. Serra R, Johnson M, Filvaroff EH, et al: Expression of a truncated, kinase-defective TGF-beta type II receptor in mouse skeletal tissue promotes terminal chondrocyte differentiation and osteoarthritis. *J Cell Biol* 1997;139(2):541-552.

16. Duan C, Ren H, Gao S: Insulin-like growth factors (IGFs), IGF receptors, and IGF-binding proteins: Roles in skeletal muscle growth and differentiation. *Gen Comp Endocrinol* 2010;167(3):344-351.

17. Eswarakumar VP, Lax I, Schlessinger J: Cellular signaling by fibroblast growth factor receptors. *Cytokine Growth Factor Rev* 2005;16(2):139-149.

18. Geiger F, Lorenz H, Xu W, et al: VEGF producing bone marrow stromal cells (BMSC) enhance vascularization and resorption of a natural coral bone substitute. *Bone* 2007;41(4):516-522.

19. Huelsken J, Birchmeier W: New aspects of Wnt signaling pathways in higher vertebrates. *Curr Opin Genet Dev* 2001;11(5):547-553.

20. Clevers H: Wnt/beta-catenin signaling in development and disease. *Cell* 2006;127(3):469-480.

21. Boland GM, Perkins G, Hall DJ, Tuan RS: Wnt 3a promotes proliferation and suppresses osteogenic differentiation of adult human mesenchymal stem cells. *J Cell Biochem* 2004;93(6):1210-1230.

22. Westendorf JJ, Kahler RA, Schroeder TM: Wnt signaling in osteoblasts and bone diseases. *Gene* 2004;341:19-39.

23. Krishnan V, Bryant HU, Macdougald OA: Regulation of bone mass by Wnt signaling. *J Clin Invest* 2006;116(5):1202-1209.

24. Borish LC, Steinke JW: 2. Cytokines and chemokines. *J Allergy Clin Immunol* 2003;111(2, suppl):S460-S475.

25. Lee YM, Fujikado N, Manaka H, Yasuda H, Iwakura Y: IL-1 plays an important role in the bone metabolism under physiological conditions. *Int Immunol* 2010;22(10):805-816.

26. Cronstein BN, Naime D, Ostad E: The antiinflammatory mechanism of methotrexate: Increased adenosine release at inflamed sites diminishes leukocyte accumulation in an in vivo model of inflammation. *J Clin Invest* 1993;92(6):2675-2682.

27. Lee SK, Lorenzo J: Cytokines regulating osteoclast formation and function. *Curr Opin Rheumatol* 2006;18(4):411-418.

28. Weber A, Wasiliew P, Kracht M: Interleukin-1 (IL-1) pathway. *Sci Signal* 2010;3(105):cm1.

29. Blanchard F, Duplomb L, Baud'huin M, Brounais B: The dual role of IL-6-type cytokines on bone remodeling and bone tumors. *Cytokine Growth Factor Rev* 2009;20(1):19-28.

30. Bird L: T-cell memory: Staying alive with IL-7. *Nat Rev Immunol* 2004;4:7.

31. Chaplin DD: Overview of the immune response. *J Allergy Clin Immunol* 2010;125(2, suppl 2):S3-S23.

32. Tang Y, Wu X, Lei W, et al: TGF-beta1-induced migration of bone mesenchymal stem cells couples bone resorption with formation. *Nat Med* 2009;15(7):757-765.

33. Boyce BF, Xing L: Functions of RANKL/RANK/OPG in bone modeling and remodeling. *Arch Biochem Biophys* 2008;473(2):139-146.

34. Takayanagi H: The role of NFAT in osteoclast formation. *Ann N Y Acad Sci* 2007;1116:227-237.

35. Weissman IL: Stem cells: Units of development, units of regeneration, and units in evolution. *Cell* 2000;100(1):157-168.

36. Ludwig TE, Levenstein ME, Jones JM, et al: Derivation of human embryonic stem cells in defined conditions. *Nat Biotechnol* 2006;24(2):185-187.

37. Zhou H, Wu S, Joo JY, et al: Generation of induced pluripotent stem cells using recombinant proteins. *Cell Stem Cell* 2009;4(5):381-384.

38. Wilmut I, Beaujean N, de Sousa PA, et al: Somatic cell nuclear transfer. *Nature* 2002;419(6907):583-586.

39. Campbell KH, McWhir J, Ritchie WA, Wilmut I: Sheep cloned by nuclear transfer from a cultured cell line. *Nature* 1996;380(6569):64-66.

40. Marie PJ: Transcription factors controlling osteoblastogenesis. *Arch Biochem Biophys* 2008;473(2):98-105.

41. Komori T: Regulation of bone development and extracellular matrix protein genes by RUNX2. *Cell Tissue Res* 2010;339(1):189-195.

42. Yoshida CA, Komori T: Role of Runx proteins in chondrogenesis. *Crit Rev Eukaryot Gene Expr* 2005;15(3):243-254.

43. Zhang C: Transcriptional regulation of bone formation by the osteoblast-specific transcription factor Osx. *J Orthop Surg Res* 2010;5:37.

44. Krawchuk D, Weiner SJ, Chen YT, et al: Twist1 activity thresholds define multiple functions in limb development. *Dev Biol* 2010;347(1):133-146.

45. Kronenberg HM: Twist genes regulate Runx2 and bone formation. *Dev Cell* 2004;6(3):317-318.

46. Satokata I, Ma L, Ohshima H, et al: Msx2 deficiency in mice causes pleiotropic defects in bone growth and ectodermal organ formation. *Nat Genet* 2000;24(4):391-395.

47. Li H, Marijanovic I, Kronenberg MS, et al: Expression and function of Dlx genes in the osteoblast lineage. *Dev Biol* 2008;316(2):458-470.

48. Meury T, Akhouayri O, Jafarov T, Mandic V, St-Arnaud R: Nuclear alpha NAC influences bone matrix mineralization and osteoblast maturation in vivo. *Mol Cell Biol* 2010;30(1):43-53.

49. Rudnicki MA, Le Grand F, McKinnell I, Kuang S: The molecular regulation of muscle stem cell function. *Cold Spring Harb Symp Quant Biol* 2008;73:323-331.

50. Black BL, Olson EN: Transcriptional control of muscle development by myocyte enhancer factor-2 (MEF2) proteins. *Annu Rev Cell Dev Biol* 1998;14:167-196.

51. Negishi-Koga T, Takayanagi H: Ca2+-NFATc1 signaling is an essential axis of osteoclast differentiation. *Immunol Rev* 2009;231(1):241-256.

52. Kawai M, Rosen CJ: PPARγ: A circadian transcription factor in adipogenesis and osteogenesis. *Nat Rev Endocrinol* 2010;6(11):629-636.

53. Tang QQ, Zhang JW, Daniel Lane M: Sequential gene promoter interactions by C/EBPbeta, C/EBPalpha, and PPAR-gamma during adipogenesis. *Biochem Biophys Res Commun* 2004;318(1):213-218.

54. Furumatsu T, Shukunami C, Amemiya-Kudo M, Shimano H, Ozaki T: Scleraxis and E47 cooperatively regulate the Sox9-dependent transcription. *Int J Biochem Cell Biol* 2010;42(1):148-156.

55. Abercrombie M: Contact inhibition in tissue culture. *In Vitro* 1970;6(2):128-142.

56. Dillon JP, Waring-Green VJ, Taylor AM, et al: Primary human osteoblast cultures, in Helfrich MH, Ralston SH, eds: *Bone Research Protocols*. New York, NY, Humana Press, 2003.

57. Beyer Nardi N, da Silva Meirelles L: Mesenchymal stem cells: Isolation, in vitro expansion and characterization. *Handb Exp Pharmacol* 2006;174:249-282.

58. Bruder SP, Jaiswal N, Ricalton NS, Mosca JD, Kraus KH, Kadiyala S: Mesenchymal stem cells in osteobiology and applied bone regeneration. *Clin Orthop Relat Res* 1998;355(355, suppl):S247-S256.

59. Bensidhoum M, Chapel A, Francois S, et al: Homing of in vitro expanded Stro-1- or Stro-1+ human mesenchymal stem cells into the NOD/SCID mouse and their role in supporting human CD34 cell engraftment. *Blood* 2004;103(9):3313-3319.

60. Gray NK, Wickens M: Control of translation initiation in animals. *Annu Rev Cell Dev Biol* 1998;14:399-458.

61. Kartsogiannis V, Ng KW: Cell lines and primary cell cultures in the study of bone cell biology. *Mol Cell Endocrinol* 2004;228(1-2):79-102.

62. Buckwalter JA, Ehrlich MG, Sandell LJ, Trippel SB: *Skeletal Growth and Development: Clinical Issues and Basic Science Advances*. Rosemont, IL, American Academy of Orthopaedic Surgeons, 1998.

63. Viguet-Carrin S, Garnero P, Delmas PD: The role of collagen in bone strength. *Osteoporos Int* 2006;17(3):319-336.

64. Katz EP, Wachtel E, Yamauchi M, Mechanic GL: The structure of mineralized collagen fibrils. *Connect Tissue Res* 1989;21(1-4):149-158.

65. Young MF, Kerr JM, Ibaraki K, Heegaard AM, Robey PG: Structure, expression, and regulation of the major noncollagenous matrix proteins of bone. *Clin Orthop Relat Res* 1992;281:275-294.

66. Fujisawa R, Wada Y, Nodasaka Y, Kuboki Y: Acidic amino acid-rich sequences as binding sites of osteonectin to hydroxyapatite crystals. *Biochim Biophys Acta* 1996;1292(1):53-60.

67. Owen TA, Aronow MS, Barone LM, Bettencourt B, Stein GS, Lian JB: Pleiotropic effects of vitamin D on osteoblast gene expression are related to the proliferative and differentiated state of the bone cell phenotype: Dependency upon basal levels of gene expression, duration of exposure, and bone matrix competency in normal rat osteoblast cultures. *Endocrinology* 1991;128(3):1496-1504.

68. Cooper MS, Hewison M, Stewart PM: Glucocorticoid activity, inactivity and the osteoblast. *J Endocrinol* 1999;163(2):159-164.

69. Feng JQ, Ward LM, Liu S, et al: Loss of DMP1 causes rickets and osteomalacia and identifies a role for osteocytes in mineral metabolism. *Nat Genet* 2006;38(11):1310-1315.

70. Bellido T, Saini V, Pajevic PD: Effects of PTH on osteocyte function. *Bone* 2012 Sep 24 (Epub ahead of print).

71. Kogianni G, Noble BS: The biology of osteocytes. *Curr Osteoporos Rep* 2007;5(2):81-86.

72. O'Brien CA, Nakashima T, Takayanagi H: Osteocyte control of osteoclastogenesis. *Bone* 2012 Aug 23 (Epub ahead of print).

73. Nakashima T, Hayashi M, Fukunaga T, et al: Evidence for osteocyte regulation of bone homeostasis through RANKL expression. *Nat Med* 2011;7(10):1231-1234.

74. Karsenty G: Transcriptional control of skeletogenesis. *Annu Rev Genomics Hum Genet* 2008;9:183-196.

75. Bilezikian JP, Raisz LG, Rodan GA: *Principles of Bone Biology*. San Diego, CA, Academic Press, 1996.

76. Teitelbaum SL: Bone resorption by osteoclasts. *Science* 2000;289(5484):1504-1508.

77. Benjamin M, Ralphs JR: The cell and developmental biology of tendons and ligaments. *Int Rev Cytol* 2000;196:85-130.

78. Schmidt A, Hall MN: Signaling to the actin cytoskeleton. *Annu Rev Cell Dev Biol* 1998;14:305-338.

79. Alberts B, Johnson A, Lewis J, Raff M, Roberts K, Walter P: *Molecular Biology of the Cell*, ed 4. New York, NY, Garland Science, 2001.

80. Aruffo A, Stamenkovic I, Melnick M, Underhill CB, Seed B: CD44 is the principal cell surface receptor for hyaluronate. *Cell* 1990;61(7):1303-1313.

81. Ekblom P, Vestweber D, Kemler R: Cell-matrix interactions and cell adhesion during development. *Annu Rev Cell Biol* 1986;2:27-47.

82. Bandorowicz-Pikula J: *Annexins: Biological Importance and Annexin-Related Pathologies*. Berlin, Germany, Plenum Publishers, 2003.

83. Goldman AS, Prabhakar BS: Immunology overview, in Baron S, ed: *Medical Microbiology*. Galveston, TX, University of Texas Medical Branch at Galveston, 1996.

84. Senolt L, Vencovský J, Pavelka K, Ospelt C, Gay S: Prospective new biological therapies for rheumatoid arthritis. *Autoimmun Rev* 2009;9(2):102-107.

85. Chen YF, Jobanputra P, Barton P, et al: A systematic review of the effectiveness of adalimumab, etanercept and infliximab for the treatment of rheumatoid arthritis in adults and an economic evaluation of their cost-effectiveness. *Health Technol Assess* 2006;10(42):iii-iv, xi-xiii, 1-229.

86. Dhimolea E: Canakinumab. *MAbs* 2010;2(1):3-13.

87. Lee SJ, Kavanaugh A: Pharmacological treatment of established rheumatoid arthritis. *Best Pract Res Clin Rheumatol* 2003;17(5):811-829.

88. Reynolds J, Shojania K, Marra CA: Abatacept: A novel treatment for moderate-to-severe rheumatoid arthritis. *Pharmacotherapy* 2007;27(12):1693-1701.

89. Evans CH, Robbins PD, Ghivizzani SC, et al: Gene transfer to human joints: Progress toward a gene therapy of arthritis. *Proc Natl Acad Sci U S A* 2005;102(24):8698-8703.

90. Moreland LW, Baumgartner SW, Schiff MH, et al: Treatment of rheumatoid arthritis with a recombinant human tumor necrosis factor receptor (p75)-Fc fusion protein. *N Engl J Med* 1997;337(3):141-147.

91. Paine PL, Moore LC, Horowitz SB: Nuclear envelope permeability. *Nature* 1975;254(5496):109-114.

92. Dundr M, Misteli T: Functional architecture in the cell nucleus. *Biochem J* 2001;356(pt 2):297-310.

93. Grosshans H, Simos G, Hurt E: Review: Transport of tRNA out of the nucleus: Direct channeling to the ribosome? *J Struct Biol* 2000;129(2-3):288-294.

94. Allmang C, Kufel J, Chanfreau G, Mitchell P, Petfalski E, Tollervey D: Functions of the exosome in rRNA, snoRNA and snRNA synthesis. *EMBO J* 1999;18(19):5399-5410.

95. Prezant TR, Agapian JV, Bohlman MC, et al: Mitochondrial ribosomal RNA mutation associated with both antibiotic-induced and non-syndromic deafness. *Nat Genet* 1993;4(3):289-294.

96. Carthew RW, Sontheimer EJ: Origins and mechanisms of miRNAs and siRNAs. *Cell* 2009;136(4):642-655.

97. Estrada de Martin P, Novick P, Ferro-Novick S: The organization, structure, and inheritance of the ER in higher and lower eukaryotes. *Biochem Cell Biol* 2005;83(6):752-761.

98. Voeltz GK, Rolls MM, Rapoport TA: Structural organization of the endoplasmic reticulum. *EMBO Rep* 2002;3(10):944-950.

99. Berridge MJ, Bootman MD, Roderick HL: Calcium signalling: Dynamics, homeostasis and remodelling. *Nat Rev Mol Cell Biol* 2003;4(7):517-529.

100. Glick BS, Nakano A: Membrane traffic within the Golgi apparatus. *Annu Rev Cell Dev Biol* 2009;25:113-132.

101. Pawelek JM, Chakraborty AK: Fusion of tumour cells with bone marrow-derived cells: A unifying explanation for metastasis. *Nat Rev Cancer* 2008;8(5):377-386.

102. Politz JC, Pederson T: Review: Movement of mRNA from transcription site to nuclear pores. *J Struct Biol* 2000;129(2-3):252-257.

103. Pfeffer SR, Rothman JE: Biosynthetic protein transport and sorting by the endoplasmic reticulum and Golgi. *Annu Rev Biochem* 1987;56:829-852.

104. Ungar D: Golgi linked protein glycosylation and associated diseases. *Semin Cell Dev Biol* 2009;20(7):762-769.

105. Luzio JP, Pryor PR, Bright NA: Lysosomes: Fusion and function. *Nat Rev Mol Cell Biol* 2007;8(8):622-632.

106. Blott EJ, Griffiths GM: Secretory lysosomes. *Nat Rev Mol Cell Biol* 2002;3(2):122-131.

107. Futerman AH, van Meer G: The cell biology of lysosomal storage disorders. *Nat Rev Mol Cell Biol* 2004;5(7):554-565.

108. Logan DC: The mitochondrial compartment. *J Exp Bot* 2006;57(6):1225-1243.

109. McBride HM, Neuspiel M, Wasiak S: Mitochondria: More than just a powerhouse. *Curr Biol* 2006;16(14):R551-R560.

110. Schapira AH: Mitochondrial disease. *Lancet* 2006;368(9529):70-82.

111. Duchen MR: Roles of mitochondria in health and disease. *Diabetes* 2004;53(suppl 1):S96-S102.

112. Zeviani M, Di Donato S: Mitochondrial disorders. *Brain* 2004;127(pt 10):2153-2172.

113. Ramaekers FC, Bosman FT: The cytoskeleton and disease. *J Pathol* 2004;204(4):351-354.

114. Saltel F, Destaing O, Bard F, Eichert D, Jurdic P: Apatite-mediated actin dynamics in resorbing osteoclasts. *Mol Biol Cell* 2004;15(12):5231-5241.

115. Crick F: Central dogma of molecular biology. *Nature* 1970;227(5258):561-563.

116. Hahn S: Structure and mechanism of the RNA polymerase II transcription machinery. *Nat Struct Mol Biol* 2004;11(5):394-403.

117. Graveley BR: Alternative splicing: Increasing diversity in the proteomic world. *Trends Genet* 2001;17(2):100-107.

118. Walsh CT, Garneau-Tsodikova S, Gatto GJ Jr: Protein post-translational modifications: The chemistry of proteome diversifications. *Angew Chem Int Ed Engl* 2005;44(45):7342-7372.

119. Arnsdorf EJ, Tummala P, Castillo AB, Zhang F, Jacobs CR: The epigenetic mechanism of mechanically induced osteogenic differentiation. *J Biomech* 2010;43(15):2881-2886.

120. Bird AP, Wolffe AP: Methylation-induced repression: Belts, braces, and chromatin. *Cell* 1999;99(5):451-454.

121. Weber WW: Epigenetics, in Taylor JB, Triggle DJ, eds: *Comprehensive Medicinal Chemistry II*. Amsterdam, The Netherlands, Elsevier, 2007, pp 251-278.

122. Barstead R: Genome-wide RNAi. *Curr Opin Chem Biol* 2001;5(1):63-66.

123. Maher SA, Hidaka C, Cunningham ME, Rodeo SA: What's new in orthopaedic research. *J Bone Joint Surg Am* 2008;90(8):1800-1808.

1: Basic Principles of Orthopaedic Surgery

124. Lambert MP, Herceg Z: Epigenetics and cancer: 2nd IARC meeting, Lyon, France, 6 and 7 December 2007. *Mol Oncol* 2008;2(1):33-40.

125. Watson JD, Gilman M, Witkowski J, Zoller M: *Recombinant DNA*, ed 2. New York, NY, Scientific American Books, 1992.

126. Pray LA: Recombinant DNA technology and transgenic animals. *Nature Education* 2008;1(1).

127. Cohen SN, Chang AC, Boyer HW, Helling RB: Construction of biologically functional bacterial plasmids in vitro. *Proc Natl Acad Sci U S A* 1973;70(11):3240-3244.

128. Evans CH, Robbins PD: Possible orthopaedic applications of gene therapy. *J Bone Joint Surg Am* 1995;77(7):1103-1114.

129. Kaplan FS, Xu M, Glaser DL, et al: Early diagnosis of fibrodysplasia ossificans progressiva. *Pediatrics* 2008;121(5): e1295-e1300.

130. Syvänen A-C: Accessing genetic variation: Genotyping single nucleotide polymorphisms. *Nat Rev Genet* 2001;2(12): 930-942.

131. Innis MA, Gelfand DH, Sninsky JJ: *PCR Strategies*. San Diego, CA, Academic Press, 1995.

132. Naylor LH: Reporter gene technology: The future looks bright. *Biochem Pharmacol* 1999;58(5):749-757.

133. Vorsanova SG, Yurov YB, Iourov IY: Human interphase chromosomes: A review of available molecular cytogenetic technologies. *Mol Cytogenet* 2010;3:1.

134. Service RF: Microchip arrays put DNA on the spot. *Science* 1998;282(5388):396-399.

135. Nath J, Johnson KL: A review of fluorescence in situ hybridization (FISH): Current status and future prospects. *Biotech Histochem* 2000;75(2):54-78.

136. Rieseberg M, Kasper C, Reardon KF, Scheper T: Flow cytometry in biotechnology. *Appl Microbiol Biotechnol* 2001; 56(3-4):350-360.

137. Johnson DS, Mortazavi A, Myers RM, Wold B: Genome-wide mapping of in vivo protein-DNA interactions. *Science* 2007;316(5830):1497-1502.

138. Park PJ: ChIP-seq: Advantages and challenges of a maturing technology. *Nat Rev Genet* 2009;10(10):669-680.

139. Pepke S, Wold B, Mortazavi A: Computation for ChIP-seq and RNA-seq studies. *Nat Methods* 2009;6(11, suppl):S22-S32.

140. Lequin RM: Enzyme immunoassay (EIA)/enzyme-linked immunosorbent assay (ELISA). *Clin Chem* 2005;51(12): 2415-2418.

141. Walker JM: The bicinchoninic acid (BCA) assay for protein quantitation. *Methods Mol Biol* 1994;32:5-8.

142. Nakasato YR, Janckila AJ, Halleen JM, Vaananen HK, Walton SP, Yam LT: Clinical significance of immunoassays for type-5 tartrate-resistant acid phosphatase. *Clin Chem* 1999; 45(12):2150-2157.

143. Goens G, Rusu D, Bultot L, Goval JJ, Magdalena J: Characterization and quality control of antibodies used in ChIP assays. *Methods Mol Biol* 2009;567:27-43.

144. Ramos-Vara JA: Technical aspects of immunohistochemistry. *Vet Pathol* 2005;42(4):405-426.

Chapter 2

Genetic Disease in Orthopaedics

P. Christopher Cook, MD FRCSC

James O. Sanders, MD

1: Basic Principles of Orthopaedic Surgery

Introduction

Many diseases commonly treated by orthopaedists have a genetic basis.[1] Despite the revolution in mapping the human genome, many diseases with strong hereditary components such as adolescent idiopathic scoliosis and osteoarthritis are still in their infancy of genetic characterization. It is likely that combinations of genetic, epigenetic, and environmental factors play an important role in many such orthopaedic diseases. Genetic disorders not only can be identified by gene expression profiling but also now by genomewide association studies allowing scanning of the entire human genome. This powerful technique compares single nucleotide DNA changes, termed single nucleotide polymorphisms (SNPs), among families who exhibit a disease with similar populations not having the disease. Algorithms can then identify particular SNPs and map them to areas of known genes. Complex diseases are now being identified with multiple SNPs, which, through the interaction with other polymorphisms and the environment, cause disease manifestation.

This chapter concentrates on only a small selection of these disorders. These examples of genetic orthopaedic disease will provide a clearer picture of how certain genetic abnormalities affect the musculoskeletal system. As a general rule, most gene polymorphisms seem to have no functional significance. Those causing the most severe manifestations of disease, particularly those manifesting severe changes before reproductive age, are unlikely to be inherited in a dominant pattern. These single gene disorders are likely to be the first ones amenable to gene therapy, though the ability to do so remains unrealized to date.

Because it is not possible for a practicing orthopaedist to be familiar with so many genetic disorders, it is important for orthopaedists to have a framework for understanding the disorders and have resources readily available. Ideally, every patient would have access to quality medical genetics evaluations. Particularly helpful resources include the Online Mendelian Inheritance in Man (OMIM) website, http://www.ncbi.nlm.nih.gov. The website is available by going to the PubMed website and selecting OMIM as the database rather than PubMed. GeneReview, also available through the National Library of Medicine, contains expert reviews of many disorders, has the advantage of delineating what additional evaluation should be completed after the diagnosis is made, and links to patient sites. GeneTest (http://www.ncbi.nlm.nih.gov/sites/GeneTests/), stays up to date with entities having specific testing available, and National Organization for Rare Disorders (http://www.rarediseases.org) has some useful expert synopses of many uncommon disorders, but the quality is quite variable.

To demonstrate the variety of disorders and how their genetics affects the skeletal system, four main categories will be discussed: syndromes, skeletal dysplasias, connective tissue disorders, and myelopathies and neuropathies.

Syndromes

Constellations of phenotypic findings in a patient constitute a syndrome. If more than one anomaly is identified, they may be syndromic. Because there are many syndromes,

Dr. Cook or an immediate family member serves as board member, owner, officer, or committee member of the Pediatric Orthopaedic Society of North America. Dr. Sanders or an immediate family member has stock or stock options in Abbott, GE Healthcare, and Hospire and serves as a board member, owner, officer, or committee member of the American Academy of Orthopaedic Surgeons, the Pediatric Orthopaedic Society of North America, and the Scoliosis Research Society.

orthopaedists should recognize some of the more common ones and consult a medical geneticist when several phenotypic abnormalities occur in the same patient.

Trisomy 21

Chromosomal disorders can include duplications, deletions, and translocations. These disorders can exhibit problems associated with either the deletion or the excessive expression of the associated genes. The sheer number of genes associated with a duplication or chromosomal deletion makes understanding the etiology of any particular phenotypic finding difficult.

The classic chromosomal disorder seen by orthopaedists is trisomy 21 or Down syndrome. It is typically a complete translocation with a risk of 1% in subsequent births. The disorder may also result from partial translocations or mosaicisms that have, typically, fewer abnormalities. Down syndrome is associated with maternal age older than 40 years. Multiple organ systems are involved; cardiac abnormalities may be severe and life threatening. Patients can have endocrine abnormalities, including diabetes and hypothyroidism and are more prone to leukemia. Adult patients are subject to premature dementia with similar findings to Alzheimer disease. Many reports indicate a higher infection and nonunion rate in patients with Down syndrome than in others.

Almost 20% of patients with Down syndrome have musculoskeletal disorders primarily associated with severe ligamentous laxity, including upper cervical instability, patellar and hip dislocations, and severe flatfoot and bunion deformities.[2-5] Generally, the deformities are asymptomatic. Polyarticular arthritis, subluxations, and swelling requiring a rheumatologic evaluation may also occur.

VATER/VACTERL Association

The VACTERL (vertebral defects, anal atresia, cardiac defects, tracheoesophageal fistula, renal malformations, and limb defects) association was first proposed with the acronym VATER, where the letter R stood for radial dysplasia. Subsequently, the acronym was expanded to include cardiac and renal defects. Both terms are used. VACTERL can be divided into upper and lower groups. The upper group is associated with heart malformations, and the lower group is associated with renal malformations.[6]

There are very few published series of patients with VACTERL in whom the clinical phenotypes have been carefully delineated. Most cases are thought to be from a disruption in embryogenesis rather than a select genetic pathway. Some, however, are perhaps associated with the sonic hedgehog pathway. Although approximately 90% of cases are sporadic, there is an approximate 10% incidence in first-degree relatives.[7]

In a patient with congenital spinal deformity or limb defect (especially radial), orthopaedists should be cognizant that other associated anomalies may exist. An echocardiogram or renal ultrasound may be required.[8]

McCune-Albright Syndrome

McCune-Albright syndrome is a heterogeneous disease with various abnormalities, including fibrous dysplasia of bone, café-au-lait lesions, and sexual precocity.[9,10] Sometimes it may have other endocrine dysfunctions, including thyroid nodules, acromegaly, or Cushing syndrome. The disorder occurs via genetic imprinting and epigenetic transmission in which gene expression is only from one allele.[11] The imprinted allele may be maternal or paternal. A classic example of imprinting is the development of the reciprocally inherited Prader-Willi syndrome and Angelman syndrome, both associated with loss of the chromosomal region 15q11-13. This region contains paternally expressed genes (*SNRPN* and *NDN*) and a maternally expressed gene (*UBE3A*). Paternal inheritance of a deletion of this region is associated with Prader-Willi syndrome (characterised by hypotonia, obesity, and hypogonadism), whereas maternal inheritance of the same deletion is associated with Angelman syndrome (characterized by epilepsy, tremors, and a perpetually smiling facial expression). In McCune-Albright syndrome, the final common pathway is early embryonic postzygotic somatic activating mutations in the *GNAS1* gene creating woven bone. The fibrous dysplasia bone is characterized by soft bone better treated with load-sharing rather than load-bearing implants. The classic lesion is the shepherd's crook deformity of hips.

Neurofibromatosis Type 1

Neurofibromatosis type 1 is caused by a mutation in the neurofibromin gene, is autosomal dominant, and is characterized by smooth café-au-lait spots and fibrous tumors of the skin. The neurofibromin gene is believed to be a tumor suppresser gene that normally functions to control cell growth and differentiation. Neurofibromin negatively regulates the gene *RAS*. Increased *RAS* activity results in cell proliferation. Neurofibromas occur if the unaffected allele coding for neurofibromin (that is, the allele not carrying the mutation causing neurofibormatosis type 1) undergoes a somatic mutation.[12,13] The major orthopaedic issues are scoliosis, which can range from an idiopathic to a dystrophic, highly progressive curve, and congenital pseudarthrosis of the tibia.[14] Patients can develop significant deformities of other bones, destructive neurofibromas, and large plexiform neurofibromas. Neurofibromatosis type 2 has no orthopaedic implications.

Skeletal Dysplasias

Although most skeletal dysplasias are rare, taken as a group they are fairly common in busy orthopaedic practices, occurring in approximately 2.4 of 10,000 births.[15] A 2010 nosology of skeletal dysplasias found 456 different skeletal dysplasias, 316 of which were associated with one or more of 226 different genes.[16] This review focuses on several illustrative disorders. Most skeletal dysplasias appear to be single-gene (mendelian) disorders.

When evaluating patients with skeletal dysplasias, it is helpful to consider the primary tissues involved (bone, articular cartilage, physeal cartilage, ligament) and how the underlying disorder affects each component.[17] For example, type I collagen disorders affect bone and ligament but only indirectly affect cartilage. Similarly, type II collagen disorders affect articular and physeal cartilage but have little effect on bone quality.

Traditionally, skeletal dysplasias have been described as short-trunk, short-limb, or short-trunk and short-limbed dwarfisms by their phenotypic classification. However, with the marked progress in molecular genetics, the phenotypic classifications are giving way to genetic classifications. The terms dysostosis and dysplasia are not interchangeable, but the language is becoming more fluid with the understanding of the various disorders improving. Dysostosis refers to malformations of single bones, alone or in combination. Dysplasia refers to developmental disorder of chondro-osseous tissue. There is broad overlap of dysostoses, dysplasias, metabolic disorders, and other syndromes.

Collagen

Type I Collagen

Type I collagen is the major structural component of bone, ligaments, and tendons. Defects in the individual chains can result in decreased levels of production or inhibit triple helix formation. The primary diseases affecting type I collagen are osteogenesis imperfecta (OI) and a couple of types of Ehlers-Danlos syndrome.[18] Ehler-Danlos is discussed later. OI is a disorder of congenital bone fragility, resulting from abnormal type I collagen. OI can result from normal but insufficient type I collagen, typically seen in type I OI. Collagen is a triple helix, and more severe forms of OI can result when one abnormal collagen monomer destabilizes the entire triple helix. Mutations in the *COL1A1* and *COL1A2* genes, coding for type I collagen, can lead to both qualitative and quantitative disturbances of this protein. Types of OI are distinguished by the severity of their manifestations. The major OI issues are fragility fractures of the spine and extremities. The limbs can become severely deformed, leading to additional fractures. The spine can develop significant scoliosis, and patients may have basilar invagination from the soft skull. Type I is the mildest form of OI, where fractures are most common in infancy. Patients have blue sclera and occasionally abnormal dentition. Long bone deformities are typically absent. Type II is often fatal in the perinatal period. In utero fractures are present, and lung hypoplasia and central nervous system malformations are common causes of death. Type III is a severe type of OI with frequent fractures, including in utero. Long bone deformities are characteristic, and muscle weakness and bone pain can be debilitating. Kyphoscoliosis may be severe enough to cause respiratory compromise, and basilar invagination may be fatal. Sclera are not typically blue. Type IV has an inheritance pattern that is not well defined but has phenotypic similarities to type I, with more severe bone involvement

and lack of blue sclera. Types V-VIII similarly have overlap with types I-III, but do not have mutations in the *COL1A1/COL1A2* genes; instead, other genetic mutations that result in altered collagen processing and secretion have been identified.

Type II Collagen

Type II collagen is the major structural protein of cartilage (articular and growth cartilage, the notocord, and the vitreous humor of the eye). Abnormalities of type II cartilage affect extremity growth (short-limbed dwarfism), the spine (short-trunk dwarfism), and the eyes, and lead to early degenerative arthrititis. Spondyloepiphyseal dysplasia, a type II collagen disorder, is autosomal dominant but most cases are sporadic. Nonorthopaedic issues include cleft palate, deafness, hernias, and eye problems (retinal conditions and cataracts), but the major orthopaedic-related issues include coxa vara, lordosis, clubfeet, genu valgum or varum, odontoid hypoplasia, and C1-C2 instability. The odontoid hypoplasia can lead to anterior-posterior C1-C2 instability and must be evaluated before any surgery. Lower extremity angular deformities can be severe, and the ligamentous laxity can make judging surgical correction difficult. Type II collagen defects may lead to early arthritis despite good alignment. Other disorders are similar to spondyloepiphyseal dysplasia and involve either type II collagen or other collagens strongly associated with the structural configuration of type II collagen such as type 11 collagen.

Kneist syndrome is similar to spondyloepiphyseal dysplasia but is associated with severe kyphoscoliosis. Stickler syndrome is associated with severe eye conditions.

Hypochondrogenesis is midway between spondyloepiphyseal dysplasia and achondrogenesis. Achondrogenesis and hypochondrogenesis are both along the spectrum of type II collagen disorders/manifestations. In both cases, the type II collagen defect results in severe growth disturbance affecting both the axial and appendicular skeleton. There is undergrowth of all regions of the skeleton that have endochondral ossification. In achondrogenesis, the defect is lethal. In hypochondrogenesis, the infant survives but has severe skeletal undergrowth, including the abnormalities noted in spondyloepiphyseal dysplasia.

Storage Diseases

Mucopolysaccharidoses include a group of disorders that manifest when specific lysosomal enzymes are deficient. Lysosomal enzymes are responsible for the degradation of glycosaminoglycans, long-chain carbohydrates comprising a major component of connective tissue. In these disorders, enzymatic abnormalities prevent the normal breakdown of glycosaminoglycans with subsequent accumulation within lysosomes.[19]

The mucopolysaccharidoses constitute a family of storage diseases with spinal abnormalities that are similar to those seen in spondyloepiphyseal dysplasia. They are quite similar orthopaedically to spondyloepiphyseal dysplasia

1: Basic Principles of Orthopaedic Surgery

Table 1

The Main Orthopaedic Mucopolysaccharidoses

Mucopolysaccharidoses	Pathophysiology	Typical Features	Treatment
Type I (Hurler syndrome)	Gene encoding α-L-iduronidase	Coarse features are evident early. Bulging fontanels, neurologic compression, corneal clouding, upper airway obstruction, pulmonary edema postoperatively, short stature; carpal tunnel	Bone marrow transplant Enzyme therapy may help Gene therapy
Type II (Hunter syndrome)	Deficient activity of iduronate 2-sulfatase X-linked; mapped to Xq27-28 Enzyme assays in cultured fibroblasts/leukocytes Increased urinary heparan and dermatan sulfate	Two forms exist (Type A – severe, type B – mild) Type A – clinical features as in type IH; onset age 1-2 years; death in adolescence, third decade Type B – may be diagnosed in adulthood; Coarse facial features; hearing loss, mental retardation (type A), absence of corneal clouding; upper airway obstruction; pulmonary edema postoperatively, hepatosplenomegaly, dysostosis multiplex, short stature, hydrocephalus; carpal tunnel, ivory skin lesions, mongolian spots, hypertrichos	Bone marrow transplant Enzyme therapy may alter disease progression; not curative Idursulfase Gene therapy may help
Type IV (Morquio syndrome) Numerous types	Type A – deficiency of galactosamine-6-sulfatase (*GALNS* gene, 16q24.3) Type B – β-galactosidase (*GLB1* gene, 3p21.33) Increased urinary excretion of keratan sulfate (cartilage/cornea); may be no excretion in mild case Enzyme-linked immunosorbent assay Enzyme assay in cultured fibroblasts/leukocytes Genetic testing to detect mutations in *GALNS*, *GLB1*	Clinically, both forms may be similar; great variability in severity within both groups Mortality related to atlantoaxial instability, myelopathy and pulmonary compromise For severe, death in second or third decade of life No coarse facial features, normal intelligence, spondyloepiphyseal dysplasia, ligamentous laxity, odontoid hypoplasia, short-trunk dwarfism, genu valgus, greater incidence of spinal involvement, bowel/bladder incontinence, obstructive sleep apnea, pulmonary infections chest wall deformity, heart valve thickening/defects, corneal clouding, enamel Less common – hearing loss, hernias	Supportive treatment

regarding their spine and long bone issues but have the addition of soft-tissue hypertrophy secondary to the metabolic product accumulation.[20]

The different types of mucopolysaccharidoses vary in severity as well as clinical manifestations. Many share features, including course facies, skeletal involvement with dysostosis multiplex and short stature, organomegaly, corneal opacification, and varying degrees of mental retardation. Table 1 lists the main orthopaedic mucopolysaccharidoses as well as

their pathophysiology, clinical manifestations, and treatment.

At birth, affected children are normal, but the accumulated glycosaminoglycan products produce soft-tissue swelling that can cause direct spinal cord compression, particularly around the craniovertebral junction and odontoid. These children pose substantial anesthesia risks because of their enlarged pharyngeal soft tissues.

Articular Cartilage Disorders

There are several disorders of cartilage resulting in early degenerative arthritis. Because physeal cartilage is also involved, these disorders often result in milder short-limbed dwarfisms without the severe spinal involvement seen in spondyloepiphyseal dysplasia.

Cartilage oligomeric matrix protein (COMP) and type IX collagen are the major cartilage genetic defects.[21] In their early stages they have a presentation similar to that of Legg-Calvé-Perthes disease, and many patients are initially confused for those with Legg-Calvé-Perthes disease.[22] Multiple epiphyseal dysplasia results in early degenerative arthritis. It has two known types: type I, which involves COMP, and type II, which involves type IX collagen. Both type IX collagen and COMP are important in the articular cartilage matrix.[23,24] They typically do not have the same effect on physeal involvement seen in the spondyloepiphyseal dysplasias. In addition, there are mild type II collagen mutations that do not result in growth deficiencies but are associated with early development of osteoarthritis with a familial genetic inheritance pattern. Pseudoachondroplasia is characterized by rhizomelic dwarfism with normal facies and without spinal stenosis. There are problems similar to those found with multiple epiphyseal dysplasia, but these conditions are worse with potential atlantoaxial instability. Symptoms are related to the inability of COMP to bind calcium. Pseudochondroplasia markedly affects type IX collagen and aggrecan.

Growth Plate Abnormalities

Some disorders affect physeal cartilage more than articular cartilage. These result in rhizomelic dwarfism, short-limbed dwarfisms with the humerus and femur affected more than the tibia and forearm because they normally grow faster. These disorders also result in spinal stenosis of the foramen magnum and lumbar spine because of poor neurocentral synchondrosis growth.

Fibroblast Growth Factor Receptor-3 Abnormalities

Achondroplasia is the most common dwarfism, is autosomal dominant, and is linked with fathers older than 36 years. Ninety percent are spontaneous mutations, and this type of dwarfism is caused by a point mutation in the gene coding for fibroblast growth factor receptor-3 (FGFR3). This mutation is almost always at the same nucleotide (nucleotide number 1138) and causes a single amino acid change (arginine to glycine) in the transmembrane portion of this cell surface receptor. This receptor is expressed in all preossified cartilage as well as diffusely in the central nervous system. The remarkable homogeneity of the phenotype in achondroplasia results from the remarkable homogeneity of the mutation in this disorder. No other autosomal dominant disorder whose gene defect is known has such a homogeneous mutation. This is the most mutable single nucleotide known in the entire human genome and there is 100% penetrance of the disease to offspring of an affected parent. The mutation results in constitutive activation of FGFR3. Thus, even in the absence of the ligand fibroblast growth factor (FGF) the receptor is turned on. The activated receptor shows proliferation of cells in the growth plate. Thus, children carrying this defect have reduced rates of growth. Malfunction of FGFR3 causes inhibition of chondrocyte proliferation in the proliferative zone of the physis. The exact mechanism is unclear.[25]

Clinically, patients have rhizomelic dwarfism, frontal bossing, bowed legs, and lumbar lordosis. Spinal stenosis can be very severe from decreased physeal growth of the neurocentral synchondrosis; foramen magnum stenosis can cause sudden death in infants, and lumbar stenosis can be problematic in adults.[26] Other FGFR3 disorders include hypochondroplasia, which results in short stature, but patients rarely have orthopaedic symptoms; and thanotophoric dwarfism, which is fatal.

Ossification Abnormalities

Two groups of skeletal dysplasias have metaphyseal ossification abnormalities: metaphyseal dysplasias and the various forms of rickets.

Metaphyseal Dysplasias

These conditions radiographically resemble rickets with poor ossification of the metaphyseal area. They are characterized by short stature, coxa vara, and bowed legs and include Schmidt (abnormal type X collagen), Jansen (parathyroid hormone [PTH]–related peptide receptor, and McKusick (cartilage-hair hypoplasia) dysplasias.

Inherited Forms of Rickets and Hypophosphatasia

Abnormal regulation of calcium and phosphate metabolism is involved in the development of rickets. There are several interrelated hormones that are important. FGF23, which is mutated in autosomal dominant hypophosphatemic rickets, is produced by osteocytes in the bone in response to elevated serum phosphatase levels. FGF23 acts systemically on the proximal tubule cells to increase the urinary secretion of phosphate. In contrast to PTH, which increases the activity of 25-hydroxyvitamin D-1-α-hydroxylase, FGF reduces the activity of this enzyme in the kidney. Thus, there are low serum levels of 1,25-dihydroxyvitamin D_3 and phosphate. 1, 25-dihydroxyvitamin D_3 is necessary for normal absorption of both calcium and phosphate from the gut. Low calcium levels in turn can elevate systemic levels of PTH, which increased calcium through bone resorption and increased activation of 1,25-hydroxyvitamin D in the kidney.

Rickets

Rickets is the most common disorder in this group, several types of which are genetic.[27] Vitamin D–dependent rickets results from deficient or abnormal function of the renal 1-α-hydroxylase, resulting in low 1,25 dihydroxyvitamin D_2

levels.[28] Vitamin D–resistant rickets is caused by a defect in the vitamin D receptor that prevents 1,25-dihydroxyvitamin D_2 binding. Both types are caused by genetic mutations and lead to hypocalcemia, secondary hyperparathyroidism, hypophosphatemia and the typical skeletal manifestations seen in vitamin D–deficiency rickets. Treatment includes pharmacologic doses of vitamin D or 1,25-dihydroxyvitamin D_2 (calcitriol), as well as calcium.

In hereditary hypophosphatemic rickets, abnormal renal phosphate reabsorption occurs, and phosphate "wasting" ensues. This is typically X-linked, but rarely, autosomal dominant inheritance occurs.[29,30] X-linked hyphophosphatemic rickets is due to a mutation in the phosphate-regulating endopeptidase homolog, X-linked (*PHEX*) gene, a metalloproteinase that is present in osteocytes. *PHEX* is involved in the catabolism of FGF23, and in the absence of *PHEX* there are elevated levels of FGF23 and excess phosphate secretion in the urine. Patients with X-linked hypophosphatemic rickets have hypophosphatemia, hyperphosphaturia, and elevated serum alkaline phosphatase; normal calcium, PTH, and 1,25-dihydroxyvitamin D_2 levels; and decreased 1,25-dihydroxyvitamin D_2 levels. Skeletal manifestations are similar to those seen with the other forms of rickets; symptoms related to hypocalcemia (seizures, tetany), however, do not occur. Interestingly, there is no evidence of increased osteoclast activity, and in treated patients, bone mass can be normal. Treatment is with large quantities of oral phosphate and calcitriol (1,25-dihydroxyvitamin D_3). However, vitamin D levels should be monitored because renal calcium stones can be caused by excess treatment with calcitriol.

Hypophosphatasia

Alkaline phosphatase is an enzyme associated with the calcification of both bone and cartilage matrix. Hypophosphatasia results from abnormally low activity of tissue-nonspecific alkaline phosphatase, which leads to rickets and/or osteomalacia. Several mutations and inheritance patterns are present and depend on the type of hypophosphatasia. The different forms of this disorder are classified by age at onset of skeletal manifestations: perinatal, infantile, childhood, and adult. Two other forms include odontohypophosphatasia and pseudohypophosphatasia. The perinatal form is lethal. The childhood form may present as delayed motor development and early loss of deciduous teeth. Many patients have severe bone pain. The adult form presents in the fourth or fifth decade of life with symptoms resulting from stress fractures or joint pain. Premature loss of deciduous teeth also occurs. Pseudohypophosphatasia is clinically indistinguishable from the perinatal form, except for normal alkaline phosphatase activity. It is thought that although tissue nonspecific alkaline phosphatase functions normally in vitro, it has abnormal activity in vivo.

All Cartilage

Some disorders affect all cartilage. An example is sulfate transport gene, which is essential for proteoglycan sulfation.

Defects result in poor articular cartilage, dwarfism, and nose and ear cartilage defects.

Diastrophic dysplasia affects all types of cartilage and is manifested by very stiff joints, cervical kyphosis, hitchhiker thumbs, and cauliflower ears. The joint abnormalities associated with this disorder result in painful osteoarthrosis at an early age. These patients, who are of normal intelligence, are severely handicapped by their joint abnormalities.

Diastrophic dysplasia is caused by a mutation in a gene coding for a sulfate transporter protein. Cartilage requires properly sulfated glycosaminoglycan side chains for normal proteoglycan function. This is impaired by diastrophic dysplasia sulfate transporter gene mutations. In normal cartilage, proper sulfation and a sufficient negative charge are necessary for proteoglycans to function properly. The gene responsible for the synthesis of this protein is expressed in virtually all cell types but its effects are most pronounced in cartilage-producing cells because of the greater requirement for sulfate in cartilage proteoglycan synthesis. Specifically, a defect in sulfate transport across the cell membrane results in inadequate intracellular sulfate and undersulfation of proteoglycans. Sulfate transport gene disorders in decreasing order of severity are achondrogenesis 1B, atelosteogenesis 2, diastrophic dysplasia, and recessive multiple epiphyseal dysplasia.

Multiple Hereditary Exostosis

Multiple hereditary exostosis is an autosomal dominant trait characterized by multiple exostosis or cartilage-capped bony prominences typically arising in the metaphyseal region of long bones. The diaphysis, spine, and ribs may also be involved. It is commonly seen by orthopaedists, perhaps because the lesions are often quite noticeable.

The osteochondromas are typically asymptomatic. The primary difficulties arise from their mass effect, physeal growth disturbance, fracture within the osseous portion, or potential malignant degeneration. Growth abnormalities are typically most significant in the two bone segments, the forearm and the leg, but can also result in deformities about any affected physis. Clinically, the exostoses occur in multiple metaphyseal areas. The patients are often shorter than normal by 0.5 to 1 standard deviation. In growing children, the lesions can cause growth disturbances, limb shortening, and significant deformities, particularly in the two bone segments of the forearm and leg. They can also cause impingement upon the joints and soft tissues, including muscles and nerves.

There are three known chromosomal loci for the disorder, EXT1 (chromosome 8q24), EXT2 (chromosome 11), and EXT3 (chromosome 19), with some evidence for an additional locus.[31] Multiple osteochondromas also occur in metachondromatosis and Langer-Giedion syndrome, also known as trichorhinophalangeal syndrome type II. The exostosis from metachondromatosis and dysplasia epiphysealis hemimelica do not come from the EXT genes. Recently, there is some evidence that EXT1 and EXT2 encode endoplasmic reticulum–resident type II transmembrane glycoproteins, which are involved in the regulation of cell-surface heparin sulfate proteoglycans that, in turn, are integral to the diffusion of several families of cell-signaling molecules. Clinically, patients with EXT1 typically have more involvement than those with other types.

A key large cartilage growth factor appears to be Indian hedgehog (Ihh). When glycosylated, Ihh has a narrow range of diffusion. In the absence of glycosylation, Ihh has an increased range of activity. Ihh has a role in the columnar organization of the growth plate, and perturbation of Ihh signaling in the setting of EXT gene mutations results in the formation of osteochondromas. The overall risk of malignant degeneration widely varies in the literature. Malignancy is thought to arise because the encoding genes are classic tumor suppressors. Multiple hereditary exostosis results in an autosomal dominant pattern when one of the genes is affected. Disruption of the other gene then allows malignant transformation. The best estimate is 0.57%, but it is very difficult to obtain an accurate estimate because it is those who develop malignancy who come to medical attention. The mean age of malignant degeneration is 31 years, and the condition rarely occurs before age 10 years or after age 50 years. Particular areas of concern are the pelvis, proximal femur, shoulder girdle, and ribs. Patients should be aware of the malignant potential and report any increased pain or size of lesions. Positron emission tomography shows some promise in distinguishing benign from malignant lesions.

Poor Bone Reabsorption

Without osteoclast remodeling, bone becomes hard and unable to remodel to stress. Osteopetrosis, a defect in osteoclastic resorption, in the severe form, results in extramedullary hematopoiesis and fractures that are difficult to fix.[32] Treatment is bone marrow transplant for the severe, malignant type.

Connective Tissue Disorders

Ehlers-Danlos Syndrome

Ehlers-Danlos syndrome is a disorder of loose joints associated with several collagen abnormalities.[33] This group of disorders is characterized by laxity and weakness of the dermis, ligaments, and blood vessels. Nine clinical and genetic subtypes have been described, and all whose etiology is known are caused by mutations in fibrillar collagen genes or genes for enzymes that modify the fibrillar collagens. Two of these disorders are type I collagen abnormalities, although they are not the most common types. Flatfoot, scoliosis, dislocated hips, and joint pain all can occur.[34] Type I is an autosomal dominant condition characterized by lax joints, hyperextensible skin, and wide, atrophic scars. Type II is a milder form with the same clinical characteristics. Both disorders result from mutation of the gene coding for collagen V. Collagen V is coexpressed with collagen I in many tissues and is important for proper formation of collagen I fibrils.

Marfan Syndrome

The disorder is caused by a mutation in the fibrillin-1 gene (*FBN1* on chromosome 15) and has autosomal dominant inheritance. Patients are characteristically tall with long arms, a long narrow face, and a high arched palate. Their fingers and toes are long (arachnodactyly). They may also have pectus deformity, scoliosis, protrusio acetabuli, flatfoot, and dural ectasia. Marfan syndrome is common in scoliosis clinics, and a high index of suspicion should be maintained. Other common features include myopia and lens dislocations, spontaneous pneumothorax, aortic dilation, and aortic rupture.[35] Clearly, making the diagnosis is extremely important for the proper treatment and prevention of serious if not fatal complications.[36]

Pathophysiologically, abnormal fibrillin-1 monomers disrupt the normal fibrillin, important in microfibril formation, and normal elastic fiber formation. Interestingly, transforming growth factor-β (TGF-β) normally interacts with latent TGF-β binding proteins in the extracellular matrix. The fibrillins also interact with the binding proteins. The abnormal fibrillin in Marfan syndrome subsequently causes abnormal TGF-β activity, which appears to cause many of the syndrome's manifestations.[37] Other related disorders include Beals syndrome or congenital contractural arachnodactyly associated with fibrillin-2, and Loeys-Dietz syndrome associated with TGF-β R1/2. Therapeutic TGF-β inhibitors are being studied to modify the disease's manifestations.

Myopathies and Neuropathies

The neuromuscular diseases discussed in this section are also described in chapter 23.

Duchenne and Becker Muscular Dystrophies

Dystrophin is an intracellular protein that is associated with two transmembrane complexes—the dystroglycan complex and the sarcoglycan complex. The sarcoglycan complex and the dystroglycan complex are part of the dystrophin-glycoprotein complex that spans the muscle membrane from the cytoskeleton to the basal lamina. Loss of dystrophin leads to loss of all components of these complexes and loss of cellular cytoskeletal structure. The dystrophin gene is the largest human gene yet identified, making it a very large target for new mutations. It is located on the X chromosome, making inheritance X-linked. One third of patients with dystrophinopathy have new mutations. Most patients can be identified by DNA testing.

Duchenne muscular dystrophy has absent dystrophin in muscle,[38,39] and the milder Becker phenotypes have decreased or abnormal dystrophin. Duchenne and Becker muscular dystrophies represent different phenotypes resulting from different mutations in a single gene. Duchenne muscular dystrophy presents in early childhood with proximal muscle weakness and calf hypertrophy. Affected boys experience a slight delay in attaining motor milestones. Toe walking may be an early manifestation of the disease. The course is one of steadily worsening weakness. The milder dystrophinopathies are varied in clinical phenotype. Affected males who present in childhood with proximal weakness, calf hypertrophy, and very high creatine kinase values, but follow a more indolent course than the patients with Duchenne muscular dystrophy, are given the diagnosis of Becker muscular dystrophy.

Carrier female patients may be symptomatic on the basis of skewed X-inactivation. They usually present with limb-girdle weakness and elevated creatine kinase levels. Cardiomyopathy can be clinically significant and occasionally is the primary manifestation of dystrophinopathy.

Autosomal Recessive Limb-Girdle Dystrophies

The autosomal recessive limb-girdle dystrophies are progressive muscular dystrophies that predominantly affect the pelvic and shoulder girdle musculature.[40] The severity ranges from severe forms manifesting weakness in the first decade of life with rapid progression (called Duchenne-like muscular dystrophy) to mild forms with late onset and slow progression. Eight genetic loci have been identified in families with this phenotype. Four loci code for proteins that are part of the sarcoglycan complex: the alpha, beta, gamma, and delta sarcoglycans. Another form is caused by a mutation in the gene coding for calpain-3, a muscle-specific proteolytic enzyme. The sixth form with an identified gene is caused by a mutation in dysferlin. Two other forms have been linked to regions on chromosomes 9 and 17 but their mechanism is not known.

Hereditary Spastic Paraplegia

The hereditary spastic paraplegias (familial spastic paraparesis, Strumpell-Lorrain syndrome) are characterized by progressive spasticity of the legs. Symptoms usually manifest during the second to fourth decades, and gait slowly and steadily worsens. These disorders have been classified by mode of inheritance and whether the lower extremity spasticity is the only finding (uncomplicated) or whether other neurologic conditions, such as optic neuropathy, dementia, ataxia, mental retardation, or deafness, are autosomal recessive, or X-linked.

Autosomal dominant forms have been linked to 11 different loci, and four causative genes have been identified. It appears that disruption of normal intracellular-trafficking dynamics may be the common link in the various gene defects causing this disorder. The clinical phenotype is similar among families with mutations at the same loci.

Charcot-Marie-Tooth Disease (Hereditary Motor Sensory Neuropathies)

The hereditary motor sensory neuropathies are a heterogeneous group of inherited peripheral neuropathies.[41-43] Charcot-Marie-Tooth (CMT) disease is the most common of these disorders. The two most common types, types 1 and 2, will be discussed.

CMT-1A is an autosomal dominant disorder and is characterized by progressive distal muscle wasting and weakness, areflexia, and foot deformities—most commonly cavovarus. Nerve conduction velocities show severe slowing, and nerve pathology reveals simultaneous demyelination and remyelination. This disorder has variable expression but usually begins in childhood. Patients with foot deformities usually present to the orthopaedic surgeon in late childhood or early adolescence. At the molecular level, 70% to 80% of affected individuals have a duplication of the gene coding for peripheral myelin protein 22 (PMP22). This protein appears to modulate cell proliferation. Rare patients with point mutations in this gene have also had the CMT-IA phenotype, providing strong evidence for the primary role of PMP22 in disease causation. CMT-1B, causing 5% of CMT-1 phenotype, is caused by a mutation in the MPZ gene, which encodes the protein myelin protein 0. This gene encodes a protein that makes up nearly 50% of all protein in peripheral myelin. Some families with the CMT-1 phenotype have a gene cause that has not been located and are designated CMT-1C. Additional families have the CMT-1 phenotype caused by a mutation in the early growth response gene (EGR2), a transcription factor involved in early myelination, and are designated CMT-1D. This gene is also involved in some cases of Dejerine-Sottas disease.

CMT type 2 is an autosomal dominant, axonal polyneuropathy with age at onset in the second or third decade of life, characterized by near-normal motor nerve conduction velocity. Nomenclature is in flux as new variants are found. Of five presently described subtypes, four have been linked to chromosomal regions. The gene cause has been identified in three. The gene encoding kinesin (KIF1B), part of a family of mitochondrial motor transport proteins, causes CMT-2A. CMT-2D is caused by mutations in the glycyl transcription RNA synthetase gene. This is the first transcription RNA synthetase enzyme known to cause a human disease. The neurofilament-light gene (NF-L), which encodes neurofilament proteins involved in axonal structure, causes CMT-2E. A few families with the CMT-2 phenotype have been found with point mutations in the MPZ gene. An autosomal recessive form of CMT-2 is caused by mutations in the LMNA gene, which encodes lamin A/C nuclear-envelope proteins—a component of the nuclear envelope.

Spinal Muscular Atrophy

Spinal muscular atrophy has been classified into three clinical forms. Werdnig-Hoffmann disease is characterized by generalized muscle weakness and hypotonia at birth, and early death. The intermediate type of spinal muscular atrophy afflicts patients who initially achieve normal motor milestones, but never gain the ability to walk. Kugelberg-Welander is the mildest type; patients have muscle weakness, which becomes evident after age 2 years. All three types of spinal muscular atrophy are characterized by anterior horn cell degeneration and result in limb and trunk paralysis with muscle atrophy. Major orthopaedic conditions include scoliosis and hip instability.

It has long been recognized that there is a continuum from the most severe early forms through the milder later-onset disease. This clinical impression has been borne out by the mapping of all forms of spinal muscular atrophy to one small region of chromosome 5. Several genes have been identified in this region, including the survival motor neuron gene (*SMN*), the neuronal apoptosis inhibitory protein, and the p44 gene. This is a very complex and unstable segment of the genome. Two copies of the *SMN* gene with very minor differences are present in this region, one centromeric and one telomeric to each other. More than 90% of patients with spinal muscular atrophy have deletions or conversion of the telomeric *SMN* to the centromeric *SMN* type in a specific portion of the telomeric *SMN* gene. Spinal muscular atrophy types II and III appear to have a conversion of the telomeric *SMN* to the centromeric *SMN* gene and have more copies of the centromeric *SMN* gene than exist in typed disease. The telomeric *SMN* gene encodes the fully functional protein, whereas the centromeric *SMN* gene encodes a transcript lacking exon 7. The neuronal apoptosis inhibitory protein may provide an additional explanation for the variations in genotype/phenotype correlation. The neuronal apoptosis inhibitory protein gene functions to inhibit motor neuron programmed cell death. Programmed cell death is a normal occurrence in the development of the nervous system. Failure to inhibit cell death at the appropriate time could be part of the explanation for the anterior horn cell loss seen in spinal muscular atrophy. In a group of patients with the most severe type of spinal muscular atrophy, a high percentage of deletions in this gene was found. However, deletion of this gene may simply be coincidentally associated with more disease because of a more severe interruption in the *SMN* gene function.

Trinucleotide Repeat Disorders

Repeated sequences of nucleotides occur throughout the human genome and are the basis for inherited polymorphisms that have allowed the dramatic increase in identification of disease-causing genes in the last decade. Expansion of certain trinucleotide repeats causes several known neurologic disorders, including Friedreich ataxia, myotonic dystrophy, fragile X syndrome, X-linked spinal and bulbar muscular atrophy, Huntington disease, spinocerebellar ataxia type 1, spinocerebellar ataxia type 2, spinocerebellarataxia type 6, spinocerebellar ataxia type 7, spinocerebellar ataxia type 3 (Machado-Joseph disease), and dentatorubral-pallidoluysian atrophy. The repeated sequences are unstable and change size in successive generations, usually becoming longer. Myotonic dystrophy and fragile X syndrome contain repeat sequences that are not within the protein coding region and, probably, cause disease by altering gene expression rather than by altering the protein product. Expansion of trinucleotide repeats (CAG repeats) in the coding region causes Huntington disease, spinal and bulbar muscular atrophy, spinocerebellar ataxia

types 1 and 6, dentatorubral-pallidoluysian atrophy, and Machado-Joseph disease. The CAG repeat results in polyglutamine amino acid sequences and evidence suggests these polyglutamine regions are specifically neurotoxic by themselves. The trinucleotide repeat expansion provides a molecular basis for "anticipation," which is the worsening of the clinical phenotype (earlier onset, more severe disease) in succeeding generations. The trinucleotide repeats tend to lengthen in succeeding generations, and the severity of the disease correlates, although not perfectly, with the length of the repeat segment.

Myotonic Dystrophy

Myotonic dystrophy is an autosomal dominant, multisystem disease with marked clinical variability with an incidence of 1 per 8,000 patients. The most severely affected patients are babies with congenital myotonic dystrophy. These children have severe hypotonia and weakness. They often require ventilatory support and nasogastric feedings. Clubfeet and dislocated hips are common. These children are almost always born to myotonic mothers rather than affected fathers. If they survive the neonatal period, these children show improvement in strength but have persistent motor disability. In addition, they are uniformly mentally retarded. At the other extreme, the only manifestation of myotonic dystrophy in the most mildly affected individuals may be cataracts. After the neonatal period, the disease presents with mild muscle weakness and myotonia exacerbated by cold. Wasting of the temporalis muscles contributes to the typical phenotype of long narrow facies with bitemporal narrowing. Cardiac conduction defects are common and may necessitate a pacemaker. Diabetes mellitus, male pattern baldness, infertility, and mental retardation are also manifestations of myotonic dystrophy. The abnormal gene, myotonia, is a protein kinase. The substrate for the kinase and the pathophysiology of the disease remain unknown. Recent data suggest that the adjacent *DMAHP* gene may play a complementary or even primary role in the pathogenesis of myotonic dystrophy. The protein location has been shown by immunoelectron microscopy to be membrane-bound in the terminal cisternae of the sarcoplasmic reticulum, mainly in the I-band. The mutation is an expansion of a trinucleotide repeat in the 3' untranslated region of the gene. The normal gene has 5 to 30 copies of this CTG repeat. This is expanded in myotonic dystrophy patients, reaching thousands of copies. The congenitally affected infants have the largest expansions, on average, and the mildest phenotypes are associated with the smallest expansions into the disease-associated range.

Friedreich Ataxia

Friedreich ataxia is the most common early-onset hereditary ataxia and occurs in approximately 2 to 4 per 100,000 patients in ethnically European populations. It is an autosomal recessive disorder characterized by progressive ataxia beginning before age 25 years. Muscle weakness, cardiomyopathy, and diabetes mellitus are frequent accompanying conditions. Scoliosis and pes cavus are common orthopaedic manifestations that often require treatment. The cause of Friedreich ataxia is a mutation of the gene *FRADA*, which codes for the protein frataxin. Friedreich ataxia is caused by a GAA repeat expansion in intron 1 of the gene *FRADA*.[44,45] The mutation appears to cause an accumulation of iron in mitochondria leading to excess free radical production and subsequent cell damage/death. Earlier age at onset and more frequent occurrence of associated conditions such as diabetes and cardiomyopathy are associated with larger repeat expansions.

Summary

The number of known genetically related orthopaedic disorders will only increase as understanding of musculoskeletal cellular and molecular biology increases. It is likely that future advancements will come from the ability to intervene more directly in these pathways rather than improved surgical techniques. The disorders discussed in this chapter are illustrative of these mechanisms and were selected because they are frequently seen by orthopaedists in practice.

References

1. Alman BA: A classification for genetic disorders of interest to orthopaedists. *Clin Orthop Relat Res* 2002;401:17-26.

2. Rossi R, Blonna D, Germano M, Castoldi F: Multidisciplinary investigation in Down syndrome: Bear in mind. *Orthopedics* 2008;31(3):279.

3. Caird MS, Wills BP, Dormans JP: Down syndrome in children: The role of the orthopaedic surgeon. *J Am Acad Orthop Surg* 2006;14(11):610-619.

4. Lana-Elola E, Watson-Scales SD, Fisher EM, Tybulewicz VL: Down syndrome: Searching for the genetic culprits. *Dis Model Mech* 2011;4(5):586-595.

5. Mik G, Gholve PA, Scher DM, Widmann RF, Green DW: Down syndrome: Orthopedic issues. *Curr Opin Pediatr* 2008;20(1):30-36.

6. Keckler SJ, St Peter SD, Valusek PA, et al: VACTERL anomalies in patients with esophageal atresia: An updated delineation of the spectrum and review of the literature. *Pediatr Surg Int* 2007;23(4):309-313.

7. Solomon BD: VACTERL/VATER association. *Orphanet J Rare Dis* 2011;6:56.

8. Maschke SD, Seitz W, Lawton J: Radial longitudinal deficiency. *J Am Acad Orthop Surg* 2007;15(1):41-52.

9. Chapurlat RD, Orcel P: Fibrous dysplasia of bone and McCune-Albright syndrome. *Best Pract Res Clin Rheumatol* 2008;22(1):55-69.

10. Collins MT, Singer FR, Eugster E: McCune-Albright syndrome and the extraskeletal manifestations of fibrous dysplasia. *Orphanet J Rare Dis* 2012;7(Suppl 1):S4.

11. Leet AI, Collins MT: Current approach to fibrous dysplasia of bone and McCune-Albright syndrome. *J Child Orthop* 2007;1(1):3-17.

12. Jett K, Friedman JM: Clinical and genetic aspects of neurofibromatosis 1. *Genet Med* 2010;12(1):1-11.

13. Jouhilahti E-M, Peltonen S, Heape AM, Peltonen J: The pathoetiology of neurofibromatosis 1. *Am J Pathol* 2011;178(5):1932-1939.

14. Feldman DS, Jordan C, Fonseca L: Orthopaedic manifestations of neurofibromatosis type 1. *J Am Acad Orthop Surg* 2010;18(6):346-357.

15. Rasmussen SA, Bieber FR, Benacerraf BR, Lachman RS, Rimoin DL, Holmes LB: Epidemiology of osteochondrodysplasias: Changing trends due to advances in prenatal diagnosis. *Am J Med Genet* 1996;61(1):49-58.

16. Warman ML, Cormier-Daire V, Hall C, et al: Nosology and classification of genetic skeletal disorders: 2010 revision. *Am J Med Genet A* 2011;155A(5):943-968.

17. Alanay Y, Lachman RS: A review of the principles of radiological assessment of skeletal dysplasias. *J Clin Res Pediatr Endocrinol* 2011;3(4):163-178.

18. Carter EM, Raggio CL: Genetic and orthopedic aspects of collagen disorders. *Curr Opin Pediatr* 2009;21(1):46-54.

19. Hendriksz CJ, Al-Jawad M, Berger KI, et al: Clinical overview and treatment options for non-skeletal manifestations of mucopolysaccharidosis type IVA. *J Inherit Metab Dis* 2012.

20. White KK: Orthopaedic aspects of mucopolysaccharidoses. *Rheumatology (Oxford)* 2011;50(Suppl 5):v26-v33.

21. Briggs MD, Chapman KL: Pseudoachondroplasia and multiple epiphyseal dysplasia: Mutation review, molecular interactions, and genotype to phenotype correlations. *Hum Mutat* 2002;19(5):465-478.

22. Sheridan BD, Gargan MF, Monsell FP: The hip in osteochondrodysplasias: General rules for diagnosis and treatment. *Hip Int* 2009;19(Suppl 6):S26-S34.

23. Unger S, Bonafé L, Superti-Furga A: Multiple epiphyseal dysplasia: Clinical and radiographic features, differential diagnosis and molecular basis. *Best Pract Res Clin Rheumatol* 2008;22(1):19-32.

24. Jackson GC, Mittaz-Crettol L, Taylor JA, et al: Pseudoachondroplasia and multiple epiphyseal dysplasia: A 7-year comprehensive analysis of the known disease genes identify novel and recurrent mutations and provides an accurate assessment of their relative contribution. *Hum Mutat* 2012;33(1):144-157.

25. Foldynova-Trantirkova S, Wilcox WR, Krejci P: Sixteen years and counting: The current understanding of fibroblast growth factor receptor 3 (FGFR3) signaling in skeletal dysplasias. *Hum Mutat* 2012;33(1):29-41.

26. Shirley ED, Ain MC: Achondroplasia: Manifestations and treatment. *J Am Acad Orthop Surg* 2009;17(4):231-241.

27. Levine BS, Kleeman CR, Felsenfeld AJ: The journey from vitamin D-resistant rickets to the regulation of renal phosphate transport. *Clin J Am Soc Nephrol* 2009;4(11):1866-1877.

28. Tosson H, Rose SR: Absence of mutation in coding regions of CYP2R1 gene in apparent autosomal dominant vitamin D 25-hydroxylase deficiency rickets. *J Clin Endocrinol Metab* 2012;97(5):E796-E801.

29. Carpenter TO: The expanding family of hypophosphatemic syndromes. *J Bone Miner Metab* 2012;30(1):1-9.

30. Bergwitz C, Jüppner H: FGF23 and syndromes of abnormal renal phosphate handling. *Adv Exp Med Biol* 2012;728:41-64.

31. Jennes I, Pedrini E, Zuntini M, et al: Multiple osteochondromas: Mutation update and description of the multiple osteochondromas mutation database (MOdb). *Hum Mutat* 2009;30(12):1620-1627.

32. Ihde LL, Forrester DM, Gottsegen CJ, et al: Sclerosing bone dysplasias: Review and differentiation from other causes of osteosclerosis. *Radiographics* 2011;31(7):1865-1882.

33. Malfait F, Wenstrup RJ, De Paepe A: Clinical and genetic aspects of Ehlers-Danlos syndrome, classic type. *Genet Med* 2010;12(10):597-605.

34. Stanitski DF, Nadjarian R, Stanitski CL, Bawle E, Tsipouras P: Orthopaedic manifestations of Ehlers-Danlos syndrome. *Clin Orthop Relat Res* 2000;376:213-221.

35. Levenson D: New guidelines for diagnosis of Marfan and Loey-Dietz syndromes. *Am J Med Genet A* 2010;152A(11).

36. Sponseller PD, Erkula G, Skolasky RL, Venuti KD, Dietz HC III: Improving clinical recognition of Marfan syndrome. *J Bone Joint Surg Am* 2010;92(9):1868-1875.

37. Munger JS, Sheppard D: Cross talk among TGF-β signaling pathways, integrins, and the extracellular matrix. *Cold Spring Harb Perspect Biol* 2011;3(11):a005017.

38. Bushby K, Finkel R, Birnkrant DJ, et al: Diagnosis and management of Duchenne muscular dystrophy, part 2: Implementation of multidisciplinary care. *Lancet Neurol* 2010; 9(2):177-189.

39. Bushby K, Finkel R, Birnkrant DJ, et al: Diagnosis and management of Duchenne muscular dystrophy, part 1: Diagnosis, and pharmacological and psychosocial management. *Lancet Neurol* 2010;9(1):77-93.

40. Nigro V, Aurino S, Piluso G: Limb girdle muscular dystrophies: Update on genetic diagnosis and therapeutic approaches. *Curr Opin Neurol* 2011;24(5):429-436.

41. Rotthier A, Baets J, Timmerman V, Janssens K: Mechanisms of disease in hereditary sensory and autonomic neuropathies. *Nat Rev Neurol* 2012;8(2):73-85.

42. Siskind CE, Shy ME: Genetics of neuropathies. *Semin Neurol* 2011;31(5):494-505.

43. Wilmshurst JM, Ouvrier R: Hereditary peripheral neuropathies of childhood: An overview for clinicians. *Neuromuscul Disord* 2011;21(11):763-775.

44. Martelli A, Napierala M, Puccio H: Understanding the genetic and molecular pathogenesis of Friedreich's ataxia through animal and cellular models. *Dis Model Mech* 2012; 5(2):165-176.

45. Koeppen AH: Friedreich's ataxia: Pathology, pathogenesis, and molecular genetics. *J Neurol Sci* 2011;303(1-2):1-12.

1: Basic Principles of Orthopaedic Surgery

Chapter 3

Biomechanics of Musculoskeletal Tissues

Jason P. Caffrey, BS
Robert L. Sah, MD, ScD

Introduction

Biomechanics is the application of the principles and methods of mechanics to biologic components and systems. Biomechanics provides a quantitative description of the behavior of biologic objects when subjected to force or displacement. Orthopaedic biomechanics addresses musculoskeletal structures at scales ranging from molecules to cells, extracellular matrix, tissues, organs, organ systems, and whole organisms. What is manifest as macroscopic loading, movement, deformation, and failure are phenomena that are dependent inherently on the multiscale hierarchy of skeletal structures, as well as interactions between multiple skeletal tissues and organs. In addition, in orthopaedic surgery, biomechanics can reflect interactions between native musculoskeletal tissues and artificial materials (see chapter 4). The analysis of musculoskeletal biomechanical function is intimately related to delineation of the structures underlying such functions.

Musculoskeletal biomechanics is relevant to a variety of clinical situations in orthopaedic surgery. For example, the motion of skeletal elements, such as the lower limbs during gait, reflects the coordinated activities of the neuromuscular activation and control system, acting upon multiple joints and supporting soft and hard tissues. At a finer scale, the local deformation of tissues can reflect their integrity in native and disease states, or after repair such as with sutures. The force on an element should be less than that tolerated, such as that on bones and affixed plates after surgical stabilization of a fracture. The articulation of tissues, such as carti-

lage in joints within the synovial fluid environment, should occur with minimal wear.

The biomechanics of musculoskeletal tissues are not static, but change over time. During the fetal, postnatal, and childhood stages of life and into adulthood, skeletal tissues grow and adapt to varying mechanical demands, often in ways that are different for males and females. However, with advancing age or traumatic injury, skeletal dysfunction, regeneration, and deterioration may occur, especially for certain types of diseases or injuries at particular skeletal sites. During the stages of growth up to early adulthood, the properties of skeletal tissues often vary, and indeed the growth process itself can be described with biomechanical formalism. With aging in the adult as well as age-associated diseases such as osteoarthritis, osteoporosis, disk degeneration, and rotator cuff degeneration, skeletal tissues exhibit a different set of biomechanical properties. Thus, individual skeletal tissues exhibit a spectrum of properties.

The changes in the biomechanical properties of musculoskeletal tissues over time reflect biologic and chemical processes that modulate the composition and structure of the tissues under tight regulation. Such processes can achieve a steady-state homeostasis, or, alternatively, a net anabolic state causing growth; or, conversely, a net catabolic state causing resorption or deterioration. Such biologic processes may be modulated by the mechanical environment itself, a closely related field termed mechanobiology. Key components of mechanobiology are an understanding of the local mechanical environment and the response of cells and tissues to such an environment.

Thus, the objective of this chapter is to introduce several biomechanical concepts that are useful for the orthopaedic surgeon. Terms for structural analysis are introduced and defined, and then used in the static analysis of elements assumed to be rigid. Then, terms for analysis of motion are

Mr. Caffrey or an immediate family member has stock or stock options held in Talon Therapeutics. Dr. Sah or an immediate family member has stock or stock options held in GlaxoSmithKline, Johnson & Johnson, and Medtronic.

provided, enabling discussion of the fields of dynamics and kinetics. Next, terms for material level analysis are defined, with a focus on their use in describing skeletal tissues as materials. With both structural and material terms introduced, elastic, viscoelastic, and strength properties are summarized, with implications for energy dissipation. Finally, topics comprising tribology, friction, wear, and lubrication are introduced. Throughout the chapter, examples relevant to clinical orthopaedics are provided.

Terms and Definitions for Structural Analyses

Throughout this chapter, the term "object" is chosen to describe a component of a biomechanical system of interest (eg, bone, tendon, or entire skeleton).[1,2] In classic mechanics and some biomechanics literature, such an object is referred to as a body, but this word will be avoided where possible to avoid confusion with the body of an organism, with a few exceptions (for example, rigid body, free body diagram).

For values of force and displacement, the International System of Units (SI) will be used. The SI system has base units including meter (m), kilogram (kg), second (s), and mole (mol) for the quantities length, mass, time, and amount of substance, respectively. The SI system also has derived units including m^2, m^3, m/s, m/s^2, for area, volume, velocity, and acceleration, respectively; as well as coherent units with special names and symbols, including radian (rad), hertz (Hz), newton (N), pascal (Pa), joule (J), degrees Celsius (°C) for plane angle, frequency, force, pressure and stress, energy and work, and Celsius temperature, respectively.

The use of relevant metric prefixes allows for concise description and order of magnitude comparison of length and time scales relevant to the biomechanical structure and event, respectively, of interest. Biomechanical analysis can be performed at a relatively large length scale (cm to m) in the case of entire bones, ligaments, and tendons to a microscale (mm) in the case of tissues, to a cellular scale (10 μm), to a nanoscale (nm) in the case of molecules. Biomechanical events may occur at time scales ranging from milliseconds in the case of impact, to seconds for ambulation, to hour and day for intervertebral disk equilibration, to weeks and months for tissue remodeling, and years for growth. Using appropriate prefixes and time scales can allow for order of magnitude comparisons of various biomechanical quantities.

Force

The basis for biomechanics is force, defined as an influence on an object that causes one of three changes to that object: translation, rotation, and deformation.[1-4] A force is characterized by its point of application, magnitude, and direction. As such, force is quantified with a vector, a mathematical expression possessing both magnitude and direction. Vectors

are diagrammed by a line segment connecting the tail, at the point of application, to the head, containing the arrow, with the direction defined as that from tail to head. Vectors have several useful properties characteristic of forces. Vectors that possess the same direction and magnitude are said to be equal. Vectors can be added commutatively, meaning that $\vec{A} + \vec{B} = \vec{B} + \vec{A}$. However, it is not necessarily true that the magnitude $|\vec{A} + \vec{B}|$ is equal to the sum of magnitude $|\vec{A}|$ and magnitude $|\vec{B}|$. This is because the resultant vector $|\vec{A} + \vec{B}|$ has a magnitude that is dependent on the direction of each vector relative to one another, while the magnitudes of individual vectors are independent of direction. The vector sum of multiple forces at a single point of application can be combined into a single vector quantity called the resultant force. Calculating resultant forces often helps to simplify force analysis.

Some specific classifications of force acting on an object depend on the direction of force. When an object is being pulled apart, the force is referred to as tension. When an object is pushed together, the force is referred to as compression. Typically tendons and ligaments are in tension, whereas bone, cartilage, and intervertebral disks are in compression.

To analyze forces in biomechanics, it is useful to draw a free body diagram, with a simplified geometry of the system of interest and all the forces acting on it. An example of a free body diagram is shown in **Figure 1, A**. In the musculoskeletal system, there are external forces, as well as internal forces. Examples of external forces include gravitational force and contact forces. Examples of internal forces include those generated by springs, passive tension of tendon, or active tension of muscle.

Torque

Whenever a force is applied to an object at a point outside of its axis of rotation (as in **Figure 1, A**), there arises a tendency for the object to rotate. An example of this is a force pushing down on the forearm while the humerus is held steady, causing the forearm to rotate about the elbow joint. The torque, also known as the moment or rotational moment, is the tendency for a force to rotate an object about an axis perpendicular to the force.[1-4] The torque, denoted as the vector $\vec{\tau}$, is computed by

$$\vec{\tau} = \vec{r} \times \vec{F},\tag{1}$$

which is the vector cross product between the lever arm $\vec{\tau}$, the displacement vector from the point of rotation to the point of applied force, and $\vec{F}$, the force vector. The direction of the resulting cross product vector, and thus the direction of torque, is governed by the right-hand rule. Using the right hand, the extended index finger is pointed in the direction of $\vec{r}$ (pointing from the point of rotation to the point of force application), the flexed middle finger is then pointed in the direction of $\vec{F}$, and consequently the direction of the extended thumb is that of $\vec{\tau}$. Similarly, if the

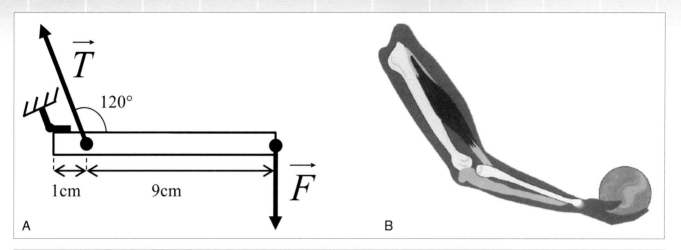

Figure 1 **A**, Mechanical analog free body diagram view. T = tension; F = force. **B**, Anatomic view of a human arm with a ball in hand. All forces and distances are labeled on the free body diagram.

right thumb is pointed in the direction of the torque, the natural curl of the fingers is in the direction of rotation. The magnitude of torque is found using the cross product magnitude equation

$$\tau = rF\sin(\theta) \qquad (2)$$

where τ is the magnitude of torque, r is the magnitude of displacement, F is the magnitude of force, and θ is the angle between the displacement and force vectors when the tails of both vectors are coincident.

One example illustrating the use of vectors, force, and torque to describe a musculoskeletal subsystem is the analysis of holding a ball in hand, shown in **Figure 1, B**. The forces include the gravitational force of the ball, arm, and forearm and the generated tension from the biceps muscle. To simplify the analysis, it can be assumed that the weight of the arm and forearm is small compared with the weight of the ball and tension in the biceps and can be ignored. Because the forearm is allowed to rotate relative to the forearm via the elbow, both forces induce torque on the elbow. The ball causes extension of the elbow, whereas the biceps force causes flexion of the elbow. In the next section, it will be shown that when these torques are equal, the forearm will not start to rotate.

Now, the torque from each of the two forces can be computed using the free body diagram in **Figure 1, A**. Suppose the gravitation force of the ball, $\vec{F}$, is 50 N and the tension generated by the muscle, $\vec{T}$, is 200 N. For the muscle, the pivot-to-force distance is 1 cm, and the angle between is 120°, giving a torque of 1.73 N*m using equation 2. Using the right-hand rule, the torque from the muscle causes counterclockwise rotation. For the ball, the pivot-to-force distance is 10 cm, and the angle between is 90°, giving a torque of 5 N*m using equation 2. Using the right-hand rule, the torque from the ball causes clockwise rotation.

Newton's Laws

The properties of forces are dictated by Newton's laws.[1-4] Newton's first law states that if the net force on an object is zero, $\Sigma\vec{F} = 0$, then the object does not accelerate. As is described in the Statics section, this is the basis for static equilibrium of rigid bodies. When rigid objects are not in static equilibrium, they are subject to translational or rotational acceleration that obeys Newton's second law, which states that force is equal to the product of mass and acceleration, $\vec{F} = m\vec{a}$. This equation is the basis for dynamics, described further below, when there is a nonzero net force on an object. Newton's third law states that for every action there is an equal and opposite reaction.

Statics

When studying biomechanics, it is often appropriate to assume that the objects are not deformed; such objects are referred to as rigid bodies. A practical rigid body in orthopaedics may be a titanium rod or plate that under normal conditions does not bend or deform appreciably. An additional example is the assumption of rigid bone in gait analysis, in which the deformation of bone is significantly less than the length scale of gait motion. Although all objects technically are under some degree of deformation when loaded, when the deformation is very small, it may be appropriate to neglect it and simplify the analysis. For purposes of analysis, rigid bodies are objects that can translate or rotate but cannot deform.

When rigid bodies remain motionless or at a constant velocity, a static analysis can be performed. Statics is the field of mechanics that involves the forces and moments in non-accelerating objects.[1,3-5] It is important to know the constraints imposed by joints between the objects in a system when analyzing a statics problem. A constraint prevents motion, which can either be a translation or rotation, in a particular direction. Joints, by virtue of their geometry and the

Joint Shape	Geometry and Motion	Sample Joint(s)	Translational Degrees of Freedom	Rotational Degrees of Freedom
Pivot	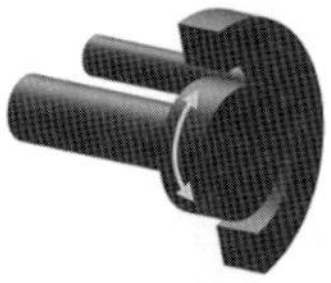	Proximal radioulnar	0	1
Hinge	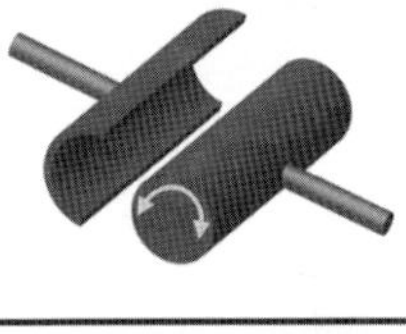	Ulnohumeral, interphalangeal	0	1
Saddle	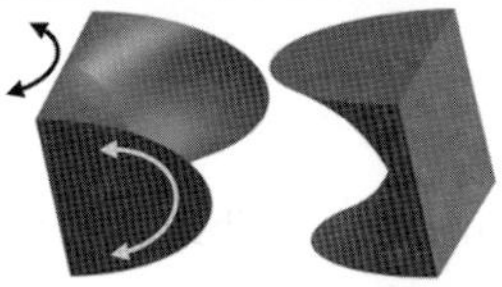	Carpometacarpal of the thumb	0	2
Spheroidal	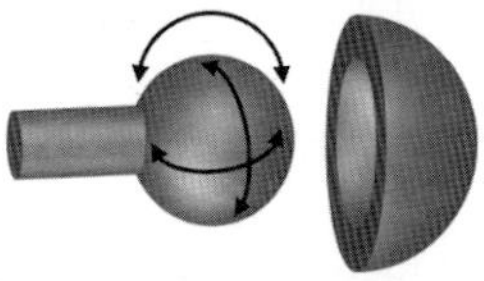	Hip, shoulder	0	3
Ellipsoidal	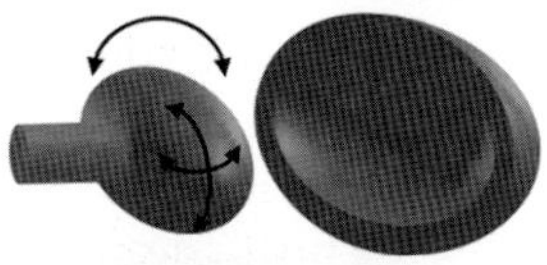	Radiocarpal	0	3
Plane	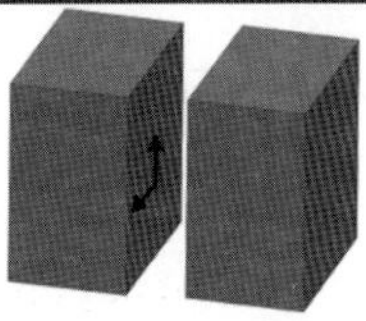	Intercarpal, intertarsal	2	0

Figure 2 Geometry and degrees of freedom for common types of orthopaedic joints.

constraints imposed on them by various tissues, are essentially limited to certain types and directions of motion (**Figure 2**). Each unconstrained translation or rotation is called a degree of freedom, such that in three-dimensional Cartesian space there are six degrees of freedom (three translation and three rotation) and in two-dimensional Cartesian space there are three degrees of freedom (two translation and one rotation). An example of a joint with one degree of freedom is the ulnohumeral (elbow) joint, which constrains translation about all three axes and rotation about two axes. One type of single rotation connection is classified as a hinge. In Cartesian coordinates, a system can have between zero and six degrees of freedom. Most bodily joints except for planar joints have zero translational degrees of freedom and between one and three rotational degrees of freedom. Most orthopaedic fixtures (screws, pins, plates, rods) have zero de-

grees of freedom, because their purpose is to restrict movement during healing or create a permanent attachment. Biologic joints of the human body have mechanical analogs, with certain types of unconstrained motions and numbers of degrees of freedom (**Figure 2**). Although joints are often classified by shape and types of motions depending on soft- and hard-tissue constraints, many variations exist, and almost all joints have small degrees of other types of motion. Although these motions are often assumed insignificant, for the purpose of classification, some joints such as the knee have complex motion.

When a force acts against a constraint, the two connected objects are considered rigid and treated as a single rigid body. When all the forces and moments on a system balance, the system does not change motion and is considered in equilibrium. Static equilibrium is defined as the state when the vector sum of forces and moments on a system is zero. Although a system in static equilibrium could be motionless, it could also be translating or rotating at a constant velocity. In those cases, the use of the kinematics equations (3 through 7) in the following section on dynamics (neglecting acceleration) may be useful.

Reconsidering **Figure 1**, the tension generated by the biceps to maintain static equilibrium can be calculated if $\vec{F}$ is known, for example, 10 N. Considering only the arm of the body, it can be assumed that the upper arm is rigidly constrained at the shoulder (zero degrees of freedom). The elbow is defined as a hinge having one degree of freedom (rotation). The forces are balanced in both the x and y directions, knowing that the elbow will also provide a translational reaction force. Because there are no translation degrees of freedom in the system, the forces are balanced by the elbow hinge. Similarly, the torques generated can be balanced by the ball and the biceps muscle using the equality (1 cm) T sin (120°) = (10 cm)(10 N) sin (90°). Solving for T, it can be shown that the biceps muscle generates 115 N of tension to maintain static equilibrium.

Dynamics

When the forces and/or torques are not balanced, the object is no longer at equilibrium and requires analysis of the change in motion and the nonzero acceleration of the system. Dynamics is the field of mechanics involving the relationship between forces and moments on objects in motion.[2-4] Kinematics describes the motion of points, objects, and systems of objects without consideration of the causes of such motion. Kinematic analysis can be useful both in the case of a static system, moving at constant linear and/or angular velocity, as well as in the case of a dynamic system. Kinetics, in contrast, is the study of motion and its causes.

Both kinematic and kinetic analyses are performed routinely in orthopaedic clinical practice. The determination of the range of motion of joints is one common and practical example of kinematic analysis. The assessment of the stability of a joint, by imposing a translational force or rotational torque and observing resultant motion, is an example of kinetic analysis. In addition, motion analysis, whether of gait or other motions, involves analyses of motion as well as load (and/or torque). Inverse dynamics refers to the method of computing forces and/or moments based on the kinematics of a body, inertial analysis, and often measurement of ground reaction forces.

If the sum of forces is not zero, a resultant motion is translational linear acceleration. As noted previously, this acceleration is described by Newton's second law, $\vec{F} = m\vec{a}$. This can be transformed into an equation of motion that can be solved for a variety of cases. For the case of constant acceleration, the resultant motion is described by the following formula:

$$\vec{r} = \vec{r}_0 + \vec{v}_0 t + \frac{\vec{a}t^2}{2} \qquad (3)$$

$$\vec{v} = \vec{v}_0 + \vec{a}t \qquad (4)$$

where $\vec{r}$ is position, $\vec{r}_0$ is initial position, $\vec{v}$ is velocity, $\vec{v}_0$ is initial velocity, $\vec{a}$ is acceleration, and t is time. Because the position, velocity, and acceleration vectors are all collinear, the vector terms can be simplified to magnitudes, each with the common direction.

The rotational analogy to the above situation is one where the sum of torques is not zero, and the resulting motion is rotational acceleration. For rotational acceleration, Newton's second law for rotation dictates acceleration by the relationship

$$\vec{\tau} = I\vec{\alpha} \qquad (5)$$

where $\vec{\tau}$ is torque as described earlier, I is the mass moment of inertia, and $\vec{\alpha}$ is the angular (rotational) acceleration. The mass moment of inertia is dependent on both the mass of the object, as well as the geometric distribution of mass relative to the axis of rotation. It can be thought of conceptually as the resistance to rotational acceleration. In general, the farther mass is distributed from the axis of rotation, the greater the mass moment of inertia. For constant rotational acceleration of an object, the following equations describe the motion of the object:

$$\vec{\theta} = \vec{\theta}_0 + \vec{\omega}_0 t + \frac{\vec{\alpha}t^2}{2} \qquad (6)$$

$$\vec{\omega} = \vec{\omega}_0 + \vec{\alpha}t \qquad (7)$$

where $\vec{\theta}$ is angular displacement, $\vec{\theta}_0$ is initial angle, $\vec{\omega}$ is angular velocity, $\vec{\omega}_0$ is initial angular velocity, $\vec{\alpha}$ is angular acceleration, and t is time (equations 6 and 7). Equations of motion for nonconstant acceleration are more complex and require extensive analysis.

A simple example of a dynamic situation is an extension of the example in **Figure 1**, of a biceps curl where the elbow is flexed. In this case, the moment about the elbow created by the tension in the biceps is greater than the moment created by the ball. Hence, there is a net nonzero torque. By Newton's second law for rotation, there is a nonzero angular acceleration.

Terms and Definitions for Material Analyses

Although skeletal objects are often treated as rigid bodies in statics and dynamics, there are several situations in which more extensive deformation of the object occurs or needs to be considered. To describe such deformation as well as the causes of such deformation, several additional biomechanical terms are used[6,7] and quantities and relationships assessed, as described in the following paragraphs. More

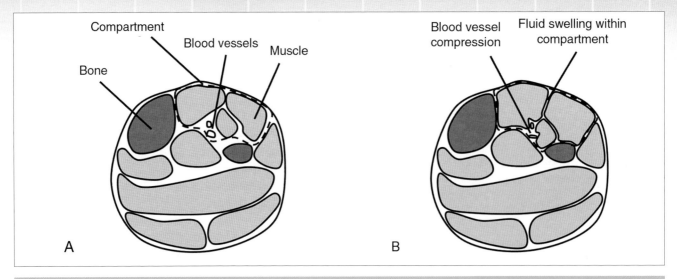

Figure 3 Cross-section of lower leg anatomy. The compartment, denoted by dotted lines, is separated by fascia layers in the normal state (**A**) and the swollen compartment syndrome state (**B**) caused by muscle swelling, edema, or internal bleeding. Compartment expansion is limited by tensile strength of fascia and skin layers, causing increased internal pressure and compressing blood vessels and nerves or causing bone fracture.

generally, this branch of biomechanics involves continuum mechanics, where the mechanical behavior of objects is modeled as a continuous deformable mass rather than as a discrete nondeformable mass or particle.

Stress

To analyze the cause of deformation of an object, force must be considered after normalization to the area of application, instead of as a point force as done in statics and dynamics. Stress is defined as the amount of force per unit area,[6,7] and in a single dimension, can be expressed as a scalar quantity,

$$\sigma = \frac{F}{A} \qquad (8)$$

where σ is stress, F is force, and A is area. However, in general, stress takes the form of a tensor, a 3×3 matrix, that can describe both normal stresses and shear stresses. A normal stress is one that acts perpendicular to a surface plane, and thus can be in three orthogonal directions. A shear stress is one that acts tangential to a surface plane and thus can comprise six components, two tangential directions to each of three surface planes. Most physiologic stresses are a combination of normal and shear stresses. It is important to note this difference, as most organic and inorganic materials have different responses to normal and shear stresses and thus, different properties in compression or tension and in shear.

It is useful to obtain a tangible feeling for stress quantities. Suppose a person is standing upright on both feet and has a mass of 70 kg. If each foot has a cross-sectional area of 100 cm², the stress is 34 kPa by equation 8. If the person stands on only one foot, the new stress is 68 kPa, twice as much.

A commonly used term for stress is pressure. In biomechanics, pressure may refer to several mechanical phenomena. Pressure may refer to the stress at a surface, especially in contacting surfaces such as joint surface, where it is denoted as contact pressure. Such pressure may be due to a combination of both solid and fluid pressure. Alternatively, pressure may refer to fluid pressure, which is defined as the average of the normal stresses in each orthogonal direction. Although this chapter primarily addresses tissues that are considered solids, it is also important to consider the fluid component of tissues and the fluid pressure that is present.

An orthopaedic example of the effects of fluid pressure is compartment syndrome. In this situation, swelling of the muscles within the compartment, bleeding into the compartment, or several other factors leads to an increase in pressure inside the limb compartment. This is due to the restraining nature of the fascia and skin, whose tension balances the pressure forces to resist the enlargement of the limb compartment (**Figure 3**). This pressurization can cause compression of the venous and lymphatic vessels that normally drain the muscle compartment. As arterial blood continues to flow in and exceed venous and lymphatic return, the volume and pressure build up. The eventual decrease in blood flow and/or compaction of muscle and nerve may cause tissue necrosis.

Deformation and Strain

When objects are subjected to external or internal stress, they change in configuration or undergo displacement. Such displacement has two components, a rigid body displacement and a deformation. The rigid body displacement is analogous to that described earlier in static and dynamic analyses. Superimposed on that is deformation, a change in

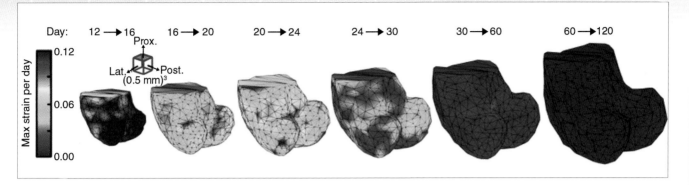

Figure 4 Distal femur shape at days 12, 16, 20, 24, 30, and 60. Color maps indicate maximum principal strain rates (per day), calculated between the age intervals indicated at the top and mapped onto the shape of the younger age point. (Reproduced with permission from Chan EF, Harjanto R, Asahara H, et al: Structural and functional maturation of distal femoral cartilage and bone during postnatal development and growth in humans and mice. *Orthop Clin North Am* 2012;43:173-185.)

shape and/or size of the object, associated with the quantity strain.[6,7] In a single dimension, strain is defined as the amount of deformation normalized to the total length. Just as in the case of stress, strain takes the form of a tensor, a 3 × 3 matrix, that can describe both normal strains and shear strains. Although many precise definitions of strain are used in continuum mechanics, a common definition is the change in length per initial length

$$\varepsilon = \frac{\Delta L}{L_0} \qquad (9)$$

where ε is strain, ΔL is a change in length, and L_0 is the initial length. The parameter ε for strain is technically appropriate when the magnitude of ε is "small," ie, <1.

Although strain is often considered to be the result of applied external loads or active muscle contraction generating internal loads, there are several situations in which internally developed stresses cause strain. A classic example of this is growth strain, associated with skeletal development and growth, in which new tissue formation causes stresses that change the size and shape of bodily structures. Such a growth strain may be represented for an object in three dimensions or at a surface in two dimensions. A two-dimensional example is the growth strain of the surface of the distal femur (**Figure 4**), varying with position and different stages of growth.

Musculoskeletal tissues, as well as orthopaedic implants, encounter a variety of stresses and strains that typically are harmless or even beneficial. In order for the musculoskeletal system to provide support and mobility, ligaments, tendons, and bone are typically loaded with characteristic values for various types of stresses and strains. Because tendons and ligaments are usually stretched, they undergo tensile stress and strain. Opposing those forces, bone is typically compressed, undergoing compressive stress and strain. Many orthopaedic implants, such as metal plates to immobilize bone, are loaded in tension, compression, or shear, depending on which type of expected movement should be re-

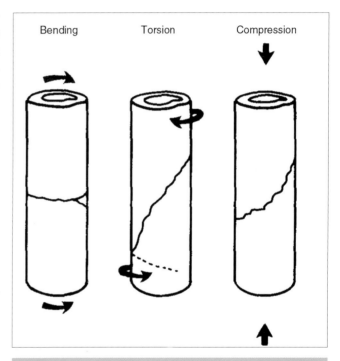

Figure 5 Typical loading schemes on a bone and typical failure fracture patterns. Arrows indicate direction of applied force. (Adapted with permission from Carter DR, Spengler DM: Biomechanics of fractures, in *Bone in Clinical Orthopaedics*. Philadelphia, PA, WB Saunders, 1982, pp 305-334.)

stricted. Orthopaedic fasteners, such as pins and screws, are often loaded in shear as well as compression.

In biomechanics, there are several common loading patterns on tissues, including tension, compression, torsion, and shear. As previously mentioned, tension is the axial elongation (positive stress and strain) that occurs in tendons, ligaments, muscle (passive), and cartilage. Active tension in muscles is characterized by a shortening of the muscle due to an internally generated force. Compression is the axial shortening (negative stress and strain) that occurs in

1: Basic Principles of Orthopaedic Surgery

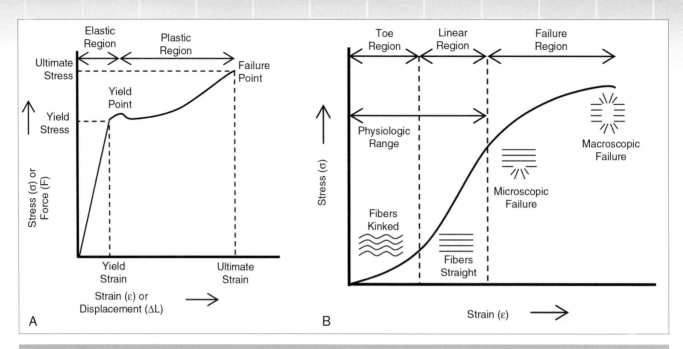

Figure 6 A, Typical stress-strain (material properties) or force-displacement (structural properties) curve for a ductile material. **B,** Typical stress-strain curve for a soft tissue, with regions and microscopic structure labeled.

bones, cartilage, intervertebral disks, and menisci. Torsion is the twisting around the axis, and shear is the loading transverse to the axis. Each of these loading cases is evident for long bones (**Figure 5**).

When considering multidimensional problems, the choice of coordinate system can be important and lead to simplified biomechanical analysis. Particular coordinate systems are naturally used for certain tissues, based on their geometry. The standard coordinate systems are Cartesian (x,y,z), cylindrical (r,θ,z), and spherical (r,θ,ϕ). In orthopaedics, Cartesian and cylindrical are typically the most common systems. One such example is the cylindrical coordinate system for bone. Most long bones are roughly hollow cylinders in shape, conforming well to cylindrical coordinates.

Elastic Properties

Structural properties describe the relationship between force and elongation, whereas material properties describe the relationship between stress and strain. For both cases, constitutive laws, such as Hooke's law, describe the relationship and are important and useful for biomechanics. To determine such properties, typically either a force (stress) or an elongation (strain) is applied while the other quantity is measured. Stress and strain may be measured with specialized sensors or deduced from measurements of force or displacement. Specimens are typically isolated intact for structural property measurements or prepared into specific geometries (such as a uniform cylinder or block) for material property measurements; these specific geometries facilitate the determination of stress and strain in orthogonal directions.[6,7]

Elastic Structural Properties

Skeletal tissues often exhibit elastic structural properties, wherein the object behaves like an energy-conserving spring.[6,7] The testing of a skeletal object in the laboratory can be done in a variety of modes, often with force being controlled and displacement being measured, or vice versa. For an elastic structure, the loading and unloading phases are identical, and the structure returns to the initial length when the load is removed, or conversely, the structure returns to a zero load state when the displacement is removed. The result of such tests are quantified by plots of force versus time, displacement versus time, and force versus displacement. In the force versus displacement plot, force and displacement are plotted against each other for each time point (**Figure 6, A**). The slope of the curve is termed stiffness, which is a structural property that is dependent on the tissue material and geometry. Several elastic tissues obey Hooke's law ($F = -kx$), especially with relatively low displacement amplitudes or forces, such that the force is directly proportional to the displacement and an elastic constant.

Elastic Material Properties

If force and displacement data are normalized to geometric parameters to obtain stress and strain equivalents, elastic material properties can be obtained.[4,6,7] From a stress-strain curve, the slope in the linear region, E, Young's modulus, is the scaling factor relating the strain, ε, to the stress, σ, according to the material form of Hooke's law,

$$\sigma = E\varepsilon \qquad (10)$$

Table 1
Material Properties of Different Orthopaedic Materials

Material	Loading Direction	Elastic Modulus (MPa)	Ultimate Strength (MPa)
Cortical bone	Compression	18,000	200
Trabecular bone	Compression	10-150	1-10
Tendons	Tension	300-600	40-60
Ligaments	Tension	300	40
Articular cartilage	Compression	0.3-1.0	N/A
Articular cartilage	Tension	3-6	5-10
Meniscus	Compression	0.1-0.6	N/A
Meniscus	Tension	50-150	1-4
Intervertebral disk	Tension	0.5	0.3
Titanium	Tension	200,000	550
Stainless steel	Tension	110,000	490-1,400
Ultrahigh-molecular-weight polyethylene	Compression	400-1,200	40

For skeletal tissues, the type of loading often markedly affects the material modulus. Young's modulus can be determined either in compression or tension. In either case, the assumption is that the test sample is free to expand or contract laterally during axial displacement. Compressive and tensile moduli can be substantially different, in large part because the load-bearing elements are not simple springs that are symmetric in compression and tension, but rather governed by a variety of extracellular matrix components (**Figure 6, B**). Analogously, the shear modulus can be determined from shear stress and shear strain and thought of as the intrinsic stiffness of a material in shear. The bulk modulus can be considered the intrinsic stiffness of a material as it expands or contracts volumetrically (ie, equally in all orthogonal directions). These moduli of elasticity represent intrinsic material properties, in contrast to structural stiffness of an object, which does depend on tissue geometry. **Table 1** shows moduli values for a range of orthopaedic tissues and other materials to illustrate the absolute and relative values, as well as for reference.[4,8-14]

Another useful elastic material property describes the inverse relationship between axial and transverse strain. Poisson's ratio, ν, describes the extent of transverse strain when an object undergoes axial strain, as given by the expression

$$\nu = \frac{-\varepsilon_{transverse}}{\varepsilon_{axial}} \quad (11)$$

where $\varepsilon_{transverse}$ is the transverse strain and ε_{axial} is the axial strain. Typically, when an object is stretched axially (positive strain), it contracts transversely (negative strain). Likewise, when an object is compressed axially (negative strain), it expands transversely (positive strain). In both these cases, ν is positive. For most materials, Poisson's ratio is positive; however, for some materials, it is zero or even negative.

Most biologic soft tissues and some polymers have nonlinear stress-strain relationships in their elastic region. Such curves are often approximately exponential and widely variable between samples, unlike the linear stress-strain curves of metals and ceramics. In contrast, most orthopaedic metals and ceramics have a distinct linear elastic region and well-defined modulus values. For biologic tissues, the initial low-strain, low modulus region is called the toe region. In tension, the toe region can be caused by kinked fibers on the microscopic level that are initially straightened, after which they stiffen from being stretched. Therefore, the main regions of soft-tissue stress-strain curves are the toe (elastic), linear (elastic), and failure (plastic) regions (**Figure 6, B**). Although the material may be nonlinear, it can be helpful to designate an approximately linear region to be able to compare modulus values.

Homogeneity of Material Properties
Up until this point, material properties have been considered uniform throughout the volume of the object, or homogeneous.[4] However, many skeletal tissues exhibit inhomogeneous material properties over a variety of length scales, reflecting variation in their composition and microstructure between different regions of interest. The relationships between local biomechanical material properties and the local composition and structure of musculoskeletal tissues can vary normally in space and also during development, growth, aging, and disease.[7-10] A material that is inhomogeneous is one whose properties vary between regions of the object. For example, cartilage has inhomogeneous compres-

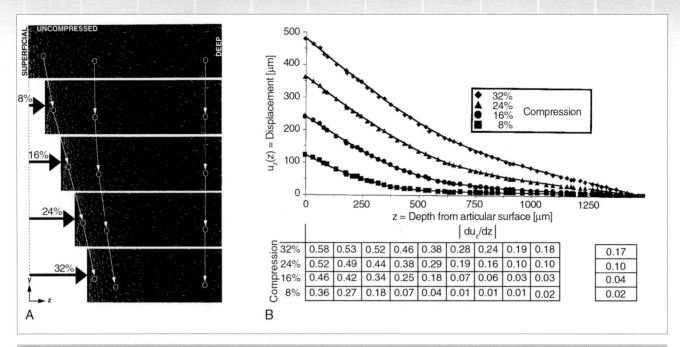

Figure 7 A, Epifluorescent micrographs of stained chondrocyte nuclei subjected to graded levels of equilibrium confined compression. Arrows and circles indicate tracking of nuclei from the reference state through each level of compression, showing the differential strain through the thickness. **B,** Typical displacement and strain (du$_z$/dz) in a full-thickness cartilage specimen. Plot of measured displacement relative to the uncompressed state versus depth from the articular surface for four compression levels (top). The chart indicates the corresponding magnitude of strain in each tissue layer for each of the four compression levels (bottom). (Reproduced with permission from Schinagl RM, Gurskis D, Chen AC, Sah RL: Depth-dependent confined compression modulus of full-thickness bovine articular cartilage. *J Orthop Res* 1997;15:499-506.)

sive properties as a function of depth from the articular surface (**Figure 7**). Conversely, steel is normally a homogeneous material, with constant properties throughout its volume.

Isotropy of Material Properties

Most skeletal tissues also have mechanical properties that vary with the direction of testing.[7] The degree of such directional uniformity is described by the term isotropy. A material is isotropic if its mechanical properties are independent of the orientation of the coordinate system (direction) at a point. If a material is not isotropic, then it is described as anisotropic. There are many lesser degrees of anisotropy, which simplify analysis of mechanical properties including orthotropy and transverse isotropy. An orthotropic material is one whose material properties are symmetric within at least two orthogonal planes, where they are independent of direction. One example of a material that is often described as orthotropic is bone, whose mechanical properties vary between the axial and transverse directions. A further simplified subset of orthotropy is transverse isotropy, in which material properties are uniform within a single plane (for example, x-y plane), but differ along the axis normal to the plane (for example, z-axis). A fully anisotropic material is one whose material properties exhibit different material properties in all testing directions.

Consideration of the length-scale of material characterization can add both complexity and precision to the analy-

sis. A material may be anisotropic at one length scale, but isotropic on a larger length scale. For example, the crystalline grain structure of steel may be anisotropic, whereas the macroscale material shows isotropic behavior. This is due to the averaging over the properties of many different grain orientations, which converge to a single overall property on a larger length scale.

Viscoelastic Properties

All of the discussion about stress-strain relationships thus far has been independent of loading time and rate. However, a characteristic material property of biologic tissues is that of viscoelasticity, in which the tissue has a time-varying relationship between stress and strain.[3,4,7] Such behavior may be due to a structural element that itself exhibits viscoelasticity. Alternatively, such behavior may be due to the interaction of elastic (solid-like) and viscous (fluid-like) components of a tissue that interact during deformation. Viscoelasticity gives rise to two experimental tissue behaviors in response to prescribed changes in stress or strain, stress relaxation and creep. Stress relaxation is a decrease in stress over time in response to a change of and then maintenance of constant strain. Creep is the increase in strain over time in response to a step increase in stress. Viscoelasticity also gives rise to energy-dissipating behavior during cyclic loading. In viscoelastic tissues, there is a loss of energy with loading, so that the loading and unloading phases are distinct, a characteristic called hysteresis (**Figure 8**).

With some tissues, continued cyclical loading will lead to smaller differences between consecutive loading or unloading curves, reflecting a phenomenon called preconditioning. In some cases, preconditioning a tissue during a laboratory test yields more reproducible biomechanical properties. In tendon transfer surgery, preconditioning an attached muscle is often done before setting the muscle length to achieve a physiologically appropriate microstructure.

Determination of viscoelastic structural or material properties can be useful for comparing tissues or determining time constants, characteristic time values such as for creep and stress relaxation. One approach to viscoelastic tissue characterization is fitting of data to one of three lumped-parameter representations: Maxwell, Voigt, and Kelvin models. In these models, the tissue is represented by combinations of elastic elements (springs) and viscous elements (dashpots – similar to shock absorbers). Such models can exhibit creep, stress relaxation, and hysteresis behaviors (**Figure 9**). Another approach to viscoelastic tissue charac-

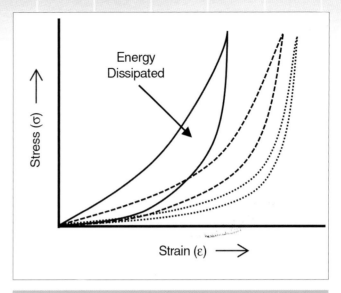

Figure 8 Hysteresis loading and unloading curves for three cycles, showing preconditioning effect. Area within loading and unloading curve represents dissipated energy.

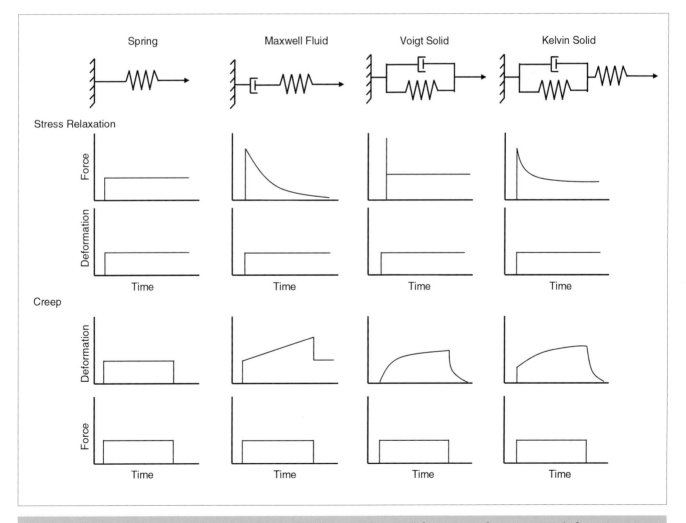

Figure 9 Time-varying force and deformation responses to a step response in deformation or force, respectively for spring, Maxwell fluid, Voigt solid, and Kelvin solid models.

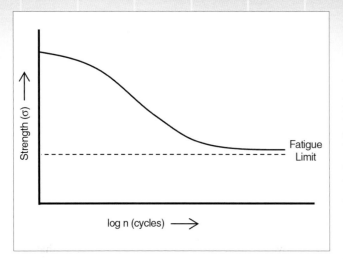

Figure 10 Typical failure strength versus cycle number for repeated loading conditions. Dotted line represents the fatigue limit strength.

terization is fitting of data to physically motivated models. For porous fluid-filled materials, viscoelastic behavior can be related to contributions from a solid-like matrix with elastic material properties and from viscous fluid flow through the porous matrix, as described by the hydraulic permeability.[8] The long viscoelastic time constant of creep compression of intervertebral disks is responsible for the gradual shortening of the spine during the day with loading, and the lengthening of the spine during the evening with off-loading.

Strength

An important biomechanical property of an object is that of failure, the loss of a structure's load-carrying capacity. There are several different modes of failure that are important in orthopaedic applications. In the stress-strain curve (**Figure 6, A**), after the low strain and elastic regions, there is often a plastic region characteristic of ductile materials. Here, deformation is permanent due to microstructural damage, and the material does not return to the original length when the load is removed. This transition point is called the yield point, characterized by the yield strength (stress) and yield strain.[4,6] The highest stress achieved is referred to as the ultimate strength (stress) and occurs at the ultimate strain. Such a mode of failure is typical of a variety of soft tissues in tension. In orthopaedic applications, it is essential to prevent tissues or implants from reaching the yield point to ensure proper structure and function.

In contrast, there can be an absence of such a plastic region with a brittle mode of failure. Such failure is due to the formation of cracks, which dissipate energy according to the increase in surface area. The tips of cracks act as effective stress concentrators leading to their propagation. The experimental failure strength of a material is often substantially less than the theoretical atomic strength of a material due to

the presence and expansion of microscale defects. When ductile materials fail under load, they yield by plastic deformation.

Another common failure mode is buckling, a sudden failure of beams under compression due to the presence of two possible equilibrium states, the undeformed state and the laterally deformed state. As compressive load increases, the stress becomes high enough that the beam becomes unstable and buckles laterally. Buckling is relevant to long, slender columns, where buckling stress can be much less than the material's failure stress. The compressive buckling force of a beam is governed by the Euler buckling equation

$$F = \frac{\pi^2 EI}{(KL)^2} \quad (12)$$

where F is the buckling force, E is the elastic modulus, I is the area moment of inertia, K is the column effective length factor (depends on the conditions of the end supports), and L is the length of the column. Under high compression, it is possible for long bones to buckle, causing loss of load-bearing capacity, and to fail in shear from lateral bending.

Although the previously discussed descriptions have assumed failure during a single bout of loading, the musculoskeletal system is subjected to cyclical loading, leading to an additional mode of failure. Fatigue is the progressive, localized structural damage to a material subjected to cyclic loading. This causes the structure's effective yield and ultimate strength to decrease as a function of cycle number (**Figure 10**). Such failure involves the formation of a microscopic crack at the material surface, leading to local stress concentration and crack propagation. Several factors affect fatigue life, such as geometry, surface roughness, size and distribution of internal defects, and material type. Some materials have a minimum strength at which the number of cycles does not cause failure, whereas others decrease in strength to very low stress values. In orthopaedics the polishing of knee replacement surfaces increases fatigue life by decreasing surface roughness, which can cause premature failure of a knee replacement. Additionally, this decreases friction between articulating surfaces, which makes for a smoother, lower resistance knee replacement.

When designing or using fixation methods or instrumentation in orthopaedic surgery, it is important to consider a safety factor, the ratio of structural load strength to expected maximum load. The structural load strength is typically the yield stress limit for the given geometric structure and loading conditions. Although it is important to have a substantial safety factor with orthopaedic fixation, such must be balanced with a micromechanical environment to encourage healing and integration with surrounding tissues. For example, if a fractured bone is repaired with a metal plate designed to support 30 kg of load and the expected normal loading is 15 kg, this would be a safety factor of two. This may be acceptable for certain cases, such as bone immobilization, where increased loading forces are highly unlikely. However, when the possibility for higher loads is likely, as in a patient fall, larger safety factors should be used.

Stress concentration is a concept related to structural failure. It is the increased stress in local regions, such as with decreased cross-sectional area typical of holes or slots. An orthopaedic example is the increased stress of a bone that has a fracture halfway across the cross-section compared with a normal bone. The presence of such stress concentrations can decrease the safety factor and hence the maximum load before the material yields. In such a situation, surgical procedures to add support with a metal plate or rod are useful. The addition of such implants with high moduli and yield strength raise the overall structural strength and prevent further bone damage. Also, the high stiffness of such implants can reduce local strain to levels that are conducive to bone healing.

Another orthopaedic example involving strength is the fixation of an anterior cruciate ligament graft such as bone–patellar tendon–bone using an interference screw. Tension from the tendon is transmitted through the small area of attachment from the screw, which may cause failure at the screw site. Here, there is substantial stress concentration around the threads of bone screws interfaced to the local bone tissue. This may cause local tissue deterioration, which if not countered by sufficiently rapid tissue healing, may lead to graft detachment.

Tribology

In the musculoskeletal system, there are a variety of tissue surfaces that normally are apposed and loaded but slide against one another. Tribology is the study of friction, wear, and lubrication between surfaces in relative motion.[15] Articulating cartilage and meniscus, as well as gliding tendons within sheaths, are examples of native tissues that exhibit low friction and wear, lubricated by fluids containing specialized lubricant molecules. However, such tribologic properties can deteriorate in aging and after injury. Thus, tribology can be useful for the clinician.

Friction is the force opposing the relative motion of two objects sliding against one another. Frictional force, F_f, is given by the equation

$$F_f = \mu F_N \qquad (13)$$

and acts parallel to the contacting surfaces, μ is the frictional coefficient, and F_N is the force normal to the surface. Static friction is the force between two nonmoving objects, opposing the direction of applied force. Dynamic friction is the force between two objects sliding along each other, opposing the direction of motion. The static friction coefficient is always greater than the dynamic friction coefficient. An orthopaedic example of beneficial static friction is the interface between the bone of an osteochondral graft and the host bone, providing stable fixation of the tissue implant. An example of dynamic friction is that present with the articulation of cartilage surfaces in synovial joints.

Components of the musculoskeletal system are typically subjected to cyclic load, so that wear properties are an important consideration. Wear is the erosion of material away from a surface from the repeated contact of an opposing surface. There are many types of wear, including adhesive, abrasive, fatigue, fretting, and erosive wear. Adhesive wear occurs by plastic deformation of microscopic fragments on surfaces in frictional contact and material transfer from one surface to another. Abrasive wear occurs when a solid surface slides against particles of a material or a rough material that is of equal or greater hardness, as in the sliding between the stainless steel and polymer surfaces in a total knee replacement. Surface fatigue is the propagation of microscopic cracks from the surface, as described earlier. Fretting wear is the removal of material from one or both surfaces that are cyclically sliding along one another. Erosive wear is caused by the mechanical effect of solid or liquid particles impacting a surface that acts to essentially cut away the surface. Each of these phenomena, individually or in combination, can cause substantial surface wear and deterioration over time.

In the skeletal system, lubrication can occur through several physical and chemical mechanisms to reduce friction and wear. Broadly, such mechanisms can be divided into two categories: fluid pressurization and surface interactions. Fluid pressurization allows substantial support of normal load with little resistance to sliding force. In contrast, surface interactions may provide relatively little load support and substantial resistance to sliding force. Lubricant molecules in synovial fluid, for example, contain proteoglycan-4 and hyaluronan molecules that minimize surface interaction to reduce friction and wear. Injury and diseases, as well as surgical procedures, may disrupt normal lubricant homeostasis and function.

Other Topics in Biomechanics

A variety of additional important topics in biomechanics were not covered in this chapter due to the need for brevity. Mass transport is important for the nutrition and metabolism of tissues, as well as the delivery of drugs systemically and locally. Fluid mechanics, especially in the microcirculation, contributes substantially to local blood flow and lymphatic clearance, and thus mass transport. Finite element models link spatially-varying material properties to complex structural behavior.

Summary

Biomechanics is the basis for musculoskeletal function, dictating movement, deformation, and loading of native tissues as well as materials. The effects of forces and displacements can be analyzed by treating the musculoskeletal system as rigid or deformable objects. In rigid body analysis, object motion is dictated by Newton's laws and laws of motion, considering the degree of freedom of all objects and connections in the system. In deformable body analysis, stresses and strains on objects are interrelated by biomechanical material properties. Biologic tissues can exhibit mechanical properties quantifying elastic or viscoelastic behavior, but are complicated by nonlinear, inhomogeneous, anisotropic, and viscoelastic properties. Musculoskeletal tissue can fail through a variety of modes, due to either a single bout or cyclic loading. Friction, wear, and lubrication are also important to the health of a variety of sliding tissue surfaces. With surgical procedures to restore skeletal function, the in vivo biomechanics need to be considered with appropriate safety margins.

References

1. Beer FP, Johnston ER Jr, Mazurek DF, Eisenberg ER: *Vector Mechanics for Engineers: Statics*, ed 9. New York, NY, McGraw-Hill, 2009.

2. Beer FP, Johnston ER Jr, Cornwell PJ: *Vector Mechanics For Engineers: Dynamics*, ed 9. New York, NY, McGraw-Hill, 2009.

3. Levangie PK, Norkin CC: *Joint Structure and Function: A Comprehensive Analysis*, ed 5. Philadelphia, PA, FA Davis, 2011.

4. Mow VC, Huiskes R, eds: *Basic Orthopaedic Biomechanics and Mechano-Biology*, ed 3. Philadelphia, PA, Lippincott Williams & Wilkins, 2004.

5. Standring S, ed: *Gray's Anatomy*, ed 40. Edinburgh, Scotland, Churchill Livingstone, 2008.

6. Beer FP, Johnston ER Jr, DeWolf JT, Mazurek DF: *Mechanics of Materials*, ed 5. New York, NY, McGraw-Hill, 2008.

7. Fung YC: *Biomechanics: Mechanical Properties of Living Tissues*, ed 2. New York, NY, Springer, 1993.

8. Maroudas A: Physicochemical properties of articular cartilage, in Freeman MAR, ed: *Adult Articular Cartilage*, ed 2. Tunbridge Wells, England, Pitman Medical, 1979:215-290.

9. Chen AC, Bae WC, Schinagl RM, Sah RL: Depth- and strain-dependent mechanical and electromechanical properties of full-thickness bovine articular cartilage in confined compression. *J Biomech* 2001;34(1):1-12.

10. Williamson AK, Chen AC, Masuda K, Thonar EJ, Sah RL: Tensile mechanical properties of bovine articular cartilage: Variations with growth and relationships to collagen network components. *J Orthop Res* 2003;21(5):872-880.

11. Reilly DT, Burstein AH: The elastic and ultimate properties of compact bone tissue. *J Biomech* 1975;8(6):393-405.

12. Johnson GA, Tramaglini DM, Levine RE, Ohno K, Choi NY, Woo SL: Tensile and viscoelastic properties of human patellar tendon. *J Orthop Res* 1994;12(6):796-803.

13. Tissakht M, Ahmed AM: Tensile stress-strain characteristics of the human meniscal material. *J Biomech* 1995;28(4):411-422.

14. Fujita Y, Duncan NA, Lotz JC: Radial tensile properties of the lumbar annulus fibrosus are site and degeneration dependent. *J Orthop Res* 1997;15(6):814-819.

15. Swanson SAV: Friction, wear, and lubrication, in Freeman MAR, ed: *Adult Articular Cartilage*, ed 2. Tunbridge Wells, England, Pitman Medical, 1979:415-460.

Chapter 4

Biomaterials in Orthopaedic Practice

Kenneth A. Mann, PhD

Matthew J. Allen, VetMB, PhD

Introduction

A natural or synthetic material used to replace part of a living system or function in intimate contact with living tissue is called a biomaterial. The biomaterials field has grown rapidly, and many active and inert biomaterials and biomaterial devices are being developed to improve human health. In orthopaedic medicine, there is a long history of using synthetic and natural materials to stabilize bone fractures, close and repair soft-tissue injuries, and replace articular joints.[1,2] The three major classes of synthetic biomaterials are metals, polymers, and ceramics (**Table 1**).

Biocompatibility

An implanted biomaterial should not have a local or systemic adverse effect on the host, and the local biologic environment should not adversely affect or degrade the biomaterial. The term biocompatibility is used to describe the integration of the biomaterial into the host environment. A biomaterial is described as inert, interactive, or viable.[3] Inert biomaterials (for example, cobalt-chromium [Co-Cr] alloys) are bulk materials having little or no adverse biologic response. Interactive biomaterials (for example, titanium porous coatings, porous tantalum) are passive materials designed to elicit a specific biologic response such as bony ingrowth. Viable biomaterials such as resorbable cell-seeded scaffolds integrate or attract cells and are subsequently resorbed or remodeled. Although a biomaterial may be inert

in bulk form, it can elicit a local adverse effect (such as osteolysis) if wear debris or corrosion develops. Therefore, it is critical to understand the mechanical, chemical, and biologic environment in which a biomaterial operates.

The Mechanical Behavior of Orthopaedic Biomaterials

The biomaterials used in orthopaedic applications usually are subjected to high loads and material stresses. The applied loads are cyclic in nature. The long-term behavior of any orthopaedic implant is determined by a combination of component geometry, material constituents, magnitude and frequency of loading, and the chemical and biologic environment in the body. Understanding the mechanical behavior of the material constituents is critical to the design process.

Standard Mechanical Testing of Biomaterials

The mechanical behavior of a solid material is determined using standard mechanical tests to measure the force and deformation of the material. Some mechanical tests are designed to determine the behavior of the material constituents (for example, the mechanical behavior of steel), and other tests are designed to determine the mechanical response of a structure (for example, the fatigue response of a femoral stem used in a total hip implant). Tensile tests illustrate some of the fundamental aspects of mechanical testing of the behavior of material components, as shown in **Figure 1**.

Stress, Strain, and Material Yielding

The stress-strain response generated by a mechanical test is useful for identifying many of the fundamental characteristics of the material. Most solid materials initially exhibit a linear stress-strain response in which the material returns to

Table 1

Biomaterials Used in Orthopaedic Surgery

Biomaterial	Typical Uses
Metal	
Cobalt-chromium alloy	Joint arthroplasty, fracture hardware
Pyrocarbon	Metacarpophalangeal joint arthroplasty
Stainless steel alloy	Fracture fixation, screws, nails
Tantalum	Joint arthroplasty, spine fusion
Titanium alloy	Joint arthroplasty, fracture hardware
Polymer	
Hydrogel (polyethylene glycol)	Fluid sealant system
Polyamide (nylon)	Monofilament and braided sutures
Polyether ether ketone (PEEK)	Spine fusion
Polyethylene	Joint arthroplasty
Polyethylene terephthalate (PET)	Braided ligaments
Polyglycolic acid	Resorbable sutures and implants
Polylactic acid	Resorbable sutures and implants
Polymethyl methacrylate (PMMA)	Bone cement
Polypropylene	Sutures, ligament augmentation
Polyurethane	Cervical disk replacement
Ceramic	
Alumina	Joint arthroplasty bearing surface
Calcium sulfate	Bone augmentation
Hydroxyapatite	Implant surface coating, bioconductive filler
Calcium phosphate	Bone augmentation
Zirconia	Joint arthroplasty bearing surface

its original length after unloading, unless the load is too great. In this linear-elastic behavior, known as the Hooke law of elasticity, no damage to the material occurs from the loading process. The ratio of stress to strain is defined as the elastic modulus and is a fundamental property of the material used in the test. This property can easily be visualized as the slope of the linear portion of the stress-strain curve.

Materials used in orthopaedic surgery span a wide range of elastic moduli[1,4-8] (**Table 2**). Materials with a relatively high elastic modulus often are described as being stiffer than other materials because they deform less under loading. For example, a Co-Cr alloy rod with an elastic modulus of 210 to 250 gigapascals (GPa) would elastically deform under tension approximately half as much as a titanium alloy rod with an elastic modulus of 110 GPa if the rods had the same dimensions. A titanium alloy rod with twice the cross-sectional area would deform under approximately as much tension as a Co-Cr rod. This example points to the in-

teraction between properties of a material and the mechanical response of the structure.

If a metal alloy rod is subjected to ever-increasing loads, local failure will begin at microscopic defects in the material. These defects grow as the load increases. If the metal rod is subsequently unloaded, the deformation will be permanent. The inelastic part of the deformation is called plastic deformation. The transition point between elastic and plastic deformation is called the yield point, and it is associated with a corresponding yield stress (**Figure 1,** A). Some materials, such as ceramics, have brittle behavior with little or no plastic deformation; instead, there is a linear stress-strain response until failure occurs. Materials such as metals and many polymers exhibit extensive plastic deformation before final failure. In these ductile materials, an inflection point from a linear stress-strain response corresponds to the yield stress. If loading continues beyond the yield point, a maximum stress is reached, called the tensile or ultimate strength.

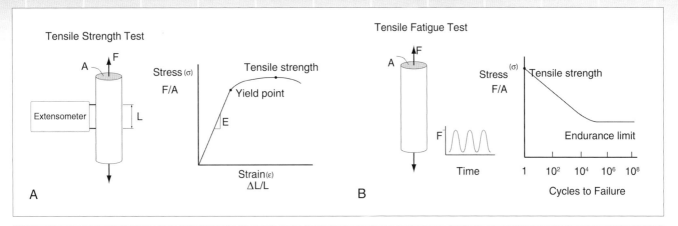

Figure 1 Schematic drawings showing the fundamental components of tests to measure tensile strength and fatigue strength. **A,** In a tensile strength test, a cylindrical metal rod with cross-sectional area (A) subjected to a tension force (F) results in a uniform tensile stress (σ) calculated as F/A. An extensometer is used to measure the deformation between two points along the length of the metal rod. The gauge length (L) is the original distance between the two reference points. After loading to tension force F, the metal rod elongates to a new length (L_f). The change in length ($\Delta L = L_f - L$) divided by the original length L is the strain ($\varepsilon = \Delta L/L$) in the material. The elastic modulus (E) can be determined from the slope of the linear portion of the stress-strain curve ($E = \sigma/\varepsilon$). Loading beyond the yield point is characterized by a reduction in the stress-strain slope. The tensile strength is defined as the largest stress the metal rod can support before failure. **B,** In a tensile fatigue test, a series of specimens is loaded cyclically to different stress levels, the number of cycles to failure is recorded, and a stress versus cycles to failure plot is constructed. The applied stress (σ) is determined from the applied force (F) divided by the cross-sectional area (A). In contrast to the strength test above, the variable applied force (F) is applied using a waveform such as the sinusoidal shape shown. The resulting stress versus number of cycles to failure curve shows that decreasing the applied stress below the tensile strength results in an increasing number of cycles to failure. The endurance limit is reached when the stress level is reduced to the point where there is no longer a failure at a high number of loading cycles (10 million to 100 million).

An analogous test performed in compression will cause a compressive yield stress and strength. The yield stress often is used as the failure criterion in the design of orthopaedic implants. The goal is to choose a component geometry that will maintain all stresses in the component below the yield stress. Uncertainties often exist with respect to the exact loads and stresses on the implant, so factors of safety must be built into a design. For example, to achieve a factor of safety of X, the allowable stress would be no more than 1/X of the yield stress.

Isotropy and Anisotropy

A material exhibits isotropic behavior if its elastic modulus does not depend on the direction of loading. Most orthopaedic biomaterials, including metals, polymers, and ceramics, are considered isotropic. In contrast, human tissues such as bone, tendon, and ligament are anisotropic. In anisotropic materials, the axis of the material aligned with the preferential loading direction has the highest modulus and strength. Synthetic fiber-matrix composite materials in which there is a preferential alignment of the fibers also have anisotropic behavior. In a composite system, the fibers often are much stiffer (have a higher modulus) than the surrounding matrix, and their fiber orientation and layup schedule can be used to create the desired anisotropy. The layup schedule describes the pattern in which sheets of directional fibers are stacked to achieve desired mechanical

properties. For an anisotropic material, the elastic modulus, yield strength, and tensile strength depend on the loading direction. It is important to understand and characterize the anisotropic behavior of the material and the loading environment for the particular orthopaedic application.

Fatigue

Most load-bearing orthopaedic biomaterials are subjected to cyclic loading during activities of daily living such as walking. Although these repetitive loads can result in stresses below the yield strength or tensile strength of a material, fatigue failure can still occur. Fatigue failure has been documented in many orthopaedic implant materials such as bone screws, femoral components of hip implants, tibial trays from knee components, fracture-fixation plates, polymethyl methacrylate (PMMA) cement used to secure an implant, implant coatings, and polyethylene articular surfaces of an arthroplasty implant. The fatigue failure process begins at stress concentration points with microscopic defects in the material, a surface scratch, or a sharp corner in an implant. Repetitive loading can cause microscopic cracks to form and subsequently grow an extremely small amount during each loading cycle. At the tip of the crack, the stresses can exceed the strength of the material over very small regions, causing local damage and crack extension. This process continues until the structure can no longer support the load, and complete and rapid fracture will occur.

Table 2
Typical Mechanical Properties of Orthopaedic Biomaterials

Biomaterial	Description	Elastic Modulus (GPa)	Yield Strength (MPa)	Ultimate Strength (MPa)	Endurance Limit (MPa)
Metal					
316L stainless steel	Annealed (ASTM F138)[4]	190	331	586	260
	30% cold worked (ASTM F139)	190	792	930	380
	Cold forged	190	1,213	1,351	820
Cobalt-chromium alloys[5]	Cast Co-Cr-Mo (ASTM F75)	210	485	770	260
	Wrought Co-Cr-Ni-Mo (ASTM F562) annealed	230	410	930	-
	Wrought Co-Cr-Ni-Mo (ASTM F562) 53% cold worked	230	2,000	2,070	790
	Wrought Co-Cr-Mo (ASTM F799) hot worked	210	930	1,370	900
	Wrought Co-Cr-W-Ni (ASTM F90) 44% cold worked	210	1,600	1,900	1,220
Titanium[1]	Commercially pure Ti (ASTM F67) cold worked	110	485	760	300
	Ti6Al4V (ASTM F136) forged	116	896	965	620
Tantalum[5]	Pure Ta	186	-	345	-
Polymer					
Polymethyl methacrylate[6]		2.3	-	35[a] 90[b]	10
Ultra-high–molecular-weight polyethylene[1]		1	25	35[a]	15
Polyether ether ketone[7]	Unfilled	4	-	93	28
	30% (weight/weight) chopped carbon fiber	20	-	170	-
Poly-L-lactic acid[8]		2.4	-	80[b]	-
Ceramic					
Alumina[1]	Aluminum oxide (Al_2O_3)	366	-	3,790[b] 310[a]	-
Zirconia[1]	Zirconium dioxide (ZrO_2)	201	-	7,500[b] 420[a]	-
Zirconia-toughened alumina		350	-	1,000[a]	-

[a]Tension test direction.
[b]Compression test direction.

Tensile fatigue tests can be performed to determine the fatigue response of a material. Identical specimens are cyclically loaded to different maximum stresses below the yield or tensile strength, and the number of cycles needed to cause failure is counted. These results can be plotted as a curve showing stress versus the number of cycles to failure (**Figure 1**, *B*). The number of cycles to failure is inversely proportional to the applied cyclic stress. The fatigue strength limit or endurance limit is the highest stress level at which no failures occur after a very high number of loading cycles (10 million to 100 million). An implant such as a hip or knee replacement device would undergo 10 to 20 million loading cycles over a 10-year period in a patient who walks 30 to 60 minutes per day. Adequate fatigue strength therefore is important for the longevity of most orthopaedic implant materials.

Wear

Wear, defined as the erosion of one material in contact with another material under repeated loading, is an important damage mechanism in orthopaedic biomaterials. Wear can occur between articulating surfaces such as the metal-on-metal, ceramic-on-metal, and metal-on-polyethylene bearing surfaces used in total joint arthroplasties. Wear also can occur in locations other than bearing surfaces, such as a fracture fixation screw-plate junction, Morse taper junction in a modular total joint component, or two-material interface such as a cement-metal interface. The debris generated by the wear process is of particular concern because it elicits a cascade of biologic responses at the cellular and tissue levels.

A material's wear performance can be characterized using relatively simple pin-on-disk experiments. In one such test, a polished Co-Cr alloy pin articulates against a spinning disk of ultra-high–molecular-weight polyethylene (UHMWPE) to determine the sliding wear properties between the Cr-Cr alloy and UHMWPE. Joint simulators are used to more fully replicate forces and bearing couple motions (kinematics) that occur during activities of daily living. The patterns of wear and debris distribution from simulator tests can be compared with retrieved components or migration measurements from clinical radiographs or in vivo radiostereometry.[9] The ability of joint simulators to recreate clinical kinematics and wear behavior is continuing to improve.[10]

Orthopaedic bearings can be described as hard-hard couples (such as metal-metal and ceramic-ceramic) and hard-soft (metal-UHMWPE and ceramic-UHMWPE) types. Hard-hard bearing couples have much lower wear rates than hard-soft bearing couples.[11] Hard-hard bearings can be polished to minimize surface roughness, and the radial clearance between components can be manufactured to permit fluid film lubrication of the bearing couple. Highly cross-linked UHMWPE has better wear characteristics than conventional UHMWPE and was found to have much lower wear rates in clinical studies.[12]

Metals
Metals in Orthopaedic Surgery

Metals for use in biomedical applications must have biologic and mechanical properties appropriate to the exposed in vivo conditions. In all cases, they should be corrosion resistant and have desirable fatigue properties, especially under cyclic loading. The alloys currently used in orthopaedic surgery evolved from materials developed for engineering, aerospace, or marine applications in which high strength and resistance to corrosion and cyclic fatigue are critical.

General Structure of Orthopaedic Metals and Alloys

The hallmark of metals is the formation of a crystalline lattice in which the positively charged nuclei are surrounded and stabilized by a cloud of negatively charged valence electrons. The electrons are loosely bound and flow easily from adjoining atoms; this characteristic imbues metals with their high thermal and electrical conductivity. The strength of the metallic bonding depends on the structure of the crystal; tightly packed crystal arrangements have the highest bond strength. In general, metals assume one of three standard crystalline arrangements, in which there is contact with 12 adjacent atoms (as in a body-centered cube or a face-centered cube) or 8 adjacent atoms (as in hexagonal packed crystals) (**Figure 2**).

Manufacturing of Orthopaedic Metal and Alloys

The pathway from raw metal ore to a finished orthopaedic implant is illustrated in **Figure 3**. Processing typically begins as the metal is melted and subsequently cooled to form a solid product called a billet. The high temperatures required for melting traditionally are generated in an electric vacuum arc furnace, but electron beam melting, in which a scanning laser is used to melt and fuse layers of metal powder into a three-dimensional structure, has been proposed as a viable option for manufacturing orthopaedic devices from certain metals (for example, titanium alloy).[13] During the melting process, small crystals combine to form a series of interconnected but irregularly arranged grains. The junction between individual grains is known as a grain boundary. The microscopic structure is best appreciated on a cut surface that has been extensively polished and acid etched to highlight the grain boundaries. In general, materials with relatively small grains are more homogeneous, more isotropic, and stronger. Clinical experience has shown that microstructural defects increase the risk of subsequent implant failure.[14] The American Society for Testing and Materials (ASTM) International publishes standards for all major orthopaedic metals and alloys, which typically dictate the minimum specifications for chemical composition, material properties, and microstructure (including grain size).

Orthopaedic alloys consist of mixtures or solutions of metals and nonmetallic elements that impart specific physical, chemical, or biologic properties to the alloy. The non-

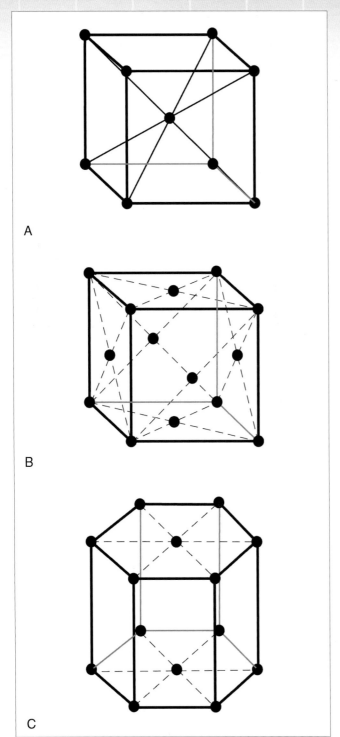

Figure 2 Schematic drawings showing three arrangements of the unit cell crystal structure in metals: the body-centered cube (**A**), face-centered cube (**B**), and hexagon (**C**).

Casting or forging typically is used to convert the metal from a raw billet into a near-final implant. The choice between these manufacturing techniques depends on the metal being used as well as the geometry and intended application of the implant. For some implants, a specific fabrication method may be necessary to achieve a complex shape. For other implants, the fabrication method can be selected based on its effect on the material's characteristics. During casting, the metal is melted, poured into a mold, and allowed to cool under controlled conditions. Many cast orthopaedic implants are fabricated using investment casting (also called lost-wax casting), in which the mold is a ceramic form fabricated by coating a wax replica of the final implant (**Figure 4**). After the metal has cooled, the investment is broken and the implant is released. Any small imperfections are removed by machining (milling, grinding, sanding, and polishing). During forging, the metal stock is compressed between two molds to fabricate the final shape. Heating to a specific temperature (the recrystallization temperature) is required to make some metals malleable enough to be pressed; this process is known as hot forging. Hot forging is commonly used to fabricate Co-Cr alloys. Cold forging, in which manipulation is at a lower temperature, can be used for some metals, such as certain stainless steels.

The advantages and limitations of casting and forging must be considered when determining the most appropriate process for a specific implant. Casting can accurately reproduce the implant's geometry as long as shrinkage is taken into account. The primary advantage of forging is that the metal is significantly strengthened by the combination of heat and pressure used during the process. Forging is more cost-effective than casting for titanium alloy, but the reverse is true for a Co-Cr alloy. For applications in which additional strength is critical, such as a femoral stem or tibial component, the cost of forged Co-Cr may be justified. Quality control of the processing conditions is especially critical for cast components. Variations in the rate of cooling, for example, can lead to air entrapment and the formation of stress risers within the microstructure of cast implants. Uncontrolled cooling also can result in the segregation of carbides, leading to a reduction in corrosion resistance. For this reason, it is common practice to check every cast implant for evidence of defects.

The mechanical properties of metals can be changed by cold working (also called strain hardening). In this process, mechanical deformation of a metal at room temperature causes permanent dislocations within the crystal structure. These dislocations increase resistance to subsequent dislocations, resulting in a net increase in strength, hardness, and stiffness. Common cold working processes include rolling, extrusion, and drawing. The most common cold-worked metal in orthopaedic practice is the extruded grade-304 stainless steel wire used for cerclage applications.

After manufacture, a series of steps can enhance the mechanical properties of the finished product. The most com-

metallic elements are added to the molten metal and allowed to mix during the process of alloy formation. In some alloys the additives become incorporated at the grain boundary, and in others the additives displace elements from the grain itself.

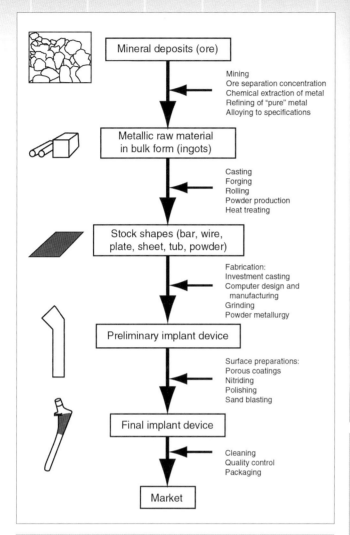

Figure 3 Schematic diagram showing the stages in the manufacture of metal orthopaedic implants. (Adapted with permission from Ratner BD, Hoffman AS, Schoen FJ, Lemons JE, eds: *Biomaterials Science: An Introduction to Materials in Medicine*, ed 2. San Diego, CA, Academic Press, 2004, p 138.)

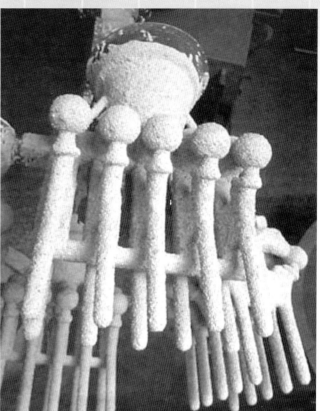

Figure 4 Photograph showing a ceramic mold used in the investment casting process for metal implants. Molten metal flows into the mold and solidifies during casting. (Reproduced with permission from Ratner BD, Hoffman AS, Schoen FJ, Lemons JE, eds: *Biomaterials Science: An Introduction to Materials in Medicine*, ed 2. San Diego, CA, Academic Press, 2004, p 138.)

mon postprocessing step is annealing, in which the metal is heated to just above its recrystallization temperature and cooled slowly under precisely controlled conditions. Annealing removes residual stresses from the material and improves its machinability. Because annealing reduces the energy required for subsequent cold working, cold working and annealing can be cycled during implant processing. In hot isostatic pressing, another heat treatment option, controlled heating of a formed, as-cast implant under high pressure (up to 200 megapascals [MPa]) results in densification of the metal, a reduction in porosity, and optimization of grain size and carbide distribution.

Additional postmanufacture treatments such as nitriding and ion implantation can be used for an orthopaedic implant, especially if the implant is intended for an articulating application. In nitriding, the surface of the implant is in-fused with nitrogen gas, leading to the creation of a thin nitride layer. This technique most often is used for a stainless steel or titanium implant to increase its wear resistance.[15,16] Ion implantation involves bombarding the implant surface with nitrogen (or other) ions generated by plasma discharge; this process results in nitrogen ion deposition without formation of a nitride layer. Nitrogen ion implantation has been shown to reduce implant wear in titanium and Co-Cr alloys that articulate against UHMWPE.[17]

Stainless Steel
Stainless steel is the most commonly used orthopaedic implant metal. Originally developed for industrial applications during the early 20th century, stainless steel has the primary advantage of being relatively resistant to corrosion. Like traditional carbon steels, stainless steels are alloys of iron and carbon, but they differ from carbon steels in that they also contain significant amounts of chromium (17% to 20%), nickel (10% to 17%), and molybdenum (2% to 4%) as well as smaller amounts of manganese, sulfur, silicon, and phosphorus (2% to 8% total). The carbon content in

medical-grade stainless steels typically is kept low to reduce the formation of chromium carbide at the grain boundaries, but corrosion resistance is thereby reduced within the bulk of the material.

Several variants of stainless steel have been evaluated in biomedical applications. Most of these materials belong to the so-called 300 series of austenitic stainless steels, which have a face-centered cube microstructure. The most widely used have a very low carbon content, typically less than 0.03% by weight. These alloys are known as 316L and 316LVM stainless steel (L refers to low carbon content, and VM refers to vacuum melt.)

Annealed stainless steel and 30% cold-worked stainless steel (ASTM F138 and F139) are the two manufactured forms of forged stainless steel commonly used in orthopaedic surgery (Table 2). The processing of stainless steel implants typically involves a passivation step in which the implant is treated with acid to produce a surface oxide layer. Over time, however, the oxide layer dissolves, leading to an increase in the rate of corrosion. The increase is exacerbated by any factor that damages the oxide layer. Although there are examples of successful long-term clinical performance by stainless steel total joint arthroplasty implants (including the original Charnley femoral stem and the bipolar Austin Moore hip replacement), stainless steel is not a good choice for a modular total joint arthroplasty implant if there is a possibility of relative motion (fretting) between the individual components. The susceptibility of stainless steel implants to crevice corrosion also limits their usefulness as a bone ingrowth surface. In addition, a stainless steel implant should not be combined with an implant component made from another alloy because of the risk of galvanic corrosion, in which the coupling of two metals with different electrochemical potentials (for example, iron and titanium) results in the flow of electrons from the metal with higher electrochemical potential (the active metal) to the metal with lower potential (the noble metal). Electron loss from the active metal results in oxidation, the products of which can be seen as corrosion, as well as the release of metal ions that can have deleterious local or systemic effects.[18]

Although medical-grade stainless steel has been replaced in many applications by a Co-Cr or titanium alloy, it still is widely used in temporary implants such as fracture plates, intramedullary pins, and screws. The ductility of stainless steel makes it an excellent choice for Kirschner wires, orthopaedic cables, and cerclage wire.

Co-Cr Alloys

Co-Cr has overtaken stainless steel as the type of alloy most commonly used in orthopaedic surgery, particularly in the context of arthroplasty. Co-Cr and titanium alloys now are the preferred implant materials for total hip and knee replacement. Because these cobalt-based alloys have extremely low ductility (Table 2), it is extremely difficult to fabricate wire or thin rods from them.

Two types of Co-Cr alloys are generally available for bio-

medical applications. Cobalt-chromium-molybdenum (Co-Cr-Mo) alloys typically are used for cast implants. Cobalt-chromium-tungsten-nickel (Co-Cr-W-Ni) and cobalt-nickel-chromium-molybdenum (Co-Ni-Cr-Mo) alloys are used for wrought implants. Cast forms of Co-Cr-Mo (ASTM F75) are widely used in dentistry as well as orthopaedic surgery. Although this form of Co-Cr alloy is hard to machine and has poorer mechanical properties than other currently used metal alloys, it continues to be popular because it is relatively inexpensive and easy to manufacture into a complex shape using investment casting. Porosity can be problematic with the as-cast material, but this effect can be reduced by the postmanufacture use of hot isostatic pressing. The warm or hot forging of cast Co-Cr-Mo billets results in a wrought product (ASTM F799) with substantially greater fatigue strength, yield strength, and ultimate tensile strength than the cast alloy (Table 2).

ASTM F90 is a 44% cold-worked wrought Co-Cr-W-Ni alloy with improved machinability. In an annealed form, its mechanical properties are similar to those of as-cast Co-Cr-Mo (ASTM F75) but these properties are dramatically improved by cold working (Table 2). Cold-worked wrought forms of Co-Cr-Ni-Mo (ASTM F562) have the best mechanical properties of all current implant alloys. Concern over the relatively high nickel content of this alloy and the role of nickel ions in metal hypersensitivity has limited its use in total joint implants, but it is a popular choice for temporary implants such as fracture repair plates.

Co-Cr alloys are well suited for use as an ingrowth-ongrowth surface and have been widely used in cementless implants such as porous-coated anatomic implants and anatomic medullary locking implants. However, the high elastic modulus of the Co-Cr alloys has been associated with the development of stress shielding and local bone pain caused by accelerated bone remodeling.[19]

The wear properties of Co-Cr alloys are superior to those of stainless steel or titanium alloy. For this reason, many modular total hip replacement systems include a Co-Cr femoral head. The coupling of Co-Cr and stainless steel is associated with an increased risk of both fretting and galvanic corrosion at the modular interface; therefore, Co-Cr femoral heads most commonly are used with titanium alloy femoral stems.

Titanium and Titanium Alloys

Titanium and titanium-based alloys have a reduced elastic modulus (100 to 110 GPa) compared with Co-Cr alloys (200 to 220 GPa) as well as excellent biocompatibility and increased resistance to corrosion. At least 38 grades of titanium alloy are recognized, of which only a few have commercial applications. Grades 1, 2, 3, and 4 are forms of commercially pure (CP) titanium. Grade 5 combines titanium with 6% aluminum and 4% vanadium and is known as Ti6Al4V or Ti 6-4. Ti6Al4V is the most commonly used form of titanium alloy, with widespread application in the aerospace, automotive, marine, and biomedical fields.

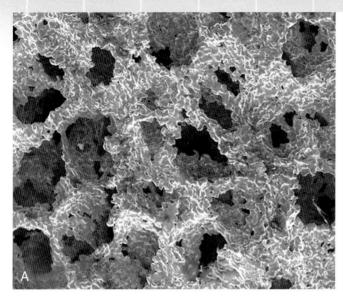
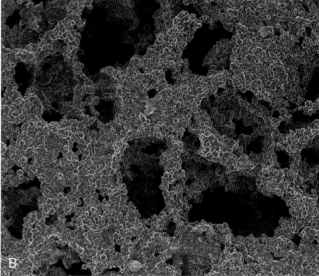

Figure 5 Scanning electron images showing three-dimensional porous titanium manufactured by two methods. **A,** The particle sintered foam method (×25 magnification). **B,** Metal injection molding (×50 magnification). (**A,** Courtesy of Stryker Orthopaedics, Mahwah, NJ; **B,** Courtesy of Praxis Technology, Queensbury, NY.)

Titanium is one of the most inert biomedical materials used in orthopaedic applications. Its excellent biocompatibility in part results from the rapid formation of a stable oxide layer on the surface of the material. This process of passivation provides a biocompatible surface with which adjacent cells and tissues can interact. The clinical interest in titanium began in dentistry, with recognition that CP titanium implants support early bone apposition and ingrowth leading to rapid osseointegration within the bone of the jaw.[20] The encouraging results of using titanium dental implants led to successful preclinical orthopaedic studies on the use of titanium as both a solid implant (for example, small bone plates) or as a coating for existing implant materials, particularly titanium alloy.[21,22]

In orthopaedics, CP titanium (ASTM F67) primarily is used as a porous bone ingrowth surface or as a textured bone apposition surface formed with a plasma spray technique. The surface finish of plasma-sprayed CP titanium typically is quite rough to facilitate immediate mechanical interlock and progressive osseointegration as bone grows up to and around the microasperities on the coating. Solid CP titanium implants are available as fracture repair plates and bone screws, but concern over the fatigue properties of CP titanium has limited its use for permanent implants in total joint arthroplasty or spine surgery. For these applications, Ti6Al4V (ASTM F136) is preferred.

Three-dimensional porous forms of CP titanium have been approved by the US Food and Drug Administration for clinical use. Two techniques have been developed under the name Tritanium (Stryker Orthopaedics, Mahwah, NJ). One of these techniques involves arc vapor deposition of CP titanium onto a polyurethane foam skeleton that is subsequently removed by heating.[23] In the second technique, particulate titanium is mixed and compacted with pore former and binder; these are subsequently dissolved in deionized water to create porosity in the titanium structure, which is then sintered[24] (**Figure 5,** *A*). In the sintering process, powdered material is consolidated under conditions of high temperature and pressure. A third fabrication method, direct metal injection molding, involves the formation of an intermediate structure consisting of powdered metal and binder; the binder is then removed by thermal, catalytic, or solvent-based methods and the final product sintered to produce the final implant (**Figure 5,** *B*).

The wear properties of Ti6Al4V are inferior to those of Co-Cr alloys. As a result, titanium alloy primarily is used for the nonarticular parts of hip and knee replacement implants (for example, metal trays in tibial components, stems of femoral components, metal shells in cementless acetabular components). The susceptibility of Ti6Al4V to fretting wear can be a concern at modular interfaces such as the femoral head-neck junction).

Bead, fiber, and mesh forms of Ti6Al4V can be used as an ingrowth surface that is sintered onto other metals to provide a fixation surface. Porous bead structures are manufactured by depositing two or three layers of beads onto the implant surface with the aid of an appropriate binding material. The implant is then heated to just below the melting point, causing the binding materials to vaporize and the beads to connect to one another and to the underlying metal substrate by the formation of contact points (called necks). Fiber metal pads are formed by compaction and diffusion bonding of titanium wire. The resulting fiber pad is highly interconnected, with a pore size of approximately 400 μm and a porosity of 50%.

Tantalum

Tantalum has excellent biocompatibility, and surface oxide formation provides an effective and durable barrier to corrosion. Tantalum most often is used as a three-dimensional open honeycomb for augmentation of cancellous bone defects.[25] A proprietary form of tantalum (Hedrocel; Zimmer, Warsaw, IN) has been approved by the US Food and Drug Administration as a means of reinforcing areas of weak or deficient bone stock. In long bone applications, the augmentation must be supplemented by internal fixation to protect the tantalum.

Tantalum also is used in the manufacture of vascular clips and the spherical marker beads used in radiostereometric analysis. The latter application takes advantage of the very high atomic number and radiopacity of tantalum, which allow markers to be seen even when they are adjacent to Co-Cr or titanium alloy implants.

Shape Memory Alloys

Shape memory alloys have the ability to return to a previously defined shape or size when exposed to an appropriate stress, most often by heating. At a structural level, the physical attributes of shape memory alloys are explained by a transition from a relatively soft martensitic (body-centered tetragonal) crystal microstructure to a high-strength austenitic (face-centered cubic) crystal microstructure. The best-known shape memory alloy is nitinol, an alloy of nickel and titanium that is widely used in cardiac stents. Although the acceptance of nitinol has been relatively slow in orthopaedic surgery, several nitinol devices have been approved. In orthopaedic trauma, nitinol is used in bone anchors and staples. Like nickel-containing Co-Cr alloys, the shape memory alloys have the potential for inducing metal sensitivity reactions, and they are not recommended for use in patients with a history of nickel sensitivity.

Polymers
PMMA Bone Cement

PMMA bone cements are widely used in orthopaedic practice to secure arthroplasty components to bone, stabilize osteoporotic fractures of the spine, and fill metastatic defects. PMMA was developed before World War II as a room-temperature polymerizing material. Sir John Charnley in 1958 initiated orthopaedic work with PMMA by using it to anchor a femoral head prosthesis to bone.[26] In this capacity, PMMA serves as a grout between the implant components and bone.

Commercial PMMA consists of powder and liquid components that are mixed together in the operating room and applied to the surgical site in a viscous state. The powder component consists of beads of PMMA or PMMA-styrene; barium sulfate or zirconium dioxide as a radiopacifier; and benzoyl peroxide as a chemical initiator. Dyes such as chlorophyll sometimes are added to the powder to alter the color of the cement. The liquid component is primarily methacrylate monomer and N,N-dimethyl-p-toluidine, which accelerates the polymerization process when the liquid and powder are mixed. Hydroquinone is added to the liquid component to prevent premature polymerization from heat or light during storage. Mixing the polymer powder and monomer liquid without the benzoyl peroxide and N,N-dimethyl-p-toluidine creates a viscous cement that does not harden at room temperature.

The polymerization of PMMA cement occurs as an exothermic reaction. Double carbon-carbon bonds of the methylmethacrylate monomer are broken so they can bond to the rapidly increasing polymer chain. The heat generated during this process (140 to 170 million joules/m^3)[27] can increase the temperature of the cement and adjacent tissue to more than 100°C. The risk of thermal damage or necrosis to bone has been raised, and it is known that prolonged exposure to temperatures above 56°C can denature collagen.[27] The amount of heat generated depends on both the mass of cement generating the heat and the ability of adjacent tissue and implant components to absorb this heat. Most cement layers used in total joint arthroplasty are relatively thin (less than 5 mm). In vivo studies measuring peak temperatures during total hip replacement found a maximum temperature of 48°C.[28] The temperature at the cement-bone interface is higher when a large volume of cement is used, as in filling a metastatic defect in metaphyseal bone, and the risk of thermal necrosis is correspondingly greater.

The handling characteristics of PMMA bone cements change after the initial mixing. Manufacturers produce cements with a variety of handling characteristics. The term viscosity refers to a cement's ability to resist shear stresses. Low-viscosity cements flow easily soon after mixing, and high-viscosity cements are much more doughlike after initial mixing. The working curve of a bone cement depicts the manner in which its handling characteristics (viscosity) change over time and with the temperature of the cement and the room.[26] The working curve often is included in the manufacturer's instructions to provide information on timing the mixing, waiting, application, and setting phases of the cement. Cements polymerize more quickly if they are mixed at a relatively high temperature and in a high humidity environment. The powder and monomer of high-viscosity cements are cooled to extend the application time after mixing. Cement injected or pressed into bone during the setting phase will not interlock well with trabecular and cortical bone and therefore has limited ability to properly secure the implant.

Improvements in the application techniques used in cemented total joint arthroplasty have had a positive effect on clinical outcomes. The Swedish Hip Registry recorded a decrease in the revision rate from 9% to 3% at 10 years postsurgery, when so-called modern cementing techniques were implemented.[29] Careful preparation of the bone bed, including the use of pulsed lavage, creates an environment favorable to good cement-bone apposition and interlock. Pressurization using a cement application system and ce-

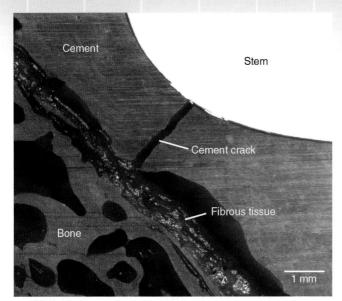

Figure 6 Schematic drawing showing a transverse section through a postmortem-retrieved cemented femoral component of a total hip implant. A crack has formed in the cement mantle surrounding the metal stem. The cement is not interdigitated with the bone, and a fibrous tissue layer has developed between the cement and bone.

ment in a sufficiently viscous state allows the cement to flow into trabecular bone spaces. Laboratory testing of postmortem-retrieved specimens found that the strength of the cement-bone interface was positively correlated with the amount of cement-bone contact.

Mixing the bulk cement in a vacuum removes porosity and entrapped air before surgical placement. However, the liquid monomer is converted to a polymer during the cement-setting process, and there is a net decrease in PMMA cement volume of approximately 7%.[30] This polymerization shrinkage may be an important source of cement porosity. Even after vacuum mixing, porosity forms in the cement mantle of cemented femoral hip components because of polymerization shrinkage.[31]

Commercial antibiotic-loaded bone cements include those premixed with tobramycin or gentamicin (as much as 1 g per 40 g of PMMA powder). Antibiotics are eluted from the surface through the water uptake of the cement. Laboratory studies offer no consensus as to whether the addition of antibiotics alters the mechanical properties of the cement, in particular those of the commercially available formulations available in the United States.[32] Diminished mechanical properties have not been reported in clinical use. Clinical data do suggest that the use of antibiotic bone cement can reduce the incidence of septic loosening.[33]

PMMA bone cements are commonly used for vertebral augmentation. The quantity of radiopacifier is increased substantially (often by a factor of 3) to improve visualization during delivery, and the reaction chemistry is modified to extend the working time. For example, Surgical Simplex P

bone cement (Stryker Orthopaedics) is designed for arthroplasty applications and has a working time of 3 minutes at 22°C. In contrast, KyphX (Medtronic Spine LLC, Sunnyvale, CA) has a working time of 8 minutes to allow sufficient time for filling the vertebral cavity and monitoring for cement extravasation.[34] A shorter working time is appropriate for arthroplasty cement because little time is needed to place an implant component.

The most common failure mechanisms in total joint arthroplasty applications are loss of fixation at the cement-bone and cement-implant interfaces and fracturing of the cement (**Figure 6**). Fixation to bone requires good cement-bone apposition and a bone bed adequate for fixation. The fixation at the implant-cement interface often does not act as a bonded interface (as when a polished stem or polyethylene component is adjacent to cement). Implant surfaces roughened with macrotexturing or an industrial blasting technique may not bond with the cement, depending on factors such as the viscosity of the cement when joined to the implant, the cement polymerization process, and shrinkage of the cement from the implant surface during polymerization.

Retrieval studies have noted fracturing of the cement associated with corners of implants, pores in the cement, or irregularities at the cement-bone interface. Cement is weaker in tension (25 to 45 MPa) than in compression (85 to 110 MPa), and it has a fatigue strength of approximately 10 MPa. Modifying cements by adding reinforcing fibers has been considered as a means of improving fatigue strength[35] and minimizing the accumulation of cement damage that could contribute to aseptic loosening.

Ultra-High–Molecular-Weight Polyethylene

UHMWPE is commonly used as half of a bearing couple that articulates with metal or ceramic in a total joint implant. Sir John Charnley's initial efforts to achieve a clinically successful low-friction arthroplasty using polytetrafluoroethylene (Teflon; Dupont, Wilmington, DE) failed because accelerated creep and wear of the polytetrafluoroethylene cup led to excessive migration of the femoral head into the cup.[1] Charnley found UHMWPE to be a much more clinically successful bearing material, and it is still being used five decades later. UHMWPE is an attractive biomaterial for total joint arthroplasty because of its low sliding friction, material toughness, wear resistance, and biologic inertness in bulk form.

UHMWPE is made up of extremely long chains of polyethylene ($[C_2H_4]_n$) in which the degree of polymerization (n) is between 71,000 (molecular weight of 2 million g/mol) and 214,000 (molecular weight of 6 million g/mol).[36] In comparison, high-density polyethylene has a molecular weight as high as 500,000 g/mol. The extension of molecular chain length from high-density polyethylene to UHMWPE increases the impact strength and wear resistance of the material dramatically. For example, there is a strong dependence of molecular weight on mechanical behavior after the

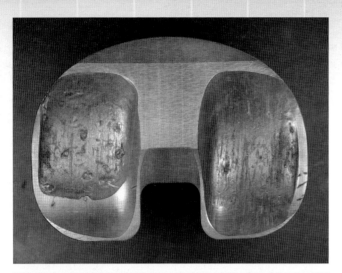

Figure 7 Photograph showing wear on the articulating surface of a retrieved UHMWPE tibial tray insert.

peak load (post-yield behavior) in specimens tested using a laboratory small punch test. Results from the small punch test show that the higher molecular weight materials require much more energy to deform after initial yielding of the material.[37]

UHMWPE is a linear, nonbranching polymer (that is, the repeating structure of polyethylene does not branch along the sides of the polymer chain). The extremely long polymer chain has crystalline and amorphous phases. The crystalline phase is formed by repeated folding of the polymer chain upon itself to create highly oriented crystalline lamellae. The amorphous phase is characterized by intertangled regions of the polymer chain with no orientation or order. In laboratory testing, higher crystallinity has been found to have a positive correlation with increased yield strength and resistance to fatigue crack propagation.[38]

Processing, sterilization, and packaging methods affect the two UHMWPE phases, which in turn affect the material's properties and mechanical performance.[37] Resin powder is consolidated into rods, sheets, or formed products using different manufacturing methods, all of which require heat above the melting point and pressure for consolidation to occur. Rods can be created by ram extrusion of the powder through a heated die. Sheets of UHMWPE can be created using a compression-molding process in which large heated platens are used for pressurization. Rods or sheets can be converted into implant components using machining operations. Direct compression molding allows the manufacturer to convert the resin into a completed part or a part that requires very little postmold machining. One benefit of direct compression molding is that the pressed surfaces are very smooth, with no machining marks at articulating surfaces. Most orthopaedic manufacturers machine components into the final form, however, to compensate for process control considerations.

Limiting wear and damage to the UHMWPE component

is critical for the long-term in vivo functioning of total joint implants (**Figure 7**). Osteolysis was found to be related to small-scale UHMWPE debris generated during articulation with the mating surface.[39] Wear can occur from adhesion, abrasion, third-body, and fatigue wear mechanisms. The stress fields are different in knee and hip components. Substantial research and development are leading to improved wear resistance in the UHMWPE articulating components.

During the 1980s and 1990s UHMWPE was commonly sterilized using gamma radiation in air. This process had the unintended consequence of initiating oxidative degradation of the polyethylene.[37] Free radicals were formed by the interaction of the radiation and the UHMWPE; they reacted with oxygen and initiated an autocatalytic process leading to further oxidation. This postirradiation aging embrittles the UHMWPE, reduces its toughness while increasing the elastic modulus, and negatively influences the clinical performance of hip and knee components. Implant manufacturers have modified their packaging and sterilization procedures to prevent oxidation. Barrier packaging prevents or reduces oxidation during long-term shelf storage. Gamma radiation sterilization in an inert gas or vacuum-packaged environment also reduces oxidative degradation. However, the free radicals created during gamma radiation still are present, and the material is subject to in vivo oxidative degradation.

Despite its negative consequences, gamma radiation has the benefit of increasing wear resistance by increasing the cross-linking of polymer chains. In so-called first-generation highly cross-linked UHMWPE, cross-linking was increased by high-dosage radiation followed by heating to a temperature below the melt transition (annealing) or above the melt transition (remelting). The thermal treatment minimizes in vivo oxidative degradation by reducing the number of nonreacted free radicals. The annealing method slightly increases crystallinity, but the UHMWPE is still susceptible to in vivo oxidation. In contrast, the remelting method reduces the crystallinity, but it also appears to reduce (but not completely eliminate) in vivo oxidation.[40]

First-generation highly cross-linked UHMWPE acetabular components have been clinically more successful in reducing wear rates than conventional UHMWPE components. Direct measurements from a series of retrieval components revealed that annealed and remelted acetabular liners from first-generation highly cross-linked UHMWPE had lower linear penetration rates (0.03 and 0.04 mm per year, respectively) than conventional inert gamma-sterilized liners (0.11 mm per year).[41] A review of a large series of studies using radiographic methods to quantify head penetration concluded that wear reduction in highly cross-linked UHMWPE ranged from 31% to 94% at 2- to 5.5-year follow-up.[42] However, increased cross-linking and in vivo oxidation can reduce the toughness of the material and may contribute to component fracture at high-stress implant locations. Retrieval studies found evidence of fracture at the rim of acetabular components; it appears that these cracks can start at the sharp notches on the backside of the cup.[43]

1: Basic Principles of Orthopaedic Surgery

Concern about the diminished mechanical properties of highly cross-linked UHMWPE has led to increased caution in total knee arthroplasty. The contact areas for a knee replacement are smaller than those for a hip replacement. Contact stresses and stresses in the material below the surface therefore are higher in the knee replacement. The movement of the contact area during gait causes cyclic loading of the material. These conditions suggest that the ability to resist fracture and crack propagation is more important for knee implants than for hip implants. Reduced knee wear rates have been found in simulations using highly cross-linked UHMWPE, but few clinical reports exist. Knee implant regions with concentrated high stress, such as a posterior stabilized tibial post or a tray-insert locking mechanism, may have an increased risk of fracture.[36]

A second generation of highly cross-linked UHMWPE has been developed in consideration of continuing concerns about in vivo oxidation and the associated risk of fracture. The general principle of the second-generation processing methods is to retain the superior wear resistance of the first-generation highly cross-linked UHMWPE as well as the strength and toughness of conventional UHMWPE.[44] Orthopaedic device manufacturers have chosen different methods to achieve this goal, including modified mechanical deformation, sequential annealing, and the addition of vitamin E as an antioxidant.[36] These new formulations have had promising results in benchtop and simulator testing, but long-term clinical studies are needed.[45]

Polyether Ether Ketone

Polyether ether ketone (PEEK) is a semicrystalline thermoplastic consisting of an aromatic molecular chain interconnected by ketone and ether functional groups. PEEK materials are used in a wide variety of industrial applications because of their high strength and resistance to chemical degradation. In orthopaedic applications, PEEK has been used for bearing surfaces, fracture fixation plates, total joint arthroplasty components, and spine implants. PEEK can be used in an unfilled state, with additives such as carbon or ceramic fibers, or with bioactive additives such as hydroxyapatite. Unfilled PEEK has an elastic modulus of 4 GPa, but, for example, adding a 30% weight fraction of chopped carbon fiber increases the elastic modulus to 20 GPa. Adding a carbon fiber weight fraction to 68% increases the modulus to 135 GPa;[7] this composite has a higher elastic modulus than titanium alloy (110 GPa). In orthopaedic surgery, PEEK is most widely used for interbody fusion cages or components in spine fixation systems. PEEK is radiolucent; this feature facilitates assessment of the surgical site with plain radiography, CT, or MRI.

Resorbable Polymers

Resorbable polymers have been synthesized to chemically and mechanically degrade in the body over time. In orthopaedic surgery, resorbable polymers are most commonly used if the permanent presence of a device is not needed or

desired, as in sutures, suture anchors, fracture fixation pins, and bone screws.[46] Resorbable implants are designed to provide initial fixation and stabilization, then resorb at a controlled rate through a process of biologic or chemical degradation. As the implant loses mechanical integrity, it becomes less stiff and loses its ability to support a load. The load increasingly is transferred through the healing tissue during the polymer resorption process. The rate at which the resorbable polymer device loses integrity is an important consideration. Resorbable polymers provide a means of releasing drugs locally to the surgery site. The rate of drug elution can be designed to correspond to factors in the healing or bone regeneration process.

Polyglycolic acid, polylactic acid, and copolymers derived from them are the most frequently used bioerodible polymers. In the body, polyglycolic or polylactic acid degrades by hydrolysis to produce glycolic acid or lactic acid, respectively. The mechanical properties and degradation times can vary widely. For example, polyglycolic acid has an elastic modulus of 7 GPa and degrades within 6 to 12 months.[46] Poly-L-lactic acid has a much lower elastic modulus (2.7 GPa) and requires more than 24 months to completely resorb.[8] Much shorter resorption times can be achieved by using copolymer formulations. A formulation of half lactic acid and half glycolic acid has a low elastic modulus (2 GPa) and very short degradation time (1 to 2 months).

Ceramics
Ceramics in Orthopaedic Surgery

Two classes of ceramic materials are in widespread use in orthopaedic surgery. Inert ceramics include alumina (dense aluminum oxide), zirconia (zirconium oxide), calcium sulfate, and pyrolytic carbon. Bioactive ceramics include hydroxyapatite, β-tricalcium phosphate, and silica-based or calcium-based bioglasses.

General Structure of Ceramic Biomaterials

Ceramics are intrinsically hard and have excellent compressive strength (**Table 2**). At the atomic level, ceramics consist of a complex lattice of metallic and nonmetallic elements held together by ionic and covalent bonds. Ceramics have a high melting point and are nonductile and brittle; hence, they are sensitive to notches and cracks. Most ceramic biomaterials have a grain-based microstructure. As with metals, variations in the processing technique can significantly affect the microstructure and mechanical properties of a ceramic product.

Manufacture of Ceramic Biomaterials

Dense inert ceramic implants are manufactured from a mixture of fine powder and water, held together by a binder and molded into the shape of the implant. The mold is heated to burn off the binder and evaporate the water, then it is sintered at a high temperature (approximately 1,600°C) to fuse the ceramic particles together into a uniformly dense structure. The strength of the final product is inversely proportional to the grain size and porosity of the material.

Thin-film bioactive ceramics are manufactured by plasma spray techniques or solution deposition. In plasma spraying, powdered ceramic is heated in gas plasma, and the resultant mist of molten ceramic is deposited onto the target, which usually is an implant. The location, thickness, and crystallinity of the coating can be precisely controlled by changes in the processing conditions. The primary advantage of plasma spray technology is that it can be applied to relatively complex geometries.

Inert Ceramics

Alumina and zirconia are formed by sintering. For implant manufacturing, the bulk material is first compacted into a form that mirrors the shape of the intended final product. Sintering times are shortened by using very fine powders and high temperatures, but the temperatures are well below the melting points of the raw material. The sintering process results in the formation of small connections (necks) between individual powder particles.

Alumina (dense aluminum oxide) has excellent biocompatibility and a very low coefficient of friction when articulated against UHMWPE. Because an alumina surface has high wettability (water remains on its surface as a film), friction is low and lubrication during articulation is improved. The combination of low friction, improved lubrication, and reduced wear has led to the popularity of alumina as a bearing surface for the femoral head in total hip replacement.[47] After alumina femoral heads were introduced in the mid 1970s, early clinical experience identified catastrophic implant failure in as many as 13% of patients.[48] Subsequent improvements in manufacturing both the dense material and the Morse tapers through which the heads connect to the metal femoral stem have resulted in a dramatic decrease in the incidence of acute fracture.[49] When alumina-on-alumina is used as a ceramic-on-ceramic articulation, wear rates have been extremely low in the laboratory setting and clinical use.[50] Several reports over the past 5 years have described squeaking from ceramic-on-ceramic hip bearings during activities of daily living in 15% to 21% of patients.[51] The cause probably is related to multiple factors involving edge loading between the head and cup, component malpositioning, and loss of lubrication. A recent laboratory investigation found that noise in the bearing coupling occurs when the fluid film between the two bearing surfaces is disrupted.[52]

Zirconia is used as a femoral bearing surface in total hip implants and in powdered form as a radiopacifier in some formulations of PMMA bone cement. Zirconia is stronger and denser than alumina, and it can be polished to a finer surface finish, resulting in lower wear rates than alumina in a laboratory setting.[53] In contrast to alumina, zirconia should not be used in ceramic-on-ceramic articulations. A high rate of early fracture of zirconia heads manufactured with a newly implemented technique led to a large recall,

and the use of zirconia as bearing surface subsequently decreased.[54] However, newer zirconia-toughened alumina matrix composites have been developed to provide greater strength and fracture toughness than alumina alone.

Bioactive Ceramics

The bioactive ceramics are extremely biocompatible, supporting intimate contact with and integration into surrounding bone. The precise nature of the chemical or physical bond that develops between bone and ceramic is not well understood, but it is known that the interface between bone and a ceramic-coated implant is stronger than that formed between bone and an uncoated implant of the same geometry.[55] Calcium phosphate–based coatings such as hydroxyapatite and β-tricalcium phosphate have been most widely studied and have been used in a variety of applications, most notably in cementless total joint arthroplasty. Over time, the ceramic coating is resorbed and replaced with new bone. The time required for complete resorption can vary from weeks to years. As with resorbable polymers, the course of ceramic resorption can be modulated by changes in the processing conditions used to fabricate the coating.[56]

Hydroxyapatite ($Ca_{10}[PO_4]_6[OH]_2$) naturally occurs in bone mineral and therefore is a logical choice for an osteophilic substrate. Hydroxyapatite coatings have been used for decades in dental as well as orthopaedic applications.[57] A large number of preclinical and clinical research studies have been completed on the optimal coating strategies for hydroxyapatite.[58-60] As is common with bioactive agents, there was initial enthusiasm for coating the entire implant with hydroxyapatite to provide strong fixation to surrounding bone. However, over time it became apparent that hydroxyapatite is best used tactically to enhance regional bone fixation. In total hip replacement implants, for example, hydroxyapatite coatings are best used around the implant shoulder, which is the most important region for robust bone apposition and implant fixation.

β-tricalcium phosphate ($Ca_3[PO_4]_2$) and bioglasses based on calcium, phosphorus, sodium, silica, and oxygen are commonly used in structural applications (for example, to fill cancellous bone defects), for bone graft replacement (as substitutes or extenders),[61,62] and particularly as an adjunct to fracture repair or fusion in the setting of trauma, orthopaedic oncology, or spine surgery. The fillers are available in forms including granules, pastes, and malleable sheets. The material properties of the ceramic are not sufficient to withstand loading, however, and supplemental internal fixation is required when these materials are placed in sites that will be exposed to significant mechanical loads. Although the use of bioglasses in orthopaedic surgery has lagged behind their use in dentistry, several products have now been approved for clinical use as bone filler materials. Additional formulations are actively being developed as fillers or bioactive bone cements.[63]

Summary

Metal, polymer, and ceramic biomaterials are synthesized, processed, formed, manufactured, and combined into engineered products that support a wide variety of uses in orthopaedic medicine. Chemical constituents, microstructure and macrostructure, and manufacturing techniques influence the mechanical behavior of a material and its biologic response after implantation. The shape and geometry of an implant structure created from a biomaterial influence the manner in which forces are transmitted through the device, and this factor can influence the integration of the implant and the host tissue. Although many biomaterials have been used for decades, new formulations and applications of metal, polymer, and ceramic materials are continually being developed. New active biomaterials intended to direct specific biologic responses are currently being developed, with the potential to improve and extend treatment options in orthopaedic practice.

References

1. Ratner BD, Hoffman AS, Schoen FJ, Lemons JE: *Biomaterials Science: An Introduction to Materials in Medicine*, ed 2. San Diego, CA, Academic Press, 2004.

2. von Recum AF: *Handbook of Biomaterials Evaluation: Scientific, Technical, and Clinical Testing of Implant Materials*, ed 2. Philadelphia, PA, Taylor & Francis, 1999.

3. Wright TM, Maher SA: *Orthopaedic Basic Science*, ed 3. Rosemont, IL, American Academy of Orthopaedic Surgeons, 2007, pp 65-85.

4. Bartel DL, Davy DT, Keaveny TM: *Orthopaedic Biomechanics: Mechanics and Design in Musculoskeletal Systems*. Upper Saddle River, NJ, Pearson Prentice Hall, 2006.

5. Spadaro JA, Clarke MT, Hasenwinkel JM: *Oncology and Basic Science*. Philadelphia, PA, Lippincott Williams & Wilkins, 2008.

6. Lewis G: Properties of acrylic bone cement: State of the art review. *J Biomed Mater Res* 1997;38(2):155-182.

7. Kurtz SM, Devine JN: PEEK biomaterials in trauma, orthopedic, and spinal implants. *Biomaterials* 2007;28(32):4845-4869.

8. Smit TH, Engels TA, Söntjens SH, Govaert LE: Time-dependent failure in load-bearing polymers: A potential hazard in structural applications of polylactides. *J Mater Sci Mater Med* 2010;21(3):871-878.

9. Bragdon CR, Martell JM, Greene ME, et al: Comparison of femoral head penetration using RSA and the Martell method. *Clin Orthop Relat Res* 2006;448:52-57.

10. Ngai V, Wimmer MA: Kinematic evaluation of cruciate-retaining total knee replacement patients during level walking: A comparison with the displacement-controlled ISO standard. *J Biomech* 2009;42(14):2363-2368.

11. Cuckler JM: The rationale for metal-on-metal total hip arthroplasty. *Clin Orthop Relat Res* 2005;441:132-136.

12. Kurtz SM, Gawel HA, Patel JD: History and systematic review of wear and osteolysis outcomes for first-generation highly crosslinked polyethylene. *Clin Orthop Relat Res* 2011;

469(8):2262-2277.

13. Marcellin-Little DJ, Cansizoglu O, Harrysson OL, Roe SC: In vitro evaluation of a low-modulus mesh canine prosthetic hip stem. *Am J Vet Res* 2010;71(9):1089-1095.

14. Rostoker W, Chao EYS, Galante JO: Defects in failed stems of hip prostheses. *J Biomed Mater Res* 1978;12(5):635-651.

15. Gil FJ, Canedo R, Padrós A, Sada E: Enhanced wear resistance of ball-and-socket joints of dental implants by means of titanium gaseous nitriding. *J Biomater Appl* 2002;17(1):31-43.

16. Derbyshire B, Fisher J, Dowson D, Hardaker CS, Brummitt K: Wear of UHMWPE sliding against untreated, TiN and hardcor-treated stainless steel counterfaces. *Wear* 1995;181-183(pt 1):258-262.

17. McKellop HA, Röstlund TV: The wear behavior of ion-implanted Ti-6A1-4V against UHMW polyethylene. *J Biomed Mater Res* 1990;24(11):1413-1425.

18. Jacobs JJ, Gilbert JL, Urban RM: Corrosion of metal orthopaedic implants. *J Bone Joint Surg Am* 1998;80(2):268-282.

19. Brown TE, Larson B, Shen F, Moskal JT: Thigh pain after cementless total hip arthroplasty: Evaluation and management. *J Am Acad Orthop Surg* 2002;10(6):385-392.

20. Albrektsson T, Brånemark PI, Hansson HA, Lindström J: Osseointegrated titanium implants: Requirements for ensuring a long-lasting, direct bone-to-implant anchorage in man. *Acta Orthop Scand* 1981;52(2):155-170.

21. Pohler OE: Unalloyed titanium for implants in bone surgery. *Injury* 2000;31(suppl 4):7-13.

22. Simmons CA, Valiquette N, Pilliar RM: Osseointegration of sintered porous-surfaced and plasma spray-coated implants: An animal model study of early postimplantation healing response and mechanical stability. *J Biomed Mater Res* 1999;47(2):127-138.

23. Allen MJ, Leone K, Quinn R, DiMaano N, Zhang R, Mann KA: Mechanical and biological performance of titanium foam (Tritanium®) as a surface for cementless fixation. *Trans ORS* 2006;31:0683.

24. Amer L, Stone TB, Warren CP, Cornwell P, Meneghini RM: Initial mechanical stability of cementless highly-porous titanium tibial components. *Proceedings of the IMAC-XXVII: Conference & Exposition on Structural Dynamics*. Orlando, FL, 2009, p 10.

25. Bobyn JD, Stackpool GJ, Hacking SA, Tanzer M, Krygier JJ: Characteristics of bone ingrowth and interface mechanics of a new porous tantalum biomaterial. *J Bone Joint Surg Br* 1999;81(5):907-914.

26. Kuehn KD, Ege W, Gopp U: Acrylic bone cements: Composition and properties. *Orthop Clin North Am* 2005;36(1):17-28.

27. Webb JC, Spencer RF: The role of polymethylmethacrylate bone cement in modern orthopaedic surgery. *J Bone Joint Surg Br* 2007;89(7):851-857.

28. Reckling FW, Dillon WL: The bone-cement interface temperature during total joint replacement. *J Bone Joint Surg Am* 1977;59(1):80-82.

29. Herberts P, Malchau H: Long-term registration has improved the quality of hip replacement: A review of the

1: Basic Principles of Orthopaedic Surgery

Swedish THR Register comparing 160,000 cases. *Acta Orthop Scand* 2000;71(2):111-121.

30. Gilbert JL, Hasenwinkel JM, Wixson RL, Lautenschlager EP: A theoretical and experimental analysis of polymerization shrinkage of bone cement: A potential major source of porosity. *J Biomed Mater Res* 2000;52(1):210-218.

31. Messick KJ, Miller MA, Damron LA, Race A, Clarke MT, Mann KA: Vacuum-mixing cement does not decrease overall porosity in cemented femoral stems: An in vitro laboratory investigation. *J Bone Joint Surg Br* 2007;89(8):1115-1121.

32. Lewis G: Properties of antibiotic-loaded acrylic bone cements for use in cemented arthroplasties: A state-of-the-art review. *J Biomed Mater Res B Appl Biomater* 2009;89(2):558-574.

33. Engesaeter LB, Lie SA, Espehaug B, Furnes O, Vollset SE, Havelin LI: Antibiotic prophylaxis in total hip arthroplasty: Effects of antibiotic prophylaxis systemically and in bone cement on the revision rate of 22,170 primary hip replacements followed 0-14 years in the Norwegian Arthroplasty Register. *Acta Orthop Scand* 2003;74(6):644-651.

34. Lewis G: Percutaneous vertebroplasty and kyphoplasty for the stand-alone augmentation of osteoporosis-induced vertebral compression fractures: Present status and future directions. *J Biomed Mater Res B Appl Biomater* 2007;81(2):371-386.

35. Kane RJ, Yue W, Mason JJ, Roeder RK: Improved fatigue life of acrylic bone cements reinforced with zirconia fibers. *J Mech Behav Biomed Mater* 2010;3(7):504-511.

36. Sobieraj MC, Rimnac CM: Ultra high molecular weight polyethylene: Mechanics, morphology, and clinical behavior. *J Mech Behav Biomed Mater* 2009;2(5):433-443.

37. Kurtz SM: *The UHMWPE Handbook: Ultra-High Molecular Weight Polyethylene in Total Joint Replacement.* San Diego, CA, Elsevier Academic Press, 2004.

38. Baker DA, Bellare A, Pruitt L: The effects of degree of cross-linking on the fatigue crack initiation and propagation resistance of orthopedic-grade polyethylene. *J Biomed Mater Res A* 2003;66(1):146-154.

39. Wright TM, Goodman SB: *Implant Wear in Total Joint Replacement: Clinical and Biologic Issues.* Rosemont, IL, American Academy of Orthopedic Surgeons, 2001.

40. Currier BH, Van Citters DW, Currier JH, Collier JP: In vivo oxidation in remelted highly cross-linked retrievals. *J Bone Joint Surg Am* 2010;92(14):2409-2418.

41. Kurtz SM, Medel FJ, MacDonald DW, Parvizi J, Kraay MJ, Rimnac CM: Reasons for revision of first-generation highly cross-linked polyethylenes. *J Arthroplasty* 2010;25(6, suppl):67-74.

42. Jacobs CA, Christensen CP, Greenwald AS, McKellop H: Clinical performance of highly cross-linked polyethylenes in total hip arthroplasty. *J Bone Joint Surg Am* 2007;89(12):2779-2786.

43. Tower SS, Currier JH, Currier BH, Lyford KA, Van Citters DW, Mayor MB: Rim cracking of the cross-linked longevity polyethylene acetabular liner after total hip arthroplasty. *J Bone Joint Surg Am* 2007;89(10):2212-2217.

44. Dumbleton JH, D'Antonio JA, Manley MT, Capello WN, Wang A: The basis for a second-generation highly cross-linked UHMWPE. *Clin Orthop Relat Res* 2006;453:265-271.

45. Lachiewicz PF, Geyer MR: The use of highly cross-linked polyethylene in total knee arthroplasty. *J Am Acad Orthop Surg* 2011;19(3):143-151.

46. Middleton JC, Tipton AJ: Synthetic biodegradable polymers as orthopedic devices. *Biomaterials* 2000;21(23):2335-2346.

47. Urban JA, Garvin KL, Boese CK, et al: Ceramic-on-polyethylene bearing surfaces in total hip arthroplasty: Seventeen to twenty-one-year results. *J Bone Joint Surg Am* 2001;83(11):1688-1694.

48. Willmann GS: Ceramic femoral head retrieval data. *Clin Orthop Relat Res* 2000;379:22-28.

49. Huet R, Sakona A, Kurtz SM: Strength and reliability of alumina ceramic femoral heads: Review of design, testing, and retrieval analysis. *J Mech Behav Biomed Mater* 2011;4(3):476-483.

50. Hamadouche M, Boutin P, Daussange J, Bolander ME, Sedel L: Alumina-on-alumina total hip arthroplasty: A minimum 18.5-year follow-up study. *J Bone Joint Surg Am* 2002;84(1):69-77.

51. Mai K, Verioti C, Ezzet KA, Copp SN, Walker RH, Colwell CW Jr: Incidence of 'squeaking' after ceramic-on-ceramic total hip arthroplasty. *Clin Orthop Relat Res* 2010;468(2):413-417.

52. Chevillotte C, Trousdale RT, Chen Q, Guyen O, An KN: "Hip squeaking": A biomechanical study of ceramic-on-ceramic bearing surfaces. *Clin Orthop Relat Res* 2010;468(2):345-350.

53. Kumar P, Oka M, Ikeuchi K, et al: Low wear rate of UHMWPE against zirconia ceramic (Y-PSZ) in comparison to alumina ceramic and SUS 316L alloy. *J Biomed Mater Res* 1991;25(7):813-828.

54. Clarke IC, Manaka M, Green DD, et al: Current status of zirconia used in total hip implants. *J Bone Joint Surg Am* 2003;85(suppl 4):73-84.

55. Cook SD, Thomas KA, Kay JF, Jarcho M: Hydroxyapatite-coated titanium for orthopedic implant applications. *Clin Orthop Relat Res* 1988;232:225-243.

56. Sun L, Berndt CC, Khor KA, Cheang HN, Gross KA: Surface characteristics and dissolution behavior of plasma-sprayed hydroxyapatite coating. *J Biomed Mater Res* 2002;62(2):228-236.

57. Søballe K, Overgaard S, Hansen ES, Brokstedt-Rasmussen H, Lind M, Bünger C: A review of ceramic coatings for implant fixation. *J Long Term Eff Med Implants* 1999;9(1-2):131-151.

58. Ban S, Maruno S, Arimoto N, Harada A, Hasegawa J: Effect of electrochemically deposited apatite coating on bonding of bone to the HA-G-Ti composite and titanium. *J Biomed Mater Res* 1997;36(1):9-15.

59. Allen MJ, Townsend KL, Bauer TW, Gabriel SM, O'Connell M, Clifford A. Evaluation of the safety of a novel knee load-bypassing device in a sheep model. *J Bone Joint Surg Am* 2012;94(1):77-84.

60. Spivak JM, Ricci JL, Blumenthal NC, Alexander H: A new canine model to evaluate the biological response of intramedullary bone to implant materials and surfaces. *J Biomed Mater Res* 1990;24(9):1121-1149.

61. Walsh WR, Vizesi F, Michael D, et al: Beta-TCP bone graft substitutes in a bilateral rabbit tibial defect model. *Biomaterials* 2008;29(3):266-271.

62. Kobayashi H, Turner AS, Seim HB III, Kawamoto T, Bauer TW: Evaluation of a silica-containing bone graft substitute in a vertebral defect model. *J Biomed Mater Res A* 2010;

92(2):596-603.

63. Koller G, Roether J, Bruce K, Deb S: Antimicrobial potential of bioactive bone cements. *J Appl Biomater Biomech* 2008; 6(1):16-22.

Chapter 5

Principles of Tissue Engineering in Orthopaedics

Tamim Diab, PhD

Nick J. Willett, PhD

Robert E. Guldberg, PhD

1: Basic Principles of Orthopaedic Surgery

Introduction

Musculoskeletal tissue damage and degeneration are the most common causes of pain and functional disability worldwide. Although tissue grafting often is effective, donor site morbidity is a significant concern. Clinical efforts to restore function to nonhealing musculoskeletal tissue defects often are complicated by high biomechanical-loading conditions, infection, ischemia, advanced age, adjacent tissue trauma, or disease. Biologic constraints specific to the individual patient and clinical condition must be considered in choosing regenerative therapies. The choice of interventional strategies to promote functional regeneration of damaged tissues may be dictated by the presence of, for example, advanced age, radiation therapy, composite tissue trauma, or a disease such as diabetes.

A vast array of biomaterial scaffolds has been developed to provide an initial structural template for cell-based extracellular matrix (ECM) synthesis. Biomaterial scaffold design variables such as material and mechanical properties, surface chemistry, porosity, pore connectivity, and degradation rate must be appropriately selected to optimize healing responses. Biomaterial scaffolds alone often are insufficient to promote regeneration, and they are used as a delivery vehicle for a biologic component. In some patients, a critically diminished endogenous progenitor cell supply may suggest the use of a cell therapy approach. In other patients, the use of a scaffold material integrated with recombinant protein may prove advantageous. In addition, there is increasing recognition that the local mechanical environment is critical in regulating the pathway of tissue regeneration. The timing, mode, and magnitude of local mechanical signals can both negatively and positively affect the key processes of inflammation, vascular growth, cellular differentiation, and tissue remodeling.

This chapter introduces the basic principles of tissue engineering in orthopaedics and summarizes the state of the art in clinical tissue regenerative strategies.

Scaffold Technology

Scaffold Materials

The scaffold material plays a critical role in the complex process of tissue regeneration. It is believed that a successful tissue-engineering strategy requires the scaffold material to mimic the natural environment of the ECM by providing temporal and spatial cues for tissue regeneration. An ideal scaffold material is highly biocompatible and does not elicit a chronic host inflammatory response;[1] supports cell adhesion, proliferation, migration, and differentiation;[2,3] degrades at a rate that approximately matches the new tissue formation rate;[3] and provides adequate mechanical stability to support tissue regeneration.[2] Finding a single material that simultaneously meets all of these criteria is one of the main challenges in the field of tissue engineering. One of the emerging paradigms in scaffold design is the use of composite materials to meet multiple functional design requirements.

Dr. Guldberg or an immediate family member is a member of a speakers' burearu or has made paid presentations on behalf of Abbott and MiMedx; serves as a paid consultant to or is an employee of MiMedx, Charles River Laboratories, and St. Joseph Translational Research Institute; has stock or stock options held in MiMedx; and has received research or institutional support from Abbott and MiMedx. Neither of the following authors or any immediate family member has received anything of value from or owns stock in a commercial company or institution related directly or indirectly to the subject of this chapter: Dr. Diab and Dr. Willett.

There are three types of materials that have been investigated for tissue-engineering applications: natural materials such as collagen, gelatin, silk fibroin, fibrin, chitosan, hyaluronan, chondroitin sulfate, and decellularized ECM; synthetic polymeric materials such as polyesters, poly(α-hydroxy) acids, and polylactones; and ceramic materials such as hydroxyapatite, tricalcium phosphate, and bioglass. Each type of material has advantages and disadvantages.

Natural Materials

The main advantage of natural materials is that typically they contain bioactive factors that may promote desirable cellular functions such as cell adhesion, proliferation, and differentiation.[4] Because they are derived from natural sources, natural materials generally are highly biocompatible, and they are more rapidly degraded by enzymes or hydrolysis (decomposition by reaction with water) compared with other types of materials.[2,4] Another important feature of natural materials is that they can be simply processed into sponges or hydrogels. Finally, the regulatory approval pathway typically is relatively straightforward for a minimally manipulated natural material such as a decellularized ECM. The disadvantages of natural materials include batch-to-batch variability, the possibility of pathogen transfer, poor mechanical properties, and limited control over physiochemical properties.[2,5] Natural materials are complex and typically not well characterized. As a result, it is difficult to determine the mechanistic basis of their effects on cell function.[4]

Synthetic Polymeric Materials

Synthetic polymeric materials are advantageous in that their physiochemical and mechanical properties can be modulated during the synthesis process to suit various applications.[2] These materials can be simply processed into sponges or hydrogels with reproducible quality and purity.[2] A major drawback of synthetic polymeric materials is that they lack integrin-binding ligands, and their inherent interaction with cells therefore is limited.[4] Poor biocompatibility and release of acidic products during degradation have been reported in several synthetic polymeric materials.[2]

Ceramic Materials

Ceramic materials are defined as solids made of inorganic nonmetallic elements.[2] They are usually produced through heat treatment followed by cooling.[2] Ceramic materials made of hydroxyapatite, a compound that has a chemical structure similar to that of the mineral component of bone matrix, are good candidates for bone tissue-engineering applications.[2,5] Ceramic materials made of hydroxyapatite integrate well with the bone tissue and possess superior osteoconductive properties (that is, they support bone formation).[5,6] Ceramic scaffolds typically are brittle and slow to degrade, however.[7]

Scaffold Designs

The structural design of the scaffold plays a vital role in determining the success of a tissue-engineering strategy. A scaffold should possess a highly interconnected porous structure to facilitate mass transport of nutrients, promote cellular and vascular invasion, and provide a large surface area (surface-to-volume ratio) for cell attachment and new matrix synthesis.[8] In load-bearing applications, a high initial mechanical strength may be required for structural stability during new tissue formation.[8] As with any porous material, the mechanical properties of a scaffold are determined by the material properties of its constituents, its porosity, and the microstructural organization (such as alignment) of the solid material. A scaffold design should balance the biologic and mechanical requirements of the intended application. For example, high porosity is advantageous for mass transport, cellular and vascular invasion, and rapid degradation but may compromise the mechanical function of the scaffold.

Fabrication Technologies

Electrospinning

Electrospinning is a process in which an electrical field is used to deposit fibers onto a targeted substance.[2] The main advantage of electrospinning is its ability to generate polymers with diameters at the nanoscale (0.5 μm) (**Figure 1, A**), to a certain extent mimicking the fibrous structure of the ECM. Other important features of electrospinning include ease of use and the broad range of natural and synthetic polymeric materials that can be used (such as collagen, fibrin, and polycaprolactone). The applications of electrospinning are hindered by poor mechanical properties, poor reproducibility, and the difficulty of controlling porosity or creating three-dimensional fabricated scaffolds.

Rapid Prototyping

Rapid prototyping is the construction of physical objects using automated systems. The major advantage of rapid prototyping is that it provides precise control of the scaffold's pore size and connectivity[3] (**Figure 1, B**). Rapid prototyping can be used in conjunction with computer-aided design and manufacturing to produce scaffolds based on radiographic studies of the individual patient.[9] Rapid prototyping has the potential to be used in fabricating scaffolds of natural materials such as chitosan, synthetic polymeric materials such as polycaprolactone, and ceramics materials such as hydroxyapatite, with controlled surface topography.[9] Controlled surface topography is known to play an important role in modulating cell-scaffold interactions.[2] Rapid prototyping has two main disadvantages: overall resolution is limited with current technologies, and only a limited selection of scaffold materials can be used with these technologies.[9]

Cellular Solid Fabrication

Scaffolds fabricated using a nonautomated system usually are classified as cellular solids.[10] Particulate leaching is a

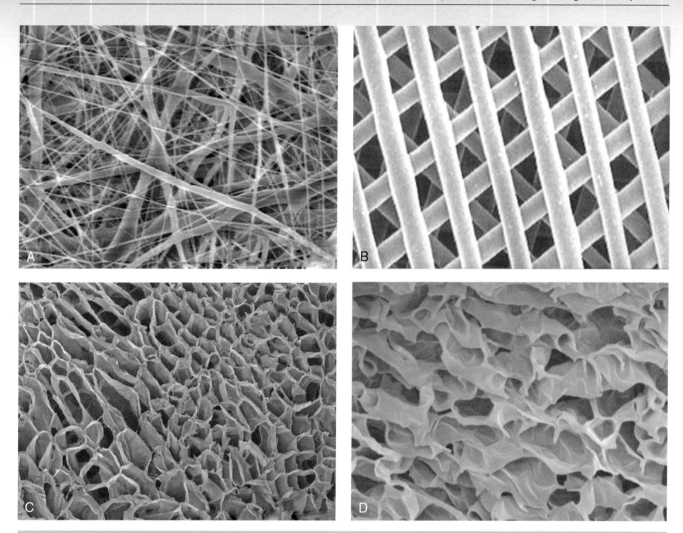

Figure 1   Scanning electron microscopic images of scaffolds created using four different fabrication technologies. **A,** Nanofiber mesh of polycaprolactone produced by electrospinning. **B,** Polycaprolactone scaffold produced by rapid prototyping. **C,** Poly-L-lactic acid scaffold produced by thermally induced phase separation, a type of cellular solid fabrication. **D,** Polyethylene glycol–peptide hydrogel synthesized by hydrogel polymerization using click chemistry. (Panel A adapted with permission from Kolambkar YM, Dupont KM, Boerckel JD, et al: An alginate-based hybrid system for growth factor delivery in the functional repair of large bone defects. *Biomaterials* 2011;32[1]:65-74; Panel B adapted with permission from Hutmacher DW: Scaffolds in tissue engineering bone and cartilage. *Biomaterials* 2000;21[24]:2529-2543; Panel C adapted with permission from Wei G, Ma PX: Structure and properties of nano-hydroxyapatite/polymer composite scaffolds for bone tissue engineering. *Biomaterials* 2004; 25:4749-4757; Panel D adapted with permission from Liu SQ, Ee PL, Ke CY, Hedrick JL, Yang YY: Biodegradable poly(ethylene glycol)-peptide hydrogels with well-defined structure and properties for cell delivery. *Biomaterials* 2009;30[8]:1453-1461.)

widely used cellular solid fabrication technology in which the scaffold material is mixed with a porogen such as salt, sugar, or paraffin spheres.[1] The solution containing the scaffold material and porogen is cast in a mold and allowed to dry. The porogen is leached out using water or an organic solvent to create a porous scaffold.[11] Thermally induced phase separation, another cellular solid fabrication technology, uses a process similar to that of particulate leaching. Instead of using a porogen, the pores are produced by thermodynamically separating the scaffold material from its solvent.[3]

Cellular solid fabrication techniques have numerous limitations. The size and connectivity of the pores in cellular solid scaffolds are not well controlled[3,10] (**Figure 1,** *C*). The use of these scaffolds may be limited in certain applications because thick cellular solid scaffolds are difficult to make. Any organic solvent used in the fabrication process must be completely removed before clinical use.[10] As with rapid prototyping, a broad range of natural materials such as collagen, synthetic polymeric materials such as poly-L-lactic acid, and ceramic materials such as hydroxyapatite can be fabricated using cellular solid techniques.

Hydrogel Polymerization

Hydrogels are a network of polymer chains capable of absorbing water from as little as 10% to as much as thousands of times their dry weight.[12] The material types that can be fabricated into hydrogels typically include a broad range of natural and synthetic polymeric materials such as collagen, alginate, and polyethylene glycol (**Figure 1,** *D*). Depending on the processing technique, hydrogels can be fabricated as premolded solids or injectable materials. The main advantage of injectable hydrogels over premolded solid hydrogels is that they can be used to fill irregularly shaped tissue defects.[3] Injectable hydrogels also can be used for minimally invasive percutaneous cell biologic delivery approaches. The limitations of hydrogels include their poor mechanical properties and the difficulty of controlling porosity.[3]

Fabrication technologies can be used in combination.[13] For example, a hybrid fabrication technology could combine electrospinning with rapid prototyping and cellular solid fabrication technology.

Surface Modification of Scaffold Materials

The surface modification of scaffold materials plays an important role in enhancing the scaffold's biologic function. Surface modification techniques can produce biomaterials that modulate specific cellular responses and guide the regeneration process. For example, surface modification by ECM-derived adhesive motifs such as arginine-glycine-aspartic acid and GFOGER (a collagen-mimicking peptide) was found to promote tissue regeneration.[2,14] Specifically, the binding of ECM-derived adhesive motifs to integrins (cell adhesion receptors) results in mechanical anchoring of cells to the biomaterial surface. After the cells adhere, specific signaling pathways can be activated because of integrin binding and clustering.[14] The activation of these signaling pathways can alter cell proliferation and/or differentiation along a particular lineage. Therefore, ECM-derived adhesive motifs have the potential to promote the regeneration process by regulating both cell attachment and function.

The two types of surface modification techniques are physiochemical alteration of the existing surface by chemical modification, etching, or mechanical roughening; and overcoating of the existing surface with a different material by direct coating, grafting, or thin film deposition.[2,15] For either physiochemical or overcoating surface modification, the modified zone should be sufficiently stable chemically and mechanically to ensure adequate biologic performance.[2,15]

The Clinical State of the Art
Bone
The clinical gold standard for osseous reconstruction relies on the use of autologous or allogeneic bone grafting. Autografts usually are harvested from the iliac crest or fibula. Autografts are nonimmunogenic and carry a low risk of disease transmission. However, autografts are associated with donor site morbidity and have limited availability for harvest. In contrast, allografts are obtained from cadaver bone and therefore are available in large quantities. Depending on the processing technique, allografts are classified as struc-

tural (bone block or segment) or morcellized (bone chip). Unlike morcellized allograft, structural allograft can withstand mechanical forces or retain a certain shape,[11] but their use can lead to late fracture because of limited revascularization and remodeling.[16] The limitations associated with bone grafting have prompted efforts to develop alternatives, including a combination of scaffolds and growth factors or cells.

One bone tissue-engineering strategy clinically used for spinal fusion or healing of a nonunited bone defect combines a biocompatible scaffold and recombinant osteoinductive (bone formation–inducing) proteins such as human bone morphogenetic protein (BMP)–2 (INFUSE; Medtronic, Minneapolis, MN). Collagen sponge has been used as a scaffold carrier for BMP-2 based on its good retention of BMP-2 as well as its favorable biocompatibility, degradation kinetics, and cell adhesion properties.[17] The drawbacks of using a collagen scaffold carrier are the necessity for implantation through an open surgical procedure and the relatively rapid release of protein.[17] Research is ongoing to develop carriers for osteoinductive proteins that could be injected percutaneously and provide sustained delivery. Improved delivery of osteoinductive proteins may reduce the incidence of clinically observed complications such as ectopic mineralization, focal osteolysis, and inflammation in adjacent tissues.[18]

Cartilage
The treatment of chondral defects is an important unresolved clinical problem in orthopaedics. None of the numerous non–tissue-engineering techniques used to treat cartilage injuries (such as microfracture and mosaicplasty) has led to successful regeneration of normal hyaline cartilage.[19] The need for a better therapy has led to the development of autologous chondrocyte implantation (ACI), in which autologous chondrocytes are injected into a chondral defect without a cell delivery matrix (**Figure 2,** *A*). Although first-generation ACI had promising results, the surgical procedure was complex, and numerous complications were noted including hypertrophy of the autologous periosteal patch and uneven distribution of the transplanted cells in the defect site. Second- and third-generation ACI eliminated the need to harvest the periosteal patch, thereby reducing disadvantages such as hypertrophy. In second-generation (collagen-covered) ACI, a collagen membrane was used rather than the autologous periosteal patch (**Figure 2,** *B*). In third-generation (matrix-induced) ACI, autologous chondrocytes are seeded onto a bilayer collagen membrane (MACI; Genzyme, Cambridge, MA; **Figure 2,** *C*) or a scaffold made of natural materials such as hyaluronan (Hyalograft; Fidia Advanced Biopolymers, Abano Terme, Italy) or collagen–chondroitin sulfate (Novocart 3D; Tissue Engineering Technologies AG, Reutlingen, Germany).[20] The main advantages of the third-generation procedure over the first- and second-generation procedures are homogenous distribution of the transplanted cells and the ability to use

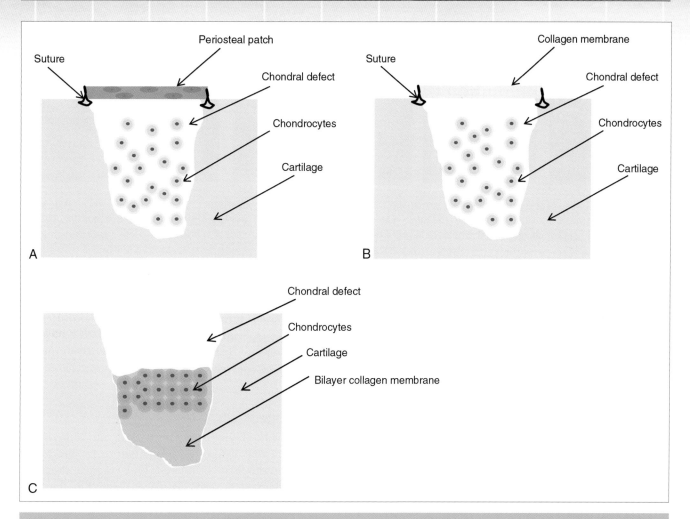

Figure 2 Schematic representations of ACI (**A**), collagen-covered ACI (**B**), and matrix-induced ACI (**C**) procedures.

surgical arthroscopic techniques. There are no conclusive clinical data showing whether ACI leads to a better clinical outcome than microfracture or mosaicplasty, which generally is more cost effective.[19] There is a clear need for development of new tissue-engineering strategies that will restore the biologic and mechanical function of injured articular cartilage.

Tendon and Ligament

The limitations of treating tendon or ligament injury with sutures or grafts include poor healing, insufficient mechanical properties, and wear (that is, the sutures or grafts will wear over time).[5] These limitations have led to the development of new clinical treatment approaches based on tissue-engineering principles for tendon and ligament regeneration. Current tendon and ligament tissue-engineering strategies primarily rely on mimicking the ECM by using acellular scaffolds made of a natural material, usually collagen (Zimmer Collagen Repair Patch; Zimmer, Warsaw, IN); or a synthetic polymeric material such as polyurethane urea (SportMesh; Biomet Sports Medicine, Warsaw, IN) or polyethylene terephthalate (Leeds-Keio; Neoligaments, Leeds,

England).[21] The natural and synthetic polymeric materials used in tendon-ligament regeneration have advantages and disadvantages. Natural materials are bioactive and have good porosity, but their mechanical properties are lower than what is desirable for tendon-ligament tissue engineering.[21] Synthetic polymeric materials have good mechanical properties but do not support robust tissue ingrowth during the tendon-ligament regeneration process. Research to improve the mechanical and biologic properties of the regenerated tissue is focused on understanding and promoting the healing of the bone–tendon-ligament junction.[21]

Muscle

The current standard of care for muscle loss relies on autologous muscle transfer, which may partially restore muscle function. The numerous drawbacks of this surgical intervention include a limited success rate, donor site morbidity, and the failure to completely restore contractile function.[22,23] Tissue engineering strategies based on acellular ECM scaffolds, such as small intestinal submucosa and abdominal muscle, with or without the addition of cultured cells, in the future may provide alternatives to autologous

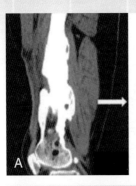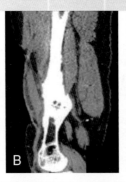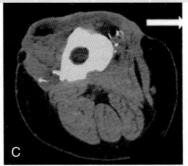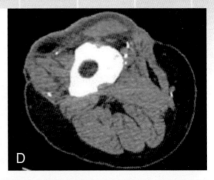

Figure 3 CT studies of the right thigh of a 19-year-old man with large volumetric muscle loss 5 months before implantation of acellular ECM scaffold derived from porcine intestinal submucosa (**A** [sagittal image] and **C** [coronal image]) and 9 months after implantation (**B** [sagittal image] and **D** [coronal image]). Arrows (in **A** and **C**) indicate the 1.9 × 4.9 × 9.4–cm area in which regenerated muscle tissue appeared after implantation (as seen in **B** and **D**). (Adapted with permission from Mase VJ Jr, Hsu JR, Wolf SE, et al: Clinical application of an acellular biologic scaffold for surgical repair of a large, traumatic quadriceps femoris muscle defect. *Orthopedics* 2010;33[7]:511.)

muscle transfer.[23] Four weeks after a 19-year-old man with large volumetric muscle loss received an acellular ECM scaffold derived from porcine intestinal submucosa (Restore; DePuy, Warsaw, IN), the patient had significant improvement in isokinetic performance. CT obtained 9 months after implantation revealed the formation of new muscle tissue[22] (**Figure 3**). The need for reinnervation for functional regeneration of volumetric muscle defects could limit the use of certain scaffolds and may prove more challenging than the formation of muscle ECM.[23]

Research Directions

Although numerous materials and fabrication technologies have been proposed for creating effective tissue-engineered scaffolds for orthopaedic applications, several key challenges remain. These include the development of a scaffold material that is highly biocompatible, does not elicit a chronic host inflammatory response, supports cell function, and has favorable mechanical and degradation properties; scaffold designs that can effectively balance the biologic and mechanical requirements of the intended application; and the fabrication of scaffolds with controlled porosity and surface topography.

Cell Technology
Cell Sources

Cell therapy represents a promising interventional strategy for promoting the functional regeneration of damaged tissues. In a successful cell-based therapy, the transplanted cells would survive after transplantation and be able to generate sufficient quantities of tissue or promote host cell–mediated tissue regeneration. An ideal cell therapy strategy should, therefore, ensure that the delivered cells possess several functional characteristics: they do not elicit an immune response or cause teratoma formation; they have a high proliferation rate to allow a sufficient number of cells to be generated for implantation; they integrate well into the regenerated tissue; and, in stem cell–based therapy, they can

differentiate into a mature cell phenotype appropriate for the intended application. In addition, the cell delivery strategy should ensure that viable cells are delivered to the injured site. Cells for transplantation are categorized as differentiated or stem progenitor.

Differentiated Cells

Differentiated cells can be obtained by in vitro differentiation of stem cells before transplantation or by direct harvesting from the tissue of interest. (For example, chondrocytes are harvested from cartilage tissue for the ACI procedure.) Although differentiation before implantation increases the proportion of cells of a specific phenotype, the lower proliferation rate of differentiated cells compared with undifferentiated cells is a major drawback. In some applications it may be desirable to allow the transplanted cells to differentiate into multiple lineages rather than being committed to a specific lineage. For example, in bone tissue-engineering applications there is emerging evidence that a mixture of osteogenesis- and angiogenesis-promoting cells may be advantageous.

Stem Cells
Adult Stem Cells

Adult stem cells typically are defined as self-renewing cells capable of generating cell types specific to the tissue in which they reside.[24] Adult stem cells have been found in almost every tissue in the body. The main advantage of adult stem cells is that autologous use improves the likelihood of cell engraftment. The ease of harvest from numerous tissue types is another important feature of adult stem cells.[25] The tumorigenic risk of an adult stem cell therapy is low in comparison with treatment using other stem cell types.[25] However, only a limited quantity of stem cells can be obtained from mature tissues. Adult stem cells can generate cell types specific to the tissue in which they reside and therefore have a restricted differentiation capacity.

The best characterized and most studied adult stem cells for musculoskeletal tissue engineering are derived from the bone marrow stroma. These mesenchymal stem cells (MSCs) have a high self-renewal capacity and can be differentiated into numerous types of tissues including bone, cartilage, and muscle.[24,26] MSCs also have the ability to secrete bioactive factors that are important in establishing a regenerative microenvironment after injury. For example, MSCs secrete angiogenic factors such as vascular endothelial growth factor (VEGF) and basic fibroblast growth factor (bFGF), which play a key role in bone regeneration. One of the challenges of using MSCs clinically is that too much time may be required to generate a sufficient number of cells, especially in older adult patients.

Embryonic Stem Cells

Embryonic stem cells are pluripotent cells that have virtually unlimited self-renewal and differentiation capacity. These characteristics suggest that embryonic stem cells could be more advantageous than adult stem cells for use in some tissue-engineering strategies. However, the use of human embryonic tissue to supply stem cells raises ethical concerns. There is a possibility that the use of embryonic stem cells could lead to teratoma formation.[24] Embryonic stem cells must be allogeneic and may elicit an immune response, although data exist to show that embryonic stem cells tend not to be rejected by the immune system.[27]

The somatic cell nuclear transfer technique has been used to overcome the risk of immune rejection with embryonic stem cells. Briefly, somatic cell nuclear transfer entails replacing the nucleus of an unfertilized human egg with a nucleus obtained from the patient.[24] After chemical or electrical stimulation, the egg cell with its new nucleus will develop into a blastocyst (an early embryo) that is genetically identical to the patient. The embryonic stem cells obtained from the blastocyst will not be rejected by the patient's immune system. Although somatic cell nuclear transfer is intriguing, its clinical application is limited by concerns about the quality of the embryonic stem cell lines it generates as well as ethical issues related to the use of human embryonic tissue.[24]

Fetal Stem Cells

Fetal stem cells isolated from the organs of aborted fetuses, umbilical cord blood, or amniotic fluid may provide a superior alternative to adult or embryonic-derived stem cells. Cultured fetal MSCs grow at a faster rate and senesce later than adult MSCs, and they have a differentiation capacity similar to that of embryonic stem cells.[5] The major concern related to using fetal stem cells is that the cells usually are from an allogeneic source. If autogenic cells are available, they will have undergone a lengthy storage period.

Induced Pluripotent Stem Cells

Induced pluripotent stem cells are adult somatic cells genetically reprogrammed to resemble patient-specific embryonic stem cells, without the use of embryonic or fetal cells.[24]

Induced pluripotent stem cells could be used in autologous cell therapy because their proliferative and differentiation characteristics are similar to those of embryonic stem cells. In 2007 it was shown that viral vectors can be used to generate induced pluripotent stem cell lines from human adult somatic cells.[2] This achievement was based on reprogramming human fibroblasts by using one of the following two combinations of transcription factors: (1) *Oct3/4, SOX2, KLF4,* and *c-Myc*; and (2) *OCT4, SOX2, NANOG,* and *LIN28*.[2] Episomal plasmid and direct protein delivery were introduced in 2009 as alternatives to viral vector delivery, but the induction efficiency of induced pluripotent stem cells is lower with these techniques than with viral vector delivery.[2]

Several concerns currently prevent induced pluripotent stem cells from being used clinically. Because viruses or recombinant reprogramming factors are used to induce genetic reprogramming from adult stem cells, the quality of the reprogrammed induced pluripotent stem cell lines must be carefully assessed before use in patients.[24] Transplantation of induced pluripotent stem cells could lead to the formation of teratoma. It is still unknown to what extent the proliferation and differentiation capacity of induced pluripotent stem cells and human embryonic stem cells are similar.[24] Reprogramming efficiency still needs to be improved. One promising strategy for this purpose is based on suppression of the p55 pathway, which leads to an increase in the number of cells undergoing induction.[2,24] Despite these limitations, there is tremendous interest in the potential of induced pluripotent stem cell–based therapies.

Cell Delivery

Systemic Cell Delivery

Systemic (intravenous) cell delivery ultimately may be a feasible and minimally invasive means of delivering cells to a site of injury. Systemic cell delivery also could be a simple method for controlling the timing of cell therapy initiation, which may be important in determining the survival rate of the delivered cells. It has been hypothesized that delayed administration of cells is necessary to avoid an initial acute inflammatory response or infection and to allow a greater number of cells to participate in the healing-regeneration process. It is unclear whether systemically delivered cells actually arrive at the injury site or become trapped in the lungs.

Local Cell Delivery

Local administration has been the method of choice for stem cell–based orthopaedic tissue-engineering applications. The main advantage of local cell delivery over systemic delivery is that it ensures that more cells arrive directly at the site of injury. This factor is particularly important if cells cannot be efficiently delivered systemically, as with compromised blood flow to the injured tissue. However, local cell delivery requires the use of scaffolds that must support cell functions and meet several other challenging requirements. Most of the current local cell deliv-

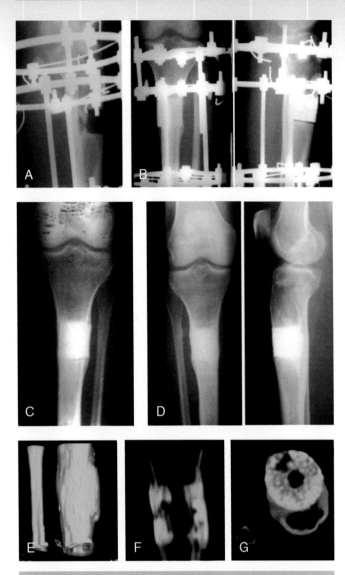

Figure 4 A macroporous hydroxyapatite scaffold seeded with autologous MSCs was used in the proximal tibia. Plain radiographs obtained before surgery (**A**) and at follow-up: 2 months (**B**), 6 months (**C**), and 2.5 years (**D**). **E**, **F**, and **G**, CT reveals new bone formation and complete integration of the scaffold with the surrounding bone at 7-year follow-up. However, CT shows that the hydroxyapatite scaffold had not degraded. (Adapted with permission from Marcacci M, Kon E, Moukhachev V, et al: Stem cells associated with macroporous bioceramics for long bone repair: 6- to 7-year outcome of a pilot clinical study. *Tissue Eng* 2007;13[5]:947-955.)

ery–based tissue-engineering strategies require an invasive surgical procedure. Research is under way to develop effective percutaneous cell delivery approaches.

Regardless of whether cell delivery is systemic or local, it is important to consider the presence of endogenous circulating adult stem cells that arrive at the injured site. These cells usually influence the regeneration process, probably by secreting bioactive factors (for example, angiogenic factors).

The Clinical State of the Art

Bone

After animal studies demonstrated the effectiveness of MSCs in bone regeneration, several small clinical studies investigated the potential of MSCs to repair bone defects in humans. One of the first such studies assessed the ability of autologous MSCs to repair nonunited bone defects.[6] Three patients received a macroporous hydroxyapatite scaffold seeded with autologous MSCs. The size and shape of the implanted scaffold was consistent with the patient's bone defect. Substantial bone regeneration as well as good integration of the scaffold with the surrounding bone was found 5 to 7 months after implantation. The limitation of hydroxyapatite as a scaffold material was revealed at 6- to 7-year follow-up, however, when the scaffold was found to have not completely degraded[7] (Figure 4). These results, as well as those of other clinical studies that found MSCs to promote bone regeneration in craniofacial defects, suggest that further research may lead to cell-based therapy becoming a viable treatment for nonhealing bone defects.

Cartilage

Several cell-based tissue-engineering strategies for repairing chondral defects in humans have had limited overall success. MSCs also have been investigated for cartilage repair. In one study, autologous MSCs embedded in a type I collagen gel construct were implanted in an articular cartilage defect and covered with autologous periosteal patch.[2,28] At 42-week follow-up, patients with a cell transplant had better histologic and arthroscopic scores than patients in the control group, but the clinical outcomes of patients in the two groups were not significantly different. This study and others that investigated the effects of cell delivery on cartilage regeneration highlight the challenges of developing a successful cartilage tissue-engineering strategy.

Tendon and Ligament

Cell-based tissue-engineering strategies for tendon and ligament have had promising results in preclinical testing but have not yet been sufficiently explored clinically.[29]

Muscle

Cell therapy has been effective in the treatment of muscular dystrophy.[30,31] In one study, patients with Duchenne muscular dystrophy received local intramuscular injections of allogeneic myogenic cells to the tibialis anterior.[31] Four weeks after transplantation, histologic and reverse transcription polymerase chain reaction analyses of muscle biopsies revealed that the transplantation of myogenic cells had resulted in a substantial increase in the expression of dystrophin, a subsarcolemmal protein that is an important indicator of the success of any treatment for Duchenne muscular dystrophy.[31] It remains to be determined whether cell therapy can be effective in the treatment of muscle defects.

Research Directions

The results of using cell technology for orthopaedic tissue-engineering applications indicate that cell-based tissue engineering may become a viable clinical treatment option. The key challenges in cell technology are identification of cell sources that possess the required characteristics, development of effective cell preconditioning or reprogramming approaches that prime the cells to withstand the harsh ischemic and inflammatory microenvironment of the injury site, and development of effective cell delivery approaches.

Biologic Regulator Delivery

Tissue-engineering strategies that deliver biologic regulators offer an alternative to cell delivery for tissue regeneration. The delivery of biologic regulators is intended to stimulate endogenous repair mechanisms by recruiting cells from the host instead of requiring the survival of implanted exogenous cells. Biologic regulators have shown substantial regenerative properties in preclinical animal models, and some techniques have now been approved by the US Food and Drug Administration (FDA) for clinical indications. The cues for tissue-engineering applications typically are categorized as recombinant proteins, gene delivery, or small molecules. The delivery techniques are somewhat similar to cell delivery in that they are local (through direct injection or a scaffold) or systemic. The optimal technique varies depending on the specific signaling molecule and the desired spatial and temporal delivery profile. Scaffold delivery of biologic regulators has a unique potential for controlled temporal release kinetics and targeted spatial delivery. Currently there is a focus on optimizing the timing of delivery and the release profile of different biologic regulators.

Recombinant Proteins

Recombinant proteins are the most common type of biologic regulator used in musculoskeletal tissue engineering, in both research and clinical applications. These proteins can be manufactured in large quantities by cells that have been genetically modified using recombinant DNA. The proteins of interest typically are native human growth factors or cytokines that can activate or attenuate specific pathways in vivo to enhance endogenous repair mechanisms.

Bone

The recombinant proteins used for bone healing primarily affect osteogenesis and angiogenesis. The goal of osteogenic techniques is to stimulate the steps that occur during endochondral or intramembranous ossification including stem cell recruitment and differentiation and bone formation. In preclinical studies, several proteins were shown to enhance bone formation: platelet-derived growth factor (PDGF), insulin-like growth factor, parathyroid hormone, and (most commonly) BMPs.[2] BMPs stimulate the differentiation of osteoprogenitor cells into chondrocytes and osteoblasts and have proangiogenic properties.[2,32] BMP-2 and BMP-7 (also

known as osteogenic protein–1) have had the most promising results in promoting bone regeneration and are commonly used clinically. In addition to bone formation, revascularization has been identified as critical to successful bone healing.

The delivery of angiogenic cues was found to increase rates of fracture healing and defect healing in preclinical animal models.[16,33] VEGF has been the primary angiogenic cue used in research to stimulate the formation of new blood vessels. Other proteins of interest include those that can increase VEGF expression or activity, such as PDGF, as well as those that can form new capillaries, such as bFGF. Many of these angiogenic and osteogenic cues have overlapping modes of action. BMPs, for example, have angiogenic capabilities, and VEGF can promote osteoblast differentiation. This overlap between angiogenic and osteogenic pathways may explain why codelivery of angiogenic and osteogenic cues (using VEGF and BMP) has not significantly improved healing over delivery of a single cue.[16,34] Further research into the timing of multiple-cue delivery may lead to better outcomes.

Cartilage

The delivery of biologic regulators for cartilage regeneration is a developing discipline. Researchers have identified transforming growth factor–β (TGF–β) superfamily members, including numerous BMPs, that can enhance chondrogenic differentiation and chondrocyte proliferation in vitro.[2] When these factors were delivered using microspheres, hydrogels, or polycaprolactone scaffolds, preclinical data showed successful chondrogenesis. However, the osteogenic properties of these cues has led to concern about ectopic bone formation.[35] Delivery of parathyroid hormone is a promising alternative because it is FDA approved for use in humans and recently was found to have in vivo chondroprotective and chondroregenerative properties.[36] Chondrogenesis was enhanced by in vitro and in vivo use of bFGF and insulin-like growth factor. This finding may provide a direction for further research.[35]

Tendon and Ligament

Recombinant proteins have been used to enhance the in vitro biomechanical properties of tendon and ligament tissue cultures and to improve healing and integration of adhesions in preclinical animal models. Studies have focused on identifying growth factors that will improve cell proliferation and migration along with production and remodeling of the ECM. In vitro cell and tissue culture studies have found improvement in mechanical properties after delivery of growth factors such as PDGF, epidermal growth factor, bFGF, TGF-β, growth differentiation factor (GDF)–5, and GDF-7.[37] In preclinical in vivo studies, GDF-5 caused ectopic tendon formation, but a recent study found robust tendonlike tissue formation after MSCs pretreated with GDF-5 were implanted into a tendon defect.[38,39] Similarly, animal studies showed that the delivery of PDGF or TGF-β can improve mechanical properties during healing of the medial collateral ligament, anterior cruciate ligament, or rotator cuff.[2,37] Another promising research direction may involve the delivery of recombinant transcription factors such as scleraxis, which is involved in tendon formation.

Muscle

Recombinant proteins delivered to muscle have not been sufficient for initiating and coordinating the regeneration response. Part of the challenge may be the complexity of the regenerative response, which requires migration and differentiation of satellite cells, fusion of myogenic progenitor cells, inhibition of fibrosis, restoration of continuity and contractile properties, and revascularization and reinnervation of the tissue. One tissue-engineering study delivered stromal cell–derived factor–1α on a collagen sponge to a surgically created volumetric muscle defect in rats.[40] Myogenesis around the wound was accelerated, although there was significant fibrosis. Better results may be achieved by early delivery of a myogenic protein followed by later delivery of an antifibrotic protein such as decorin.[41]

Gene Delivery

Gene therapy offers the potential to achieve sustained delivery of a therapeutic protein through genetic modification of cells. Transgenes typically are encoded for proteins that have been well studied and often are approved for clinical use, such as BMPs, VEGF, and PDGF. Although significant progress has been made in gene delivery techniques, safety concerns remain, and a challenging regulatory process has limited clinical translation.

The two categories of vectors for gene delivery are viral and nonviral. Viral vectors offer high transduction efficiency and are easy to produce. Adenovirus and adenoassociated virus are the most commonly used viral vectors because of relatively low safety concern, although there is still some potential for an immunogenic response. Nonviral vectors typically are naked DNA vectors. These vectors are easily produced and highly stable, but typically they have poor transfection efficiency.

Genes that promote tissue regeneration can be delivered after ex vivo genetic modification or through direct vector delivery in vivo. During traditional ex vivo gene transfer, monolayer cells (typically marrow-, muscle-, or adipose-derived cells) are expanded, and a transgene is introduced into the cells. The translation of this technique to clinical use has been limited because the process is lengthy and prohibitively expensive, and typically it requires two invasive procedures. An expedited ex vivo gene transfer technique has been developed in which cells are harvested, genetically modified, and reimplanted, all within a single surgical procedure.[42] Both ex vivo techniques require cell delivery to the injured area. Ex vivo techniques have had beneficial results in preclinical osteogenic models that used adenovirus-delivered BMP-2 in bone marrow stromal cells to heal critically sized defects in rats.[42] Ex vivo delivery of adenovirus-

based delivery of BMP-2 to cells in an autologous tendon graft was shown to enhance the strength of the tendon-bone interface in a rabbit model of anterior cruciate ligament injury.[43]

Direct vector delivery of genes traditionally was through direct injection, often with low transfection efficiency and transient gene expression. This method did lead to successful bone healing when BMP-2 transgenes were delivered to defect regions in rats, rabbits, and horses.[42] An alternative technique for direct delivery uses gene-activated matrices (GAMs), in which vectors are embedded in a scaffold. GAMs have been used to deliver transgene-encoding factors such as parathyroid hormone, BMP-2, or VEGF, all of which have improved bone healing in segmental defect models.[42,44] One of the most promising GAM technologies uses allograft bone coated with an adenoassociated virus encoding angiogenic or osteoinductive factors.[42,45] GAM technologies for delivery of PDGF in collagen gels are being clinically studied for ulcer healing, and this technology may be translated to the treatment of soft tissues such as tendon and ligament.[46]

Small Molecules

The use of small molecules is a promising alternative to protein delivery. Many small molecules have been approved for clinical use and could be translated into musculoskeletal tissue-engineering applications. Small molecules can be easily manufactured and quickly screened in large quantity to search for matches to the desired target. Pathways can be targeted in a manner similar to that of protein delivery. The more nonspecific binding effects of small molecules can lead to undesirable adverse effects, however. The use of small interfering RNAs (siRNAs) is a promising approach having high specificity. The delivery of siRNAs is particularly challenging, however, as they must be delivered into the target cell. The systemic delivery of small molecules could complement the use of a tissue-engineered construct. Researchers also are investigating the use of tissue-engineering technologies for local delivery. A key challenge is achievement of sustained-release kinetics, which is complicated by the size of the small molecules.

Bone

Some FDA-approved small molecules, including prostaglandin 2 and statins, have osteogenic properties. Statins are particularly promising because they are already widely used as a cholesterol-lowering drug, but a recent clinical study found that orally administered statins did not enhance radial fracture healing.[47] Further research is needed to develop methods for delivering statins locally or bypassing liver metabolism.[47] Similarly, siRNAs have been used to promote osteogenesis by targeting pathway inhibitors such as noggin.[48] Small molecules such as those targeting the hypoxia-inducible factor–1 pathway can be used to promote angiogenesis. Small molecules that activate this pathway have been shown to accelerate fracture healing in small animal models.[16] Adhesion peptides such as the arginine-glycine-aspartic acid amino sequence or binding motifs from heparin or collagen can promote cell binding to a tissue-engineered construct and can lead to improved osteogenesis.[35]

Tendon and Ligament

Matrix metalloproteinase inhibitors such as tetracycline and doxycycline have a potential for use in tendon or ligament healing. Preclinical animal studies of rotator cuff tears found enhanced healing with doxycycline treatment.[37]

Muscle

Antioxidants and angiotensin receptor blockers have shown early potential in tissue-engineering applications for muscle regeneration. Antioxidants such as the glutathione peroxidase mimetic ebselen were found in rats to positively affect muscle healing after injury, possibly by protecting injured muscle from secondary damage.[37] Other preclinical studies found that delivery of angiotensin receptor blockers such as losartan led to accelerated muscle regeneration.[49] Angiotensin receptor blockers are believed to act through TGF-β inhibition to reduce fibrosis during healing. The relationship between TGF-β and musculoskeletal healing clearly is complex, and the timing of delivery may play an important role.[37]

The Clinical State of the Art
Bone

Two factors for biologic regulator delivery in orthopaedics, BMP-2 and BMP-7, are FDA approved for clinical use. The FDA has approved recombinant BMP-2 (INFUSE) for four procedures: spinal fusion for patients with degenerative disk disease between L4 and S1, intramedullary nail fixation for acute open tibial shaft fracture, sinus augmentation, and localized alveolar ridge augmentation for defects associated with extraction sockets.[2,32,50] The BMP-7 product (OP-1 Putty; Stryker, Mahwah, NJ) is approved for use in spinal fusion and treatment of recalcitrant tibial nonunion or persistent pelvic ring instability.[50] The results of using BMP are comparable to those of autograft treatment. BMPs require delivery at supraphysiologic doses, however, with resulting safety concerns about heterotopic bone formation and inflammation of adjacent soft tissues.[18] Recombinant human PDGF has been used for periodontal regeneration.[51]

Cartilage, Tendon and Ligament, and Muscle

Biologic regulators for cartilage, tendon and ligament, and muscle have had promising results when delivered in preclinical tests, but biologic factor delivery using tissue-engineering techniques has not been sufficiently explored clinically. GAM delivery of PDGF in collagen gel is a promising technology undergoing clinical testing for wound healing of diabetic ulcers.[46]

Research Directions

The intent of therapies using biologic regulators is to stimulate endogenous repair mechanisms through delivery of recombinant proteins, genes, or small molecules. The key research challenges in biologic regulator delivery are to identify the optimal cue or combination of cues to be delivered and to optimize delivery techniques for specific cues, particularly with regard to the spatial and temporal delivery profile.

Biomechanical Factors

It is widely accepted that mechanical stimuli trigger a cascade of biologic signals that profoundly influence the tissue regeneration process. For instance, cyclic loading on myoblasts embedded in a type I collagen gel construct upregulates the mechanogrowth factor, which is an important contributor to muscle regeneration.[5] A biomechanical stimulus is classified as in vitro or in vivo based on whether it is applied before or after transplantation, respectively.

In Vitro Biomechanical Stimulation

The intent of a tissue-engineering approach based on the production of a functional tissue in vitro is to replace damaged tissues in vivo. A successful in vitro tissue-engineering strategy should involve expanding cells on a scaffold under controlled culture conditions that support cell viability and possibly cell differentiation. Several bioreactor systems have been developed to meet these requirements, such as spinner flask, rotating wall vessel, and perfusion bioreactor systems. Although design specifications vary from one bioreactor system to another, an ideal system must allow both the application of a mechanical stimulus and the control of environmental factors such as pH and oxygen.

Bone

A perfusion bioreactor system was used to investigate the effects of shear flow on osteogenic differentiation of MSCs seeded on titanium fiber mesh scaffolds in the presence or absence of dexamethasone, an osteogenic differentiation factor.[52] In comparison with static (no-perfusion) culture conditions, shear flow was found to induce osteogenic differentiation of MSCs, even without the use of dexamethasone, but the effect of shear flow was enhanced in the presence of dexamethasone. The study concluded that shear loading alone can promote bone regeneration and that the addition of a chemical stimulus may have an added or synergistic effect on bone regeneration.

Cartilage

To examine the effect of intermittent hydrostatic pressure on MSC chondrogenesis, MSCs were seeded on type I collagen scaffolds and cultured in a mixed medium containing osteogenic and chondrogenic differentiation factors.[53] The goal of using multiple differentiation factors was to mimic in vivo conditions in which cells are exposed to multiple dif-

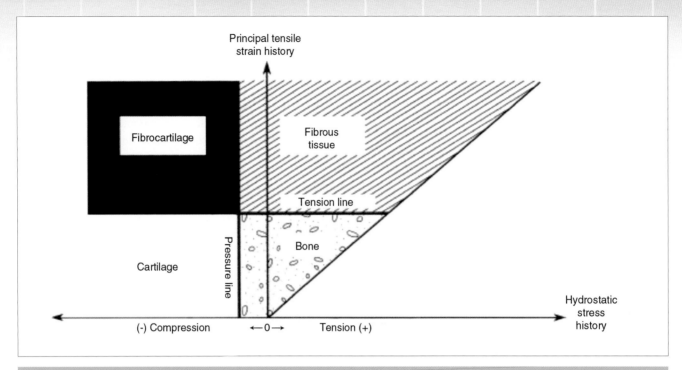

Figure 5 Schematic diagram showing the Carter and Beaupré semiquantitative mechanoregulation theory of the effects of mechanical stimulation on tissue differentiation. (Adapted with permission from Carter DR, Beaupré GS: *Skeletal Function and Form: Mechanobiology of Skeletal Development, Aging, and Regeneration.* Cambridge, England, Cambridge University Press, 2001.)

ferentiation cues.[53] It was found that intermittent hydrostatic pressure induced MSC differentiation toward the chondrogenic lineage and not toward the osteogenic lineage. This finding is consistent with the view presented by Pauwel and the semiquantitative mechanoregulation theory of Carter and Beaupré regarding the effects of mechanical stimulation on tissue differentiation[54] (**Figure 5**).

Tendon and Ligament

MSCs embedded in a type I collagen gel construct were subject to multiaxial (compressive-tensile and torsional) loading to promote the formation of tissues resembling tendon and ligament.[55] The application of a load induced the differentiation of MSCs into a ligament cell lineage without the presence of a ligament differentiation factor. The change in cell phenotype was associated with changes in cell morphology and alignment. The cells had ligamentlike cell morphology and were aligned in the direction of loading. The absence of upregulation of osteogenic- or chondrogenic-specific differentiation markers suggests that multiaxial loading can selectively differentiate MSCs into the ligament lineage.[55]

In Vivo Biomechanical Stimulation

Despite the consensus that the local mechanical environment plays an important role in tissue repair and remodeling, the effects of in vivo mechanical stimuli on tissue regeneration have not been extensively studied. The most important reason is the complexity of identifying and con-

trolling the in vivo mechanical loading conditions that promote tissue regeneration. Both the magnitude of the mechanical stimulus and the timing of load application onset are critical. Abnormally low- or high-magnitude mechanical stimuli might elicit a catabolic response and have deleterious effects on tissue regeneration and function.[2] It may be advantageous to delay the load application onset when regenerating a vascularized tissue, for example, so that the mechanical forces will not disrupt the early angiogenesis phase of the regeneration process.[56]

Joint distraction is one promising technique for cartilage repair. In one study, 73% of patients with severe ankle osteoarthritis reported significant clinical benefits after joint distraction.[57] The mechanistic basis of the beneficial effects of joint distraction on cartilage repair is still unknown. It has been suggested that unloading the joint prevents further cartilage wear and tear while maintaining synovial fluid pressure sufficient for articular cartilage nutrition, thus allowing the cartilage to repair itself without inducing further damage.[57]

Research Directions

Preclinical data indicate that biomechanical factors have a strong influence on the regeneration of orthopaedic tissues. The key challenges before biomechanical factors can be considered a viable clinical treatment option include improving the understanding of the effects of mechanical stimuli on tissue regeneration and remodeling and developing load application systems that can be clinically used.

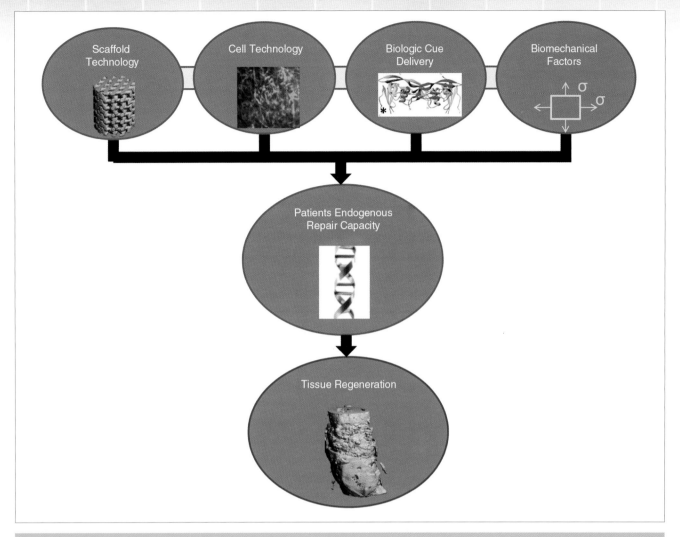

Figure 6 Schematic diagram showing the factors that contribute to tissue regeneration. (Biologic cue delivery image adapted from Nickel J, Dreyer MK, Kirsch T, Sebald W: The crystal structure of the BMP-2:BMPR-IA complex and the generation of BMP-2 antagonists. *J Bone Joint Surg Am* 2001;83[suppl 1, pt 1]:S7-S14.)

Preclinical Studies Using Animal Models

Preclinical studies using animal models are critical to the successful development and translation of tissue-engineering technologies in orthopaedics. Osteocompatability and grafting models are used to investigate bone tissue-engineering applications. Osteocompatability models are used in determining whether a material is compatible with bone healing in vivo and often in assessing cell survival or cell fate to determine the potential of cell implantation techniques. Osteocompatability studies cannot accurately predict whether a technology can be successfully translated from small animals to large animals, however. Small animal (rat, mouse) and large animal (pig, dog, goat, sheep) models are used in studies of bone grafts and bone substitutes. Small animal models typically are used for screening intervention techniques, and large animal models usually are required for clinical translational proof of concept. The major

considerations in grafting model studies include variability in the structure of bones (load bearing or non–load bearing), the type of injury or defect (segmental or intraosseous), and the remodeling process in different species.

Animal cartilage studies focus on articular cartilage but also include intervertebral disks. Articular cartilage studies include osteoarthritis, temporomandibular joint, and chondral or osteochondral defect models. These models can be used to assess resurfacing interventions and the repair of focal defects. As with animal models for bone, there are species-specific differences in cartilage architecture, particularly in chondrocyte density and cartilage thickness.

Animal tendon and ligament models are defined in relation to the synovium (intrasynovial or extrasynovial) and type of damage (full or partial tear). A full tear model may or may not include the formation of a gap between the ends. Tissue-engineered constructs are particularly useful as tissue replacements in full tear models with gap formations,

1: Basic Principles of Orthopaedic Surgery

such as an anterior cruciate ligament, a rotator cuff, or a flexor tendon tear.

Preclinical muscle injury models can broadly be categorized as exercise induced or trauma induced. Interventions designed to enhance muscle regeneration in these models typically focus on direct injection or systemic delivery of biologic regulators and cells. Recently, researchers have developed models of large volumetric muscle loss that can be used to test the efficacy of tissue-engineered muscle interventions.[58]

Summary

The interdisciplinary field of tissue engineering has emerged as a promising alternative to conventional methods for the repair of nonhealing musculoskeletal defects. Numerous challenges remain before tissue-engineering strategies can be widely used clinically. There is a need to better understand how the factors that contribute to tissue regeneration (scaffold technology, cell technology, biologic regulator delivery, biomechanical factors) interact with the patient's endogenous repair capacity to promote tissue regeneration (**Figure 6**). Future research directed toward understanding how aging, diabetes and other diseases, radiation therapy, and composite tissue trauma affect endogenous repair mechanisms will further the development of more effective tissue-engineering approaches. Despite these challenges, tissue-engineering strategies have tremendous promise for improving musculoskeletal tissue regeneration. A limited number of applications have been successfully translated into clinical practice.

References

1. Shi D: *Introduction to Biomaterials*. Singapore, World Scientific Publishing, 2006.

2. Atala A, Lanza R, Nerem R, Thomson JA: *Principles of Regenerative Medicine*, ed 2. San Diego, CA, Academic Press, 2011.

3. Ma PX: Scaffolds for tissue fabrication. *Mater Today* 2004; 7(5):10-40.

4. Tibbitt MW, Anseth KS: Hydrogels as extracellular matrix mimics for 3D cell culture. *Biotechnol Bioeng* 2009;103(4): 655-663.

5. Meyer U, Meyer T, Handschel J, Wiesmann HP: *Fundamentals of Tissue Engineering and Regenerative Medicine*. New York, NY, Springer, 2009.

6. Quarto R, Mastrogiacomo M, Cancedda R, et al: Repair of large bone defects with the use of autologous bone marrow stromal cells. *N Engl J Med* 2001;344(5):385-386.

7. Marcacci M, Kon E, Moukhachev V, et al: Stem cells associated with macroporous bioceramics for long bone repair: 6- to 7-year outcome of a pilot clinical study. *Tissue Eng* 2007; 13(5):947-955.

8. Hollister SJ: Porous scaffold design for tissue engineering. *Nat Mater* 2005;4(7):518-524.

9. Yang S, Leong KF, Du Z, Chua CK: The design of scaffolds for use in tissue engineering: Part II. Rapid prototyping techniques. *Tissue Eng* 2002;8(1):1-11.

10. Hutmacher DW: Scaffold design and fabrication technologies for engineering tissues: State of the art and future perspectives. *J Biomater Sci Polym Ed* 2001;12(1):107-124.

11. Ma PX, Elisseeff J: *Scaffolding in Tissue Engineering*. Boca Raton, FL, Taylor & Francis, 2005.

12. Hoffman AS: Hydrogels for biomedical applications. *Adv Drug Deliv Rev* 2002;54(1):3-12.

13. Kim G: Hybrid process for fabricating 3D hierarchical scaffolds combining rapid prototyping and electrospinning. *Macromol Rapid Commun* 2008;29(19):1577-1581.

14. Ducheyne P, Healy K, Hutmacher DW, Grainger DW, Kirkpatrick CJ: *Comprehensive Biomaterials*. Oxford, England, Elsevier, 2011.

15. Ratner BD, Hoffman AS, Schoen FJ, Lemons JE: *Biomaterials Science: An Introduction to Materials in Medicine*, ed 2. San Diego, CA, Elsevier Academic Press, 2004.

16. Guldberg RE: Spatiotemporal delivery strategies for promoting musculoskeletal tissue regeneration. *J Bone Miner Res* 2009;24(9):1507-1511.

17. Geiger M, Li RH, Friess W: Collagen sponges for bone regeneration with rhBMP-2. *Adv Drug Deliv Rev* 2003;55 (12):1613-1629.

18. Carragee EJ, Hurwitz EL, Weiner BK: A critical review of recombinant human bone morphogenetic protein-2 trials in spinal surgery: Emerging safety concerns and lessons learned. *Spine J* 2011;11(6):471-491.

19. Iwasa J, Engebretsen L, Shima Y, Ochi M: Clinical application of scaffolds for cartilage tissue engineering. *Knee Surg Sports Traumatol Arthrosc* 2009;17(6):561-577.

20. Brittberg M: Cell carriers as the next generation of cell therapy for cartilage repair: A review of the matrix-induced autologous chondrocyte implantation procedure. *Am J Sports Med* 2010;38(6):1259-1271.

21. Chen J, Xu J, Wang A, Zheng M: Scaffolds for tendon and ligament repair: Review of the efficacy of commercial products. *Expert Rev Med Devices* 2009;6(1):61-73.

22. Mase VJ Jr, Hsu JR, Wolf SE, et al: Clinical application of an acellular biologic scaffold for surgical repair of a large, traumatic quadriceps femoris muscle defect. *Orthopedics* 2010; 33(7):511.

23. Grogan BF, Hsu JR, Skeletal Trauma Research Consortium: Volumetric muscle loss. *J Am Acad Orthop Surg* 2011; 19(suppl 1):S35-S37.

24. Hipp J, Atala A: Sources of stem cells for regenerative medicine. *Stem Cell Rev* 2008;4(1):3-11.

25. Gates CB, Karthikeyan T, Fu F, Huard J: Regenerative medicine for the musculoskeletal system based on muscle-derived stem cells. *J Am Acad Orthop Surg* 2008;16(2):68-76.

26. Bianco P, Robey PG, Simmons PJ: Mesenchymal stem cells: Revisiting history, concepts, and assays. *Cell Stem Cell* 2008; 2(4):313-319.

27. Li L, Baroja ML, Majumdar A, et al: Human embryonic stem cells possess immune-privileged properties. *Stem Cells* 2004;22(4):448-456.

28. Wakitani S, Imoto K, Yamamoto T, Saito M, Murata N, Yoneda M: Human autologous culture expanded bone marrow mesenchymal cell transplantation for repair of cartilage

defects in osteoarthritic knees. *Osteoarthritis Cartilage* 2002; 10(3):199-206.

29. Roberts SJ, Howard D, Buttery LD, Shakesheff KM: Clinical applications of musculoskeletal tissue engineering. *Br Med Bull* 2008;86:7-22.

30. Tedesco FS, Dellavalle A, Diaz-Manera J, Messina G, Cossu G: Repairing skeletal muscle: Regenerative potential of skeletal muscle stem cells. *J Clin Invest* 2010;120(1):11-19.

31. McNally EG: The development and clinical applications of musculoskeletal ultrasound. *Skeletal Radiol* 2011;40(9):1223-1231.

32. Axelrad TW, Einhorn TA: Bone morphogenetic proteins in orthopaedic surgery. *Cytokine Growth Factor Rev* 2009;20(5-6):481-488.

33. Axelrad TW, Kakar S, Einhorn TA: New technologies for the enhancement of skeletal repair. *Injury* 2007;38(suppl 1): S49-S62.

34. Kempen DH, Lu L, Heijink A, et al: Effect of local sequential VEGF and BMP-2 delivery on ectopic and orthotopic bone regeneration. *Biomaterials* 2009;30(14):2816-2825.

35. Ericka M, Bueno J: *Biologic Foundations for Skeletal Tissue Engineering*. San Francisco, CA, Morgan & Claypool, 2011.

36. Smith J, Finnoff JT: Diagnostic and interventional musculoskeletal ultrasound: Part 2. Clinical applications. *PM R* 2009; 1(2):162-177.

37. Rodeo SA, Delos D, Weber A, et al: What's new in orthopaedic research. *J Bone Joint Surg Am* 2010;92(14):2491-2501.

38. Ohashi K, El-Khoury GY: Musculoskeletal CT: Recent advances and current clinical applications. *Radiol Clin North Am* 2009;47(3):387-409.

39. Wolfman NM, Hattersley G, Cox K, et al: Ectopic induction of tendon and ligament in rats by growth and differentiation factors 5, 6, and 7, members of the TGF-beta gene family. *J Clin Invest* 1997;100(2):321-330.

40. Grefte S, Kuijpers-Jagtman AM, Torensma R, Von den Hoff JW: Skeletal muscle fibrosis: The effect of stromal-derived factor-loaded collagen scaffolds. *Regen Med* 2010;5(5):737-747.

41. Zhu J, Li Y, Shen W, et al: Relationships between transforming growth factor-beta1, myostatin, and decorin: Implications for skeletal muscle fibrosis. *J Biol Chem* 2007;282(35): 25852-25863.

42. Evans CH: Gene therapy for bone healing. *Expert Rev Mol Med* 2010;12:e18.

43. Martinek V, Latterman C, Usas A, et al: Enhancement of tendon-bone integration of anterior cruciate ligament grafts with bone morphogenetic protein-2 gene transfer: A histological and biomechanical study. *J Bone Joint Surg Am* 2002; 84(7):1123-1131.

44. Nauth A, Miclau T III , Li R, Schemitsch EH: Gene therapy for fracture healing. *J Orthop Trauma* 2010;24(suppl 1):S17-S24.

45. Dupont KM, Boerckel JD, Stevens HY, et al: Synthetic scaffold coating with adeno-associated virus encoding BMP2 to promote endogenous bone repair. *Cell Tissue Res* 2012; 347(3):575-588.

46. Blume P, Driver VR, Tallis AJ, et al: Formulated collagen gel accelerates healing rate immediately after application in patients with diabetic neuropathic foot ulcers. *Wound Repair Regen* 2011;19(3):302-308.

47. Marsell R, Einhorn TA: Emerging bone healing therapies. *J Orthop Trauma* 2010;24(suppl 1):S4-S8.

48. Ramnath RR: 3T MR imaging of the musculoskeletal system: Part II. Clinical applications. *Magn Reson Imaging Clin N Am* 2006;14(1):41-62.

49. Bedair HS, Karthikeyan T, Quintero A, Li Y, Huard J: Angiotensin II receptor blockade administered after injury improves muscle regeneration and decreases fibrosis in normal skeletal muscle. *Am J Sports Med* 2008;36(8):1548-1554.

50. Giannoudis PV, Dinopoulos HT: BMPs: Options, indications, and effectiveness. *J Orthop Trauma* 2010;24(suppl 1): S9-S16.

51. Kaigler D, Avila G, Wisner-Lynch L, et al: Platelet-derived growth factor applications in periodontal and peri-implant bone regeneration. *Expert Opin Biol Ther* 2011;11(3):375-385.

52. Holtorf HL, Jansen JA, Mikos AG: Flow perfusion culture induces the osteoblastic differentiation of marrow stroma cell-scaffold constructs in the absence of dexamethasone. *J Biomed Mater Res A* 2005;72(3):326-334.

53. Wagner DR, Lindsey DP, Li KW, et al: Hydrostatic pressure enhances chondrogenic differentiation of human bone marrow stromal cells in osteochondrogenic medium. *Ann Biomed Eng* 2008;36(5):813-820.

54. Carter DR, Beaupré GS: *Skeletal Function and Form: Mechanobiology of Skeletal Development, Aging, and Regeneration.* Cambridge, England, Cambridge University Press, 2001.

55. Altman GH, Horan RL, Martin I, et al: Cell differentiation by mechanical stress. *FASEB J* 2002;16(2):270-272.

56. Boerckel JD, Uhrig BA, Willett NJ, Huebsch N, Guldberg RE: Mechanical regulation of vascular growth and tissue regeneration in vivo. *Proc Natl Acad Sci U S A* 2011;108(37): E674-E680.

57. Klauser AS, Peetrons P: Developments in musculoskeletal ultrasound and clinical applications. *Skeletal Radiol* 2010; 39(11):1061-1071.

58. Merritt EK, Hammers DW, Tierney M, Suggs LJ, Walters TJ, Farrar RP: Functional assessment of skeletal muscle regeneration utilizing homologous extracellular matrix as scaffolding. *Tissue Eng Part A* 2010;16(4):1395-1405.

Chapter 6

Basic Science of Immunology in Orthopaedics

Kofi A. Mensah, MD, PhD

Regis J. O'Keefe, MD, PhD

1: Basic Principles of Orthopaedic Surgery

Basic Components of the Immune System

There are two major components of the immune system, the innate immune system and the adaptive immune system.[1] The innate immune system is an ancient primordial system that is found in plants, insects, multicellular organisms, and animals and is the first line of defense against infection.[2] It nonspecifically recognizes common molecular structural patterns (for example, flagella) and has no immunologic memory—that is, the ability to "remember" previous agents and mount a faster and more specific response.[2] In contrast, the adaptive immune system is a highly specific network of cells and processes that is characteristic of vertebrate organisms. The adaptive immune system is considered the secondary line of defense. The adaptive immune response is based on highly specific recognition of particular aspects of molecular structures (antigens), for example, specific peptide sequences in flagella proteins.[3] Another hallmark of adaptive immunity is immunologic memory for quicker and more robust response on a future encounter with the antigen. The activation of the adaptive immune system is de-

Dr. O'Keefe or an immediate family member has stock or stock options held in LaGET and serves as a board member, owner, officer, or committee member of the American Board of Orthopaedic Surgery, the Orthopaedics Research Society, the National Institute of Arthritis, Skin, and Musculoskeletal Diseases Advisory Council, the NIH Council on Councils, the Shriners Hospital Research Advisory Board, and the Brown University NIH COBRE Grant Advisory Board. Neither Dr. Mensah nor any immediate family member has received anything of value from or owns stock in a commercial company or institution related directly or indirectly to the subject of this chapter.

pendent on the delivery of antigens and specific signals by the innate immune system.[1] Thus, these two systems are intimately interwoven.

Myeloid Lineage Cells of the Immune System

Understanding the nature of the adaptive and innate immune systems requires knowledge of the various cell types of the immune system. The leukocyte population includes all of the white blood cells; this is a major component of the immune system. Leukocytes are produced in the bone marrow and then are released into the circulation, providing access to numerous organs and tissues. Thus, these cells are unique in that they are not associated with a particular organ.

There are two broad classes of leukocytes. Myeloid cells are involved in inflammatory response and primarily initiate both the innate and adaptive immune responses. There are several types of myeloid cells.[2] Monocytes are circulatory cells that can gain residence in different types based on tissue (such as peritoneal macrophages or splenic macrophages). They are highly proficient phagocytes and producers of cytokines. Dendritic cells reside within specific tissues and are involved in phagocytosis, antigen processing, and activation of the adaptive immune system. Several other cell subtypes (antigen-presenting cells [APCs]) also have a role in antigen presentation. There are three types of granulocytes. Neutrophils are phagocytic, and often the first responders to the site of infection. Eosinophils kill immunoglobulin E (IgE) antibody-coated parasites but can also play a role in allergy. Basophils play a role in histamine release during allergy. Mast cells also play a role in histamine release during allergy.

Table 1

Subtypes of Lymphocytes and Specific Markers

Cell Type	T_h1	T_h2	T_h17	T_{reg}	T_c	B cell
Markers	CD4	CD4	CD4	CD25	CD8	CD19
	IFNγ	IL4	IL17	CD4		CD20

Table 2

Classes of Immunoglobulins and Relative Concentrations

Immunoglobulin Class	Percentage of Total Immunoglobulins	Heavy Chain	Comments
75%	IgG	γ	Presence usually indicates chronic immunity; involved in complement activation
15%	IgA	α	Can form dimmers or trimers
10%	IgM	μ	Earliest presence usually indicates acute immunity; involved in complement activation; can form a pentamer; largest Ig in size
0.2%	IgD	δ	Involved in B-cell activation signaling
0.002%	IgE	ε	Involved in mast cell and basophil degranulation during allergic reaction

Lymphoid Lineage Cells of the Immune System

The other broad class of immune cells is in the lymphoid cell lineage.[4] These cells can "learn" and adapt; therefore, they are primarily involved in adaptive immunity. Like the myeloid family, lymphocytes come in different cell types. There are three main classes of lymphocytes: T cells, B cells, and natural killer cells. T cells and B cells are both involved in the innate immune response.[3,4]

T cells are produced in the bone marrow, undergo maturation in the thymus, and are involved in the cell-mediated innate immune response. In the thymus, T cells undergo a selection process to ensure survival of T cells that recognize self-HLAs and are not strongly reactive to self-antigen. Errors in the selection process that allow survival of T cells that are reactive to native proteins result in the development of some autoimmune diseases. T-cell membranes have proteins that recognize specific antigens. These T-cell receptors (TCRs) are encoded by random splicing of a fixed number of gene segments to create a wide range of diversity among the TCRs. Thus, each TCR is unique and each has different binding affinities for the small peptide fragments that are presented by the HLA proteins on the surface of APCs. It is this random recombination of gene segments (rather than one gene per antigen-specific TCR) that allows the ability to generate the number of TCRs capable of recognizing millions of different possible antigens a person may encounter in a lifetime.

T cells are further divided into many subtypes[3] (**Table 1**). There are T helper (T_h) cells and cytotoxic T(T_c) cells. T_h cells produce cytokines that modulate the immune response and regulate other cell populations involved in the inflammatory response. T_c cells contain granules that release enzymes that kill cells containing foreign antigens. There are also regulatory T cells (T_{reg}) and T cells defined by their stimulation with various cytokines (for example, T_h17 cells are stimulated by interleukin (IL)-17, a cytokine).

B cells are another class of lymphocytes that are involved in antigen recognition and presentation. B cells may differentiate into plasma cells that are able to produce and secrete immunoglobulins/antibodies. Thus, similar to T cells, B cells become antigen specific. B cells also undergo random gene rearrangements to generate distinct B-cell receptors (BCRs) that recognize millions of unique antigens. The BCR is an immunoglobulin bound to the membrane. Immunoglobulins are composed of two distinct polypeptide chains — a light chain and a heavy chain. They also consist of a variable and a constant region, which have antigen-binding and effector functions, respectively. There are five classes of secreted antibodies: IgM, IgG, IgD, IgA, and IgE (**Table 2**).

Exposure to antigens causes both T cells and B cells to differentiate into effector cells that drive the adaptive immune response. Both T cells and B cells have the capacity to develop into memory cells that persist for extended periods of time in the tissues and systemic circulation. Memory cells enable a more rapid response to repeat challenge with the same antigen in the future.

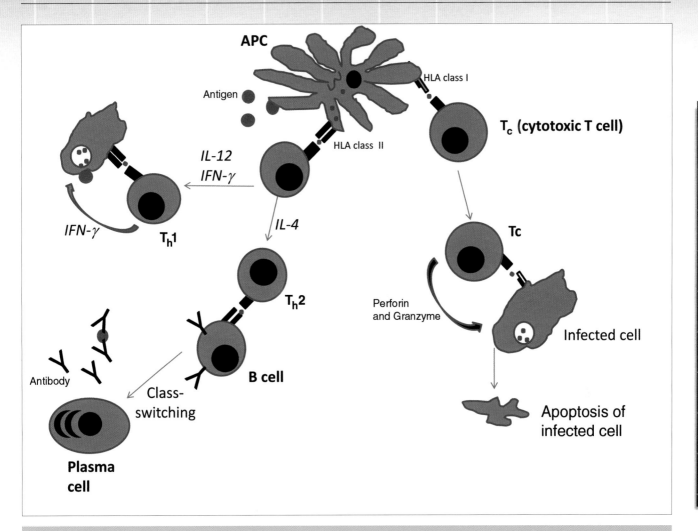

Figure 1 APCs activate T cells and stimulate the adaptive immune response. IFN = interferon.

A Typical Immune Response

To illustrate the sequence of events that occurs in an immune response, consider the reaction to infection with *Staphylococcus aureus* in the setting of osteomyelitis. The initial response involves activation of the innate immune system. Bacteria are "engulfed" or phagocytosed by macrophages and neutrophils patrolling the bone tissue. The neutrophils engage in phagocytic bactericidal actions to help clear the invading bacteria. Macrophages also engulf the bacteria where they are killed in the intracellular organelle called the phagolysosome. Activation of these processes in neutrophils and macrophages stimulates the release of cytokines and chemokines (chemotactic cytokines) and results in vasodilation and migration of more immune system cells, such as neutrophils, to the site of infection. Inflammation develops in the site with characteristic findings of rubor (redness), calor (heat), tumor (swelling), and dolor (pain).

Immature dendritic cells residing in the tissue also phagocytose the bacteria and process portions of bacterial proteins (antigens). Antigen processing involves digesting

the antigen into an 8 to 14 amino acid peptide fragment that is displayed on the surface of the APC, where it is bound to one of two types of surface proteins (**Figure 1**). These proteins are called HLAs and are sometimes also referred to as major histocompatibility complexes. Class I HLAs (HLA-A, -B, -C) process endogenous antigens. These are antigens produced using the host cell's protein-manufacturing organelles. This includes not only host cell proteins but also viral proteins that are made when the virus uses the host cell protein-manufacturing organelles to make more viral proteins. Class I HLAs are present on the surface of all nucleated cells. They are involved in self versus nonself responses and are very important in transplantation immunology.

In contrast, class II HLAs (HLA-DP, -DQ, -DR) process exogenous antigens not made by the host cell protein machinery, such as the proteins from *Staphylococcus*. The main class II HLAs encoded by six genes (*HLA-DPA1, HLA-DPB1, HLA-DQA1, HLA-DQB1, HLA-DRA,* and *HLA-DRB1*), Class II HLAs are present primarily on APCs such as dendritic cells and macrophages. They are also present on B cells, which can also present antigen but less efficiently than dendritic cells or macrophages. Class II HLAs also have minimal expression on T cells. The binding site or "cleft" for the antigens on class I HLAs is relatively narrow compared with that on the class II HLAs. The exogenous versus endogenous dichotomy is not a strict one, as some exogenous antigens can be presented on class I HLAs via a process called cross-presentation.

Myeloid cells and tissue-specific dendritic cells travel from the site of inflammation to the regional lymph node. In the lymph node, the myeloid cells present antigens (8 to 14 amino acid peptide fragments) that are loaded onto the class II HLA molecules to T lymphocytes in the regional lymph node (**Figure 1**). Although the mature dendritic cells in the lymph node expressing a particular antigen on a class II HLA molecule interact with many different T lymphocytes, only an interaction with a T cell that uniquely recognizes the antigen in the HLA binding site results in stimulation of the adaptive immune response.

Thus, once the mature dendritic cell bearing the bacterial antigen-class II HLA complex encounters a T cell with the appropriate antigen-specific TCR, the adaptive phase of the immune response begins. Interaction between the antigen-presenting dendritic cell and the T cell must involve two molecular pairings. First, the T cell must recognize the HLA. There is a rule for this pairing: T cells expressing CD4 (T_h cells) recognize class II HLAs, whereas T cells expressing CD8 (T_c cells) recognize class I HLAs. A helpful mnemonic is the rule of 8: multiply the HLA class number by the CD number and the answer must be 8 to have the right match, for example, class II with CD4 = $2 \times 4 = 8$, class I with CD8 = $1 \times 8 = 8$. The second interaction that must take place is between the TCR and the antigen. Once these two pairings are successful, the rest of the adaptive response can proceed. Class I HLAs present native/host proteins, whereas class II HLAs present foreign proteins.

The successful pairing of class II HLA and CD4+ antigen-specific T cell is followed by the interaction of co-stimulatory molecules. This results in the release of cytokines to stimulate maturation of the CD4+ T cell. The stimulated CD4+ T cell can become a T_h1 cell upon stimulation with IL-12 and interferon-γ, or a T_h2 cell upon stimulation with IL-4. Once the appropriate cytokine stimulation is received, the antigen-specific T cell undergoes IL–mediated clonal expansion where the initial antigen-specific T cell is induced to proliferate into clones expressing the same TCRs of equivalent specificity and affinity, thereby amplifying the number of T cells that can mount a response specific for the antigen. The T_h1 cells are involved in cell-mediated immunity where they secrete interferon-γ to stimulate macrophages to kill phagocytosed bacteria. Memory T cells, which will survive for decades and serve as a source for clonal expansion in the event of future contact with the antigen, are also produced. T_h2 cells stimulate B cells and the humoral immune response.

Humoral Immune Response

B lymphocytes bind antigens via the antigen-specific BCR and internalize the antigen-BCR complex for processing. Thus, B cells can function as APCs similar to dendritic cells and macrophages. Antigen-specific T_h2 cells help to amplify the immune response by secreting IL-4, IL-5, and IL-13. These cytokines stimulate the proliferation, expansion, and differentiation of antigen-specific B cells into antibody-secreting plasma cells (**Figure 1**). Plasma cells secrete antibodies that bind to proteins that are a target of the immune response. In the humoral immune response, secreted antibodies can bind to the antigen and neutralize it, or they can activate complement factors to lyse bacteria, or they can opsonize the bacteria and make them more susceptible to phagocytosis. The first type of antibody secreted is IgM. Subsequent encounters lead to class switching of the antibody heavy chain by DNA recombination to produce IgG, which is still specific for the antigen. The IgG class is the most abundant class of immunoglobulin. As with T cells, memory B cells are also produced to allow a faster response the next time the individual encounters the antigen.

Cell-Mediated Immune Response

In addition to the humoral immune response, there is also cell-mediated adaptive immunity (**Figure 1**). Dendritic cells infected with virus or dendritic cells that have taken up viral antigens display them on class I HLAs via the endogenous pathway. Cytotoxic CD8+ T cells specific for the viral antigen recognize the class I HLA–viral antigen complex. Like B lymphocytes, CD8+ T lymphocytes require help from CD4+ T cells to mature. This help is provided by interactions between CD4+ T cells and dendritic cells. The dendritic cell presents endogenously produced (using the host cell protein-producing machinery) viral antigens on the HLA class I molecules. The class I–presented antigens are recognized by CD8+ T lymphocytes. In addition to the interaction with cytotoxic CD8+ T cells, the dendritic cells also interact with CD4+ T cells via HLA class II molecules. The CD4+ cell activates the dendritic cell, and when the CD8+ T cell encounters this dendritic cell to interact with the class I HLA–expressing viral antigen, the dendritic cell secretes IL-12 and other molecules to activate maturation of the CD8+ T cell into mature T_c cells (**Figure 1**). The mature CD8+ T cells can then move on to encounter virus-infected cells that display viral antigen on their class I HLAs and kill them via secretion of perforin to make holes in the plasma membranes of the infected cells, through which granzymes enter and mediate killing of the infected cell. Memory T_c cells are also created for future responses (**Figure 1**).

Bone Tissue and the Immune System

Although osteoblasts primarily function to maintain bone mass through deposition and formation of bone and regulation of osteoclasts and bone resorption, these cells also function to regulate the hematopoietic stem cell population.[5] The interaction of osteoblasts and osteoblast precursor cells with hematopoietic stem cells is regulated in part by parathyroid hormone (PTH). PTH induces a membrane-bound protein called Jagged 1 on osteoblasts. Jagged 1 stimulates Notch receptors on the membrane of hematopoietic stem cells and results in cell proliferation. Thus, osteoblastic cells are a regulatory component of the hematopoietic stem cell niche and thereby influence the development of immune cells.

Osteoclasts are derived from the myeloid-monocyte branch of hematopoietic cells.[5] Thus, macrophages, dendritic cells, and osteoclasts are derived from a similar precursor cell.[6] The microenvironment to which the common myeloid precursor cell is exposed determines whether it differentiates into innate immune cells or bone-resorbing cells. The presence of a protein called macrophage colony stimulating factor (M-CSF) converts the early-stage myeloid-monocyte precursor cells to late-stage precursors by increasing the expression of a cell surface receptor, RANK (receptor-activator of nuclear factor-κB), that is necessary for osteoclast differentiation. Osteoblasts regulate osteoclast formation by expression of the RANK ligand (RANKL). RANKL is a protein expressed on the surface of osteoblasts. When RANKL binds to the receptor RANK on myeloid osteoclast precursor cells it initiates a series of signaling events that lead to fusion of cells and differentiation into a bone-resorbing osteoclast.[6] Recently it has been shown that osteocytes embedded in the calcified bone matrix can express high levels of RANKL and are important modulators of bone metabolism and resorption.[7] Osteocytes respond to physical stress in the bone. In the absence of physical forces on bone, increased expression of RANKL on osteocytes is one of the factors that result in disuse-mediated bone loss.[7]

In addition to monocytes, macrophages are another innate immune system cell type that can also serve as a source of osteoclasts.[5] Macrophages become osteoclasts when exposed to RANKL. Another multinucleated cell is the giant cell, which is also involved in foreign-body reactions, chronic inflammatory granulomas, and immune responses. Macrophages that are exposed to the lymphocyte-secreted protein IL-4 differentiate into giant cells. Thus, how a macrophage determines whether to become a giant cell or an osteoclast upon fusion is governed by the local cytokine milieu with RANKL-inducing bone marrow–derived macrophages to form osteoclasts while IL-4 drives giant cell formation.[8]

A molecule that has recently gained importance in the fusion process and also serves as another pivotal molecule in the field of osteoimmunology is the dendritic cell–specific transmembrane protein (DC-STAMP).[9] DC-STAMP was initially identified in myeloid DCs. DC-STAMP has also been found in macrophages and osteoclasts. Its ligand and its function in myeloid dendritic cells are still under investigation; however, in bone marrow–derived macrophages, DC-STAMP is essential for multinucleation to form giant cells in the presence of IL-4, as well as osteoclasts in the presence of RANKL and M-CSF. Mice lacking DC-STAMP are osteopetrotic and they do not have osteoclasts. That DC-STAMP plays a potential role in autoimmunity and is essential for osteoclastogenesis further shows the link between the skeletal and immune systems.

The Immune System, Periprosthetic Bone Loss, and Implant Loosening

Implant loosening from wear-debris osteolysis accounts for a considerable percentage of implant failure (more than 70% in some estimates) and is a main factor that limits longevity of implants. The major findings in patients are a combined adaptive and innate immune response with marked soft-tissue inflammation that results in tissue destruction and pseudomembrane formation.[10-12] These findings have been observed in up to 10% of patients with total hip arthroplasty and to a lesser extent in patients with total knee arthroplasty. Implant loosening from wear-debris osteolysis is secondary to local and systemic inflammatory responses to particles in the prosthetic articulating surfaces. The local inflammatory response involves activation of monocyte-macrophages, which phagocytose wear particles and stimulate an immunologic cascade involving macrophage secretion of proinflammatory cytokines such as tumor necrosis factor (TNF)–α, IL-1, IL-6, and prostaglandin E_2. In addition, there are delayed-type T-cell–mediated hypersensitivity responses to the metals in the implants. Thus, wear-debris osteolysis involves activation of both the innate and adaptive immune systems through mechanisms similar to the pathways involved during a bacterial infection, as described earlier in this chapter. This immunologic cascade results in expression of RANKL and increased osteoclast differentiation. At the same time, there is decreased osteoblast differentiation, which is likely due to the presence of TNF-α. TNF-α has been shown to decrease the ability of osteoblast precursor cells to differentiate into osteoblasts. One mechanism involved in the TNF-α–mediated reduction in bone formation involves the suppression of bone morphogenetic protein (BMP) signaling by TNF-α.[13] Wear-debris particles can also inhibit osteoblast collagen synthesis and lead to osteoblast programmed cell death. The net effect of the activation of the immune system by wear-debris particles is decreased bone formation and increased bone resorption as well as local soft-tissue damage, which all lead to loosening of the implant.

Metal-on-metal articulations were broadly introduced over the past 5 to 10 years as a method to reduce the generation of wear debris particles and limit osteolysis adjacent to hip replacements. The metal-on-metal articulation involves the interface of two hard surfaces that are resistant to volumetric wear, in contrast to the metal-on-polyethylene articulation. However, although the metal-on-metal articulation reduces the total amount of volumetric wear, it generates an enormous number of metal particles in the submicron size range and also results in marked increases in serum metal ion levels. It is now recognized that these smaller metal particles and systemic ions result in the activation of a hypersensitivity type of reaction. The synovial membrane that forms in response to metal-on-metal hip replacements is composed of granulation tissues with a distinctive perivascular lymphocytic infiltration.[14]

Inflammatory Arthritis: A Paradigm for Osteoimmunology

Inflammatory arthritis is a paradigm for interactions between the immune and skeletal systems. Cytokines upregulated during inflammatory immune responses play a role in determining the fate of osteoclast precursor cells. One of the most important is TNF-α. The link between deregulation of TNF-α and inflammatory arthritis came out of observations that this cytokine is elevated in the synovial fluid and synovial membrane of rheumatoid and psoriatic arthritis patients.[15] In this context, TNF-α can cause joint inflammation and trigger cartilage destruction and can also stimulate osteoclast development.[15] One of the important advances in the treatment of inflammatory arthritis was the clinical use of TNF-α blocking agents. Several different biologic agents have been successfully used in patients with rheumatoid arthritis and psoriatic arthritis including infliximab, etanercept, adalimumab, and golimumab.

The importance of bone to lymphocytes has long been recognized, as the early development of lymphocytes is known to take place in the bone marrow. However, the idea that lymphocytes could be involved in bone remodeling was not appreciated until the discovery of RANKL. T cells express RANKL, and it has been confirmed that T-cell–derived RANKL is responsible for pathologic osteoclastogenesis and focal bone and cartilage erosion. Activated T cells can directly trigger osteoclastogenesis through RANKL, and systemic activation of T cells in vivo leads to a RANKL-mediated increase in osteoclastogenesis and bone loss.

T_h17 cells have been found to play a critical role in the pathogenesis of rheumatoid arthritis. IL-17, produced by T_h17 cells, is involved in promoting the expression of many proinflammatory cytokines, matrix metalloproteinases, and other mediators that contribute to inflammation and the erosion of cartilage and bone in rheumatoid arthritis.[16] It was also found that IL-17 in synovial fluid from patients with rheumatoid arthritis was significantly higher than that from patients with osteoarthritis. IL-17 in synovial fluid is a potent stimulator of osteoclastogenesis.[17]

Unlike T cells that directly influence osteoclastogenesis by expressing RANKL, B cells influence skeletal health primarily through indirect mechanisms. One important role of B cells in rheumatoid arthritis is that they are the source of autoantibodies such as rheumatoid factor (RF) that can form immune complexes that contribute to the disease process. Activated B cells with RF specificity are abundant in rheumatoid synovial membrane, and RF is detected in approximately 75% of patients with RA. Although RF is con-

sidered a serologic marker of rheumatoid arthritis, approximately 20% of patients with rheumatoid arthritis do not have RF in their blood. Large studies show a tendency for a slight increase in disease severity in patients with RF expression, and these patients have a higher mortality resulting from cardiovascular and respiratory diseases.[18,19] B cells may function as APCs to present antigen to CD4+ T cells, and they provide signals for T cell maturation and function. B cells in RA synovial membrane may also function by secreting proinflammatory cytokines that amplify T cell reactions.[4] Under normal conditions B cells can reduce basal bone turnover by producing osteoprotegerin, which is a natural inhibitor of RANKL.[20] Laboratory animals lacking B cells exhibit significant reductions in osteoprotegerin levels and elevated bone resorption. However, in inflammatory conditions, B cells express RANKL and participate in the pathogenesis of bone loss.[4]

Ankylosing spondylitis (spondyloarthritis) is unique among the inflammatory joint disorders in that the disorder involves both inflammation and bone formation.[21,22] A key feature is ankylosis of the axial joints with formation of a rigid spine and a strong association with inheritance of HLA-B27.[21] There is some evidence that the inflammation and bone formation may be in disequilibrium (not linked). The inflammation of spondyloarthritis is an osteitis that occurs in the bone marrow of the axial spine. This results in vertebral body bone loss, osteopenia, and an increased risk of fracture. Simultaneously there is a process of syndesmophyte at the enthesis where capsule, tendons, and ligaments attach to the bone. The subsequent bone formation typically results in fusion of adjacent vertebral bodies. Although anti–TNF-α therapies prevent osteitis, the bone formation is affected in patients with spondyloarthritis, suggesting that the inflammation and bone formation are not directly linked.[22]

Chronic Recurrent Multifocal Osteomyelitis

Chronic recurrent multifocal osteomyelitis (CRMO) occurs in children and is now considered part of a spectrum of related inflammatory bone diseases. Other entities include synovitis-acne-pustulosis-hyperostosis-osteitis syndrome, Majeed syndrome, deficiency of IL-1 receptor antagonist, and cherubism.[23,24] These conditions have the shared features of activation of the innate immune system with spontaneous inflammation and with the absence of autoantibodies and T cell activation.[25-27] Sterile bone inflammation presents as a lytic lesion with a sclerotic border.[23] Lesions are often multifocal and occur in the metaphysis of the long bones, spine, and ribs and are painful, particularly at night. The clavicle is a common site of involvement, whereas the pelvis is less frequently involved.[23] Pathology evaluation shows subacute or chronic osteomyelitis with neutrophils, lymphocytes and plasma cells, and areas of fibrosis and sclerosis.[23-25] Fever is rare and there is typically minimal elevation of the erythrocyte sedimentation rate and C-reactive protein level.[25] Up to 25% of cases are associated with a family history of inflammatory conditions, including psoriasis and inflammatory bone disease.[24]

The standard treatment is the use of NSAIDS,[24] which lead to symptom relief in up to 80% of children with CRMO.[25] In cases of recalcitrant pain following the use of NSAIDs, bisphosphonates have been effective in some cases. The most experience has been obtained with pamidronate, but the evidence to date is limited to small case reports.[25] Finally, there are several case reports of use of biologic agents in children with recalcitrant CRMO.[25,28] Both anti-TNF therapy and anti–IL-1 therapy has been used with moderate success.[28] The use of recombinant IL receptor antagonist protein (anakira) in particular may be highly effective in deficiency of IL-1 receptor antagonist, a condition with sterile chronic multifocal osteomyelitis lesions that occur secondary to a genetic defect resulting in deficiency of IL receptor antagonist protein.[29]

Biologic Agents and the Treatment of Inflammatory Conditions

The development of biologic agents that target specific components of the immune system to reduce the autoimmune response has transformed the treatment of rheumatoid arthritis and other inflammatory conditions.[30] The biologic agents are developed by genetic engineering in which gene fragments to make a recombinant protein are artificially assembled and then inserted into nonhuman cell cultures to make a large amount of the desired protein. Biologic agents that are used clinically for rheumatoid arthritis include various monoclonal antibodies and fusion proteins (**Table 3**). Fusion proteins are artificial proteins produced by genetic rearrangement of the coding region of two different genes to make a novel protein. One method used in the development of fusion proteins is the fusion of the Fc (constant portion) of the IgG1 antibody to a binding site of another protein that specifically identifies the immune target. The Fc region of IgG1 provides stability and increases the half-life of the recombinant protein, whereas the binding region performs the drug function. This approach has been used to construct TNF-α inhibitors (etanercept) and an inhibitor of T-cell activation (abatacept). More common is the production of recombinant monoclonal antibodies. Certolizumab pegol is composed of the Fab fragment (binding portion) of an anti-TNF monoclonal antibody that is covalently attached to polyethylene glycol. The polyethylene glycol component reduces immunogenicity, increases half-life, and prevents the drug from crossing the placenta.

Because it is very expensive to make and purify recombinant proteins, they are typically used in rheumatoid arthritis as second-line therapies after failure of initial treatment.[30,31] The initial treatment of rheumatoid arthritis involves the use of disease-modifying antirheumatic drugs, which include combinations of methotrexate, leflunomide,

hydroxychloroquine, minocyclinem, and sulfasalazine.[30] A large number of biologic agents have been developed and approved for the treatment of rheumatoid arthritis. The first line of biologic therapy for patients in whom treatment with disease-modifying antirheumatic drugs has failed is use of the TNF-α inhibitors.[30] These include agents such as adalimumab, certolizumab pegol, etanercept, golimumab, and infliximab (**Table 3**). Approximately 20% of patients do not respond to anti-TNF therapy and are candidates for other biologic agents that target IL-1 (anakinra), IL-6 (tocilizumab), B cells (rituximab), or T cells (abatacept).[30]

Rheumatoid arthritis is a model for the potential of biologic agents and recombinant proteins as modulators of the immune response. Currently there are fewer biologic agents available to modulate other diseases, such as systemic lupus erythematosus (**Table 4**) and osteoporosis and inflammatory bone loss (**Table 5**). Belimumab, a monoclonal antibody that binds to and blocks the activity of B-cell–activating factor, is the only biologic agent approved to date for systemic lupus erythematosus;[32] interferon-γ is involved in its pathogenesis. B-cell–activating factor is secreted from a variety of cells in response to interferon-γ.[32] The receptors for B-cell–activating factor receptors are present on mature B cells. Denosumab, a monoclonal antibody that binds to and blocks RANKL, is the only biologic agent approved to date for the treatment of osteoporosis[33] (**Table 5**) RANKL is secreted by osteoblasts and stromal cells. The binding of RANKL to RANK receptors present on macrophages stimulates osteoclastogenesis. RANKL and the receptor are also expressed by and on T cells and dendritic cells. Thus, denosumab may have some immunomodulatory effects.[33]

Transplant Immunology

Advancements in surgical techniques and tissue preservation have made it possible to consider transplantation of allograft limbs.[34] More than 45 hand transplantations have been performed around the world.[34] Graft survival is dependent on the immune response to the transplanted tissue and the success of immunosuppressive therapy.[34] The major immunologic stimulus in composite tissue grafts is skin, which is highly immunogenic.[35]

The basis of graft survival is dependent on matching HLA/major histocompatibility haplotypes between donor and recipient.[36] There are numerous immunosuppressive agents designed to suppress the immune reaction and rejection of nonself, donor tissue. Some of the common immunosuppressive agents are cyclosporine, which inhibits IL-2 production by T_h cells; FK-506 (tacrolimus), which is similar to cyclosporine but more potent; muromonab-CD3, which is an antibody against CD3 (which is expressed on T cells); and azathioprine and mycophenolate mofetil, which both inhibit nucleic acid synthesis and therefore inhibit lymphoid proliferation.[34,36]

The major adverse effect of immunosuppressive agents is the risk of chronic viral or fungal infections, such as cytomegalovirus. There are four types of transplant rejection

Table 3

Biologic Therapies Used for the Treatment of Rheumatoid Arthritis

Biologic Agent/Drug	Binding Target	Biologic Effect	Recombinant Drug Structure	Indications
Abatacept	CD80 protein on surface of APCs	Blocks costimulatory signal necessary for APC activation of T cells	Fusion protein of extracellular domain of CTLA-4 to IgG1 Fc region (human)	Inadequate response to anti-TNF therapy
Adalimumab	Soluble TNF-α	Blocks immune modulation by TNF	Human anti-TNF monoclonal antibody	Insufficient response to DMARDs
Anakinra	Soluble IL-1	Blocks immune modulation by IL-1	Recombinant IL-1 receptor antagonist (human)	Inadequate response to anti-TNF therapy
Certolizumab pegol	Soluble TNF-α	Blocks immune modulation by TNF	PEGylated Fab fragment of anti-TNF monoclonal antibody	Insufficient response to DMARDs. PEG does not cross the placenta so theoretically safer in pregnancy
Etanercept	Soluble TNF-α	Blocks immune modulation by TNF	Fusion protein of TNF receptor 2 to IgG1 Fc region (human)	Insufficient response to DMARDs
Golimumab	Soluble TNF-α	Blocks immune modulation by TNF	Human anti-TNF monoclonal antibody	Insufficient response to DMARDs
Infliximab	Soluble TNF-α	Blocks immune modulation by TNF	Mouse/human chimeric anti-TNF monoclonal antibody	Insufficient response to DMARDs
Rituximab	CD20 on surface of B cells	Causes apoptosis of immature B cells	Mouse/human chimeric anti-CD20 monoclonal antibody	Inadequate response to anti-TNF therapy
Tocilizumab	Soluble IL-6	Blocks immune modulation by IL-6	Human anti–IL-6 monoclonal antibody	Inadequate response to anti-TNF therapy and in RA with severe structural joint damage

These agents are approved for the treatment of rheumatoid arthritis and are used in a variety of other inflammatory conditions, including psoriatic arthritis, ankylosing spondylitis, and inflammatory bowel disease. The first line of biologic therapy involves use of anti-TNF-α inhibitors. Patients with an insufficient response to these agents may respond to subsequent treatment with the non–TNF-α agents that target, IL-1, IL-6, T cells, and B cells, respectively. APC = antigen-presenting cell, CTLA = cytotoxic T-lymphocyte antigen, DMARDs = disease-modifying antirheumatic drugs, IL = interleukin, PEG = polyethylene glycol, RA = rheumatoid arthritis, TNF = tumor necrosis factor.

mediated by both humoral and cell-mediated arms of the adaptive immune system: hyperacute, accelerated acute, acute, and chronic. The hyperacute type of rejection occurs in the operating room as the host circulation perfuses the grafted tissue. It is based on humoral immunity and is mediated by antibodies in the host that react immediately with antigens in the tissue. This results in rapid necrosis of the newly transplanted tissue. Treatment of hyperacute graft rejection is to remove the grafted tissue. The accelerated acute mode of transplant rejection involves cell-mediated immune mechanisms involving T cells. Acute rejection of transplanted tissue is the most common form of transplant rejection. It also involves a T-cell–mediated response to the grafted tissue. Chronic transplant rejection occurs several

Table 4

Biologic Therapy Used for the Treatment of Systemic Lupus Erythematosus

Biologic Agent/Drug	Binding Target	Biologic Effect	Recombinant Drug Structure	Indications
Belimumab	Soluble BAFF	Blocks B cell activation by BAFF. BAFF receptors are present on mature B cells	Human anti-BAFF monoclonal antibody	SLE

Belimumab is the only biologic agent approved to date for systemic lupus erythematosus (SLE). Interferon gamma is involved in the pathogenesis of SLE. B-cell–activating factor (BAFF) is secreted from a variety of cells in response to interferon-γ. The BAFF receptors are present on mature B cells. In contrast, rituximab, which is approved for rheumatoid arthritis treatment, targets CD20, a protein that is found only on immature B cells.

Table 5

Biologic Therapy Used for the Treatment of Osteoporosis

Biologic Agent/Drug	Binding Target	Biologic Effect	Recombinant Drug Structure	Indications
Denosumab	RANKL	Blocks binding to RANK receptor on macrophages and prevents osteoclast formation	Human anti-RANKL monoclonal antibody	Osteoporosis and solid bone metastasis; ongoing trials to assess bone loss multiple myeloma, giant cell tumor, and rheumatoid arthritis

Denosumab is the only biologic agent approved to date for osteoporosis. RANKL is secreted by osteoblasts and stromal cells. The binding of RANKL to RANK receptors present on macrophages stimulates osteoclastogenesis. RANKL and the receptor are also expressed by and on T cells and dendritic cells. Thus, denosumab may have some immunomodulatory effects. RANK = receptor-activator of nuclear factor- κB, RANKL = receptor-activator of nuclear factor- κB ligand.

years after the initial transplant, and it can involve both cell-mediated and humoral immunity. Use of immunosuppressive agents has helped reduce the effect of acute rejection in hand transplantation. Chronic rejection appears to be rare.

Because of the lack of cellular components in processed allograft bone, there is minimal if any allogeneic reaction. Cartilage allograft transplantations also have minimal allogeneic reaction, primarily because the transplanted articular cartilage is avascular.

Immune Reaction to BMPs

BMP-2 and BMP-7 have both been approved for human conditions with delayed bone healing. BMP-2 has been approved for use in acute open tibia fractures treated with intramedullary nailing and for use in lumbar spine fusions in association with cages. BMP-7 has been authorized for humanitarian use in long bone nonunions when autograft is unfeasible and other methods have failed. The BMPs have been frequently used for other indications in which bone healing is potentially compromised.

There is an increasing number of reports regarding the development of an acute inflammatory soft-tissue reaction in patients treated with BMPs. There are several reports of acute swelling in association with use in cervical spine surgery with compromise of the airway.[37] Several other reports document severe soft-tissue inflammation and swelling in pediatric patients who have received BMPs.[38,39] A recent study in rats demonstrated formation of a granuloma in animals treated with BMP with a dose-dependent increase in the levels of several inflammatory cytokines, including IL-6 and TNF-α.[40] However, the manner in which BMPs cause these inflammatory reactions remains unclear.

References

1. Schenten D, Medzhitov R: The control of adaptive immune responses by the innate immune system. *Adv Immunol* 2011; 109:87-124.

2. Mahbub S, Brubaker AL, Kovacs EJ: Aging of the innate immune system: An update. *Curr Immunol Rev* 2011;7(1):104-115.

1: Basic Principles of Orthopaedic Surgery

3. Winer S, Winer DA: The adaptive immune system as a fundamental regulator of adipose tissue inflammation and insulin resistance. *Immunol Cell Biol* 2012; 90(8):755-762.

4. Horowitz MC, Fretz JA, Lorenzo JA: How B cells influence bone biology in health and disease. *Bone* 2010;47(3):472-479.

5. Lorenzo J, Horowitz M, Choi Y: Osteoimmunology: Interactions of the bone and immune system. *Endocr Rev* 2008; 29(4):403-440.

6. Miyamoto T, Ohneda O, Arai F, et al: Bifurcation of osteoclasts and dendritic cells from common progenitors. *Blood* 2001;98(8):2544-2554.

7. Xiong J, Onal M, Jilka RL, Weinstein RS, Manolagas SC, O'Brien CA: Matrix-embedded cells control osteoclast formation. *Nat Med* 2011;17(10):1235-1241.

8. Helming L, Gordon S: The molecular basis of macrophage fusion. *Immunobiology* 2007;212(9-10):785-793.

9. Yagi M, Miyamoto T, Sawatani Y, et al: DC-STAMP is essential for cell-cell fusion in osteoclasts and foreign body giant cells. *J Exp Med* 2005;202(3):345-351.

10. Cobelli N, Scharf B, Crisi GM, Hardin J, Santambrogio L: Mediators of the inflammatory response to joint replacement devices. *Nat Rev Rheumatol* 2011;7(10):600-608.

11. Catelas I, Jacobs JJ: Biologic activity of wear particles. *Instr Course Lect* 2010;59:3-16.

12. St Pierre CA, Chan M, Iwakura Y, Ayers DC, Kurt-Jones EA, Finberg RW: Periprosthetic osteolysis: Characterizing the innate immune response to titanium wear-particles. *J Orthop Res* 2010;28(11):1418-1424.

13. Mukai T, Otsuka F, Otani H, et al: TNF-alpha inhibits BMP-induced osteoblast differentiation through activating SAPK/JNK signaling. *Biochem Biophys Res Commun* 2007;356(4):1004-1010.

14. Haddad FS, Thakrar RR, Hart AJ, et al: Metal-on-metal bearings: The evidence so far. *J Bone Joint Surg Br* 2011;93(5):572-579.

15. Schett G, Coates LC, Ash ZR, Finzel S, Conaghan PG: Structural damage in rheumatoid arthritis, psoriatic arthritis, and ankylosing spondylitis: Traditional views, novel insights gained from TNF blockade, and concepts for the future. *Arthritis Res Ther* 2011;13(Suppl 1):S4.

16. van Hamburg JP, Asmawidjaja PS, Davelaar N, et al: Th17 cells, but not Th1 cells, from patients with early rheumatoid arthritis are potent inducers of matrix metalloproteinases and proinflammatory cytokines upon synovial fibroblast interaction, including autocrine interleukin-17A production. *Arthritis Rheum* 2011;63(1):73-83.

17. Okamoto K, Takayanagi H: Osteoclasts in arthritis and Th17 cell development. *Int Immunopharmacol* 2011;11(5):543-548.

18. Klaasen R, Cantaert T, Wijbrandts CA, et al: The value of rheumatoid factor and anti-citrullinated protein antibodies as predictors of response to infliximab in rheumatoid arthritis: An exploratory study. *Rheumatology (Oxford)* 2011; 50(8):1487-1493.

19. Gonzalez A, Icen M, Kremers HM, et al: Mortality trends in rheumatoid arthritis: The role of rheumatoid factor. *J Rheumatol* 2008;35(6):1009-1014.

20. Li Y, Toraldo G, Li A, et al: B cells and T cells are critical for the preservation of bone homeostasis and attainment of peak bone mass in vivo. *Blood* 2007;109(9):3839-3848.

21. Tam LS, Gu J, Yu D: Pathogenesis of ankylosing spondylitis. *Nat Rev Rheumatol* 2010;6(7):399-405.

22. Schett G: Independent development of inflammation and new bone formation in ankylosing spondylitis. *Arthritis Rheum* 2012; published online ahead of print February 21.

23. Iyer RS, Thapa MM, Chew FS: Chronic recurrent multifocal osteomyelitis: Review. *AJR Am J Roentgenol* 2011;196(6, Suppl):S87-S91.

24. Hashkes PJ, Toker O: Autoinflammatory syndromes. *Pediatr Clin North Am* 2012;59(2):447-470.

25. Twilt M, Laxer RM: Clinical care of children with sterile bone inflammation. *Curr Opin Rheumatol* 2011;23(5):424-431.

26. Chitu V, Ferguson PJ, de Bruijn R, et al: Primed innate immunity leads to autoinflammatory disease in PSTPIP2-deficient cmo mice. *Blood* 2009;114(12):2497-2505.

27. Galeazzi M, Gasbarrini G, Ghirardello A, et al: Autoinflammatory syndromes. *Clin Exp Rheumatol* 2006;24(1, Suppl 40):S79-S85.

28. Eleftheriou D, Gerschman T, Sebire N, Woo P, Pilkington CA, Brogan PA: Biologic therapy in refractory chronic nonbacterial osteomyelitis of childhood. *Rheumatology (Oxford)* 2010;49(8):1505-1512.

29. Schnellbacher C, Ciocca G, Menendez R, et al: Deficiency of interleukin-1 receptor antagonist responsive to anakinra. *Pediatr Dermatol* 2012; published online ahead of print April 4.

30. Singh JA, Furst DE, Bharat A, et al: 2012 update of the 2008 American College of Rheumatology recommendations for the use of disease-modifying antirheumatic drugs and biologic agents in the treatment of rheumatoid arthritis. *Arthritis Care Res (Hoboken)* 2012;64(5):625-639.

31. Fautrel B: Economic benefits of optimizing anchor therapy for rheumatoid arthritis. *Rheumatology (Oxford)* 2012; 51(Suppl 4):iv21-iv26.

32. Lo MS, Tsokos GC: Treatment of systemic lupus erythematosus: New advances in targeted therapy. *Ann N Y Acad Sci* 2012;1247:138-152.

33. Sinningen K, Tsourdi E, Rauner M, Rachner TD, Hamann C, Hofbauer LC: Skeletal and extraskeletal actions of denosumab. *Endocrine* 2012;42(1):52-62.

34. Tobin GR, Breidenbach WC III, Ildstad ST, Marvin MM, Buell JF, Ravindra KV: The history of human composite tissue allotransplantation. *Transplant Proc* 2009;41(2):466-471.

35. Thaunat O, Badet L, El-Jaafari A, Kanitakis J, Dubernard JM, Morelon E: Composite tissue allograft extends a helping hand to transplant immunologists. *Am J Transplant* 2006; 6(10):2238-2242.

36. Schneeberger S, Gorantla VS, Hautz T, Pulikkottil B, Margreiter R, Lee WP: Immunosuppression and rejection in human hand transplantation. *Transplant Proc* 2009;41(2):472-475.

37. Yaremchuk KL, Toma MS, Somers ML, Peterson E: Acute airway obstruction in cervical spinal procedures with bone

morphogenetic proteins. *Laryngoscope* 2010;120(10):1954-1957.

38. MacDonald KM, Swanstrom MM, McCarthy JJ, Nemeth BA, Guliani TA, Noonan KJ: Exaggerated inflammatory response after use of recombinant bone morphogenetic protein in recurrent unicameral bone cysts. *J Pediatr Orthop* 2010; 30(2):199-205.

39. Ritting AW, Weber EW, Lee MC: Exaggerated inflammatory response and bony resorption from BMP-2 use in a pediatric forearm nonunion. *J Hand Surg Am* 2012;37(2):316-321.

40. Lee KB, Taghavi CE, Song KJ, et al: Inflammatory characteristics of rhBMP-2 in vitro and in an in vivo rodent model. *Spine (Phila Pa 1976)* 2011;36(3):E149-E154.

1: Basic Principles of Orthopaedic Surgery

Section 2

Physiology of Musculoskeletal Tissues

Section Editor

Joshua J. Jacobs, MD

Chapter 7

Thromboembolic Disease and Fat Embolism Syndrome

Vincent D. Pellegrini Jr, MD

Introduction

Venous thromboembolic disease (VTED) and fat embolism syndrome have a similar underlying pathophysiology that depends on intravasation of the adipose tissue of the bone marrow into the vascular tree. In both conditions the lung acts as an essential filter in clearing the embolic material from the bloodstream and determining the nature of the body's response to the embolic insult. The differences in the clinical presentation of the two conditions depend upon the size and aggregate volume of the embolus as well as the nature of the embolic material invoking a response from the lung. The embolic material in VTED primarily is clotted blood, and in fat embolism syndrome it consists of fat globules enmeshed in platelets.

Considering that musculoskeletal injury, disease, and related surgical procedures frequently involve disruption of the marrow contents and associated fat, it is no wonder that these clinical conditions can complicate the course of orthopaedic treatment. Orthopaedic surgeons need to understand the pathophysiology and treatment of these conditions, not only for effective patient care and communication with consulting physicians but also (and even more importantly) to place the specific treatment of these complications into the context of overall orthopaedic management of the patient.

Dr. Pellegrini or an immediate family member has received royalties from DePuy; serves as a paid consultant to or is an employee of Covidien and DePuy; and serves as a board member, owner, officer, or committee member of the American Orthopaedic Association, the Hip Society, the University of Maryland Medical Center, the Council of Academic Societies of the Association of American Medical Colleges, and the Residency Review Committee for Orthopaedic Surgery of the Accreditation Council for Graduate Medical Education.

For instance, appropriate prophylaxis for VTED after total joint arthroplasty cannot be thoughtfully prescribed without a balanced consideration of the perioperative bleeding risk inherent to the arthroplasty procedure. The orthopaedic surgeon is much more likely to be familiar with this risk than a pulmonologist who is consulting on anticoagulant choice and administration.

Venous Thromboembolic Disease

The most significant perioperative threat to the life of a patient undergoing arthroplasty is VTED, and specifically pulmonary embolism (PE). In a series of 7,959 total hip arthroplasties (THAs) from 1962 to 1973, the overall incidence of PE was 7.89% and the incidence of fatal PE was 1.04%.[1] As Charnley[2] stated, "The possibility of fatal pulmonary embolism after total hip replacement is a hip surgeon's constant worry...no matter how rare this might be." In addition, bleeding complications related to VTED prophylaxis have become the most common cause of hospital readmission after hip or knee replacement. VTED remains one of the most controversial topics in contemporary orthopaedics.

Deep venous thrombosis (DVT) is the most common precursor of PE. The predominant form of DVT after total knee arthroplasty (TKA) is in the calf distal to the trifurcation, probably as initiated by stasis. Proximal DVT after TKA typically results from propagation of a clot originating in the calf (**Figure 1**). Proximal thrombi, specifically segmental clots in the femoral vein at the level of the lesser trochanter, predominate after THA and probably are initiated by intimal injury resulting from torsion of the vein during femoral preparation (**Figure 2**). PE traditionally was diagnosed by pulmonary arteriography (**Figure 3**) but now is most sensitively identified by CT of the chest. The prevalence of PE is difficult to quantify, and its clinical importance is difficult to ascertain. In the general population, the

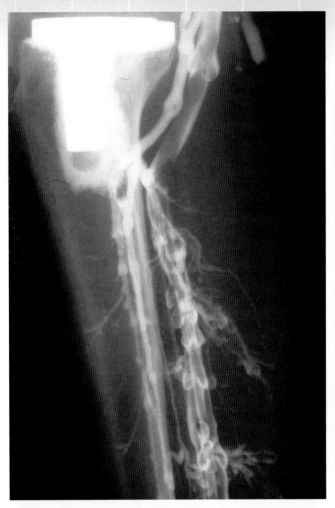

Figure 1 Contrast venogram showing calf thrombosis extending proximally into the popliteal vein after TKA. (Courtesy of Vincent D. Pellegrini, Jr, MD, Baltimore, MD.)

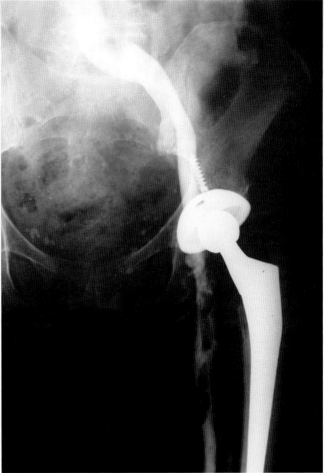

Figure 2 Contrast venogram showing segmental proximal femoral vein thrombosis at the level of the lesser trochanter after THA. (Courtesy of Vincent D. Pellegrini, Jr, MD, Baltimore, MD.)

frequency of autopsy-proven fatal PE is 2.5 times that of symptomatic nonfatal PE. In addition, DVT may be solely responsible for morbidity related to chronic venous insufficiency. Five years after surgery, signs and symptoms of postthrombotic syndrome were found in 67% of patients with asymptomatic, venographically confirmed postoperative DVT, compared with 32% of patients who had a negative postoperative venogram.[3] Postthrombotic morbidity is more common after idiopathic DVT than after postoperative DVT,[3] probably because most postoperative thrombosis is nonocclusive, and flow past the thrombus is maintained.

Epidemiology
Before Routine Prophylaxis
Historically, the risk of DVT in an unprotected patient was 70% to 84% after THA or TKA; the risk of symptomatic PE approached 15%, and the risk of fatal PE was 1% to 3.4%.[4,5] Coventry et al[4] reported a 3.4% fatal PE rate after 2,012 consecutive THAs from 1969 to 1971; the average duration of surgery was 2.4 hours, the average blood loss was 1,650 mL, patients were on bed rest for 1 week, and the mean postoperative hospital stay was 3 weeks. Since that time, the incidence of DVT after total joint arthroplasty has been reduced. The reasons for the decrease are widely accepted as being the implementation of several pharmacologic and mechanical prophylactic regimens as well as improved surgical techniques and anesthetic management.[6,7] Data from two studies with a 3- to 6-month follow-up revealed a fatal PE rate as low as 0.12% to 0.35% in 4,594 patients who underwent THA without any type of chemoprophylaxis.[7-9] Compared with patients in earlier studies, these patients benefited from more rapid postoperative mobilization and a shorter length of hospital stay. However, the rarity of fatal PE increases the difficulty of showing a statistically convincing reduction in the rate. With further decreases in the likelihood of fatal PE, it will be necessary to balance the incremental benefit of eliminating PE by using potent anticoagulants against the risk of bleeding complications induced by these anticoagulants.[9] In 1977, Johnson, Green, and Charnley[1] reported a 1.68%

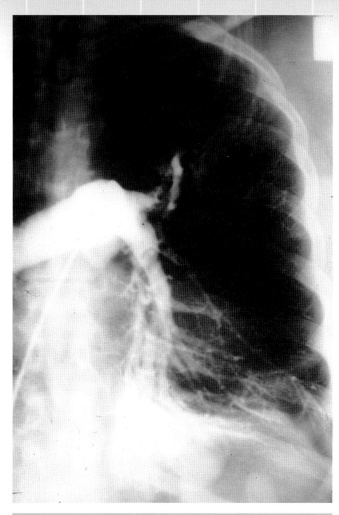

Figure 3 Pulmonary arteriogram revealing the presence of pulmonary emboli. (Courtesy of Vincent D. Pellegrini, Jr, MD, Baltimore, MD.)

overall perioperative mortality after 7,959 THAs, in the absence of VTED prophylaxis. Two later studies involving a total of 12,769 patients undergoing THA found a 1.71% overall mortality rate without VTED prophylaxis.[7,8] Not surprisingly, the current management of VTED risk is as variable as the underlying perceptions of the prevalence of VTED.

Knowledge concerning the mechanisms of venous thrombosis and patient predisposition to the condition has increased along with the understanding of the basic science of coagulation. At the same time, the relative risks and benefits of prophylaxis, the choice and duration of specific agents in the face of abbreviated hospitalization, the role of routine diagnostic surveillance, and guidelines for treatment of established VTED have come under renewed scrutiny.

After Routine Prophylaxis

Routine prophylaxis for VTED after THA or TKA became the standard of care in North America after it was recommended by the National Institutes of Health (NIH) Consen-

sus Conference in 1986.[10] Low-intensity warfarin is the agent most commonly used by orthopaedic surgeons during the past three decades.[11,12] Although warfarin use has considerably reduced the incidence of DVT, screening venography reveals asymptomatic venous system thrombi in 15% to 25% of patients after THA and in 35% to 50% after TKA.[6] A similarly smaller reduction in venographic DVT after TKA than after THA has been observed with the use of newer anticoagulant agents.[6] The overall risk of DVT is two to three times greater after TKA than after THA with the use of current prophylactic agents.[6] The frequency of clinically significant bleeding events in patients treated with warfarin was found to be reduced with acceptance of low-intensity anticoagulation; the frequency was 8% to 12% when a prothrombin time index of 2.0 was routinely targeted, but it was 1% to 2% when the targeted prothrombin time index was 1.3 to 1.5 (International Normalized Ratio [INR] 2.0 to 2.5).[13] Although these data suggest that VTED is more refractory to standard prophylaxis after TKA than after THA, 85% to 90% of thrombi after TKA occur below the venous trifurcation in the deep calf veins, and the immediate risk of embolization is much smaller.[5] In contrast, the distribution of DVT after THA historically was 40% proximal and 60% distal.[4,6] It has been reported for newer prophylactic agents that fewer than 10% of thrombi after THA are located proximal to the trifurcation, with the remainder occurring in the calf.[14] Because 85% to 90% of all DVTs after THA or TKA occur in the calf when current prophylaxis is used, greater attention is being given to distal thrombotic disease. Longitudinal surveillance studies found that 17% to 23% of these distal thrombi extend to the more proximal veins of the thigh, where they acquire considerable embolic potential.[15,16] The relationship between asymptomatic nonocclusive calf clots and late postthrombotic syndrome appearing as chronic venous insufficiency is unclear, but the considerable embolic potential of postoperative calf thrombi means that anticoagulant therapy with extended prophylaxis should be continued for several weeks after surgery.[14] DVT in the calf was reported to have a proximal propagation rate of almost 25% in general surgical patients, and symptomatic PE was reported in as many as 31% of patients with untreated deep calf thrombosis after THA.[15,16] Spontaneous calf DVT in a patient who is ambulatory and has not recently undergone a surgical procedure is unlikely to be a precursor of PE, however.

Pathogenesis

The Virchow triad, consisting of stasis, hypercoagulability, and damage to the intimal wall, remains the basis of the conceptual understanding of the mechanism of coagulation. Perturbations in elements of the triad are responsible for the abnormalities of thrombosis after musculoskeletal injury, disease, or surgery. Recent discoveries and improved understanding of the clotting cascade form the basis of new therapeutic approaches to preventing and treating thrombotic disease (**Figure 4**).

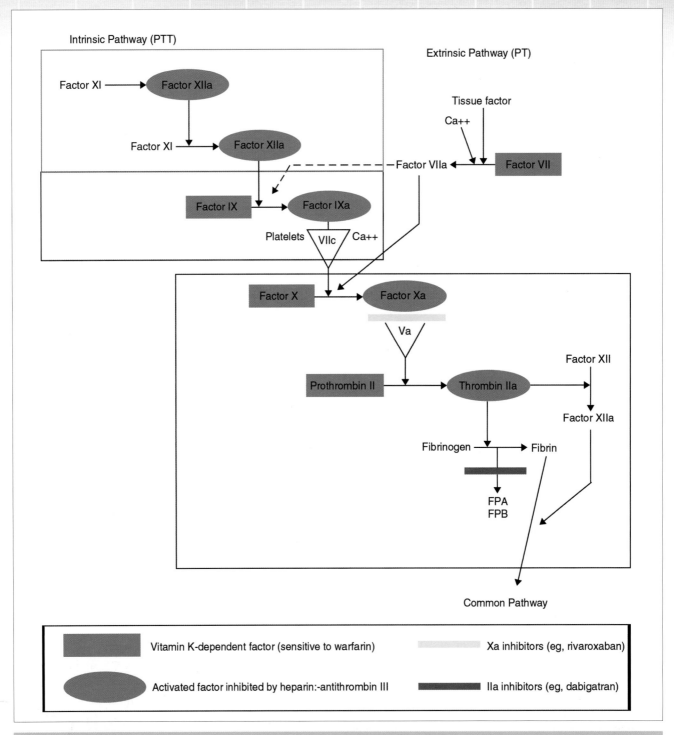

Figure 4 Schematic diagram showing the clotting cascade, with critical points of interference by anticoagulant agents. FPA = fibrinopeptide A, FPB = fibrinopeptide B, PT = Prothrombin time, PTT= partial thromboplastin time. (Adapted with permission from Stead RB: Regulation of hemostasis, in Golhaber SZ, ed: *Pulmonary Embolism and Deep Venous Thromboembolism.* Philadelphia, PA, WB Saunders, 1995, p 32.)

Familial Thrombophilia and Factor V Leiden

Familial thrombophilia is the heritable tendency to develop severe and recurrent VTED, often spontaneously. This condition has not been adequately explained by any deficiency of circulating anticoagulants; levels of proteins C and S as well as antithrombin III were rarely found to be low in patients with familial thrombophilia. Mutations in genetic material encoding proteins C and S or antithrombin III were found to account for fewer than 5% of all incidences of familial thrombophilia.[17] In 1994, a single amino acid substitution of glutamine for arginine in the protein C cleavage region of factor V was reported to occur in 50% of patients with familial thrombophilia, compared with 3% to 7% of the general population.[18] This single nucleotide substitution, known as factor V Leiden, is responsible for resistance of activated factor V to cleavage inactivation by protein C, which normally provides a physiologic check on the clotting cascade.

Variable phenotypic expression of factor V Leiden subsequently was found to be responsible for a host of clinical disease states related to thrombosis. In more than half of all individuals with factor V Leiden, DVT will develop in the presence of a single additional risk factor, such as a long bone fracture or total joint arthroplasty. The presence of factor V Leiden predicts a 60% occurrence of DVT during the first trimester of pregnancy.[19] The Physicians' Health Study followed approximately 15,000 men for cardiovascular events and observed a 4% to 6% prevalence of factor V Leiden among those not experiencing myocardial infarction, stroke, or another related event; in contrast, factor V Leiden was found among 11.6% of those with PE or DVT (increased relative risk, 3.5 times).[20] Similarly, the incidence of factor V Leiden was 26% among men older than 60 years with primary spontaneous DVT. Mixed findings have been reported from preliminary investigations of activated protein C resistance and VTED after total joint arthroplasty. Two North American studies of patients who had undergone THA or TKA found no correlation between the presence of factor V Leiden (or depletion of any other circulating anticoagulant) and the occurrence of VTED.[21,22] This negative observation can be explained by the effect of a thrombogenic stimulus associated with violation of the medullary canal during total joint arthroplasty, which is intense enough to overshadow any heritable predisposition to thrombosis imparted by factor V Leiden.

Thrombogenesis After Musculoskeletal Injury

It has long been recognized that VTED is more refractory to standard prophylaxis after orthopaedic procedures than after general surgical procedures. This phenomenon was first recognized as the inefficacy of subcutaneous heparin for DVT prevention after THA, despite the successful use of subcutaneous heparin after major abdominal or chest surgery. The discrepancy was found to be secondary to a decline in circulating levels of antithrombin III (a binding intermediary necessary for the heparins to be clinically effective) that occurred in conjunction with a decline in several other acute-phase reactants after skeletal injury or manipulation of the medullary canal (as occurs during total joint arthroplasty).[23]

The findings of a study by Geerts et al[24] of patients with multiple injuries and an injury severity score higher than 9 underscores the influence of skeletal trauma on the clotting cascade. Contrast venography of 349 patients showed an overall DVT prevalence of 58% and a proximal DVT rate of 18%. Like patients who undergo total joint arthroplasty, most of these patients were asymptomatic; only 3 of 201 DVTs (1.5%) were clinically evident. The overall incidence of DVT associated with specific single-system trauma was 41% for injury to the face, chest, or abdomen; 39% for closed head injury; 66% for lower extremity fracture; and 68% for spinal cord injury. The overwhelming influence of fracture on the clotting cascade was shown by a DVT incidence of 61% with pelvic fracture, 77% with tibial shaft fracture, and 80% with femoral shaft fracture; isolated femoral or tibial shaft fracture was associated with a relative DVT risk almost five times as high as that of the overall group. Spinal cord injury was associated with an 81% incidence of DVT and an odds ratio of 8.5, compared with the total group.[24]

The same investigators subsequently studied the effect of VTED prophylaxis on 344 patients with polytrauma who were randomly assigned to one of two anticoagulant protocols.[24] Patients receiving unfractionated heparin had an overall DVT incidence of 44% (60 of 136 patients), compared with 31% of those receiving enoxaparin (40 of 129 patients, $P = 0.014$); the rates for proximal DVT were 15% (20 of 136) and 6% (8 of 129), respectively ($P = 0.012$). These findings highlight the relative ineffectiveness of unfractionated heparins for clinical thromboprophylaxis when circulating levels of antithrombin III have been reduced. Major bleeding complications were five times more common with enoxaparin therapy (2.9%) than with heparin (0.6%, $P = 0.12$). Because of their propensity for causing increased bleeding, fractionated heparin should be used cautiously for VTED prophylaxis in patients with polytrauma, and especially in those with closed head trauma, a visceral injury, or an expectation of delayed surgical fracture repair (especially if the pelvis is involved).

Thrombogenesis During Anesthesia and Total Joint Arthroplasty

It is now accepted that the principal thrombogenic stimulus associated with THA occurs intraoperatively. More specifically, femoral preparation is closely linked with intense activation of the clotting cascade as well as torsion or complete obstruction of the femoral vein. Sharrock et al[25] measured markers of thrombin generation and fibrin formation in circulating blood during THA and found that the process of thrombosis does not begin immediately but is delayed until preparation of the femoral canal. Elevation of prothrombin F1.2, thrombin-antithrombin complexes, fibrinopeptide A, and D-dimer was most pronounced during insertion of the cemented femoral component and continued to increase throughout the first hour after surgery. Mean values for three of the four markers were significantly higher after insertion of a cemented femoral component than after insertion of a cementless component. Mean pulmonary artery pressures peaked and central venous oxygen tension reached a nadir after reduction of the hip. These measurements at-

2: Physiology of Musculoskeletal Tissues

test to the delayed collection of embolic medullary contents in the lung resulting from kinking of the femoral vein during component insertion. Mechanical manipulation while the limb is being positioned for femoral preparation also is likely to cause local intimal injury to the femoral vein, may cause the unique finding of segmental femoral thrombi after THA, and completes an across-the-board disturbance in the Virchow triad (along with hypercoagulability and stasis) in this high-risk scenario.

A subsequent investigation of the efficacy of short-acting anticoagulants for blunting the intraoperative activation of the clotting cascade during THA found that standard heparin administered intravenously after socket implantation significantly inhibited fibrin formation at 10 units/kg and completely suppressed fibrin formation at 20 units/kg.[26] With a 30- to 40-minute half-life, the dose of unfractionated heparin in theory briefly increased the bleeding risk, but no additional intraoperative bleeding was clinically evident. This anticoagulation strategy targets primary prevention of intraoperative clot formation rather than secondary prevention of the postoperative extension of existing thrombi. In 1,947 patients undergoing 2,032 primary THAs, an average intraoperative dose of 1,200 units of heparin was intravenously administered before preparation of the femur, in conjunction with hypotensive epidural anesthesia. The nonfatal PE rate was 0.6% (12 of 1,947) and the incidence of proximal thrombus was only 2.6% (51 of 1,947) as determined by duplex ultrasonography, resulting in an overall readmission rate for venous thromboembolic disease of 3.2% (63 of 1,947 patients).[26] No untoward bleeding was observed. To mitigate the continued risk of hypercoagulability for weeks after total joint arthroplasty, 80% of the patients also received postoperative aspirin, and the 20% of patients considered to be at high risk received warfarin as VTED prophylaxis after hospital discharge.

Antiplatelet agents such as aspirin traditionally were not believed to influence thrombosis in the venous circulation, but accumulating observational data suggest that aspirin can have a meaningful role in reducing the embolic risk of existing thrombi despite the failure of aspirin to reduce venographic thrombosis in clinical studies.[26-30]

Epidural anesthesia, when evaluated by contrast venography as an outcome measure for DVT, has a similarly beneficial influence on thrombogenesis and VTED prophylaxis.[26,31] The mechanism for reducing the risk of VTE with epidural anesthesia or epidural analgesia has been the subject of much conjecture. Inhibition of platelet and leukocyte adhesion and stimulation of endothelial fibrinolysis have been proposed as valid mechanisms but have not been substantiated by controlled studies. Rather, the sympathectomy effect of epidural blockade, resulting in increased lower extremity blood flow and mitigating the adverse effects of stasis, is most likely to be responsible for reducing the risk of venous thrombosis. Regardless of the type of anticoagulant prophylaxis, a 40% to 50% reduction in the risk of venographic DVT was found when regional anesthesia was used,

compared with general anesthesia.[32] The incidence of fatal PE also is reduced when epidural anesthesia is used rather than general anesthesia; a retrospective review of THA and TKA by Sharrock et al[33] reported a 0.12% rate of fatal in-hospital PE (7 of 5,874 patients) when general anesthesia was used between 1981 and 1986, compared with a 0.02% rate (2 of 9,685 patients, $P = 0.03$) when epidural anesthesia was used between 1987 and 1991. The addition of controlled hypotension to the epidural anesthetic reduces blood loss and secondary vasoconstriction. An overall venographic DVT rate of 10.3% and a proximal DVT rate of 4.3% were reported after 2,037 THAs in which patients also received aspirin or warfarin prophylaxis. Of the 22 PEs (1.1%), 11 (0.54%) occurred after hospital discharge and 10 of the 11 patients had negative screening venograms while in hospital. Fatal PE occurred in one patient (0.04%). Continued use of the epidural catheter for postoperative analgesia was found to benefit VTED prophylaxis. In another study that used warfarin exclusively as VTE prophylaxis, 322 consecutive patients undergoing THA who received epidural anesthesia and 48-hour postoperative epidural analgesia demonstrated an overall venographic DVT rate of 8.9%, with proximal thrombi in 2.3% of patients.[31] Both aspirin, as an antiplatelet agent, and regional anesthesia have been observed to modify expression of VTED (in particular, clinically evident PE) after total joint arthroplasty.[26-29,32,33]

Thromboprophylaxis

Methods for preventing VTE can be categorized as mechanical or pharmacologic. In the second category, the three categories of chemoprophylaxis are aspirin, warfarin, and the newer anticoagulants. The most recent NIH-sponsored consensus conference on VTE (in 1986) recommended prophylaxis "for high-risk orthopedic patients undergoing elective hip surgery or knee reconstruction...low-dose warfarin, dextran, or adjusted dose-heparin...for at least 7 days."[10] The NIH panel noted that these regimens were believed to reduce the rate of clinical PE, but that "the lowered death rate from pulmonary embolism, while suggestive, is not statistically significant." The panel cautioned that "warfarin and dextran in commonly used doses can cause complications of operative bleeding and wound hematomas...[that] can be a significant problem in joint replacement patients."[10] During the past 25 years, many relatively selective anticoagulant drugs have been introduced, but the evidence for prevention of fatal PE after THA and TKA has changed very little. The Institute of Medicine has identified this area as a priority for comparative effectiveness research, and an Agency for Healthcare Research and Quality Evidence-based Practice Center project is in progress; nonetheless, the Joint Commission and Surgical Care Improvement Project now mandate VTE prophylaxis for all patients undergoing THA or TKA, according to prevailing guidelines.[34]

The guidelines of the American College of Chest Physicians (ACCP) historically have been based on the goal of reducing the frequency of DVT (as a surrogate for fatal PE), using prospective randomized clinical studies for the underlying data set.[35] As of the 2008 edition, the ACCP guidelines endorsed the use of fractionated heparins, full-intensity warfarin (INR 2.0 to 3.0), and synthetic pentasaccharide; and specifically recommended against the use of aspirin for VTE prophylaxis. The guideline of the American Academy of Orthopaedic Surgeons (AAOS) is intended to reduce the incidence of clinical PE while avoiding bleeding that could result in wound hematoma and secondary infection, both of which can require reoperation and prosthesis removal. In the first AAOS clinical practice guideline on the subject, released in 2007[36] and published in 2009,[37] patients were stratified into four risk groups, with a recommendation for the elective use of ACCP-recommended agents.[36,37] The use of aspirin or low-intensity warfarin was endorsed for patients with standard risk of VTE and bleeding as well as those with elevated risk of bleeding and either standard or elevated risk of VTE (because the rates of clinical PE with these agents are comparable to those of ACCP-recommended agents, and rates of bleeding are lower). Both ACCP and AAOS supported the use of adjunctive pneumatic compression.[36,37]

These disparate recommendations are predicated on studies using vastly different scientific methodologies.[38] Prospective randomized clinical trials found a reduction in the incidence of lower limb clots with the use of potent new anticoagulants but were unable to confirm a commensurate reduction in fatal PEs.[14,30] These studies were insufficiently powered for discerning a difference in bleeding events, however, and may have had bias related to industry funding. Observational studies found low PE event rates, comparable to those with newer ACCP-endorsed agents, with the use of aspirin, low-intensity warfarin (INR 2.0), and multimodal prophylaxis regimens predicated on use of mechanical compression devices.[26-30] In 2011 the AAOS released the second version of its clinical practice guideline for VTE prophylaxis after THA and TKA,[39] and less than 6 months later the ACCP released the ninth edition of its guidelines for antithrombotic therapy and thrombosis prevention.[40] The disagreement between earlier guidelines originated in surgeons' concern about perioperative bleeding coupled with observational data supporting the efficacy of aspirin for preventing clinical PE, despite its failure to reduce radiographic thrombosis in venographic end point studies. In their current guidelines, the AAOS and ACCP have moved toward a loosely defined middle ground; the AAOS no longer specifically endorses aspirin, and the ACCP awards aspirin the same level of recommendation as every other form of chemoprophylaxis, including unfractionated heparin. Both guidelines now leave the choice to the practitioner. The AAOS provides no preference or strength of recommendation for any chemoprophylaxis agent, and the ACCP's level-1B endorsement of all agents considered evidence of efficacy in preventing clinical thromboembolic events mitigated by a new valuation of patient-perceived importance of bleeding. The absence of a clear endorsement of one che-

moprophylaxis regimen by either organization and the passive acceptance of aspirin by both organizations has calmed the turbulent medicolegal waters surrounding PE after total joint arthroplasty and is a welcome reprieve for surgical practitioners. Nonetheless, the generic recommendations in the new guidelines leave room for debate and further study. The ideal prophylaxis has yet to be determined, but it must represent a balance between the risk of fatal PE and the morbidity of anticoagulation-associated bleeding. In many respects the optimal prophylaxis for fatal PE after musculoskeletal injury or surgery is less clear currently than it was in 1986 after the last NIH consensus conference. This scenario creates fertile ground for a large randomized clinical study to investigate the efficacy and safety of thromboprophylaxis after THA or TKA under a single protocol.

Mechanical Modalities

External pneumatic compression devices are inherently attractive because they increase venous return, decrease stasis, and enhance endothelium-derived fibrinolysis without creating a bleeding risk. Sequential calf and thigh sleeves were associated with a reduction in calf DVT but had a variable effect on high-risk proximal clots; it has been suggested that pneumatic compression used alone is more likely than warfarin prophylaxis to lead to high-risk proximal DVT after THA.[41,42] Plantar foot compression combined with aspirin was found to reduce the incidence of proximal DVT after TKA when compared with aspirin alone. External pneumatic devices alone have not been shown to be as effective as pharmacologic prophylaxis after THA, but they may offer an advantage when used in combination with pharmacologic prophylaxis. Although the use of graduated compression stockings is widely accepted, a comparison of warfarin with pneumatic compression sleeves after THA found a complementary decrease in distal DVT and a worrisome increase in proximal DVT when pneumatic sleeves were used.[6,41,42] This finding suggests that thigh-high pneumatic compression sleeves alone are less efficacious for specifically preventing proximal thrombosis than warfarin prophylaxis.

The 2008 ACCP guidelines endorse the use of pneumatic compression during the acute postoperative period as the sole means of thromboprophylaxis after TKA or THA (a level 1B or level 1A recommendation, respectively), if the bleeding risk with pharmacologic agents is unacceptably high.[35] The ACCP guidelines further recommend that chemoprophylaxis be added to or substituted for mechanical modalities as soon as the period of elevated bleeding risk has passed.

The recent release of a portable pneumatic compression device that is synchronized in phase with respiratory effort to optimize venous return has attracted considerable attention. One study found a greater bleeding risk only when enoxaparin was used, compared with pneumatic compression alone (6% versus 0%, $P = 0.0004$).[43] This study had fewer than 200 patients per group and a 5% incidence of clinical thrombotic events in each group; however, it was

2: Physiology of Musculoskeletal Tissues

grossly underpowered for providing meaningful insight into the device's efficacy for preventing VTE. The current enthusiasm among surgeons about the potential role of mobile pneumatic compression systems far exceeds the level justified by data available to support their use as the sole modality for VTED prophylaxis.

Chemoprophylaxis

Aspirin

The 1986 NIH Consensus Conference concluded that aspirin "has not been shown to be beneficial" in VTE prophylaxis.[10] This conclusion was based on conflicting data from published studies that comingled general and regional anesthetics, reported variable efficacy (better for men than women), and used a range of dosages. The NIH statement, coupled with long-standing conventional wisdom among thrombosis experts that antiplatelet agents are not effective on the venous side of the circulation, essentially eliminated any enthusiasm for aspirin in orthopaedic VTE prophylaxis. Subsequently, during the 1990s, the use of aspirin for VTE prophylaxis regained popularity among orthopaedic surgeons. This development was not based on new efficacy data but was largely attributable to the greater safety and lower bleeding risk associated with aspirin in comparison with the fractionated heparins introduced during the same decade. Some authors found that all-cause mortality among patients who received potent anticoagulants such as low-molecular-weight heparin (LMWH) after THA or TKA was more than twice that of patients treated with aspirin, pneumatic compression devices, and regional anesthesia.[44] In the absence of any extensive clinical event data for PE, almost 15% of orthopaedic surgeons preferred aspirin for inpatient prophylaxis, and as many as 35% used aspirin for extended prophylaxis after hospital discharge.[11,12]

Since 2006, observational data from three large single-center studies and a national joint arthroplasty registry analysis have provided credence to the belief that aspirin can effectively prevent clinically evident PE after total joint arthroplasty, especially when used in conjunction with regional anesthesia.[26,28,29] More than 2,000 patients undergoing THA were managed with hypotensive epidural anesthesia, intravenous heparin during femoral preparation, and in-hospital pneumatic compression, followed by 6 weeks of aspirin (325 mg twice daily, in 82% of patients) or low-intensity warfarin (in 18% of patients).[26] The clinical PE rate was 0.6%; there was no fatal PE, and the overall VTE-related readmission rate was 3.2%. Similarly, more than 3,400 TKAs were performed under regional anesthesia administered for 36 hours and followed by aspirin (325 mg twice daily for 6 weeks), with the 2% of patients considered to be at high risk receiving warfarin.[29] The fatal PE rate was 0.1%, the nonfatal PE rate was 0.26%, and the overall VTE-related readmission rate was 0.5%. In the third study, 2,203 consecutive primary THAs and 2,050 consecutive primary TKAs were performed under spinal anesthesia and followed by aspirin (150 mg daily for 6 weeks), with less than 2% of patients considered to be at high risk receiving warfarin or fractionated heparin.[28] The fatal PE rate was 0.07%, the nonfatal PE rate was 0.7%, and the overall VTE-related readmission rate was 1.1%. Perhaps the most striking data, from the National Joint Registry of the United Kingdom in 2009, suggested that 20% of surgeons use aspirin as primary VTE prophylaxis for THA and TKA.[45] A cohort subanalysis of 22,942 patients who received aspirin matched with the same number of patients who received fractionated heparin revealed no difference in 90-day outcomes related to clinical PE (0.7%), DVT (0.95%), stroke or gastrointestinal bleeding (0.75%), or reoperation (0.35%). Patients who received fractionated heparin had an advantage in all-cause mortality compared with those who received aspirin (0.49% versus 0.65%, relative risk = 0.75, $P = 0.02$).

Reexamination of data from the Pulmonary Embolism Prevention (PEP) study recently resulted in an endorsement of aspirin in the 9th edition of the ACCP practice guidelines for thromboprophylaxis after THA and TKA.[40] The PEP study primarily involved 13,356 patients with hip fracture but also included 4,088 patients undergoing elective THA or TKA.[30] Prophylaxis consisted of aspirin (160 mg daily for 35 days) or placebo, and outcome measures were in-hospital clinical PE-VTE morbidity and 35-day mortality. Aspirin use resulted in a 34% reduction in the overall incidence of PE and DVT compared with placebo (2.3% versus 1.6%, $P = 0.003$) after hip fracture, but there was no difference in overall PE-DVT incidence or mortality in the patients undergoing arthroplasty. Since its publication in 2000, the PEP study has been interpreted as not supporting the use of aspirin for VTE prophylaxis after THA or TKA. This original interpretation was based on perceived critical methodologic flaws in the PEP study including failure to control or report anesthetic type, the additional use of a fractionated heparin for thromboprophylaxis in 35% of patients, and the incompatibility of patients with fracture or arthroplasty. A more recent assessment of the study considered comparative clinical effectiveness, was more tolerant of the methodologic impurities, and validated the study as having sound methodology.[40] In the patients with hip fracture, aspirin use resulted in a 43% reduction in PE and a 29% reduction in DVT, and it prevented four fatal PEs for every 1,000 patients.[30] In the patients undergoing arthroplasty, aspirin use resulted in an overall 19% reduction in aggregate VTE end points (1.15% versus 1.4%). Nonetheless, most thrombosis experts continue to favor nonaspirin-based regimens for pharmacoprophylaxis. There is an increasingly compelling need for a randomized clinical study to rigorously investigate the effectiveness of aspirin for orthopaedic VTE prophylaxis.

Warfarin

Warfarin has remained the single most commonly used agent for total joint arthroplasty thromboprophylaxis in the United States for the past three decades (interrupted only by a transient surge in popularity of the fractionated heparins during the 1990s).[11,12] Warfarin is an orally administered vitamin K antagonist that blocks synthesis of related procoagulant factors (factors II, VII, IX, and X) and physiologic anticoagulants (proteins C and S) in the liver. Despite the need for regular monitoring, warfarin represents the best therapeutic compromise between efficacy and safety and between VTE prevention and bleeding, compared with other chemoprophylaxis agents. The critics of warfarin have been more concerned about untoward bleeding associated with its use than with its efficacy.

Early warfarin studies reported bleeding rates of 8% to 12%, with occasional life-threatening events. In a landmark study, Coventry et al[4] delayed prophylactic anticoagulation therapy until the fifth postoperative day, presumably because of a concern over bleeding during the early postoperative period, but still observed untoward bleeding in 4.1% of patients on warfarin. In a similar report, Amstutz et al[46] administered warfarin prophylaxis for 3 weeks postoperatively and observed overall bleeding complications in 1.5% of 3,000 patients undergoing THA. Bleeding was noted in 4.7% of the first 405 patients, but closer monitoring and lowering of the target prothrombin time from between 18 and 20 seconds to between 16 and 18 seconds resulted in a reduction in the bleeding rate to 1% in the subsequent patients. Of the 44 major bleeding complications, 36 were wound hematomas and 8 involved the gastrointestinal or genitourinary tracts. Cementless stems were associated with a bleeding rate of 2.3%. More recent recommendations favoring reduced-intensity anticoagulation with a prothrombin time ratio of 1.3 to 1.5 times control (INR 2.0 to 2.5) have been associated with markedly lower rates of bleeding, ranging from 1.2% to 3.7%.[6] Similarly, medical patients newly started on outpatient warfarin had a major bleeding rate of 3% during the first month after hospital discharge, with an increase in the bleeding rate of 0.8% for each subsequent month of anticoagulation therapy.[47,48] In a meta-analysis of DVT prophylaxis after hip replacement, Imperiale and Speroff[49] identified a six times greater risk of clinically important bleeding with the use of LMWH compared with no chemoprophylaxis and a 50% greater risk compared with warfarin. Colwell et al[50] compared clinically evident VTE after THA in patients receiving adjusted-dosage warfarin or LMWH (enoxaparin 30 mg every 12 hours) for an average of 6.5 days; clinically important bleeding was significantly more frequent with enoxaparin (1.3%) than with warfarin (0.5%).

Low-intensity warfarin prophylaxis (INR 2.0) resulted in overall venographic DVT rates of 9% to 26% and proximal clot rates of 2% to 5% after THA[51,52] and in overall DVT rates of 35% to 55% and proximal clot rates of 2% to 14% after TKA.[53] Moreover, warfarin was shown to have a peculiar propensity for reducing the incidence of proximal DVT compared with distal calf thrombosis after THA. Consistent with most reports on the effects of regional anesthesia, recent evidence suggests that 48 hours of warfarin combined with continuous epidural anesthesia-analgesia is associated with an additional 50% reduction in residual DVT rates in comparison with a combination of warfarin and general anesthesia.[6,31]

Most convincing are observational data from centers using extended low-intensity warfarin prophylaxis. A two-decade review studied 3,293 patients undergoing THA or TKA for a 6-month period after hospital discharge.[52,53] Contrast venography was used for routine surveillance before discharge, and all patients with negative venograms were discharged home without further prophylaxis. Patients with documented VTE received standard heparin and warfarin therapy. During the first decade of the study, patients not completing venography were discharged without further anticoagulant prophylaxis. Because of observed readmissions related to embolic events in these patients, during the second decade all patients not completing venography received empirical low-intensity warfarin for 6 weeks after discharge. Readmissions for VTE, DVT, PE, or a bleeding complication within 6 months of surgery were audited by communication with the patient or primary care physician. The overall readmission rate for VTE was 1.6% in patients who underwent THA (32 of 1,972 patients, including 14 with PE and 18 with DVT),[52] compared with 0.6% after TKA (8 of 1,321 patients, including 3 with PE and 5 with DVT, $P = 0.009$).[53] The readmissions affected 2.2% of the patients who underwent THA and had negative venography with no further anticoagulation therapy (19 of 880 patients), compared with 0.28% of patients who underwent THA and received outpatient warfarin (1 of 360 patients, $P = 0.013$). In the combined population of patients undergoing THA or TKA, 6 weeks of warfarin therapy eliminated the risk of PE (0 of 844 patients versus 17 of 2,449 patients, $P = 0.01$) and significantly reduced the VTE-related readmission rate (2 of 844 patients [0.2%] versus 38 of 2,449 patients [1.6%], $P = 0.0015$) compared with patients who did not continue warfarin therapy after hospital discharge. Three bleeding events (in 3 of 3,292 patients [0.1%]) led to one death from intracranial bleeding while on warfarin and two reoperations necessitated by hematoma while on fractionated heparin. Routine surveillance, even with contrast venography, was a poor predictor of the need for continued anticoagulant prophylaxis after discharge. Extended warfarin as a method of secondary prophylaxis eliminated PE-related deaths and reduced the rate of VTE-related readmission after THA or TKA.

Extending low-intensity warfarin (INR 1.5 to 2.0) for 4 to 6 weeks after surgery is a highly effective and time-honored method of prophylaxis; VTE-related readmission is necessary in only 0.3% of patients after THA and only 0.2% after TKA, the major bleeding rate is 0.1%, and the residual incidence of DVT is less than 10% in conjunction with sustained epidural anesthesia after THA.[51-53] The optimal use of warfarin begins the evening before surgery because of its 48-hour latency to onset of anticoagulant effect. The combination of preoperative warfarin and epidural anesthesia has been found safe and effective.[52,53] Moreover, warfarin use prevents VTE-related morbidity and mortality, as judged by late PE-related readmission or death, even in patients with a tendency to form thrombi despite primary warfarin prophylaxis.[52,53]

Newer Selective Anticoagulants

Newer anticoagulants (fractionated heparins,[54,55] synthetic pentasaccharide, factor Xa,[56-59] and direct thrombin inhibitors[60]) all have greater demonstrated efficacy than older agents for reducing venographic thrombosis when used as primary chemoprophylaxis after THA or TKA. However, the newer agents are uniformly associated with a considerably increased risk of perioperative bleeding.[61,62] In contrast, low-intensity warfarin (INR 2.0) and aspirin have been associated with an incidence of residual venographic clotting as much as five times higher than that of the newer agents, but with a comparable clinical PE rate. The risk of major bleeding complications with low-intensity warfarin and aspirin is two to three times less than with the more potent anticoagulants.[49]

Heparin is a mixture of glycosaminoglycans with a molecular weight ranging from 3,000 to 40,000 d (average, 12,000 to 15,000 d) that naturally occurs in mammalian tissues including the liver, lung, and intestine. LMWH (fractionated heparin) has a molecular weight ranging from 3,000 to 15,000 d (average, 5,000 lcd). Heparins bind to a five-sugar site on antithrombin III, which promotes steric transformation of a second binding site on antithrombin III. Although the fractionated heparin–antithrombin III complex can bind to either factor X or factor II (thrombin), it has a much greater affinity for factor X. The upstream position of factor X in the clotting cascade, compared with thrombin, and the strong propensity of fractionated heparin–antithrombin III to bind to factor X rather than to thrombin mean that LMWH is a much more potent anticoagulant than unfractionated heparin. Fractionated heparin has less antiplatelet effect and is less bound by plasma proteins than unfractionated heparin, and so there is a tenfold reduction in the risk of heparin-induced thrombocytopenia (prevalence of 0.2%) and a nearly threefold increase in bioavailability compared with conventional unfractionated heparin. LMWH is an injectable preparation given as a fixed dose without monitoring; peak plasma concentrations are reached in 90 minutes, with a half-life of 4 to 6 hours, and it is excreted by the kidneys. The advantages of fractionated heparin over unfractionated heparin therefore include a more predictable and rapid dose response, a longer half-life, and a smaller hemorrhagic effect, with the same antithrombotic efficacy.

LMWH in the form of enoxaparin was compared with unfractionated heparin (5,000 IU) administered subcutaneously) twice daily in patients with multiple trauma (an injury severity score higher than 9 and likely survival of more than 7 days).[24] Patients were stratified for the presence of lower extremity fractures, and those with intracranial bleeding, uncontrolled hemorrhaging, coagulopathy, or contrast allergy were excluded. Bilateral venography was performed in 265 patients, including 129 receiving enoxaparin and 136 receiving heparin, on or before day 14. No fatal PEs occurred in either group; the overall DVT rate was 44% with regular heparin and 31% with LMWH (P = 0.014). The rates of proximal DVT were 15% for unfractionated heparin and 6% for LMWH (P = 0.017), respectively. There were only six major bleeding incidents (1.7%). LMWH was clearly superior with respect to venographic thrombi in this high-risk population, with the advantages of rapid onset and decline of action as well as parenteral administration.

In studies comparing unfractionated heparin in THA using a venographic end point, the use of LMWH led to lower rates of venographic DVT, symptomatic PE, and major bleeding.[54,55] Studies comparing LMWH and warfarin (INR 2.0 to 3.0) after THA had less compelling results. Lower venographic clot rates and comparable symptomatic PE rates were offset by higher rates of bleeding complications.[62] Colwell et al[50] compared clinically evident VTED after THA in 1,494 patients receiving adjusted-dose warfarin and 1,517 patients receiving enoxaparin (30 mg every 12 hours). The pharmacologic prophylaxis was administered for an average of 6.5 days in both groups of patients, and VTE events were monitored for 3 months after hospital discharge. At 3-month review, all-cause mortality was 0.8% in each group, and confirmed VTE was found in 3.6% of the patients receiving enoxaparin and 3.8% of those receiving warfarin. Clinically evident VTE events were more common during hospitalization in patients receiving warfarin (1.1% versus 0.3%) and more frequent after hospital discharge in those receiving enoxaparin (3.3% versus 2.7%). Clinically important bleeding occurred in 20 patients receiving enoxaparin (1.3%) and 8 receiving warfarin (0.5%). A study of 1,472 patients undergoing THA compared warfarin (INR 2.0 to 3.0) with two dalteparin (fractionated heparin) regimens (beginning 2 hours before or 4 hours after surgery), using a venographic end point. The incidences of total and proximal DVT were significantly less in the patients in both dalteparin groups. The incidence of symptomatic DVT was reduced only in patients in the preoperative dalteparin group compared with patients in the warfarin group (1.5% versus 4.4%, P = 0.02), but patients in the preoperative dalteparin group also had twice the frequency of major bleeding events (8.9% versus 4.5%, P = 0.01) and surgical site bleeding events (8.3% versus 3.9%, P = 0.03) in comparison with patients receiving warfarin. It has become increasingly evident that bleeding complications, especially those related to the surgical wound, occur at considerably higher rates with the use of fractionated heparins at dosages sufficient for significantly reducing the incidence of DVT than with low-dosage warfarin regimens.[50,61,62] In patients undergoing TKA, venographic DVT rates are lower with the use of LMWH than with warfarin, bleeding complications are more common with LMWH, and there appear to be no significant differences in clinical PE event rates between the prophylaxis types. Although the reduction in venographic thrombi after THA and TKA is undeniable, there is no convincing evidence that a reduction in clinical PE events can justify the perioperative use of fractionated heparins, which is accompanied by an increased frequency of bleeding events.

Fondaparinux is a completely synthetic five-sugar chain (pentasaccharide) that precisely corresponds to the heparinoid binding site on ATIII. This compound provides highly selective indirect inhibition of the clotting cascade at the level of factor X. Pentasaccharide carries no risk of disease transmission, has no activity against thrombin, and does not induce platelet aggregation. A greater than 50% reduction in overall venographic DVT was found after THA, TKA, and hip fracture repair with fondaparinux compared with enoxaparin.[63] Specifically, fondaparinux was the first agent to reduce the rate of venographic thrombi below 20% after TKA and is the most rigorously studied agent for use after hip fracture repair. When fondaparinux was compared with enoxaparin in patients undergoing hip fracture surgery, there were reductions in the rates of total venographic DVT (19.1% versus 8.3%, $P = 0.001$) and proximal venographic DVT (4.3% versus 0.9%, $P = 0.001$). The bleeding event rates of approximately 3% to 6% with fondaparinux were equal to or greater than the rates with enoxaparin.

Rivaroxaban, an orally administered direct inhibitor of activated factor X (factor Xa), is used for thromboprophylaxis in several countries throughout the world but was only recently approved for use in the United States. It was studied extensively (in 12,729 patients) after both THA and TKA in direct comparison with enoxaparin, using clinical event end points and venographic screening.[56-59] A pooled analysis of two hip arthroplasty studies (7,050 patients) and two knee arthroplasty studies (5,679 patients) showed a 58% reduction in combined all-cause mortality and symptomatic VTE (0.6% versus 1.3%, $P < 0.001$).[64] However, the use of rivaroxaban was associated with an increase in major or clinically relevant nonmajor bleeding events (3.2% versus 2.6%, $P = 0.039$). Initial efforts to gain approval for rivaroxaban use in the United States were unsuccessful. Apixaban, another direct oral factor Xa inhibitor, showed superior efficacy for reducing all-cause mortality and total VTE incidence (1.4% versus 3.9%, $P < 0.001$) in 3,866 patients undergoing THA, with rates of major or clinically relevant nonmajor bleeding comparable to those of enoxaparin.[65] Dabigatran, an oral direct inhibitor of activated factor II (thrombin), is in use for thromboprophylaxis around the world and is approved in the United States for cardiovascular anticoagulation, specifically atrial fibrillation. It was widely studied (in 8,210 patients) after both THA and TKA in direct comparison with enoxaparin, using a screening contrast venography end point.[60] Dabigatran (220 mg or 150 mg once daily) had efficacy comparable to that of enoxaparin for all-cause mortality, total VTE prevention, and major bleeding rates after THA, when compared with enoxaparin (40 mg once daily). Dabigatran had similar efficacy and safety after TKA when compared with the European dosage of enoxaparin (40 mg once daily) but was inferior in efficacy to the North American enoxaparin regimen (30 mg twice daily). A study of dabigatran for atrial fibrillation found that it had comparable efficacy to warfarin with respect to stroke and systemic embolism, with reduced bleeding risk at a reduced dabigatran dose (110 mg twice daily).[66]

Despite their superior efficacy, these newer, more specific agents have been associated with a risk of bleeding equal to or greater than that of fractionated heparin, which itself carries a greater bleeding risk than low-intensity warfarin or aspirin. In one study, patients receiving fractionated heparin prophylaxis had a rate of nonfatal PE 60% to 70% greater than those receiving only aspirin and mechanical compression,[44] indicating that PE occurs despite prophylaxis with potent anticoagulants and should not be considered a "never event." Another study specified that LMWH prophylaxis was a failure because the risk of complications exceeded the risk of the disease being prevented: symptomatic DVT (3.8%), nonfatal PE (1.3%), persistent wound drainage resulting in readmission (4.7%), and reoperation (3.4%) occurred at rates exceeding the experience with a low-intensity warfarin regimen.[61] The adjunctive use of pneumatic compression to augment venous return and increase fibrinolysis has become widespread in orthopaedics because of its favorable safety profile, with no known increase in bleeding risk. An observational report of 1,048 consecutive patients undergoing THA or TKA in the United Kingdom found that patients treated with rivaroxaban prophylaxis had more than double the rate of reoperation for wound complications of those treated with fractionated heparin (3.9% versus 1.8%).[67]

Accordingly, orthopaedic surgeons have been slow to routinely use these newer agents and have favored a more balanced strategy that offers a lower bleeding risk while protecting against thromboembolic events. Despite variable dosing and the need for monitoring, low-intensity warfarin (INR 1.5 to 2.0) remains the chemoprophylaxis of choice for almost 50% of all orthopaedic surgeons performing total joint arthroplasty in North America. Despite a paucity of clinical event data for PE, almost 15% of orthopaedic surgeons prefer aspirin prophylaxis, largely on the basis of its negligible bleeding risk. Therefore, approximately two thirds of THA and TKA surgeons favor VTE prophylaxis regimens that do not utilize the newer more potent anticoagulant agents as favored by the most recent ACCP guidelines, which recommend the use of warfarin with a target INR of 2.0 to 3.0. Indeed, the likelihood that an arthroplasty surgeon will choose a potent new anticoagulant for thromboprophylaxis is inversely related to the number of joint arthroplasties the surgeon performs.[12] It is important to note that all of the large-scale clinical studies have been funded by the pharmaceutical industry. The pharmaceutical industry also sponsored each of the prior ACCP clinical guidelines (through the eighth edition), which endorsed the newer anticoagulants that are unpopular among surgeons because of the associated bleeding risk. The recently released ninth edition of the ACCP guidelines was free of in-

2: Physiology of Musculoskeletal Tissues

dustry sponsorship and panel member conflict of interest and awarded all the agents a 1B rating. Even a highly ethical pharmaceutical company has a financial interest in promoting the sale of an expensive newer agent, despite increased risks. As evidence accumulates for the effectiveness of aspirin and low-intensity warfarin (INR 1.5 to 2.0) regimens in preventing clinically meaningful PE, it is increasingly evident that a large investigator-initiated, independently funded randomized clinical study is required for objectively assessing the safety and efficacy of the available regimens and reconciling divergent guideline recommendations.

Fat Embolism Syndrome

Posttraumatic fat embolization, specifically the fat embolism syndrome, has been a source of interest since the original description by Zenker in 1861 in a patient with a thoracoabdominal crush injury.[68] The fat embolism syndrome can be practically defined as a complex alteration in coagulation homeostasis that occurs as an infrequent complication of fracture of the pelvis and long bones and is clinically manifested as acute respiratory insufficiency. The full-blown clinical syndrome is evident in 0.5% to 2% of patients after an isolated long bone fracture and in 5% to 10% of patients with multiple fractures and pelvic injury after polytrauma.[68] In contrast, fat embolization occurs as a subclinical event after every fracture and every instrumentation of the medullary canal with release of fatty marrow during total joint arthroplasty. The likelihood of fat embolization resulting in the clinical syndrome characterized by florid respiratory failure is determined by the quantity of fat intravasated into the systemic circulation and the ability of the patient's cardiopulmonary system to withstand the filtration of this material by the lung. Fat embolization also can result from metabolic conditions but typically is of little clinical significance and is an incidental postmortem finding.

Pathophysiology

Disruption of the intramedullary canal, whether accidentally through trauma or iatrogenically during surgical instrumentation, results in liberation of marrow fat from its protected position within the long bones. Neutral fat and tissue thromboplastin released from the fracture site enter the systemic circulation and activate the clotting cascade and platelet aggregation. Suppression of the fibrinolytic system in the injured patient aggravates the ongoing accumulation of aggregates of fat macroglobules, marrow elements, platelets, erythrocytes, fibrin, and leukocytes. These heterogeneous emboli passively concentrate in the lung as a result of the filtering action of the lung on venous blood before it returns to the systemic circulation (**Figure 5**).

When the fat emboli become lodged in the pulmonary bed, a biphasic reaction ensues within the lung.[68] The pulmonary circulation normally is a low-pressure, low-resistance system; observations from acute PE suggest that 80% of the pulmonary circulation must be obstructed to create a significant hemodynamic effect. Massive fat embolization to the lungs therefore can result in elevation of right heart pressures and, in extreme circumstances, acute cor pulmonale and death. Such a dramatic circulatory collapse has been found in animals but is rare in humans. The situation can be further aggravated if the patient has a patent foramen ovale, in which a right-to-left shunt bypassing the lung filter allows immediate systemic embolization of fat to the arterial circulation with clinical consequences such as stroke and digital ischemia (**Figure 6**).

The subacute or delayed clinical manifestations of fat embolization most commonly are seen in patients with the fat embolism syndrome.[69,70] The primary defect is in arterial oxygenation, with severe hypoxemia resulting from a large ventilation-perfusion shunt. This clinical scenario has been reproduced in animals immediately after injection of fatty acids or within 72 hours after injection of neutral fat; a rise in serum lipase is observed concurrent with the lung changes after neutral fat injection.[71] Peltier[70] promoted a theory of pulmonary failure after fracture in humans, in which neutral marrow fat becomes lodged in the lung, where is it broken down by lipase produced locally by pneumatocytes in response to the embolic material. The resulting free fatty acids chemically inactivate existing surfactant and are toxic to the alveolar type II cells that synthesize surfactant in the lung. This theory of free fatty acid liberation in the lung is controversial, but it is supported by an observed increase in serum lipase and free fatty acids before a decrease in oxygenation in patients with fulminant fat embolism syndrome. It is not necessary to implicate the local conversion of neutral marrow fat to free fatty acids in the lung to explain the profound respiratory collapse characteristic of fat embolism syndrome. Aggregates of fat, fibrin, platelets, and leukocytes by themselves are capable of disturbing oxygen diffusion in the lung by inciting release of numerous vasoactive substances that result in increased pulmonary capillary permeability and impaired gas exchange. Regardless of the particular insult to the lung, whether by fatty acid conversion and toxicity, leukocyte lysosomal enzymes, or complement activation from intravascular marrow fat, it is evident that the final common pathway of pulmonary injury leads to acute respiratory distress syndrome, which is characterized by so-called wet lung and life-threatening impairment of oxygen exchange.

Clinical Presentation and Treatment

It is important to distinguish between fat embolization, which is a common subclinical event occurring after fracture or medullary canal instrumentation, and fat embolism syndrome, which is a rare clinical event of respiratory failure after fracture or polytrauma. Clinical fat embolism syndrome develops in children nearly 100 times less commonly than adults, presumably because children have a paucity of fatty marrow and a prevalence of hematopoietic (so-called red) marrow. Conditions that increase the size and fatty content of the marrow cavity, such as collagen vascular dis-

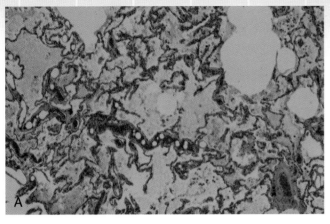

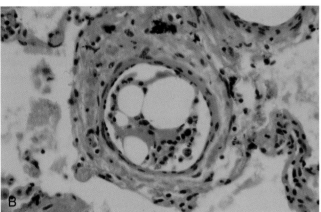

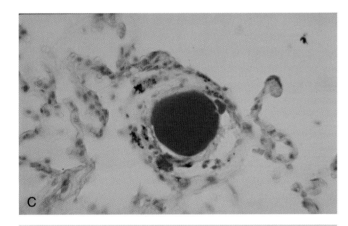

Figure 5 Postmortem embolic material from the lung of a patient with fatal fat embolism syndrome. **A,** Fat globules in a pulmonary arteriole, with prominent exudate in the air spaces (17× magnification). **B,** Embolic marrow elements and fat in a pulmonary arteriole (110× magnification). **C,** Oil Red O stain showing fat in a pulmonary arteriole (110× magnification). (Courtesy of Vincent D. Pellegrini, Jr, MD, Baltimore, MD.)

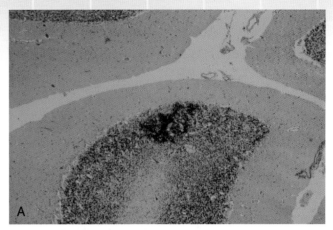

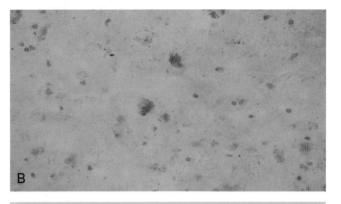

Figure 6 Postmortem brain tissue from a patient with systemic fat embolization. **A,** Petechial hemorrhage in the cerebellum (17× magnification). **B,** Oil Red O stain showing fat in the brain (43× magnification). (Courtesy of Vincent D. Pellegrini, Jr, MD, Baltimore, MD.)

eases and osteoporosis, increase the risk of developing fat embolism syndrome.

The initial insult after embolic fat reaches the lungs is characterized by increased right heart pressures and cardiovascular collapse. Although this condition rarely is clinically evident in humans,[68] it has been reported after cementation of the femoral component during THA[72] (especially for femoral neck fracture in an elderly osteoporotic patient) or after intramedullary nailing of the femur for an impending pathologic fracture with concurrent filling of the medullary canal with methyl methacrylate cement. Embolic marrow elements have been found postmortem in the capillary bed of the brain in such patients, suggesting that an overwhelmed lung filter allowed overflowing of embolic material into the systemic circulation.[60] Transient aphasia and even death have been observed after major orthopaedic procedures in patients later found to have a patent foramen ovale with a documented embolic intracerebral event.[73]

The typical fat embolism syndrome is delayed in its appearance. Clinical signs and symptoms develop in 60% of patients within 24 hours and in 85% of patients within 48 hours after fracture or medullary canal instrumentation.[68-70] This delay is believed to be secondary to the evolving effects of vasoactive substances in the lung and the resulting decrement in gas exchange. The clinical manifestations are primarily cardiopulmonary in nature and include arterial hypoxemia; oxygen desaturation, sinus tachycardia, and fever are the classic triad of early findings.[69,70] Nonspe-

2: Physiology of Musculoskeletal Tissues

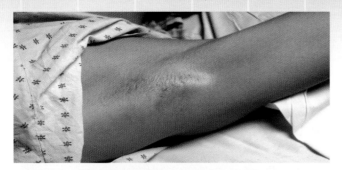

Figure 7 Photograph showing petechiae, as are commonly seen in the axilla, in a patient with a fat embolism syndrome after a closed femoral shaft fracture. (Courtesy of Vincent D. Pellegrini, Jr, MD, Baltimore, MD.)

cific changes of pulmonary congestion can be seen on the chest radiograph in one third of patients, and the electrocardiogram may show ST segment elevation consistent with ischemia or right heart strain. Alterations in cognition are common, ranging from lethargy to delirium and possibly seizures; it is unclear whether these findings are more related to hypoxemia or fat embolization to the brain. Petechiae develop in 50% to 60% of patients, typically in the axilla (**Figure 7**), over the chest and base of the neck, and in the conjunctivae; often they appear after 24- to 48-hour delay and are transient in nature. Some believe that thrombocytopenia is the cause, but embolic fat in capillaries with local hemorrhage has been found on skin biopsies. Despite the frequency of abnormalities in laboratory coagulation markers, a clinical bleeding disorder rarely is a component of fat embolism syndrome.[69,70] This constellation of findings is uncommon after musculoskeletal trauma, but the mortality rate approaches 10% to 15% in patients in whom full-blown fat embolism syndrome develops, and a high index of suspicion is necessary for early identification and proper treatment.

A discussion of fat embolism syndrome is most relevant to the fields of orthopaedic trauma, arthroplasty, and orthopaedic oncology. The timing and method of fracture fixation after skeletal trauma, especially in a patient with polytrauma, is controversial and has received considerable attention in recent years. In economically developed countries, traction for the treatment of femoral shaft fracture has been replaced by intramedullary nailing. Nailing soon after injury has been promoted as critical for early mobilization and avoidance of the pulmonary and thromboembolic complications of recumbency.[74-76] Some investigators have challenged this doctrine of early fracture nailing as adding insult to lung injury in a patient with polytrauma, and they have recommended delaying intramedullary fixation if the patient has compromised pulmonary function from the index injury. The consensus in North America is that patients with isolated long bone fracture or polytrauma without lung injury should be treated with early intramedullary nailing to facilitate mobilization but that intramedullary fracture fixa-

tion should be delayed 5 days, or until pulmonary function improves, for patients with polytrauma and lung dysfunction. Preparation of the femoral canal during total hip arthroplasty or intramedullary nailing for an impending pathologic fracture has been associated with cardiopulmonary dysfunction, especially if cement is being used.[72] In the operating room, clinically important fat embolization leading to cardiopulmonary dysfunction may be manifested as hypotension, right heart strain, bradycardia, and cardiovascular collapse, and postoperatively it typically appears as hypoxemia and self-limiting confusion and changes in cognition. Distal venting of the femoral canal with direct suction is advisable, particularly during cementing of a long stem for fracture fixation or nailing of the femur in a patient with metastatic disease and multiple lytic lesions. The purpose is to reduce intramedullary pressures and subsequent embolization of fat to the lungs and thereby to reduce the likelihood of pulmonary complications. During bilateral TKA, when the medullary canals of four bones are instrumented and the volume of intravasated fat can be large, it is unwise to operate on both knees concurrently.[77] Instead, it is more prudent to complete the arthroplasty on one knee and note whether there is a substantial drop in oxygen saturation or systolic pressure after tourniquet release; if so, the second-knee operation should be deferred. Bilateral TKA with extramedullary instrumentation that did not violate the medullary canals was not found to offer an advantage over intramedullary instrumentation related to observed fat embolization and pulmonary function.[78] In elective surgery, the most effective treatment is to avoid substantial fat embolization. It also is advisable to delay intramedullary nailing of fractures in the presence of lung dysfunction, to vent the femur when cementing a stem or nail in a patient with osteoporosis or metastatic disease, and to perform sequential rather than concurrent bilateral TKAs. Supportive care is critical for a patient with florid respiratory failure secondary to fat embolism syndrome. The mainstays of treatment are mechanical ventilation with airway pressure support, volume repletion, and judicious use of steroids to stabilize the pulmonary capillary and improve gas exchange.[79] Notwithstanding considerable research on fat embolism syndrome, specific therapies have yet to be developed.

Summary

Thromboembolic phenomena resulting from instrumentation of the intramedullary canal of long bones are common and potentially serious complications of major orthopaedic procedures that must be understood by every orthopaedic practitioner. Intravasation of marrow fat activates the clotting cascade and is responsible for the uniquely high prevalence of venous thromboembolism observed after THA and TKA as well as hip fracture repair. In its most severe form, massive pulmonary embolism may result in sudden death after any of these procedures as well as long bone fixation, repair of ankle fracture, and even anterior cruciate ligament reconstruction. Although there is consensus on the routine use of prophylaxis for venous thromboembolism after THA and TKA as well as hip fracture, there is no agreement on which agents or methods provide the optimal balance between efficacy in preventing fatal PE, and safety in avoiding excessive bleeding complications. Likewise, massive embolization of marrow fat droplets from the medullary canal to the pulmonary capillary bed may cause acute cardiovascular collapse as well as late manifestations of hypoxemia attributable to the adult respiratory distress syndrome. Optimal timing of long bone fracture fixation is the best way to avoid this condition, and high-dosage steroids may blunt life-threatening signs and symptoms once the fat embolism syndrome is evident.

References

1. Johnson R, Green JR, Charnley J: Pulmonary embolism and its prophylaxis following the Charnley total hip replacement. *Clin Orthop Relat Res* 1977;127(127):123-132.

2. Charnley J: *Low Friction Arthroplasty of the Hip: Theory and Practice.* Berlin, Germany, Springer-Verlag, 1979.

3. Prandoni P, Lensing AW, Prins MR: The natural history of deep-vein thrombosis. *Semin Thromb Hemost* 1997;23(2):185-188.

4. Coventry MB, Nolan DR, Beckenbaugh RD: "Delayed" prophylactic anticoagulation: A study of results and complications in 2,012 total hip arthroplasties. *J Bone Joint Surg Am* 1973;55(7):1487-1492.

5. Stulberg BN, Insall JN, Williams GW, Ghelman B: Deep-vein thrombosis following total knee replacement: An analysis of six hundred and thirty-eight arthroplasties. *J Bone Joint Surg Am* 1984;66(2):194-201.

6. Pellegrini VD Jr, Sharrock NE, Paiement GD, Morris R, Warwick DJ: Venous thromboembolic disease after total hip and knee arthroplasty: Current perspectives in a regulated environment. *Instr Course Lect* 2008;57:637-661.

7. Seagroatt V, Tan HS, Goldacre M, Bulstrode C, Nugent I, Gill L: Elective total hip replacement: Incidence, emergency readmission rate, and postoperative mortality. *BMJ* 1991;303(6815):1431-1435.

8. Warwick D, Williams MH, Bannister GC: Death and thromboembolic disease after total hip replacement: A series of 1162 cases with no routine chemical prophylaxis. *J Bone Joint Surg Br* 1995;77(1):6-10.

9. Murray DW, Britton AR, Bulstrode CJ: Thromboprophylaxis and death after total hip replacement. *J Bone Joint Surg Br* 1996;78(6):863-870.

10. Prevention of venous thrombosis and pulmonary embolism. *Natl Inst Health Consens Dev Conf Consens Statement* 1986;6(2):1-8.

11. Markel DC, York S, Liston MJ Jr, et al: Venous thromboembolism: Management by American Association of Hip and Knee Surgeons. *J Arthroplasty* 2010;25(1):3-9, e1-e2.

12. Anderson FA Jr, Huang W, Friedman RJ, et al: Prevention of venous thromboembolism after hip or knee arthroplasty: Findings from a 2008 survey of US orthopedic surgeons. *J Arthroplasty* 2012;27(5):659-666, e5.

13. Hirsh J: Oral anticoagulant drugs. *N Engl J Med* 1991;324(26):1865-1875.

14. Eikelboom JW, Quinlan DJ, Douketis JD: Extended-duration prophylaxis against venous thromboembolism after total hip or knee replacement: A meta-analysis of the randomised trials. *Lancet* 2001;358(9275):9-15.

15. Kakkar VV, Howe CT, Flanc C, Clarke MB: Natural history of postoperative deep-vein thrombosis. *Lancet* 1969;2(7614):230-232.

16. Pellegrini VD Jr, Langhans MJ, Totterman S, Marder VJ, Francis CW: Embolic complications of calf thrombosis following total hip arthroplasty. *J Arthroplasty* 1993;8(5):449-457.

17. De Stefano V, Leone G, Mastrangelo S, et al: Clinical manifestations and management of inherited thrombophilia: Retrospective analysis and follow-up after diagnosis of 238 patients with congenital deficiency of antithrombin III, protein C, protein S. *Thromb Haemost* 1994;72(3):352-358.

18. Bertina RM, Koeleman BP, Koster T, et al: Mutation in blood coagulation factor V associated with resistance to activated protein C. *Nature* 1994;369(6475):64-67.

19. Martinelli I, Mannucci PM, De Stefano V, et al: Different risks of thrombosis in four coagulation defects associated with inherited thrombophilia: A study of 150 families. *Blood* 1998;92(7):2353-2358.

20. Ridker PM, Glynn RJ, Miletich JP, Goldhaber SZ, Stampfer MJ, Hennekens CH: Age-specific incidence rates of venous thromboembolism among heterozygous carriers of factor V Leiden mutation. *Ann Intern Med* 1997;126(7):528-531.

21. Woolson ST, Zehnder JL, Maloney WJ: Factor V Leiden and the risk of proximal venous thrombosis after total hip arthroplasty. *J Arthroplasty* 1998;13(2):207-210.

22. Ryan DH, Crowther MA, Ginsberg JS, Francis CW: Relation of factor V Leiden genotype to risk for acute deep venous thrombosis after joint replacement surgery. *Ann Intern Med* 1998;128(4):270-276.

23. Gabay C, Kushner I: Acute-phase proteins and other systemic responses to inflammation. *N Engl J Med* 1999;340(6):448-454.

24. Geerts WH, Jay RM, Code KI, et al: A comparison of low-dose heparin with low-molecular-weight heparin as prophylaxis against venous thromboembolism after major trauma. *N Engl J Med* 1996;335(10):701-707.

25. Sharrock NE, Go G, Harpel PC, Ranawat CS, Sculco TP, Salvati EA: Thrombogenesis during total hip arthroplasty. *Clin Orthop Relat Res* 1995;319:16-27.

26. González Della Valle A, Serota A, Go G, et al: Venous thromboembolism is rare with a multimodal prophylaxis protocol after total hip arthroplasty. *Clin Orthop Relat Res* 2006;444:146-153.

27. Collaborative overview of randomised trials of antiplatelet therapy—III: Reduction in venous thrombosis and pulmonary embolism by antiplatelet prophylaxis among surgical and medical patients. Antiplatelet Trialists' Collaboration. *BMJ* 1994;308(6923):235-246.

28. Cusick LA, Beverland DE: The incidence of fatal pulmonary embolism after primary hip and knee replacement in a consecutive series of 4253 patients. *J Bone Joint Surg Br* 2009;91(5):645-648.

29. Lotke PA, Lonner JH: The benefit of aspirin chemoprophylaxis for thromboembolism after total knee arthroplasty. *Clin Orthop Relat Res* 2006;452:175-180.

30. Prevention of pulmonary embolism and deep vein thrombosis with low dose aspirin: Pulmonary Embolism Prevention (PEP) trial. *Lancet* 2000;355(9212):1295-1302.

31. Dalldorf PG, Perkins FM, Totterman S, Pellegrini VD Jr: Deep venous thrombosis following total hip arthroplasty: Effects of prolonged postoperative epidural anesthesia. *J Arthroplasty* 1994;9(6):611-616.

32. Sharrock NE, Ranawat CS, Urquhart B, Peterson M: Factors influencing deep vein thrombosis following total hip arthroplasty under epidural anesthesia. *Anesth Analg* 1993;76(4):765-771.

33. Sharrock NE, Cazan MG, Hargett MJ, Williams-Russo P, Wilson PD Jr: Changes in mortality after total hip and knee arthroplasty over a ten-year period. *Anesth Analg* 1995;80(2):242-248.

34. Centers for Medicare and Medicaid Services: Medicare and Medicaid move aggressively to encourage greater patient safety in hospitals and reduce never events [press release]. July 31, 2008. http://www.cms.gov/apps/media/press/release.asp?Counter=3219. Accessed March 27, 2012.

35. Geerts WH, Bergqvist D, Pineo GF, et al: Prevention of venous thromboembolism: American College of Chest Physicians evidence-based clinical practice guidelines (8th edition). *Chest* 2008;133(6, Suppl):381S-453S.

36. American Academy of Orthopaedic Surgeons: *Clinical Guideline on Prevention of Symptomatic Pulmonary Embolism in Patients Undergoing Total Hip or Knee Arthroplasty.* Rosemont, IL, American Academy of Orthopaedic Surgeons, 2007.

37. Johanson NA, Lachiewicz PF, Lieberman JR, et al: Prevention of symptomatic pulmonary embolism in patients undergoing total hip or knee arthroplasty. *J Am Acad Orthop Surg* 2009;17(3):183-196.

38. Eikelboom JW, Karthikeyan G, Fagel N, Hirsh J: American Association of Orthopedic Surgeons and American College of Chest Physicians guidelines for venous thromboembolism prevention in hip and knee arthroplasty differ: What are the implications for clinicians and patients? *Chest* 2009;135(2):513-520.

39. American Academy of Orthopaedic Surgeons: *Clinical Guideline on Preventing Venous Thromboembolic Disease in Patients Undergoing Elective Hip and Knee Arthroplasty.* September 2011. http://www.aaos.org/research/guidelines/VTE/VTE_guideline.asp. Accessed March 27, 2011.

40. Falck-Ytter Y, Francis CW, Johanson NA, et al: Prevention of VTE in orthopedic surgery patients: Antithrombotic Therapy and Prevention of Thrombosis, 9th ed: American College of Chest Physicians Evidence-Based Clinical Practice Guidelines. *Chest* 2012;141(2, Suppl):e278S-e325S.

41. Francis CW, Pellegrini VD Jr, Marder VJ, et al: Comparison of warfarin and external pneumatic compression in prevention of venous thrombosis after total hip replacement. *JAMA* 1992;267(21):2911-2915.

42. Paiement G, Wessinger SJ, Waltman AC, Harris WH: Low-dose warfarin versus external pneumatic compression for prophylaxis against venous thromboembolism following total hip replacement. *J Arthroplasty* 1987;2(1):23-26.

43. Colwell CW Jr, Froimson MI, Mont MA, et al: Thrombosis prevention after total hip arthroplasty: A prospective, randomized trial comparing a mobile compression device with low-molecular-weight heparin. *J Bone Joint Surg Am* 2010;92(3):527-535.

44. Sharrock NE, Gonzalez Della Valle A, Go G, Lyman S, Salvati EA: Potent anticoagulants are associated with a higher all-cause mortality rate after hip and knee arthroplasty. *Clin Orthop Relat Res* 2008;466(3):714-721.

45. Jameson SS, Charman SC, Gregg PJ, Reed MR, van der Meulen JH: The effect of aspirin and low-molecular-weight heparin on venous thromboembolism after hip replacement: A non-randomised comparison from information in the National Joint Registry. *J Bone Joint Surg Br* 2011;93(11):1465-1470.

46. Amstutz HC, Friscia DA, Dorey F, Carney BT: Warfarin prophylaxis to prevent mortality from pulmonary embolism after total hip replacement. *J Bone Joint Surg Am* 1989;71(3):321-326.

47. Landefeld CS, Goldman L: Major bleeding in outpatients treated with warfarin: Incidence and prediction by factors known at the start of outpatient therapy. *Am J Med* 1989;87(2):144-152.

48. Landefeld CS, Rosenblatt MW, Goldman L: Bleeding in outpatients treated with warfarin: Relation to the prothrombin time and important remediable lesions. *Am J Med* 1989;87(2):153-159.

49. Imperiale TF, Speroff T: A meta-analysis of methods to prevent venous thromboembolism following total hip replacement. *JAMA* 1994;271(22):1780-1785.

50. Colwell CW Jr, Collis DK, Paulson R, et al: Comparison of enoxaparin and warfarin for the prevention of venous thromboembolic disease after total hip arthroplasty: Evaluation during hospitalization and three months after discharge. *J Bone Joint Surg Am* 1999;81(7):932-940.

51. Lieberman JR, Wollaeger J, Dorey F, et al: The efficacy of prophylaxis with low-dose warfarin for prevention of pulmonary embolism following total hip arthroplasty. *J Bone Joint Surg Am* 1997;79(3):319-325.

52. Pellegrini VD Jr, Donaldson CT, Farber DC, Lehman EB, Evarts CM: Prevention of readmission for venous thromboembolic disease after total hip arthroplasty. *Clin Orthop Relat Res* 2005;441:56-62.

53. Pellegrini VD Jr, Donaldson CT, Farber DC, Lehman EB, Evarts CM: Prevention of readmission for venous thromboembolism after total knee arthroplasty. *Clin Orthop Relat Res* 2006;452:21-27.

54. Bergqvist D, Benoni G, Björgell O, et al: Low-molecular-weight heparin (enoxaparin) as prophylaxis against venous thromboembolism after total hip replacement. *N Engl J Med* 1996;335(10):696-700.

55. Planes A, Vochelle N, Darmon JY, Fagola M, Bellaud M, Huet Y: Risk of deep-venous thrombosis after hospital discharge in patients having undergone total hip replacement: Double-blind randomised comparison of enoxaparin versus placebo. *Lancet* 1996;348(9022):224-228.

56. Eriksson BI, Borris LC, Friedman RJ, et al: Rivaroxaban ver-

sus enoxaparin for thromboprophylaxis after hip arthroplasty. *N Engl J Med* 2008;358(26):2765-2775.

57. Kakkar AK, Brenner B, Dahl OE, et al: Extended duration rivaroxaban versus short-term enoxaparin for the prevention of venous thromboembolism after total hip arthroplasty: A double-blind, randomised controlled trial. *Lancet* 2008;372(9632):31-39.

58. Lassen MR, Ageno W, Borris LC, et al: Rivaroxaban versus enoxaparin for thromboprophylaxis after total knee arthroplasty. *N Engl J Med* 2008;358(26):2776-2786.

59. Turpie AG, Lassen MR, Davidson BL, et al: Rivaroxaban versus enoxaparin for thromboprophylaxis after total knee arthroplasty (RECORD4): A randomised trial. *Lancet* 2009; 373(9676):1673-1680.

60. Eriksson BI, Dahl OE, Rosencher N, et al: Dabigatran etexilate versus enoxaparin for prevention of venous thromboembolism after total hip replacement: A randomised, double-blind, non-inferiority trial. *Lancet* 2007;370(9591): 949-956.

61. Burnett RS, Clohisy JC, Wright RW, et al: Failure of the American College of Chest Physicians-1A protocol for lovenox in clinical outcomes for thromboembolic prophylaxis. *J Arthroplasty* 2007;22(3):317-324.

62. Francis CW, Pellegrini VD Jr, Totterman S, et al: Prevention of deep-vein thrombosis after total hip arthroplasty: Comparison of warfarin and dalteparin. *J Bone Joint Surg Am* 1997;79(9):1365-1372.

63. Turpie AG, Bauer KA, Eriksson BI, Lassen MR: Fondaparinux vs enoxaparin for the prevention of venous thromboembolism in major orthopedic surgery: A meta-analysis of 4 randomized double-blind studies. *Arch Intern Med* 2002;162(16):1833-1840.

64. Turpie AG, Lassen MR, Eriksson BI, et al: Rivaroxaban for the prevention of venous thromboembolism after hip or knee arthroplasty: Pooled analysis of four studies. *Thromb Haemost* 2011;105(3):444-453.

65. Lassen MR, Gallus A, Raskob GE, et al: Apixaban versus enoxaparin for thromboprophylaxis after hip replacement. *N Engl J Med* 2010;363(26):2487-2498.

66. Connolly SJ, Ezekowitz MD, Yusuf S, et al: Dabigatran versus warfarin in patients with atrial fibrillation. *N Engl J Med* 2009;361(12):1139-1151.

67. Jensen CD, Steval A, Partington PF, Reed MR, Muller SD: Return to theatre following total hip and knee replacement, before and after the introduction of rivaroxaban: A retrospective cohort study. *J Bone Joint Surg Br* 2011;93(1):91-95.

68. Gossling HR, Pellegrini VD Jr: Fat embolism syndrome: A review of the pathophysiology and physiological basis of treatment. *Clin Orthop Relat Res* 1982;165:68-82.

69. Gurd AR: Fat embolism: An aid to diagnosis. *J Bone Joint Surg Br* 1970;52(4):732-737.

70. Peltier LF: Fat embolism: A current concept. *Orthop Clin Relat Res* 1969;66:241-253.

71. Tornabene VW, Fortune JB, Wagner PD, Halasz NA: Gas exchange after pulmonary fat embolism in dogs. *J Thorac Cardiovasc Surg* 1979;78(4):589-599.

72. Herndon JH, Bechtol CO, Crickenberger DP: Fat embolism during total hip replacement: A prospective study. *J Bone Joint Surg Am* 1974;56(7):1350-1362.

73. Della Valle CJ, Jazrawi LM, Di Cesare PE, Steiger DJ: Paradoxical cerebral embolism complicating a major orthopaedic operation: A report of two cases. *J Bone Joint Surg Am* 1999;81(1):108-110.

74. Bone LB, Johnson KD, Weigelt J, Scheinberg R: Early versus delayed stabilization of femoral fractures: A prospective randomized study. *J Bone Joint Surg Am* 1989;71(3):336-340.

75. Pell AC, Christie J, Keating JF, Sutherland GR: The detection of fat embolism by transoesophageal echocardiography during reamed intramedullary nailing: A study of 24 patients with femoral and tibial fractures. *J Bone Joint Surg Br* 1993;75(6):921-925.

76. Pinney SJ, Keating JF, Meek RN: Fat embolism syndrome in isolated femoral fractures: Does timing of nailing influence incidence? *Injury* 1998;29(2):131-133.

77. Kim YH: Incidence of fat embolism syndrome after cemented or cementless bilateral simultaneous and unilateral total knee arthroplasty. *J Arthroplasty* 2001;16(6):730-739.

78. O'Connor MI, Brodersen MP, Feinglass NG, Leone BJ, Crook JE, Switzer BE: Fat emboli in total knee arthroplasty: A prospective randomized study of computer-assisted navigation vs standard surgical technique. *J Arthroplasty* 2010; 25(7):1034-1040.

79. Habashi NM, Andrews PL, Scalea TM: Therapeutic aspects of fat embolism syndrome. *Injury* 2006;37(Suppl 4):S68-S73.

2: Physiology of Musculoskeletal Tissues

Chapter 8

The Development and Growth of the Skeleton

Maurizio Pacifici, PhD

Introduction

The skeleton can be thought of as the ultimate morphogenetic machine determining the overall shape, size, organization, and features of the body. Paleontologists and biologic anthropologists have long used bone fragments to envision and reconstruct the anatomic features of distant human ancestors, down to the level of facial composition and expression. Thus, the formation, sculpting, and growth of the skeletal elements must be regarded as a feat of development, structure, organization, and evolution.[1,2] Biomedical research over recent decades has provided many important insights into the mechanisms by which the skeletal tissues form and their major cell types (chondrocytes, osteoblasts, osteocytes, and osteoclasts) acquire their diversified phenotypic functions.[3-8] However, the understanding of skeletal morphogenesis remains primitive. Most skeletal elements, including the cranial base, vertebrae, ribs, pelvis, and long bones, are formed through endochondral ossification. During this process mesenchymal cells differentiate into chondrocytes that produce and assemble the initial cartilaginous skeletal anlage, which serves as the blueprint for the adult skeleton. The chondrocytes become organized into growth plates that represent the major engine of skeletal growth. In the growth plates, the chondrocytes proliferate, accumulate large amounts of extracellular matrix, and undergo hypertrophy. The hypertrophic chondrocytes mineralize their matrix, undergo apoptosis, provide the mineralized scaffold onto which osteoprogenitor cells differentiate, and produce endochondral bone tissue.[5] The remaining skeletal elements

including the calvaria, mandible, and a portion of the clavicle form through intramembranous ossification.[3] Ectomesenchymal cells differentiate directly into bone cells during this process.

Though distinct in many respects, the endochondral and intramembranous processes are more intimately connected than might be apparent. The first bone tissue to form in a developing long bone is intramembranous and is called the bone collar because it surrounds the incipient diaphysis. Likewise, the mandible forms in intimate association with the Meckel cartilage. The mandibular condyle, which articulates with the glenoid fossa to form the temporomandibular joint, is entirely endochondral. Research has also revealed that cells similar to chondrocytes are transiently present during the early stages of calvaria bone formation.[9]

Cartilage and bone form and work intimately together at multiple places and times during prenatal and postnatal life to bring about skeletogenesis and skeletal growth and morphogenesis. This chapter describes the key steps in the formation of the craniofacial, axial, and appendicular skeleton, discusses recent data on the mechanisms regulating the behavior and function of skeletal cells and the growth of skeletal elements, and illustrates the manner in which defects in basic growth and developmental mechanisms can lead to congenital skeletal conditions.

Craniofacial Development

The progenitor cells responsible for formation of the craniofacial skeletal elements derive from the ectodermal neural crest and the neighboring mesoderm.[2] Between the first and second month of gestation (the embryonic period), the cells migrate from their points of origin, assemble, proliferate to form cell condensations at appropriate sites and times, and give rise to the primordium of the intramembranous and endochondral elements of the skull. The in-

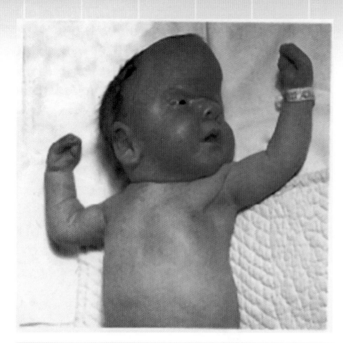

Figure 1 Photograph of an infant with craniosynostoses and considerable skull deformity. (Reproduced with permission from Schoenwolf GC, Bleyl SB, Brauer PR, Francis-West PH: *Larsen's Human Embryology*, ed 4. Philadelphia, PA, Churchill Livingstone Elsevier, 2009.)

tramembranous elements include the frontal and parietal cranial vault bones, the squama of the occipital and temporal bones, the zygomatic bone, the maxilla, and the mandible. The endochondral elements include the occipital bone, the cranial base, the mandibular condyle, and the nasal bone. The skull elements can also be classified as neurocranial or viscerocranial. The neurocranium includes the elements that surround and protect the brain and sensory organs. The viscerocranium includes the elements of the face and pharyngeal arches. Thus, this classification is anatomic and functional and does not take into account whether the elements are intramembranous or endochondral or whether they derive from the neural crest, the mesoderm, or both.

Three-dimensional growth of the intramembranous elements continues through the remaining months of gestation (the fetal period) and into early childhood. The process occurs mostly by apposition, during which progenitor cells differentiate into osteoblasts and are apposed onto the preexisting bone tissue. The progenitor cells responsible for appositional growth of cranial vault elements are part of the fibrous connective and mesenchymal tissue masses called sutures and are connected at the fontanelles located at the corners where the elements meet. Progenitor cell function and differentiation in the sutures are controlled by various mechanisms. Chief among these mechanisms is signaling by members of the fibroblast growth factor (FGF) family through interactions with their high-affinity cell surface receptors FGF-R1, FGF-R2, and FGF-R3.[7] FGF-R3 signaling primarily regulates proliferation of the progenitor cells, and

FGF-R1 signaling regulates osteogenic differentiation. This proliferation-differentiation balance must be maintained for normal vault development. Growth and expansion of the cranial vault and the underlying brain are anatomically and temporally regulated. The posterior and anterolateral fontanelles close during the first 3 months after birth; the other fontanelles remain open and close at approximately 2 years of age. In comparison, the endochondral elements grow not by apposition but through the activities of the growth plate including chondrocyte proliferation, matrix accumulation, and chondrocyte hypertrophy. Much is known about the regulation of chondrocyte behavior and function in growth plates in the skull as well as the trunk and limbs, and this information is described further in the next paragraphs.

The growth plates act not only as the engines of growth but also as morphogenetic instruments. This factor is most apparent in the base of the skull, one of the most anatomically complex and finely shaped skeletal structures in the body, which is designed to accommodate and support the different portions of the brain and neighboring organs. The base of the skull, called the chondrocranium because all of its elements are endochondral, has numerous independent growth plates oriented in different directions and of different sizes. These growth plates support growth and ossification in distinct spatiotemporal directions. Thus, the growth plates can fine-tune morphogenesis in three dimensions and can create exquisite skeletal shapes and molds such as the sella turcica of the sphenoid bone, which accommodates the pituitary gland. The base of the skull, encompassing the region from the ethmoid bone to the foramen magnum, derives from three pairs of cartilaginous plates: the prechordal, hypophyseal, and parachordal cartilages. These pairs of cartilages fuse at midline and give rise to the ethmoid bone, the body of the sphenoid, and the occipital bone, respectively. The cranial base contains unique growth plates called the intrasphenoidal, sphenooccipital, and intraoccipital synchondroses. Each synchondrosis consists of two opposing, mirror-image growth plates that share a central reserve chondrocyte zone, display two proliferative, two prehypertrophic, and two hypertrophic zones, and sustain bidirectional growth along the naso-occipital axis. Despite their unique arrangement and configuration, the synchondrosis dual growth plates are regulated by many of the mechanisms that regulate the single growth plates in all other locations in the developing skeleton.[10] One key set of mechanisms is under the jurisdiction of the signaling secreted molecule Indian hedgehog (Ihh), which is produced by prehypertrophic chondrocytes. Research has shown that another hedgehog family member, sonic hedgehog (Shh), also participates in synchondrosis and skull element development.[11] Under normal circumstances, the intraoccipital synchondroses close at age 1 to 3 years, and the sphenooccipital synchondrosis closes at puberty.

Defects in synchondrosis function and growth rates can cause hypoplasia of the cranial base, as is seen in Apert and

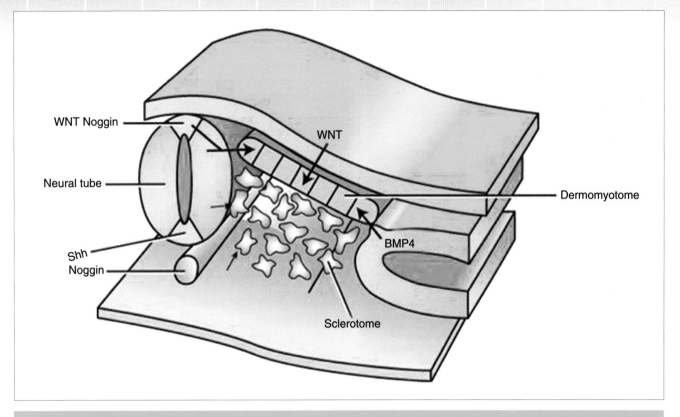

Figure 2 Schematic drawing showing the migration of somite-derived sclerotome cells toward the notochord to form a vertebral primordium. The migration of companion sclerotome cells from the contralateral somite is not depicted. (Adapted with permission from Schoenwolf GC, Bleyl SB, Brauer PR, Francis-West PH: *Larsen's Human Embryology*, ed 4. Philadelphia, PA, Churchill Livingstone Elsevier, 2009.)

Crouzon syndromes, and can have negative repercussions on overall skull growth.[12,13] Likewise, defects in suture function and the timing of suture closure can lead to craniosynostoses that have pathologic repercussions for the cranial base. Craniosynostoses are caused by gain-of-function mutations in the *FGF-R1, FGF-R2,* or *FGF-R3* genes that alter the fine balance between proliferation and differentiation of progenitor cells, cause premature closure of the sutures, and can cause significant skull deformation[14] (**Figure 1**). Craniosynostoses also are associated with mutations in the transcription factors *TWIST* and MSH homeobox 2 (*MSX2*), which also have an important role in cell differentiation. Holoprosencephaly is a devastating condition caused by loss-of-function mutations in the *SHH* gene or its receptor *PATCHED1.*[15] Hedgehog signaling is mediated by primary cilia on the surface of many cell types, and human syndromes affecting the skeleton and other organs, such as Meckel-Gruber syndrome, are caused by malfunction of primary cilia-associated proteins.[16]

Somitogenesis and Axial Skeleton Specification

Beginning at approximately the third week of gestation, the mesoderm flanking the notochord (the paraxial mesoderm)

begins to locally condense, undergoes a mesenchymal-to-epithelial transformation, and produces the first pair of somites near the incipient anatomic border of the future head and trunk and flanking the developing neural tube.[2] Additional pairs of somites form by the same process at short, regular intervals along the cranial-to-sacral axis. Somitogenesis is completed in approximately 1 week with the formation of more than 40 pairs of somites each located to the left and the right of the neural tube. Formation of each somite pair is driven by rapid cycles of expression of Notch family members such as the lunatic fringe gene (*Lnfg*). Examples of this segmentation clock include the formation of a new pair of somites every 90 minutes in chick embryos and every 20 minutes in zebrafish embryos.[17] Soon thereafter, the cells constituting the ventral portion of each somite pair (and collectively known as the sclerotome) undergo an inverse process of epithelial-to-mesenchymal transformation, and migrate toward and gather around the notochord, which is located immediately below the neural tube (**Figure 2**). These processes are directed by Shh secreted by the notochord and the adjacent ventral portion of the neural tube, which diffuses to create a concentration gradient in its surroundings. The cells constituting the dorsal portion of each somite represent the dermomyotome; these

2: Physiology of Musculoskeletal Tissues

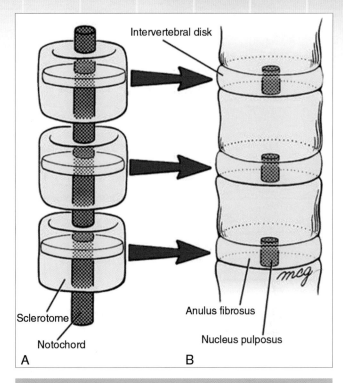

Figure 3 Schematic drawing showing the formation of the intervertebral disks and the vertebrae. **A,** The intervertebral disk is derived from the intersegmental sclerotome and associated notochord segment. **B,** The vertebra is formed by the fusion of the caudal and cranial portions of the neighboring sclerotomes gathered around the notochord. (Adapted with permission from Schoenwolf GC, Bleyl SB, Brauer PR, Francis-West PH: *Larsen's Human Embryology*, ed 4. Philadelphia, PA, Churchill Livingstone Elsevier, 2009.)

cells produce tissues including the dermis and skeletal muscles in the trunk and limbs.

The sclerotomal cells gathering around the notochord are responsible for generating the vertebrae and ribs. The sclerotomal cells deriving from the cranial portion of each somite express Ephrine-B receptor 3 (EphB3), and the cells deriving from the caudal portion express the ligand Ephrin-B1.[18] This differential gene expression is linked to the role of each subpopulation in vertebral formation. Each vertebra is formed by the condensation around the notochord of cranial cells from one somite pair and caudal cells from the preceding somite pair (**Figure 2**). The border between the cranial and caudal subpopulations is called the intersegmental boundary or von Ebner fissure. This border is where the intervertebral disks will form and the spinal nerves will leave the spinal cord. The condensed sclerotomal cells corresponding to each vertebra undergo chondrogenesis and produce three-dimensionally complex cartilaginous templates corresponding to the diverse portions and typical morphologies of each vertebra, such as the vertebral body, neural arches enclosing the vertebral foramen, and transverse processes. The notochord segment present within the developing vertebral body undergoes involution and disappears.

The newly formed chondrocytes become organized into distinct growth plates, undergo hypertrophy and endochondral ossification, and produce the definitive bony vertebrae. Spared from these maturation and hypertrophic processes are the chondrocytes located near the developing intervertebral disk that remain cartilaginous and produce the articulating end plates. More than 40 somite pairs initially form. The sclerotomes of the four occipital somites and the first cervical sclerotome aggregate to produce the two parachordal cartilages that fuse at midline and produce the occipital bone of the skull base. In addition, many pairs of sacral somitic sclerotomes fuse to produce the sacrum and the coccyx.[2] As development and growth of the 24 vertebrae proceed, the spine acquires its typical species-specific curvature, as required for normal biomechanical function and movement. Very little is known of the mechanisms that subtend the spatiotemporal acquisition of normal spine curvature.

The intervertebral disks are critical for spine movement. Each disk is composed of a central nucleus pulposus and the surrounding anulus fibrosus (**Figure 3**). These two components have distinct embryologic origins. The progenitor cells producing the anulus fibrosus are sclerotome cells located along the intersegmental boundary. The cells gather around the notochord but undergo differentiation into fibrocartilaginous cells and produce the collagen I- and II-rich, relatively stiff, and tensile strength–endowed matrix typical of the anulus fibrosus. The progenitor cells of the nucleus pulposus are notochord cells, specifically those around which the intersegmental sclerotome cells gather. Unlike the developing vertebral body notochord cells, which disappear, these notochord cells persist, differentiate into chondrocyte-like nucleus pulposus cells, and produce and accumulate a large amount of extracellular matrix. The extracellular matrix is rich in aggrecan and other proteoglycans but poor in collagen; it attracts a large quantity of water and ions and establishes a very high osmotic pressure, which is believed to be essential for establishing the functional elasticity of the disk. The intervertebral disk (anulus fibrosus plus nucleus pulposus) and flanking vertebral end plates together make up the joints of the spine, which, like typical synovial joints in the limbs, are characterized by local production of lubricating molecules such as lubricin (proteoglycan 4) that sustain movement and minimize mechanical friction (**Figure 4**).

Small lateral sclerotome-derived mesenchymal cell condensations form along the arches of all developing vertebrae at approximately the fifth week of embryogenesis, and those in the thoracic region continue to grow and curve ventrally to produce the ribs. The growing ribs reach the developing sternum by embryonic day 45. Five additional lumbar ribs form and are called false ribs; they are short and do not articulate with the sternum. All ribs are endochondral elements; they develop and elongate through the activities of a single growth plate that progressively shifts in relative position from dorsal toward ventral. The most ventral tips of the

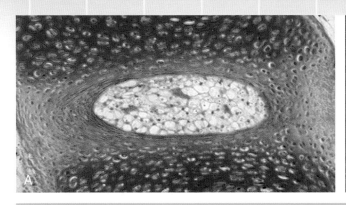
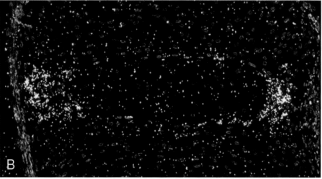

Figure 4 Lubricin gene expression in the developing mouse intervertebral disk. **A,** Bright field microscopic image showing the nucleus pulposus surrounded by the anulus fibrosus. **B,** In situ hybridization signal image showing lubricin transcripts along the nucleus pulposus–anulus fibrosus boundary. (Courtesy of E. Koyama, DDM, PhD, Philadelphia, PA.)

true ribs maintain a cartilaginous character to provide articulation with the sternum.

Given the multiplicity and complexity of the developmental and specification processes regulating the development of the axial skeleton, it is not surprising that a malfunction can lead to numerous pathologies. Spina bifida occulta is caused by defects in the specification, induction, and growth of vertebral arches. Rib defects can result from an absence or misspecification of vertebral identity (called homeotic transformation) or a defect in number, as in spondylocostal dysostoses, Alagille syndrome (caused by mutations in *JAGGED1*), Klippel-Feil syndrome, and other anomalies.[19] The physiologically important spine curvature is affected in patients with scoliosis or excessive kyphosis or lordosis. These conditions include both idiopathic and congenital forms, but their underlying mechanisms are largely unknown. **Figure 5** shows a PA standing radiograph of a patient with adolescent idiopathic scoliosis. The main clinical forms of adolescent idiopathic scoliosis are distinguished using the Lenke classification system which consists of a curvature type, a lumbar spine modifier, and a sagittal thoracic modifier.[20] Low back pain affects a large proportion of the population, particularly older adults, and is associated with progressive loss of the structural arrangements and features of the intervertebral disks, including thinning and stiffening of the tissues, loss of extracellular matrix and water, and, ultimately, loss of functional resilience.[21] It is believed that a major cause of this condition is excessive loss of notochord-derived nucleus pulposus cells because of apoptosis and action by reactive oxygen species, with consequent loss of the proteoglycan-rich matrix and possibly of lubricin and lubrication.

Limb Patterning and Skeletogenesis

The upper and lower limb buds begin to emerge at approximately 3 weeks of embryogenesis as small protrusions at specific locations along the embryonic trunk. The mesenchymal cells present in the limb buds derive from the lateral mesoderm, the somitic dermomyotome, and the neural

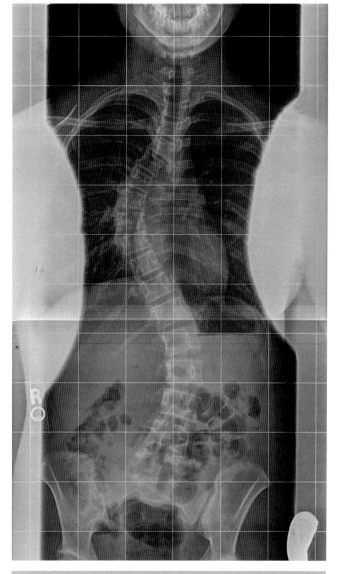

Figure 5 PA standing radiograph of a patient with adolescent idiopathic scoliosis. (Courtesy of John P. Dormans, MD, Philadelphia, PA.)

2: Physiology of Musculoskeletal Tissues

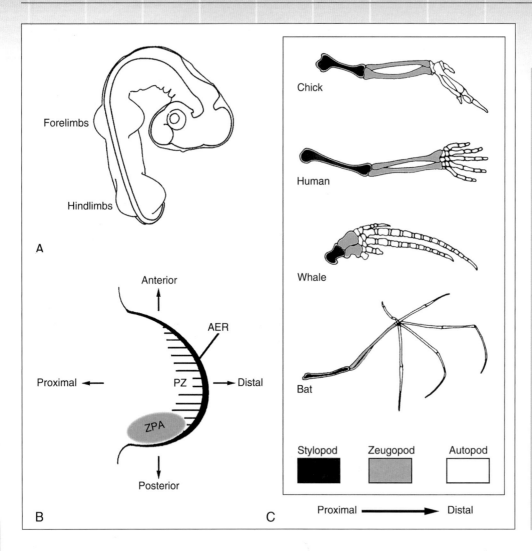

Figure 6 Schematic drawings showing limb bud and skeletal patterning and development. **A,** The location of forelimb and hindlimb buds. **B,** The apical ectodermal ridge (AER) and zone of polarizing activity (ZPA) regulate the proximal-distal and posterior-anterior axes of development and the function of the mesenchymal progress zone (PZ) cells. The dorsal-ventral axis is perpendicular to the plane of this image and is not shown. **C,** Stylopod (proximal), zeugopod (medial), and autopod (distal) portions of the limb skeleton in four species. (Reproduced with permission from Capdevila J, Izpisúa Belmonte JC: Patterning mechanisms controlling vertebrate limb development. *Annu Rev Cell Dev Biol* 2001;17:87-132.)

crest.[2] The lateral mesoderm cells will produce all limb skeletal elements, connective tissues, and ligaments; the somitic dermomyotome cells will produce all the limb skeletal muscles and endothelial cells; and the neural crest cells will produce melanocytes and Schwann cells. Limb outgrowth continues rapidly and is oriented and propelled by three key signaling centers along the proximal-distal, posterior-anterior, and dorsal-ventral axes of symmetry[22,23] (**Figure 6**). The apical ectodermal ridge is located at the very tip of the limb bud and regulates patterning and outgrowth along the proximal-distal axis. The apical ectodermal ridge cells produce Fgf-4, Fgf-8, Fgf-9, and Fgf-17, which diffuse and stimulate proliferation of the underlying mesenchymal cells (collectively known as the progress zone), resulting in further limb outgrowth. Limb outgrowth and development stop if the ectodermal ridge is experimentally removed, but they can resume with application of exogenous FGFs. The zone of polarizing activity regulates patterning along the posterior-anterior axis. This zone consists of mesenchymal cells located at the posterior margin of each limb bud, which produce Shh. Shh diffuses from the zone of polarizing activity, forms a concentration gradient along the

posterior-anterior axis, and regulates patterning and skeletal element identity. For example, the high posterior concentrations of Shh favor small finger formation, and the low anterior concentrations of Shh favor thumb development. If the zone of polarizing activity is removed microsurgically, the posterior-anterior axis of symmetry is completely disrupted. On the other hand, if an additional zone of polarizing activity is transplanted to the anterior margin of a host limb bud (so that the host limb has two zones of polarizing activity and two opposite sources of Shh), limb skeletal development is duplicated in a mirror-image fashion along the posterior-anterior and anterior-posterior axes. In addition, cells present in the dorsal ectoderm regulate limb patterning and growth along the dorsal-ventral axis and produce factors such as wingless-type family member 7A (Wnt-7A). When the dorsal ectoderm is microsurgically removed and transplanted to the ventral side, the dorsal-ventral axis is reversed 180° (for example, foot pads form on the dorsal side). A similar axis inversion is seen in *Wnt-7a* null mice. *Wnt-7a* function is mediated by the homeobox-containing transcription factor Lmx1b. Mice that are mutant for *Lmx1b* in the limbs lack dorsal structures; they also have defects along the posterior-anterior axis because *Lmx1b* regulates *Shh* expression in the zone of polarizing activity.[24]

The three main signaling centers (the apical ectodermal ridge, zone of polarizing activity, and dorsal ectoderm) and signals from flanking structures such as the somites[25,26] closely interact, and they mutually sustain and influence their respective functions. Through these actions, they sustain limb patterning and outgrowth, in particular the progressive formation of mesenchymal condensations corresponding to the humerus and femur (the stylopod region of the limb), the radius and ulna, the tibia and fibula (the zeugopod), and the wrist, ankle, and digit skeletal elements (the autopod) (**Figure 6**). The signaling centers also probably influence formation of all additional tissues and structures specific for each portion of the limb, including skeletal muscles and ligaments. Once formed, the preskeletal mesenchymal condensations undergo chondrogenic cell differentiation that requires the action of transcription factors such as Sox-5, Sox-6, and Sox-9 as well as signaling proteins including bone morphogenetic proteins (BMPs). The resulting chondrocytes assemble the initial cartilaginous anlage that serve as a blueprint of the limb skeleton and can be seen in the proximal region of the limb at approximately the fifth week of embryogenesis and in the distal region at approximately the sixth and seventh weeks.

In addition to the generation of new cells for growth, the normal development of the limb requires the elimination of certain populations of cells by programmed cell death (apoptosis). An important example of this mechanism can be seen in the autopod during the sixth and seventh weeks of embryogenesis, when the interdigit tissues are progressively eliminated to free the developing fingers and toes (the digit rays). Interdigit cell death depends on the action of members of the BMP family,[27] and an increase or decrease in this function can lead to excessive or suboptimal cell death. Interdigit cell death is evolutionary and developmentally controlled; it does not occur in an animal such as a duck, which needs interdigit tissue for swimming.

Limb rotation is another critical aspect of limb development.[2] Initially, the limb buds emerge from the flank at a 90° angle with respect to the main cranial-caudal axis of the embryo. By the fifth week of embryogenesis, however, the outgrowing limbs begin to rotate in a differential manner to eventually position the future arms and legs in their final functional orientation. Thus, the forelimb buds begin to rotate dorsally and bend ventrally so that the future arms will face each other and be able to meet along the ventral midline. The hindlimb buds begin to rotate caudally and align themselves to each other so that the legs will develop caudally and parallel to each other. Despite the critical importance of limb rotation, its underlying mechanisms are essentially unknown.

The early stages of limb development can be affected by many pathologies. For instance, in polydactyly the extra digits are caused by excessive activity of Shh-dependent mechanisms that control the posterior-anterior axis of limb bud development as well as digit number and type.[28] A mutation in the mouse gene *Lmx1b* causes an inversion of the dorsal-ventral axis and limb aberrations; there is a correlation with the mutation in LIM homeobox transcription factor 1β (*LMX1B*) that causes nail-patella syndrome in humans. Normally, the absence of interdigit tissue is regulated by apoptosis. Conditions including Pfeiffer, Apert, and Jackson-Weiss syndromes are caused by gain-of-function mutations in *FGF-R2;* the resulting constitutive activation of FGF signaling triggers excessive survival mechanisms in the interdigit tissues, resulting in webbing and syndactyly.[29]

Formation and Functioning of the Growth Plate

As described in the previous paragraphs, mesenchymal and ectomesenchymal progenitor cells gather at specific sites and times during early embryonic development to produce the condensations of future skeletal elements. Those destined to produce endochondral elements are the most numerous and undergo chondrogenic cell differentiation, thus producing the cartilaginous primordia and the overall blueprint of the future endochondral skeleton. Soon after they form, the chondrocytes further develop and assemble into growth plates. This process has been most studied during the development of limb long bones and will be used here as a paradigm of growth plate formation, functioning through embryogenesis and postnatal life and to closure by the end of puberty.

Once the chondrocytes have differentiated and the cartilaginous long bone anlagen have become apparent by the fourth to fifth week of embryogenesis, the chondrocytes occupying the incipient diaphyseal region begin to mature, slightly enlarge into prehypertrophic chondrocytes, and begin to express Ihh (**Figure 7**). The Ihh-expressing chondrocytes interact with the incipient epiphyseal periarticular chondrocytes and induce them to express parathyroid hormone–related protein (PTHrP).[30] The resulting positive Ihh-PTHrP loop stimulates mitotic activity in underlying chondrocytes together with cyclin-D1 and Sox9, thus establishing the proliferative zone of the growth plate and sustaining the initial elongation of the anlagen. Shortly thereafter, the chondrocytes in the diaphysis further mature into collagen X–producing hypertrophic chondrocytes (the hypertrophic zone). These chondrocytes become flanked by two sets of Ihh-producing prehypertrophic chondrocytes that maintain the Ihh-PTHrP loop with each opposing epiphyseal end. The Ihh-PTHrP loops continue to regulate the rates of proliferation and the rates at which the chondrocytes leave the proliferative zone and irreversibly proceed toward hypertrophy.[5,30] The formation of hypertrophic chondrocytes requires the action of Runt-related transcription factors Runx2 and Runx3 as well as myocyte enhancer factors Mef2C and Mef2D; is stimulated by BMP, Wnt/β-catenin, retinoid signaling, and action by thyroid hormone;[31-35] and is aided by factors including CCAAT en-

2: Physiology of Musculoskeletal Tissues

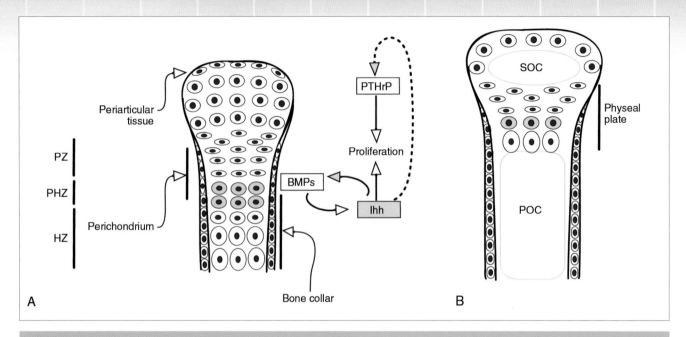

Figure 7 Schematic diagrams showing long bone development. **A,** In the early stage, Ihh produced by prehypertrophic chondrocytes functionally interacts with PTHrP produced by periarticular cells to regulate chondrocyte proliferation and rates of maturation. Ihh also diffuses laterally to induce bone collar formation, with BMPs. **B,** In the late stage after formation of the secondary ossification center, the typical physeal growth plate becomes defined and is flanked by bone on each side. PZ = proliferative zone; PHZ = prehypertrophic zone; HZ = hypertrophic zone; POC = primary ossification center, SOC = secondary ossification center. (Courtesy of E. Koyama, DDM, PhD, Philadelphia, PA.)

hancer–binding protein C/Ebpβ, panexxin-3, histone deacetylase-4 (Hdac4), and stromal cell-derived factor–1 (Sdf-1).[6] The hypertrophic chondrocytes finally reach the terminal developmental stage, at which they mineralize their matrix. This is an essential step because only mineralized matrix can serve as a suitable substrate for ossification. Matrix mineralization is closely and topographically controlled by the hypertrophic chondrocytes that produce and release matrix vesicles.[36] The vesicles bud from the surface of the cells and already contain small preformed hydroxyapatite-rich crystals in their interior; calcium channel proteins on their surface including annexins II, V, and VI; and alkaline phosphatase. Although the exact sequence of mineralization steps is not fully clear, it is believed that the calcium channels facilitate ingress of calcium and further growth of the crystals, then puncture the membrane, spread onto the surrounding matrix, and self-propagate. Counteracting mechanisms limit and contain the mineralization process, including pyrophosphate and proteins such as matrix GLA protein (Mgp). Alkaline phosphatase can aid mineralization by hydrolyzing inhibitors such as pyrophosphate. Mice lacking Mgp exhibit excessive mineralization at ectopic sites including the aorta.[4]

The first bone tissue that forms in developing long bones is intramembranous. Formation is induced by lateral diffusion of Ihh from the prehypertrophic zone into the adjacent metaphyseal perichondrium, resulting in formation of the so-called bone collar[37,38] (**Figure 7**). In the meantime, the hypertrophic chondrocytes located in the diaphysis begin to produce factors including vascular endothelial growth factor A (Vegf-A) and matrix metalloproteases (MMPs) such as Mmp-9 and Mmp-13, which stimulate the recruitment, growth, and invasion of vessels and associated osteoprogenitor and osteoclastogenic cells into the hypertrophic mineralized matrix and promote tissue and matrix remodeling and formation and deposition of endochondral bone (primary spongiosa).[39] Recent genetic cell tracing-tracking research indicates that perichondrial cells form the bone collar and constitute the main source for formation of cortical bone, whereas the progenitor cells associated with the invading blood vessels represent the main source of endochondral bone in primary spongiosa and additional trabecular bone.[40] The research also confirmed that the hypertrophic chondrocytes undergo apoptosis, are eliminated, and do not become bone cells themselves. The phenotypes of mouse mutants are concordant with the above mechanisms. Mice lacking Ihh fail to produce the bone collar and have severe defects in chondrocyte proliferation and endochondral ossification. This finding attests to the essential nature and broad relevance of the Ihh signaling factor.[41] Mice lacking Mmp-9 and/or Mmp-13 exhibit a delay in endochondral ossification as well as significant thickening and expansion of the hypertrophic zone.[39]

Additional mechanisms exist to regulate and fine-tune these complex processes. Prominent among these mechanisms are Fgf-R3, which is expressed by chondrocytes in the proliferative zone, and Fgf-R1, expressed in the hypertrophic zone.[7] The search for possible ligands has led to the identification of Fgf-18, which is produced in the perichondrium, diffuses into the growth plate, and exerts an inhibitory effect on chondrocyte proliferation. The perichondrium also produces members of the transforming growth factor–β (Tgf-β) family that are believed to diffuse into the growth plate, affect PTHrP production by epiphyseal periarticular cells, and thus influence the Ihh-PTHrP loop, which regulates the proliferation of and rate at which the chondrocytes exit the proliferative zone and become irreversibly committed to hypertrophy.[42] Finally, the perichondrium expresses members of the BMP family, specifically *BMP-2, BMP-3, BMP-4, BMP-5* and *Bmp-7. BMP-7* also is expressed in the proliferative zone of growth plate, and *BMP-6* and *BMP-7* are expressed in the hypertrophic zone.[35] It is not clear what function the members of the BMP family play in the perichondrium; one possibility is that they are reserve factors mobilized in case of need, for example during fracture repair. In the growth plate, BMP signaling has a positive role in *IHH* expression and chondrocyte proliferation as well as a positive role in hypertrophy through stimulation of the Runx2 factor.

Development of the Secondary Ossification Center and Physeal Plate Definition

Toward the end of embryogenesis and early postnatal life, the cartilaginous epiphyseal ends of the long bone anlage undergo endochondral ossification, resulting in the formation of a secondary ossification center (**Figure** 7). Chondrocytes located in the central, deepest portion of the epiphysis begin to enlarge, and they mature into hypertrophic chondrocytes reached by blood vessels penetrating from specific sites in surrounding tissues. The arrival of blood vessels initiates endochondral bone formation that spreads radially at 360°. Most long bones have two secondary ossification centers, although the metacarpals and metatarsals have only one. Spared from maturation, hypertrophy, and ossification, the epiphyseal articular chondrocytes that abut the synovial cavity retain a permanent cartilaginous phenotype and sustain joint function throughout life.

The formation of a secondary ossification center leads to the definition of the growth plate as a classic physeal plate flanked by bone on both sides. Most long bones have two growth plates located at each epiphyseal end. Interestingly, the growth plates have distinct rates of elongation even within the same skeletal element, as seen in the proximal and distal growth plates in the radius and ulna. It is not at all clear whether these divergent rates of growth activity are solely influenced by intrinsic mechanisms such as the Ihh-PTHrP loop or Fgf signaling or are directed by systemic factors also well known for their overall roles in growth plate function. Overall, the most prominent of these systemic factors are growth hormone, liver-derived insulin-like growth factor–1, thyroid hormone, and vitamin D. Chondrocyte hypertrophy is the main propeller of skeletal growth, with

chondrocyte proliferation and cartilaginous matrix accumulation acting as additional important contributors. Notably, long bone growth and elongation are not continuous but are most prominent at night. This recumbency pattern suggests that the growth plates can pause in their activity and that biomechanical and circadian mechanisms and circuits play major roles in their activity and in skeletal growth rates.[43] This is in keeping with the fact that biomechanical loading and compression forces across the growth plate are known to reduce growth (the Heuter-Volkmann law) and increases in tensile forces to stimulate growth (the Delpech law). Thus, the relatively prominent growth during recumbency is likely to reflect a relaxation of compression. Under normal circumstances, the growth plates continue to operate under the influence of all of the above complex local and systemic factors through the end of puberty, when skeletal growth is complete and the growth plates close under the influence of mechanisms including estrogen, which acts through its receptor α.[44]

Growth Plate Pathologies

Given the multitude of mechanisms regulating the development and functioning of growth plates, it is not surprising that many defects can affect them, leading to a broad spectrum of human pathologies. Achondroplasia is one example; it is caused by activating mutations in Fgf-R3, resulting in a severe suppression of chondrocyte proliferation, precocious chondrocyte hypertrophy, and dwarfism. Short limbs and dwarfism also are seen in Jansen-type metaphyseal chondrodysplasia caused by activating mutations in the PTH/PTHrP receptor 1, which cause a severe retardation of chondrocyte maturation and hypertrophy as well as matrix mineralization and are associated with hypercalcemia. Rickets is caused by a vitamin D deficiency that disturbs calcium and phosphate homeostasis, causes defects in growth plate mineralization, and leads to broadening of the hypertrophic zone. Because phosphate has a role in apoptosis of hypertrophic chondrocytes,[45] it is likely that the broadening of the hypertrophic zone in rickets is caused by inhibition of apoptosis. Hypophosphatasia, a related condition, is caused by missense mutations in the tissue-nonspecific alkaline phosphatase gene (*ALPL*).[46] Its clinical expression ranges from prenatal death with severe hypomineralization to an adult propensity to fracture, probably related to the severity of the mutation and loss of function. Deficient propagation of mineralization in hypertrophic cartilage and bone typically causes rickets or osteomalacia. Mutations in *IHH* that reduce its bioactivity are associated with brachydactyly type A1 and other skeletal growth deficiencies that reflect the broadly relevant roles of *IHH* in skeletal development and growth plate function. Hereditary multiple exostoses syndrome is caused by loss-of-function mutations in the exostosin genes *EXT1* or *EXT2* that are Golgi-associated glycosyltransferases responsible for heparan sulfate polymerization.[47] The resulting deficiency in heparan sulfate may cause widespread distribution of growth

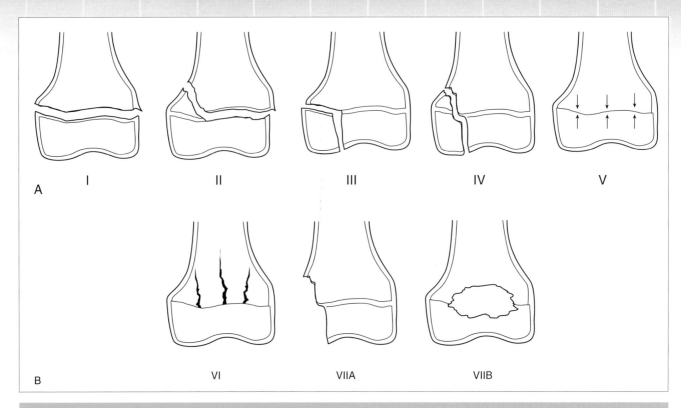

Figure 8 Schematic drawings showing physeal fractures in pediatric patients. **A,** Types I through V, as classified using the Salter-Harris system. **B,** Types VI, VIIA, and VIIB, as classified using the Peterson system. (Adapted with permission from Dormans JP: *Pediatric Orthopaedics: Core Knowledge in Orthopaedics*. Philadelphia, PA, Elsevier Mosby, 2005.)

plate–associated heparan sulfate–binding signaling proteins such as the hedgehogs and BMPs, and it may trigger exostosis formation.

Growth Plate Fractures

Pediatric fractures involving the growth plate require particular attention. Cartilage tissue, especially growth plate cartilage, is largely avascular and is composed of a single cell type (the chondrocyte). Cartilage tissue is precisely demarcated from its surroundings by a unique, specific tissue, the perichondrium. This organizational structure is required for the normal functioning of the growth plate and the permanent cartilages. When the organizational arrangement is violated, as it can happen after a fracture, the growth plate can be seriously damaged or irreversibly compromised if it is invaded by blood vessels, connective tissues, and body fluids that normally are excluded from cartilage. Growth arrest, limb-length discrepancies, and skeletal deformities can occur after growth plate fracture. Their likelihood and the seriousness of the clinical consequences depend on the type of fracture.[48]

Growth plate fractures are classified using the Salter-Harris and Peterson systems (types I through V and VI through VII, respectively) (**Figure 8**). A type I fracture can be caused by shearing forces and can run through and parallel to the physeal plate. This type of fracture does not compromise the neighboring bone and usually does not cause growth disturbance. A type II fracture is similar but extends into the underlying physeal bone to produce a metaphyseal triangular tissue fragment. A type II fracture can lead to growth disturbance, particularly at the junction, and may require reduction and fixation. A type III injury involves a right-angle fracture through the joint that continues laterally through the physeal plate to reach the perichondrium. These injuries are semistable and can cause growth defects. A type IV injury involves the joint and continues through the underlying physeal plate and metaphyseal bone. The fracture usually is low risk if it is anatomically reduced. A type V injury is caused by compression or crush of the physeal plate. This rare type of fracture is potentially serious if crushing is particularly severe. A type VI injury consists of a metaphyseal fracture extending to the physeal plate. In a type VII fracture, there is partial loss of the epiphyseal-metaphyseal region of the skeletal element (type VIIA) or complete central or peripheral loss of the physis (type VIIB). These classifications provide a framework for diagnosis and treatment but can vary greatly depending on the extent of trauma (**Figure 9**). Predictably, the outcome is influenced by factors including the patient's overall health, age, sex, and nutritional status.

Joint Diversity and Formation

The skeletal elements of the body are connected and articulate with one another by means of three main types of joints. The fibrous joints connect neighboring bones but allow little or no movement; an example is the fibrous joints of the skull and pelvis. The cartilaginous joints connect bones and allow some movement; an important example is the costochondral joints. Finally, the synovial joints interconnect and allow full movement of skeletal elements in the limbs and spine. The temporomandibular joint is a specialized example of a synovial joint. The cavity between adjacent bones is filled with synovial fluid rich in lubricating molecules including lubricin and hyaluronan and is enclosed by a synovial capsule to insulate it from surrounding tissues. Most current information on joint development is related to the formation of limb synovial joints and is thus described in detail in the next paragraphs.

Limb joint formation becomes apparent with the emergence of the so-called mesenchymal interzone at each prescribed joint site, first proximally and then distally (**Figure 10**). The interzone at the elbow and knee locations forms at approximately the fifth week of gestation, and the interzones between phalangeal elements appear at approximately the sixth week. The interzone is composed of flat, tightly packed mesenchymal cells that initially define and delineate the anatomic boundary between the adjacent cartilaginous anlagen. It has been found that several signaling molecules converge on the interzone cells to establish and preserve their mesenchymal character at these early stages of joint formation. These signaling molecules include members of the Wnt signaling protein family (Wnt-9A and Wnt-4), the BMP signaling inhibitor noggin, the hedgehog signaling modulator Hip-1, members of the nuclear retinoic acid receptor family, and members of the transforming growth factor–β family.[49]

Classic experiments in which microsurgical removal of the interzone led to joint ablation and fusion showed that the interzone is not merely a transient mesenchymal boundary but is needed for joint formation. However, it was unclear what specific roles the mesenchymal interzone cells have and whether these cells can directly contribute to joint tissue formation. Clear answers to these long-held questions were provided by recent genetic cell tracing-tracking studies involving mice expressing a reporter transgene (β-galactosidase) under the direction of regulatory DNA sequences derived from the interzone master gene growth and differentiation factor 5. The interzone cells were found to persist at the joint sites over time and give rise only to the joint tissues, including articular cartilage, intrajoint ligaments, synovial lining, and inner capsule[50] (**Figure 10**). Thus, interzone cells represent a specialized subset of limb mesenchymal cells that are endowed early in development with a unique capacity to produce joint tissues. What remains unclear is how the interzone cells enter specific differentiation paths and lineages to produce the diverse joint tissues. Some promising studies have indicated that the formation of articular chondrocytes from interzone cells is aided by Pthrp (which is strongly expressed in early periarticular cells) and transcription factor Erg.[51,52] Both Pthrp

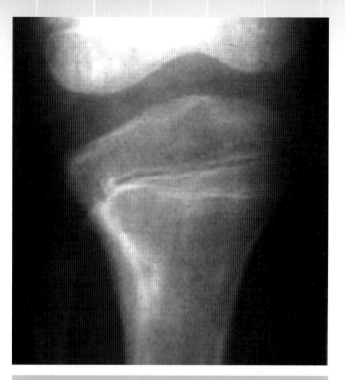

Figure 9 AP radiograph of a patient with a growth arrest line at the knee after a type II or IV physeal fracture. (Reproduced with permission from Dormans JP: *Pediatric Orthopaedics: Core Knowledge in Orthopaedics*. Philadelphia, PA, Elsevier Mosby, 2005.)

and Erg have the ability to maintain chondrocytes in a stable, differentiated, and functional state while preventing the cells from undergoing maturation and hypertrophy, as seen in growth plate chondrocytes. These Pthrp- and Erg-mediated mechanisms could be crucial to endowing articular chondrocytes with their unique and critical ability to maintain a permanent phenotype and sustain joint function for years, thus avoiding the hypertrophy and apoptosis characteristic of growth plate chondrocytes.

Classic embryologic studies involving limb nerve transection or the use of paralyzing agents found that muscle-driven movement in the incipient joints is needed for the progress and completion of joint formation. Recent studies provided further evidence to this effect in mice in which genes responsible for skeletal muscle development (*MyoD* and *Myf5*) were deleted.[53] The resulting mutant embryos displayed limb joints with profound defects and near fusion. Thus, as seen in long bone and growth plate development, a multitude of biomechanical, signaling, and transcriptional mechanisms intervene to bring about the development of synovial joints. A great deal remains unknown, particularly with regard to the means by which each joint acquires its unique shape and three-dimensional configuration, the interzone cells produce the different joint tissues, and the different types of joints form. If available, this type of information could have very important translational medicine implications. For example, if it was known exactly

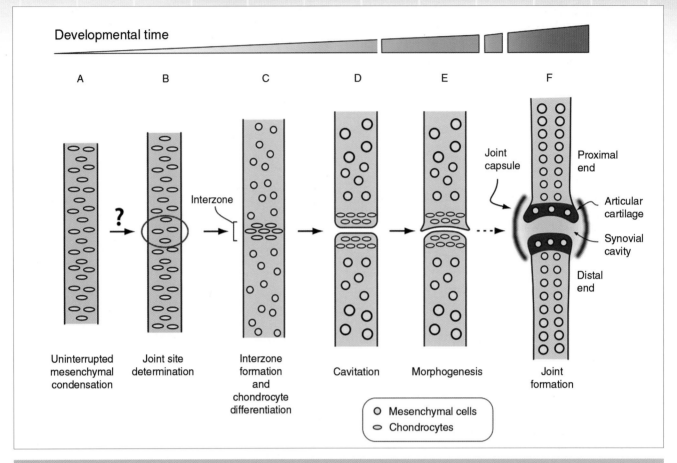

Developmental time

A   B   C   D   E   F

Interzone

Joint capsule

Proximal end

Articular cartilage

Synovial cavity

Distal end

Uninterrupted mesenchymal condensation

Joint site determination

Interzone formation and chondrocyte differentiation

Cavitation

Morphogenesis

Joint formation

O Mesenchymal cells
⊖ Chondrocytes

Figure 10 Schematic diagrams showing the major stages (A to F) in the formation of limb synovial joints. Joint formation is initiated with the emergence of the mesenchymal interzone, whose cells solely give rise to all joint tissues over developmental time. The question mark between stages A and B signifies that the mechanisms of joint site determination are totally unknown at present. Stages A to F span approximately week 4 to week 6 of human gestation. (Adapted with permission from Pacifici M, Koyama E, Iwamoto M: Mechanisms of synovial joint and articular cartilage formation: Recent advances, but many lingering mysteries. *Birth Defects Res C Embryo Today* 2005;75(pt C):237-248.)

how interzone cells produce articular cartilage, the mechanisms could be used to program generic stem-progenitor cells with such developmental capacity and to use such cells for joint repair and regeneration.

Joints are affected by conditions including chronic age-related osteoarthritis and genetic conditions. Joint ablation and fusion can be observed in mouse embryos lacking *noggin*, *Wnt9a*, or *Wnt4*. Significant joint defects occur in patients with proximal symphalangism or multiple synostoses syndrome caused by loss-of-function mutations in noggin or gain-of-function mutations in the growth differentiation factor–5 gene (*GDF-5*). Other conditions affect joint morphogenesis, in particular the process by which the opposing sides of a given joint acquire their reciprocal and ball-and-socket shapes. Developmental dysplasia of the hip is a common pathology that occurs in varying degrees of severity; a recent study linked a familial form to a 4-Mb region in chromosome 17q21 in one multigeneration family.[54]

Summary

This outline of skeletal development and growth in the skull, trunk, and limbs summarizes the remarkable features of these processes as well as their complexities, multiple levels of regulation and modulation, and susceptibility to varied pathologies. The work of many biomedical and clinical research groups has led to critical information on the cellular, biochemical, molecular, and biomechanical regulation of skeletal development and growth and the use of this information to develop and implement therapies. Such coordinated efforts of skeletal researchers and clinician scientists will continue to broaden basic information and improve the diagnosis and treatment of congenital and acquired skeletal conditions.

References

1. Hall BK: *Bones and Cartilage: Developmental and Evolutionary Skeletal Biology*. San Diego, CA, Elsevier Academic Press, 2005.

2. Schoenwolf GC, Bleyl SB, Brauer PR, Francis-West PH: *Larsen's Human Embryology*, ed 4. Philadelphia, PA, Churchill Livingstone Elsevier, 2009.

3. Helms JA, Schneider RA: Cranial skeletal biology. *Nature* 2003;423(6937):326-331.

4. Karsenty G: The complexities of skeletal biology. *Nature* 2003;423(6937):316-318.

5. Kronenberg HM: Developmental regulation of the growth plate. *Nature* 2003;423(6937):332-336.

6. Marino R: Growth plate biology: New insights. *Curr Opin Endocrinol Diabetes Obes* 2011;18(1):9-13.

7. Ornitz DM, Marie PJ: FGF signaling pathways in endochondral and intramembranous bone development and human genetic disease. *Genes Dev* 2002;16(12):1446-1465.

8. Bonewald LF: The amazing osteocyte. *J Bone Miner Res* 2011;26(2):229-238.

9. Nah H-D, Pacifici M, Gerstenfeld LC, Adams SL, Kirsch T: Transient chondrogenic phase in the intramembranous pathway during normal skeletal development. *J Bone Miner Res* 2000;15(3):522-533.

10. Shum L, Wang X, Kane AA, Nuckolls GH: BMP4 promotes chondrocyte proliferation and hypertrophy in the endochondral cranial base. *Int J Dev Biol* 2003;47(6):423-431.

11. Koyama E, Young B, Nagayama M, et al: Conditional Kif3a ablation causes abnormal hedgehog signaling topography, growth plate dysfunction, and excessive bone and cartilage formation during mouse skeletogenesis. *Development* 2007; 134(11):2159-2169.

12. Jensen BL, Kreiborg S: Development of the skull in infants with cleidocranial dysplasia. *J Craniofac Genet Dev Biol* 1993; 13(2):89-97.

13. Mooney MP, Losken HW, Tschakaloff A, Siegel MI, Losken A, Lalikos JF: Congenital bilateral coronal suture synostosis in a rabbit and craniofacial growth comparisons with experimental models. *Cleft Palate Craniofac J* 1993;30(2):121-128.

14. Marie PJ, Coffin JD, Hurley MM: FGF and FGFR signaling in chondrodysplasias and craniosynostosis. *J Cell Biochem* 2005;96(5):888-896.

15. Roessler E, Belloni E, Gaudenz K, et al: Mutations in the human Sonic Hedgehog gene cause holoprosencephaly. *Nat Genet* 1996;14(3):357-360.

16. Badano JL, Mitsuma N, Beales PL, Katsanis N: The ciliopathies: An emerging class of human genetic disorders. *Annu Rev Genomics Hum Genet* 2006;7:125-148.

17. Aulehla A, Johnson RL: Dynamic expression of lunatic fringe suggests a link between notch signaling and an autonomous cellular oscillator driving somite segmentation. *Dev Biol* 1999;207(1):49-61.

18. Durbin L, Brennan C, Shiomi K, et al: Eph signaling is required for segmentation and differentiation of the somites. *Genes Dev* 1998;12(19):3096-3109.

19. Zelzer E, Olsen BR: The genetic basis for skeletal diseases. *Nature* 2003;423(6937):343-348.

20. Lenke LG, Edwards CC II, Bridwell KH: The Lenke classification of adolescent idiopathic scoliosis: How it organizes curve patterns as a template to perform selective fusions of the spine. *Spine (Phila Pa 1976)* 2003;28(20, 20S):S199-S207.

21. Tsai T-T, Guttapalli A, Agrawal A, Albert TJ, Shapiro IM, Risbud MV: MEK/ERK signaling controls osmoregulation of nucleus pulposus cells of the intervertebral disc by transactivation of TonEBP/OREBP. *J Bone Miner Res* 2007;22(7): 965-974.

22. Capdevila J, Izpisúa Belmonte JC: Patterning mechanisms controlling vertebrate limb development. *Annu Rev Cell Dev Biol* 2001;17:87-132.

23. Zeller R, López-Ríos J, Zuniga A: Vertebrate limb bud development: Moving towards integrative analysis of organogenesis. *Nat Rev Genet* 2009;10(12):845-858.

24. Yang Y, Niswander L: Interaction between the signaling molecules WNT7a and SHH during vertebrate limb development: Dorsal signals regulate anteroposterior patterning. *Cell* 1995;80(6):939-947.

25. Mercader N, Leonardo E, Piedra ME, Martínez-A C, Ros MA, Torres M: Opposing RA and FGF signals control proximodistal vertebrate limb development through regulation of Meis genes. *Development* 2000;127(18):3961-3970.

26. Cooper KL, Hu JK, ten Berge D, Fernandez-Teran M, Ros MA, Tabin CJ: Initiation of proximal-distal patterning in the vertebrate limb by signals and growth. *Science* 2011; 332(6033):1083-1086.

27. Zou H, Niswander L: Requirement for BMP signaling in interdigital apoptosis and scale formation. *Science* 1996; 272(5262):738-741.

28. Lettice LA, Heaney SJ, Purdie LA, et al: A long-range Shh enhancer regulates expression in the developing limb and fin and is associated with preaxial polydactyly. *Hum Mol Genet* 2003;12(14):1725-1735.

29. Wilkie AO, Morriss-Kay GM, Jones EY, Heath JK: Functions of fibroblast growth factors and their receptors. *Curr Biol* 1995;5(5):500-507.

30. Vortkamp A, Lee K, Lanske B, Segre GV, Kronenberg HM, Tabin CJ: Regulation of rate of cartilage differentiation by Indian hedgehog and PTH-related protein. *Science* 1996; 273(5275):613-622.

31. Enomoto-Iwamoto M, Kitagaki J, Koyama E, et al: The Wnt antagonist Frzb-1 regulates chondrocyte maturation and long bone development during limb skeletogenesis. *Dev Biol* 2002;251(1):142-156.

32. Grimsrud CD, Romano PR, D'Souza M, et al: BMP signaling stimulates chondrocyte maturation and the expression of Indian hedgehog. *J Orthop Res* 2001;19(1):18-25.

33. Koyama E, Golden EB, Kirsch T, et al: Retinoid signaling is required for chondrocyte maturation and endochondral bone formation during limb skeletogenesis. *Dev Biol* 1999; 208(2):375-391.

34. Robson H, Siebler T, Stevens DA, Shalet SM, Williams GR: Thyroid hormone acts directly on growth plate chondrocytes to promote hypertrophic differentiation and inhibit clonal expansion and cell proliferation. *Endocrinology* 2000; 141(10):3887-3897.

35. Yoon BS, Pogue R, Ovchinnikov DA, et al: BMPs regulate multiple aspects of growth-plate chondrogenesis through opposing actions on FGF pathways. *Development* 2006; 133(23):4667-4678.

2: Physiology of Musculoskeletal Tissues

36. Kirsch T, Harrison G, Golub EE, Nah H-D: The roles of annexins and types II and X collagen in matrix vesicle-mediated mineralization of growth plate cartilage. *J Biol Chem* 2000;275(45):35577-35583.

37. Koyama E, Leatherman JL, Noji S, Pacifici M: Early chick limb cartilaginous elements possess polarizing activity and express hedgehog-related morphogenetic factors. *Dev Dyn* 1996;207(3):344-354.

38. Nakamura T, Aikawa T, Iwamoto-Enomoto M, et al: Induction of osteogenic differentiation by hedgehog proteins. *Biochem Biophys Res Commun* 1997;237(2):465-469.

39. Page-McCaw A, Ewald AJ, Werb Z: Matrix metalloproteinases and the regulation of tissue remodelling. *Nat Rev Mol Cell Biol* 2007;8(3):221-233.

40. Maes C, Kobayashi T, Selig MK, et al: Osteoblast precursors, but not mature osteoblasts, move into developing and fractured bones along with invading blood vessels. *Dev Cell* 2010;19(2):329-344.

41. St-Jacques B, Hammerschmidt M, McMahon AP: Indian hedgehog signaling regulates proliferation and differentiation of chondrocytes and is essential for bone formation. *Genes Dev* 1999;13(16):2072-2086.

42. Mukherjee A, Dong SS, Clemens T, Alvarez J, Serra R: Coordination of TGF-beta and FGF signaling pathways in bone organ cultures. *Mech Dev* 2005;122(4):557-571.

43. Noonan KJ, Farnum CE, Leiferman EM, Lampl M, Markel MD, Wilsman NJ: Growing pains: Are they due to increased growth during recumbency as documented in a lamb model? *J Pediatr Orthop* 2004;24(6):726-731.

44. Weise M, De-Levi S, Barnes KM, Gafni RI, Abad V, Baron J: Effects of estrogen on growth plate senescence and epiphyseal fusion. *Proc Natl Acad Sci U S A* 2001;98(12):6871-6876.

45. Mansfield K, Rajpurohit R, Shapiro IM: Extracellular phosphate ions cause apoptosis of terminally differentiated epiphyseal chondrocytes. *J Cell Physiol* 1999;179(3):276-286.

46. Mornet E: Hypophosphatasia: The mutations in the tissue-nonspecific alkaline phosphatase gene. *Hum Mutat* 2000;15(4):309-315.

47. Zak BM, Crawford BE, Esko JD: Hereditary multiple exostoses and heparan sulfate polymerization. *Biochim Biophys Acta* 2002;1573(3):346-355.

48. Dormans JP: *Pediatric Orthopaedics: Core Knowledge in Orthopaedics.* Philadelphia, PA, Elsevier Mosby, 2005.

49. Pacifici M, Koyama E, Iwamoto M: Mechanisms of synovial joint and articular cartilage formation: Recent advances, but many lingering mysteries. *Birth Defects Res C Embryo Today* 2005;75(3, pt C):237-248.

50. Koyama E, Shibukawa Y, Nagayama M, et al: A distinct cohort of progenitor cells participates in synovial joint and articular cartilage formation during mouse limb skeletogenesis. *Dev Biol* 2008;316(1):62-73.

51. Chen X, Macica CM, Nasiri A, Broadus AE: Regulation of articular chondrocyte proliferation and differentiation by indian hedgehog and parathyroid hormone-related protein in mice. *Arthritis Rheum* 2008;58(12):3788-3797.

52. Iwamoto M, Tamamura Y, Koyama E, et al: Transcription factor ERG and joint and articular cartilage formation during mouse limb and spine skeletogenesis. *Dev Biol* 2007;305(1):40-51.

53. Kahn J, Shwartz Y, Blitz E, et al: Muscle contraction is necessary to maintain joint progenitor cell fate. *Dev Cell* 2009;16(5):734-743.

54. Feldman G, Dalsey C, Fertala K, et al: The Otto Aufranc Award: Identification of a 4 Mb region on chromosome 17q21 linked to developmental dysplasia of the hip in one 18-member, multigeneration family. *Clin Orthop Relat Res* 2010;468(2):337-344.

Chapter 9

Form and Function of Bone

Oran D. Kennedy, PhD
Robert J. Majeska, PhD
Mitchell B. Schaffler, PhD

Introduction

Bones come in a variety of shapes, sizes, and internal organizational patterns, all of which appear well suited to their physiologic roles in providing support, leverage, and protection to other tissues; and in serving as repositories of calcium and phosphate to help maintain mineral homeostasis. High mechanical strength, resistance to fracture, and a high surface-to-volume ratio are specific structural/architectural features of bone related to these functions. Moreover, these features are evident at all levels of structural hierarchy, from overall tissue shape through intermediary organization—the relationships among cellular cohorts and their extracellular matrix (ECM)—to molecular associations among matrix constituents. Yet the relationship between form and function in bone is even more complex (and interesting) because the architecture of bone is dynamic. The rigidity of bone structure and its persistence far beyond the average person's lifetime has led to the mistaken impression that bone is largely inert. Bone has the ability to alter its structure in response to both mechanical and metabolic stimuli, and indeed that capability not only underlies some of bone's distinctive and advantageous mechanical features, but also many diseases whose pathologic signatures involve the skeleton.

This chapter will discuss what makes bone so distinctive and how it is formed during development, its structural fea-

tures at all hierarchical levels (from macroscopic size and shape through tissue-level organization to ECM composition and microstructure), and the major cell types in bone. Also discussed are issues of tissue mechanics, mechanical regulation, and the clinical consequences that ensue when bone structure and function are altered.

Bone Structure

Bone is a connective tissue (similar to cartilage, tendon, dentin, and dermis, for example) and contains an abundance of ECM relative to cells. The properties of that ECM are responsible in large part for the physical, chemical, and biologic features of the tissue itself.[1-5] The properties of a connective tissue's ECM, including whether it will mineralize, are in turn determined by the cells that produce it—osteoblasts for bone, chondrocytes for cartilage, and fibroblasts for various fibrous connective tissues, for example. Features such as size and shape are determined by control mechanisms operating at a different hierarchical level to determine where and when the tissue will be formed or broken down. Those morphogenetic "decisions" are based on the relationship of the newly forming bone to other tissues, on inherent morphogenetic programming of the bone cells, and on environmental cues that include physical as well as chemical signals.

Bones initially form by the differentiation of embryonic progenitor cells into osteoblasts that synthesize and secrete bone ECM.[6,7] As this process continues, the bone grows. The size and shape of the bone are determined by controlling when and where progenitors can be recruited to differentiate into osteoblasts and produce bone, and also when and where other cells (osteoclasts) can be recruited to degrade bone. These sets of anabolic and catabolic processes combine to sculpt the unique shapes ultimately achieved by each bone. The specific aspects of bone formation and degradation will be discussed in detail later in the chapter.

Dr. Majeska or an immediate family member serves as a paid consultant to or is an employee of Medtronic Sofamor Danek and has stock or stock options held in Pfizer. Neither of the following authors or any immediate family member has received anything of value from or owns stock in a commercial company or institution related directly or indirectly to the subject of this chapter: Dr. Kennedy and Dr. Schaffler.

2: Physiology of Musculoskeletal Tissues

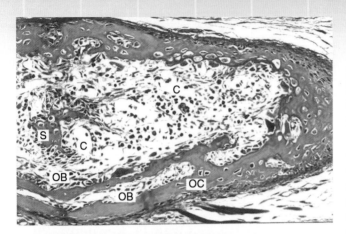

Figure 1 Intramembranous bone formation. Section of a growing flat bone showing the outer cortex of newly formed bone containing osteocytes (OC) with osteoblasts (OB) lining the bony surfaces. A core of mesenchymal tissue, which is supplied by capillaries (C), can be seen. New spicules (S) of bone can also be seen, which will become the individual trabeculae. (Courtesy of Yale, School of Medicine, Developmental Histology, New Haven, CT.)

Bones form by two distinct developmental pathways.[2,5,7] In intramembranous bone formation (**Figure 1**), small concentrations of cells form within regions of embryonic mesenchyme and differentiate into osteoblasts, which secrete bone ECM. Clusters of osteoblasts directly form small spicules of bone and these regions of bone coalesce into bone plates. Bones formed by the intramembranous path include the flat bones of the cranium and small portions of the postcranial skeleton. The second pathway of osteogenesis, termed endochondral bone formation (**Figure 2**), is more complex and is the pathway used to form long bones such as the femur and tibia, as well as vertebral bodies and most small bones of the postcranial skeleton. Endochondral bone formation begins with the formation of a cartilage model (anlage) within embryonic mesenchyme. A collar of bone forms around the central region of the cartilage rod as other mesenchymal cells differentiate into osteoblasts and begin to produce bone ECM. Subsequently both bone and cartilage grow in a coordinated way as the tissue expands. In addition, degradation of both cartilage and bone also occurs. These processes shape the bone and moreover cause the regions of growing cartilage to become restricted to narrow zones near the ends of the growing bone. The combination of formation and breakdown continues until the bone reaches its ultimate size at skeletal maturity. At this point, cartilage growth ceases and the remaining cartilage is removed and replaced by bone. Details of these developmental processes are available in most anatomy texts. However, a few points should be noted here. First, the growth in length of long bones depends not so much on the recruitment and activity of osteoblasts but on the growth of cartilage in the growth zones. Second, as long as endochondrally formed bones are growing in length, regions of cartilage will be ev-

ident. Third, this endochondral bone formation process begins in utero during the first trimester of development and continues until the cessation of skeletal growth in late adolescence. In addition, even after skeletal maturity, a few islands of cartilage that have not been completely replaced by bone may be apparent. These features are not seen in intramembranous bone.

CLINICAL NOTE: The development of bones by the endochondral pathway depends critically on the control of cartilage differentiation and growth throughout the developmental process. As a result, a large number of orthopaedic pathologies characterized by skeletal malformations arise from genetic or developmental deficiencies in cartilage rather than bone per se. These include instances of defective skeletal patterning (for example, polydactyly) due to altered expression of transcription factors controlling chondrocyte differentiation and various forms of dwarfism due to impaired function of chondrocytes in growth zones.

In addition, the fundamental architecture of cancellous bone (discussed later) is formed from the growth plate. Thus, the structure and mechanical function of cancellous bone are largely established during growth and development, and these cannot be "fixed" easily if the tissue is not laid down correctly the first time.

Anatomy

Bones are often categorized roughly as being either long or flat.[1-4] As noted, long bones, which include those of the appendicular skeleton such as the humerus, femur, and tibia, generally form endochondrally, whereas flat bones, like those of the cranium, arise via intramembranous ossification. All bones contain an outer layer of dense compact, or cortical, bone that surrounds a network of thin trabecular, or cancellous, bone and an interior space filled with marrow. Like size and shape, the relative amounts and spatial distributions of cortical bone, cancellous bone, and marrow differ greatly among bones. These differences generally reflect functional differences (for example, in load bearing or support of hematopoiesis). Cortical bone accounts for approximately 80% of adult skeletal mass, predominates in bones of the appendicular skeleton (arms, legs, digits) rather than the axial skeleton (cranium, spine), and plays major roles in mechanical support and protection. Cancellous bone consists of a lattice of struts and plates whose organization and orientation tend to reflect its mechanical environment. Indeed, the organization and orientation of cancellous bone provided much of the basis for the Wolff laws of bone remodeling. Cancellous bone has a greater amount of surface relative to its mass than cortical bone (approximately 20:1 versus 4:1, respectively), and because bone cell activities are surface based, cancellous bone turns over about three to five times more rapidly. Cortical bone and cancellous bone often respond differently to physical and chemical perturbations. As an example, bone loss that results from aging or gonadal steroid depletion can differ between cortical and cancellous bone, just as for bones from

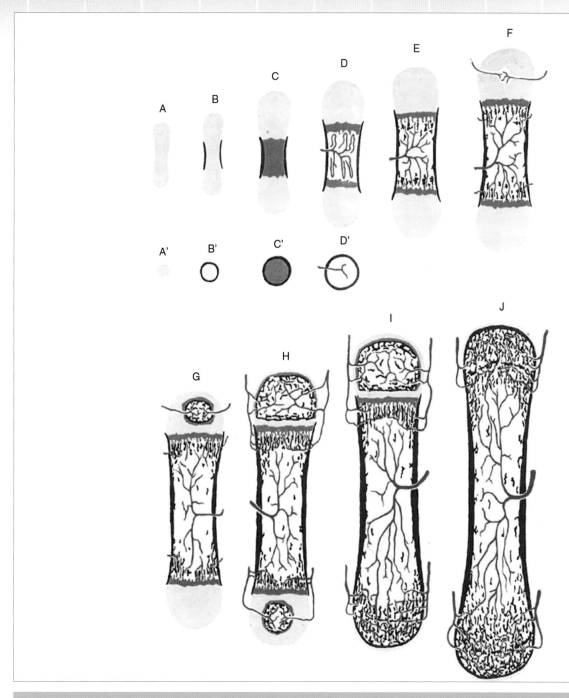

Figure 2 Schematic representation of each of the steps of endochondral ossification from the entirely cartilaginous anlage through to the fully vascularized mature long bone. **A** through **J** show longitudinal sections of the developing bone. **A**' through **D**' show cross sections through the centers of their respective images. Cartilage is shown in blue, calcified cartilage in purple, bone in black, blood vessels in red, and marrow (within the bone) in white. **A,** Cartilage model. **B,** Cartilage with bony collar. **C,** Hypertrophy and mineralization of cartilage in the central region beneath bony collar. **D,** Invasion of blood vessels and removal of calcified cartilage in the central region. **E,** Formation of bone on trabeculae of calcified cartilage, which is subsequently removed. **F** through **H,** Invasion of blood vessels near ends of developing tissue and formation of secondary ossification centers. **I** and **J,** Continued growth in length and diameter, expansion of marrow cavity, and restriction of growth to epiphyseal plates. **J,** Closure of epiphyseal growth plates; cartilage is seen at articular surfaces. (Adapted with permission from Bloom W, Fawcett D: Bone, in *A Textbook of Histology.* Philadelphia, PA, WB Saunders, 1969, p 247.)

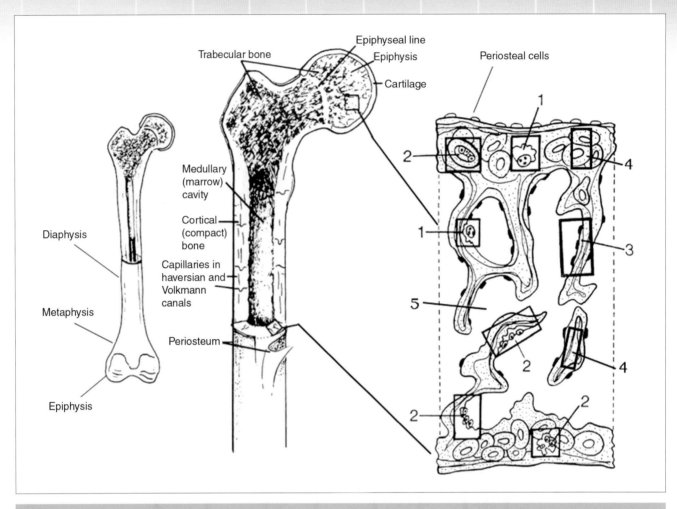

Figure 3 Schematic diagram of cortical and trabecular bone showing the different structures and cell types. 1 = osteoclasts, 2 = osteoblasts, 3 = bone lining cells, 4 = osteocytes, 5 = marrow space. (Reproduced with permission from Hayes WC: Biomechanics of cortical and trabecular bone: Implications for assessment of fracture risk, in *Basic Orthopaedic Biomechanics*. New York, NY, Raven Press, 1991, pp 93-142.)

different anatomic sites (for example, spine versus hip).

Most features of bone can be illustrated by the femur, a prototypical long bone that roughly resembles a cylinder with fluted ends (**Figure 3**). The middle region (diaphysis) is flanked by the metaphyses and the epiphyses. The diaphysis consists of a thick shell of compact cortical bone enclosing a marrow cavity with little or no cancellous bone. In the metaphyses and epiphyses, the cortices are thinner and surround a more extensive network of cancellous bone. Marrow occupies the internal spaces of the bone. As noted previously, the growth plate, or physis, separates the epiphysis from the metaphysis in growing bones, but cartilage disappears from the physeal region after growth ceases.

Both the external and internal (marrow) surfaces of bone are covered by some form of nonmineralized connective tissue. Externally, the ends of bones that form joint surfaces are covered by articular cartilage, whereas the remainder of bone is covered by the periosteum, a somewhat elastic sleeve of dense fibrous connective tissue. The periosteum includes a layer of cells near the bone surface (the cambium layer)

that contains progenitor cells capable of forming new bone and cartilage when necessary, for example, during growth or in response to injury. Internally, surfaces of both cortical and cancellous bone are covered by the bone marrow stroma, a fibrous connective tissue more loosely organized than the periosteum. Cells of the marrow stroma comprise a heterogeneous group that plays several roles in maintaining both the hematopoietic system and connective tissues. Hematopoietic stem cells that give rise to all blood cell types reside physically in or around the stroma, whereas connective tissue cell populations within marrow stroma produce growth factors needed to sustain the hematopoietic stem cells and to support their differentiation. In addition, bone marrow stroma contains a population of nonhematopoietic adult stem cells (termed mesenchymal stem cells or MSCs) capable of differentiating into bone, cartilage, tendon, and muscle cells, among others. As a result, bone marrow stroma has been a focus of considerable interest in the search for cells for use in tissue engineering and regenerative medicine.

Like all tissues, bone is supplied by blood vessels and nerves.[8] These are more extensively distributed throughout the periosteum and the bone marrow than in bone itself. Vessels and nerves that supply the marrow pass through cortical bone only at limited entry points (nutrient foramina). Smaller vessels and nerves are distributed throughout cortical bone, passing through channels in the tissue termed haversian canals and Volkmann canals (discussed in the next paragraphs). The extent of intracortical vasculature varies considerably among individual bones and certainly among species. In bones that lack haversian systems, primary vascular canals are still present, running in both longitudinal and transverse directions.

Blood vessels in both the periosteum and the marrow combine to maintain cortical bone. The outer third of the cortex is supplied by periosteal vessels, whereas the inner portion is supplied by vessels emanating radially from within the marrow compartment. Bone marrow vasculature also services trabecular bone, which itself does not contain vessels. There is a second so-called circulatory system in bone—the extravascular movement of fluids and solutes through the pericellular space between osteocytes and their processes and their bony lacunar and canalicular walls; fluid in this space moves under convective flow driven by blood pressure and by mechanical loading. Finally, the question of whether bone has lymphatic drainage remains unresolved.

Tissue-Level Organization

Tissue-level (or intermediate) organization considers the way cells and ECM are arranged within bone tissue at the microscopic length scale, and its description is historically based largely on microscopy and histologic staining methods.[1,6,9] Most cortical and cancellous bone can be characterized as either woven or lamellar. Woven bone is a poorly organized tissue in which neither the bone cells nor the fibers in their surrounding matrix exhibit a regular, periodic arrangement. Most notably, the collagen fibers in woven bone matrix are randomly oriented. Woven bone is produced during periods of rapid bone formation, for example, during development, in fracture callus, and in primary bone tumors (osteosarcomas). In nonpathologic circumstances, woven bone is a temporary or provisional tissue that is removed and replaced by more highly organized lamellar bone, which comprises effectively all adult cortical and cancellous bone tissue. Lamellar bone consists of tissue layers (lamellae) approximately 3 to 5 μm thick, in which the collagen fibers run mainly in the same direction. The orientation of fibers in adjacent lamellae, however, differs by as much as 90°, giving lamellar bone a "cross-ply" or plywood-like appearance that is particularly evident under polarized light microscopy. This arrangement of fibers in successive lamellae is illustrated in **Figure 4**. The interfaces between successive lamellae are not understood, but may have mechanical significance.

In cortical bone, lamellae are generally organized in one of several ways. (1) Circumferential lamellae extend continuously around some or all of a bone's circumference. The most prominent example is the deposition of effectively complete circumferential sheets on the periosteal surface of bone during radial growth of diaphyses ("outer circumferential lamellae"). (2) Circumferentially oriented lamellae are added to parts of the endosteal surface as well ("inner circumferential lamellae"), although these often do not extend the full extent of the inner surface of the bone. (3) Osteonal or haversian lamellae are concentric rings of tissue that lie inside an osteon or haversian system—a cylindrical region that surrounds a vascular channel within bone. (4) Interstitial lamellae are remnants of lamellae that lie between haversian systems and can be composed of fragments of circumferential lamellar bone from earlier times in a bone's growth, or of fragments of preexisting haversian systems.

Haversian systems or secondary osteons are formed after the initial bone is laid down, and arise by bone remodeling—the sequential removal and replacement of a region of bone, a process that will be discussed in greater detail later in the chapter. During osteonal remodeling, a new blood vessel buds from an existing vessel—either in periosteum, marrow, or within the bone—and grows within the remodeling region to keep pace with the excavation process.[5] It then remains in place within the newly formed bone, in a central vascular canal, after remodeling is complete. The vascular canals that are roughly aligned with the long axis of the bone are termed haversian canals, whereas those that run transversely are called Volkmann canals. The borders of each osteon are delineated by a thin layer of distinctive matrix that is termed a cement line. The cement line is a bonding layer formed after the old matrix has been removed during remodeling and before new bone matrix is deposited.

In cancellous bone, lamellae are organized comparably to cortical bone. The lamellae are present as unremodeled layers, crescent-shaped remodeling packets, or interstitial lamellae between these packets. Remodeling packets are formed because remodeling of trabeculae occurs along the surface. This process has been termed hemiosteonal remodeling. Cement lines separate the hemiosteonal packets of remodeled bone from the interstitial regions.

The organizational patterns of osteons, lamellae, struts, and plates discussed so far reflect the way that ECM is distributed in bone, but has not addressed the cellular components of the tissue.[1,5,6,9] In both woven and lamellar bone, four types of cells can be found either on bone surfaces or distributed throughout the matrix. Osteoblasts (bone-forming cells), osteoclasts (bone-resorbing cells), and bone-lining cells are present on the surfaces (lining cells covering the quiescent surfaces of bone). Osteocytes, by contrast, are embedded within the mineralized bone matrix. The osteocytes extend numerous dendritic processes that connect to each other, forming an extensive cellular network. The spaces in the mineralized matrix occupied by osteocyte cell bodies are termed lacunae, and are roughly ellipsoidal and 300 to 500 μm³ in volume; the tiny canals surrounding the cell processes are approximately 0.3 μm in diameter and ap-

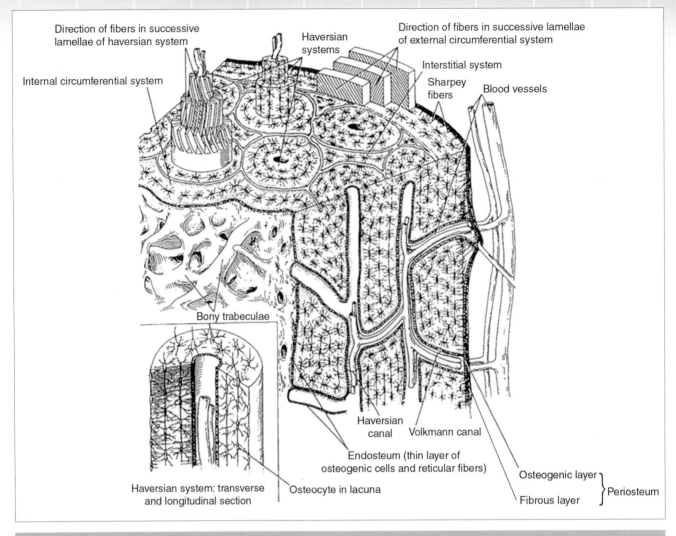

Direction of fibers in successive
lamellae of haversian system

Haversian
systems

Direction of fibers in successive lamellae
of external circumferential system

Interstitial system

Internal circumferential system

Sharpey
fibers

Blood vessels

Bony trabeculae

Haversian
canal

Volkmann canal

Endosteum (thin layer of
osteogenic cells and reticular fibers)

Osteogenic layer
⎫
⎬ Periosteum
⎭
Fibrous layer

Haversian system: transverse
and longitudinal section

Osteocyte in lacuna

Figure 4 Diagram of the structure of cortical bone, showing the types of cortical lamellar bone: the internal circumferential system, interstitial system, osteonal lamellae, and outer circumferential system. The diagram also shows the intraosseous vascular system that serves the osteocytes and connects the periosteal and medullary blood vessels. The haversian canals run primarily longitudinally through the cortex, whereas the Volkmann canals create oblique connections between the haversian canals. Cement lines separate each osteon from the surrounding bone. Periosteum covers the external surface of the bone and consists of two layers: an osteogenic (inner) cellular layer and a fibrous (outer) layer. (Adapted from Miller JD, McCreadie BR, Alford AI, et al: Form and function of bone, in Einhorn TA, O'Keefe RJ, Buckwalter JA, eds: *Orthopaedic Basic Science*, ed 3. Rosemont, IL, American Academy of Orthopaedic Surgeons, 2007, pp 129-159.)

propriately named canaliculi. In lamellar bone, the lacunae are regularly arranged and consistent with the organization of the lamellae; in woven bone, lacunae are arranged randomly. The lacunar-canalicular system, the interconnected pericellular space surrounding osteocytes and their processes, provides the major route through which fluids, nutrients, signaling molecules, wastes, and other molecules move through bone. Recent studies suggest that this fluid movement may be how osteocytes sense mechanical loading that drives the Wolff Law. In addition, the lacunae, together with the vascular channels, comprise the void spaces or pores of bone, the distribution of which is a major factor determining tissue mechanical properties.

Extracellular Matrix

ECM accounts for the overwhelming majority of bone mass and volume and as such is the principal determinant of bone's material/mechanical properties. Moreover, as a major repository of calcium and phosphate in the body, bone ECM also contributes to systemic mineral metabolism.[1,3,4,10] Bone ECM can be considered a composite material with an organic phase consisting mainly of fibers plus a lesser amount of nonfibrous organic material, and an inorganic phase consisting of mineral crystals precipitated within and around the fibers. The organic phase accounts for approximately 20% to 25% of bone tissue by weight while the inorganic phase accounts for 60% to 70%; the re-

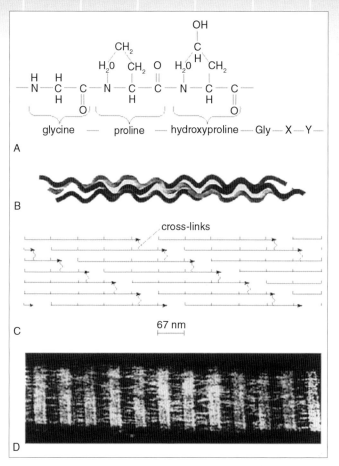

Figure 5 Type I collagen structure. **A,** Chemical structure of the repeated tripeptide sequence (– glycine – proline – 3-hydroxyproline –) found within the helical region of type I and other fibril-forming collagens. **B,** Schematic diagram showing the triple helix formed by two α1 chains and one α2 chain within a tropocollagen molecule. **C,** Side-by-side alignment of tropocollagen molecules in a collagen fibril. All tropocollagen molecules are oriented in the same direction and staggered by approximately 25% of their length, resulting in gaps or holes within the fibril. As a result, collagen fibrils present a banded appearance with a period of approximately 67 nm in negatively stained electron micrographic images. Cross-links are shown between tropocollagen molecules within the collagen fibril. Cross-links can also form between adjacent fibrils (not shown in this diagram). **D,** Electron microscopic image of a collagen fibril illustrating the banding periodicity. (Courtesy of Collagen, Encyclopedia. AccessScience. http://accessscience.com. Accessed Dec. 1, 2012.)

mainder is water.[1,11] Broadly speaking, the fibrous matrix governs the tissue's tensile properties and fracture toughness whereas the mineral phase confers rigidity and compressive strength; however, this is clearly an oversimplification. The organic constituents of bone matrix can have substantial effects on bone's mechanical properties, such as resistance to fracture, and on its physiologic activities in mineral metabolism.[10,12]

Typical of mineralized tissues across the phylogenetic spectrum, the organic matrix of bone is laid down first and the inorganic phase is deposited later. The organic matrix serves as a template that constrains the space available to the inorganic phase and also, by less well-understood mechanisms, may regulate the formation, deposition, and orientation of mineral crystals. In addition, interactions between organic matrix constituents and existing mineral can influence both the exchange of ions with extracellular fluid and the way that the mineral phase contributes to tissue mechanical properties.

Organic Matrix Constituents
Collagen
Type I collagen is the most abundant constituent of the organic matrix of bone; it accounts for approximately 90% of all the organic material in bone and is the nearly exclusive component of bone matrix fibers.[1,5,11] Other collagen types that are found in bone in substantial amounts are not part of bone matrix per se, but rather belong to distinct tissue types such as cartilage remnants from endochondral ossification (mainly types II and X), fibrous tissues of periosteum and marrow (type III), or blood vessels (type IV). Small amounts of other collagen types, including types III, V, and XI, have been identified in bone ECM, but under restricted circumstances and in association with type I fibers.

Type I collagen is the prototypical member of the collagen family, whose known members number close to 30 different collagens.[11,13] Like bone, the structure of collagen is complex and hierarchical (**Figure 5**). The structural unit of type I collagen is termed tropocollagen, and is a trimer composed of three polypeptide chains. Two are α1 (I) chains, encoded by the *col1a1* gene, whereas the third polypeptide of the trimer, α2 (I), is encoded by the *col1a2* gene. The three chains form a distinctive unit in which the polypeptides wrap around each other for most of their length, forming a tight triple helical braid. This triple helical structure, which is not the same as the α-helix that is formed by a single polypeptide chain, is the defining structural feature of all collagens. In other collagens (for example, type III) three copies of the α1 (III) chain form the trimer unit. The triple helical region of collagen comprises the central region of the trimeric molecule; the remainder of the molecule includes nonhelical N- and C-telopeptides flanking the helical region on each side, as well as N- and C-terminal propeptides that are cleaved during posttranslational processing. Because the long helical region makes up most of the sequence of mature collagen molecules, each tropocollagen unit resembles a fairly stiff rod with a consistent length of approximately 300 nm.

The collagen triple helix forms because both the α1 and α2 chains contain repeated sequences of the amino acid sequence (-gly-X-Y-) where gly represents glycine, X is proline, and Y is frequently hydroxyproline. Both proline and hydroxyproline are imino acids; that is, the nitrogen that combines with adjacent amino acid to form the polypeptide

2: Physiology of Musculoskeletal Tissues

backbone exists as part of a five-membered ring and is not able to rotate freely. This constrained structure imparts a tight kink in the polypeptide chain at each proline or hydroxyproline residue. The positioning of glycine, which lacks a side chain, at every third position along this repeating tripeptide sequence (and adjacent to a proline) is essential to prevent steric hindrance that would otherwise impair wrapping of the helical braid.

Type I collagen (and others including types II and III) are fibril-forming collagens. Fibril formation is a self-assembly process; in vivo (and in vitro as well), at physiologic pH, temperature, and ionic strength; monomeric tropocollagen in solution spontaneously aggregates in a regular fashion to form fibrils. The spontaneous nature of fibril formation suggests that most or all tropocollagen will exist as part of a fibril, and moreover that mechanisms must exist in vivo to ensure that the fibrils are of the appropriate dimensions, and that fibril formation only occurs under the correct circumstances. The control of collagen fibrillogenesis remains incompletely understood, although some likely regulatory mechanisms have been identified (see the next paragraphs). However, it is clear that collagen fibril size and organization in vivo are regulated, as evidenced by consistent tissue-specific patterns.

Collagen fibrils are organized in a distinctive manner that has several critical physiologic implications. In the fibrils, the rodlike tropocollagen monomers are aligned in the same direction, but with the ends of the monomers offset by approximately 25% of their length—a quarter-stagger configuration relative to the collagen monomers immediately laterally. Thus, the tips of each tropocollagen molecule do not contact each other; rather, there are gaps (holes) between successive tropocollagen units in a line. This regular arrangement of monomers and gaps accounts for the characteristic banding patterns observed in electron microscopic images of collagen fibrils. Because of this arrangement, the addition of each new tropocollagen monomer to a growing fibril via this staggered, side-to-side interaction of monomers results in changes to the width as well as the length of the fibril. The fibrils formed by collagen can be very long, but are roughly circular in cross section and have a limited distribution of diameters that is tissue type dependent. Collagen fibril diameter appears to depend on many factors, including the association of other collagen types (minor collagens such as type V collagen), proteoglycans, or noncollagenous proteins with the fibrils.

The presence of holes within the fibril structure of collagen also has implications for the distribution of noncollagenous elements, especially the mineral crystals, in bone ECM. The hole zones between the ends of tropocollagen molecules define a network of spaces that extends throughout the three-dimensional extent of the collagen fibrils and is also continuous with interfibrillar space. Consequently, tissue fluid and its soluble components, including noncollagenous proteins and inorganic ions, are able to permeate regions within as well as between collagen fibrils. Because of

this accessibility, bone mineral crystals are closely integrated into the fibrils of bone ECM.

Biosynthesis and Posttranslational Modifications of Collagen

Collagen biosynthesis and assembly make up a complex process that entails several forms of posttranslational modification (**Figure 6**). These include proteolytic cleavage of propeptides, hydroxylation of proline and lysine side chains, glycosylation of hydroxylated amino acids, and the formation of covalent cross-links between collagen chains. Both α1 and α2 chains of collagen are initially translated as proforms, with peptide sequences at both their N- and C-termini that are removed during the maturation process. Typical of secreted proteins, the chains are directly translocated from ribosomes into the lumen of the endoplasmic reticulum, where they assemble into their triple helical form.

One function of the propeptides is to ensure proper alignment of the collagen molecules to permit correct trimer assembly. Interestingly, unlike most proteins, assembly of procollagen trimers occurs beginning from the C-termini—the most recently translated segments of the chains. Folding and braiding of the chains then proceeds toward the N-termini.

Hydroxylation of Proline and Lysine

Proline and lysine molecules undergo enzyme-mediated hydroxylation within the endoplasmic reticulum and Golgi apparatus, before formation of the triple helix is complete. Prolyl-3-hydroxylase and prolyl-4-hydroxylase catalyze hydroxylation reactions at the 3- and 4-positions of the proline ring, respectively. Hydroxylation of lysine side chains results from the action of a family of lysyl hydroxylases. These hydroxylation sites on lysines are the sites of intermolecular cross-links between collagen molecules that are essential to stabilize collagen fibrils. Lysine hydroxylation occurs at residues located in both the helical and nonhelical (telopeptide) regions, and the degree of hydroxylation in these regions differs among tissues (for example, between bone and skin). Hydroxylysine residues are also sites of presecretory glycosylation. The nature and extent of collagen glycosylation depends on several factors, including the availability of carbohydrate substrates and the site specificity of glycosylating enzymes. These factors likely contribute to observed tissue-specific differences in collagen glycosylation.

CLINICAL NOTE: The functional consequences of normal tissue-specific differences in collagen glycosylation are unclear. However, differences in glycosylation during intracellular collagen processing have been noted in certain cases of osteogenesis imperfecta where a single amino acid change in one of the collagen chains was found to alter the rate of protein folding. Changes in the glycosylation pattern would be expected in such circumstances, because potential sites of posttranslational modification may become unavailable as the three procollagen chains form the triple helix. It is possible that pathologic glycosylation differences could contribute to altered fibril formation or packing capability of

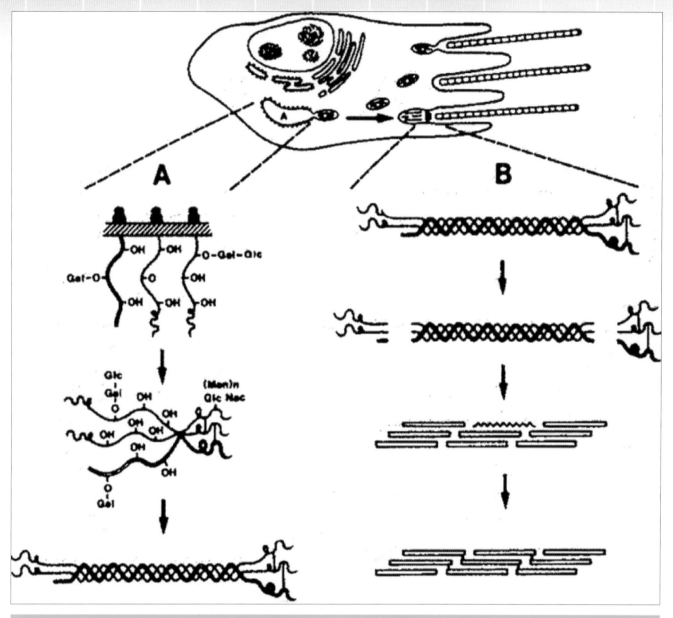

Figure 6 Collagen biosynthesis and assembly. **A,** Intracellular events. Top: Posttranslational insertion into the endoplasmic reticulum and hydroxylation of proline and lysine. Middle: Glycosylation of hydroxylated amino acids. Bottom: Formation of procollagen by folding of the three collagen chains beginning from the C-terminal propeptide. **B,** Extracellular events. Top: Procollagen (as in part A) now at the point of secretion from the cell. Top middle: Cleavage of N- and C-propeptides from procollagen. Lower middle: Self-assembly of collagen fibrils. Bottom: Formation of cross-links between tropocollagen molecules.

mutant tropocollagen monomers in these instances of osteogenesis imperfecta. Addition of carbohydrates to collagen chains after they are part of an established ECM also has pathologic consequences, as described in the following paragraphs.

Proteolytic Removal of N- and C-Propeptides
Removal of the N- and C-terminal collagen propeptides occurs by cleavage of all three collagen chains by specific N- and C-propeptidases, respectively. This occurs as the proteins are secreted from the cell, leaving mature tropocolla-

gen molecules with intact N- and C-telopeptides flanking the triple helix. A major role of the N-propeptide may be to suppress self-assembly, thereby preventing cellular damage or destruction from the premature aggregation of collagen monomers. Following cleavage, the procollagen peptides do not remain as part of the ECM; rather, they are washed out and eventually appear in the serum and finally are excreted in urine.

CLINICAL NOTE: The appearance in serum and urine of detectable amounts of collagen propeptide fragments, which are produced in equimolar amounts to collagen, has made them highly useful as biomarkers to assess collagen synthesis in vivo under normal and pathologic circumstances. Immunoassays are currently available to detect N- and C-procollagen peptides from types I and III and other collagens in serum and urine.

Collagen Cross-linking

Although intracellular modifications (hydroxylation of proline and lysine) prepare tropocollagen molecules for subsequent cross-linking needed to stabilize the collagen fibrils, the cross-linking process itself occurs outside the cell.[14] Lysyl oxidase, an extracellular enzyme that converts the ε-amino groups of lysine and hydroxylysine into aldehydes via oxidative deamination, typically initiates the cross-linking process. Several nonenzymatic reactions can then occur, depending on the availability and nature of reactive side chains. For example, allysine or hydroxyallysine (the oxidative products of lysyl oxidase action on lysine and hydroxylysine, respectively) can react with nearby lysine or hydroxylysine to form divalent crosslinks. These divalent cross-links are unstable, but do help to stabilize immature collagen fibers. These divalent cross-links can then be converted to extremely stable trivalent cross-links by additional (nonenzymatic) reaction with a third aldehyde-bearing side chain. Again, the nature of the cross-links depends on the number and nature of side chains (for example, lysine versus hydroxylysine) in proximity to each other, and so cross-linking patterns will vary depending on collagen type, tissue, and age.

CLINICAL NOTE: When any collagenous matrix is broken down as part of bone resorption or remodeling of other tissues such as tendon, ligament, or skin, the chemically complex segments of collagen chains that contain the cross-links are resistant to cleavage by protease. These resistant fragments, which contain chemically distinctive interchain links (such as pyridinoline) coupled to a few amino acids, move into the circulation and eventually are excreted in urine, similar to the propeptide products of collagen synthesis. In addition, like the procollagen peptides, the ability to detect and quantitate collagen cross-links in plasma/serum and urine has allowed them to be used as biomarkers to assess rates of collagen degradation in vivo. The limitation of these biomarker assays, of course, is that they reflect the levels of collagen synthesis or degradation from all tissues, not just bone; as a result, it is difficult to obtain specific and unambiguous information about bone matrix metabolism from these assays alone.

Glycation

In addition to posttranslational modifications that are part of normal collagen processing, mature collagen is subject to nonenzyme-mediated addition of carbohydrates to their side chains (nonenzymatic glycation) through the Maillard reaction, the chemical process underlying carmelization. The presence of additional carbohydrate groups on collagen molecules makes them susceptible to excessive and potentially pathologic cross-linking. Glycation occurs gradually, progressively, and irreversibly, so that the level of glycated collagen increases with age. Moreover, resulting sugar-based cross-links decrease compliance and energy-absorbing capacity of connective tissues. In addition, because the rate of nonenzymatic glycation depends on the concentrations of available carbohydrate in circulation, it is increased whenever glucose levels in tissue fluids are elevated, as in poorly controlled diabetes.

Genetic Alterations of Collagen Structure

Our understanding of the way collagen contributes to the organization and function of bone matrix has been aided enormously by studies of genetically altered collagens, both in animal models and in human patients. In this respect, long-standing clinical and biochemical investigations of patients with osteogenesis imperfecta have been especially productive. Osteogenesis imperfecta comprises a set of genetic disorders whose hallmarks include fragility of the skeleton and other type I collagen–based connective tissues. The wide range of osteogenesis imperfecta severity reflects diverse changes in the structure of *col1a1* or *col1a2* genes, from complete ablation to single base changes in one or both copies of the collagen genes. These studies of human disease have more recently been supplemented by the use of transgenic mouse models, beginning with *mov-13*, produced by insertion of a transgene into the *col1a1 gene*, and resulting in a mild osteogenesis imperfecta–like phenotype in the heterozygote and embryonic lethality in the homozygote. These examples are only a few of many human diseases affecting connective tissues (including, but not limited to, Ehlers-Danlos syndrome, Marfan syndrome, and a host of chondrodysplasias) where this combination of approaches has been used productively. Information about specific conditions has been cataloged and is readily available in hardcopy or online in databases such as Online Mendelian Inheritance in Man.

Noncollagenous Proteins

Although type I collagen makes up most bone matrix, it cannot alone account for the distinctive features of that matrix, because it also serves as the structural framework of numerous tissues, both nonmineralized (dermis, tendon, ligament) and mineralized (dentin). This responsibility falls to the broad array of noncollagenous proteins that also compose bone ECM. Moreover, the uniqueness of bone matrix structure appears to be a combinatorial phenomenon, dependent on all of the matrix constituents, with no single molecular species playing a dominant and tissue-specific role. Early speculations (and perhaps hopes) that the unique nature of bone matrix might be attributable to one or two bone-specific molecules have been disabused by the accumulation of data demonstrating that virtually all of the bone noncollagenous proteins are expressed in many tissues.[15-17]

Bone noncollagenous proteins encompass a variety of structures, functions, and cellular origins (**Table 1**). Struc-

Table I
Bone ECM Constituents (Partial List)

Collagens[29]
Type I
Type V, type III (trace)
Proteoglycans
Biglycan
Decorin
Fibromodulin
Perlecan
Osteoglycin/mimecan
Osteoadherin
SIBLING Proteins
Osteopontin (2ar, spp1)
Bone sialoprotein
DMP-1 (dentin matrix protein-1)
Dentin sialophosphoprotein
MEPE
Glycoproteins
BAG-75
Alkaline phosphatase
Osteonectin
Tetranectin
Serum Proteins
Serum albumin
A2HS-glycoprotein
Vitamin K–Dependent Proteins (gla-proteins)
Osteocalcin
Matrix gla-protein
RGD-Containing Proteins
Fibronectin
Thrombospondins
Fibrillins (1 and 2)
Extracellular Enzymes
Lysyl oxidase
Alkaline phosphatase ("tissue-nonspecific" isoenzyme, TNSALP)
Matrix metalloproteinases
PHEX
Growth Factors/Cytokines
Bone morphogenetic proteins (BMPs)
BMP antagonists (noggin, chordin)

Table I (continued)

Growth Factors/Cytokines
Insulin-like growth factors (IGF-1, IGF-2, and IGF-binding proteins)
TGF-βs and binding proteins
Fibroblast growth factors
Sclerostin
Wnts, coactivators (eg, LRP5) and antagonists (eg, Dkk1)

This noncomprehensive list includes molecules isolated from bone and/or produced by bone cells either in vivo or in vitro. Extracellular enzymes such as alkaline phosphatase and MMP-14 are mostly associated with cell surfaces.

turally, they represent several non–mutually exclusive molecular families, among which are proteoglycans, glycoproteins, SIBLING (Small, Integrin-Binding LIgand, N-linked Glycoproteins), and vitamin K–dependent (gla) proteins. Functionally, these molecules act as structural elements, enzymes, and/or diffusible signals (cytokines), categories that can also be considered to overlap. For example, it has become clear that ECM itself has informational content that can be interpreted by its resident cells and that changes in matrix composition or organization can regulate cell behavior. Finally, noncollagenous proteins of bone arise from a variety of cellular sources, both within and outside of bone. For example, some ECM proteins are synthesized and secreted by osteoblasts before mineral deposition while others are produced by osteocytes after the mineral phase is deposited. Other proteins found in bone matrix, like serum albumin and α2HS glycoprotein, are produced by remote tissue like liver, reach the bone extracellular fluid via the circulation, and subsequently become adsorbed on the surfaces within the matrix.

A common feature of many noncollagenous proteins of bone ECM is the ability to interact simultaneously with multiple binding partners. These partners may include cell surface receptors, other matrix macromolecules, soluble ions (in particular Ca^{2+}), and the surfaces of mineral crystals. This capacity is in part genetically determined, based on the presence of multiple binding motifs encoded in their primary structure (such as the arg-gly-asp sequence recognized by certain integrins) or the presence of regions enriched in acidic amino acid residues (asp, glu) that promote binding to cations or positively charged surfaces. Nongenetic factors, principally differences in the nature and degree of posttranslational modifications, also help determine the interactive capacity of bone ECM molecules. Notable modifications include phosphorylation, glycosylation (where the presence of sulfated residues or sialic acid in the modifying carbohydrates is of particular interest), and the

2: Physiology of Musculoskeletal Tissues

vitamin K–dependent gamma-carboxylation of glutamate residues in osteocalcin. Also of note, posttranslational modification depends on many factors, including age and metabolic circumstance. Consequently, a single species of ECM molecule may exhibit structural polydispersity and a range of functionality.

Proteoglycans

Proteoglycans are an extremely diverse macromolecular family sharing a fundamental structural motif: a single polypeptide chain (the core protein) with one or more of its amino acid side chains modified by members of a specific disaccharide family, the glycosaminoglycans (GAGs). The most common GAGs are chondroitin sulfate, heparan sulfate, and keratan sulfate. The structures and key functions of proteoglycans and GAGs are discussed in greater detail in chapter 10. Not all proteoglycans are present in bone, and those that have been detected are present at fairly low abundance. Three proteoglycans specifically identified in bone are decorin, biglycan, and perlecan. Decorin and biglycan, two members of the small, leucine-rich proteoglycan family, contain only one and two GAG chains per molecule, respectively, and have been suggested to regulate collagen fibril diameter. Perlecan has a larger core protein and more extensive GAG modifications and has been identified in the pericellular space of the lacunar-canalicular system. Canalicular diameter and pericellular matrix around osteocytes were found to be mildly altered in perlecan-deficient mice, but the specific role of the proteoglycan remains to be established clearly.

SIBLING Proteins

Members of the SIBLING family present in bone ECM include bone sialoprotein (BSP), osteopontin (OPN), dentin matrix protein-1 (DMP-1), and matrix extracellular phosphoglycoprotein (MEPE).[11,16,17] These structurally related proteins possess cell-binding capability via arg-gly-asp (RGD) sequences recognized by integrin adhesion receptors, most notably integrin αVβ3. They are also subject to several forms of posttranslational modification, including glycosylation, phosphorylation and, particularly in the cases of DMP-1 and MEPE, proteolytic processing.

OPN (also known as secreted phosphoprotein-1/spp1 and 2ar) is produced by osteoblasts, hypertrophic chondrocytes, and osteoclasts, as well as nonskeletal cell types. Its name stems from its potential to "bridge" cells (via RGD interactions) with the mineralized matrix (via sequences enriched in acidic amino acids). The ability of OPN to bind calcium and to interact with mineral surfaces has suggested roles both in mineralization and in bone resorption. OPN was shown to inhibit mineralization in vitro, and recent studies have suggested that formation of complexes between OPN and mineral crystals may impart material toughness. One role proposed for OPN was to mediate the adhesion of osteoclasts to bone surfaces during resorption, and interestingly mice genetically deficient in OPN fail to lose bone in response to hindlimb suspension and ovariectomy. However, OPN-deficient mice are not osteopetrotic, indicating that its role is likely not essential to osteoclast function.

BSP, while similar in molecular size and overall structural organization to OPN, is more restricted in its expression, being found mainly in mineralizing tissues that include bone, hypertrophic cartilage, and cementum. BSP also differs functionally from OPN. In vitro studies have shown that BSP, unlike OPN, can nucleate mineral deposition, although it inhibits later growth of mineral crystals. Also in contrast to OPN, mice lacking BSP lose bone following hindlimb suspension, similar to wild-type animals.

Osteoblasts produce several other ECM proteins that are not exclusive to bone, but are common to most connective tissue matrices.[11] These include fibronectin, osteonectin (also termed SPARC, or Secreted Protein, Acidic, and Rich in Cysteine) and thrombospondin. Fibronectin is not an abundant protein in bone, but it is a major mediator of adhesion between many of the cells in bone to collagenous matrices. Fibronectin has also been recognized as a participant in the organization of pericellular matrix by cells and is essential to the formation of several tissues during development. Fibronectin-deficient mice die during gestation, even before the development of skeleton. OPN, members of the thrombospondin family, and other proteins that have the ability to interact simultaneously with other ECM proteins and with cell surface receptors have been described as "matricellular" proteins. Overexpression and deletion of thrombospondin isoforms in mice lead to alterations in skeletogenesis and wound healing but overall the phenotypes are mild.

In addition to OPN and BSP, bone matrix contains several other proteins that are both glycosylated and substantially phosphorylated, including bone acidic glycoprotein-75 (BAG-75), DMP-1, and MEPE. BAG-75 is characterized by an ability to self-associate into complexes that can sequester phosphate ions and so may regulate mineral deposition and/or ion exchange. DMP-1 and MEPE, in contrast to OPN and BSP, are produced in bone mainly by osteocytes rather than osteoblasts. In addition, both are subject to proteolytic cleavage. Only a small fraction of the DMP-1 in bone is intact. DMP-1 deficiency in humans and in knockout mouse models is characterized by defective bone mineralization, suggesting that it may play multiple roles in regulating the deposition and maintenance of bone mineral. MEPE overexpression in mice results in deficient mineralization, whereas MEPE deletion leads to increased bone formation. MEPE is of particular interest in that its cleavage to yield a phosphorylated, mineralization-inhibiting peptide (the ASARM peptide) is regulated by PHEX (phosphate-regulating gene with homologies to endopeptidases on the X chromosome) – a protein also produced by osteocytes and implicated in genetic diseases of phosphate metabolism, including X-linked hypophosphatemic rickets, which results when PHEX is inactivated.

Vitamin K–Dependent Proteins

Certain bone ECM proteins contain a distinctive posttranslational modification also found in the clotting protein prothrombin: gamma carboxyglutamic acid (gla), which results from the addition of a carboxyl group to the gamma position on some of its glutamic acid residues. The most abundant gla-containing protein in bone is osteocalcin (also known as bone gla-protein). A second, termed matrix gla-protein, is found primarily in calcified cartilage, whereas a third, periostin, is produced by osteoblasts in intramembranous bone, and localized mainly in periosteum and periodontal ligament. Addition of the extra carboxyl group is enzymatic, requires vitamin K, and confers on these molecules the ability to form complexes with calcium and to bind readily to hydroxyapatite – properties not shared by nongamma-carboxylated forms. The vitamin K dependency of this mineralization regulatory makes it susceptible to the action of the anticoagulant warfarin.

Osteocalcin is produced mainly by mature osteoblasts and osteocytes and is a frequently used marker of the osteoblast phenotype, but its function in bone is still uncertain. It is not essential for mineralization, because genetically osteocalcin-deficient mice and rabbits whose bones are rendered osteocalcin-depleted by vitamin K antagonists exhibit only modest skeletal phenotypes. Osteocalcin has also been suggested to have a systemic signaling role in neuroendocrine control of energy metabolism.

α2HS-Glycoprotein

α2HS-glycoprotein is a highly acidic protein synthesized in liver. It has the capacity to bind large quantities of calcium ions and is thought to act systemically as an inhibitor of ectopic calcification. α2HS-glycoprotein is abundant in bone, where it is likely adsorbed onto the surfaces of mineral crystals, and modulates the exchange of calcium ions with tissue fluid.

Other proteins found in bone matrix include a variety of signaling molecules and enzymes necessary to carry out local modifications of matrix structure. Perhaps the best known examples of signaling molecules are the bone morphogenetic proteins (BMPs), whose activities were first identified in demineralized bone matrix; others include the BMP antagonist noggin, other members of the transforming growth factor–β (TGF-β) superfamily, the TGF-β binding proteins, fibroblast growth factors (FGFs), and sclerostin. Examples of bone matrix enzymes include alkaline phosphatase (ALP), members of the matrix metalloproteinase (MMP) family, notably MMP-2, MMP-13, and MMP-14, tissue inhibitor of metalloproteinase (TIMP), and PHEX.

Inorganic Matrix Constituents – The Mineral

The inorganic phase of bone ECM consists of mineral crystals whose structure approximates hydroxyapatite $[Ca^{2+}_{10}(PO_4^{3-})_6(OH^-)_2]$ that is variably substituted by other ions, mainly Mg^{2+} and CO_3^{2-}.[11] Other cations such as aluminum, lead, and strontium (as well as heavy isotopes such as thorium, plutonium, and barium) and anions such as F- may also become incorporated into bone mineral (usually in trace amounts) due to diet or environmental exposure, and the first mineral crystals that form under physiologic conditions are likely to differ from hydroxyapatite in structure and composition. Furthermore, crystal size and perfection may depend on metabolic circumstances (such as rate of bone turnover). However, most mineral, even in embryonic bone, is apatitic.

Bone mineral is distributed throughout the organic matrix—not only between collagen fibrils but also within the hole zones described earlier. However, the accumulation of mineral in substantial amounts does not begin until some time after the organic matrix is deposited, and at a distance apart from the bone surface and its active osteoblasts. How bone mineral forms, how it is deposited so completely within the interstices of collagen fibrils, and how it is organized in a consistent fashion have yet to be fully answered. The minimum requirement for precipitation of a mineral salt is that the concentrations of its constituents are high enough so that they interact in the proper orientation to form a crystal nucleus. Subsequent growth by addition of new molecules to an existing crystal lattice is less energetically demanding. Formation and growth of crystals can be facilitated by increasing the concentrations of its constituents (either directly or by removing inhibitors that might bind to the ions and thereby reduce their effective concentration), or by heterogeneous nucleation – provision of a separate molecular entity (such as a catalyst) whose surface is a crystal nucleus and allows ions to bind in a regular arrangement and grow in a crystalline array. Mineralization of bone uses several of these mechanisms.

Bone mineralization is regulated mainly at the local level by osteoblasts and perhaps osteocytes.[16-18] Systemic levels of Ca and Pi (inorganic orthophosphate, found principally as HPO_4^{2-} and $H2PO_4^-$ at physiologic pH) are homeostatically maintained and their overall levels in bone and other tissues are relatively constant. Pathologic changes in systemic Ca or Pi levels will affect mineralization of bone, but under normal conditions the process is regulated locally, principally by osteoblasts. Osteoblasts produce both metabolites and macromolecules that can either favor or inhibit mineral crystal nucleation and growth. Osteoblasts produce an endogenous inhibitor of mineralization, pyrophosphate (PPi, $P_2O_7^{4-}$), by hydrolysis of trinucleotides such as adenosine triphosphate (ATP) (for example, ATP → adenosine monophosphate + PPi) by enzymes that are found both within the cytoplasm and on the cell surface. Movement of PPi from the cytoplasm to the extracellular space is performed via a transmembrane protein, ANKH, the human homolog of the mouse *ank* gene product that, when mutated, results in a progressive ankylosing spondylitis. On the other hand, osteoblasts also express two phosphatases, ALP on cell surfaces and PHOSPHO1 (phosphatase orphan 1) intracellularly, that cleave PPi to yield two molecules of orthophosphate (Pi, PO_4^{3-}). These enzymes promote mineralization by two mechanisms, simultaneously removing the inhibitor PPi and generating two molecules of Pi that are required for bone mineral crystal formation. The balance of Pi to PPi thus is a critical determinant of matrix mineralization. In addition to these mechanisms, production and phosphorylation of matrix proteins such as osteopontin and BAG-75, which can interact with Ca ions and also with crystal surfaces, may also modulate the mineralization process. OPN, in particular, has been shown both to promote and inhibit mineral precipitation in vitro. The appearance of mineralized matrix in newly forming bone does not occur simultaneously with the deposition of the organic matrix. There is always a region of unmineralized matrix at sites of new bone formation, termed an "osteoid seam." In pathologic circumstances such as osteomalacia, where bone matrix is produced but does not mineralize, the osteoid seams are wide and remain so until the condition is remedied. The analogous condition in cartilage, rickets, is similarly characterized by widened, unmineralized growth plates. Once bone formation ceases, mineralization continues until the osteoid seam disappears and virtually the entire matrix is mineralized. The time course of mineral accumulation in bone is biphasic. Roughly 70% of mineral deposition at a site occurs in an exponential fashion within 5 to 10 days, whereas the remaining 30% is added over the following 3 to 6 months.

CLINICAL NOTE: Several diseases are associated with either impaired or excessive mineralization. Impaired mineralization of growth plate cartilage (rickets) or bone (osteomalacia) despite normal production of organic matrix often results from endocrine disorders of mineral metabolism that affect circulating levels of Ca and Pi. The classic example is decreased Ca absorption due to vitamin D deficiency. In addition, hypophosphatasia, a group of genetic diseases characterized by deficiencies in the enzyme ALP, leads to impaired mineralization that is sometimes fatal, and was a major factor in implicating this enzyme as a regulator of skeletal mineralization. Excessive mineralization, on the other hand, is exemplified by the deposition of mineral in tissues that otherwise would not mineralize. Formation of kidney or bladder stones is often associated with metabolic diseases of Ca metabolism (hyperparathyroidism, hypercalcemia of malignancy). Other examples include vascular calcification associated with coronary artery disease, heterotopic ossification that occurs after trauma or surgery, and the rare but severe genetic disease fibrodysplasia ossificans progressiva (FOP). In these conditions, inappropriate mineralization appears to be part of an aberrant phenotypic change in nonskeletal tissue–resident cells. In particular, FOP was recently shown to result from mutations in the protein ACVR1, a subunit of the receptor for BMPs, potent inducers of bone and cartilage cell differentiation (discussed in greater detail in the following sections). As a result of these mutations, nonskeletal cells become activated, often in the absence of ligand, and trigger the focal and sporadic differentiation of their cells and subsequently the progressive formation of cartilage and bone tissue.[19]

Bone Cells

Bone cells are classified by their relationships with bone matrix. Initial histologic observations extended by advances in cell and molecular analysis—both in vitro and in vivo — have greatly increased our understanding of their functions, origins, and fates. Briefly stated, the osteoblasts produce bone matrix and the osteoclasts degrade (resorb) it, whereas the osteocytes and bone-lining cells reside, respectively, inside of and on the quiescent surfaces of bone and act to maintain the tissue throughout life.[1,2,6] These cells will be the major focus of this section. Many other cell types also exist in bone, as part of distinct or specialized tissues, such as cartilage, marrow, vasculature, periosteum, and tendon or ligament insertions. Although these latter cells play important roles in various aspects of overall bone function, they will mainly be discussed in relation to the four principal bone cell types.

Bone cells belong to two distinct lineages[1,6,9]: osteoblastic and osteoclastic (**Figure 7**). The osteoblastic lineage, including the osteocytes and lining cells, which are in fact "retired" osteoblasts that have stopped producing bone matrix and either have become buried within the matrix (osteocytes) or have spread out to cover the bone surface (lining cells), are of connective tissue–mesenchymal stem origin. Osteoclasts, by contrast, are of hematopoietic origin, derived from the myeloid (monocyte-macrophage) family. They are recruited to sites of incipient bone resorption from pools of monocyte-macrophage progenitors resident in marrow or circulating in the blood. Osteoblasts and osteoclasts have been the most studied, not only because of their obvious functional importance as the effector cells that change bone shape and control bone mass, but also because they were more amenable to study, both in situ and in cell culture model systems, than cells either entombed within the matrix or flattened almost to the point of invisibility against "quiescent" bone surfaces. Many of these technical difficulties have been overcome, permitting recent studies to shed much light on the properties and functions of osteocytes; however, lining cells remain less well understood.

Osteoblasts

Osteoblasts are mesenchyme-derived cells that synthesize the distinctive ECM of bone.[1,6,9,20] Morphologically, osteoblasts are characterized by their location on bone surfaces and by their overtly secretory appearance: they are mononucleate, cuboidal cells, often with an eccentric nucleus shifted away from the bone surface and extensive protein synthetic machinery (rough endoplasmic reticulum, Golgi apparatus, secretory vesicles) nearer to it (**Figure 8**). The molecular signature of osteoblasts, in vivo and in vitro, includes expression (at the mRNA and protein levels) of bone matrix proteins (type I collagen, osteopontin, osteonectin, bone sialoprotein, osteocalcin) as well as the enzyme ALP, whose association with osteoblasts and other cells directly involved in biomineralization (hypertrophic chondrocytes, odontoblasts) has been known and studied since the 1920s.

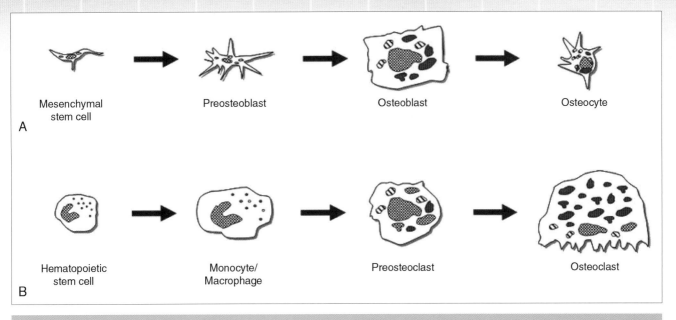

A
Mesenchymal stem cell → Preosteoblast → Osteoblast → Osteocyte

B
Hematopoietic stem cell → Monocyte/ Macrophage → Preosteoclast → Osteoclast

Figure 7 Diagram showing cell lineage from mesenchymal stem cells through osteoblasts (**A**) and osteocytes and pathway from hematopoietic stem cells through osteoclasts (**B**). (Adapted with permission from Marquis ME, Lord E, Bergeron E, et al: Bone cells biomaterials interactions. *Biosci* 2009; 14[1]:1023-1067.)

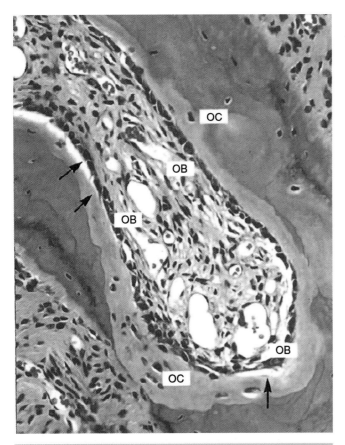

Figure 8 Stained histologic image of an infilling bone multi-cellular unit showing osteoblasts (OB, arrows) on bone-forming surfaces, some of which have become embedded to form osteocytes (OC). (Courtesy of Yale, School of Medicine, Developmental Histology, New Haven, CT.))

CLINICAL NOTE: Of these molecules, osteocalcin and ALP are often used as osteoblast phenotypic markers in vivo and in vitro—both to identify the osteoblasts in heterogeneous cell populations and to assess the effects of various perturbations on osteoblast function. ALP, a cell surface enzyme, is upregulated early in osteoblast differentiation and remains present in mature osteoblasts but is lost when the cells become osteocytes. ALP is a convenient marker to assay because it can be detected by both biochemical and histochemical activity assays; however, it is not cell type–specific (osteoblasts express the tissue-nonspecific ALP gene). Although ALP is absent or minimally expressed in most fibroblastic cells, it is expressed by certain leukocytes and other cells in bone marrow. Osteocalcin, although not as easy to assay as ALP, is considered specific for the osteoblast lineage. It appears later in the differentiation process than ALP—that is, in mature osteoblasts. Both ALP and osteocalcin can be measured in serum.

In postembryonic bone, osteoblasts form by differentiation of progenitor cell populations that reside in the periosteum and bone marrow stroma or are associated with skeletal blood vessels (perivascular fibroblasts, or pericytes). These progenitors are probably adult stem cells (MSCs) also capable of differentiating into other connective tissue lineages. MSCs have also been isolated from sources such as deciduous teeth, adipose tissue, skin, and peripheral blood. The ability of cells in diverse, nonskeletal sites to differentiate along an osteoblastic path has both positive and negative implications. On the one hand, this property may underlie several pathologic conditions of ectopic calcification like that which occurs in vascular plaques, posttraumatic heterotopic ossification, and FOP. On the other hand, the potential

Table 2
Direct Regulators of Bone Cell Function (Partial List)

Endocrine regulators produced in nonskeletal tissues, act on bone cells

Peptides/proteins	Parathyroid hormone, calcitonin, growth hormone, insulin-like growth factor–1 (IGF-1), binding proteins
Steroids, secosteroids, others	Estrogens/androgens, corticosteroids, vitamin D (1,25(OH)$_2$-vitamin D$_3$, other forms), thyroid hormones, retinoids

Autocrine/paracrine produced locally (by bone and/or nonbone cells), act on bone cells

Peptides/proteins	BMPs (antagonists, noggin/chordin, etc), TGF-βs, IGF-1 + IGF-binding proteins, PDGF (platelet-derived growth factor), FGFs, vascular endothelial growth factors (VEGF), TNF-α, interleukins and interleukin receptor antagonists, Wnts, epidermal growth factor, PTH-related peptide , ephrins, sclerostin, periostin, RANK ligand/OPG
Small molecules and metabolites	Adrenergic hormones (epinephrine, norepinephrine), prostaglandins, leukotrienes, sphingosine-1-phosphate, lysophosphatidic acid, ATP, nucleotdes, nitric oxide

All listed regulators have been reported to act directly on one or more "bone cells", that is, osteoblasts, osteoclasts, or osteocytes, in vivo and/or in vitro.
Binding proteins or antagonists, where identified, do not necessarily bind directly to bone cells, but may interact with the appropriate regulator to alter its function or availability.

to obtain osteoblast progenitors from more readily accessible tissue sources than bone marrow may prove useful in developing convenient cell-based approaches to engineering of skeletal tissues.

Differentiation of osteoblasts, like that of all cell types, is controlled primarily at the level of gene expression, and specification of the osteoblastic lineage among potential progenitor populations is dependent on particular sets of transcriptional regulators.[1,5,20,21] Two transcription factors active during differentiation of osteoblasts are osterix and Runx2 (previously identified as CBFA1). The specific requirement for Runx2 in osteogenesis was dramatically illustrated in Runx2 knockout mice, where cartilage forms but bone does not. The human condition resulting from Runx2 haploinsufficiency is cleidocranial dysplasia. The best

known molecular triggers that stimulate cells to differentiate along an osteoblastic pathway are members of the TGF-β superfamily, in particular the BMPs. TGF-βs and BMPs are structurally related and bind to homologous receptor types that act by phosphorylating members of the Smad family of intracellular signaling molecules. Both BMPs and TGF-β are autocrine/paracrine factors; osteoblasts produce these factors as well as respond to them. In addition, once secreted they remain within bone ECM. The BMPs were originally identified in extracts of bone matrix and named for their ability to induce bone and cartilage formation in ectopic sites. However, subsequent work established that BMP regulation of morphogenesis is much more widespread and begins in the earliest phases of embryonic development. The activities of BMPs and TGF-β are regulated by interactions with specific extracellular molecules. Latent TGF-β–binding protein (LTBP) binds TGF-β and sequesters it in the ECM. Proteolytic cleavage of LTBP then releases functional TGF-β as needed, for example, at sites of matrix turnover or cellular invasion. BMPs are regulated by stoichiometric binding of specific soluble antagonists, among which are noggin and chordin, which compete with membrane receptors for the morphogens.

Most aspects of osteoblastic cell activity, from proliferation and differentiation of progenitors to matrix production to their eventual life span and fate, are regulated by many factors, both local and systemic (**Table 2**). Cells within the osteoblastic lineage express receptors for calcitropic hormones that regulate bone turnover and calcium metabolism, most notably parathyroid hormone (PTH), the PTH-related peptide and 1,25-(OH)$_2$-vitamin D. Although these agents are known for their specific effects on the skeleton, osteoblastic cells also respond to regulators with more widespread actions. These include systemic hormones (glucocorticoids, estrogens, androgens, thyroid hormone) as well as locally acting factors such as IGFs, epidermal growth factor (EGF), FGFs, vascular endothelial growth factors (VEGFs), and several interleukins. Many of these local regulators are also produced by cells of the osteoblast lineage.

Recent studies have focused considerable attention on osteoblast regulation by the Wnt family of regulatory molecules.[20,22] Wnts are secreted proteins that are widely expressed and act on target cells via the Frizzled (Frz) receptor and a coreceptor protein, low-density lipoprotein receptor-like protein (LRP5/6), which are expressed on the cell surface. Members of the Wnt family operate via multiple intracellular signaling pathways. In the best known pathway, referred to as the "canonical" Wnt pathway, Wnt binding to its receptor suppresses the degradation of intracellular β-catenin, which is then able to translocate to the nucleus and regulate the transcription of specific target genes. Wnts also act via alternative pathways, not directly linked to β-catenin; these "noncanonical" pathways involve separate sets of intracellular regulators (for example, members of the MAPK, or mitogen-activated protein kinase, family) and a different spectrum of intracellular regulatory responses. The canonical Wnt signaling pathway in cells of the osteoblast lineage activates genes associated with bone formation and also suppresses bone resorption by upregulating expression of the RANKL antagonist osteoprotegerin (OPG). The importance of this pathway was first established when gain-of-function mutations in LRP5 in humans were shown to produce a skeletal phenotype characterized by high bone mass and strong bones that are exceptionally resistant to fracture, whereas loss of LRP5 function was found to be the basis for osteoporosis-pseudoglioma syndrome. Subsequently, numerous alterations in the Wnt signaling pathway were found to result in a range of skeletal phenotypes of varying magnitude. For example, the dramatic suppression of bone formation in multiple myeloma has been associated with overproduction of the Wnt antagonist Dkk1. In addition, sclerostin, a protein produced by osteocytes, was recently shown to be a potent Wnt antagonist and an essential contributor to the inhibition of osteoblast activity at the end of a bone formation cycle. Furthermore, continued expression of sclerostin appears to be necessary to keep bone formation suppressed, and bone formation is initiated when sclerostin production ceases. Antibodies directed against sclerostin have been found to be potent bone anabolic agents, and are currently being developed as treatments to prevent or reverse bone loss (see next paragraphs for further discussion).

Once osteoblasts form, they have a lifespan of approximately 100 days, after which they follow one of three potential fates: (1) entombment as osteocytes within the bone matrix produced by themselves and their neighbors; (2) quiescence as bone-lining cells on the bone surface at the end of the bone formation phase at a given site; or (3) death by apoptosis. The latter appears to be the fate of most (60% to 80%) osteoblasts; 10% to 20% of osteoblasts ultimately become osteocytes, and a similar number become bone-lining cells.

CLINICAL NOTE: Attempts to develop therapeutic approaches to stimulate osteogenesis have been directed toward two types of applications — local and systemic. Local applications are aimed at facilitating healing at specific sites, such as problematic fractures (for example, complex fractures or nonunions) or acute surgical reconstructions that use bone grafts. The second concerns longer term and systemic enhancement of bone growth to prevent or reverse bone loss due to aging, gonadal insufficiency, or chronic glucocorticoid treatment. Virtually every growth factor, hormone, or cytokine shown to act on osteoblasts in vitro or on bone in vivo has been investigated in the search for useful bone anabolic effectors.[20,21,23]

Recombinant BMP products have been approved for clinical use in local skeletal healing (for example, spinal fusion), but have encountered complications. As a systemic agent, PTH has long been known as an extremely potent anabolic agent in vivo when administered intermittently in low doses, although it can also acutely stimulate resorption when given at high doses. Recently, a recombinant 1-34 PTH peptide (teriparatide) was approved for treatment of osteoporosis. Additional systemic bone anabolic agents are also under development for osteoporosis treatment. Sclerostin, a cytokine produced by osteocytes, suppresses osteoblast function by suppressing canonical Wnt signaling. A monoclonal antibody against sclerostin has shown strong positive anabolic effects in vitro and in vivo. It should be noted that the bone anabolic agents used to date are all peptides, which have potential drawbacks in terms of expense, mode of administration (injection) and the possibility of developing immune reactions. Presumably one of the goals for the next generation of skeletal pharmaceuticals will be the development of more convenient small molecules that mimic the actions of anabolic proteins or peptides.

Osteoclasts

The catabolic counterpart to the osteoblast is the osteoclast, which carries out bone resorption – the wholesale removal of a localized packet of bone tissue.[1,2,6,9,24-29] Osteoclasts are large, multinucleated cells with numerous morphologic and biochemical features designed to carry out this unique excavation function (**Figure 9**). Resorption is a specialized phagocytic process that dissolves bone mineral and degrades its organic matrix constituents simultaneously (unlike formation, where matrix deposition and mineralization are sequential). The specialized features of the osteoclast are most evident at its apical surface, where it interacts with the bone matrix (or, in vitro, with the surface of the vessel upon which it is cultured). This region consists of a ruffled border surrounded by an attachment, or sealing, zone. At the ruffled border, the plasma membrane exhibits numerous infoldings and the adjacent cytoplasm contains numerous lysosomes and other vesicular organelles, indicating a high level of membrane activity as part of active exocytosis and endocytosis.

The sealing zone surrounding the ruffled border is the site of osteoclast attachment to the bone surface, and forms a gasket-like ring to create an enclosed extracellular compartment within which bone matrix degradation takes place. Osteoclast attachment to bone appears to be mediated largely through $\alpha_V\beta_3$ integrins, whose expression de novo is a hallmark of osteoclast differentiation. Occupation of the $\alpha_V\beta_3$ integrin binding site by ligands on the bone surface also appears to trigger additional cellular activities associated with resorption. $\alpha_V\beta_3$ integrins bind to the arg-gly-asp tripeptide sequence which is found in many matrix proteins, including osteopontin. The ability of osteopontin and its relatives to mediate osteoclast attachment is consistent with the previously discussed capacity of certain matrix proteins to interact simultaneously with multiple partners, in this case with bone mineral (via acidic amino acids or posttranslational modifications) and osteoclast integrins (via RGD sequences). It should also be noted that osteoclast attachment to bone can likely be mediated by several matrix proteins or by alternate mechanisms. As an example, osteopontin-deficient mice fail to exhibit increased osteoclastic bone loss upon mechanical unloading; however, the

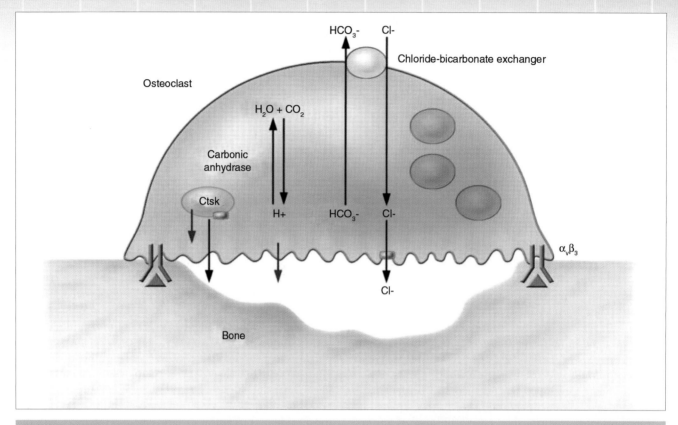

Figure 9 Diagram illustrating how the osteoclast adheres to bone via binding of RGD-containing proteins (green triangles) to the integrin $\alpha_v\beta_3$, initiating signals that lead to insertion into the plasma membrane of lysosomal vesicles that contain cathepsin K (Ctsk). Consequently, the cells generate a ruffled border above the resorption lacuna, into which is secreted hydrochloric acid and acidic proteases such as cathepsin K. The acid is generated by the combined actions of a vacuolar H^+ ATPase (red arrows), its coupled Cl^- channel (pink boxes), and a basolateral chloride–bicarbonate exchanger. Carbonic anhydrase converts CO_2 and H_2O into H^+ and HCO_3-. Solubilized mineral components are released when the cell migrates; organic degradation products are partially released similarly and partially transcytosed to the basolateral surface for release. (Reproduced with permission from Ross FP, Christiano AM: Nothing but skin and bone. *J Clin Invest* 2006;116:1140-1149.)

mice do not exhibit a phenotype characteristic of marked osteoclast dysfunction, such as osteopetrosis.

The cytoplasmic region above the sealing zone is largely devoid of membranous organelles and is termed a clear zone. However, osteoclasts contain an extensive network of actin-based cytoskeletal filaments in this region. Actin filaments can bind, either directly or via adaptor molecules, to the cytoplasmic domains of integrins, and these interactions have been shown to play crucial roles in regulating the shape and migration of numerous cell types. The importance of integrin-based adhesion and of the actin cytoskeleton to osteoclast function is illustrated by demonstrations that osteoclast activity in vitro and in vivo can be inhibited by agents that disrupt integrin-based adhesion (for example, the snake venom echistatin) and the integrity of the actin cytoskeleton (for example, high-potency amino-bisphosphonates, which inhibit cellular guanosine triphosphatases that regulate actin filament formation).

The space between the ruffled border and the bone surface is functionally a large, extracellular lysosome. The os-

teoclasts generate protons by the action of carbonic anhydrase within their cytoplasm, they then pump those protons into the resorption space via transport molecules in the ruffled border membrane. Intracellular pH and ionic balance are maintained by additional ion transport systems located in portions of the plasma membrane outside the ruffled border. The secreted protons, which render the resorption space acidic, begin to dissolve the apatite mineral salts and disrupt intramolecular and intermolecular interactions of organic constituents. (These reactions use up some of the secreted protons; however, the overall pH of the resorption space remains low). In addition, the osteoclasts secrete lysosomal enzymes, including tartrate-resistant acid phosphatase (TRAP, an enzyme that has served as a convenient, histochemical marker to specifically identify osteoclasts) and proteases (most notably cathepsins B, L, and K). Cathepsin K (CatK) is particularly important to the resorption process. High expression of CatK is a specific feature of osteoclasts, and genetic deficiency of CatK results in pycnodysostosis, a disease of impaired osteoclastic resorption

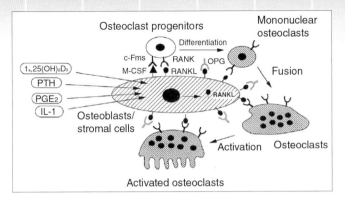

Figure 10 Illustration of osteoclast differentiation and function regulated by RANKL and M-CSF. Osteoclast progenitors and mature osteoclasts express RANK, the receptor for RANKL. Osteotropic factors such as $1\alpha,25(OH)_2D_3$, PTH, and IL-1 stimulate expression of RANKL in osteoblasts/stromal cells. Membrane- or matrix-associated forms of both M-CSF– and RANKL-expressed stromal cells are responsible for the induction of osteoclast differentiation in the coculture. RANKL also directly stimulates fusion and activation of osteoclasts. Mainly osteoblasts/stromal cells produce OPG, a soluble decoy receptor of RANKL. OPG strongly inhibits the entire differentiation, fusion, and activation processes of osteoclasts induced by RANKL. IL-1 = interleukin 1; (Adapted from Miller JD, McCreadie BR, Alford AI, et al: Form and function of bone, in Einhorn TA, O'Keefe RJ, Buckwalter JA, eds: *Orthopaedic Basic Science*, ed 3. Rosemont, IL, American Academy of Orthopaedic Surgeons, 2007, pp 129-159.)

characterized by increased bone mass. Interestingly, osteoclast activity is not completely impaired in pycnodysostosis, and so the phenotype is rather mild in comparison to the more severe condition, osteopetrosis. The proteolytic activity of CatK-deficient osteoclasts likely results from other cathepsins; in addition, certain MMPs (MMP-9) also may contribute to osteoclastic bone resorption. During resorption, calcium and phosphate are taken up by cells and subsequently released to the extracellular fluid, whereas organic matrix molecules are degraded more completely via lysosomes within the osteoclast.

The activity of mature osteoclasts is exquisitely sensitive to inhibition by the hormone calcitonin, which operates via an adenylate cyclase–coupled, G-protein–based receptor, similar to PTH and adrenergic hormones in osteoblasts and other cell types. However, calcitonin appears to have little effect on activity of existing osteoclast or ongoing bone resorption in vivo; rather, physiologic control of bone resorption appears to occur more at the level of osteoclast formation, via progenitor recruitment and differentiation. Calcitonin effects are transient and subject to escape due to receptor desensitization. Nevertheless, administration of exogenous calcitonin has been used clinically to achieve effective, if temporary, inhibition of osteoclast activity in cases similar to Paget disease, where resorption can be extremely active.

Osteoclasts originate from progenitor cells within the hematopoietic system—specifically, the monocyte/macrophage lineage.[24-29] The differentiation process includes fusion of mononuclear cells to form multinucleated osteoclasts. Once recruited to sites where bone is to be resorbed, these osteoclast progenitors begin to undergo changes in phenotype, including expression of TRAP; multinucleation occurs late in the differentiation process from fusion of the mononuclear cells, not as a result of nuclear division. In vivo, the number of nuclei appears to change during the working lifetime of an osteoclast, as individual nuclei are lost and new mononuclear cells are incorporated. Osteoclast differentiation and its regulation have been extensively investigated in vitro, and several models exist that mimic the process. Often these systems comprise mixed cell cultures of hematopoietic cells (from bone marrow, spleen, or established cell lines), which serve as sources of osteoclast progenitors, and supporting cells (osteoblasts, marrow stromal cells, or permanent cell lines derived from these populations) that provide some or all of the requisite cytokines (see below). Osteoclast differentiation is monitored by counting the number of TRAP-positive multinucleated cells with a microscope, usually after 3 to 7 days. The osteoclast-like cells formed in vitro resemble authentic osteoclasts, including the ability to resorb mineralized matrices in vitro.

Osteoclasts are not permanent cells; they are formed on demand only where and when bone resorption is demanded. The formation of osteoclasts, and subsequent bone resorption, can be triggered by a wide variety of chemical and physical stimuli. A highly incomplete list includes inflammation, hyperparathyroidism, deficiency of gonadal steroids, and both mechanical overloading (causing physical damage to the matrix) and underloading of the skeleton. Nevertheless, formation of new osteoclasts appears to require the activation of monocytic progenitor cells by a very restricted set of critical regulatory factors (**Figure 10**). Two in particular, receptor activator of nuclear factor κB ligand (RANKL) and macrophage colony-stimulating factor (M-CSF), have been shown to be necessary and sufficient to stimulate differentiation of monocytic precursors into osteoclasts. RANKL is expressed by a variety of connective tissue cell types, including endothelial cells and cells of the osteoblast lineage (osteoblasts and osteocytes). In addition, cells that produce RANKL also produce an antagonist of RANKL named OPG. OPG binds stoichiometrically to RANKL, and in doing so prevents it from activating RANK in target cells. As a result, activation of osteoclastogenesis through RANKL may be regulated by upregulating its expression, by reducing levels of OPG, or by a combination of the two. The ratio of RANKL to OPG thus serves as a convenient index of whether or not osteoclastogenesis is favored. M-CSF, or CSF-1, is also produced by cells of the osteoblast lineage as well as by several marrow cell types, including those of the marrow stroma. Absence of M-CSF has been identified as the basis for certain rodent models of osteopetrosis.

2: Physiology of Musculoskeletal Tissues

CLINICAL NOTE: The osteoclast has long been a focal point of research directed against skeletal diseases characterized by bone loss or elevated bone turnover. Increased net osteoclastic bone resorption drives the osteoporosis resulting from mechanical underloading, gonadal insufficiency (for example, estrogen loss), and metastatic disease, as well as Paget disease. The following paragraphs briefly describe some of the principal osteoclast-directed antiresorptive drugs now in use or under development. Some of the clinical consequences of these and other skeletally active drugs are discussed in a later section of this chapter.

Bisphosphonates

The bisphosphonates are analogs of pyrophosphate ($P_2O_7^{4-}$) in which the P-O-P phosphodiester bonds are replaced by P-C-P phosphonate bonds that cannot be hydrolyzed by phosphatases.[30] The carbon atom linking the two P atoms also has two additional bonds that must be occupied (the simplest case would be two H atoms, making the structure [$P-CH_2-P$]), and so a range of structurally and functionally diverse bisphosphonate compounds have been synthesized. The P-C-P motif allows bisphosphonates to bind to bone mineral crystals, so they will selectively target regions of bone where mineral is exposed (for example, sites of formation or resorption). Originally it was thought that bisphosphonates could inhibit resorption by purely physicochemical means, by making it more difficult for osteoclasts to dissolve mineral crystals with bisphosphonates covering their surfaces. The first-generation bisphosphonates were either ineffective or produced physiologic complications that limited their usefulness. However, new generations of amine-containing bisphosphonates, beginning with alendronate, were found to inhibit osteoclastic activity by direct action, and these are now the standard clinical bisphosphonates. Subsequent investigations established that the osteoclast inhibitory potency of several amino bisphosphonates was related to their ability to inhibit an enzyme (farnesylpyrophosphate synthase) involved in regulation of the actin cytoskeleton, thereby interfering with the ability of osteoclasts to adhere to bone. Osteoclast inhibition by bisphosphonates thus has two key elements. Bisphosphonates bind stably to bone mineral, and can accumulate in bone. Initiation of bone resorption by osteoclasts then releases some of the bisphosphonate locally, which suppresses further osteoclast action. Many bisphosphonates are now in routine clinical use and compose the main line of antiresorptive therapy. However, because of their high binding affinity for bone mineral these compounds are thought to have very functional long half-lives in vivo, which coupled with their efficacy at suppressing bone turnover has raised concerns about long-term bone health.

CatK Inhibitors

Although the mechanism of bisphosphonate action in inhibiting osteoclasts was not what was originally anticipated when the drugs were developed, the path of CatK inhibitor development remained closer to the expected findings. Development was based on the following observations: CatK is the principal lysosomal enzyme used by osteoclasts to degrade bone matrix; CatK is selectively expressed in osteoclasts, unlike several other cathepsins; and genetic deficiency of CatK in humans and animal models resulted in pycnodysostosis, a high bone mass condition associated with impaired osteoclast function. A chemical inhibitor of CatK activity (odanacatib) is currently in clinical trials.

Calcitonin

Calcitonin, produced by cells of the thyroid, dramatically suppresses osteoclast activity through a specific adenylate cyclase–coupled G-protein–linked receptor. Its activity is short-lived, however, as calcitonin receptors undergo desensitization. Calcitonin has been effective in suppressing the extremely high turnover of bone in Paget disease on a temporary basis. The need for injection as a means of delivery for this peptide hormone has largely been overcome by the availability of a nasally delivered inhalant form of calcitonin.

RANKL Inhibitors

The discovery that RANKL was essential for the differentiation of osteoclasts and that its decoy receptor, OPG, existed, has led to the development of agents designed to block RANKL action.[31] Denusomab is a humanized anti-RANKL monoclonal antibody that binds to RANKL and blocks its function. Biologic inhibitors such as denusomab have a potential advantage over bisphosphonates in that they do not accumulate in bone and so their on-off actions can be titrated more effectively by controlling the administration regimen.

Osteocytes

Osteocytes are the most abundant cell type in mature bone, and the longest lived.[1,3,32-34] Unlike osteoblasts and osteoclasts, which have life spans of days to weeks, osteocytes are more permanent tissue residents that can remain viable for decades. Also, unlike all other bone cell types, they reside completely inside the matrix of both cortical and cancellous bone (**Figure 11**). Morphologically, osteocytes have much smaller cell bodies than their immediate progenitors (osteoblasts), and they extend a large number of thin, dendritic cell processes throughout the matrix; these processes connect with neighboring cells—either the processes of adjacent osteocytes or the lining cells or osteoblasts on the nearest bone surface. At the points where cell processes contact nearby cells or processes, gap junctions formed by the junction of two cell process membranes permit direct movement of ions and small molecules between the cytoplasms of the linked cells. As a result, cohorts of gap junction–connected cells compose functional syncitia. The ability to communicate by direct cytoplasmic transfer of signals through gap junctions has led to the concept that there is a functional syncitial network among osteocytes that may sense, inte-

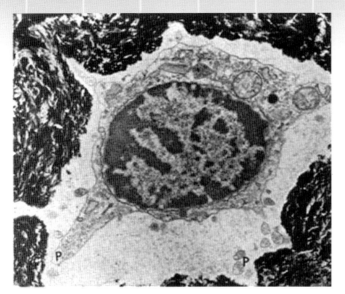

Figure 11 An electron microscope image of an osteocyte within its lacuna in bone. Although the nucleus is prominent, the cytoplasm and organelles are greatly reduced in comparison with an osteoblast, its immediate progenitor. The principal cytoplasm components are abundant ribosomes and rough endoplasmic reticulum. Elongated cell processes (P) extend from the cell and penetrate into the matrix via canaliculi. (Reproduced with permission from Cooper RR: The cell, in Albright JA, Brand RA: *The Scientific Basis of Orthopedics*. New York, NY, Appleton Century Crofts, 1979, pp 1-19.)

grate, and respond to environmental signals in a coordinated fashion. However, additional communication mechanisms may operate within a network of osteocytes. For example, extracellular (secreted) signals may be propagated by diffusion or by convection through the lacunar-canicular system. These pathways of osteocyte connectivity are also the preferred routes through which fluids and small or moderately sized solutes (up to about 50 to 70 kD) travel through bone outside of vascular channels.

Osteocyte processes not only contact other cells, but electron microscopic evidence demonstrates that they periodically make contact with canalicular walls, both directly and via "tethering fibers" that span the canalicular space.[34] The molecular identity of the tethers, and whether or not their connections with the osteocyte process or with the canalicular wall are covalent, have yet to be established. Proteoglycans may be candidates for this role, because they are present within the lacunar-canalicular system and their dimensions are consistent with such a function. The proteoglycan perlecan, for example, has been implicated in maintaining the pericellular space around osteocytes and their processes, but whether it also has a tethering function is not known. Direct contacts between the membrane of osteocyte processes and the canalicular walls occur at discrete points along the canaliculi. These contacts appear to be mediated by β3 integrins, which also exhibit a punctuate distribution in bone that is not associated with the osteocyte cell bodies

or lacunar spaces. By contrast, β1 integrins (a more diverse family whose members include the fibronectin receptor) were only seen in association with osteocyte cell body in lacunae, where they appear to attach to molecules in the pericellular matrix rather than the bony lacunar wall.

Like their morphology, the gene expression pattern of osteocytes is distinct from that of osteoblasts, their direct progenitors. Although osteoblasts produce type I collagen and express ALP, osteocytes synthesize DMP-1 and MEPE and are negative for ALP. Osteocytes also express proteases that degrade matrix proteins (for example, PHEX and various MMPs) as well as signaling molecules with activities at both local and systemic levels. Sclerostin, for example, is a recently discovered osteocyte product that suppresses osteoblast function, and appears to act as a signal to inhibit bone formation at a particular site. Moreover, osteocyte sclerostin levels in vivo appear to be proportional to mechanical demand, such that osteocytes in low-strain regions produce the highest levels of sclerostin, whereas those in high-strain regions stop producing the inhibitor, allowing osteoblasts to form bone where needed. FGF-23 is also produced by osteocytes and acts on the kidney to regulate phosphate and vitamin D metabolism. Finally, osteocytes express RANKL and may be major contributors to the recruitment and differentiation of osteoclasts. The role of osteocytes in bone resorption and remodeling will be discussed in greater detail in the following paragraphs.

Of the numerous cellular activities that occur during the transition (differentiation) of osteoblasts into osteocytes, perhaps the most intriguing and poorly understood is the way that dendritic processes form and establish connections with the processes of neighboring cells. Formation of the osteocyte originates before the newly formed bone matrix becomes mineralized and is not a passive event. Osteocytes begin to extend processes toward the mineralization front soon after becoming engulfed in matrix. Osteocyte process development may be regulated by podoplanin, the product of the same *E11* gene responsible for dendrite formation in the neurons, and formation of the canalicular space around the process appears to require the membrane-bound protease MMP-14.

Although osteocytes are generally assumed to have the responsibility for maintaining bone throughout life, their specific functions remain incompletely understood, due largely to technical difficulties associated with studying a cell population effectively buried in a calcium phosphate cement. However, numerous recent advances have improved the understanding of the role these cells may play in mechanosensation, damage monitoring, tissue remodeling, and mineral homeostasis.

Mechanosensation

Osteocytes are now widely thought to be the mechanosensing elements of bone.[33] The interactions of osteocyte processes with canalicular walls, both by direct contact and by tethering fibers, have strong implications for the role of osteocytes as mechanoreceptors in bone. Osteocytes, osteoblasts, and other adherent cells are sensitive to substrate deformations and to fluid shear stresses generated when bone is loaded, and these have been directly demonstrated. However, the stimuli needed to evoke cellular responses in vitro by direct substrate strain would require corresponding in vivo load levels that would fracture bone, so direct mechanical strain on osteocytes seems an unlikely player. Both forms of contact between osteocyte processes and rigid canalicular walls would act as stress concentrations on the cell process membrane, enhancing the sensitivity of osteocytes to shear stresses produced by movement of fluid through the lacunar-canalicular system. In these circumstances, fluid movements produced by physiologic activity levels would produce stresses on osteocyte process membranes comparable to those needed to evoke cellular responses in vitro. The pericellular space around the cell body is much larger (approximately 1μm) so the rate of fluid flow around cells in lacunae will be lower than that around the processes within canaliculae. Moreover, the distance between the osteocyte cell body and the lacunar wall is too large to permit extensive direct attachment via candidate mechanotranduction molecules such as integrins. The signal transduction pathways activated in osteocytes by mechanical stimulation in vivo have yet to be fully established. Similarly, the pathways by which mechanical signals are transmitted from the cells that initially sense them (that is, osteocytes within the bone) to the cells at bone surfaces where formation or resorption must be initiated, remain unclear. However, in vitro evidence has demonstrated that mechanical stimulation regulates ionic (notably Ca) movements in osteocytic cells, and also leads to the release of diffusible signaling molecules like prostaglandins and nucleotides (for example, ATP) that are small enough to pass readily through the lacunar-canalicular system.

Another mechanosensory mechanism imputed to osteocytes involves primary cilia,[32] which are microtubule-based structures found in virtually all cell types (they are related to centrioles and linked to establishment of polarity of the mitotic spindle during cell division). Primary cilia are logical candidates for fluid flow-based mechanosensors because they use such a mechanism to sense fluid movement around auditory hair cells and in distal renal tubules. However, their presence in mature osteocytes appears to be quite limited. Moreover, in humans, genetic defects in primary cilia have been shown to underlie polycystic kidney disease, but affected patients have only a mild skeletal phenotype (mild osteopenia). More evidence is needed to determine the extent to which primary cilia may influence osteocyte mechanosensation.

Damage Recognition and Tissue Remodeling

Like all tissues (and all materials), bone sustains wear and tear, which in the case of bone results largely from mechanical fatigue and is evidenced by physical damage (microscopic cracks). Osteocytes play an essential role in recognizing certain forms of matrix damage, specifically linear microcracks, and initiating a bone remodeling response that resorbs the damaged region and replaces it with new bone.[34] In particular, formation of linear microcracks leads to regulated (apoptotic) death of osteocytes in the region of the crack. Dying osteocytes trigger expression of RANKL by neighboring surviving osteocytes that is essential for osteoclast formation and bone resorption.

Mineral Metabolism

In addition to its mechanical function, bone is its own major mineral storehouse, particularly for calcium and phosphate reserves. The osteocyte lacunar-canalicular system contributes an enormous amount of bone surface, estimated to be more than an order of magnitude greater surface than presented in trabecular bone, with the potential to exchange mineral with tissue fluid and the systemic circulation, and osteocytes are directly associated with all of it. Although the concept that osteocyte action contributes significantly to bone loss in diseases such as osteoporosis (via osteocytic osteolysis) has been discredited in favor of a dominant role for osteoclastic resorption and bone remodeling, recent evidence has shown that mineral is indeed moved in and out from the osteocyte lacunar-canalicular space. Osteocytes are now known to play a role in systemic mineral metabolism in a different way, particularly related to phosphate transport. Osteocytes express PHEX, the bone matrix protease described earlier in this chapter whose substrates include MEPE. PHEX deficiency was shown to underlie cases of familial hypophosphatemia. Recently, another osteocyte product, FGF-23, was shown to act on the kidney to regulate vitamin D metabolism and phosphate homeostasis; moreover, FGF-23 appears to be the culprit in vitamin D–resistant hypophosphatemic rickets. Thus, osteocytes now appear to be established as regulators of systemic phosphate metabolism by endocrine as well as paracrine pathways.

Bone-Lining Cells

The surface of normal quiescent bone tissue (bone that is neither forming or resorbing) is lined by a 1- to 2-μm–thick layer of unmineralized matrix (lamina limitans) on which there is a layer of flat, elongated cells called bone-lining cells that form when the last osteoblasts on a surface flatten out.[1,2,6,9] Lining cells are much less metabolically active than osteoblasts and have reduced cell volume and matrix synthetic machinery, though they remain effectively polarized cells by virtue of their environment, existing between bone and its so-called investing fibrous membrane of periosteum or bone marrow stroma. The fluid space beneath the lining cells appears to be continuous with that of the osteocyte lacunar-canalicular system. Although the full physiologic role of this cell type is not yet known, it has been suggested that it is vital in signaling osteoclasts to bone sites that require resorption, because they provide the cellular interface layer to the marrow compartment. Furthermore, os-

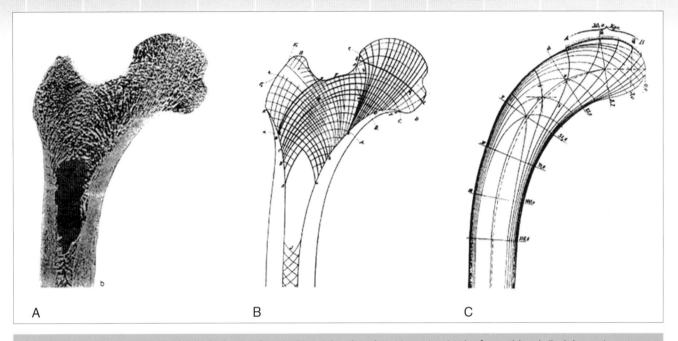

Figure 12 **A,** An illustration of the similarities between actual trabecular orientation in the femoral head. **B,** Schematic representation drawn by Meyer (1967). **C,** Stress trajectories in a model analyzed by Culmann using graphical statics. Stress trajectories are curves representing the orientations of the maximal and minimal principal stresses in the material under load. (Reproduced from Miller JD, McCreadie BR, Alford AI, et al: Form and function of bone, in Einhorn TA, O'Keefe RJ, Buckwalter JA, eds: *Orthopaedic Basic Science,* ed 3. Rosemont, IL, American Academy of Orthopaedic Surgeons, 2007, pp 129-159.)

teoclasts cannot easily attach to the unmineralized surface layer of bone so it is also thought that bone-lining cells secrete collagenase (MMP-1) at the required site to aid this process. Finally, these cells can dedifferentiate into functional osteoblasts under appropriate circumstances.

Regulation of Bone Form and Function

Although its rigidity and relatively sparse cellular population in comparison to its overall volume suggest a static structure, bone is in fact a remarkably dynamic tissue that modulates its external and internal structure throughout life and is exquisitely sensitive to mechanical and systemic cues. A classic example of the similarity between the structure of trabeculae in the femoral neck and the theoretical stress lines in a mechanical crane are shown in **Figure 12**. These responses fall into two categories of metabolic processes, both of which involve formation and resorption: modeling and remodeling. Although these terms are sometimes used interchangeably in the orthopaedic community, these processes use the same cells in fundamentally different spatial and temporal sequences and relationships, exert different controls on osteoblasts and osteoclasts, and have different results on whole bone and tissue architecture.

Modeling

Modeling of bone involves formation and resorption of tissue at different surfaces, resulting in the relative movement or "drift" of a bone surface over time.[1-3] The two processes may occur at the same time, or one process may occur with-

out the other; however, the net result is an overall change in the shape of the tissue. Modeling occurs principally during development, as the bones grow and their shapes change through cortical drifts. An example of modeling during development is the growth in diameter of a long bone, where expansion of the marrow cavity occurs by resorption at the endocortical surface of the diaphysis, whereas growth of the cortex in diameter results from bone formation at the periosteal surface. In early development, both resorption and formation occur in a largely uniform fashion around the inner and outer diameters of the cortex, respectively. However, with time, different areas of both surfaces undergo formation and resorption, resulting in modeling drifts that change the overall shape of the tissue, not simply its size (consider the shapes of the femur in a newborn and an adult). Modeling as the major driver of bone shape change effectively ceases at skeletal maturity except for very limited circumstances. For example, a small amount of periosteal apposition continues throughout life, mainly in men, and this occurs through low-level modeling. If chronically elevated loads become dangerously high (several thousand microstrain), modeling can be become reactivated, often starting with woven bone formation. Anabolic use of PTH also appears to activate modeling. Modeling patterns are determined by multiple factors that are not yet fully understood. These include genetics and chemical signals from morphogens responsible for establishing the general overall size and shape of a bone, and also dominant influences from mechanical forces generated by muscle action and by weight bearing that are responsible for the precise functional adjustments of bone shape, cortical dimensions, and trabecular architecture. For example, a congenitally paralyzed femur will have the basic shape of the bone (diaphyses, condyles, femoral head) but it will be too small and lack the normal curvatures, trochanters, linea aspera, and so on. Because mechanosensation is crucial to modeling, osteocytes appear to play central roles in processing the modeling signals and determining the appropriate anabolic and catabolic responses.

Shape changes in bone resulting from mechanical demands were first described in detail in the 19th century. With our current understanding of bone adaptation, it is now known that such changes are effected through modeling processes, not bone remodeling processes. The nature of the physical signals driving bone's mechanical adaption has been the subject of decades of research with mechanical strain, strain-generated electrical (streaming) potentials, piezoelectricity, and microscopic fluid flow. All have been posited as potential mechanisms, although some, such as piezoelectricity, have effectively been discredited. Recent studies point to the osteocyte as the cell responsible for sensing mechanical loading changes to bone, although the specific local signals have yet to be conclusively established. However, most studies now point to microscopic fluid movement within the lacunar-canalicular system as the major physical stimulus that osteocytes "see" as a result of mechanical loading.[33-36]

Remodeling

Bone remodeling is a tissue turnover process characterized by the sequential removal of a discrete packet of bone by osteoclastic resorption and its replacement with new bone at the same site by osteoblastic bone formation.[1-3,9] Resorption and formation always occur sequentially, and formation follows resorption in a tightly anatomically and temporally coupled fashion within each remodeling packet. These focal remodeling packets that remove and replace bone within a microscopic location are now commonly referred to as basic multicellular units (BMUs). Each remodeling unit causes no overall net change in the shape of the tissue, although the process often results in a small change in the amount of tissue at the site, such that slightly more bone is removed than is replaced within a BMU. These small bone balance changes in each remodeling unit sum together and these summations can result in larger scale changes in bone loss (endocortical thinning, increased porosity, trabecular bone loss). Bone remodeling is the principal metabolic activity occurring in the adult skeleton, and is performed to replace tissue that has become damaged or otherwise lost its usefulness. Replacement of damaged bone is necessary because age-related changes in bone increase its susceptibility to fracture. Progressive increases in bone mineral content make the tissue more brittle, whereas daily wear and tear causes microscopic cracking in the tissue that, if left unremodeled, could propagate, causing failure of the structure.

As a result of remodeling, the skeletal bone mass of an average human can be completely turned over every 15 to 20 years. Complete turnover, of course, only occurs in a statistical sense; the presence of circumferential lamellae in specimens of aged bone indicates that some parts of the bone remain in place (with viable osteocytes) for decades.

Bone remodeling in BMUs is traditionally divided into four phases characterized by their central biologic events: activation, resorption, reversal, and formation. The activation phase involves the steps needed to recruit osteoclast progenitors (monocytes) to a site of incipient bone remodeling and cause them to differentiate into osteoclasts. Studies of osteoclastogenesis in vitro and in vivo indicate that the appearance of multinucleated osteoclasts takes at least 3 to 7 days following a resorptive stimulus. More rapid changes in indicators of bone resorption in vivo (for example, increases in serum calcium or levels of collagen cross-links) result from effects of a stimulus on ongoing bone resorption. Once the resorption phase begins, it continues for 2 to 4 weeks as osteoclasts completely tunnel out the resorption space within cortical bone, or erode in from the surfaces of trabeculae or the endosteal or periosteal surfaces of bone. The reversal phase denotes the interval of time and space between the end of resorption and the beginning of osteoblastic bone formation. During this time, material that comprises the cement line, a distinct but narrow strip of organic material that separates the old mineralized matrix from newly deposited matrix, is deposited on the recently exposed bone surface. Mononuclear cells have been observed in the reversal zone, but their nature remains uncertain. They have been speculated to be either osteoclast progenitors or even mononuclear bone-resorbing cells that finish off the surface and perhaps create the initial cementing surface for the ensuing osteoblast once the heavy excavation cell (the osteoclast) has completed its work. Finally, during the formation phase, osteoblasts move in and deposit new osteoid upon the cement line, filling up the void formed by the osteoclasts. Formation proceeds as it does during initial bone formation: first the osteoid is laid down, after which it is mineralized; some of the osteoblasts are buried within the matrix and becoming osteocytes while others either continue to produce matrix or die by apoptosis; and finally once the osteoblasts have completed the formation phase, the last surviving osteoblasts flatten out and become lining cells, covering the newly formed bone surface (**Figure 13**).

As noted previously, resorption and formation are spatially and temporally coupled during the bone remodeling cycle at both intracortical and surface sites. Furthermore, all of the bone cells and attendant angiogenic elements in the area of tissue where remodeling is under way are readily recognized as a distinct morphologic entity of the BMU.[1,9] Yet while the cellular and molecular processes involved in intracortical and surface-based bone remodeling are the same, the structural arrangement of BMUs is different. In intracortical (osteonal) remodeling, the remodeling process tun-

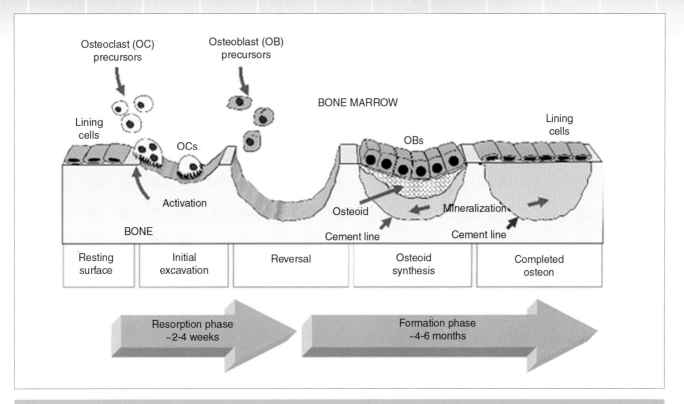

Figure 13 The remodeling cycle. An illustration showing the different stages of cellular activity that a remodeling cycle passes through temporally from the resorption of old bone by osteoclasts and the subsequent formation of new bone by osteoblasts. For simplicity, the illustration shows remodeling in only two dimensions, whereas in vivo it occurs in three dimensions, with the osteoclasts continuing to enlarge the cavity at one end and osteoblasts beginning to fill it in at the other end. (Reproduced from Miller JD, McCreadie BR, Alford AI, et al: Form and function of bone, in Einhorn TA, O'Keefe RJ, Buckwalter JA, eds: *Orthopaedic Basic Science*, ed 3. Rosemont, IL, American Academy of Orthopaedic Surgeons, 2007, pp 129-159.)

nels out from an internal blood vessel, and then tunnels longitudinally. When osteoblasts fill in the resorption space with concentric lamellar bone, except for a central channel that contains blood vessels and vasomotor nerves, the end result is identifiable as a secondary osteon or haversian system. The morphology of this BMU viewed longitudinally is comparable to a tunnel boring within the bone (**Figure 14**). The front end consists of a cutting cone or resorption front, where osteoclasts are actively resorbing and advancing through the bone. The resorbed area widens behind the osteoclasts, reaching a diameter in the reversal zone that will be the same as that of the completed osteon. Immediately behind the reversal zone, osteoblasts begin to lay down new matrix, resulting in a closing cone of new bone with osteocytes buried inside it. The central region of the BMU contains the growing blood vessel or capillary bud, whose tip extends to a point shortly behind the osteoclasts at the tip of the cutting cone. Viewed in cross section, the BMU is roughly circular, with a diameter that varies depending on the point at which the BMU is viewed, and a cellular makeup that reflects the activity (resorption, reversal, formation) at that location.

By contrast, remodeling that occurs on open bone surfaces (periosteal, endocortical, or trabecular) resembles digging and filling a trench along the surface rather than tunneling. In these BMUs, osteoclasts dig along the surface and osteoblasts fill the trench in behind them with new bone. Because remodeling occurs on surfaces adjacent to periosteum or marrow, a supply of blood vessels is available in these overlying tissues to supply osteoclast progenitors. Thus, BMUs on bone surfaces resemble half of an intracortical BMU, and remodeling on trabecular, periosteal, and endocortical bone surfaces has been referred to as hemiosteonal.

After bone resorption occurs, a brief reversal phase ensues before osteoblasts occupy the site and begin to deposit new osteoid. During this period, mononuclear cells of indeterminate identity lie near the bone surface. Some of these cells likely belong to the monocyte-macrophage lineage and form additional osteoclasts. Others of these mononuclear cells appear to play a direct role in finishing off the resorption surface and preparing the surface for the adhesion of osteoblasts for the formation phase. The thin covering of matrix distinct from osteoid that is laid down over the recently resorbed bone surface, the cement line that demarcates the border of an osteon, may be produced by these mononuclear cells.

The tight coupling of osteoclasts and osteoblasts within BMUs is a fascinating phenomenon, and its basis is also not

2: Physiology of Musculoskeletal Tissues

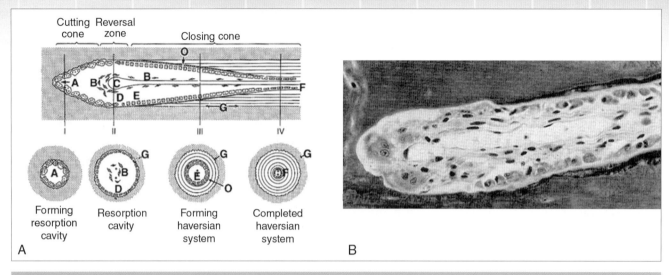

Figure 14 Cortical remodeling. **A,** Diagram showing a longitudinal section through a cortical remodeling unit with corresponding transverse sections below. A = multinucleated osteoclasts in Howship lacunae advancing longitudinally from right to left and radially to enlarge a resorption cavity. B = perivascular spindle-shaped precursor cells. C = capillary loop delivering osteoclast precursors and pericytes. D = mononuclear cells (osteoblast progenitors) lining the reversal zone. E = osteoblasts apposing bone centripetally in radial closure and its perivascular precursor cells. F = flattened cells lining the haversian canal of completed haversian system or osteon. Transverse sections at different stages of development: resorption cavities lined with osteoclasts; completed resorption cavities lined by mononuclear cells, the reversal zone; forming haversian system or osteons lined with osteoblasts that had recently apposed three lamellae; and completed haversian system or osteon with flattened bone cells lining canal/cement line (G); osteoid (stippled) between osteoblast (O) and mineralized bone. **B,** Cortical cutting cone. Osteoclasts resorbing a tunnel and osteoblasts filling it. (Reproduced from Miller JD, McCreadie BR, Alford AI, et al: Form and function of bone, in Einhorn TA, O'Keefe RJ, Buckwalter JA, eds: *Orthopaedic Basic Science*, ed 3. Rosemont, IL, American Academy of Orthopaedic Surgeons, 2007, pp 129-159.)

fully resolved.[1,36] Growth factors released from the matrix during resorption (for example, BMPs, TGF-β) could stimulate the recruitment and differentiation of osteoblast osteoprogenitors, and have been proposed to do so. Similarly, factors produced by osteoclasts themselves could stimulate osteoblastic cells (osteoclast ephrin B2 acting on osteoblastic EphB4 provides one example). Vascular tissue may also play one or more roles in resorption-formation coupling. As a source of progenitor cells for both osteoclasts (from the circulation) and osteoblasts, local changes in vascular function (for example, permeability) could regulate the availability of both populations at remodeling sites. In addition, because vascular cells and cells of the osteoblast lineage have many cytokine signaling pathways in common, reciprocal cross-talk between them likely aids in coordinating local patterns of osteoblast progenitor migration and differentiation.

The key point about coupling in remodeling is that it is effectively the default situation, comprising the overwhelmingly dominant physiologic activity in the adult skeleton. Resorption is followed by formation in almost every instance examined, whether it is normal remodeling, or diseases of increased remodeling (such as postmenopausal and disuse osteoporosis), where both resorption and formation are elevated due to an increase in the number of BMUs activated – albeit with the bone balance in each BMU shifted more heavily toward bone resorption. The few exceptions to the rule of resorption-formation coupling in the adult skeleton are noteworthy. Glucocorticoids both increase osteoclastic activity and lead to osteoblast death, so that resorption is not followed by any infilling and the resulting osteoporosis develops rapidly and severely. In bone metastases, high TNF-α levels drive aggressive resorption and suppress osteoblast recruitment. Multiple myeloma interferes with Wnt signaling and prevents osteoblast recruitment to sites of resorption.

CLINICAL NOTE: Because bone remodeling is the principal metabolic activity that occurs in the adult skeleton, most skeletal diseases, whether intrinsic to bone (such as age-related bone loss) or extrinsic (such as metabolic bone diseases due to endocrinopathy), disrupt the remodeling process. Similarly, most of the drugs and devices designed to treat skeletal disorders also modulate the remodeling process in some way. Rapid bone remodeling leads to bone loss because even properly coupled bone formation lags behind bone resorption. Moreover, in osteonal bone remodeling, the new tissue always contains a vascular pore that did not exist previously. On the other hand, it has been argued that failure to remodel can also lead to deleterious effects on bone. Because normal remodeling removes bone that has been rendered defective (as evidenced by the death of some of its osteocytes), suppression of normal remodeling would be expected to result in an accumulation of the defective bone, potentially leading to increased propensity to accumulate damage and ultimately to fail mechanically (that is, undergo fracture). With the widespread use of potent antiresorptive agents (bisphosphonates) to combat bone loss, increased incidence of unusual skeletal pathologies (initially, osteonecrosis of the jaw and more recently rare, atraumatic subtrochanteric femoral fractures) has lent support to that assertion. Although these concerns may only apply to a subpopulation of patients undergoing antiresorptive therapy, the use of antiresorptive agents has been increasingly examined to determine who may be at particular risk for these complications and whether the risk can be minimized by improving bisphosphonate treatment regimens, by developing new bisphosphonates, or by using alternative strategies such as inhibitors of RANKL or CatK, or anabolic agents.

Fracture Healing

Unlike bone remodeling, which replaces small areas of bone that have become damaged or otherwise outlived their usefulness, fracture healing repairs major tissue damage due to severe traumatic injury. The process is beyond the scope of this chapter, so only a few comments will be made here.

First, fracture healing is a fascinating and unique form of tissue repair in that it involves a true regeneration of the preinjury tissue, rather than simply formation of scar tissue. Following the acute hemostatic response, fracture healing activates both intramembranous and endochondral pathways of osteogenesis that largely replicate the intramembranous and endochondral bone formation processes that occur in the tissue during embryonic development. Although a scarlike tissue (fracture callus) is produced initially, it is ultimately replaced by a combination of modeling and remodeling to yield a tissue that is virtually identical in its composition and overall structure to that which was present before the injury. Thus, bone is unique and privileged among all connective tissues in that it can heal postnatally without scar. Second, fracture healing is under normal circumstances a highly effective process, often more so than soft-tissue healing. Nevertheless, nonunions or delayed unions occur at a frequency that makes them a significant public health problem, and demands efforts to understand their basis and to develop effective countermeasures.

Mechanical Properties of Bone

Mechanical function is one of bone's two dominant physiologic functions (the other being calcium-endocrine). Thus, understanding the behavior of bone under habitual loads, as well as those involved in traumatic and pathologic events, is critical for the development of an accurate framework of bone's mechanical and physiologic function. Bone mechanical properties are subject to the same principles as those of conventional engineering materials, and thus can be characterized in much the same way.[37] However, the ability of bone to adapt to mechanical demands, via specific cellular activities, sets it apart from inert engineering materials. It is clinically important to understand how conditions of bone loss, excessive mineralization, and implant instability can affect the mechanical performance of bone tissue.[38]

The lexicon of biomechanics is based on that of mechanical engineering. The concepts of stress (σ) and strain (ε) are central and fundamental to bone biomechanics. Stress is normalized force (force per unit area) and has units of newtons (N/mm^2) or pascals, which allow for comparison between individual units of a given material that may differ in size. Forces/loads can be applied to materials in a variety of ways (such as compression, tension, torsion, or bending), and stresses also can be expressed in this way. The common terminologies used to describe those modalities in terms of stress are compressive (material becomes shorter, so stress values are given a negative sign, for example, 10 N), tensile (material becomes longer, so stress values are given a positive sign, for example, 10 N), shear (planes try to slide relative to each other, like a deck of cards), and torsion (material is twisted around an axis).

In real-life situations, complex stresses arise as some combination of these simple load or stress cases. Consider the example of a structure that experiences a bending load; imagine that a standardized beam of bone is created such that it has a uniform square cross section along its length. Now the beam is put into a loading apparatus whereby both ends are supported from underneath and a load is applied on top to one point directly at its center, such that it deflects toward the floor. Even without rigorous analysis it is apparent that the material nearest the bottom of the specimen is being pulled apart (experiences tension), whereas the material toward the top is being pressed together (experiences compression); thus, bending is a combination of the two. It is worth noting that if two opposing surfaces experience positive (tensile) and negative (compressive) stresses, then somewhere in the middle of the structure that value must pass through zero. The location of this zero-stress plane in a structure experiencing a bending load is called the neutral axis.

When a structure or material is subjected to external load it is almost a certainty that some deformation in or of the material will result at the microscopic or molecular levels. Strain is the concept that deals with this deformation of material under load. In its simplest form, strain is defined as a percentage change in length, that is change in length (ΔL) divided by original length (L). As a ratio of lengths, strain has no units and is normally stated as a relative deformation or in terms of microstrain. If something of length 100 mm has been stretched to 101 mm, then by the given formula ($\Delta L/L$) we calculate $1/100 = 0.01$. As noted, this is a dimensionless value and as such would be stated as 0.01 strain, in terms of relative deformation this number would be multiplied by 100 and referred to as a percentage, in this case 1% deformation. When strains are particularly low, as they typically are in relatively stiff materials such as bone, it is useful

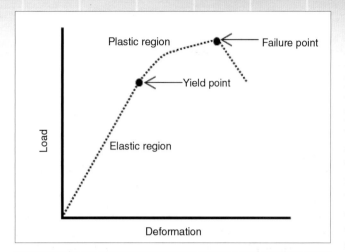

Figure 15 Representative load-deformation curve showing elastic and plastic regions as well as yield and failure points.

to speak in terms of microstrain. The micro- prefix simply means that the number in question is multiplied by 1×10^{-6} as per standard scientific notation, so in this example 1/100 = 0.01 strain = 10,000 microstrain = 1% deformation. To put these numbers into a clinical context, peak habitual loading activity, which might be experienced by athletes and military recruits during rigorous training, would result in peak cortical bone strains in the range of 2,500 to 3,000 microstrain in their bone tissue – approximately 20% to 25% of the typical yield strain in cortical bone. Physiologic strains in cancellous bone are thought to be greater, but they cannot be measured in vivo.

Visualization and characterization of a structure's mechanical properties are most effectively achieved by analyzing a load-deformation curve (**Figure 15**). This curve can be broadly separated into two parts, the elastic and the plastic regions.[39] If a bone is loaded within the former, it behaves like a spring — that is, when load is removed it will "spring" back to its original shape unchanged. However, once the latter region is reached the bone will not return to its original shape on removal of load. This is because permanent damage in the form of microcracks or some other nano/microstructural disruption has been caused. These two regions are separated by what is known as the yield point, accordingly the elastic and plastic regions are sometimes referred to as the preyield and postyield regions, respectively. The slope of the elastic region of the load-deformation curve represents the stiffness of the structure; the peak load carried at the point of fracture is widely considered the strength, and the area beneath the curve is the work-to-fracture. Recent studies of bone mechanics have also emphasized the importance of the postyield displacement (the displacement length from yield to fracture on a load-displacement curve) as a practical and effective way to gauge the relative brittleness of bone, which in turn can be interpreted as an estimation of fracture toughness. Fracture toughness is a particularly important property in relation to

bone tissue, and it will be discussed in more detail in subsequent sections.

Consider load-displacement tests of this type performed on two sets of bones, one group containing bones from large individuals and the other from small individuals. The values of load and stiffness would likely be considerably higher in the first group. However, if the load and deformation data sets were converted (by the normalizations, as described previously) and replotted as a stress-strain curve, the slope of the elastic portion of that curve, reflecting the intrinsic stiffness or Young modulus of the bone material, would be quite similar, because their sizes had been accounted for. All aspects of the load-displacement curve have corresponding aspects on a stress-strain curve (ultimate stress, yield), but like the stiffness versus Young modulus example just mentioned, reflect intrinsic values of the material.

Bone Matrix: Structure and Mechanical Function

Because the ECM of bone is composed of both organic and inorganic phases, it is important to consider the contribution of each phase to the overall tissue mechanical properties. For example, under compressive loads, in the elastic region, the inorganic mineral phase dominates in terms of contribution to tissue strength and stiffness.[40] This can be illustrated by what is known about the changes in bone mechanical properties during the aging process. As bone tissue gets older, more mineral crystals are deposited along and between the collagen fibers — thus the tissue as a whole becomes more mineralized than "normal" younger bone. Mechanical testing of aging bone has shown that indeed there is increased bone matrix stiffness compared with younger tissue, when the increases in porosity are accounted for. However, although this may seem like an improvement in structural integrity, often it is not. This is because increased elastic (preyield) properties are often coupled with decreased plastic (postyield) properties (increased brittleness), which are of particular importance because bone fracture is a postyield phenomenon. A primary clinical example of this is a so-called greenstick fracture in children, where less mineralized, lower-stiffness bone actually resists overt fracture.

Once the yield point has been reached, the relative contribution of each phase is altered, with the organic phase (collagen fibers) assuming a larger role in postyield behavior. An interesting clinical example of this can be found with osteogenesis imperfecta, a disease characterized by a collagen defect. This defect gives rise to reduced postyield properties, whereas the elastic stiffness, mostly governed by the mineral phase, is relatively normal. It is also important to note that bone tissue is more than the sum of its parts in terms of the mechanical contribution of each phase individually. The interplay between phases at the nanoscale as well as their arrangement into lamellae and osteons at the micron level serve as toughening mechanisms that inhibit crack propagation. This allows for dissipation of energy and improves the fracture toughness of the material consider-

2: Physiology of Musculoskeletal Tissues

ably. The ability of a material to resist the initiation and propagation of internal cracks over time is worthy of particular attention because these characteristics strongly influence fracture risk. From the engineering perspective, these considerations can be treated under a general heading of a material's fatigue properties.

Bone Fatigue Properties

The habitual physiologic loading that bone experiences, despite being considerably lower in magnitude than that involved in trauma or outright fracture, is applied repetitively and causes bone to fatigue.[3] As noted previously, peak habitual loading activity, which might be experienced by athletes and military recruits, results in peak cortical bone strains that are approximately 20% to 25% of the yield strain in cortical bone, whereas moderate activity strains are even lower. Cyclic loading of bone causes microscopic cracking and damage accumulation, with typical microcracks on the size order of tens of microns or smaller.[41] Unlike metals where a single crack will lead to fracture, bone matrix is a composite structure of solid phase mineral and reinforcing fibers. In composites, like bone or fiber reinforced graphite, small cracks are trapped by the internal interfaces in the matrix. Composites can tolerate a large number of microcracks before cracks accumulate sufficiently to weaken the material. Thus, the metal component of a prosthesis must be engineered to resist the start of a crack. A single fatigue crack will directly cause fracture, whereas bone is designed by nature as a damage-tolerant material.

Another unique aspect of bone as a composite material is that when microcracks do form at this scale in bone, a biologic response ensues. Specifically, bone remodeling is activated in a highly targeted manner such that osteoclasts remove the damage focus and osteoblastic infilling replaces the damaged bone with healthy new matrix. Thus, bone remodeling plays a central role in maintaining bone material properties. Recent data indicate that microcracks injure osteocytes and cause focal cell death providing the cellular triggers for the activation and targeting of bone remodeling units to microdamage foci.

CLINICAL NOTE: Failure to remodel microcracks or weakened bone tissue effectively will cause damage to accumulate, compromising the strength and fracture resistance of the bone and potentially leading to fracture due to weakened material. Fatigue damage may accumulate from overuse, such that damage occurs more rapidly than bone remodeling can repair (for example, stress fractures of athletes, dancers, and military recruits). In situations where the applied loads are normal but the tissue quality is impaired (for example, osteoporosis), fatigue damage accumulation can be accelerated. Finally, with suppression of bone remodeling, which occurs with antiresorptive drugs (bisphosphonates, anti-RANKL antibody) or aging, fatigue microdamage will accumulate in bone due to lack of remodeling-repair in bone; this phenomenon is thought to underlie both osteonecrosis of the jaw and atypical fractures in patients on long-term antiresorptive therapy.

Mechanical Properties of Cortical Versus Trabecular Bone

In general terms, cortical and trabecular bone are composed of the same basic material — both at the matrix and lamellar tissue levels. However, because of their vastly different organizations their respective mechanical properties vary accordingly. There are various tests that can be performed to assess the basic mechanical properties of cortical bone. The most common approach is to use direct loading in a materials testing system; however, other alternatives include ultrasound or indirect methods such as radiographic or densitometric imaging. The tissue level value of Young modulus (E) in cortical bone in the longitudinal direction is approximately 17 to 19 GPa and ultimate strength is approximately 100 to 150 MPa, whereas in the transverse directions (both radial and tangential) those values are approximately 8 to 10 GPa and 9 to 11 MPa, respectively. This illustrates that cortical bone is highly directional in its behavior under load. In engineering terms a material has anisotropic properties if it behaves differently depending on the direction that the load is applied. Maximum strength and stiffness of cortical bone is obtained in the osteonal direction, which is roughly parallel to the long axis of the bone. Thus, its microstructure, particularly in the diaphyseal region, is optimized to bear the loads it habitually experiences.[37]

Another important mechanical property of bone is its viscoelasticity.[42] This means that the mechanical response of the tissue is dependent on the loading rate applied to it. The phenomenon of viscoelasticity occurs because there is fluid present within bone tissue, within pores of various length-scales. If a load is applied at a slow rate, that fluid has time to move through the porosities of the tissue in the direction of the changing pressure gradient. However, when the loading rate is high, the fluid has insufficient time to move and thus has the effect of stiffening the material. Despite the appearance of higher stiffness and strength, loading at a high rate may cause more brittle failure if loaded beyond yield. Although the viscoelastic effect in bone is relatively small in comparison with soft tissue it is nonetheless an important consideration to characterize the tissue fully, especially with regard to high-rate loading failures such as those that can occur during motor vehicle accidents.

The lattice-like microstructure of trabecular bone, with its interconnected network of struts and plates, each approximately 100 to 150 μm in width, has properties vastly different from those of cortical bone.[43] It can be argued that its microarchitecture is really the primary determinant of its mechanical properties. This is why, at least in part, the direct measurement of trabecular bone mechanical properties is much more difficult than for cortical tissue. The range of reported values for Young modulus in trabecular bone is 0.5 to 1.5 GPa, whereas strength is typically on the order of 5 to 10 MPa. Although the osteon is the basic repeating micro-

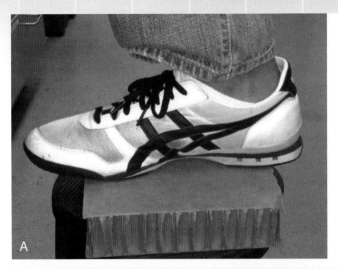
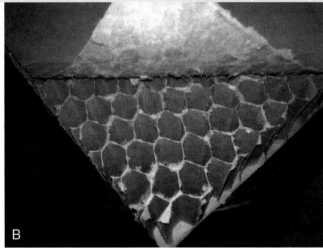

Figure 16 **A**, Paperboard cellular material supporting an individual's full body weight (approximately 200 lb). **B**, Internal structure showing cellular structures formed by thin (approximately 200 μm) paper septae.

structural unit of cortical bone, in trabecular bone it is the individual trabeculum. Various approaches have been used to directly assess these structures in isolation; however, the results reported vary widely due to the challenges of defining, extracting, and mechanically testing "single" trabeculae. Therefore, mechanical properties of trabecular bone are typically measured from bulk specimens at least 5 mm in diameter.

From a mechanical perspective, the design criteria of trabecular bone makes it particularly well suited for efficient impact/energy absorption and stress redistribution/load transfer under compressive loads. In contrast, it is not especially well designed for handling bending or torsional loads and thus does not perform particularly well under those circumstances. Trabecular bone can be referred to as a cellular material or cellular foam; the term cellular in this description does not refer to anything biologic but rather the array of geometric structures created by the individual struts and plates. The mechanical behavior of this structure is often compared with that of other cellular solids and foams. Many everyday materials, such as corrugated paperboard, have an analogous reinforced lattice structure to trabecular bone and function in a similar way from a mechanical perspective. **Figure 16, A** shows a piece of paperboard packing material being subjected to compressive loads that are generated by the full weight of the 200-lb individual standing on top of it. The bulk dimensions of this structure are 200 × 200 × 50 mm, while its weight is only 100 g. **Figure 16, B** shows the internal structure of the paperboard with its array of interconnected paper septae, each of which has a wall thickness of approximately 200 μm. This illustrates the efficient way in which cellular solids can handle considerable compressive loads. However, much like trabecular bone this structural example would not perform as well in a bending or torsional environment.

From a clinical standpoint, the mechanical properties of trabecular bone are particularly important because aging and osteoporosis are known to have pronounced effects on this tissue. Interestingly much of the material that is lost during these processes seems to be preferentially removed from struts and plates, which bear stresses in the nonhabitual loading direction (transverse or horizontal trabeculae). Thus, over time the structure becomes more vulnerable to loads that come from unusual or unexpected directions, such as those experienced during a fall, when fractures often occur. Fatigue loading and viscoelastic effects may also play a role in the mechanics and physiology of this tissue type.

Whole Bone Properties

Throughout the skeleton, great variety exists in the sizes and shapes of individual bones, from femora to vertebrae to the small bones of the hand, wrist, and foot.[44] A general common form exists in the structure of each, which includes an outer shell of cortical bone surrounding an internal trabecular component. For example, in the femur most of the central diaphysis is cortical bone alone, whereas the contribution of trabeculae is mostly restricted to the area beneath the articulating surfaces and in the metaphyses. In contrast, the vertebrae and small bones of the wrist and foot are made up mostly of trabecular bone, surrounded by a thin cortical shell. Flat bones like the cranium and sesmoidal bones such as the patella also follow this general pattern. Although consideration of cortical and trabecular bone separately is important to understanding their properties at a fundamental level, it is also important to remember that they are interdependent in the in vivo situation. At the macro level, the geometric properties of a bone play a major role in its mechanical response to load.[45] In long bones, parameters such as cortical thickness, moment of inertia, and overall volume fraction will be of particular mechanical importance. Although for vertebrae, which are composed mostly of trabecular bone, considerations of heterogeneity, asymmetry, and microarchitecture would be more relevant.

In all cases, the material composition of the tissue will also contribute significantly to the properties of the whole bone. Another issue that illustrates how whole bones mechanically function as more than the sum of their parts is hydraulic stiffening. In principle, hydraulic stiffening represents a mechanism that can increase the upper range of dynamic loads tolerated by the skeleton. The contained (mostly fluid) cellular tissues that comprise the bone marrow likely play a role in stiffening the entire structure under certain conditions.

It is instructive to think about the structure of whole bones from an engineering design standpoint. The relevant design criteria for the construction of any mammalian long bone would be largely similar: the central shaft should be particularly efficient at bearing compressive, bending, and torsional stresses. For all of these loading modes, sharp angles would not be optimal due to the possibility of generating stress concentrations. For resisting bending and torsion, having material located centrally would not be as important as having it toward the outer surface. Thus, a hollow cylindrical structure would be a suitable design. Toward the ends of the bone, having a wider profile and good impact/energy absorption properties beneath the joint surface would be advantageous. Furthermore, the ability to distribute and channel those loads toward the stiffer denser tissue in the shaft of the bone would also be desirable. Thus, it seems that nature has followed classic engineering principles in the design of many whole bones in the mammalian skeleton.

Clinical Implications of Bone Properties

Aging and Osteoporosis

Clinically, it is well-known that bone fragility increases with age as well as in disease states such as osteoporosis. Clinical knowledge of these processes from a mechanical standpoint, as well as from a physiologic perspective, is important to achieve accurate predictions of fracture risk. Osteoporosis is the most common metabolic bone disorder and is a growing health care problem as the global population continues to age and thus become susceptible. This condition often is underrecognized and thus undertreated because it often manifests without warning in the form of sudden fracture. To a large extent, the definition of bone fragility in aging and osteoporosis is focused on whether or not bone is strong enough to bear normal loads, a logical extension of the fact that bone mineral density (BMD) and strength are well correlated. However, in response to mechanical loading, there is more than just strength alone that must be considered.[46] As described previously, bone under load exhibits a region of elastic deformation (where strength and stiffness are important parameters), followed by a region of plastic deformation (in which strength and stiffness are less dominant) where permanent damage begins to initiate and accumulate. Thus, materials can be strong and stiff and yet be relatively poor at resisting fracture, and failure can occur in a brittle

manner once yield point has been reached. Important material properties that help to describe fracture resistance are work to fracture, postyield compliance, and crack propagation parameters. These properties are generally independent of elastic properties or strength, and thus are not indexed at all in bone mass or density measurements. Accordingly, a global definition of bone fragility must take into account bone's fracture resistance as well as its strength determinants.

Pharmacologic Treatments

Bisphosphonates are the most common pharmacologic treatment used in situations of reducing, or reduced, bone mass. When they are prescribed and used correctly, bisphosphonates can reduce the risk of osteoporotic fracture by preventing or slowing the rate of bone loss.[46] The fracture reduction reported following treatment is often considerably more than would be expected based solely on measured changes in BMD. Thus, the precise mechanism by which these drugs actually operate has still not been fully clarified. As described earlier in this chapter, bone is continually being turned over by the removal of bone via osteoclasts and its subsequent replacement by osteoblasts. With the onset of aging, and in particular the loss of estrogen in women at menopause, this balance is disrupted such that osteoclasts remove more bone than osteoblasts can replace. Bisphosphonates inhibit the action of the osteoclasts and reduce the rate of bone destruction. It is known that this suppression of remodeling occurs site specifically, and it most likely does not have a direct effect on osteoblasts or bone formation. It is also known that the commercially available bisphosphonates tend to vary with respect to speed of onset, duration of effect, and magnitude of suppression. However, in a clinical sense, it is still not clear which combination of effects is optimal. Ongoing research seeks to address precisely how much remodeling is sufficient, what is the optimal duration of treatment, and how long is required to restore remodeling to pretreatment levels following withdrawal. It has also come to light in recent years that suppression of remodeling is related to microdamage accumulation. The action of these agents on osteoclasts prevents their targeted repair of damaged tissue, which is essential to maintain healthy tissue. The effects of bisphosphonates on the fatigue properties of bone are also currently unknown, but the topic has become the focus of research in recent years.

Atypical Fractures

Long-term treatment with bisphosphonates has recently been linked with the occurrence of "atypical femoral fractures." These differ from regular, more commonly observed femur fractures for several reasons in that (1) they often occur with little or no trauma, (2) they tend to occur in the femoral diaphysis rather than as the more commonly seen fractures of the femoral neck, (3) they often exhibit cortical thickening and a "beaking" pattern is often evident at the fracture site, and (4) the fracture paths they tend to travel

2: Physiology of Musculoskeletal Tissues

are usually transversely across the cortex rather than in a spiral or oblique, consistent with a more brittle fracture mode fashion. Although it is not certain that bisphosphonates are the cause, these unusual femur fractures have been predominantly reported in patients taking bisphosphonates.[47] Although these fractures are very uncommon and currently account for less than 1% of all hip and femur fractures overall, their occurrence raises important biomechanical questions in terms of the long-term effects of bisphosphonates on bone tissue. However, the broad view on this issue is that the bisphosphonates are clearly extremely useful in the clinical setting; they have demonstrable potency in reducing the rate of bone loss and can be powerful tools in reducing the risk of fracture in certain patients.

Summary

Bone is a highly complex hierarchical tissue that has a multifunctional role in the physiologic and mechanical performance of the skeleton. Mechanically, bone tissue serves to protect vital internal organs from harmful external forces and also, by acting as a system of levers, forms the basis of the locomotive system. In physiologic terms, the skeleton is integral to mineral homeostasis through calcium storage and also contains bone marrow, which is the source of new blood cells for the cardiovascular system. Structurally, bones are designed to carry out their specific roles in a highly efficient manner. This efficiency is achieved by using lightweight solutions to load bearing, while also remaining highly fracture resistant due to their composite makeup. When damage does occur in bone, a remodeling response is activated that has the capacity to locate and remove damaged areas of tissue. The primary mechanosensory role in bone is performed by osteocytes, which form a complex and active cell network throughout the matrix. The functions of bone tissue are finely balanced for optimal performance; a deep understanding of the fundamental form and function of this tissue is necessary to address potential issues that arise from aging and disease from a clinical perspective.

References

1. Jee WS: Integrated bone tissue physiology: Anatomy and physiology, in Cowin SC, ed: *Bone Mechanics Handbook*, ed 2. Boca Raton, FL, CRC Press, 2001, pp 1.1-1.68.

2. Hancox NM: *Biology of Bone*. London, England, Cambridge University Press, 1972, pp 10-40.

3. Martin RB, Burr DB, Sharkey NA: *Skeletal Tissue Mechanics*. London, England, Springer-Verlag, 1998, pp 127-223.

4. Currey JD: *Bones: Structure and Mechanics*. Princeton, NJ, Princeton University Press, 2002, pp 54-124, 194-245.

5. Morgan EF, Barnes G, Einhorn TA: The bone organ system: Form and function, in Marcus R, Feldman D, Nelson DA, Rosen CJ, eds: *Osteoporosis*, ed 3. Waltham, MA, Elsevier Academic Press, 2008, pp 3-22.

6. Kerr JB: *Atlas of Functional Histology*. London, England, Mosby, 1999, pp 163-184.

7. Yang Y: Skeletal morphogenesis and embryonic development, in Rosen CJ, ed: *Primer on the Metabolic Bone Diseases and Disorders of Mineral Metabolism*. Washington, DC, American Society for Bone and Mineral Research, 2009, pp 2-10.

8. Brookes M, Revell WJ: *Blood Supply of Bone*. London, United Kingdom, Springer-Verlag, 1998, pp 142-175.

9. Eriksen EF, Axelrod DW, Melsen F: *Bone Histomorphometry*. New York, NY, Raven Press, 1994, pp 3-12.

10. Burr DB: The contribution of the organic matrix to bone's material properties. *Bone* 2002;31(1):8-11.

11. Robey PG, Boskey AL: The composition of bone, in Rosen CJ, ed: *Primer on the Metabolic Bone Diseases and Disorders of Mineral Metabolism*, ed 7. Washington, DC, American Society for Bone and Mineral Research, 2009, pp 32-38.

12. Viguet-Carrin S, Garnero P, Delmas PD: The role of collagen in bone strength. *Osteoporos Int* 2006;17(3):319-336.

13. Gordon MK, Hahn RA: Collagens. *Cell Tissue Res* 2010; 339(1):247-257.

14. Eyre DR, Weis MA, Wu J-J: Advances in collagen cross-link analysis. *Methods* 2008;45(1):65-74.

15. Kalamajski S, Oldberg A: The role of small leucine-rich proteoglycans in collagen fibrillogenesis. *Matrix Biol* 2010;29(4): 248-253.

16. Gorski JP: Biomineralization of bone: A fresh view of the roles of non-collagenous proteins. *Front Biosci* 2011;16:2598-2621.

17. Murshed M, McKee MD: Molecular determinants of extracellular matrix mineralization in bone and blood vessels. *Curr Opin Nephrol Hypertens* 2010;19(4):359-365.

18. Sapir-Koren R, Livshits G: Bone mineralization and regulation of phosphate homeostasis. *IBMS BoneKEy* 2011;8:286-300.

19. Shore EM, Kaplan FS: Insights from a rare genetic disorder of extra-skeletal bone formation, fibrodysplasia ossificans progressiva (FOP). *Bone* 2008;43(3):427-433.

20. Long F: Building strong bones: Molecular regulation of the osteoblast lineage. *Nat Rev Mol Cell Biol* 2012;13(1):27-38.

21. Harada S, Rodan GA: Control of osteoblast function and regulation of bone mass. *Nature* 2003;423(6937):349-355.

22. Monroe DG, McGee-Lawrence ME, Oursler MJ, Westendorf JJ: Update on Wnt signaling in bone cell biology and bone disease. *Gene* 2012;492(1):1-18.

23. Baron R, Hesse E: Update on bone anabolics in osteoporosis treatment: Rationale, current status, and perspectives. *J Clin Endocrinol Metab* 2012;97(2):311-325.

24. Ross FP: Osteoclast biology and bone resorption, in Rosen CJ, ed: *Primer on the Metabolic Bone Diseases and Disorders of Mineral Metabolism*, ed 7. Washington, DC, American Society for Bone and Mineral Research, 2009, pp 16-22.

25. Tanaka S, Miyazaki T, Fukuda A, et al: Molecular mechanism of the life and death of the osteoclast. *Ann N Y Acad Sci* 2006;1068:180-186.

26. Nakamura I, Takahashi N, Jimi E, Udagawa N, Suda T: Regulation of osteoclast function. *Mod Rheumatol* 2012;22(2): 167-177.

27. Suda T, Takahashi N, Udagawa N, Jimi E, Gillespie MT, Martin TJ: Modulation of osteoclast differentiation and function by the new members of the tumor necrosis factor receptor and ligand families. *Endocr Rev* 1999;20(3):345-357.

28. Teitelbaum SL, Ross FP: Genetic regulation of osteoclast development and function. *Nat Rev Genet* 2003;4(8):638-649.

29. Boyle WJ, Simonet WS, Lacey DL: Osteoclast differentiation and activation. *Nature* 2003;423(6937):337-342.

30. Russell RG: Bisphosphonates: The first 40 years. *Bone* 2011;49(1):2-19.

31. Lewiecki EM: New targets for intervention in the treatment of postmenopausal osteoporosis. *Nat Rev Rheumatol* 2011;7(11):631-638.

32. Bonewald LF: The amazing osteocyte. *J Bone Miner Res* 2011;26(2):229-238.

33. Fritton SP, Weinbaum S: Fluid and solute transport in bone: Flow-induced mechanotransduction. *Annu Rev Fluid Mech* 2009;41:347-374.

34. Schaffler MB, Kennedy OD: Osteocyte signaling in bone. *Curr Osteoporos Rep* 2012;10(2):118-125.

35. Ehrlich PJ, Lanyon LE: Mechanical strain and bone cell function: A review. *Osteoporos Int* 2002;13(9):688-700.

36. Tamma R, Zallone A: Osteoblast and osteoclast crosstalks: From OAF to Ephrin. *Inflamm Allergy Drug Targets* 2012;11(3):196-200.

37. Guo XE: Mechanical properties of cortical bone and cancellous bone tissue, in Cowin SC, ed: *Bone Mechanics Handbook*, ed 2. Boca Raton, FL, CRC Press, 2001, pp 10.1-10.23.

38. Katz JL: Composite material models for cortical bone, in Cowin SC, ed: *Mechanical Properties of Bone*. New York, NY, American Society of Mechanical Engineers, 1981.

39. Turner CH, Burr DB: Basic biomechanical measurements of bone: A tutorial. *Bone* 1993;14(4):595-608.

40. Lucchinetti E: Composite models of bone properties, in Cowin SC, ed: *Bone Mechanics Handbook*, ed 2. Boca Raton, FL, CRC Press, 2001, pp 12.1-12.19.

41. Frost HL: Presence of microscopic cracks in vivo in bone. *Henry Ford Hosp Med Bull* 1960;8:25.

42. Lakes R: Viscolelastic properties of cortical bone, in Cowin SC, ed: *Bone Mechanics Handbook*, ed 2. Boca Raton, FL, CRC Press, 2001, pp 11.1-11.12.

43. Keaveny TM, Morgan EF, Yeh OC: Bone mechanics, in Kutz M, ed: *Standard Handbook of Biomedical Engineering and Design*. New York, NY, McGraw-Hill, 2003, pp 8.1-8.17.

44. Nordin M, Frankel VH: *Basic Biomechanics of the Musculoskeletal System*, ed 3. New York, NY, Lippincott, Williams & Wilkins, 2001.

45. Bouxsein ML, Jepsen KL: Etiology and biomechanics of hip and vertebral fracture, in Orwoll ES, ed: *Atlas of Osteoporosis*, ed 2. Philadelphia, PA, Current Medicine Inc, 2003, pp 166-172.

46. Allen MR, Burr DB: Bisphosphonate effects on bone turnover, microdamage, and mechanical properties: What we think we know and what we know that we don't know. *Bone* 2011;49(1):56-65.

47. Shane E, Burr D, Ebeling PR, et al: Atypical subtrochanteric and diaphyseal femoral fractures: Report of a task force of the American Society for Bone and Mineral Research. *J Bone Miner Res* 2010;25(11):2267-2294.

2: Physiology of Musculoskeletal Tissues

Chapter 10

Form and Function of Articular Cartilage

Susan Chubinskaya, PhD

Anne-Marie Malfait, MD, PhD

Markus A. Wimmer, PhD

Overview

Definition and Primary Function of Articular Cartilage Tissue

The three major types of cartilage tissue in the body are distinguished by their composition, structure, and mechanical properties. Hyaline cartilage is the tissue found in diarthroidial joints, also called articular cartilage when it covers articulating surfaces of long bones. In synovial joints, hyaline articular cartilage tissue faces the joint cavity (the space in which synovial fluid accumulates) on one side and is linked to the subchondral bone plate via a layer of calcified cartilage tissue on the other.[1] Together with bone, menisci, ligament, tendon, and synovium, hyaline articular cartilage ensures the integrity of articular joints. It is originated from mesenchymal stem cells and in its mature state is a highly complex stratified tissue. In the immature state, articular cartilage is much thicker and unstratified, with cells (called chondrocytes) being distributed in a random isotropic pattern. In addition, hyaline cartilage forms the growth plate by which long bones grow during childhood. In this case, it is called growth plate cartilage. The key functions of articular

Dr. Chubinskaya or an immediate family member has received research or institutional support from Zimmer, Joint Restoration Foundation, and Regentis and serves as a board member, owner, officer, or committee member of the Orthopaedic Research Society, the Osteoarthritis Research Society International, and the International Cartilage Repair Society. Dr. Malfait or an immediate family member is a member of a speakers' bureau or has made paid presentations on behalf of Pfizer and has stock or stock options held in Pfizer. Dr. Wimmer or an immediate family member serves as an unpaid consultant for Endolab GmbH and has received research or institutional support from Zimmer.

cartilage are to transmit applied load across surfaces, permit smooth articulation within the joint with lubrication and low friction, and absorb shock. To perform its main functions, cartilage must have the high tensile strength and elasticity that is provided by the composition of its extracellular matrix (ECM).[2] The thickness of articular cartilage varies between the joints and the exact location on the articular surface and ranges from a fraction of a millimeter in the hand joints to up to 5 to 7 mm in the knee joint. It is, in general, thicker in larger joints and on joints receiving higher relative stresses. Articular cartilage thickness is not dependent on body size or body mass index, but rather varies with individual genetics. Articular cartilage is an avascular, aneural, and alymphatic tissue with limited potential for self-repair. It receives its nutrients by diffusion from the synovial fluid[2] controlled by the charge, the size, and steric configuration of the diffusing solutes and molecules.[3]

Fibrocartilage is a transitional tissue between dense regular connective tissue and cartilage or bone that is temporarily present at fracture sites. It is present as a permanent tissue in three major locations in the body: the intervertebral disks, a covering of the mandibular condyle in the temporomandibular joint, and the meniscus.

Elastic cartilage (yellowish and opaque, more flexible than hyaline), exists in the epiglottis and the eustachian tube. It has the same basic organization as hyaline cartilage, containing chondrocytes in lacunae, cell nests, and perichondrial layer, but the major difference between these two tissues is that the matrix of elastic cartilage contains large amounts of elastin.

Supramolecular Organization of Articular Cartilage

Morphologically, human articular cartilage can be described as a tissue with one cell type, chondrocytes, embedded in an

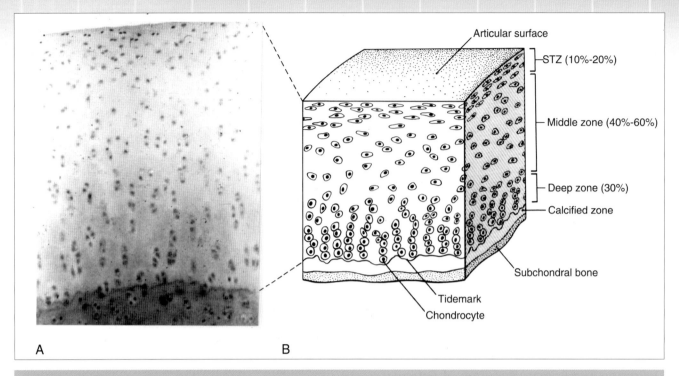

Figure 1 **A**, Histologic section of normal adult articular cartilage showing even safranin staining and distribution of chondrocytes. **B**, Diagram of chondrocyte organization in the three major zones of the uncalcified cartilage, the tidemark, and the subchondral bone. STZ = superficial tangential zone. (Reproduced with permission from Mow VC, Proctor CS, Kelly MA: Biomechanics of articular cartilage, in Noordin M, Frankel VH, eds: *Basic Biomechanics of the Musculoskeletal System*, ed 2. Philadelphia, PA, Lea and Febiger, 1989, pp 31-57.)

abundant ECM that consists mainly of a collagen type II network, containing the high-molecular-weight proteoglycan, aggrecan, and water. The aggrecan molecule consists of a core protein to which chondroitin sulfate and keratan sulfate glycosaminoglycan chains are attached. Under normal homeostasis, articular cartilage undergoes controlled turnover, with the chondrocytes being responsible for the production, organization, and maintenance of the extensive extracellular matrix. There are four zones identified horizontally in adult cartilage: the superficial zone, representing approximately 10% to 20% of the full thickness; the middle or transitional zone, representing 40% to 60% of the tissue; the deep zone that constitutes approximately 30% of the entire thickness; and the calcified zone that separates the cartilage tissue from the underlying subchondral bone (**Figure 1**). The junction between the deep and calcified layers is defined by a smoothly undulating tidemark, a distinct basophilic line that is critical for the transmission of load from the cartilage to the bone. Each cartilage zone is distinguished by the orientation of collagen fibers, the composition of matrix components, and the properties of residing chondrocytes. In the superficial zone, the collagen fibrils are arranged parallel to the articular surface and the amount of proteoglycans is reduced in comparison with other zones. Chondrocytes residing in the superficial zone have an elongated shape; they are small in size, present in higher density, and are distributed parallel to the surface as single cells (**Figure 1**). The middle zone of cartilage is characterized by randomly arranged collagen fibrils that are less densely packed, by reduced fibril concentration and high levels of aggrecan and water. Middle zone chondrocytes are randomly distributed throughout the matrix as single rounded cells. In the deep zone, the collagen fibrils are arranged radially, perpendicular to the joint surface; they cross the tidemark to enter the calcified zone,[2] allowing a stable anchor between soft and hard tissues, specifically the deep layer of the cartilage and hard, calcified cartilage and subchondral bone. The water content is the lowest in the deep zone, whereas the concentration and density of proteoglycans is the highest. Chondrocytes in the deep zone are rounded and arranged in columns in the same vertical direction as collagen fibers. The deep zone chondrocytes form functional structural units called chondrons.[4]

Collagen organization is also differentially arranged within these concentric subdivisions. Collagen fibers adjacent to the cell form a tightly woven (consisting exclusively of type VI collagen), densely compacted nest-like enclosure around each chondrocyte, called pericellular matrix. In the territorial matrix (the 5-μm– to 10-μm–wide matrix immediately outside the pericellular matrix),[4] collagen fibers are thicker and form radial bundles. Territorial matrix can surround a single chondrocyte or a group/column of chondrocytes. The interterritorial matrix is characterized by the largest collagen fibers where their compact organization and

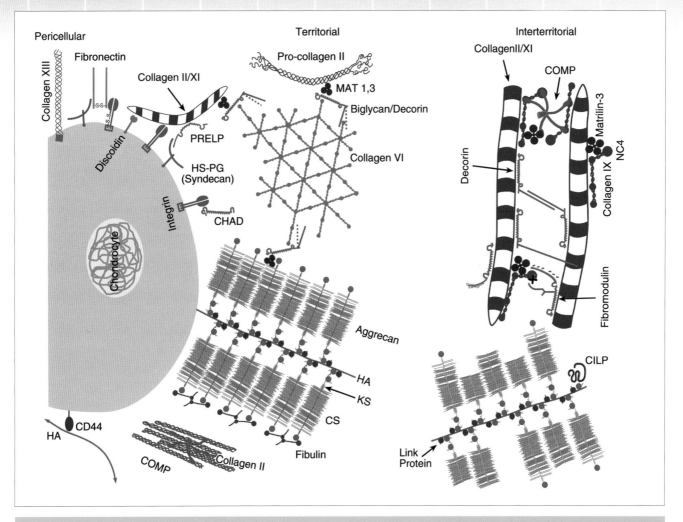

Figure 2 Schematic illustration of molecular constituents in cartilage and their arrangement into large multimolecular assemblies. The different compositions and organizations at the cell surface with several receptors interacting with specific matrix molecules, at the interterritorial matrix closer to the cells and the interterritorial matrix at a distance are indicated. CHAD = chondroadherin; CILP = cartilage intermediate layer protein, encoded by the *CILP* gene; CS = chondroitin sulfate; COMP = cartilage oligomeric matrix protein; HA = hyaluronan; HS-PG = heparan sulfate proteoglycan; KS = keratan sulfate; MAT = matrilin; PRELP = prolargin, a protein encoded by the *PRELP* gene. (Reproduced with permission from Heinegärd D, Saxne T: The role of cartilage matrix in osteoarthritis. *Nat Rev Rheumatol* 2011;7[1]:50-56).

radial alignment defines the collagen bundles, which were classically described as arcades by Benninghoff.[5] The interterritorial matrix occupies most of the volume of articular cartilage and fills the space between territorial matrices of individual or a group of cells. The interterritorial matrix is also called ECM. Thus, articular chondrocytes are surrounded by a complex pericellular microenvironment, which, in the middle and deep zones, is integrated with a territorial matrix, separated from adjacent territories by the interterritorial matrix[6] (**Figure 2**). This structural organization of adult articular cartilage defines biomechanical properties of the tissue and recognizes chondrocytes as key regulators of both catabolic and anabolic events necessary for cartilage homeostasis.

Biomechanical Function of Articular Cartilage

The intricate architecture of articular cartilage is a prerequisite to fulfill its function as a load-bearing and low-friction tissue. The specific material properties allow cartilage to carry high contact forces, dampen force spikes, and dispense the resulting compressive stresses to the underlying subchondral bone. To keep the shear stresses low, a very sophisticated lubrication mechanism is facilitated during articulation. This keeps friction and wear low when the joint surfaces glide on each other.

From a structural perspective, cartilage is biphasic with a fluidal and a solid phase, whereby the solid phase can be perceived similar to that of a fiber-reinforced composite solid matrix (**Figure 3**). As mentioned previously and reviewed in more detail in the following paragraph, the fibers are collagen type II and comprise more than 50% of the dry

2: Physiology of Musculoskeletal Tissues

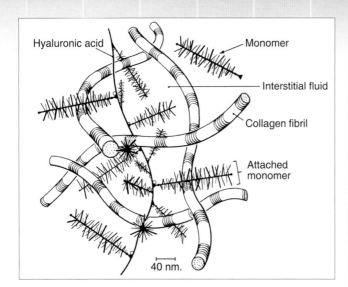

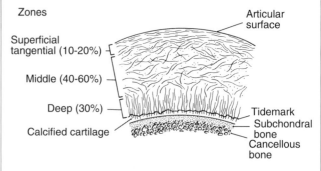

Figure 4 The collagen fiber architecture of articular cartilage is often categorized into three different zones: superficial, middle, and deep. Note that the fiber orientation is tangential in the superficial zone and radial in the deep zone, while it is less oriented in the middle zone. (Reproduced with permission from Mow VC, Proctor CS, Kelly MA: Biomechanics of articular cartilage, in Noordin M, Frankel VH, eds: *Basic Biomechanics of the Musculoskeletal System*, ed 2. Philadelphia, PA, Lea and Febiger, 1989, pp 31-57.)

Figure 3 Solid matrix organization of articular cartilage. The collagen fibers resist the tensile stresses, whereas the proteoglycans attract water molecules exerting swelling pressure onto the matrix. (Reproduced with permission from Mow VC, Proctor CS, Kelly MA: Biomechanics of articular cartilage, in Noordin M, Frankel VH, eds: *Basic Biomechanics of the Musculoskeletal System*, ed 2. Philadelphia, PA, Lea and Febiger, 1989, pp 31-57.)

weight of cartilage. They act as a scaffold to impart the shape of the tissue and immobilize the proteoglycans within the ECM. Mechanically, they provide the tensile strength necessary to resist the shear loads during articulation. Initial studies of their macro-organization presumed an arrangement of arcades with the superior aspect of the arches placed most superficially.[5] It was thought that this arrangement allows compression with subsequent return to its original shape. More recent studies, however, show that the fibers have a less ordered organization, in particular in the middle zone (**Figure 4**). Within the fiber network, the water-laden proteoglycans exert swelling pressure and keep the previously described scaffold inflated and the collagen fibers prestressed.[7] This is what provides articular cartilage with the capability to first dispense focal contact stresses evenly to the underlying bone and, second, due to the water-laden tissue, to generate a lubricating film on the gliding surfaces.[8] Because of the structural arrangement of its constituents, during dynamic loading well over 90% of the load is carried through pressurized fluid in healthy cartilage, keeping the stresses on the solid phase to a minimum.

Articular Chondrocytes

Chondrocytes as Unique Cells That Perform Multiple Functions

Chondrocytes are responsible for the growth and maintenance of the tissue. In the mature state, they occupy approximately 5% of the tissue volume, yet these unique cells control multiple functions, including matrix synthesis and matrix degradation. In other tissues and cells, these functions are performed by different types of cells (for example in bone, osteoblasts are responsible for bone matrix synthesis, whereas osteoclasts control bone resorption).[9] The formation, degradation, and remodeling/regeneration of cartilaginous tissues require regulated cell proliferation, growth, synthesis of ECM proteins, production and activation of matrix-degrading enzymes, and in some cases matrix calcification and cell death. Chondrocytes are the only cells that control these processes and conversely, a large number of signaling pathways regulate their activity.

Mechanical Properties

The mechanical properties of chondrocytes essentially differ from the macroscopic properties of the ECM. They are much softer than the ECM and their elastic modulus is approximately three orders of magnitude smaller (0.6 kPa versus 0.5 to 0.7 MPa). The matrix stiffness around the chondrocyte is still orders of magnitude lower than the ECM but somewhat stiffer than the embedded cell itself.[10] This difference in elastic modulus considerably alters the stresses and strains in the microenvironment of the cell and leads to more heterogeneous stress-strain fields than what is observed macroscopically[11] (**Figure 5**).

Chondrocyte Properties in Relation to Cartilage Zones

Though all cells within articular cartilage are called chondrocytes, they are heterogeneous in their morphology, genotype, phenotype, metabolism, and signaling, depending on the cartilage zone in which they reside. In articular cartilage, chondrocytes are embedded in a specialized matrix microenvironment (discussed later in this chapter). Because chondrocytes elaborate and maintain this complex matrix, the zonal variations in the extracellular matrix result from metabolic differences between the cells.[12] The characteristic feature of the chondrocyte embedded in cartilage matrix is its rounded or polygonal morphology. The exception occurs at tissue boundaries, such as the articular surface of joints, where chondrocytes may be flattened or discoid. It has been calculated[13] that the cell density of full-thickness, human, adult, femoral condyle cartilage is maintained at 14.5 ($\pm$ 3.0) $\times$ 10^3 cells/mm^2 from age 20 to 30 years. Adult articular chondrocytes are nonmitotic cells that survive at low oxygen tension in the absence of a vascular supply; thus it could be anticipated that with aging, chondrocyte density is perhaps diminished, as a result of cell death occurring due to a process called "senescence" (discussed in the following paragraphs).[14]

Changes in depth in the tissue are gradual, not abrupt, and even within one zone there may be considerable cellular heterogeneity. The morphology and metabolism of articular chondrocytes was primarily studied in vitro, when subpopulations of cells were isolated from different zones of the cartilage and culture conditions favored a chondrocytic phenotype.[12] Significant differences between chondrocytes derived from the superficial and deep zones of cartilage have been reported in multiple studies and in various species including humans.[12,15,16] These cells expressed distinct phenotypic stability, gene expression profile, responsiveness to various stimuli, metabolic activity, and the type of matrix they synthesize. Thus, chondrocytes from the superficial zone, when cultured in agarose gel, became irregular in shape with numerous processes and in a liquid medium formed clusters covered by flattened cells resembling a perichondrium;[12,15] they also produced very little ECM. In contrast, chondrocytes from the deep zone retained a rounded shape and morphologic features typical for mature chondrocytes. They produced extensive ECM rich in proteoglycans and containing collagen fibrils. The proliferation rate of isolated bovine or porcine chondrocytes in fetal serum cultures was also different between the two zones, with the cells from the deep zone having a higher proliferative activity. However, these differences were diminished in human chondrocytes cultured in the presence of human serum containing lower concentration of growth factors than fetal bovine serum.[15] Zonal differences in metabolism have been demonstrated not only in isolated chondrocytes, but also when the cells remained in their original undisrupted matrix cultured as tissue explants. With regard to matrix synthesis, chondrocytes from both cartilage zones predominantly synthesize aggrecan as a major aggregated proteoglycan and type II collagen as a major collagen; deep zone chondrocytes synthesize these matrix components in much greater quantities. One of the key differences between chondrocytes from the superficial and deep zones is that the former produce a glycoprotein, called proteoglycan-4, also known as lubricin or superficial zone protein (SZP), homologous to megakaryocyte stimulating factor and encoded by the gene *PRG4*. It is a

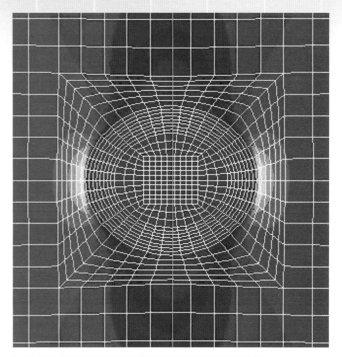

Figure 5 Note that the microscopic stress/strain fields around chondrocytes are heterogeneous, even if the macroscopic field is homogeneous as shown by this finite element model. The stresses have been calculated following a multiscale finite element model approach. (Reproduced with permission from Görke UJ, Günther H, Wimmer MA: Multiscale FE-modeling of native and engineered articular cartilage tissue. *European Congress and Computational Methods in Applied Sciences and Engineering (ECCOMAS)*. Jyväskylä, Finland, 2004, pp 1-20.)

multifunctional proteoglycan that is required for a smooth articulation of articular joints (discussed in the following paragraphs).[17,18] Numerous in vitro and in vivo studies are focused on the properties of lubricin in normal joint homeostasis and in posttraumatic osteoarthritis. It has also been produced as recombinant protein and used as a joint supplement in experimental studies on osteoarthritis.

Further differences between the superficial zone chondrocytes and the deep zone chondrocytes were found in response to catabolic mediators, particularly interleukin-1 (IL-1). IL-1 induced more severe inhibition of proteoglycan synthesis and a lower ratio of secreted tissue inhibitor of metalloproteinase-1/stromelysin in chondrocytes from superficial cartilage than those from deeper cartilage, whereas interleukin receptor antagonist blocked responses to IL-1 more effectively in chondrocytes from the deep cartilage zone than in superficial zone chondrocytes.[12,19] These responses were due, at least in part, to a higher number of IL-1 receptors on the surface of the superficial zone chondrocytes. Therefore, chondrocytes from the surface of articular cartilage show a greater vulnerability to the harmful effects of catabolic mediators and are less responsive to the

2: Physiology of Musculoskeletal Tissues

potential therapeutic effects aimed at blocking IL-1–mediated responses.

Chondrocytes are distinct not only between cartilage zones, but also between different diarthrodial joints, for instance, knee and ankle joints.[20,21] In addition to anatomic, structural, and biomechanical differences, biochemical differences in the strength of the responses to catabolic and anabolic stimuli of chondrocytes from knee and ankle joints have been demonstrated. Thus, knee chondrocytes showed a stronger response to the factors that increase damage to the cartilage matrix (IL-1 or fibronectin fragments). This response by knee chondrocytes resulted in enzymatic damage to the matrix that may be difficult for the cells to repair, whereas the weaker response of ankle chondrocytes may allow the cells to repair their damaged matrix. In contrast, ankle chondrocytes have been shown to be more responsive to anabolic stimuli, for example the growth factor osteogenic protein-1, especially after the removal of IL-1.[20,21] These differences in metabolic activity between the cartilages of the two joints could in part help to explain their differences in susceptibility to osteoarthritis.

Motility
One of the emerging fields in chondrocyte biology is the migration of chondrocytes within the surrounding ECM and the potential to overcome the density and pressure of the matrix under nonpathologic conditions, that is, without adversely affecting tissue structure and function. This question is particularly important for tissue engineering and cartilage repair and regeneration. Several pioneering studies have shown that isolated chondrocytes are able to migrate under the direction of different stimuli on or within various planar and three-dimensional matrices. For example, it has been reported that chondrocytes move in response to various growth factors, such as bone morphogenetic protein, hepatocyte scatter factor, urokinase plaminogen activator, insulin-like growth factor–1, transforming growth factor–β, platelet-derived growth factor, and fibroblast growth factor.[21] The cells have also been shown to move when seeded on natural polymeric matrices, such as sulfated hyaluronic acid, fibronectin, fibrin, collagen I, and alginate, and even polarize and move toward cathodic electrical fields. Chondrocyte movement has been observed through three-dimensional collagen I gels or polymer scaffolds, such as alginate. After 7 days in alginate bead culture in the presence of serum or growth factors, the cells moved out of the bead and formed a monolayer on the bottom of the culture dish. Importantly, these actions apparently did not cause changes in chondrocyte phenotype and they continued to synthesize type II collagen.[22,23] In vivo, few studies have shown outgrowth of cells from human cartilage explants, especially in cases of matrix damage or disruption of the collagen network by extensive cutting, collagenase digestion, or defect drilling. It is unclear whether the exit of chondrocytes from the cartilage is solely due to a robust proliferative response of cells close to or on the edge of the wounds followed by

their attachment to outer planar surfaces and subsequent migration. However, there are indications that in certain models, cells polarize, and elaborate extensions while still within cartilage. Current data on cartilage in vitro and in vivo raise the possibility that chondrocytes may display regulated movements during growth and remodeling. This phenomenon can specifically be observed when the remodeling activity of the cell results in loosened matrix and reduced matrix stiffness, thus allowing cell passage.[22]

Low-Oxygen Environment
Normal articular cartilage, unlike other tissues, is a hypoxic tissue with oxygen levels between 0.5% and 5%, dependent on tissue depth. It has been shown that hypoxia is a strong promoter of ECM matrix synthesis by chondrocytes with production of key cartilage-specific matrix components (such as aggrecan and collagen types II, VI, IX, and XI) and key transcription factors (Sox 9).[24] The chondrocytes can sense surrounding oxygen levels through hypoxia–inducible transcription factors (initially named HIF1-a), whose expression and function are regulated posttranslationally, mainly by hydroxylation reactions. Hypoxia triggers essential signals, affecting many aspects of chondrocyte biology, and is also involved in the maintenance of chondrocyte phenotype. With regard to differences between superficial and deep zone chondrocytes, it has been shown that the deep cells had greater oxygen consumption than the superficial cell and this is consistent with the differences in their mitochondrial volume.[25]

Senescence and Aging
It has been suggested that cellular aging is a cumulative result of repetitive minor damage to cellular structures, which culminates in a state of cellular growth arrest called senescence. Although senescent cells remain viable for a certain period of time (from months to years), their normal function is perturbed. Senescence is induced by damage to DNA or mitochondria caused by oxidative stress and exposure to mutagens, but it is also an inevitable consequence of cell division. Two forms of senescence are known: replicative senescence linked to DNA replication[26] and extrinsic or stress-induced senescence.[27] Replicative senescence occurs in differentiated viable cells due to irreversible cell cycle arrest, which happens when cells have reached a set limit of both population doublings and telomere length. Correlation has been found between chronologic age of human donors and markers of senescence detected in cartilage specimens (decline in DNA synthesis, senescence-associated β-galactosidase expression, and telomere erosion), which suggests that replicative senescence occurs not only in vitro during cell culture, but also in vivo in cartilage and other connective tissues. Extrinsic or stress-induced senescence[27] could be more suitable for explanation of senescence in postmitotic cells such as neurons or chondrocytes. Stress-induced senescence can occur from diverse stimuli, including ultraviolet radiation, oxidative damage, activated onco-

genes, and chronic inflammation. Oxidative damage to DNA can directly contribute to stress-induced senescence and, because the ends of chromosomes are particularly sensitive to oxidative damage, can result in telomere shortening similar to that seen with replicative senescence.[27] Due to oxidative stress, stress-induced senescence fits well with a theory of aging that refers to free radicals as mediators of aging. Senescent cells have a complex, metabolically active phenotype characterized by irreversible cell division/cell cycle arrest; resistance to apoptosis, which may result in accumulation of senescent cells in tissues; secretion of proteases, cytokines, or growth factors; and reduced responsiveness to growth factors, all of which may contribute to or are associated with tissue aging.[26] As mentioned previously, in vivo cell senescence could be documented by the presence of specific markers, such as histologic staining for senescence-associated β-galactosidase and heterochromatin; increased p53, p21, and p16; and reduced Wnt2.[27]

Biochemical Composition of the Cartilage ECM

Proteins of the Cartilage ECM

The remarkable biomechanical properties of articular cartilage are in large part derived from its unique molecular organization and the specialized biochemical characteristics of its major constituents (listed in **Table 1**). In healthy cartilage, assembly and tissue distribution of ECM molecules vary according to the vicinity of the matrix to chondrocytes. Essentially, the cartilage matrix can be divided into three areas: the pericellular, the territorial, and the interterritorial matrix, each with its unique molecular organization (**Figure 2**).

Water

Normal cartilage has a water content ranging from 65% (deep zones) to 80% (surface) of its wet weight. The flow of water through the tissue is governed by mechanical and physicochemical laws, and it is this flow that allows the transport of nutrients through this avascular tissue, in addition to providing cartilage with its biomechanical properties (please refer to the section on biomechanics). Articular cartilage holds water with avidity, through contact with the major macromolecules in cartilage, type II collagen, and proteoglycans.

Collagens

The shape of articular cartilage and its material strength depend heavily on its extensively cross-linked collagen network and characteristic fibrillar organization, which varies with tissue depth and distance from the cell.

Type II Collagen

The main collagen in articular cartilage is type II collagen, a triple helix composed of three identical α chains synthesized from the *COL2A1* gene. Two splice variants of procollagen exist, with type IIA characteristic for chondroprogenitors and type IIB the predominant type II collagen in adult

Table 1

Proteins of the Cartilage Matrix

Collagens

Type II (75% of total in fetal, 90% in adult collagen)

Type III (>10% in adult human cartilage)

Type IX (covalently fibril-associated collagen; 10% fetal, 1% adult)

Type X (only in hypertrophic cartilage)

Type XI (part of the fibril; 10% fetal, 3% adult)

Type VI (chondron, microfilaments; < 1%)

Type XII/XIV

Type XIII (transmembrane)

Proteoglycans

Aggrecan (95% of total proteoglycan)

Biglycan

Decorin

Fibromodulin

Lumican

Asporin

Chondroadherin

Osteoadherin

Prolargin (PRELP)

Noncollagenous Proteins

Fibronectin

Thrombospondins, mainly thrombospondin 5 (COMP)

Matrilin 1 (previously cartilage matrix protein)

Matrilin 2

Matrilin 3

Anchorin

Tenascin-C

Thrombomodulin

Chondroadherin

Cartilage intermediate layer protein (CILP)

Fibulin

Membrane Proteins

Syndecan

CD44

Integrins (α1, 2, 3, 5, 6, 10; β1, 3, 5)

(Section on collagens adapted with permission from Eyre DR, Weis MA, Wu JJ: Articular cartilage collagen: An irreplaceable framework? *Eur Cell Mater* 2006;12:57-63.)

2: Physiology of Musculoskeletal Tissues

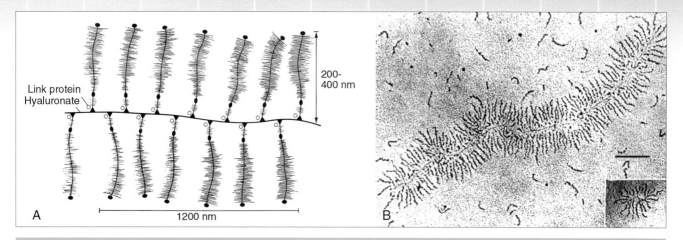

Figure 6 **A**, A diagram of the aggrecan molecules arranged as a proteoglycans aggregate. Many aggrecan molecules can bind to a chain of hyaluronate, forming macromolecular complexes that effectively are immobilized within the collagen network. **B**, Electron micrographs of bovine articular cartilage proteoglycans aggregates from (skeletally immature calf (larger figure) and skeletally mature steer (inset). These show the aggregates to consist of a central hyaluronic acid filament and multiple attached monomers (bar = 500 μm). (Reproduced with permission from Buckwalter JA, Kuettner KE, Thonar EJ: Age-related changes in articular cartilage proteoglycans: Electron microscopic studies. *J Orthop Res* 1985;3:251-257.)

Table 2

Function of Types IX, XI, III, VI Collagen

Type IX collagen	Decorates the surface of type II collagen fibers and forms bridges with other molecules in the ECM (for instance, fibronectin). Contributes to matrix assembly.
Type XI collagen	Forms a template that constrains the lateral growth of type II collagen heterofibrils.
Type III collagen	Plays a role in response of articular cartilage to matrix damage—may add cohesion to a weakened type II collagen network (in aging and in osteoarthritis).
Type VI collagen	These microfilaments are tightly woven to form a nest-like enclosure around each chondrocyte, called the chondron, thus providing communication between the cell and its microenvironment.

cartilage. During biosynthesis, three identical α chains wind around each other to form collagen molecules, which then associate in a staggered alignment to form long, unbranched, banded fibrils that provide tensile strength. Transmission electron microscopy has revealed patterns of preferred fibril orientation;[28] in the surface zone of cartilage (0 to 2 mm), fibrils are thin and tend to run primarily parallel to the articular surface. In the middle zones, a greater range of fibril diameters exists, and their organization appears more random. The thickest fibrils are in the deep zone, where they are perpendicular to the cartilage surface and anchored in the subchondral bone.

Other Collagens

Type II collagen fibrils contain other types of collagen within the fibril or surrounding it. These collagens are often referred to as "minor" collagens because of their relative amount, not their functional importance.[29] The main functions of these minor collagens[30,31] are listed in **Table 2**. Collagens II, IX, and XI form cross-linked heterotypic fibrils that lay out the backbone template of the collagen network in developing articular cartilage. As articular cartilage matures, the collagen framework consists mainly of collagen II. With age, chondrocytes start to produce type III collagen, which gets superimposed in varying amounts on the original collagen fibril network. Type III collagen molecules with unprocessed N-propeptides are extensively cross-linked to type II collagen in aged joints. Because type III collagen is known to be prominent at sites of healing and repair in skin and other tissues, it has been postulated to act as a covalent modifier that may add cohesion to a weakened collagen type II fibril network as part of a chondrocyte healing response to matrix damage.[30, 32]

Aggrecan

The hydrophilic nature of proteoglycans is what gives cartilage its affinity for water. The major proteoglycan in cartilage is aggrecan, which consists of a 220- to 250-kDa protein core, containing three globular domains, G1, G2, and G3. G1 and G2 are near the N terminus and separated by a short interglobular domain. The third globular domain, G3, is near the C terminus of the core protein, and the long stretch between G2 and G3 is heavily substituted with keratin sulfate and approximately 100 chondroitin sulfate glycosaminoglycan (GAG) chains[6] (**Figure 6**). All GAGs have repeating carboxyl (COOH) and sulfate (SO_4) groups, which are ionized ($COO-$ and SO_3-) in solution and give the cartilage its negative charge. Aggrecan monomers form very large aggregates through interaction with the polysaccharide, hyaluronan. The G1 domain associates noncovalently with hyaluronan, an interaction stabilized by a third molecule, the 45-kDa link protein, to form high-molecular-weight aggregates (> 200 MDa). Because these negatively charged aggregates are tightly packed in the collagen fibrillar network, their fixed charges are spaced only 10 to 15 Å apart, which results in extreme charge-to-charge repulsive forces. Thus, the constraining forces developed within the collagen network surrounding the trapped proteoglycan aggregates ensure a strong and cohesive matrix, which holds water avidly. The aggrecan gel further protects cartilage collagen fibrils from degradation by collagenases. It has been demonstrated that collagen in freeze-thawed cartilage depleted of aggrecan is completely degraded after incubation with matrix metalloproteinase (MMP)-1, whereas collagen in cartilage with intact aggrecan is not. Additionally, selective aggrecanase inhibitors that do not block MMP activity protect against aggrecan degradation as well as against collagenolysis in cartilage explants exposed to catabolic cytokines. These data suggest that aggrecan plays a protective role in preventing pathologic degradation of collagen fibrils.[33]

Other Matrix Molecules

Other noncollagenous molecules in the cartilage ECM provide functions for tissue assembly and for maintaining cartilage properties. For instance, the assembly of the collagen type VI network in the pericellular matrix is regulated by small leucine-rich proteoglycans (SLRPs) such as decorin, biglycan, lumican, and fibromodulin. These small proteoglycans are nonaggregating and have shorter protein cores than aggrecan and, unlike aggrecans, they do not fill a large volume of the tissue. Biglycan is glycosylated with two chondroitin or dermatan sulfate chains. Decorin is glycosylated with a single chondroitin or dermatan sulfate chain, and fibromodulin with up to five keratan sulfate chains. Both decorin and fibromodulin have been found to bind to collagens type I and II and may have a role in organizing and stabilizing the collagen meshwork.[6] SLRPs can further interact with other molecules, including cartilage oligomeric matrix protein (COMP) and matrilins. Matrilin-1 to -4 form a family of widely distributed proteins containing von Willebrand Factor A (vWFA) domains that are often present in proteins involved in protein interactions.[34] In cartilage, matrilins-1 and -3 are predominantly present, where they bind different types of collagen as well as aggrecan, so they essentially support matrix assembly by connecting fibrillar components and establishing interactions between collagen networks and aggrecan (**Figure 7**). COMP (also known as thrombospondin 5) is also a part of

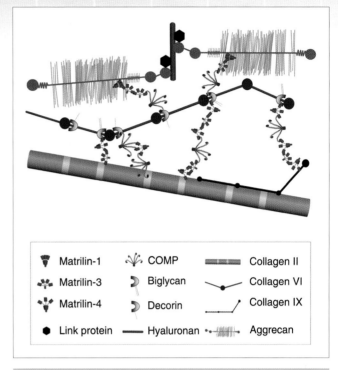

Figure 7 Model for the role of matrilins in the formation of supramolecular networks in cartilage. Matrilin-1, -3, and -4 and COMP act as adaptor molecules that interconnect D-periodically banded collagen II–containing cartilage fibrils with collagen VI–containing beaded filaments and aggrecan aggregates to generate a complex macromolecular network. The interactions may be mediated either by matrilins binding directly to the collagenous COL3 domain of collagen IX or via COMP that associates with the NC4 domain of collagen IX. The contacts of matrilin-1, -3, and -4 with collagen VI filaments are mediated by the small LRR proteoglycans decorin and/or biglycan, which preferentially bind to the filaments in the vicinity of the collagen VI N-termini, themselves acting as adaptor molecules. Note that the size of the molecules is not to scale. (Reproduced with permission from Klatt AR, Becker AK, Neacsu CD, Paulsson M, Wagener R: The matrilins: Modulators of extracellular matrix assembly. *Int J Biochem Cell Biol* 2011;43:320-330.)

this ingenious assembly. It consists of five identical subunits held together close to their N terminus by a coiled coil domain, whereas the C-termini have a globular domain that binds other matrix molecules (**Figure 7**). Most notably, through this fivefold binding capacity, one COMP molecule can rapidly bring together five collagen molecules and thus act as a catalyst for early collagen fibril formation. In osteoarthritis, COMP levels are dramatically increased, so that a single COMP molecule can occupy all binding sites on one collagen molecule, thereby hampering fibril formation and effectively hindering tissue repair.[6]

In addition to matrix assembly, it is becoming clear that matrix molecules (or fragments thereof) play a key role in modulating cell behavioral responses, including cell metabolism, differentiation, and survival. The past decade has de-

2: Physiology of Musculoskeletal Tissues

livered many new insights into the role of members of the SLRP gene family as signaling molecules.[35] Soluble SLRPs can engage various cell surface receptors, including insulin-like growth factor–1 receptor and epidermal growth factor receptor, triggering downstream signaling events that regulate cell behavior. In addition, these glycoproteins bind and sequester various cytokines, growth factors, and morphogens (for example, transforming growth factor–β)[36] involved in multiple signaling pathways. In the pericellular matrix, matrix molecules interact with cell surface receptors; for example, fibronectin can bind integrins and heparan sulfate proteoglycans such as syndecan, collagen binds discoidin domain receptors, and CD44 acts as a hyaluronan receptor (**Figure 5**). Many molecules that can bind these receptors on the surface of chondrocytes also interact with molecules in the territorial matrix, establishing communication between the matrix (sometimes far removed from the cell) and the chondrocyte. The chondrocyte can thus sense what is going on in the matrix and respond accordingly. Recently, it has been suggested that the content of matrilins in the pericellular matrix can alter the mechanical sensitivity of chondrocytes.[32] Other proteins in the cartilage matrix (listed in **Table 1**) fulfill important roles, many of which are the subject of active research. Fibulin has been shown to be important in the supramolecular organization of the cartilage matrix, through binding of the G3 domain of aggrecan.[6] Some proteins, such as tenascin C, are present in small amounts, but their expression goes up dramatically in osteoarthritis.

As the matrix undergoes changes as part of aging or as part of a pathologic process (arthritis), molecular interactions and subsequent cellular responses can be dramatically altered, resulting in a changed metabolic environment and often leading to a compromised function of the cartilage tissue. Furthermore, molecules released from the matrix can be biologically active and have been linked to inflammation through at least two mechanisms. First, matrix molecules such as fibromodulin and COMP can activate complement and thus contribute to inflammation, which in turn generates more degradation of the matrix.[6] Second, matrix components such as tenascin-C, fibronectin, and fragments of hyaluronic acid can activate toll-like receptors, expressed by many cells including chondrocytes, synoviocytes, and macrophages, resulting in the release of numerous chemokines and cytokines.[37]

Lubricin

To help withstand biomechanical shear forces due to articulation, articular cartilage surfaces possess an inherently low coefficient of friction, which is facilitated in part by localization of the boundary lubricant, lubricin, secreted by chondrocytes and synoviocytes. One of the primary functions of lubricin is the maintenance of joint lubrication and the prevention of cellular adhesion. Lack of lubricin expression has been connected to premature joint failure, as in the camptodactyly-arthropathy-coxa vara-pericarditis

syndrome in humans, in which genetic mutations elicit a lubricin deficit,[38] and the use of recombinant lubricin as an intra-articular biotherapeutic for osteoarthritis is currently explored.[39] Interestingly, joint articulation stimulates the expression of lubricin, whereas pure compressive loading does not.[40] It has been speculated that the oscillating joint drags fluid into the joint space, thereby causing biophysical effects similar to those of fluid flow. Velocity magnitude of the oscillating bodies (and thus the dragged fluid) is a critical determinant for the cellular response. Also, the complexity of the motion pattern seems to play a role, as suggested by studies using isolated chondrocytes in a scaffold.[41]

Matrix Fragmentation

In healthy cartilage, matrix turnover is slow, and the half-life of the major constituents, collagen and aggrecan, is very long. The half-life of type II collagen has been reported to be more than 100 years.[42] Using aspartic acid racemization as a marker of molecular age, it has been proposed that the half-life of the large aggrecan monomer in human cartilage is 3.4 years, whereas the free hyaluronan-binding region fragments have a half-life of 25 years. This suggests that the rate of formation and turnover of the large monomer is much more rapid than the final degradation of the free binding region fragments, which explains the accumulation of these fragments in cartilage during aging (discussed in the following paragraphs).[43] During arthritic disease, factors such as cytokines induce chondrocytes to secrete proteolytic enzymes that degrade the matrix. The aggrecanases, primarily A disintegrin and metalloproteinase with thrombospondin motif (ADAMTS)-4 and ADAMTS-5,[44] cleave the aggrecan core protein at five distinct cleavage sites, thus generating multiple fragments that diffuse from the matrix into the synovial fluid. Cleavage between the amino acids Glu^{373} and Ala^{374} in the interglobular domain of the aggrecan core protein results in the loss of the bulk of the GAG-bearing portion of aggrecan from the cartilage matrix, thereby compromising its function.[45] ADAMTS-4 has been reported to cleave matrilin-3, and ADAMTS-7 and -12 have been reported to cleave COMP, which may all contribute to destabilization of the ECM.[46] As these events occur, the collagen network becomes increasingly vulnerable to the action of collagenases, in particular MMP-13. The specific cleavage products that are thus generated can be monitored in the synovial fluid, and even in the urine, which has generated invaluable information on the pathogenesis of osteoarthritis. There are ongoing efforts in standardizing methods to measure levels of specific matrix fragments (including fragments of collagen, aggrecan, and COMP) in biologic fluids, so that they can be used as biomarkers of disease. Importantly, matrix fragments are not biologically inactive, and they may further contribute to the pathologic process. For instance, fibronectin, a multimeric glycoprotein found in plasma and tissues, is a minor component of normal cartilage. However, osteoarthritic cartilage contains up to tenfold more fibronectin (through synthesis and accumulation), and this is accompanied by increased levels in the synovial fluid. Products of fibronectin fragmentation are able to induce a catabolic phenotype in chondrocytes, and fragments have been shown to induce enzymes such as MMP-13 and ADAMTS-4/5.[47] In osteoarthritic cartilage, the enzyme responsible for generating specific fibronectin fragments was recently shown to be ADAM-8.[48]

Aging of the ECM

Joint tissues change with age, thus contributing to increased risk for development of osteoarthritis. Cartilage changes include chondrocyte senescence (discussed previously) and changes in the ECM. These matrix changes include formation of advanced glycation end products (AGE), which affect mechanical properties of cartilage through increased cross-linking of the collagen network (which makes the cartilage too stiff) and changes in the GAG composition, which not only affect biomechanical properties of cartilage but also dramatically alter the susceptibility of the aggrecan core protein to cleavage by aggrecanases.[44,49] Also, aggrecan cleavage by aggrecanases between the amino acids Glu[373] and Ala[374] in the interglobular domain generates small fragments that are retained in the matrix through the interaction of the G1 domain with hyaluronan and thus accumulate in cartilage during the lifetime of the individual. These aggrecan fragments bound to hyaluronan occupy the binding sites where newly synthesized complete aggrecan molecules should bind and thus result in smaller proteoglycan aggregates being present with increasing age.

Genetic Variability in Matrix Proteins

Mutations in genes encoding cartilage matrix proteins are not uncommon, especially for collagen. For example, mutations in COLII, COLIX, and COLXI lead to chondrodysplasias and premature osteoarthritis.[50] Recent genetic association studies attempting to understand how genetic variation in population cohorts is associated with osteoarthritis have uncovered novel insights in the role of some cartilage molecules.[51] For instance, the strongest genetic association with knee osteoarthritis identified by a genome-wide association study to date was found with double von Willebrand factor A in an Asian population, although this finding could not be replicated in a European cohort. This newly identified gene was then found to encode the collagen VI α 4 chain. Other polymorphisms of interest are being discovered, including an association between knee osteoarthritis and a polymorphism in the gene encoding the matrix molecule, asporin, which suppresses transforming growth factor–β–mediated expression of aggrecan and type II collagen. An association between a mutation in the gene encoding matrilin-3 is linked to osteoarthritis of the hand. This particular mutation (T298M) was found to have a pronounced influence on the formation of cartilage collagen fibrils in in vitro assays.[32] Finally, among the genes that have been linked to hip osteoarthritis, a highly heritable disease, are several that are involved in the development and maintenance of joint shape, including members of the Wingless (Wnt) and the bone morphogenetic protein family. Several features of hip joint architecture, such as acetabular dysplasia, pistol grip deformity, wide femoral neck, and altered femoral neck-shaft angle, appear to play an important role in the pathogenesis of osteoarthritis and may predate the development of clinical osteoarthritis by decades.[52]

Biomechanics of Articular Cartilage
Load Transfer

At the joint level, articular cartilage is primarily loaded in compression and less in shear (due to a highly sophisticated lubrication mechanism that keeps the tangential loads low, as discussed in the next section). In the human hip joint, contact pressures have been measured at approximately 1 MPa during static standing, ranging from 0.1 to 5.6 MPa while walking, and up to 7 MPa while stair climbing.[53,54] Loading peaks have been reported in the range of 20 MPa. To deal with these high contact stresses, articular cartilage relies on its internal architecture. The presence of water within the tissue allows the support of most of the load through pressurized fluid, which is important to minimize friction and wear. This fluid support is not uniform between the different zones of the tissue, with the superficial zone having a higher support (95% of applied load) than the deep zone (70% of applied load).[55] In addition, the interstitial fluid support is short-term and decreases quickly over time. The decreased interstitial fluid support causes increased loading of the solid phase, including chondrocytes. Hence, prolonged loading of the tissue on a single spot can cause nonphysiologic forces on the chondrocytes, resulting in cell death. This is why in a healthy joint the contact area migrates on each of the cartilage surfaces in contact. Even in ball-and-socket joints, such as the hip joint, the contact area migrates not only at the femoral head but also within the acetabular socket during daily activity (such as walking). In that sense, the architecture of the natural hip joint differs from the design of artificial hip replacements, which typically prohibit a displacement of the ball due to tight clearance tolerances of the cup.

With 1- to 3-mm thickness, cartilage is surprisingly thin and relatively soft (aggregate modulus of 0.5 to 1 MPa) to withstand the high compressive loads. This is only possible because cartilage is supported by the underlying subchondral bone, which provides structural support at a much higher stiffness (elastic modulus of approximately 10 GPa).[56] The mechanical properties of cartilage are typically described as nonlinear and viscoelastic, meaning that the tissue response upon deformation cannot be compared with a simple coil spring. Due to frictional interactions between the fluid and solid components of the tissue (arising when the fluid is pressed through the small pores of the tissue network), the force response is nonlinear and depends on loading speed and frequency. Hence, cartilage shows more resistance to deformation with increasing loading speed. During this process, energy is dissipated and the loading and unloading curves follow different stress-strain characteristics. Mechanically, a biphasic, porous model consisting of a solid phase and a fluid phase can be used to describe such properties. When two cartilage layers are pressed together, pressure is generated in its pores and is referred to as interstitial fluid pressure.

Recent investigations have shown that, due to the distinct orientation of the collagen fibrils, the solid matrix of the cartilage tissue must be considered as an anisotropic elastic material.[57] Often the rate-dependence of biphasic material behavior is exclusively attributed to the fluid flow through the solid matrix. However, next to the flow-dependent viscoelasticity due to the fluid-solid interaction,[58] the typical time-dependent response of the material is also caused by the intrinsic viscoelastic behavior of the solid skeleton.[59]

In addition to the roles of solid and fluid phases of articular cartilage, dissolved electrolytes together with the fixed charges of the solid matrix bring about mechanoelectrochemical phenomena adding to the load-bearing capacity of the tissue.[60,61] This has been discussed in the literature as a third phase, the ion phase, and led to the development of triphasic theory.[62] The negatively charged groups of the proteoglycans (ionized carboxyl and/or sulfate groups) require positive ions of the fluid phase (such as sodium and calcium) to maintain electroneutrality. These freely mobile counterions induce the Donnan osmotic pressure effect, in that a larger ion concentration within cartilage causes water to flow into the tissue and exert swelling pressure (which is counterbalanced by the stress generated in the collagen matrix). In the absence of neutralizing counterions, the negative fixed charges along the proteoglycan molecule generate repulsive electrostatic forces because proteoglycans are packed so tightly within the collagen matrix taking only one fifth of their free solution volume.

Apart from distinct nonlinear stress-strain characteristics under finite deformations, articular cartilage shows a different response with respect to tension and compression. This behavior has been described as bimodular material behavior[63] and is caused by the microscopic properties of the collagen fibrils, which are much stiffer in tension than in compression, as well as the macroscopic properties of structural orientation. All these characteristics provide the tissue with quite remarkable properties to withstand multiple body weights and provide a low coefficient of friction during compression.

Friction and Lubrication

Articular cartilage provides a low-friction interface between the articulating surfaces. The coefficient of friction against glass can be as low as 0.01 but may rise up to 0.3 with increasing load share of the solid phase. This finding was first described by McCutchen,[64] who demonstrated experimentally that the friction coefficient of cartilage against glass rises over time under a constant applied load, and challenged the theory of a hydrodynamic lubrication mecha-

nism where the pressurization of the fluid film occurs due to the relative velocity of the bearing surfaces (a more recent study using stringent engineering principles supports such arguments against a hydrodynamic lubrication mode[65]). Hence, in newer experiments such findings were related to interstitial fluid load support and the lubrication mode was termed 'biphasic' to account for the observation that the friction force at the articular surface increases with decreasing fluid load support.[66] Given the porous nature of cartilage matrix, compressive loads exude interstitial fluid from the tissue over time and dissipate the interstitial fluid pressurization. The load distribution changes and more load is shifted to the solid matrix. Without sufficient interstitial fluid pressurization, alternative lubrication mechanisms such as mixed or boundary lubrication come into play.

In boundary lubrication the load is supported by direct surface contact between the two opposing surfaces. Proteins, like lubricin, play a role in the boundary lubrication mode. It is thought that lubricin alters the physical and chemical attributes of the cartilage surface by binding to the surface to generate mutual repulsion between the opposing surfaces. However, the exact lubrication mechanism is unclear and a matter of current research. Although it has been proposed that lubricin binds ionically to the cartilage surface, it has also been observed that lubricin decreases the coefficient of friction in artificial bearings, suggesting a lubricating effect of soluble lubricin. Another theory attributes the boundary-lubricating ability to surface-active phospholipid and reduces the role of lubricin to a macromolecular watersoluble carrier of surface-active phospholipid.[67] The authors argue that lubricin would render the outermost lining of cartilage hydrophilic, whereas in healthy cartilage the surface is very hydrophobic, indicating a fatty constituent. In any case, the boundary lubrication mode, although less effective than the biphasic lubrication mode, plays an important role in cartilage homeostasis and health. It acts at low sliding speeds (up to 1 mm/s) without any pressure buildup in the lubricant[63] and supports low friction and wear at the joint during multiple start-stop procedures of daily activity. Although boundary lubrication is less effective than biphasic lubrication in lowering the coefficient of friction (the difference is in the order of a magnitude), its presence is important to keep the joint healthy. Lubricin knockout mice, for instance, have shown early signs of cartilage breakdown with subsequent joint failure.[68]

Another lubrication mode that is currently under debate is the so-called brush lubrication. In technical applications it has been shown that polymer brushes reduce friction between sliding surfaces onto which they are attached. It was found that polyzwitterionic brushes that were polymerized directly from the surface can have friction coefficients as low as 0.0004 at pressures as high as 7.5 MPa in aqueous solutions.[69] The charged polymer brushes repel each other when compressed and sustain significant pressure due to a socalled hydration lubrication mechanism: the water dipoles hold strongly onto the charged brushes, reluctant to be squeezed out, and thus carry high load while providing low friction at the same time. Macromolecules in the natural joint, for example, hyaluronan, aggrecan, and lubricin, emanating from the surface of the cartilage into the joint space could replicate such a brush and lead to friction coefficients of 0.001 or lower.

Tissue Wear

It can be expected that the sophisticated lubrication regimes largely protect cartilage from wear. Although very little is known about the acting wear mechanisms during normal homeostasis, it must be assumed that the wear process itself is noncontinuous and any lost tissue will be rapidly replaced with newly synthesized material. However, once tissue degrades with age or injury, lubrication becomes less effective, and mechanical wear will have a major role in the tissue degradation process.

Summary

This chapter has provided basic information on articular cartilage physiology, structure, composition, and biomechanical and biochemical properties. Articular cartilage is a marvelously complex tissue where one cell type, the chondrocyte, elaborates and manages an abundant avascular and aneural extracellular matrix. The biochemical characteristics of the macromolecules that build up this matrix provide the cartilage with its remarkable biomechanical properties. The past decade has witnessed significant new findings in the understanding of the fine assembly of this molecular meshwork, which has important implications for lubrication and friction of the joint. In this context, the role of interstitial fluid pressurization and lubricin has been highlighted. This chapter also introduces emerging areas of study in cartilage biology such as chondrocyte motility, senescence, effect of hypoxia, and genetics that collectively point toward the future of the field. In addition, considerable knowledge about the changing properties of chondrocytes and their matrix with aging and in arthritic disease has been gained. Enzymatic degradation of the matrix generates fragments that are biologically active and can serve as signals to chondrocytes or other cells in the joint. These fragments can also be monitored in the synovial fluid, and hopefully, in the near future may be developed as functional biomarkers of cartilage health. The role of mechanical wear in the overall degradation process, particularly when the tissue has been compromised due to aging or injury, has yet to be elucidated and will be an area of ongoing investigation.

References

1. Hunziker EB: Articular cartilage structure in humans and experimental animals, in Kuettner KE, Schleyerbach R, Peyron JG, Hascall VC (eds): *Articular Cartilage and Osteoarthritis*. New York, NY, Raven Press, 1991, pp 183-199.

2. Guilak F, Setton LA, Kraus VB: *Principles and Practice of Orthopaedic Sports Medicine*. Philadelphia, PA, Lippincott Williams & Wilkins, 2000, pp 53–73.

3. Nimer E, Schneiderman R, Maroudas A: Diffusion and partition of solutes in cartilage under static load. *Biophys Chem* 2003;106(2):125-146.

4. Poole CA: Articular cartilage chondrons: Form, function and failure. *J Anat* 1997;191(Pt 1):1-13.

5. Benninghoff A: Form und Bau der Gelenkknorpel in ihren Beziehungen zur Funktion. *Anat Entwicklungsgesch* 1925; 76:43.

6. Heinegård D: Proteoglycans and more: From molecules to biology. *Int J Exp Pathol* 2009;90(6):575-586.

7. Nagel T, Kelly DJ: The influence of fiber orientation on the equilibrium properties of neutral and charged biphasic tissues. *J Biomech Eng* 2010;132(11):114506.

8. Roughley P, Martens D, Rantakokko J, Alini M, Mwale F, Antoniou J: The involvement of aggrecan polymorphism in degeneration of human intervertebral disc and articular cartilage. *Eur Cell Mater* 2006;11:1-7.

9. Beier F, Loeser RF: Biology and pathology of Rho GTPase, PI-3 kinase-Akt, and MAP kinase signaling pathways in chondrocytes. *J Cell Biochem* 2010;110(3):573-580.

10. Guilak F, Jones WR, Ting-Beall HP, Lee GM: The deformation behavior and mechanical properties of chondrocytes in articular cartilage. *Osteoarthritis Cartilage* 1999;7(1):59-70.

11. Görke UJ, Günther H, Wimmer MA: Multiscale FE-modeling of native and engineered articular cartilage tissue. *European Congress on Computational Methods in Applied Sciences and Engineering (ECCOMAS)*. Jyväskylä, Finland, 2004, pp. 1-20

12. Aydelotte MB, Schumacher BL, Kuettner KE: Heterogeneity of articular chondrocytes, in Kuettner KE, Schleyerbach R, Peyron JG, Hascall VC, eds: *Articular Cartilage and Osteoarthritis*. New York, NY, Raven Press, 1991, pp 237-249.

13. Stockwell RA, Meachim G: *Adult Articular Cartilage*. Tunbridge Wells, England, Pitman Medical, 1979, pp 69-144.

14. Goldring MB: Cartilage and chondrocytes, in Ferinstein GS, Budd RC, Harris ED Jr, McInnes IB, Ruddy S, Sergent JS eds: *Kelley's Textbook of Rheumatology*, ed 8. Philadelphia, PA, Saunders, 2008.

15. Archer CW, McDowell J, Bayliss MT, Stephens MD, Bentley G: Phenotypic modulation in sub-populations of human articular chondrocytes in vitro. *J Cell Sci* 1990;97(Pt 2): 361-371.

16. Aydelotte MB, Kuettner KE: Differences between sub-populations of cultured bovine articular chondrocytes: I. Morphology and cartilage matrix production. *Connect Tissue Res* 1988;18(3):205-222.

17. Flannery CR, Hughes CE, Schumacher BL, et al: Articular cartilage superficial zone protein (SZP) is homologous to megakaryocyte stimulating factor precursor and is a multifunctional proteoglycan with potential growth-promoting, cytoprotective, and lubricating properties in cartilage metabolism. *Biochem Biophys Res Commun* 1999;254(3): 535-541.

18. Schumacher BL, Block JA, Schmid TM, Aydelotte MB, Kuettner KE: A novel proteoglycan synthesized and secreted by chondrocytes of the superficial zone of articular cartilage. *Arch Biochem Biophys* 1994;311(1):144-152.

2: Physiology of Musculoskeletal Tissues

19. Hauselmann HJ, Flechtenmacher J, Michal L, et al: The superficial layer of human articular cartilage is more susceptible to interleukin-1-induced damage than the deeper layers. *Arthritis Rheum* 1996;39(3):478-488.

20. Cole AA, Kuettner KE: Molecular basis for differences between human joints. *Cell Mol Life Sci* 2002;59(1):19-26.

21. Eger W, Schumacher BL, Mollenhauer J, Kuettner KE, Cole AA: Human knee and ankle cartilage explants: Catabolic differences. *J Orthop Res* 2002;20(3):526-534.

22. Morales TI: Chondrocyte moves: Clever strategies? *Osteoarthritis Cartilage* 2007;15(8):861-871.

23. Chubinskaya S, Huch K, Schulze M, Otten L, Aydelotte MB, Cole AA: Gene expression by human articular chondrocytes cultured in alginate beads. *J Histochem Cytochem* 2001; 49(10):1211-1220.

24. Lafont JE: Lack of oxygen in articular cartilage: Consequences for chondrocyte biology. *Int J Exp Pathol* 2010; 91(2):99-106.

25. Heywood HK, Knight MM, Lee DA: Both superficial and deep zone articular chondrocyte subpopulations exhibit the Crabtree effect but have different basal oxygen consumption rates. *J Cell Physiol* 2010;223(3):630-639.

26. Mollano AV, Martin JA, Buckwalter JA: Chondrocyte senescence and telomere regulation: Implications in cartilage aging and cancer (a brief review). *Iowa Orthop J* 2002;22:1-7.

27. Loeser RF: Aging and osteoarthritis: The role of chondrocyte senescence and aging changes in the cartilage matrix. *Osteoarthritis Cartilage* 2009;17(8):971-979.

28. Chen MH, Broom N: On the ultrastructure of softened cartilage: A possible model for structural transformation. *J Anat* 1998;192(Pt 3):329-341.

29. Eyre DR, Weis MA, Wu JJ: Articular cartilage collagen: An irreplaceable framework? *Eur Cell Mater* 2006;12:57-63.

30. Parsons P, Gilbert SJ, Vaughan-Thomas A, et al: Type IX collagen interacts with fibronectin providing an important molecular bridge in articular cartilage. *J Biol Chem* 2011; 286(40):34986-34997.

31. Aigner T, Bertling W, Stöss H, Weseloh G, von der Mark K: Independent expression of fibril-forming collagens I, II, and III in chondrocytes of human osteoarthritic cartilage. *J Clin Invest* 1993;91(3):829-837.

32. Wu JJ, Weis MA, Kim LS, Eyre DR: Type III collagen, a fibril network modifier in articular cartilage. *J Biol Chem* 2010; 285(24):18537-18544.

33. Pratta MA, Yao W, Decicco C, et al: Aggrecan protects cartilage collagen from proteolytic cleavage. *J Biol Chem* 2003; 278(46):45539-45545.

34. Klatt AR, Becker AK, Neacsu CD, Paulsson M, Wagener R: The matrilins: Modulators of extracellular matrix assembly. *Int J Biochem Cell Biol* 2011;43(3):320-330.

35. Iozzo RV, Schaefer L: Proteoglycans in health and disease: Novel regulatory signaling mechanisms evoked by the small leucine-rich proteoglycans. *FEBS J* 2010;277(19):3864-3875.

36. Hildebrand A, Romarís M, Rasmussen LM, et al: Interaction of the small interstitial proteoglycans biglycan, decorin and fibromodulin with transforming growth factor beta. *Biochem J* 1994;302(Pt 2):527-534.

37. Loeser RF, Goldring SR, Scanzello CR, Goldring MB: Osteoarthritis: A disease of the joint as an organ. *Arthritis Rheum* 2012;64(6):1697-1707.

38. Jay GD, Torres JR, Rhee DK, et al: Association between friction and wear in diarthrodial joints lacking lubricin. *Arthritis Rheum* 2007;56(11):3662-3669.

39. Flannery CR, Zollner R, Corcoran C, et al: Prevention of cartilage degeneration in a rat model of osteoarthritis by intraarticular treatment with recombinant lubricin. *Arthritis Rheum* 2009;60(3):840-847.

40. Grad S, Lee CR, Gorna K, Gogolewski S, Wimmer MA, Alini M: Surface motion upregulates superficial zone protein and hyaluronan production in chondrocyte-seeded three-dimensional scaffolds. *Tissue Eng* 2005;11(1-2):249-256.

41. Wimmer MA, Alini M, Grad S: The effect of sliding velocity on chondrocytes activity in 3D scaffolds. *J Biomech* 2009; 42(4):424-429.

42. Verzijl N, DeGroot J, Thorpe SR, et al: Effect of collagen turnover on the accumulation of advanced glycation end products. *J Biol Chem* 2000;275(50):39027-39031.

43. Maroudas A, Bayliss MT, Uchitel-Kaushansky N, Schneiderman R, Gilav E: Aggrecan turnover in human articular cartilage: Use of aspartic acid racemization as a marker of molecular age. *Arch Biochem Biophys* 1998;350(1):61-71.

44. Tortorella MD, Malfait AM: Will the real aggrecanase(s) step up: Evaluating the criteria that define aggrecanase activity in osteoarthritis. *Curr Pharm Biotechnol* 2008;9(1):16-23.

45. Little CB, Fosang AJ: Is cartilage matrix breakdown an appropriate therapeutic target in osteoarthritis? Insights from studies of aggrecan and collagen proteolysis. *Curr Drug Targets* 2010;11(5):561-575.

46. Tortorella MD, Malfait F, Barve RA, Shieh HS, Malfait AM: A review of the ADAMTS family, pharmaceutical targets of the future. *Curr Pharm Des* 2009;15(20):2359-2374.

47. Ding L, Guo D, Homandberg GA: The cartilage chondrolytic mechanism of fibronectin fragments involves MAP kinases: Comparison of three fragments and native fibronectin. *Osteoarthritis Cartilage* 2008;16(10):1253-1262.

48. Zack MD, Malfait AM, Skepner AP, et al: ADAM-8 isolated from human osteoarthritic chondrocytes cleaves fibronectin at Ala(271). *Arthritis Rheum* 2009;60(9):2704-2713.

49. Shane Anderson A, Loeser RF: Why is osteoarthritis an age-related disease? *Best Pract Res Clin Rheumatol* 2010;24(1): 15-26.

50. Horton WA, Hecht JT: Disorders of cartilage matrix proteins, in Royce P, Steinmann B, eds: *Connective Tissue and Its Heritable Disorders* ed 2. New York, NY, Wiley-Liss, 2002, pp 909-937.

51. Valdes AM, Spector TD: Genetic epidemiology of hip and knee osteoarthritis. *Nat Rev Rheumatol* 2011;7(1): 23-32.

52. Baker-LePain JC, Lane NE: Relationship between joint shape and the development of osteoarthritis. *Curr Opin Rheumatol* 2010;22(5):538-543.

53. Hodge WA, Fijan RS, Carlson KL, Burgess RG, Harris WH, Mann RW: Contact pressures in the human hip joint measured in vivo. *Proc Natl Acad Sci U S A* 1986;83(9):2879-2883.

54. Tackson SJ, Krebs DE, Harris BA: Acetabular pressures during hip arthritis exercises. *Arthritis Care Res* 1997;10(5):308-319.

55. Park S, Krishnan R, Nicoll SB, Ateshian GA: Cartilage interstitial fluid load support in unconfined compression. *J Biomech* 2003;36(12):1785-1796.

56. Jin ZM, Dowson D, Fisher J: Stress analysis of cushion form bearings for total hip replacements. *Proc Inst Mech Eng H* 1991;205(4):219-226.

57. Schinagl RM, Gurskis D, Chen AC, Sah RL: Depth-dependent confined compression modulus of full-thickness bovine articular cartilage. *J Orthop Res* 1997;15(4):499-506.

58. Mow VC, Kuei SC, Lai WM, Armstrong CG: Biphasic creep and stress relaxation of articular cartilage in compression: Theory and experiments. *J Biomech Eng* 1980;102(1):73-84.

59. Hayes WC, Bodine AJ: Flow-independent viscoelastic properties of articular cartilage matrix. *J Biomech* 1978;11(8-9):407-419.

60. Grodzinsky AJ, Lipshitz H, Glimcher MJ: Electromechanical properties of articular cartilage during compression and stress relaxation. *Nature* 1978;275(5679):448-450.

61. Gu WY, Lai WM, Mow VC: A mixture theory for charged-hydrated soft tissues containing multi-electrolytes: Passive transport and swelling behaviors. *J Biomech Eng* 1998;120(2):169-180.

62. Lai WM, Hou JS, Mow VC: A triphasic theory for the swelling and deformation behaviors of articular cartilage. *J Biomech Eng* 1991;113(3):245-258.

63. Huang CY, Mow VC, Ateshian GA: The role of flow-independent viscoelasticity in the biphasic tensile and compressive responses of articular cartilage. *J Biomech Eng* 2001;123(5):410-417.

64. McCutchen CW: The frictional properties of animal joints. *Wear* 1962;5:1-17.

65. Gleghorn JP, Bonassar LJ: Lubrication mode analysis of articular cartilage using Stribeck surfaces. *J Biomech* 2008;41(9):1910-1918.

66. Ateshian GA: The role of interstitial fluid pressurization in articular cartilage lubrication. *J Biomech* 2009;42(9):1163-1176.

67. Hills BA, Crawford RW: Normal and prosthetic synovial joints are lubricated by surface-active phospholipid: A hypothesis. *J Arthroplasty* 2003;18(4):499-505.

68. Rhee DK, Marcelino J, Baker M, et al: The secreted glycoprotein lubricin protects cartilage surfaces and inhibits synovial cell overgrowth. *J Clin Invest* 2005;115(3):622-631.

69. Chen M, Briscoe WH, Armes SP, Klein J: Lubrication at physiological pressures by polyzwitterionic brushes. *Science* 2009;323(5922):1698-1701.

2: Physiology of Musculoskeletal Tissues

Form and Function of the Knee Meniscus

Johannah Sanchez-Adams, PhD

Farshid Guilak, PhD

Anatomy

The menisci are wedge-shaped and semilunar tissues anchored within the medial and lateral sides of the knee joint by a network of ligaments (**Figures 1** and **2**). Although once thought to be a vestigial tissue, the meniscus is now known to play an integral role in increasing congruence between articulating bones, stabilizing joint movement, and distributing joint loads. Loss or injury of the meniscus leads to alterations in joint loading as well as local biochemical alterations that are strongly associated with joint degeneration and osteoarthritis (OA).

Due to the wedge-shaped cross-section of the menisci, they are well suited to stabilize the femoral condyle as it articulates against the tibial plateau by increasing congruence between the two surfaces. The size and shape of the meniscus varies slightly between individuals, but the general geometry is often conserved. The geometry of the medial and lateral menisci is measured anteroposteriorly (lengthwise) and mediolaterally (widthwise). Typical dimensions for the medial meniscus is 40.5 to 45.5 mm in length and 27 mm in width, whereas length and width dimensions of the lateral meniscus are typically 32.4 to 35.7 mm and 26.6 to 29.3 mm, respectively.[1] The circumferential length of the medial meniscus is approximately 90 to 110 mm, whereas the lateral meniscus is slightly shorter at 80 to 100 mm. These dimensions change with the age of the individual and closely match the growth of the femur and tibia. Significant sex differences exist in the size of the menisci, with male menisci being approximately 17% larger than female menisci.[2]

The specialized function of the meniscus is dependent on its complex mechanical properties and its attachments within the joint.[3] Specifically, as load is applied across the joint, the unique shape of the meniscus results in radial stresses that deform the tissue, thereby bearing some of the load. This radial displacement is opposed by posterior and anterior attachments on the tibial plateau, resulting in a hoop stress in the tissue. There are several ligamentous attachments that aid in stabilizing the meniscus within the knee joint during loading (**Figure 2**). In the posterior region, the ligaments of Humphry and Wrisberg connect the posterior horn of the lateral meniscus to a lateral insertion site on the medial femoral condyle and are located anteriorly and posteriorly, respectively, to the posterior cruciate ligament. Interestingly, studies on human cadaver knees have shown that although most joints (93%) present at least one of these ligaments, only an estimated 50% of knees have both.

Anteriorly, the medial and lateral menisci are joined together by the transverse ligament, and each meniscus is anchored to the tibial plateau via anterior and posterior meniscal horns. These horns connect the meniscus to the underlying bone, thereby maintaining its position within the joint. The insertion sites of the horns are highly innervated and can be classified into four different zones: ligamentous, uncalcified fibrocartilage, calcified fibrocartilage, and bone. Peripherally, the medial meniscus is connected to the medial collateral ligament and coronary ligaments also run along the periphery of each meniscus, providing additional attachment to the tibial plateau. This complex network of attachments forms an important part of the overall

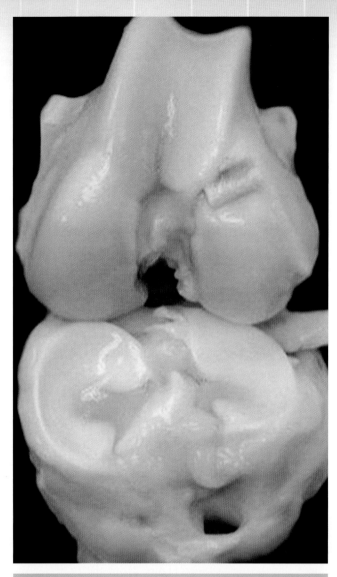

Figure 1 The native knee meniscus. Knee joint (bovine) showing the white, semicircular cartilages that make up the knee meniscus. The meniscus increases congruence between the femoral condyle and tibial plateau, and aids in normal joint function.

function of the meniscus, holding the tissue in place in some areas, and allowing its deformation elsewhere.

Regional Variations

During development, the meniscus shows dramatic changes in vascularity, size, and cellularity, which eventually lead to large regional variations in tissue composition and properties. When first formed in the body, both the medial and lateral menisci are completely vascular and have a high degree of cellularity. This widespread vascularity diminishes rapidly from gestation to birth and then more gradually to adulthood, when it is estimated that 10% to 25% of the lateral meniscus and 10% to 30% of the medial meniscus contain blood vessels.[4] The peripheral region of each meniscus

is innervated, with large nerve fibers running circumferentially along the tissue and smaller fibers positioned radially.

Because the adult meniscus contains blood vessels and nerves only peripherally in the tissue, it is generally classified radially by the presence of vascularity. The vascularized and innervated (red) region is located exclusively in the outer periphery, and the nonvascularized (white) region makes up the inner portion of the tissue (**Figure 3**). These two regions are joined by the transitional red-white region, which exhibits only limited vasculature and innervation. The repair capacity of these regions appears to be dependent on the presence of vasculature, giving the red region the most regenerative potential and the white region the least. The red and white regions also differ greatly in terms of structure, biochemical content, cell type, and mechanical properties.

Biochemical Content

Overall, the meniscus is composed of approximately 70% water. Of the solid phase, approximately 75% is collagen. Although collagen is present throughout the meniscus, different types are prevalent in different regions. The outer region of the meniscus contains 80% collagen by dry weight and is almost exclusively type I, with less than 1% of other collagen types.[5] In contrast, the inner region of the meniscus is 70% collagen by dry weight. Of this collagen, approximately 60% is type II and 40% is type I.[5] Therefore, the outer portion of the meniscus is found to be more fibrous, and the inner portion of the meniscus, containing collagen type II, displays hyaline cartilage-like properties. Other collagens present in the meniscus include types III, IV, V, VI, and XVIII, but to a much smaller degree than types I and II.[6]

As the largest fraction of the extracellular matrix, collagen has an important role in the overall function of the meniscus. The fibrillar collagens (primarily types I and II) are highly organized in the meniscus and contribute significantly to the mechanical properties of the tissue. The alignment of collagen fibers in the meniscus varies with depth in the tissue, imparting both tensile stiffness and resistance to splitting.[7] In particular, collagen organization can be considered in three layers: superficial, lamellar, and deep, which describe the tissue from surface to core. As illustrated in **Figure 4**, collagen fibers are amorphous in the superior superficial layer, but can be radially oriented in the inferior superficial layer, closest to the tibial plateau.[8] Amorphous collagen organization persists through the lamellar layer, but is distinguished from the superficial layer in that it contains short, radially oriented fibers only at the posterior and anterior horns.[9] In the deep layer, collagen is predominantly oriented circumferentially, with a few radially oriented fibers.[8,10,11] This predominantly circumferential collagen alignment allows for the meniscus to withstand the high hoop stresses that are generated by axial loading of the tissue.

Although most fibers in the meniscus are collagens, elastin has also been found in the matrix, although it comprises

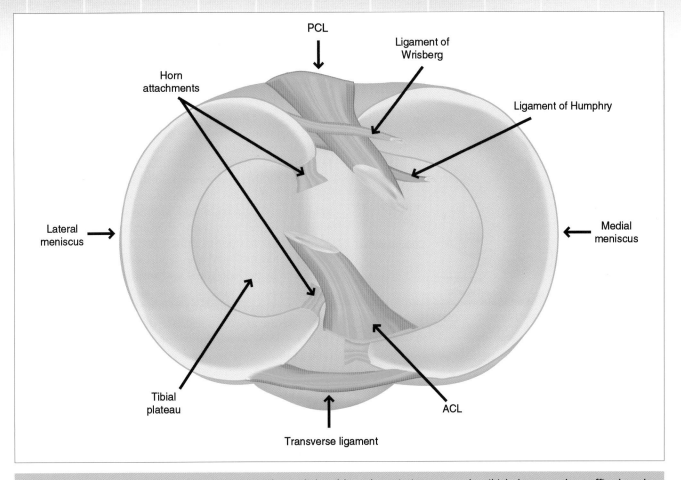

Figure 2 Meniscal attachments (superior view). The medial and lateral menisci rest atop the tibial plateau and are affixed to the tibia via horn attachments and to each other via the transverse ligament. Other ligaments in the joint space help to restrict movement, such as the anterior and posterior cruciate ligaments (ACL and PCL) and ligaments of Wrisberg and Humphry.

only about 1% or less of the dry weight. The presence of elastin is thought to provide resiliency to the tissue, as elastin is known for being able to recover its original shape after large strains. It has also been proposed that elastin interacts directly with the collagen network during loading to impart elasticity to the matrix.[12]

The remaining 25% of the solid content of the human meniscus is primarily composed of proteoglycans (approximately 15%) and cells (approximately 2%), and this breakdown can vary regionally.[6,13] Proteoglycans consist of a core protein that is decorated with glycosaminoglycans (GAGs), and are commonly classified based on the GAGs present. Of the GAGs that are found in the meniscus, 40% are chondroitin-6-sulfate, 10% to 20% are chondroitin-4-sulfate, 20% to 30% are dermatan sulfate, and 15% are keratan sulfate.[13] GAGs are negatively charged and therefore play a central role in attracting water into the tissue, imparting both hydration and compressive stiffness.[14] Cells from the inner two-thirds of the meniscus produce more proteoglycans than the outer third.[15] Biglycan, which is theorized to protect cells during loading, is at its highest concentration in the inner third of the meniscus.[15] In addition, deco-

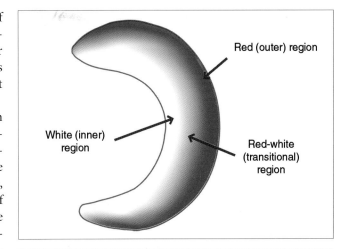

Figure 3 Regional variation in the meniscus. Vascularity defines regions radially in the meniscus. Closest to the synovial membrane is the red (outer) region, which is highly vascularized. Moving toward the center of the joint space, blood vessels become more sparse in the red-white (transitional) region, and are absent in the white (inner) region.

2: Physiology of Musculoskeletal Tissues

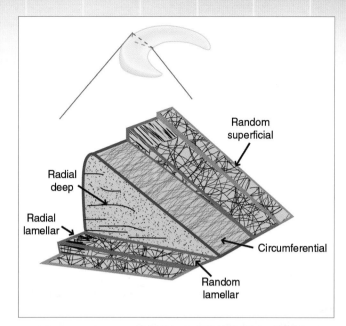

Figure 4 Collagen organization. From core to surface, collagen arrangement changes from structured to unstructured. Collagen orientations in the meniscus are of three main types: circumferential, radial, and random. Circumferential fibers are the most abundant in the tissue and are found in the deep zone. Radial fibers are dispersed throughout the deep zone and are present on the periphery and at the horns of the meniscus in the lamellar zone. Despite the presence of radial fibers, random fiber orientation dominates the lamellar zone. In the superficial zone, fiber orientation is typically random in the superior region and more radially oriented in the inferior region.

rin, which aids in collagen fibril organization, is found primarily in the outer third of the tissue, where collagen organization is most pronounced.[15] Due to its wedge shape, compressive loading in the meniscus is mostly borne by the inner region, whereas the outer region experiences mainly tensile loads.[16] The spatial organization of proteoglycans within the meniscus may therefore allow the tissue and the cells within it to withstand compressive loading and may also help organize collagen fibrils to bear tensile loads.

In addition to proteoglycans, collagen, and cells, the meniscus also contains a small amount of adhesion glycoproteins that comprise less than 1% of the organic matter. Adhesion glycoproteins are a specialized class of molecules that aid in binding matrix molecules to one another and to cells. Within the meniscus, type VI collagen, fibronectin, and thrombospondin have been identified.[11] All of these molecules contain the arginine-glycine–aspartic acid amino acid sequence that aids in cell attachment and also allows for cellular and extracellular matrix connections.

Cells of the Meniscus

Development of the meniscus begins with the condensation of a vast number of cells that are largely indistinguishable from one another. After the tissue has matured, however, the cells in the different meniscal layers become morphologically distinct. In the superficial layers of the meniscus, cells appear oval and fusiform, similar to fibroblasts.[17,18] In the deeper zones, however, cells are found to be more rounded and similar to articular chondrocyte morphology.[17] These variations have made the classification of meniscal cells difficult. As a result, researchers have used various terms to describe them including fibroblasts, fibrocytes, chondrocytes, fibrochondrocytes, and meniscal cells.[17,19]

Since the first morphologic distinctions were observed, meniscal cells have been further characterized by their unique gene expression and protein synthetic profiles. In particular, it has been found that inner meniscal cells stain positively for α-smooth muscle actin, which imparts contractile behavior,[20] and also tend to produce more proteoglycans than the polygonal and fusiform cells of the outer region.[21] Inner region cells can also be characterized by higher gene expression and production of collagen type II and aggrecan, as well as negative staining for the cell surface marker CD34, which functions in cell-to-cell adhesion.[22] Cells in this region also have high gene expression for nitric oxide synthase, which is implemented in nitric oxide production and has been shown to regulate meniscal cell biosynthesis.[23,24] The cells in the outer zone are distinct from inner zone cells because they contain gap junctions, produce predominantly collagen type I, and also produce proteases matrix metalloproteinase (MMP) 2 and MMP3, which can aid in cell migration and matrix remodeling.[17,23] Thus, the characteristics of inner and outer meniscal cells differ in multiple aspects aside from basic morphology.

Meniscal cells mainly produce the collagens and GAGs described in the various regions of the tissue. Although the different meniscal cells produce different types of collagen, total collagen production does not vary among the regions of the meniscus. In addition to types I and II, the cells of the meniscus also produce collagen types III, IV, V, and VI.[21] The GAGs produced by meniscal cells are predominantly chondroitin sulfate and, to a lesser degree, keratan sulfate.[25] Cells of the meniscus are responsive to a variety of growth factors and cytokines that regulate their anabolic and catabolic activities.[25-27]

In addition to fibrochondrocytes, the meniscus also contains endothelial cells, which are needed for maintaining the microvasculature of the outer meniscus.[28] These cells are distinct from fibrochondrocytes because they are found only in the lumen of meniscal vasculature in the outer zone.

Functional Aspects of the Meniscus

Under normal loading conditions the femur compresses the meniscus, creating radial displacement in the tissue that is opposed by anterior and posterior anchors. This displacement is translated into hoop stresses, radial tension, shear, and compression, which are borne by a network of collagen fibers (**Figure 5**) and proteoglycans. In the superficial and lamellar layers, amorphous and radial collagen fibers act to resist mediolateral splitting of the meniscus, and in the deep zone circumferentially oriented fibers work in tension as a result of hoop stresses.[29] Shear forces generated by the joint loading are opposed by matrix molecule interactions, and negatively charged proteoglycans in the meniscus impart compressive properties by resisting fluid loss.[6]

During normal activities such as walking or ascending stairs, the knee joint experiences loads of up to five times body weight.[30] Overall, it is estimated that the knee meniscus bears anywhere from 45% to 75% of this total joint load, varying with degree of joint flexion, animal model, and health of the tissue.[31] As the knee flexes, the contact area between the bones in the joint decreases by 4% for every 30°, accounting for some of the variability in load-bearing capacity of the meniscus.[32] It has been shown that at full extension, the lateral meniscus bears the majority of the load on the lateral side, whereas the medial meniscus bears approximately 50% of the medial load.[33] The meniscus not only acts to increase congruence in the joint, it also acts as a spacer to create approximately 1 mm of space between most of the articulating femoral and tibial surfaces and allowing only about 10% of these surfaces to contact.[33] In the absence of a functional meniscus, support of the femoral condyles is dramatically reduced and the joint force is concentrated, increasing the stress on the articular cartilage two to three times higher than normal.[34] These observations suggest that the load-bearing capacity of the normal meniscus plays an important role in protecting the hyaline cartilage surfaces of the femur and tibia. Both geometry and anatomic anchors play an important role in the stabilizing, load-bearing, and protective functions of the meniscus.

Mechanical Behavior of the Meniscus

Biomechanically, the meniscus displays highly complex properties that are inhomogeneous (depend on location), anisotropic (depend on direction), nonlinear (stress-strain properties are not linear), and viscoelastic (dependent on rate or time). The viscoelastic behavior of the meniscus is primarily attributed to the biphasic (solid/fluid) properties of the tissue. The first phase of the tissue consists of the porous and permeable collagen and proteoglycan solid matrix, whereas the second phase is made up of water and salts that are present throughout the matrix.[35,36] It is the interaction between the solid and fluid phases that is primarily responsible for the viscoelastic properties to the meniscus[37] (**Figure 6**). Compression of the tissue leads to pressurization of the interstitial fluid, and frictional drag is produced by fluid being forced through the tissue during loading, producing creep and stress-relaxation responses.[35] When subjected to a step load, the meniscus first displays elastic-like properties immediately after loading (**Figure 7**). This initial behavior is controlled by the hydrostatic pressure developed in the interstitial fluid portion of the tissue. After this initial response, the tissue continues to deform under the constant stress, but at a slower rate. As the fluid phase is expelled from the matrix, over time the solid matrix is responsible

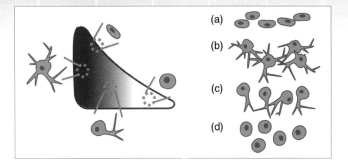

Figure 5 Cell types of the meniscus. Superficial zone cells are flattened (a), red zone cells display many cell processes (b), red-white zone cells display some cell processes (c), and white zone cells are rounded and chondrocyte-like (d).

for resisting more of the load. This deformational behavior under a constant step load is called the creep response of the tissue.[36]

A similar behavior can be observed when a step strain or displacement is placed on meniscal tissue, resulting in a stress-relaxation response.[36] Initially, the solid matrix responds elastically by creating a reaction force that is linearly related to the applied displacement. Over time, this reaction force diminishes in an exponential manner as the fluid is expelled from the matrix and the load is shared by both fluid and solid components. Eventually, the fluid flow reaches equilibrium and only the solid matrix supports the applied load.

Following load removal within the joint, the fluid that was expelled during loading is reimbibed by the tissue, initiated by the negatively charged proteoglycans in the matrix that provide for a gradient in osmotic pressure between the tissue and the surrounding synovial fluid. This results in the tissue's recovery behavior and also functions to transport nutrients throughout the tissue and surrounding hyaline cartilage, remove waste, and aid in lubrication.[38] Thus, the mechanical behavior of the meniscus is not only vital to ensure proper load distribution, but also contributes to the overall health and lubrication of the joint.

Biomechanical Evaluation of Meniscal Properties

Several different biomechanical tests have been used to quantify the properties of meniscal tissue under tension, compression, and shear. The tests are generally performed on geometrically defined specimens to allow normalization to the sample size, allowing determination of the material properties of the tissue rather than the overall structural properties of the meniscus. Due to the variation in collagen alignment and the asymmetrical shape of the meniscus, a complete evaluation of the mechanical properties of the meniscus has involved specimens that vary spatially within the tissue and are oriented along, and perpendicular to, the direction of collagen alignment. The most common

2: Physiology of Musculoskeletal Tissues

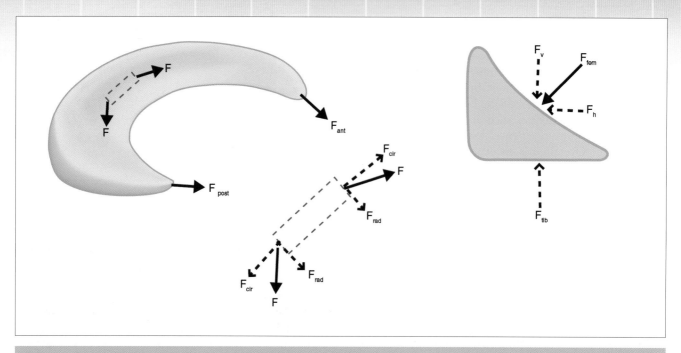

Figure 6 Forces acting on the meniscus during loading. As the femur presses down on the meniscus during normal loading, the meniscus deforms radially but is anchored by its anterior and posterior horns (F_{ant} and F_{post}). During loading, tensile, compressive, and shear forces are generated. A tensile hoop stress (F_{cir}) results from radial deformation, while vertical (F_v) and horizontal (F_h) forces result from the femur pressing on the curved superior surface of the tissue. A radial reaction force (F_{rad}) balances the femoral horizontal force (F_h).

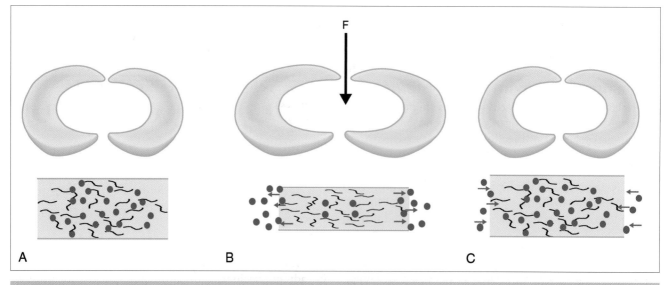

Figure 7 Biphasic behavior of the meniscus. **A**, GAGs (black lines) and water (blue dots) coexist in the matrix. **B**, As the meniscus is loaded (F), water is forced from the matrix. **C**, When the load is released, the negatively charged GAGs attract water back into the matrix, rehydrating the tissue.

methods used to characterize the mechanical properties of meniscal tissue are tensile and compressive tests. It is important to note that as the availability of human tissue is limited, some mechanical characterization data are only offered for animals such as the cow, pig, or sheep.

Tensile Properties

The tensile properties of meniscal tissue vary with orientation and tissue depth. Considering specimens from the anterior, central, and posterior meniscus, the circumferential Young's modulus varies spatially, and the lateral meniscus has a higher average tensile circumferential modulus (vary-

Chapter 11: Form and Function of the Knee Meniscus

ing from approximately 159 to 294 MPa) than the medial meniscus (93 to 159 MPa).[38] In the radial direction, the modulus of the bovine meniscus is highest closest to the posterior region of the meniscus, and decreases moving toward the anterior horn.[9] There is evidence that the tie fibers in the posterior region of the bovine meniscus are closely packed and form sheets, which may explain the higher modulus found there.[9] Tensile properties of the meniscus also change from being isotropic on its surface to anisotropic in deeper layers due to the variation in collagen fiber alignment. Compared with the deep zone, the radial stiffness of meniscal tissue is about sixfold higher in the superficial zone (approximately 71 MPa) where isotropic collagen alignment dominates.[39] Additionally, in the deeper zones the tensile modulus in the circumferential direction can be threefold to tenfold higher than in the radial direction, because of the abundance of circumferentially oriented collagen fibers relative to radially oriented ones.[9,38]

Compressive Properties

Methods for compressive testing of meniscal tissue include confined or unconfined compression and creep indentation.[39-42] Both bulk compressive testing and creep indentation can yield the aggregate modulus and permeability. Creep indentation provides a more local measurement but allows for the additional calculation of the Poisson ratio, and thus, the shear modulus of the tissue. This type of testing has shown that different regions in the meniscus have varying compressive properties, as a result of their biochemical makeup and extracellular matrix organization. Using the creep indentation apparatus, the aggregate modulus of the human meniscus has been found to be greatest in the anterior region (approximately 150 kPa), as compared with the central and posterior regions (approximately 100 kPa).[42] Also notable is that the permeability and shear modulus measured within the meniscus are relatively constant among all regions.[42] Using a different compression test, unconfined compression at 20% strain, the meniscus also displays anisotropic behavior with the highest compressive Young modulus (in the axial direction) being twice as high as in the circumferential and radial directions.[41] This higher axial compressive stiffness is likely related to the collagen organization, which is highly anisotropic. The compressive properties of the meniscus allow for resistance to axial loading, and because of the geometry of the tissue, this load is also translated into circumferential, radial, and shear stresses.

Shear Properties

For testing the meniscus in shear, dynamic oscillatory or constant shear strain is applied to the specimen, yielding the dynamic shear modulus as well as the transient shear modulus relaxation function.[37] It has been shown that the dynamic shear modulus of the meniscus is frequency dependent and anisotropic. The frequency dependence indicates the viscoelastic nature of the tissue that is independent of fluid flow, whereas the anisotropy of the modulus suggests that collagen organization and interactions between collagen and proteoglycans are central to shear resistance.[37] The normal human meniscus has a shear modulus on the order of 120 kPa at 1.5 Hz and 10% strain.[38] As with compressive properties, the meniscus shows anisotropy in shear properties, but this anisotropy can only be detected at low compressive tissue strains (less than 10%). Specifically, the shear modulus calculated for a sample under dynamic shearing in the circumferential direction is 20% to 36% higher than in the radial direction.[37]

Pathology

Normal geometric, biochemical, and biomechanical characteristics of the meniscus are all essential to stress distribution in the knee as well as overall joint function.[43] Importantly, there is overwhelming clinical evidence that the menisci are critical to the function of the knee joint, as patients without healthy menisci will develop signs of OA such as articular cartilage fibrillation and erosion, bone remodeling, and joint-space narrowing.[44,45] Furthermore, animal models of meniscal injury or meniscectomy consistently exhibit degenerative changes in joint tissues such as articular cartilage, subchondral bone, and synovium that are consistent with posttraumatic arthritis.[46-48] These changes are believed to be due to a combination of biomechanical and biochemical changes in the joint environment following injury.

Unfortunately, various deviations from these normal characteristics occur as a result of abnormal development, disease, degeneration, or traumatic injury. Regardless of their cause, meniscal pathologies are often painful and debilitating, and can significantly reduce a patient's quality of life. Developmental abnormalities of the meniscus often affect the geometry of the tissue. A discoid meniscus is one form of developmental abnormality in which the inner portion of the meniscus extends and the tissue is disk-like in shape. This most commonly affects the lateral meniscus and can be complete, in which the meniscus covers almost the entire articulating surface, or incomplete, covering more surface area than normal. The incidence of the discoid abnormality is unclear, but population estimates range from 0.4% to 5%.[49] Although many cases are thought to be asymptomatic and therefore undiagnosed, some discoid menisci can cause knee locking and pain.[49]

The meniscus may also be affected by metabolic diseases, including calcium pyrophosphate crystal deposition, hemochromatosis, and ochronosis. Diseases such as these can cause calcification, gross discoloration, and interference with the overall consistency of the tissue.[50] These symptoms heavily compromise the functionality of the meniscus, but cannot be treated locally as they stem from systemic changes in the body.

Meniscal tissue is also prone to degenerative changes and although little is known about the causes of meniscal degeneration, with degeneration the meniscus becomes more prone to injury.[51] In particular, OA can cause widespread degenerative changes in the meniscus as well as the

2: Physiology of Musculoskeletal Tissues

© 2013 American Academy of Orthopaedic Surgeons

205

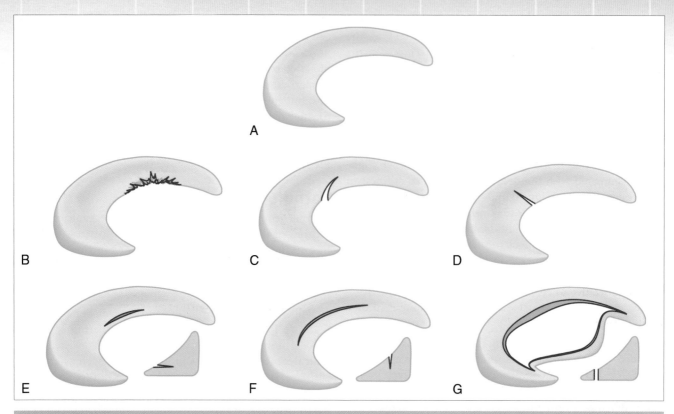

Figure 8 Classes of meniscal tears. The normal meniscus (**A**) is smooth, wedge-shaped, and semicircular. Complex (degenerative) tears (**B**) result in a jagged edge and combine many different types of tears. Oblique tears (**C**) and radial tears (**D**) typically propagate from the inner portion of the meniscus to its periphery. Horizontal tears (**E**) split the tissue into superior and inferior parts and also typically propagate outward. Vertical longitudinal tears (**F** and **G**) split the meniscus along the direction of collagen orientation. When a vertical longitudinal tear passes through the tissue's thickness it becomes a bucket-handle tear (**G**).

surrounding hyaline cartilage, and has been implicated in promoting meniscal injury. Although in the early 1980s meniscal pathology was found to be only weakly correlated with OA, researchers have more recently identified meniscal injury in approximately 75% of patients with symptomatic OA.[52]

OA affects meniscal geometry and biochemistry, compromising the tissue's functionality. Geometric changes include thickening of the medial posterior and lateral anterior horns, which may affect the biomechanics of the meniscus and make it more prone to injury.[53] OA changes in the biochemical makeup of the meniscus may also play a role in promoting injury, as induced OA in dogs causes an increase in meniscal water content as well as changes in GAG content and type over time.[54] OA may also be associated with calcification of the meniscus, but causality has yet to be confirmed.[55] Additionally, it has also been shown that severe OA causes medial joint-space narrowing as the medial meniscus displaces radially, which acts to preserve the tissue at the horns slightly, but the load-bearing function of the tissue is lost and widespread meniscal degeneration is apparent.[56] Therefore, OA degeneration can be an important contributor to meniscal injuries.

Meniscal Injury

Traumatic injuries resulting in meniscal tears also compromise the overall structural integrity of the joint, as well as cause symptoms such as locking and catching of the knee, a sensation of giving way, and joint pain.[57] According to one study surveying 1,000 patients, meniscal tears occurred more often in the right knee (56.5%).[58] Overall, meniscal tears affect men more often than women, with 70% to 80% of meniscal tears occurring in men.[57] Afflicted men are most often 21 to 30 years of age, whereas this pathology affects women most often between the ages of 11 and 20 years.[57] Traumatic injuries also dominate in younger patients, whereas older patients are more prone to degenerative changes.

Various types of meniscal tears can occur as a result of degeneration and/or trauma. There are four main types of meniscal tears: vertical longitudinal, oblique, radial, and horizontal[57,59] (**Figure 8**). Additionally, there are degenerative (complex) tears that describe an overall fraying of the inner meniscal edge consisting of many different types of tears. The vertical longitudinal tear occurs when the meniscus is split along a circumferential line. These tears can either span the entire thickness of the meniscus vertically (called a bucket-handle tear), or only a portion of it.[57]

When a bucket-handle tear occurs, the inner portion of the meniscus is free to intrude into the joint space, causing mechanical opposition to joint movement. The length of vertical longitudinal tears ranges from less than 1 mm to almost the entire circumference of the tissue.[57] Oblique tears are also vertical in nature but extend inward from the inner meniscus in a slanted fashion.[57] These tears are often referred to as parrot beak or flap tears. The free end of this type of tear can catch within the joint, inhibiting joint movement. Radial tears are similar to oblique tears but propagate radially, cleaving the circumferential collagen fibers.[57] These tears often exist without any symptoms as their free ends are not as prone to catching within the joint space as other tear geometries. However, radial tears can be especially damaging to the overall function of the tissue if left to propagate. Horizontal tears cut the meniscus into superior and inferior parts. They begin in the inner portion of the meniscus and extend outward, and are often associated with the formation of fluid-filled cysts.[57] Horizontal tears are thought to be a result of shear forces within the joint and are more common in older patients.[57]

Common tears in the medial meniscus differ from those in the lateral meniscus. Of medial meniscal lesions, most (75%) are found to be vertical longitudinal tears and 23% are horizontal tears.[58] In the lateral meniscus the tears are more diverse, with 54% being vertical longitudinal tears and the rest divided among oblique and complex pathologies.[58]

The intact meniscus is also heavily reliant on the ligamentous attachments of the knee. Joint laxity (instability of the joint) as a result of a ruptured anterior cruciate ligament (ACL) can have a profound effect on the meniscus as it has been estimated that the ACL contributes 85% to the restraint of anterior displacement of the tibia.[60,61] Clinically, meniscal tears are common in patients with torn ACLs, highlighting the codependence of the meniscus with surrounding ligaments for normal joint function.[57,62,63] Nonlinear finite element modeling of knee joints confirms this clinical finding, showing that without the ACL, the medial meniscus is subjected to higher loads from 0° to 30° flexion.[64] Although the biomechanics of the knee are altered by an ACL tear, the types of tears that the meniscus endures are indistinguishable from those of an ACL-intact knee. This evidence suggests that meniscal tears are more frequent when knee stability is compromised, and that meniscal tears follow certain patterns regardless of ligament health.

Healing and Repair

In general, the adult meniscus shows little capacity for self-repair. Although lesions or tears that occur in the outer periphery of the tissue can regenerate in certain cases due to the high degree of vasculature there, damage to the inner nonvascularized portion of the tissue is usually unable to heal.[6,57,65,66] Following injury in the vascular portion of the meniscus, the defect site is filled with a fibrin clot that uses proinflammatory factors to recruit blood vessels from the surrounding areas.[66] After this initial response, and depending on proximity to abundant blood vessels, fibrous scar tissue can take as little as 10 weeks to form.[66,67] After a few months, the scar tissue will then mature into tissue with inferior mechanical properties to the native meniscus.[66] This timeline is extended with distance from the peripheral blood supply, and does not occur for injuries in the inner meniscus. For inner meniscal injuries, some reorganization of the matrix may take place due to the changed mechanical environment, but a healing response is absent.[66,68] Some research has focused on creating vascular access channels from the outer to the inner meniscus to allow healing factors from the blood to reach the damaged white zone, which has helped heal longitudinal tears in the avascular region of dogs and goats and has reduced symptoms in patients.[69,70] As a result, proximity to blood vessels is the best predictor of a meniscal healing response, but the minimal extent of healing that takes place generally does not restore tissue functionality.

Although the outer portion of the meniscus may heal to some degree, the new repair tissue is quite different from native tissue. Repair tissue in the outer portion of the meniscus is distinct from normal meniscal tissue in that it may contain calcified regions, cysts, unattached collagen fragments, and pools of proteoglycans.[10] This is in stark contrast to normal tissue in which the collagen matrix is highly aligned with proteoglycans throughout and no calcification or void spaces. In torn menisci it is twice as common for the tissue to become calcified over time, and this is often found in conjunction with OA.[71]

Functionally, meniscal repair tissue is weaker than normal tissue. Repair tissue in rabbits has been measured to require approximately 75% less energy (0.8 to 0.9 mJ) to fail than normal tissue at 12 weeks postinjury.[72] The strength of this tissue increases only marginally with the use of sutures or fibrin glue to hold the torn edges together, and does not reach normal values.[72] Therefore, even in the region of the meniscus that undergoes some repair, the tissue is either lacking in quantity or insufficient in strength and there is an inhibitory environment for new tissue formation. This evidence points to the need for tissue engineering or other technologies to heal or replace a damaged meniscus and prevent calcification or other unwanted changes from taking place.

Future of Meniscal Repair

Treating meniscal injuries has long been a challenge for clinicians due to the mechanically demanding environment of the tissue and its limited intrinsic healing capacity. Currently, a variety of arthroscopic techniques such as suturing or abrasion are used to reduce pain and increase functionality of a compromised meniscus. Unfortunately, these techniques are not always effective and may not protect against further degenerative changes in the joint due to altered meniscal function. However, there are several emerging technologies that may provide better alternatives for restoring the tissue's unique role in the knee joint. These technologies

2: Physiology of Musculoskeletal Tissues

can be roughly categorized as biologic and nonbiologic, and have the potential to provide significant advances to the current standard of care.

In vitro studies on meniscal repair have allowed for a more complete understanding of the factors influencing successful meniscal regeneration. Recent evidence suggests that the reparative response of the meniscus is inhibited by inflammatory mediators, including interleukin-1 (IL-1) and tumor necrosis factor α (TNF-α). IL-1 and TNF-α are both upregulated following joint injury and have significant catabolic and antianabolic effects on meniscus tissue, including increased proteoglycan release, inhibition of collagen synthesis, and upregulation of MMPs.[73,74] However, anabolic factors such as transforming growth factor β1 (TGF-β1), inhibitors of IL-1 and TNF-α, and dynamic loading of the tissue have been shown to limit these effects. These observations indicate that certain biologic factors may enhance the integrative repair of the meniscal following injury, and that some loading of the meniscal following injury may also be beneficial.[75,76] Although these biologic factors hold significant promise for enhanced meniscal repair, further investigation is needed to determine their safety and efficacy in vivo.

In addition to investigating factors influencing the intrinsic healing capacity of the meniscal, researchers are developing tissue-engineered alternatives for meniscal repair. These technologies are often directed toward the repair of large defects, and eventually aim to reconstruct the whole meniscal as a biologic replacement option. To achieve this, researchers typically follow the tissue-engineering paradigm in which cells are self-assembled or seeded onto a scaffold, and biochemical and/or biomechanical factors are used to stimulate tissue formation. Currently, a variety of cell types are used, including meniscal cells, articular chondrocytes, embryonic stem cells, and adult stem cells. A wide range of scaffold materials are also used, such as hydrogels, synthetic polymers, and extracellular matrix components. Even without the use of a scaffold, researchers have been able to recreate meniscal-like properties. In particular, by using meniscal cells and articular chondrocytes in a scaffoldless approach and stimulating with TGF-β1, the wedge-shaped morphology of the meniscal and similar biochemical properties can be achieved.[77] However, although enhanced by growth factor application, the mechanical properties and spatial organization of matrix molecules still need to be improved. In contrast, scaffold-based approaches often meet or exceed the mechanical properties of native meniscal tissue before matrix deposition by seeded cells. Moreover, when scaffold-based approaches are combined with growth factors and mechanical stimulation, they can also produce constructs with biochemical properties similar to native tissue.[78,79] It is important to note, however, that degradation products produced by some of these scaffolds and the overall biocompatibility of these constructs need further investigation before their successful implementation. Despite some obstacles yet to be overcome, tissue-engineering technologies are approaching many of the native characteristics necessary for the successful repair of damaged meniscal tissue.

Aside from sutures and other fixation devices for meniscal repair, nonbiologic materials are currently being used to develop meniscal replacements instead of biologic alternatives. Although allografts have been used as replacements for the meniscal, they remain a scarce resource and are known to shrink following implantation. Additionally, whereas researchers are making significant advances toward a biologic meniscal replacement using tissue-engineering principles, current research is often limited to small animal models and the effects of scaling up these methods are uncertain. Therefore, nonbiologic replacements for the meniscal present a desirable option for more immediate clinical applications. Polycarbonate-urethane implants have recently been engineered to recapitulate the morphology and chondroprotective role of the meniscal within the knee joint. These implants have been designed with and without the need for attachment to the tibial plateau.[80,81] In vitro and in vivo findings have shown that polycarbonate-urethane implants may be able to restore normal joint movement and slow the progression of degenerative changes in the joint cartilages. These are encouraging outcomes, as one main debilitating aspect of meniscal degeneration is the progression of OA.

Summary

Advances in the understanding of meniscal structure have revealed the complexity of biochemical constituents, cell types, and matrix architecture that allow this tissue to function in load bearing and stabilization within the knee joint. Despite this wealth of knowledge, injuries to the meniscus are common and treatment options are insufficient to restore full tissue functionality. Careful characterization of normal meniscal structure and function, however, is essential to form a groundwork for studying and enhancing meniscal healing.

Whether it is supplying biologic factors to enhance or allow meniscal repair, implanting tissue-engineered constructs, or replacing a damaged meniscal with a nonbiologic substitute, current research on meniscal repair will likely result in improved clinical outcomes. Recent advances in the understanding of agonists and antagonists to meniscal repair and the role of meniscal biomechanics in the knee joint have aided these emerging technologies and will continue to inform the pursuit of treatment options. Although further refinement and investigation are necessary to determine the precise design characteristics for successful implementation of these repair options, the results of current research offers promise for the future.

References

1. McDermott ID, Sharifi F, Bull AM, Gupte CM, Thomas RW, Amis AA: An anatomical study of meniscal allograft sizing. *Knee Surg Sports Traumatol Arthrosc* 2004;12(2):130-135.

2. Elsner JJ, Portnoy S, Guilak F, Shterling A, Linder-Ganz E: MRI-based characterization of bone anatomy in the human knee for size matching of a medial meniscal implant. *J Biomech Eng* 2010;132(10):101008.

3. Hauch KN, Villegas DF, Haut Donahue TL: Geometry, time-dependent and failure properties of human meniscal attachments. *J Biomech* 2010;43(3):463-468.

4. Clark CR, Ogden JA: Development of the menisci of the human knee joint: Morphological changes and their potential role in childhood meniscal injury. *J Bone Joint Surg Am* 1983;65(4):538-547.

5. Cheung HS: Distribution of type I, II, III and V in the pepsin solubilized collagens in bovine menisci. *Connect Tissue Res* 1987;16(4):343-356.

6. Sweigart MA, Athanasiou KA: Toward tissue engineering of the knee meniscus. *Tissue Eng* 2001;7(2):111-129.

7. Gabrion A, Aimedieu P, Laya Z, et al: Relationship between ultrastructure and biomechanical properties of the knee meniscus. *Surg Radiol Anat* 2005;27(6):507-510.

8. Aspden RM, Yarker YE, Hukins DW: Collagen orientations in the meniscus of the knee joint. *J Anat* 1985;140(pt 3): 371-380.

9. Skaggs DL, Warden WH, Mow VC: Radial tie fibers influence the tensile properties of the bovine medial meniscus. *J Orthop Res* 1994;12(2):176-185.

10. Ghadially FN, Lalonde JM, Wedge JH: Ultrastructure of normal and torn menisci of the human knee joint. *J Anat* 1983;136(Pt 4):773-791.

11. McDevitt CA, Webber RJ: The ultrastructure and biochemistry of meniscal cartilage. *Clin Orthop Relat Res* 1990;252:8-18.

12. Höpker WW, Angres G, Klingel K, Komitowski D, Schuchardt E: Changes of the elastin compartment in the human meniscus. *Virchows Arch A Pathol Anat Histopathol* 1986;408(6):575-592.

13. Herwig J, Egner E, Buddecke E: Chemical changes of human knee joint menisci in various stages of degeneration. *Ann Rheum Dis* 1984;43(4):635-640.

14. Sanchez-Adams J, Willard VP, Athanasiou KA: Regional variation in the mechanical role of knee meniscus glycosaminoglycans. *J Appl Physiol* 2011;111(6):1590-1596.

15. Scott PG, Nakano T, Dodd CM: Isolation and characterization of small proteoglycans from different zones of the porcine knee meniscus. *Biochim Biophys Acta* 1997;1336(2):254-262.

16. Upton ML, Guilak F, Laursen TA, Setton LA: Finite element modeling predictions of region-specific cell-matrix mechanics in the meniscus. *Biomech Model Mechanobiol* 2006;5(2-3): 140-149.

17. Hellio Le Graverand MP, Ou Y, Schield-Yee T, et al: The cells of the rabbit meniscus: Their arrangement, interrelationship, morphological variations and cytoarchitecture. *J Anat* 2001;198(Pt 5):525-535.

18. Nakata K, Shino K, Hamada M, et al: Human meniscus cell: Characterization of the primary culture and use for tissue engineering. *Clin Orthop Relat Res* 2001;(391, suppl):S208-S218.

19. Ghadially FN, Thomas I, Yong N, Lalonde JM: Ultrastructure of rabbit semilunar cartilages. *J Anat* 1978;125(pt 3): 499-517.

20. Mueller SM, Schneider TO, Shortkroff S, Breinan HA, Spector M: α-Smooth muscle actin and contractile behavior of bovine meniscus cells seeded in type I and type II collagen-GAG matrices. *J Biomed Mater Res* 1999;45(3):157-166.

21. Tanaka T, Fujii K, Kumagae Y: Comparison of biochemical characteristics of cultured fibrochondrocytes isolated from the inner and outer regions of human meniscus. *Knee Surg Sports Traumatol Arthrosc* 1999;7(2):75-80.

22. Verdonk PC, Forsyth RG, Wang J, et al: Characterisation of human knee meniscus cell phenotype. *Osteoarthritis Cartilage* 2005;13(7):548-560.

23. Upton ML, Chen J, Setton LA: Region-specific constitutive gene expression in the adult porcine meniscus. *J Orthop Res* 2006;24(7):1562-1570.

24. Cao M, Stefanovic-Racic M, Georgescu HI, Miller LA, Evans CH: Generation of nitric oxide by lapine meniscal cells and its effect on matrix metabolism: Stimulation of collagen production by arginine. *J Orthop Res* 1998;16(1):104-111.

25. Gruber HE, Mauerhan D, Chow Y, et al: Three-dimensional culture of human meniscal cells: Extracellular matrix and proteoglycan production. *BMC Biotechnol* 2008;8:54.

26. Imler SM, Doshi AN, Levenston ME: Combined effects of growth factors and static mechanical compression on meniscus explant biosynthesis. *Osteoarthritis Cartilage* 2004; 12(9):736-744.

27. Shin SJ, Fermor B, Weinberg JB, Pisetsky DS, Guilak F: Regulation of matrix turnover in meniscal explants: Role of mechanical stress, interleukin-1, and nitric oxide. *J Appl Physiol* 2003;95(1):308-313.

28. Miller RR, Rydell PA: Primary culture of microvascular endothelial cells from canine meniscus. *J Orthop Res* 1993; 11(6):907-911.

29. Ghosh P, Taylor TK: The knee joint meniscus: A fibrocartilage of some distinction. *Clin Orthop Relat Res* 1987;224: 52-63.

30. Paul JP: Force actions transmitted by joints in the human body. *Proc R Soc Lond B Biol Sci* 1976;192(1107):163-172.

31. Shrive NG, O'Connor JJ, Goodfellow JW: Load-bearing in the knee joint. *Clin Orthop Relat Res* 1978;131:279-287.

32. Walker PS, Hajek JV: The load-bearing area in the knee joint. *J Biomech* 1972;5(6):581-589.

33. Walker PS, Erkman MJ: The role of the menisci in force transmission across the knee. *Clin Orthop Relat Res* 1975; 109:184-192.

34. Kurosawa H, Fukubayashi T, Nakajima H: Load-bearing mode of the knee joint: Physical behavior of the knee joint with or without menisci. *Clin Orthop Relat Res* 1980;149: 283-290.

35. Favenesi JA, Shaffer JC, Mow VC: Biphasic mechanical properties of knee meniscus. *Trans Orthop Res Soc* 1983;8:57.

36. McDermott ID, Masouros SD, Amis AA: Biomechanics of the menisci of the knee. *Curr Orthop* 2008;22(3):193-201.

37. Zhu W, Chern KY, Mow VC: Anisotropic viscoelastic shear properties of bovine meniscus. *Clin Orthop Relat Res* 1994; 306:34-45.

2: Physiology of Musculoskeletal Tissues

38. Fithian DC, Kelly MA, Mow VC: Material properties and structure-function relationships in the menisci. *Clin Orthop Relat Res* 1990;252:19-31.

39. Proctor CS, Schmidt MB, Whipple RR, Kelly MA, Mow VC: Material properties of the normal medial bovine meniscus. *J Orthop Res* 1989;7(6):771-782.

40. Joshi MD, Suh JK, Marui T, Woo SL: Interspecies variation of compressive biomechanical properties of the meniscus. *J Biomed Mater Res* 1995;29(7):823-828.

41. Leslie BW, Gardner DL, McGeough JA, Moran RS: Anisotropic response of the human knee joint meniscus to unconfined compression. *Proc Inst Mech Eng H* 2000;214(6):631-635.

42. Sweigart MA, Zhu CF, Burt DM, et al: Intraspecies and interspecies comparison of the compressive properties of the medial meniscus. *Ann Biomed Eng* 2004;32(11):1569-1579.

43. Bedi A, Kelly NH, Baad M, et al: Dynamic contact mechanics of the medial meniscus as a function of radial tear, repair, and partial meniscectomy. *J Bone Joint Surg Am* 2010; 92(6):1398-1408.

44. Fairbank TJ: Knee joint changes after meniscectomy. *J Bone Joint Surg Br* 1948;30(4):664-670.

45. Roos H, Laurén M, Adalberth T, Roos EM, Jonsson K, Lohmander LS: Knee osteoarthritis after meniscectomy: Prevalence of radiographic changes after twenty-one years, compared with matched controls. *Arthritis Rheum* 1998; 41(4):687-693.

46. Moskowitz RW, Davis W, Sammarco J, et al: Experimentally induced degenerative joint lesions following partial meniscectomy in the rabbit. *Arthritis Rheum* 1973;16(3):397-405.

47. LeRoux MA, Arokoski J, Vail TP, et al: Simultaneous changes in the mechanical properties, quantitative collagen organization, and proteoglycan concentration of articular cartilage following canine meniscectomy. *J Orthop Res* 2000; 18(3):383-392.

48. Glasson SS, Blanchet TJ, Morris EA: The surgical destabilization of the medial meniscus (DMM) model of osteoarthritis in the 129/SvEv mouse. *Osteoarthritis Cartilage* 2007; 15(9):1061-1069.

49. Washington ER III, Root L, Liener UC: Discoid lateral meniscus in children: Long-term follow-up after excision. *J Bone Joint Surg Am* 1995;77(9):1357-1361.

50. Bjelle A: Cartilage matrix in hereditary pyrophosphate arthropathy. *J Rheumatol* 1981;8(6):959-964.

51. DeHaven KE: Meniscectomy versus repair: Clinical experience, in Mow VC, Arnoczky SP, Jackson DW, eds: *Knee Meniscus: Basic and Clinical Foundations.* New York, NY, Raven Press, 1992, p 132.

52. Berthiaume MJ, Raynauld JP, Martel-Pelletier J, et al: Meniscal tear and extrusion are strongly associated with progression of symptomatic knee osteoarthritis as assessed by quantitative magnetic resonance imaging. *Ann Rheum Dis* 2005;64(4):556-563.

53. Bamac B, Ozdemir S, Sarisoy HT, Colak T, Ozbek A, Akansel G: Evaluation of medial and lateral meniscus thicknesses in early osteoarthritis of the knee with magnetic resonance imaging. *Saudi Med J* 2006;27(6):854-857.

54. Adams ME, Billingham ME, Muir H: The glycosaminoglycans in menisci in experimental and natural osteoarthritis. *Arthritis Rheum* 1983;26(1):69-76.

55. Hough AJ Jr, Webber RJ: Pathology of the meniscus. *Clin Orthop Relat Res* 1990;252:32-40.

56. Sugita T, Kawamata T, Ohnuma M, Yoshizumi Y, Sato K: Radial displacement of the medial meniscus in varus osteoarthritis of the knee. *Clin Orthop Relat Res* 2001;387:171-177.

57. Greis PE, Bardana DD, Holmstrom MC, Burks RT: Meniscal injury: I. Basic science and evaluation. *J Am Acad Orthop Surg* 2002;10(3):168-176.

58. Dandy DJ: The arthroscopic anatomy of symptomatic meniscal lesions. *J Bone Joint Surg Br* 1990;72(4):628-633.

59. Smillie IS: The current pattern of the pathology of meniscus tears. *Proc R Soc Med* 1968;61(1):44-45.

60. Noyes FR, Grood ES, Butler DL, Malek M: Clinical laxity tests and functional stability of the knee: Biomechanical concepts. *Clin Orthop Relat Res* 1980;146:84-89.

61. Roberts D, Andersson G, Fridén T: Knee joint proprioception in ACL-deficient knees is related to cartilage injury, laxity and age: A retrospective study of 54 patients. *Acta Orthop Scand* 2004;75(1):78-83.

62. Allen CR, Wong EK, Livesay GA, Sakane M, Fu FH, Woo SL: Importance of the medial meniscus in the anterior cruciate ligament-deficient knee. *J Orthop Res* 2000;18(1):109-115.

63. Belzer JP, Cannon WD Jr: Meniscus tears: Treatment in the stable and unstable knee. *J Am Acad Orthop Surg* 1993;1(1): 41-47.

64. Moglo KE, Shirazi-Adl A: Biomechanics of passive knee joint in drawer: Load transmission in intact and ACL-deficient joints. *Knee* 2003;10(3):265-276.

65. Brindle T, Nyland J, Johnson DL: The meniscus: Review of basic principles with application to surgery and rehabilitation. *J Athl Train* 2001;36(2):160-169.

66. Arnoczky SP: Gross and vascular anatomy of the meniscus and its role in meniscal healing, regeneration, and remodeling, in Mow VC, Arnoczky SP, Jackson DW, eds: *Knee Meniscus: Basic and Clinical Foundations.* New York, NY, Raven Press, 1992, pp 6-12.

67. Arnoczky SP, Warren RF: The microvasculature of the meniscus and its response to injury: An experimental study in the dog. *Am J Sports Med* 1983;11(3):131-141.

68. McAndrews PT, Arnoczky SP: Meniscal repair enhancement techniques. *Clin Sports Med* 1996;15(3):499-510.

69. Zhang Z, Arnold JA: Trephination and suturing of avascular meniscal tears: A clinical study of the trephination procedure. *Arthroscopy* 1996;12(6):726-731.

70. Zhang Z, Arnold JA, Williams T, McCann B: Repairs by trephination and suturing of longitudinal injuries in the avascular area of the meniscus in goats. *Am J Sports Med* 1995;23(1):35-41.

71. Noble J, Hamblen DL: The pathology of the degenerate meniscus lesion. *J Bone Joint Surg Br* 1975;57(2):180-186.

72. Roeddecker K, Muennich U, Nagelschmidt M: Meniscal healing: A biomechanical study. *J Surg Res* 1994;56(1):20-27.

73. LeGrand A, Fermor B, Fink C, et al: Interleukin-1, tumor necrosis factor alpha, and interleukin-17 synergistically up-regulate nitric oxide and prostaglandin E2 production in explants of human osteoarthritic knee menisci. *Arthritis Rheum* 2001;44(9):2078-2083.

74. Ferretti M, Madhavan S, Deschner J, Rath-Deschner B, Wy-pasek E, Agarwal S: Dynamic biophysical strain modulates proinflammatory gene induction in meniscal fibrochondro-cytes. *Am J Physiol Cell Physiol* 2006;290(6):C1610-C1615.

75. McNulty AL, Estes BT, Wilusz RE, Weinberg JB, Guilak F: Dynamic loading enhances integrative meniscal repair in the presence of interleukin-1. *Osteoarthritis Cartilage* 2010;18(6):830-838.

76. McNulty AL, Moutos FT, Weinberg JB, Guilak F: Enhanced integrative repair of the porcine meniscus in vitro by inhibition of interleukin-1 or tumor necrosis factor alpha. *Arthritis Rheum* 2007;56(9):3033-3042.

77. Huey DJ, Athanasiou KA: Maturational growth of self-assembled, functional menisci as a result of TGF-β1 and enzymatic chondroitinase-ABC stimulation. *Biomaterials* 2011;32(8):2052-2058.

78. Aufderheide AC, Athanasiou KA: Comparison of scaffolds and culture conditions for tissue engineering of the knee meniscus. *Tissue Eng* 2005;11(7-8):1095-1104.

79. Mueller SM, Shortkroff S, Schneider TO, Breinan HA, Yan-nas IV, Spector M: Meniscus cells seeded in type I and type II collagen-GAG matrices in vitro. *Biomaterials* 1999;20(8):701-709.

80. Elsner JJ, Portnoy S, Zur G, Guilak F, Shterling A, Linder-Ganz E: Design of a free-floating polycarbonate-urethane meniscal implant using finite element modeling and experimental validation. *J Biomech Eng* 2010;132(9):095001.

81. Zur G, Linder-Ganz E, Elsner JJ, et al: Chondroprotective effects of a polycarbonate-urethane meniscal implant: Histopathological results in a sheep model. *Knee Surg Sports Traumatol Arthrosc* 2011;19(2):255-263.

2: Physiology of Musculoskeletal Tissues

Chapter 12

Form and Function of Tendon and Ligament

Katherine E. Reuther, BS
Chancellor F. Gray, MD
Louis J. Soslowsky, PhD

Introduction

Tendons and ligaments are complex connective tissues and essential components of the musculoskeletal system, aiding in locomotion and assisting in both dynamic and static joint stabilization. Musculoskeletal injuries are estimated to cost approximately $250 billion annually, and with an aging and progressively more active population, this cost is likely to increase.[1] Because tendon and ligament disorders are especially common and are significant contributors to musculoskeletal injury, a clear understanding of their function in health, as well as their dysfunction in pathology and treatment mechanisms, is essential.

Tendon and ligament are frequently discussed together because of the many similarities they share and despite their significant differences. Both have elastic and viscoelastic properties that contribute to their ability to resist a variety of loading scenarios. These behaviors are a result of their complex composition and structural characteristics at each level of organization that lead to their response to joint function.

This chapter will provide an overview of the basic science concepts behind clinical conditions involving tendon and ligament, highlighting anatomic considerations; gross morphology, microanatomy, and biology; their biomechanical function in the body; relevant injuries; considerations in tendon and ligament repair; and current concepts in tissue engineering for tendon and ligament injuries.

Ms. Reuther or an immediate family member has stock or stock options held in Pfizer. Neither of the following authors or any immediate family member has received anything of value from or owns stock in a commercial company or institution related directly or indirectly to the subject of this chapter: Dr. Gray and Dr. Soslowsky.

Tendon

Classification and Anatomy

Tendons can be classified through multiple schema, according to anatomic considerations: specifically, shape (round or flat), anatomic location (intra-articular or extra-articular; intra-articular soft-tissue injuries have a lower likelihood of healing),[2] or the surrounding layer of connective tissue (paratenon or synovium, which acts to reduce friction and allows for tendon gliding).

Gross Morphology, Histology, Microanatomy, and Cell Biology

The connection of the tendon between muscle and its point of origin or insertion at the bone requires several complex anatomic and morphologic characteristics that are continued through the microscopic and molecular level. Primarily, this connection allows for the transfer of force from muscle to bone and enables highly specific motion by the musculoskeletal system. Not all muscles have a tendon; those that do primarily provide motion at a joint or need to provide force either over a distance or in a tightly confined space. Tendons provide a mechanical advantage for muscle by focusing or redirecting force, lengthening a lever arm, or acting around a pulley (such as in the flexor hallucis longus tendon).

The round or flat shape of the tendon is associated with specific functional consequences. Classic examples of round tendons include the flexor digitorum tendons of both the upper and lower extremities; flat tendons include the rotator cuff tendons and the Achilles tendon. Most round tendons behave similarly and are biomechanically subjected to a consistent environment. They are accustomed to high tensile loads and are capable of a high degree of motion, or gliding. The flat tendons are less easily categorized. They are generally subject to less glide, but are capable of bearing

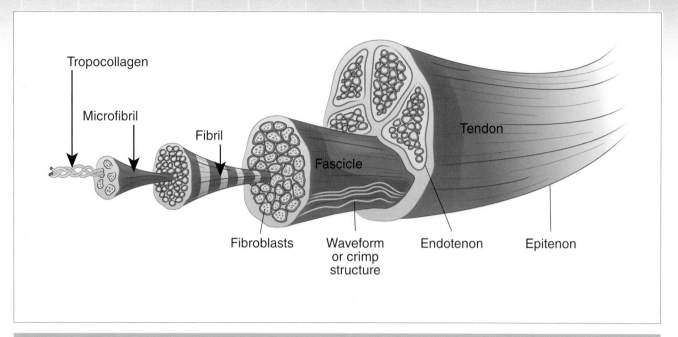

Figure I Tendon has a hierarchical structure, with collagen molecules assembled into progressively larger bundles, until the level of the tendon itself is reached. Note the endotenon (surrounding the fascicle) and epitenon (surrounding the tendon), containing the neurovasculature of the tendon.

high tensile loads (as in the quadriceps tendon) in addition to more complex loads such as compression and shear. Consequently, these different functions are represented in the structure of these tendons.

Further investigation of tendons reveals a complex composition with more functional implications. At the most basic level, tendon composition is organized consistently throughout the body, despite its often-differing superstructure. Like most connective tissue, the main functional components of tendon are water and collagen. Water is the primary constituent, comprising approximately 50% to 60% of tendon weight. Collagen makes up approximately 75% of the dry weight with 95% type I collagen and a small amount of type III and other collagens. Tendon is also composed of tendon cells, referred to as tenocytes, and proteoglycans. Proteoglycans are composed of a core protein covalently bound to one or more glycosaminoglycan (GAG) chains. GAGs are thought to play an important role in mechanics, specifically viscoelastic properties, through their association with water. The main proteoglycans in tendon are decorin and biglycan, members of the small leucine-rich proteoglycan family (SLRPs). These molecules have been shown to bind to collagen and mediate fibril assembly in tendon and other tissues.[3] Several investigators have suggested a role for these proteins in tendinopathy, although the specific mechanisms of this relation remain unclear.

At the molecular level, tendons are arranged in a hierarchy starting with the triple helix of collagen, then microfibrils, fibrils, fascicles, and ultimately the tendon itself (**Figure 1**). The mediated assembly and cross-linking of collagen into these microfibrils is critical for the mechanical strength

of the tissue. This process is largely dependent on the family of extracellular SLRPs, which can dictate the overall thickness and quality of fibril assembly.[4] Another important element of collagen assembly and structure is crimp. Crimp is evident ultrastructurally, and appears as "crimped" lines in the tendon when viewed at the microscopic level. This crimping results from the specific orientation of the microfibrils in the tendon and contributes important mechanical properties that are discussed later in this chapter.

The superstructure of tendons is the progressive organization of fibrils into larger fascicles that group to yield a functional tendon, as well as supporting connective tissue that preserves local anatomic and physiologic relationships. These groups of fascicles are separated and bound together by a thin connective tissue layer known as the endotenon. Contiguous with the endotenon is the epitenon, which envelops the entire tendon. Some tendons are then wrapped with a paratenon (for example, Achilles tendon), and some are covered with synovium (for example, flexor tendons), depending on the degree of gliding required. The endotenon and epitenon serve to permeate the tendon with vasculature, lymphatics, and nerves.

Another aspect of tendon's morphology and functional relationships are its origin and insertion (its junctions). As the tissue that bridges muscle to bone, tendon has two junction regions: the myotendinous junction, where the muscle transitions to tendon, and the bone-tendon junction, where the tendon transitions to bone. Each is differentially organized and contributes to the varying properties along the length of the muscle-tendon-bone unit. The myotendinous junction is composed of the interdigitations of end sarcom-

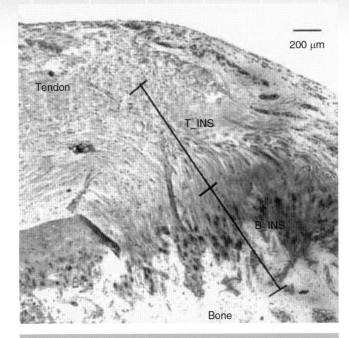

200 μm

Tendon

T_INS

B_INS

Bone

Figure 2 The four transition zones that make up the direct tendon insertion: tendon, uncalcified fibrocartilage, calcified fibrocartilage, and bone, as seen in a rat supraspinatus tendon insertion site. This transition enables transfer of load from a compliant (tendon) to a stiff (bone) material (T_INS = tendinous insertion, B_INS = bony insertion). (Reproduced with permission from Thomopoulos S, Williams GR, Gimbel JA, Favata M, Soslowsky LJ: Variation of biomechanical, structural, and compositional properties along the tendon to bone insertion site. *J Orthop Res* 2003;21[3]:413-419.)

eres and connective tissue elements. An end portion of the sarcomere, known as the z-line, which is arranged in a staggered organization with the next sarcomere, splits and gives rise to myofilament bundles that insert directly onto collagen fibrils. This arrangement minimizes stress to the myotendinous junction with forceful contractions.

At the bone-tendon junction, known as the enthesis, there are two typical arrangements with different biomechanical roles: direct or indirect insertions. Direct, or fibrocartilaginous, insertions have been classically characterized by a four-layer transition from tendon to bone: tendon, fibrocartilage, mineralized fibrocartilage, and bone (**Figure 2**). These insertions are typical in regions where the tendon-bone unit is subject to high tensile loads (such as the rotator cuff).[5,6] In an indirect insertion, which is less common than the direct insertion, the tendon fibers insert directly into the periosteum. The fibers that interdigitate with the periosteal tissue have commonly been referred to as Sharpey fibers. These transitions are more common in areas where tensile loading at the tendinous insertion does not predominate (such as the distal head of the rectus femoris).

At the cellular level there are also considerations that have implications for structure and function. Tendon is of-

ten classified as relatively hypocellular, yet recent evidence connects tenocytes with a highly defined role in maintenance of tendon structure.[7] Tenocytes maintain the extracellular milieu that allows the normal function of tendon by secreting the extracellular matrix, synthesizing collagen and the proteoglycans. They possess long cellular processes that envelop and interdigitate with the collagen fibrils and other tenocyte processes and cell bodies. They are responsive to mechanical loading, and can communicate with adjacent tenocytes through gap junctions at their interface as well as by production of inflammatory mediators under stress.[7]

Blood Supply and Innervation

Although tendon is considered largely hypovascular, blood flow has important consequences for tendon in health and disease. The blood supply and innervation of tendon, as mentioned previously, is primarily through the endotenon and epitenon. The tendon is fed primarily through vasculature that enters through the paratenon or at the bony insertions, and continues to travel throughout the endotenon. The situation is more complex in sheathed tendons, in which blood supply must enter the tendon through mesotenon in vincula, defined as redundancies of the synovium that tether the tendon to its sheath in certain locations, analogous to the mesentery of the peritoneum (**Figure 3**). Sheathed tendon is also thought to receive some nutrition through diffusion via the synovial fluid. In addition to tendon's hypovascularity, there are specific regions of relative avascularity between vascular zones, which are thought to be at particular risk for rupture. These hypovascular areas have been identified in the supraspinatus tendon, long head of the biceps tendon, Achilles tendon, and patellar tendon, all of which are prone to rupture.[8]

Innervation in tendon includes several types of nerve endings with different functions. A tendon is typically innervated by the same nerve as its muscle. The various special organs include Golgi organs, which provide steady-state information when undergoing large stimulations for prolonged periods; Pacini corpuscles, which are considered sensitive, fast-adapting mechanoreceptors; and Ruffini endings, which are also very sensitive but can relay information for prolonged periods similar to Golgi organs. These end-organs are typically localized to the myotendinous region. Free nerve endings, responsible for nociception, on the other hand, tend to be clustered at the enthesis.

Tendon Functions

Tendon serves the primary purpose of allowing the transmission of force from muscle to bone, providing the capacity for locomotion, as well as allowing dynamic joint stability in concert with ligament, which provides more static restraint to joint translation. This is accomplished through an intricately designed and executed structure that enables these certain biomechanical properties. The relationship between structure and function is paramount.

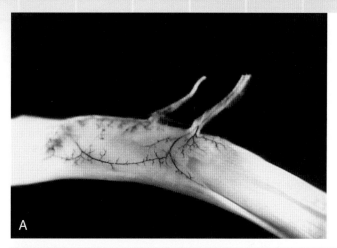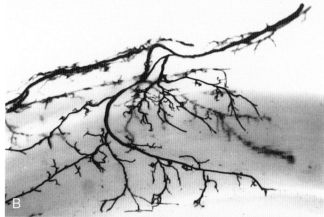

Figure 3 **A,** Human flexor digitorum profundus tendon, injected with India ink, highlighting the contribution of the vinculum (a bandlike structure connecting the flexor tendon and the phalanges) to tendon blood supply. **B,** Close-up of the tendon demonstrating the extent of the vinculum blood supply, (Reproduced with permission from Woo SL, An KN, Frank CB, et al: Anatomy, biology, and biomechanics of tendon and ligament, in Buckwalter JA, Einhorn TA, Simon SR, eds: *Orthopaedic Basic Science*, ed 2. Rosemont, IL, American Academy of Orthopaedic Surgeons, 2000, p 585.)

Mechanical

The mechanical function of tendon is to orchestrate a fine balance between mobility and stability. The most obvious aspect of this function is the transmission of muscle-derived force to bone, which provides volitional control of the skeleton. Tendon also possesses the ability to elastically store and transfer energy. This dual ability has protective implications for the musculoskeletal system, as tendon can help absorb force and protect surrounding tissue. The composition of tendon as primarily water and collagen enables it to function viscoelastically, with its stiffness changing in response to loading. This viscoelastic behavior will be discussed later in the chapter.

Another important mechanical function of tendon is to provide secondary restraint to joint motion and add stability to the musculoskeletal system. The insertion of a tendon just distal to the joint on which it primarily acts enables the tendon to buttress against translation of the articular surfaces. A classic example of this function is the hamstring mechanism as a secondary stabilizer of the knee, protecting against anterior tibial translation in the setting of anterior cruciate ligament (ACL) deficiency.

These functional properties of tendon are derived from material and structural properties of the constituents, from intrinsic tendon properties as well as the characteristics of the muscle-tendon-bone interface. The intrinsic tendon properties are referred to as material properties because they describe characteristics that are specific to the tendon material itself. This differentiates material properties from the structural properties, which are not normalized by tendon area or length, and thus describe qualities of the whole structure.

Three essential components of tendon function, and both its material and structural properties, are its nonlinear anisotropy and its elastic and viscoelastic behavior. The term nonlinear anisotropy means that tendon mechanical properties differ depending on the direction of applied force, and have different values depending on the magnitude of force applied. Viscoelasticity describes a propensity of many biologic tissues, in which a tissue's mechanical properties are different depending on the time and recent history of loading the tissue.

Nonlinear anisotropic properties that are important when discussing tendon can be derived from two experimental scenarios. The first, representing structural properties, is called a load-elongation study. In this setting, the tendon-bone unit is elongated while the resultant load developed in the construct is measured (**Figure 4,** *A*). At low loads, the tendon is stretched easily (low slope) with nonlinear behavior; this is known as the toe region. This stretching has been attributed to the recruitment and realignment of crimped collagen fibrils (**Figure 5**). Following the toe region, there is a linear region, where rate of load development is constant. Finally, there is a failure region, at which point load drops off, and stretching is easily accomplished. From this test, the following properties can be derived: stiffness, represented by the slope of the curve in the linear region; ultimate load, represented by the load value at failure; and energy absorbed to failure, represented by the area under the curve. These parameters are useful in understanding the overall performance of the enthesis in a given experimental setting.

A more refined measure of the tendon material properties is obtained by the normalization of these structural properties to tendon area and length. This analysis yields a curve known as a stress-strain curve (**Figure 4,** *B*). Strain, which represents change in length of the tendon relative to total tendon length, is derived in several ways, the discussion

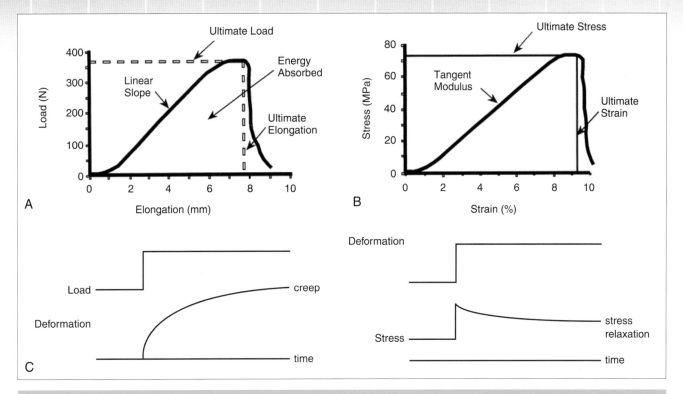

Figure 4 Load-elongation curve of tendon, with load as the dependent variable and elongation as the independent variable. **A,** Various material properties can be derived from this curve. **B,** Stress-strain curve of tendon. This curve normalizes properties to tendon parameters, including length and area. (Reproduced with permission from Woo SL, Debski RE, Withrow JD, Janaushek MA: Biomechanics of knee ligaments. *Am J Sports Med* 1999;27(4):533-543.) **C,** Viscoelastic behavior of tendon, demonstrating the response to load history. For a creep test (left), load is held constant, and amount of deformation is measured. For a stress relaxation test (right), the deformation is held constant while developed stress is measured. (Adapted with permission from Brinker MR, O'Connor DP, Almekinders LC, et al: Physiology of injury to musculoskeletal structures, in Drez D Jr, DeLee JC, Miller MD, eds: *Orthopaedic Sports Medicine: Principles and Practice.* Philadelphia, PA, WB Saunders, 2007.)

of which is beyond the scope of this chapter. This curve is also nonlinear and represents uniaxial tensile loading of the tendon per area. Several parameters can be determined, including modulus, which is the slope of the curve; tensile strength, which is the stress value at failure; ultimate strain; and strain energy density, represented by the area under the curve.

Both structural and material properties are important in experimental evaluation of tendon and its enthesis, especially when considering tendon repair and healing. It should be recognized that an increase in stiffness alone might not be a positive indicator of repair strength; if there has been a substantial increase in cross-sectional area of the tendon, stiffness may increase while modulus decreases. This is a scenario indicative of an increase in quantity, not quality, of tendon tissue and may not represent successful reconstitution of tendon properties.

Viscoelastic

The viscoelastic properties of tendon are essential to understanding how tendon structure contributes to its function. Viscoelasticity can be defined as mechanical behavior that is time- and history-dependent, with material characterized by

both viscous properties (resisting deformation under stress) and elastic properties (indicating a tendency to resume its original shape when stress is removed). Stated differently, a viscoelastic material subjected to stress will undergo an initial deformation but the same stress will cause less deformation with time. Tendon behavior tends to be dominated by viscous properties at low loads and more elastic behavior at high loads.

Viscoelastic behavior can be characterized by creep, stress relaxation, hysteresis, and strain rate sensitivity parameters (**Figure 4,** *C*). Under a constant applied load, tendon will undergo initial deformation and then continue to elongate at a much slower rate, without any further increase in applied load. This tendency is known as creep. Another aspect of this phenomenon can be seen in the case of a constant elongation. In this scenario, the elongation is the independent variable, held constant. The load in the tendon is the measured, dependent variable. With time, the load will decrease. This behavior is known as stress relaxation. Tendon also displays a behavior responsive to its loading history. If tendon is cyclically elongated to a set length and allowed to relax, and the load is measured, the tendon will unload along a different curve than in loading. The area between the two curves rep-

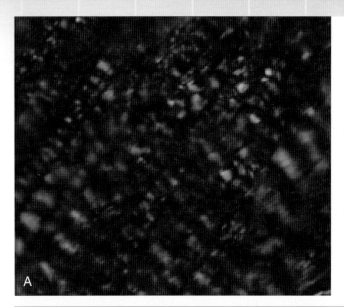
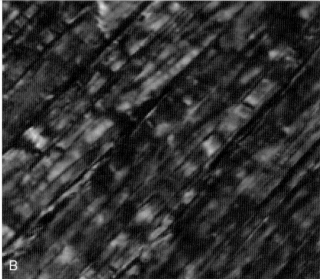

Figure 5 Polarized light microscopy of collagen fibril crimp in mouse supraspinatus tendon (90 days old) (**A**). Under applied tensile loading, the collagen fibrils become uncrimped (**B**). Reproduced with permission from Miller K, Connizzo B, Feeney E, Soslowsky L: Characterizing local collagen fiber re-alignment and crimp behavior throughout mechanical testing in a mature mouse spraspinatus tendon model. *J Biomech* 2012;45[11]:1861-2060.)

resents dissipated energy and is known as hysteresis. Furthermore, repeated cycling will give rise to progressively smaller loads in the tissue, consistent with stress relaxation, in a pattern known as cyclic load relaxation. In addition, when a repeated stress is applied, nonlinear changes occur in the deformation, resulting in cyclic creep.

Proprioception

Tendon has been shown to have excellent innervation for the purpose of proprioception, or the sensing of joint position in space. This ability enables tendon to contribute more effectively to biomechanical function. Clinically, an appreciation of proprioception is relevant because of tendon repair and transfer surgeries. If proprioception is not reestablished, tendon repair outcomes seem to be diminished. As an example, the outcome of teres major transfer to the supraspinatus insertion for massive rotator cuff tear is dramatically improved if the teres can be retrained to function as an arm abductor, which requires preservation of proprioception in the teres tendon.[9]

Biologic Factors Influencing Tendon Properties

Several biologic factors have significant effects on tendon properties, including age, presence of comorbidities, activity level, and anatomic location. Specifically, studies have shown that tendons from older individuals are prone to increased incidence of tendon injury.[10,11] Additionally, medical comorbidities can lead to in vivo degradation of tendon; diabetes, hypercholesterolemia, and kidney disease each have been identified. Exercise can also profoundly affect tendon, with exercised tendons showing increased modulus compared with age-matched control tendons.[12] Anatomic

location also significantly affects tendon tensile strength. As shown previously, tendon from the erector spinae muscles have modulus values an order of magnitude higher than the rotator cuff tendons.[13] These factors apply to most connective tissue and will be discussed in more detail in the section of this chapter on ligament.

Experimental Factors Influencing Tendon Properties

Several technical aspects must be considered when performing experimental measurements as a method to determine tendon mechanical properties. These include the appropriate testing environment, specimen type and orientation, strain rate, and specimen storage, as well as biologic conditions; samples must be similar in age at the moment of harvest and these must be similar in size and diameter.

Testing Environment

The environment for testing has a significant effect on mechanical properties. Specifically, the hydration and temperature of the tissue should be taken into consideration. For example, studies have shown that tendon stiffness decreases with increased temperature.[13]

Specimen Type and Orientation

As described previously, tendon is composed of a bone-tendon-muscle complex. To examine the structural properties, the entire complex is often tested experimentally. The specimen is typically positioned in an anatomic orientation, so that the amount of fibers engaged along the longitudinal axis during loading is maximized. In addition, to examine material properties, the attachments to the tendon are often removed and the tendon is tested independently of the bone. In each of these situations, the specimens must be gripped differently to determine tensile properties. To minimize the error as a result of slipping and stress concentrations at the grips, the tendon should have a high length versus width ratio, defined as an aspect ratio.

Finally, the rate of loading applied experimentally and proper specimen storage also have significant effects on tendon properties. These factors are characteristic of most soft tissues and will be discussed in more detail in the ligament section.

Clinically Relevant Injuries

Tendon injuries are an important aspect of musculoskeletal medical conditions. There are several types of tendon injury, ranging from overuse injuries (such as tendinosis) to rupture, with different clinical consequences. Tendon ruptures are classified into direct and indirect ruptures based on mechanism: direct injuries involve direct trauma to the tendon causing a tear, whereas indirect injuries result from forceful loading of the muscle-tendon-bone unit to the point of tendon failure.

Tendinopathy is an umbrella term for a group of syndromes on the same spectrum, considered to be overuse injuries, resulting in pain and varying degrees of loss of function of the tendon. Tendinosis has largely replaced the term tendinitis in the orthopaedic literature to describe the chronic overuse injury to tendon, as true inflammation is generally absent in these patients. These injuries are characterized by persistent pain and radiographic evidence of intrasubstance tendon degeneration.[14] Upon histologic examination, the hallmarks of tendinosis include disrupted and disorganized collagen, increased extracellular matrix, increased tenocyte population, and neovascularization. Tendinosis, in addition to being a clinical problem itself, can lead to more severe injury, such as complete tendon rupture. Direct and indirect ruptures of tendons remain an important orthopaedic problem, with ongoing management challenges. Injury to the flexor tendons of the upper extremity is the most common and highly characterized of the direct tendon injuries. Penetrating trauma is usually responsible, with stab wounds making up a large portion of these injuries. These tendons typically have no preexisting condition that predisposes them to injury. The tendon is lacerated and retracts because of its muscular attachment. Additionally, the tendon sheath is violated, introducing the risk of infection into a hypovascular space and depriving the tendon of synovial fluid, through which it obtains a portion of its nutrition.[15]

By contrast, indirect tendon injuries are more common and occur through overloading of the bone-tendon-muscle unit. The underlying tendon is predisposed to injury from a variety of etiologies.[16] As described previously, tendinosis has been identified as a likely factor predisposing to rupture, in addition to location in a hypovascular zone, which is also a likely etiology. Several tendons are prone to indirect rupture and are a common orthopaedic injury, including the rotator cuff tendons, long head and distal biceps tendons, hamstring tendon, quadriceps and patellar tendons, and Achilles tendon.

As discussed previously, the material and structural properties of tendon are finely organized to maximize stability and mobility at minimal risk of injury. In the setting of tendinosis, the behavior of tendon is disturbed, and injury becomes a threat. The mechanism of this injury is classically an eccentric contraction, in which there is forced lengthening of the myotendinous unit during contraction. This condition puts maximum stress through the tendon and leads to rupture at a site of weakening, disabling the naturally protective qualities of tendon discussed previously, including viscoelastic behaviors.

Tendon Repair
Healing Processes, Principles, and Deficiencies

Tendon healing processes are characterized by a reactive scar formation that results in tissue that is biologically and mechanically inferior to native tissue. In some instances the healing is functional, producing tissue that adequately substitutes for native tissue, whereas in other instances the tissue is nonfunctional, leading to further tendon injury and sometimes joint instability and altered joint function.

Paratenon-covered tendon healing primarily follows the generalized healing process for connective tissues, occurring in three overlapping phases: inflammation, proliferation, and remodeling. During the inflammatory phase, inflammatory cells and erythrocytes migrate to the site of injury and the gap between the tendon ends is filled. Next, resorption of the initial hematoma is initialized by monocytes and macrophages that enter the lesion. Various vasoactive and chemotactic factors increase vascularity and recruit more inflammatory cells, triggering both degradative and reparative processes, to remove and replace damaged material. During the final stages of inflammation, tenocytes begin to migrate to the injury site and the synthesis of type III collagen begins.[17]

The proliferative phase follows. Within a few days after injury, matrix and cellular proliferation predominate at the injury site. This stage is characterized by continuous collagen production and deposition, creating a scarlike fibrous tissue (**Figure 6,** *A*). The synthesis of type III collagen is maximal during this stage, and cellularity remains high.

The remodeling phase begins approximately 6 weeks following injury and is characterized by a gradual decrease in cellularity and vascularity and the continually increasing organization and maturation of scar tissue over time. During this phase, collagen fibers, along with fibroblasts, attempt to reorient themselves along the length of the tendon (**Figure 6,** *B*). In addition, the synthesis of type I collagen, the main collagen present in uninjured tendons, predominates.[17] Each of these steps in the remodeling phase represents a significant attempt during the healing process to return to normal tendon characteristics (**Figure 6,** *C*). Tendon healing occurs by two mechanisms, each of which has both drawbacks and benefits to function. As previously mentioned, tendons

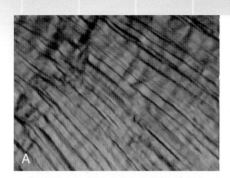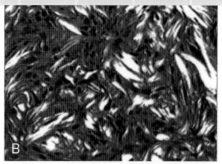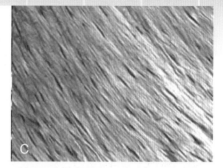

Figure 6   Polarized light histology of the supraspinatus tendon in the rat for uninjured control (**A**), 1 week postinjury (**B**), and 16 weeks postinjury (**C**). The uninjured control demonstrates aligned collagen fibers and collagen crimp, as observed in normal tendon. After 1 week postinjury, the tendon displays an increase in collagen disorganization and by 16 weeks, the collagen organization improves. (Reproduced with permission from Gimbel JA, Van Kleunen, JP, Mehta S, Perry SM, Williams GR, Soslowsky LJ: Supraspinatus tendon organizational and mechanical properties in a chronic rotator cuff tear animal model. *J Biomech* 2004; 37[5]:739-749.)

heal by deposition of scar tissue at the site of injury. Although this scar tissue may allow for functional healing, deposition of scar tissue is often harmful to the tissue when it impedes tendon gliding and ultimately tendon function. This is particularly apparent in tendons encapsulated with a synovial sheath, such as zone II in the flexor tendon system of the hand. Two mechanisms of tendon healing have been proposed: intrinsic and extrinsic. The extrinsic mechanism involves cells from the periphery invading the injury site whereas the intrinsic mechanism involves cells within the tendon itself (**Figure 7**). It is likely that a combination of the two mechanisms occurs clinically; however, the extrinsic mechanism has been implicated as the primary source of adhesions between the tendon and surrounding structures. Therefore, it is hypothesized that suppression of the extrinsic mechanism may improve the healing capability of the tissue, particularly for sheath-covered tendons.[15]

Clinically Relevant Variables Affecting Tendon Repair

Optimization of tendon repair by enhancing both stability and mobility is essential for adequate joint function. Rehabilitation regimens, specifically immobilization and early postoperative motion, are important factors in enhancing stability and mobility, respectively. However, these regimens are conflicting, with immobilization leading to increased stiffness that limits mobility and early postoperative motion potentially disrupting the initial stability of the repair. Thus, optimal treatment must consider careful balance of the two.

Numerous suture techniques, including various configurations, quantities, and materials of sutures, have also been developed in an attempt to optimize the mechanical strength of the tendon.[15] Increasing the strength of the construct may allow for a more aggressive prescribed postoperative protocol.

As mentioned previously, tendons are extremely sensitive to their mechanical environment and therefore specific rehabilitation protocols for injured tendons are critical for healing. For uninjured tendons, the mechanical properties

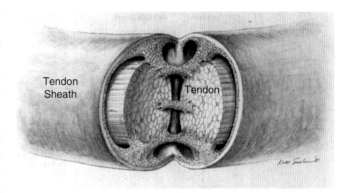

Figure 7   Illustration of extrinsic and intrinsic healing processes in a sheathed tendon. Adhesions may result from activation of the extrinsic process, inhibiting tendon gliding within the synovial sheath. (Adapted with permission from Gelberman RH, Vande Berg JS, Lundborg GN, Akeson WH: Flexor tendon healing and restoration of the gliding surface: An ultrastructural study in dogs. *J Bone Joint Surg Am* 1983;65[1]:70-80.)

tend to increase with increased loading (during exercise) and decrease with decreased loading (during immobilization). However, conflicting evidence exists regarding the optimal rehabilitation treatment of healing tissues. Several studies have shown benefits to increased loading,[18] whereas others have shown negative effects. In general, low loading regimens seem to promote healing, whereas high-intensity loading regimens may have detrimental effects, such as decreased mechanical properties.[19]

Chronic tendon injuries caused by overuse and excessive loading have limited propensity for healing because of irrecoverable degeneration of the tendon tissue. Previous work has shown that tendons with chronic injuries demonstrate decreased collagen organization, increased cellularity, altered cell shape (for example, more rounded), and decreased mechanical properties, indicative of a degenerative tissue.[20]

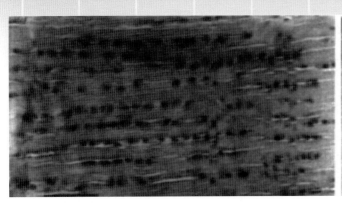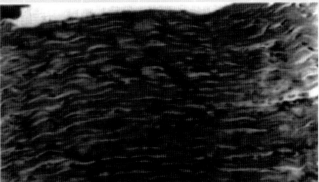

Figure 8 Differing morphology of intra-articular ACL cells (**A**) and extra-articular MCL cells (**B**) in the New Zealand white rabbit. ACL cells are chondroid in appearance while the MCL cells appear more elongated. (Reproduced with permission from Frank CB: Ligament injuries: Pathophysiology and healing, in Zachazewski JE, Magee DJ, Quillen WS, eds: *Athletic Injuries and Rehabilitation*. Philadelphia, PA, WB Saunders, 1996.)

In addition, chronic rotator cuff tears are clinically characterized by fatty degeneration and atrophy of the rotator cuff muscles, which alter the healing response and limit the success of rotator cuff tendon repairs. The difficulties associated with healing of chronic injuries may be a result of the lack of inflammation and the failed healing response associated with the degenerative tissue.[21,22] As a result of these findings, the quality of the tissue should be assessed before prescribing both surgical treatment and postoperative protocols.

Ligament

Classification and Anatomy

Like tendons, ligaments are classified as dense bands of fibrous connective tissue characterized by closely packed collagen fibers. Despite their gross similarities, ligaments and tendons differ in their function, mechanical properties, and biochemical composition. Most noticeably, ligaments both originate and insert onto bone whereas tendons connect muscle to bone. Ligaments also have different inherent properties based on their function and anatomic location. In general, the basic function of ligaments is to guide joint kinematics, maintain joint stability, and prevent abnormal displacement of bones. Anatomically, they are classified according to their attachment sites on bone, which are critical for the distribution and dissipation of joint forces. Capsular ligaments, which are located within the articular capsule that surrounds synovial joints, are anatomically less discrete than extracapsular ligaments but also function to provide stability to the joint.

Gross Morphology, Histology, Microanatomy, and Cell Biology

Ligament is composed of collagenous connective tissue arranged in a hierarchical manner, as in tendon. In general, ligament is characterized as relatively avascular. A thin layer of connective tissue, the epiligament, surrounds the ligament and is analogous to the tendon epitenon. Similar to tendon, the epiligament carries nerves, blood vessels, and lymphatics and is thought to play a role in ligament healing.

Morphologically, collagen fiber interactions in ligaments are defined as being more highly cross-linked than tendon and more intertwined in comparison with the generally parallel-oriented tendon fibers. Ligaments also contain more metabolically active fibroblast cells that are incorporated between the collagen fibers. In addition to differences in cell morphology, ligaments also have more type III collagen than tendon but in general have less total collagen.

Different ligaments have different properties and structure according to their anatomic location, based on their interaction with joint synovial fluid (whether they are intra-articular or extra-articular). For example, the intra-articular ACL has cells that are more chondroid in appearance and are classified as less biologically active than those of the medial collateral ligament (MCL), which is extra-articular (**Figure 8**).

Within a ligament, there are also important regional differences in collagen fiber orientation and composition and cell shape between the midsubstance and bony insertion sites. The morphology of the insertion site has two different forms, direct and indirect. As with tendon, direct insertions are most common and are characterized by four zones: ligament, fibrocartilage, calcified fibrocartilage, and bone. Indirect insertions, such as the tibial insertion site of the MCL, are anchored directly to the bone by calcified collagen fibers, called Sharpey fibers, that merge with the periosteum and bone. In the midsubstance, cells appear elongated in shape whereas at the insertion the cells appear to be more rounded. This cellular transition and change in collagen composition is a reflection of the distribution and dissipation of stresses during loading.

The composition of ligament is similar to that of tendon. The primary constituents are water, collagen, elastin, proteoglycans, and cells. Water comprises approximately 60%

2: Physiology of Musculoskeletal Tissues

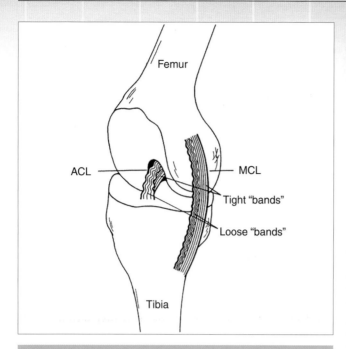

Figure 9 Schematic of the distinct, functional bands in the ACL and MCL of the knee. Positioning of the joint determines which band is under tension, and each contributes specifically to joint rotation and translation. (Reproduced with permission from Frank CB: Ligament injuries: Pathophysiology and healing, in Zachazewski JE, Magee DJ, Quillen WS, eds: *Athletic Injuries and Rehabilitation*. Philadelphia, PA, WB Saunders, 1996.)

to 70% of the total weight whereas approximately 80% of the dry weight is attributed to collagen. Type I collagen is the main collagen present in ligaments (approximately 90% of the collagen present). A significantly smaller portion is type III collagen with the addition of many other types including V, VI, XI, and XIV. Proteoglycans represent approximately 1% of the ligament dry weight and function in ligament hydration and viscoelastic behavior. The relative proportions of proteoglycans vary according to ligament anatomic location and function, specifically whether there is a significant compressive load-bearing responsibility in addition to its primary tensile load-bearing function. Another component that appears in ligament in a small proportion (approximately 1% of dry weight) is the fibrillar protein elastin. Elastin functions in ligament elasticity and in its return to a prestretched length after loading. The primary cell type found in ligament is fibroblasts, which are oriented longitudinally within the collagen fiber framework. These cells synthesize the collagen and extracellular matrix that constitute ligament structure.

Blood Supply and Innervation

Vascularity is crucial for nutrient supply and healing of ligaments. Despite its generally sparse vasculature, ligament has an organized and distinct microvasculature system. As described previously, the epiligamentous plexus, surrounding the ligament, gives rise to most ligament vasculature; in general, ligaments exhibit regional differences, with a denser distribution near the insertion sites.[23] Ligaments also accommodate different sensory nerve endings near their insertion sites. These nerves have different capabilities as nociceptive pain sensors as well as proprioceptive position sensors, which both contribute to the functional stability of the joint.[24]

Ligament Functions
Mechanical

Ligaments serve as the primary static stabilizers in joints. They connect bone to bone and act as passive restraints, guiding joint motion. In addition, ligaments are also characterized as having both dominant and load-sharing functions. For example, the knee joint is stabilized by the interaction of several ligaments, particularly the ACL and MCL, which have an interdependent load-sharing relationship. When one structure is deficient, the force in the complementary structure increases significantly to compensate.[25] However, in general, individual ligaments can be characterized by their dominant functions and their ability to resist unique abnormal displacements (for example, the role of the ACL in resisting anterior tibial translation).

Ligament mechanical properties are directly influenced by their structure, collagen composition, and fiber orientation. As in tendon at low loads, ligaments tend to behave in a nonlinear viscous-dominated manner, whereas at high loads ligaments are more elastic-dominated. As previously mentioned, ligaments have a more disorganized collagen orientation compared with the highly aligned tendon. Thus, the toe region is typically elongated in ligament because it takes more time to align the ligament collagen fibers in the direction of loading.

Some individual ligaments also have a unique functional anatomy, consisting of distinct bands serving specific functions (**Figure 9**). These bands are recruited differently throughout the entire joint range of motion. For example, the ACL can be divided into two distinct bands, the anteromedial and posterolateral, with dominant roles in preventing anterior tibial translation and resisting rotation in knee extension, respectively.[26] Thus, the position of the joint determines which band is most tightly engaged and therefore most susceptible to damage.

Viscoelastic

As in tendon, ligaments also express viscoelastic behavior (time- and history-dependent behavior). This is due in part to the complex interaction between collagen, water, and other extracellular matrix components. Proteoglycans and associated negatively charged GAGs play a major role in water retention and have been identified as factors that contribute to soft-tissue viscoelasticity. However, the role of GAGs remains controversial—some studies have shown that

GAGs may have no direct contribution to ligament viscoelasticity.[27] The primary viscoelastic properties of ligaments are measured, as with tendon, during a stress relaxation test, where under constant elongation, the tissue will relax and the load will decrease over time, and during a creep test, where under constant load, the deformation will increase over time.

Proprioception

As previously mentioned, ligaments have proprioceptive nerve endings that play a key role in joint function and dynamic stability. Histologic evidence in the knee and shoulder has identified the presence of mechanoreceptors in the ligaments. In addition, several techniques have been used to quantify joint proprioceptive function in vivo, including joint position sense and threshold to detection tests. Specifically, it has been shown that in an ACL-deficient knee, proprioceptive function is less than that found in a normal knee and that in general, decreased proprioceptive function correlates with a decreased amount and subsequent disruption of mechanoreceptors.[28] Thus, these mechanoreceptors may play an afferent role in providing the central nervous system with joint proprioceptive information.[29]

Biologic Factors Influencing Ligament Properties

As in tendon, many biologic factors influence ligament properties. Biologic factors that lead to ligament variation include skeletal maturation and aging, anatomic location, and sex, as well as variation in tissue response associated with immobilization and exercise.

Skeletal Maturation and Aging

The tensile properties of both skeletally immature and mature ligaments have also been examined. In general, ligament structural properties, including stiffness, ultimate load, and energy absorbed at failure, increase over time but remain relatively constant after skeletal maturation. In addition, the mode of failure in skeletally mature specimens is typically localized to the midsubstance whereas immature specimens often undergo avulsion-type failure, most likely a result of the weaker open epiphyses.[30]

In addition, ligament properties are also found to change with aging. In human cadaver knees and shoulders, studies have shown that the structural properties, including stiffness, ultimate load, and energy absorbed at failure, of the ligaments decrease with aging. In addition, older specimens have a higher incidence of midsubstance failure than younger specimens.[31,32]

Anatomic Location

Ligaments also have different properties based on anatomic location. For example, the shoulder joint experiences a larger range of motion than the knee joint, and therefore the mechanical behavior of these ligaments varies as a result of their different functions.

Sex

Sex-specific and hormone-related variables have also been implicated as potential biologic factors influencing ligament properties. Studies have shown that females are two to eight times more likely to damage their ACL than males.[33,34] This is due, in part, to the increased dynamic valgus and abduction loads experienced by females during physical activity,[35] which may be a result of anatomic differences between males and females. Changes in hormone levels have also been implicated, although evidence suggests that ligament mechanical properties are not influenced by alterations in estrogen, the primary female sex hormone.[36] Recent evidence found that another female hormone, relaxin, which has been reported to affect collagen synthesis, may decrease connective tissue mechanical properties, including load to failure and stiffness.[37] One study demonstrated that when treated with excess relaxin hormone, the ACL was found to be significantly weaker.[38] These results suggest that reduced mechanical properties caused by increased serum relaxin levels may place the joint at higher risk for injury.

Immobilization

As previously mentioned, stress deprivation due to immobilization has profound morphologic, biochemical, and biomechanical effects on synovial joints. Some changes include the development of synovial adhesions (which leads to increased joint stiffness), disruption of ligament collagen and cellular organization, disruptions in the ligament insertion sites (caused by osteoclastic resorption of bone), and in general, decreased ligament structural properties.[39] As in tendon, remobilization in the ligament reveals a slow but significant improvement of the detrimental effects following immobilization. However, incomplete recovery occurs at the insertion sites and ligament properties do not return to normal.[40]

Exercise

Ligament properties following exercise have also been extensively evaluated, and evidence suggests that short-term exercise regimens increase ligament mechanical and structural properties, including strength and stiffness.[41-43] For example, one study demonstrated that failure load of the MCL was significantly increased in an exercise group compared with a decreased activity group.

Experimental Factors Influencing Ligament Properties

Similar to tendon, many experimental factors, including strain rate, specimen storage, and appropriate testing environment, in addition to the unique bone-ligament-bone complex specific to ligaments, also influence ligament properties. In general, the tensile properties of ligaments slightly increase with increased extension rates.[44] In addition, the effect of freezing ligaments, which is necessary to preserve ligament tissue, has displayed no significant difference in the ligament structural or mechanical properties in comparison with fresh ligament tissue.[45] In contrast to tendon, structural properties of ligaments are characterized by the bone-ligament-bone complex. When tested in various orientations, the structural properties and modes of failure significantly differ in the ligament,[32,46] suggesting that a standard for experimental testing should be followed.

Clinically Relevant Injuries

Ligament injuries are typically the result of traumatic joint injury and are often classified according to severity of the injury (grade I, II, or III). Grade I injuries are characterized as a mild sprain in which fibers are overstretched but not actually torn, grade II injuries are classified as partial disruption of ligament fibers, and grade III injuries involve complete rupture of the ligament. Grade II and III ligament tears may have serious implications, putting patients at an increased risk for recurrent injury (with an incidence as high as 75% in patients with ACL tears[47]) and with few returning to their preinjury activity levels. One study evaluated patients with isolated partial ruptures of the ACL and found that only 30% resumed preinjury activities.[48] In addition, ligament tears are associated with increased joint instability and in some cases, the development of debilitating chronic conditions.[49]

Traumatic joint injuries often involve multiple ligaments, such as the combination of ACL and MCL ruptures in the knee. Combined ligamentous injuries cause dramatic instability in the joint, decreasing the propensity for spontaneous healing. Ligament replacement or repair is often required to prevent or delay the progression of damage to the joint, caused by chronic joint laxity and instability.

Ligament Repair
Healing Processes, Principles, and Deficiencies

The healing process of ligaments is analogous to that of the tendons, occurring in three phases: inflammation, matrix and cellular proliferation, and remodeling and maturation. In general, severe (complete) ligament injuries lead to poor healing due to retraction of torn ends. Various biologic alterations occur during ligament healing including the alteration of proteoglycan and collagen content, specifically increased expression of types III and V collagen.[50] Healing ligaments are also characterized by their increased vascularization[51] and discontinuities within their cellular connections and organization.[52]

Despite the various healing challenges, experimental evidence suggests that in some cases natural healing is possible. When the gap created by the retraction of the torn ligament ends is minimal, certain ligaments have the potential to develop local repair responses, in an attempt to "bridge the gap." Cellular components recruited to the area synthesize collagen and other extracellular matrix components at the injury site. The result is the formation of a collagen-rich scar and matrix that slowly remodel to align with the ligament tissue. Ultimately, the healed ligament is mechanically inferior to native tissue, reaching only 30% to 50% of native tissue quality.[53]

Clinically Relevant Variables Affecting Ligament Repair: Strategies to "Heal"

Because of the MCL's ability to heal spontaneously, it has often been used as a model system to understand ligament healing and the effect of various treatment modalities on ligament repair. For instance, nonsurgical treatment of an isolated MCL injury has been found in some studies to produce better results than surgical intervention.[53] In addition, immobilization after ligament injury was found to lead to increased collagen disorganization as well as decreased structural and mechanical properties, including ultimate load and maximum energy adsorbed and stress-strain behavior, respectively.[40] As a result of these findings, clinical management of MCL tears has shifted to nonsurgical treatment with early controlled remobilization.[2]

Biochemical interventions have also been evaluated as potential methods to improve scar tissue quality and composition. Extrinsic factors including growth factors, hyaluronic acid, platelet-rich plasma, and prolotherapy have all been implicated as potential strategies to assist in ligament healing. However, controversy exists over the quality of evidence to support these interventions and therefore their effectiveness has not been clearly defined. As previously mentioned, gap size is another clinically relevant variable affecting ligament repair. Evidence suggests that the natural healing ability of ligament is variable and that the amount of retraction by the torn ends can be highlighted as a causative factor.

Tendon and Ligament Grafting and Replacement
Overview: Repair Versus Reconstruction

As discussed previously, tendon and ligament injuries occur as a result of acute trauma or chronic overuse and are among the most common musculoskeletal injuries. The understanding of the pathogenesis of these conditions continues to improve; however, treatment regimens remain suboptimal. Both ACL and rotator cuff tendon tears do not heal spontaneously and the success of nonsurgical management in active patients is limited. Therefore, these soft tissues must undergo either repair or reconstruction to prevent joint instability, which may lead to the development of chronic pain, disability, and osteoarthritis.

Several factors influence the standards for surgical treatment including the tissue's anatomic location and the severity of the injury. Typically, intrasynovial tissues have limited ability to heal and therefore the common standard for surgical treatment is reconstruction with a local autograft or allograft. The standard treatment of extrasynovial tissues, on the other hand, is often direct repair. For instance, ACL tears are typically treated by reconstruction whereas rotator cuff tendon tears are usually treated with direct repair. In addition, the severity of the injury must also be taken into consideration when determining the appropriate surgical treatment. In cases where the tissue has a chronic or massive tear,

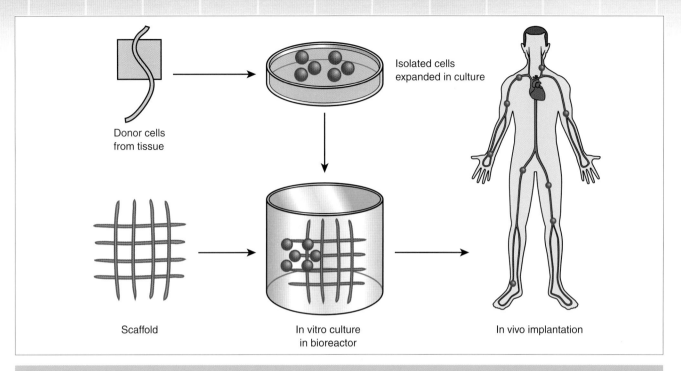

Donor cells
from tissue

Isolated cells
expanded in culture

Scaffold

In vitro culture
in bioreactor

In vivo implantation

Figure 10 Functional tissue-engineering approaches for tendon and ligament include the use of biologic scaffolds and methods to replicate the native tissue properties using cell seeding and mechanical stimulation techniques.

Grafting Using Normal Tissues

Currently, the gold standard for tendon and ligament repair and reconstruction is grafting connective tissue within the same individual (autograft) or from another individual postmortem (allograft). These tissues have become main sources for harvestable grafts because of their potentially expendable roles. Xenografts (taken from a different species) are also useful for tissue grafting but currently have no clinical use in tendon or ligament reconstruction.

For reconstruction, the primary role of the replacement graft is to reproduce the anatomy and function of the native tissue. The most commonly used grafts for reconstruction include the bone–patellar tendon–bone complex and the semitendinosus or gracilis of the hamstring. For repair, the primary role of the graft is to augment the natural healing process while maintaining the mechanical properties of the native tissue. The primary sources for repair materials include the small intestine submucosa, dermis, and tensor fascia lata.

In addition to material type, graft placement, initial graft tension, and graft fixation are significant factors that will alter joint kinematics, graft forces in situ, and articular compressive loads. For ACL reconstruction, various graft/fixation combinations include bone–patellar tendon–bone grafts and free porcine tendon grafts, fixed by various methods, including interference screws, pin fixation, or an Endobutton (Acufex, Microsurgical Inc, Mansfield, MA). Additionally, the amount of graft tensioning prior to fixation could decrease the amount of graft elongation following fixation and therefore its optimization for ACL reconstruction remains a heavily researched and controversial topic.[54] Despite the increased understanding of ideal techniques for grafting, the results are still suboptimal and under cyclic loading, grafts have a tendency to elongate and migrate leading to deterioration of the initial stability of the reconstruction.[55] In addition, no grafting technique has been able to mimic the function of the native tissue and as a result, the standard for grafting using normal tissues remains a highly debated and heavily researched topic.

Functional Tissue Engineering: Current Concepts

Studies have shown that neither spontaneous healing nor soft-tissue repair or reconstruction has the ability to generate native quality tissue after injury; as a result, restoring the normal function remains a significant challenge. Therefore, new treatment modalities are being considered to improve the properties of healing ligaments and tendons. As tissue engineering and regeneration techniques become more readily available, increased focus has been placed on utilization of these techniques as tools to enhance ligament and tendon healing.

With recent advances in tissue engineering, tendon and ligament grafts have taken a comprehensive role, acting as both a source of mechanical stability and a biologic environment with the ability to regenerate and incorporate living tissue (**Figure 10**). A variety of biologic and synthetic materials can act as scaffolds, however, regardless of type; each of these scaffolds should have specific characteristics.

These characteristics include biocompatibility and high porosity to permit cell permeation and growth. Some biologic materials used include collagen derivatives and as mentioned in the previous section, normal tissues such as allografts, autografts, and xenografts. In addition, current synthetic materials being considered include resorbable polyesters, such as poly(lactic-co-glycolic)acid and silk, and nonresorbable materials, such as carbon, polytetraethylene, and polytetrafluroethylene. Ultimately, the goal of the tissue-engineered construct is to replicate the mechanical and biologic properties of the native tissue.

In addition to scaffold material, with advances in molecular biology and biochemistry, several novel therapeutic approaches have been identified for both in vitro and in vivo augmentation of tendon and ligament grafts. These techniques include the incorporation of growth factors (such as transforming growth factor–β, platelet-derived growth factor, fibroblast growth factor, and endothelial growth factor), the incorporation of native cells (such as mesenchymal stem cells and fibroblasts), and gene therapy (which involves altering protein synthesis to induce expression of specific proteins). To prepare the graft for the appropriate mechanical environment, mechanical stimulation techniques have been used to align the collagen fibers and fibroblasts in a physiologic manner. In addition, various vascularization strategies (including the application of vascular endothelial growth factor, basic fibroblast growth factor) have been used to replicate the native vascularized biologic environment.

Despite recent advances in functional tissue engineering, optimal constructs have not been developed for tendon or ligament and further progress must be made. Alternatively, successful tissue-engineering approaches have been developed in a related connective tissue, the skin. Skin substitutes such as Integra (Integra Lifesciences, Plainsboro, NJ), Dermagraft (Smith and Nephew, Largo, FL), and Apligraf (Organogenesis, Canton, MA) have been approved by the US Food and Drug Administration to treat burn victims and/or heal skin wounds, and each has proved successful.

The recent advances in functional tissue-engineering approaches and successes achieved by marketed skin substitutes elucidate the potential of connective tissue constructs in general. With further improvements, tissue-engineered products have the potential to provide immediate, economical treatments of ligament and tendon injuries.

Summary

Tendons and ligaments are connective tissues that are functionally and biologically diverse. As with most connective tissues, tendons and ligaments have a complex structure that affects their mechanical behavior. In addition, tendons and ligaments are capable of biologically adapting to altered loading and disease states. However, in chronic conditions or after severe injury, the modified tissue is often inadequate and fails to restore joint function. As a result, increased focus has been placed on reconstruction and regenerative techniques such as functional tissue engineering in an attempt to enhance tendon and ligament healing. In the near future, research and clinical trials will help in the understanding of pathologic and physiologic events after nonsurgical or surgical treatment.

References

1. Praemer A, Furner S, Rice DP: *Musculoskeletal Conditions in the United States.* Rosemont, IL, American Academy of Orthopaedic Surgeons, 1999.

2. Indelicato PA: Isolated medial collateral ligament injuries in the knee. *J Am Acad Orthop Surg* 1995;3(1):9-14.

3. Merline R, Schaefer RM, Schaefer L: The matricellular functions of small leucine-rich proteoglycans (SLRPs). *J Cell Commun Signal* 2009;3(3-4):323-335.

4. Kalamajski S, Oldberg A: Homologous sequence in lumican and fibromodulin leucine-rich repeat 5-7 competes for collagen binding. *J Biol Chem* 2009;284(1):534-539.

5. Thomopoulos S, Genin GM, Galatz LM: The development and morphogenesis of the tendon-to-bone insertion: What development can teach us about healing. *J Musculoskelet Neuronal Interact* 2010;10(1):35-45.

6. Cooper RR, Misol S: Tendon and ligament insertion: A light and electron microscopic study. *J Bone Joint Surg Am* 1970;52(1):1-20.

7. Cook JL, Feller JA, Bonar SF, Khan KM: Abnormal tenocyte morphology is more prevalent than collagen disruption in asymptomatic athletes' patellar tendons. *J Orthop Res* 2004;22(2):334-338.

8. Cheng NM, Pan WR, Vally F, Le Roux CM, Richardson MD: The arterial supply of the long head of biceps tendon: Anatomical study with implications for tendon rupture. *Clin Anat* 2010;23(6):683-692.

9. Steenbrink F, Nelissen RG, Meskers CG, van de Sande MA, Rozing PM, de Groot JH: Teres major muscle activation relates to clinical outcome in tendon transfer surgery. *Clin Biomech (Bristol, Avon)* 2010;25(3):187-193.

10. Langberg H, Olesen J, Skovgaard D, Kjaer M: Age related blood flow around the Achilles tendon during exercise in humans. *Eur J Appl Physiol* 2001;84(3):246-248.

11. Abate M, Silbernagel KG, Siljeholm C, et al: Pathogenesis of tendinopathies: Inflammation or degeneration? *Arthritis Res Ther* 2009;11(3):235.

12. Arnoczky SP, Lavagnino M, Egerbacher M, Caballero O, Gardner K, Shender MA: Loss of homeostatic strain alters mechanostat "set point" of tendon cells in vitro. *Clin Orthop Relat Res* 2008;466(7):1583-1591.

13. Mow VC, Rik AH: *Basic Orthopaedic Biomechanics and Mechano-Biology.* Philadelphia, PA, Lippincott Williams & Wilkins, 2005.

14. Mishra A, Woodall J Jr, Vieira A: Treatment of tendon and muscle using platelet-rich plasma. *Clin Sports Med* 2009;28(1):113-125.

15. Beredjiklian PK: Biologic aspects of flexor tendon laceration and repair. *J Bone Joint Surg Am* 2003;85(3):539-550.

16. McMaster PE: Tendon and muscle ruptures: Clinical and experimental studies on the causes and location of subcutaneous ruptures. *J Bone Joint Surg Am* 1933;15(3):18.

17. Sharma P, Maffulli N: Tendon injury and tendinopathy: Healing and repair. *J Bone Joint Surg Am* 2005;87(1):187-202.

18. Gelberman RH, Woo SL, Lothringer K, Akeson WH, Amiel D: Effects of early intermittent passive mobilization on healing canine flexor tendons. *J Hand Surg Am* 1982;7(2):170-175.

19. Thomopoulos S, Williams GR, Soslowsky LJ: Tendon to bone healing: Differences in biomechanical, structural, and compositional properties due to a range of activity levels. *J Biomech Eng* 2003;125(1):106-113.

20. Dourte LM, Perry SM, Getz CL, Soslowsky LJ: Tendon properties remain altered in a chronic rat rotator cuff model. *Clin Orthop Relat Res* 2010;468(6):1485-1492.

21. Kovacevic D, Rodeo SA: Biological augmentation of rotator cuff tendon repair. *Clin Orthop Relat Res* 2008;466(3):622-633.

22. Carpenter JE, Thomopoulos S, Flanagan CL, DeBano CM, Soslowsky LJ: Rotator cuff defect healing: A biomechanical and histologic analysis in an animal model. *J Shoulder Elbow Surg* 1998;7(6):599-605.

23. Bray RC, Fisher AW, Frank CB: Fine vascular anatomy of adult rabbit knee ligaments. *J Anat* 1990;172:69-79.

24. Johansson H, Sjölander P, Sojka P: A sensory role for the cruciate ligaments. *Clin Orthop Relat Res* 1991;268:161-178.

25. Lujan TJ, Dalton MS, Thompson BM, Ellis BJ, Weiss JA: Effect of ACL deficiency on MCL strains and joint kinematics. *J Biomech Eng* 2007;129(3):386-392.

26. Petersen W, Zantop T: Anatomy of the anterior cruciate ligament with regard to its two bundles. *Clin Orthop Relat Res* 2007;454:35-47.

27. Lujan TJ, Underwood CJ, Jacobs NT, Weiss JA: Contribution of glycosaminoglycans to viscoelastic tensile behavior of human ligament. *J Appl Physiol* 2009;106(2):423-431.

28. Adachi N, Ochi M, Uchio Y, Iwasa J, Ryoke K, Kuriwaka M: Mechanoreceptors in the anterior cruciate ligament contribute to the joint position sense. *Acta Orthop Scand* 2002;73(3):330-334.

29. Grandis A, Spadari A, Bombardi C, Casadio Tozzi A, De Sordi N, Lucchi ML: Mechanoreceptors in the medial and lateral glenohumeral ligaments of the canine shoulder joint. *Vet Comp Orthop Traumatol* 2007;20(4):291-295.

30. Woo SL, Ohland KJ, Weiss JA: Aging and sex-related changes in the biomechanical properties of the rabbit medial collateral ligament. *Mech Ageing Dev* 1990;56(2):129-142.

31. Lee TQ, Dettling J, Sandusky MD, McMahon PJ: Age related biomechanical properties of the glenoid-anterior band of the inferior glenohumeral ligament-humerus complex. *Clin Biomech (Bristol, Avon)* 1999;14(7):471-476.

32. Woo SL, Hollis JM, Adams DJ, Lyon RM, Takai S: Tensile properties of the human femur-anterior cruciate ligament-tibia complex: The effects of specimen age and orientation. *Am J Sports Med* 1991;19(3):217-225.

33. Arendt E, Dick R: Knee injury patterns among men and women in collegiate basketball and soccer: NCAA data and review of literature. *Am J Sports Med* 1995;23(6):694-701.

34. Stevenson H, Webster J, Johnson R, Beynnon B: Gender differences in knee injury epidemiology among competitive alpine ski racers. *Iowa Orthop J* 1998;18:64-66.

35. Krosshaug T, Nakamae A, Boden BP, et al: Mechanisms of anterior cruciate ligament injury in basketball: Video analysis of 39 cases. *Am J Sports Med* 2007;35(3):359-367.

36. Warden SJ, Saxon LK, Castillo AB, Turner CH: Knee ligament mechanical properties are not influenced by estrogen or its receptors. *Am J Physiol Endocrinol Metab* 2006;290(5):E1034-E1040.

37. Pearson SJ, Burgess KE, Onambélé GL: Serum relaxin levels affect the in vivo properties of some but not all tendons in normally menstruating young women. *Exp Physiol* 2011;96(7):681-688.

38. Dragoo JL, Padrez K, Workman R, Lindsey DP: The effect of relaxin on the female anterior cruciate ligament: Analysis of mechanical properties in an animal model. *Knee* 2009;16(1):69-72.

39. Akeson WH, Amiel D, Abel MF, Garfin SR, Woo SL: Effects of immobilization on joints. *Clin Orthop Relat Res* 1987;219:28-37.

40. Woo SL, Gomez MA, Sites TJ, Newton PO, Orlando CA, Akeson WH: The biomechanical and morphological changes in the medial collateral ligament of the rabbit after immobilization and remobilization. *J Bone Joint Surg Am* 1987;69(8):1200-1211.

41. Tipton CM, James SL, Mergner W, Tcheng TK: Influence of exercise on strength of medial collateral knee ligaments of dogs. *Am J Physiol* 1970;218(3):894-902.

42. Cabaud HE, Chatty A, Gildengorin V, Feltman RJ: Exercise effects on the strength of the rat anterior cruciate ligament. *Am J Sports Med* 1980;8(2):79-86.

43. Noyes FR, Torvik PJ, Hyde WB, DeLucas JL: Biomechanics of ligament failure: II. An analysis of immobilization, exercise, and reconditioning effects in primates. *J Bone Joint Surg Am* 1974;56(7):1406-1418.

44. Woo SL, Peterson RH, Ohland KJ, Sites TJ, Danto MI: The effects of strain rate on the properties of the medial collateral ligament in skeletally immature and mature rabbits: A biomechanical and histological study. *J Orthop Res* 1990;8(5):712-721.

45. Viidik A, Lewin T: Changes in tensile strength characteristics and histology of rabbit ligaments induced by different modes of postmortal storage. *Acta Orthop Scand* 1966;37(2):141-155.

46. Figgie HE III, Bahniuk EH, Heiple KG, Davy DT: The effects of tibial-femoral angle on the failure mechanics of the canine anterior cruciate ligament. *J Biomech* 1986;19(2):89-91.

47. Noyes FR, Mooar LA, Moorman CT III, McGinniss GH: Partial tears of the anterior cruciate ligament: Progression to complete ligament deficiency. *J Bone Joint Surg Br* 1989;71(5):825-833.

48. Bak K, Scavenius M, Hansen S, Nørring K, Jensen KH, Jørgensen U: Isolated partial rupture of the anterior cruciate ligament: Long-term follow-up of 56 cases. *Knee Surg Sports Traumatol Arthrosc* 1997;5(2):66-71.

49. Jones L, Bismil Q, Alyas F, Connell D, Bell J: Persistent symptoms following non operative management in low grade MCL injury of the knee: The role of the deep MCL. *Knee* 2009;16(1):64-68.

2: Physiology of Musculoskeletal Tissues

50. Niyibizi C, Kavalkovich K, Yamaji T, Woo SL: Type V collagen is increased during rabbit medial collateral ligament healing. *Knee Surg Sports Traumatol Arthrosc* 2000;8(5):281-285.

51. Bray RC, Leonard CA, Salo PT: Correlation of healing capacity with vascular response in the anterior cruciate and medial collateral ligaments of the rabbit. *J Orthop Res* 2003; 21(6):1118-1123.

52. Lo IK, Ou Y, Rattner JP, et al: The cellular networks of normal ovine medial collateral and anterior cruciate ligaments are not accurately recapitulated in scar tissue. *J Anat* 2002; 200(pt 3):283-296.

53. Weiss JA, Woo SL, Ohland KJ, Horibe S, Newton PO: Evaluation of a new injury model to study medial collateral ligament healing: Primary repair versus nonoperative treatment. *J Orthop Res* 1991;9(4):516-528.

54. Figueroa D, Calvo R, Vaisman A, Meleán P, Figueroa F: Effect of tendon tensioning: An in vitro study in porcine extensor tendons. *Knee* 2010;17(3):245-248.

55. Staerke C, Möhwald A, Gröbel KH, Bochwitz C, Becker R: ACL graft migration under cyclic loading. *Knee Surg Sports Traumatol Arthrosc* 2010;18(8):1065-1070.

2: Physiology of Musculoskeletal Tissues

Chapter 13

Form and Function of Skeletal Muscle

Adam Wright, MD

Burhan Gharaibeh, PhD

Johnny Huard, PhD

Introduction

Muscle injuries are extremely common, and they tend to recur. The development of regeneration-restrictive fibrotic tissue at the original site of injury may lead both to limitations in force production and reinjury. This chapter reviews the basic anatomy and physiology of skeletal muscle, with a description of the basic mechanisms of muscle growth and adaptation, the types of muscle injuries, and the stages of the healing process. Recent achievements in biologic muscle healing after injury include methods for improving muscle regeneration and reducing muscle fibrosis.

Types of Skeletal Muscle

Skeletal muscles can be categorized based on the distribution of myofibers and their insertion into the tendons. Muscles with parallel fibers are most common. These parallel fibers can produce a substantial change in length with relatively little force, but their relatively small cross-

Dr. Gharaibeh or an immediate family member has received research or institutional support from Cook MyoSite, Inc. Dr. Huard or an immediate family member serves as a paid consultant to or an employee of Cook MyoSite, Inc; and serves as a board member, owner, officer, or committee member of Journal of Surgical Science, Journal of Tissue Science & Engineering, World Journal of Orthopaedics, World Journal of Biological Chemistry, Gene Review Letters, Journal of Stem Cell Reviews, Journal of Histology and Histopathology, Journal of Molecular Therapy, Journal of Current Genomics, and the Journal of Cell Transplantation: The Regenerative Medicine Journal. Neither Dr. Wright nor any immediate family member has received anything of value from or owns stock in a commercial company or institution related directly or indirectly to the subject of this chapter.

sectional area means that total force production is relatively small. A unipennate muscle has fibers that insert on only one side of a tendon, thus creating a relatively large cross-section and greater strength but less change in length. Fibers in a bipennate muscle consolidate on two sides of the inserting tendon, increasing relative cross-section, allowing greater strength than a unipennate muscle, with smaller changes in length.

The Structure of Skeletal Muscle

Gross Structure

Skeletal muscle is enclosed by fascia (a smooth sheath of connective tissue that allows the muscle to slide past surrounding tissues). A muscle is composed of bundles of muscle fibers called fascicles, which are connected by a delicate connective tissue called epimysium. Fascicles are composed of hundreds of muscle fibers enclosed by perimysium, and each individual fiber (myofiber) is enveloped by endomysium. Each myofiber is a long, thin, tubular structure, often many centimeters long and usually running the entire length of the muscle (**Figure 1**).

Cell Structure

The skeletal muscle cell has a plasma membrane called the sarcolemma, which is surrounded by several layers of tissue including a connective tissue basement membrane, a reticular layer, and the extracellular matrix. These surrounding layers make up the endomysium (**Figure 1**). The skeletal muscle fiber contains multiple nuclei, typically situated at the periphery of the cell just beneath the sarcolemma. The unique structure of the sarcolemma makes the muscle fiber an efficient contractile apparatus. The sarcolemma extends into the cell, surrounding the contractile elements of the muscle cell (myofibrils) and forming transverse tubules.

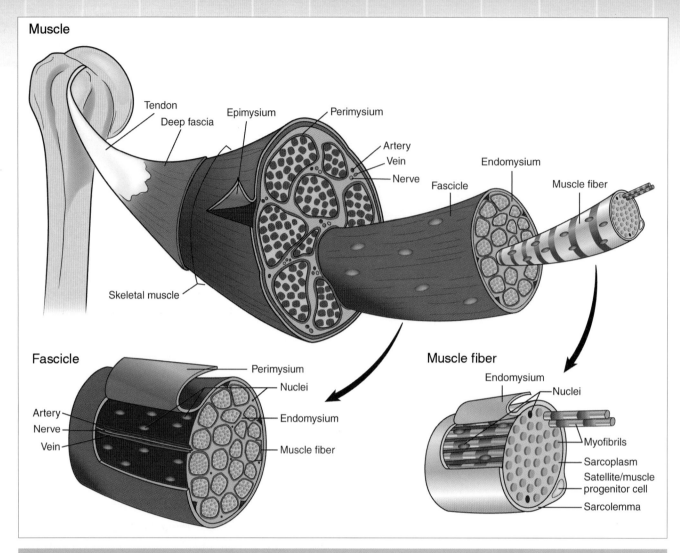

Muscle

Fascicle

Muscle fiber

Figure 1   Structure of the skeletal muscle.

Smaller longitudinal tubules extend from the transverse tubules to interact with the sarcoplasmic reticulum, which is a system of membrane-bound organelles that stores calcium. The sarcoplasmic reticulum contains several enzymes to regulate calcium sequestration and release; the intracellular concentration of calcium turns the contractile apparatus on and off. The permeating design of the sarcolemma and sarcoplasmic reticulum increases the cross-sectional area, permits quick transmission of action potentials to the contractile elements, and provides a reservoir of calcium ions close to the contraction.

Sarcomeres

The myofibrils are a highly ordered set of proteins arranged in parallel along the axis of the cell. This arrangement ensures a cumulative effect of contractions. A distinct banding pattern produces the characteristic striated appearance of alternating light and dark bands seen under the microscope. Myofibrils are divided into contractile units called sarco-

meres (**Figure 2**). The dark band (the A band) represents thick filaments centered around interconnecting proteins (the M line). The thick filaments are primarily composed of myosin, which is a large protein made up of a long, insoluble helical portion and two globular portions called crossbridges. The globular portions are capable of binding the thin filaments and hydrolyzing high-energy adenosine triphosphate (ATP) to release stored chemical energy. The thick filaments also contain C protein, M protein, myosin, titin, and creatine kinase.

The thin filaments attach to an interconnecting set of structural proteins (called the Z line or Z disk) and extend into the middle of the sarcomere. The thin filaments are primarily composed of the protein actin as well as troponin and tropomyosin. Additional proteins at the Z disk include desmin, α-actinin, and filamin. The overlap of actin and myosin allows binding between the proteins and subsequent contraction of the myofibrils.

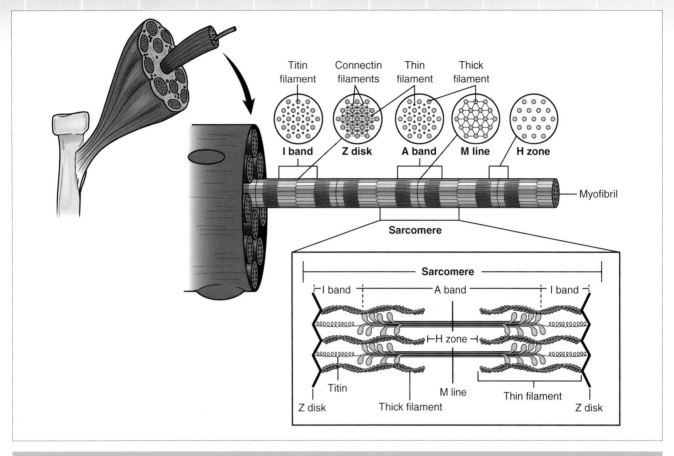

Figure 2 Structure of the myofibril.

Muscle Contraction

The Sliding Filament Theory

Muscular contraction is produced by interaction between the thick and thin filaments. The myosin molecules in the thick filaments form cross-bridges with the actin molecules of the thin filaments. The globular domain of the myosin molecule hydrolyzes ATP to adenosine diphosphate, causing a conformational change in the myosin molecule that pushes the filaments past each other. The myosin molecule quickly releases the actin molecule and returns to its original conformation. This ATP-dependent cycle repeats in rapid succession to cause the thick and thin filaments to pull toward each other. Because of the relative polarities of the thick and thin filaments, active cross-bridging results only in a sliding of the thick and thin filament complexes toward each other and a shortening or resistance to stretching of the sarcomere.

Cross-bridge cycling is modulated by intracellular calcium through the regulatory proteins troponin and tropomyosin. Tropomyosin is a molecule on the thin filament that prevents myosin-actin interaction. Troponin is a calcium-dependent regulatory protein with three domains: the troponin-C subunit binds calcium, troponin-T binds tropomyosin, and troponin-I is inhibitory to the actin-

myosin interaction. When troponin-C binds calcium, the molecule changes conformation, relieving the troponin-I and tropomyosin inhibition of myosin-actin cross-bridging. Therefore, when intracellular calcium levels are high, cross-bridge cycling is active, and the myofibrils contract.

The Motor Unit

Each myofiber is stimulated by one nerve axon, but one axon can branch and stimulate multiple myofibers. All of the myofibers contacted by one axon constitute a motor unit. When the motor unit is activated, all of its muscle fibers contract. The number of muscle fibers in a motor unit ranges from approximately 10 to thousands; in general, muscles that require fine motor control have relatively few fibers per motor unit. The neuromuscular junction is the site at which the nervous system controls muscular contraction. The neuromuscular junction is composed of the presynaptic axon, the synaptic cleft, and the postsynaptic muscle cell.

The Action Potential

During the conversion of neuronal depolarization to muscular contraction, an action potential from the motor neuron reaches the axon terminal, releasing acetylcholine into

2: Physiology of Musculoskeletal Tissues

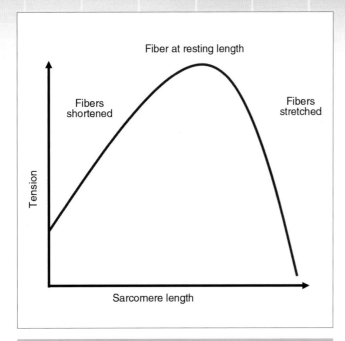

Figure 3 The relationship between tension and sarcomere length. The greatest tension is attained at the normal muscle fiber length, when the overlap between actin and myosin is greatest.

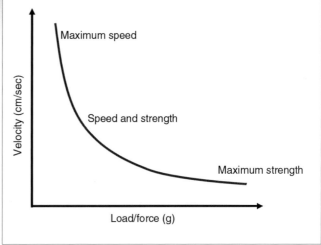

Figure 4 The relationship between force and velocity in isometric skeletal muscle contraction. The smaller the load, the more rapid is the muscle response.

the synaptic cleft. Acetylcholine binds to postsynaptic receptors, which respond by increasing permeability to sodium and depolarizing the sarcolemma. This depolarization spreads through the transverse tubules, stimulating the sarcoplasmic reticulum to release calcium into the cell. Calcium binds to the protein troponin, allowing myosin filaments to slide past actin filaments in an ATP-dependent process and shorten the muscle fiber. Contraction ceases when acetylcholine is degraded at the postsynaptic receptor, the membrane repolarizes, and calcium is pumped back into the sarcoplasmic reticulum.

A single action potential results in a quick contraction followed by relaxation. The length of the contraction ranges from approximately 7.5 ms (for fast myofibers) to 100 ms (for slow myofibers). Unlike nerve tissue, muscle tissue has no refractory period for the contractile mechanism; a rapid sequence of depolarizations results in a continuous, tetanic contraction.

Types of Contractions

Muscular contractions typically are described as shortening the muscle in a concentric contraction. Several other types of contractions also exist. In an eccentric contraction, myosin-actin cross-bridges are formed, but the opposing force is greater than the force created by the muscle, and the muscle therefore lengthens. In an isometric contraction, the force of contraction equals the opposing force, and the length does not change.

The Relationship Between Length and Tension

The structural makeup of skeletal muscle creates unique properties of force production based on muscle length (**Figure 3**). The length of the sarcomere at the time of contraction affects the amount of force produced, due to the amount of overlap between actin and myosin molecules. The overlap is greatest at resting length; as a result, more cross-bridging occurs, and greater force is achieved. The force of contraction drops off exponentially as a muscle fiber is shortened or lengthened. These anatomic properties of skeletal muscle are significant in determining biomechanical strength, running speed, and jumping height.

The Relationship Between Force and Velocity

The force-velocity relationship also is a property of skeletal muscle mechanics. As originally described in isometrically stimulated amphibian muscle, the velocity of a muscle contraction is related to the load placed on the muscle (**Figure 4**). The larger the load, the lower is the velocity at which the muscle can contract. In contrast, muscle velocity increases with a light load. This relationship applies only to the initial concentric action after isometric stimulation. In eccentric contraction, the force-velocity curve is different; an eccentrically loaded muscle lengthens rather than shortens. Because muscle becomes more stiff when it resists shortening, a large change in load results in a smaller change in velocity. Eccentric contractions produce more force at the same movement velocity and therefore require less energy expenditure. This difference is clinically important. For example, in normal gait the quadriceps is most active eccentrically during heel strike, while the knee is flexing, and is most active concentrically during knee extension.

Table 1

Sources of Energy for Skeletal Muscle Contraction

Activity Duration (Approximate)	Type of Pathway	Energy Substrate
< 10 sec	Anaerobic	ATP + creatine phosphate
10 to 30 sec	Anaerobic	ATP + creatine phosphate + glycogen
30 sec to 1 min	Anaerobic	Glycogen
1 to 4 min	Aerobic + anaerobic	Glycogen + lactic acid
> 4 min	Aerobic	Glycogen + fatty acids

Stretch Receptors

Muscle spindles are stretch receptors within the muscle that sense a change in muscle length and relay this information to the spinal cord. Muscle spindles are part of the feedback loops that monitor and control muscle stiffness by way of afferent (type I or II) and efferent (γ, α, or β) innervation. When the muscle is shortened, the muscle spindle relays the change in length by decreased afferent discharge. This action causes increased efferent activity that resets the sensitivity of the muscle spindle at a new tension. Another type of stretch receptor, the Golgi tendon organ, is located at the musculotendinous junction and detects tendon lengthening to prevent excessive tendon stretch.

Fiber Types

Skeletal muscle is a heterogeneous tissue. The myofibers frequently are grouped based on their contraction speed and predominant energy pathways. This heterogeneity is the result of different structural and metabolic properties of the fibers. Variability in isoforms of the contractile and structural proteins can result in different fiber types. Most important are the types of myosin ATP, which produce different shortening speeds (the fast and slow forms of myosin). The three general fiber types are slow oxidative (type I), fast oxidative-glycolytic (type IIA), and fast glycolytic (type IIB). Type I fibers are smaller, contract more slowly, and produce less force than type II fibers, but they are fatigue resistant. Type II fibers are larger, contract more quickly and forcefully, and are more easily fatigued. Type IIA is considered intermediate; type IIB is the fastest, most powerful, and most fatigable type. When motor units are activated by the central nervous system, the smallest motor units (predominantly type I), are recruited first; the larger type IIA and IIB units are recruited when more intense contractions are required.

Energy Pathways

ATP is the common energy source for muscle contraction. The intracellular stores of ATP are limited, however. ATP is regenerated to supply energy for contracting muscle through three pathways. Creatine phosphate is dephosphorylated by mitochondrial creatine kinase to convert adenosine diphosphate to ATP. Creatine phosphate reserves are adequate for short-duration (10 to 20 s), high-intensity contractions, as required for sprinting. After a maximum of 30 seconds of exercise, muscle glycogen is converted to ATP through anaerobic glycolysis, and lactate is produced. In sustained exercise of more than approximately 1 minute, aerobic oxidation of glucose and fatty acids predominates, allowing a much more efficient energy yield. Although anaerobic oxidation yields 2 ATP per molecule of glucose, aerobic oxidation yields 32 per molecule (**Table 1**). Cardiac output and total ventilation increase dramatically to provide the oxygen required to support aerobic oxidation. The endurance limit (approximately 370 W in elite athletes) is the maximum sustainable energy output, as restricted by the rate of oxygen delivery and aerobic oxidation. Beyond this limit, anaerobic glycolysis can temporarily compensate through the rapid production of lactate. Increasing lactate and H^+ ion production causes a systemic drop in pH, inhibiting the reactions that drive muscular contraction. At a plasma lactate level of approximately 4 mmol/L, the anaerobic threshold is reached; at this point, performance declines and rapid fatigue ensues.

Muscle Growth and Adaptation

Development

Skeletal muscle arises from mesodermal somite tissue. Early muscle progenitor cells are called myoblasts, and the fusiform cells that eventually fuse into multinucleated cells are called myotubes. Many contractile elements appear in the cell at the approximate time of myotube formation. Further differentiation occurs with muscle-specific expression of contractile proteins, elements of the metabolic pathways, and connections to the extracellular matrix.

Growth

During normal development, skeletal muscle grows in volume and length. To accommodate skeletal growth, total muscle length increases but sarcomere length remains constant. Additional sarcomeres are added in series near the region of the myotendinous junction. This mechanism persists at skeletal maturity, when muscles immobilized under stretch increase in length. Initially, the myofibrils and sar-

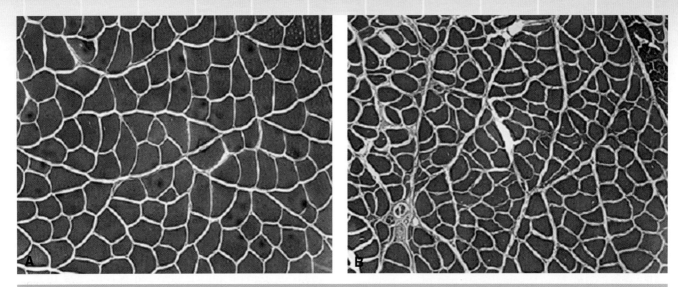

Figure 5   Effect of denervation on mouse skeletal muscle anatomy. **A,** Eosin staining of normal gastrocnemius muscle with intact innervation. **B,** The effect of a 5 mm gap in the sciatic nerve. At 4 weeks postdenervation, fiber diameter has become significantly smaller than that of the control muscle (**A**).

comeres of a stretched muscle are lengthened. Over a period of weeks, additional sarcomeres are added so that resting sarcomere length is restored but the entire muscle remains at the new, stretched length. The mechanical properties of a lengthened muscle also change; the length-tension curve shifts to produce peak tension at a greater length and to produce less passive force when stretched. Conversely, greater passive force is generated by the same stretch if a muscle is shortened for a prolonged period of time. Clinically, the mutability of muscle length has been advantageously applied in surgical limb-lengthening and muscle transfer procedures.

Immobilization

Muscle undergoes several changes in response to immobilization or disuse. When skeletal muscle is immobilized, atrophy quickly ensues because of many factors, including reduced protein synthesis and hormonal contributions. The result is a loss of cross-sectional area, leading to decreased muscle strength. Fatigability increases, partly because of diminished energy stores and metabolic efficiency. The response to immobilization depends on muscle length, however. Atrophy, loss of extensibility, and loss of force production are more pronounced in muscle immobilized without tension than in muscle immobilized under stretch. When muscles are stretched in immobilization, the loss of strength is partially compensated for by the growth in length, with formation of new sarcomeres and contractile proteins. Stretched muscle also produces less tension from stretch and maintains its extensibility. Although prolonged immobilization should be avoided, attention to joint position and muscle length can optimize future function.

Training

Under the demands of physical training, the skeletal musculature undergoes a range of adaptations to improve muscle performance. The types of training and their primary effects can be simplified into three categories: motor learning, endurance training, and resistance training. Motor learning to improve the accuracy and performance of motor skills primarily results in nervous system adaptations such as the timing and rate of contractions. Endurance training (for example, in distance running) focuses on increasing the oxidative capacity of slow-twitch (type I) fibers, mainly by increasing mitochondrial density and cardiac output. Resistance training (for example, in weight lifting) uses relatively short, powerful contractions and requires training the fast-twitch (type II) fibers. Adaptations result from increases in the cross-sectional area of the muscle as well as improved neural activation.

Atrophy

Skeletal muscle atrophies during periods of decreased muscle stimulation or systemic illness, as during immobilization or bed rest (for example, in burn treatment or surgery). The mechanisms driving disuse atrophy are a decrease in muscle protein synthesis and an increase in muscle protein breakdown, along with denervation[1] (**Figure 5**). As the body ages, skeletal muscle atrophies, and muscle function gradually declines, with decreased force production, contraction velocity, and impaired relaxation.[2] Sarcopenia (degenerative loss of skeletal muscle) was found in approximately 25% of people age 65 to 70 years, and 40% of those older than 80 years.[3] Resistance exercise training and nutritional supplementation have been shown to improve the results of rehabilitation and to reduce muscle wasting in disuse, aging, or

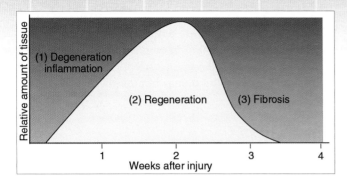

Figure 6 The general process of skeletal muscle repair.

disease states.[4]

Muscle Injury

Muscle injury commonly occurs during physical activities and almost always with skeletal trauma. Muscle injury usually is found with a strain, contusion, or laceration. Regardless of the mechanism of injury, the pattern of biologic response is muscle destruction and inflammation followed by regeneration and fibrous scar formation (**Figure 6**).

Destruction and Inflammation

In a contusion or laceration injury, a compressive force or direct tear causes tissue destruction close to the injury site. In a muscle strain injury, tensile force along the muscle typically causes rupture near the musculotendinous junction.[5] Mechanical injury usually disrupts the myofiber across its entire cross-section, and necrosis can develop along the entire length of the long, threadlike cell. However, condensations of cytoskeleton, called contraction bands, contain the injury at regular intervals.[6] The plasma membrane defect is sealed off within hours. Blood vessels are also damaged, and hematoma develops. Inflammatory cells enter the injury site directly through the damaged blood vessels and are recruited via chemoattractants.[7] The extracellular matrix stores growth factors that are released when the extracellular matrix is disrupted.[8] Local macrophages and fibroblasts produce growth factors, cytokines, and chemokines in response to injury. Neutrophils are the predominant inflammatory cell during the acute period, and an influx of monocytes follows 1 day after the injury. These monocytes mature into macrophages that phagocytose the necrotic tissue before tissue repair.

Regeneration

Myofiber regeneration occurs approximately 1 to 4 weeks after the injury. Myofibers are terminally differentiated, but skeletal muscle also contains cell populations capable of forming new muscle tissue. Satellite cells are a well-defined population of undifferentiated cells found underneath the basal lamina of myofibers. The proliferation of satellite cells is stimulated when inflammatory cells release stimulatory growth factors such as the fibroblast growth factors, insulin-like growth factor–1 (IGF-1) and hepatocyte growth factor.[9] These cells differentiate into myoblasts, which fuse with the injured myofibers. Additional progenitor cells have been found to contribute to regeneration, including cells present in muscle tissue (muscle-derived stem cells), as well as cells from bone marrow, neuronal tissues, and mesenchymal tissues.[5]

Fibrosis

Fibrosis (the formation of a connective tissue scar) begins with the cross-linking of fibrin and fibronectin within the hematoma to create early granulation tissue. Fibroblasts anchor to the granulation tissue and synthesize extracellular matrix components. Early strength and elasticity are provided to the granulation tissue by fibronectin, followed by type III collagen. After several days, fibroblasts produce type I collagen, the major component of mature scar, thereby increasing the tensile strength of the muscle. The connective tissue scar ceases to be the weakest point in the muscle after approximately 10 days. Any rupture that occurs later is at the scar-myofiber interface.[5]

Revascularization and Reinnervation

The vascular supply must be restored to allow full recovery of the injured muscle. Early myotubes possess few mitochondria and function largely on anaerobic metabolism. In late regeneration, however, aerobic metabolism is predominant. New capillary ingrowth appears to be necessary to provide the level of oxygen required for aerobic metabolism and full regeneration.[10] Similarly, new myofibers require reinnervation for full recovery after nerve injury. After myotubes are formed in denervated muscle, the new myofibers will atrophy in the absence of subsequent innervation.[11] When the nerve axon is disrupted, regrowth of the distal axon segment must be completed to ensure full reinnervation and muscle regeneration.

Approaches to Improving Muscle Repair

Treatment of Muscle Injury

The acute treatment of muscle injuries generally includes rest, ice, compression, and elevation (the RICE protocol). These immediate measures reduce bleeding at the injury site. Immobilization prevents retraction of the muscle edges, reduces further hematoma formation, and reduces the size of the fibrotic scar.[12] Although immobilization is beneficial immediately after injury, after more than a few days it is detrimental to muscle regeneration. Immobilization causes muscle fiber atrophy, loss of strength, and excessive connective tissue deposition. In a mouse laceration model, 5 days of immobilization decreased histologic and functional healing.[13] Return to function can be maximized by relatively early mobilization (approximately 3 to 5 days after injury), followed by progressive strengthening, stretching, and a graduated return to activity.

NSAIDs are commonly used to control pain after muscle injury, but their effect on muscle healing is not well understood. In vitro mouse studies indicate that disruption of the cyclooxygenase-2 pathway may delay muscle regeneration and increase fibrotic deposition.[14,15] The use of NSAIDs in muscle injuries should be carefully considered because of the possibility of impairing the healing process.

Biologic Approaches to Modulate Muscle Repair

Although the established treatments of muscle injury are limited, biologic approaches to improving muscle repair are evolving. These approaches include the addition of stimulatory growth factors, gene therapies, and antifibrotic agents. Growth factors serve a variety of roles during muscle regeneration.[16] In mice, direct injections of the stimulatory growth factors IGF-1, basic fibroblast growth factor, and (to a lesser extent) nerve growth factor were found to enhance muscle regeneration and muscle strength after laceration, contusion, or strain.[17-19] Direct injection of recombinant growth factors is safe and easy. However, a high concentration of these recombinant proteins is required to generate a substantial effect, and therefore they have limited efficacy. Growth factors have a dose-dependent effect on myoblast proliferation and differentiation in vitro, but measurable enhancement of skeletal muscle healing in mice usually requires multiple consecutive injections of a relatively high concentration of IGF-1, basic fibroblast growth factor, and nerve growth factor (100 ng/injection for each growth factor).[17-19] Short biologic half-life and rapid clearance from the bloodstream may explain the need for high concentrations of growth factor.

The injection of platelet-rich plasma (PRP), which provides local delivery of a wide variety of growth factors, is increasingly common in treating musculoskeletal injury but has not been well studied in muscle injury. PRP injection in a rat model of muscle strain led to functional improvement as well as elevated myogenesis.[20] Animal and early clinical data provide limited scientific support for the use of PRP in muscle strain injuries.[21] Gene therapy may be an effective method of delivering high, steady concentrations of growth factor to injured muscle. Adenovirus-based delivery of IGF-1 improved muscle healing in a laceration model, although muscle fibrosis remained at the injury site and functional recovery was incomplete.[22] The formation of connective tissue scar at the site of muscle injury interferes with complete muscle regeneration. TGF-β1 plays a role in the formation of fibrosis in some tissues and muscle diseases, and strong expression of TGF-β1 has been observed in injured skeletal muscle.[23,24] TGF-β1 probably plays an important role in the development of fibrosis after muscle injury. Antifibrotic agents that block the effects of TGF-β1 include a neutralizing TGF-β1 antibody or receptor blocker,[25] decorin,[27] relaxin,[28] interferon-γ,[29] and losartan (an angiotensin-II blocker).[30] By blocking the stimulation of TGF-β1 production by angiotensin II, the US Food and Drug Administration–approved antihypertensive drug losartan has been shown to significantly decrease fibrosis and increase muscle fiber regeneration in mice.[30] These agents and others that disrupt the fibrotic cascade, at points such as collagen deposition, may improve healing after skeletal muscle injury.

Summary

The skeletal muscles represent a large part of body mass and can efficiently regenerate after injury because of the presence of endogenous progenitor cells (called satellite cells). However, the regeneration process declines with aging or the progression of muscle diseases such as muscular dystrophies. The phases of muscle recovery are remarkably similar after different injuries. The interrelated and overlapping stages of muscle repair involve degeneration of injured muscle fibers, an inflammatory phase, myofiber regeneration, and the development of fibrosis. Acute muscle injuries usually are treated with the RICE protocol, and NSAIDs often are used to control pain. Muscle healing may be impaired by the use of NSAIDs. Biologic approaches to modulating muscle repair use a combination of stem cell populations including muscle-derived stem cells; cell growth–promoting biologic products such as IGF-1, basic fibroblast growth factor, and PRP; antifibrotic agents such decorin, suramin, and losartan; tissue-engineered scaffolding and slow-release beads; and gene therapy. These therapies may become effective for improving muscle healing. However, basic science and preclinical studies must be performed to ensure the safety of such therapies before they can become part of standard orthopaedic care.

References

1. Marimuthu K, Murton AJ, Greenhaff PL: Mechanisms regulating muscle mass during disuse atrophy and rehabilitation in humans. *J Appl Physiol* 2011;110(2):555-560.

2. Ryall JG, Schertzer JD, Lynch GS: Cellular and molecular mechanisms underlying age-related skeletal muscle wasting and weakness. *Biogerontology* 2008;9(4):213-228.

3. Baumgartner RN, Koehler KM, Gallagher D, et al: Epidemiology of sarcopenia among the elderly in New Mexico. *Am J Epidemiol* 1998;147(8):755-763.

4. Phillips SM: Physiologic and molecular bases of muscle hypertrophy and atrophy: Impact of resistance exercise on human skeletal muscle (protein and exercise dose effects). *Appl Physiol Nutr Metab* 2009;34(3):403-410.

5. Järvinen TA, Järvinen TL, Kääriäinen M, Kalimo H, Järvinen M: Muscle injuries: Biology and treatment. *Am J Sports Med* 2005;33(5):745-764.

6. Hurme T, Kalimo H, Lehto M, Järvinen M: Healing of skeletal muscle injury: An ultrastructural and immunohistochemical study. *Med Sci Sports Exerc* 1991;23(7):801-810.

7. Tidball JG: Inflammatory cell response to acute muscle injury. *Med Sci Sports Exerc* 1995;27(7):1022-1032.

8. Rak J, Kerbel RS: bFGF and tumor angiogenesis: Back in the limelight? *Nat Med* 1997;3(10):1083-1084.

9. Chargé SB, Rudnicki MA: Cellular and molecular regulation of muscle regeneration. *Physiol Rev* 2004;84(1):209-238.

10. Järvinen M: Healing of a crush injury in rat striated muscle: 3. A micro-angiographical study of the effect of early mobilization and immobilization on capillary ingrowth. *Acta Pathol Microbiol Scand A* 1976;84(1):85-94.

11. Rantanen J, Ranne J, Hurme T, Kalimo H: Denervated segments of injured skeletal muscle fibers are reinnervated by newly formed neuromuscular junctions. *J Neuropathol Exp Neurol* 1995;54(2):188-194.

12. Järvinen MJ, Lehto MU: The effects of early mobilisation and immobilisation on the healing process following muscle injuries. *Sports Med* 1993;15(2):78-89.

13. Menetrey J, Kasemkijwattana C, Fu FH, Moreland MS, Huard J: Suturing versus immobilization of a muscle laceration: A morphological and functional study in a mouse model. *Am J Sports Med* 1999;27(2):222-229.

14. Shen W, Li Y, Tang Y, Cummins J, Huard J: NS-398, a cyclooxygenase-2-specific inhibitor, delays skeletal muscle healing by decreasing regeneration and promoting fibrosis. *Am J Pathol* 2005;167(4):1105-1117.

15. Shen W, Prisk V, Li Y, Foster W, Huard J: Inhibited skeletal muscle healing in cyclooxygenase-2 gene-deficient mice: The role of PGE2 and PGF2alpha. *J Appl Physiol* 2006;101(4):1215-1221.

16. Huard J, Li Y, Fu FH: Muscle injuries and repair: Current trends in research. *J Bone Joint Surg Am* 2002;84(5):822-832.

17. Kasemkijwattana C, Menetrey J, Somogyl G, et al: Development of approaches to improve the healing following muscle contusion. *Cell Transplant* 1998;7(6):585-598.

18. Kasemkijwattana C, Menetrey J, Bosch P, et al: Use of growth factors to improve muscle healing after strain injury. *Clin Orthop Relat Res* 2000;370:272-285.

19. Menetrey J, Kasemkijwattana C, Day CS, et al: Growth factors improve muscle healing in vivo. *J Bone Joint Surg Br* 2000;82(1):131-137.

20. Hammond JW, Hinton RY, Curl LA, Muriel JM, Lovering RM: Use of autologous platelet-rich plasma to treat muscle strain injuries. *Am J Sports Med* 2009;37(6):1135-1142.

21. Wright-Carpenter T, Klein P, Schäferhoff P, Appell HJ, Mir LM, Wehling P: Treatment of muscle injuries by local administration of autologous conditioned serum: A pilot study on sportsmen with muscle strains. *Int J Sports Med* 2004;25(8):588-593.

22. Lee CW, Fukushima K, Usas A, et al: Biological intervention based on cell and gene therapy to improve muscle healing after laceration. *J Musculoskelet Res* 2000;(4):265-277.

23. Li Y, Huard J: Differentiation of muscle-derived cells into myofibroblasts in injured skeletal muscle. *Am J Pathol* 2002;161(3):895-907.

24. Li Y, Foster W, Deasy BM, et al: Transforming growth factor-beta1 induces the differentiation of myogenic cells into fibrotic cells in injured skeletal muscle: A key event in muscle fibrogenesis. *Am J Pathol* 2004;164(3):1007-1019.

25. Burks TN, Cohn RD: Role of TGF-β signaling in inherited and acquired myopathies. *Skelet Muscle* 2011;1(1):19.

26. Li Y, Li J, Zhu J, et al: Decorin gene transfer promotes muscle cell differentiation and muscle regeneration. *Mol Ther* 2007;15(9):1616-1622.

27. Nozaki M, Li Y, Zhu J, et al: Improved muscle healing after contusion injury by the inhibitory effect of suramin on myostatin, a negative regulator of muscle growth. *Am J Sports Med* 2008;36(12):2354-2362.

28. Li Y, Negishi S, Sakamoto M, Usas A, Huard J: The use of relaxin improves healing in injured muscle. *Ann N Y Acad Sci* 2005;1041:395-397.

29. Foster W, Li Y, Usas A, Somogyi G, Huard J: Gamma interferon as an antifibrosis agent in skeletal muscle. *J Orthop Res* 2003;21(5):798-804.

30. Bedair HS, Karthikeyan T, Quintero A, Li Y, Huard J: Angiotensin II receptor blockade administered after injury improves muscle regeneration and decreases fibrosis in normal skeletal muscle. *Am J Sports Med* 2008;36(8):1548-1554.

2: Physiology of Musculoskeletal Tissues

Chapter 14

Peripheral Nerves: Form and Function

Wesley M. Jackson, PhD

Edward Diao, MD

Introduction

Many significant breakthroughs in clinical medicine have occurred during military conflicts. In particular, the combat operations in Afghanistan and Iraq since 2003 have necessitated advancements in musculoskeletal research and clinical orthopaedic medicine. The extensive use of body armor and widespread exposure to improvised explosive devices are among the combat-related factors that have led to an intense research focus on extremity reconstruction.[1] These conflicts began just as new methods in tissue engineering and regenerative medicine were being developed in the laboratory. Advanced treatment strategies and surgical techniques are being applied to the treatment of injured service personnel in an effort to provide them with the highest level of medical care.

One consistent factor limiting the clinical success of tissue repair strategies is the inability to effectively reinnervate the distal extremity.[2] Often the decision to salvage or amputate an injured limb must be made by a military forward surgical team, and one of the primary considerations is whether regeneration of the damaged peripheral nerves can reasonably be expected, within the current limits of technology and surgical technique. The functional success of the extremity reconstruction will partly depend on the patient's motor and sensory function in that limb. Failure of reinner-

vation after extremity reconstruction can contribute to soft-tissue fibrosis, adipose tissue accumulation, neuropathic dermal injuries, heterotopic ossification, and ankylosis. These pathologic tissue repair processes are likely to lead to complications during the patient's rehabilitation.

Clinical experience underscores the importance of peripheral nerve form and function to orthopaedic surgery. End-organ innervation is important to almost every orthopaedic procedure to ensure patient satisfaction and prevent surgical complications. This chapter provides an overview of the anatomy and physiology of peripheral nerves as well as an update on recent research advances relevant to the practice of orthopaedic surgery.

Cellular Anatomy

Peripheral Neurons

The neuron is the basic functional unit of both the peripheral nervous system and the central nervous system (CNS). Neurons are highly polarized cells containing a cell body and one or more axons that connect the neuron to the spinal cord or an end organ (Figure 1). Cell bodies contain the nucleus and most of the organelles necessary for cellular metabolism (such as the mitochondria) and for protein synthesis (such as the ribosomes and Golgi apparatus). Specialized cytoplasmic extensions called dendrites may protrude from the cell body and serve as receptors for upstream neurologic signaling. The cell body tapers into the axon in the axon hillock; this region is a narrow cellular process that may extend 1 m or more away from the cell body. Neurons communicate with one another through a synapse, which contains specialized cell membrane structures for biochemical signaling through neurotransmitters or for electrical conduction through ion exchange. A typical interneuron communication is initiated by the terminus of the axon,

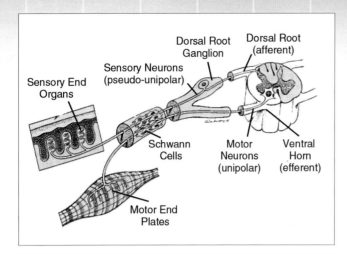

Figure 1 Schematic drawing showing the peripheral nervous system. Peripheral nerves carry afferent information from the sensory organs to the CNS and efferent information from the CNS to the skeletal muscles. (Adapted with permission from Lundborg G: Intraneural microcirculation. *Orthop Clin North Am* 1988;19:1-12.)

crosses the synapse, and is received by the dendrites of an adjacent cell.

The axon contains a highly specialized cytoskeletal network to facilitate intracellular transport and signal transduction. Bundles of microtubules and actin filaments run parallel to the direction of the axon. The microtubules provide a scaffold and support a variety of microtubule-associated proteins that carry out the intracellular transport functions of the axon. Specialized microtubule-associated proteins connect the microtubules to adjacent actin filaments and to a specialized class of cytoskeletal proteins called neurofilaments. The neurofilaments are oriented perpendicular to the axis of the axon and maintain the appropriate spacing between adjacent microtubules. Thus, the neurofilaments are required to allow intracellular movement of vesicles along the microtubules and through the axon.

Afferent signals are carried to the CNS through sensory neurons. These cells are pseudounipolar cells; they contain a single axon that branches immediately after extending away from the cell body. The cell bodies of the sensory neurons are bundled within the dorsal root ganglia, which are cellular nodules adjacent to the spinal cord containing specialized glial cells to support the sensory neuron cell bodies. The central branch of the sensory neuron extends away from the medial end of the dorsal root ganglion and is connected to the spinal cord by the dorsal horn. The peripheral branch emerges from the lateral end of the dorsal root ganglion and extends through the body. The axon terminal connects with sensory receptors primarily located in the muscular and cutaneous tissues.

Efferent signals from the CNS are transmitted to the muscles through motor neurons. These neurons are unipolar, consisting of cell bodies located in the ventral horn of the spinal cord and axons that exit the CNS and travel through the body. Dendrites within the spinal cord connect to neurons of the CNS and receive the efferent signals, which are transmitted along the axons to the end organs. At specialized synapses called neuromuscular junctions, alpha motor neurons innervate the extrafusal muscle fibers, which are capable of contraction to generate muscle movement. The terminal region of the motor axon typically branches several times and interfaces with the motor end plate, which is a highly excitable region of extrafusal muscle fiber where the neurotransmitters produced by the motor neuron are translated into a muscle contraction. A second class of motor neurons, called gamma motor neurons, are involved in the control of muscle contraction by providing proprioception to provide the brain with information about the position of the body. Although the anatomy of all motor neurons is similar, the conduction velocity of the gamma motor neurons is three to four times slower than that of the alpha motor neurons. This difference in conduction speed can be attributed to the smaller diameter of the gamma motor neurons (as explained in the section on nerve physiology).

Schwann Cells

The Schwann cell is the principal glial cell type in the peripheral nervous system. Schwann cells arise in the neural crest during fetal development, and they migrate with the extending neurites of the peripheral nervous system as they lengthen through the body, branch, and reach their terminal organs. Schwann cells play an important role in the process of radial sorting, in which they infiltrate the bundles of axons that innervate the soma to fully separate and associate with individual axons. By random interaction, Schwann cells adjacent to large-diameter axons become myelinating, but all other Schwann cells remain nonmyelinating. The myelinating Schwann cells wrap themselves tightly around the axon, forming as many as 100 revolutions, and then begin to produce myelin, a lipid-rich membrane, to insulate the axon. The footprint of each Schwann cell along the axon is approximately 100 μm. The spaces between Schwann cells are called the nodes of Ranvier. The nonmyelinating Schwann cells, also known as ensheathing Schwann cells, gather smaller-diameter axons into groups called Remak bundles and folds of the Schwann cells, inserted between the axons prevent the axons from touching.

Schwann cells have several functions in healthy nerves.[3] Myelinating Schwann cells are recognized for their effect on signal transduction, but all Schwann cells have important functions that are required to maintain normal nerve function. Like epithelial tissues, Schwann cells are connected by tight junctions and produce a basal lamina that separates the neuronal cells from the surrounding mesenchymal tissues. This structure generates a blood-nerve barrier. As an extension of the blood-brain barrier, the blood-nerve barrier tightly regulates which proteins are able to interact with the peripheral neurons. The Schwann cells produce a variety of neurotrophic factors including nerve growth factor–β,

Table 1
The Classification of Peripheral Nerve Fibers

Classification System					
Letter (Afferent and Efferent Fibers)	Numeral (Afferent Fibers)	Myelination	Central Axon Diameter (μm)	Conduction Velocity (m/s)	Typical Functions
Aα	Ia	Yes	13-22	70-120	Motor neurons, primary muscle spindle
Aα	Ib	Yes	13-22	70-120	Golgi tendon organs
Aβ	II	Yes	8-13	40-70	Touch, kinesthesia, secondary muscle spindle
Aγ		Yes	4-8	15-40	Motor neurons
Aδ	III	Yes	1-4	5-15	Pain (sharp or prickling), touch, temperature (cold), pressure
C	IV	No	0.1-1	0.2-2	Pain (aching or throbbing), temperature (heat)

brain-derived growth factor, insulin-like growth factor–1, and erythropoietin, which promote the survival of adjacent Schwann cells and the neurons they ensheath after routine minor damage. The Schwann cells are the primary cells responsible for coordinating regeneration of the nerve after traumatic injury.

Nerve Fibers
The neurons ensheathed by Schwann cells form a functional unit called a nerve fiber. Running through the center of these threadlike extensions is the axon of a single neuron. The axon is surrounded by the axolemma, which is a specialized membrane that maintains the membrane potential of the neuron. The Schwann cells surround the axolemma and may be myelinated to form a myelin sheath. The outermost layer of the Schwann cells is the neurolemma, which generates the basal lamina and the outside boundary of the nerve fiber.

Nerve fibers are classified based on the diameter of the central axon. One classification system uses Roman numerals to refer to afferent fibers only, and a second system uses letters of the Roman and Greek alphabets to refer to both afferent and efferent fibers (Table 1). By convention, the Roman numeral classification is used to describe sensory nerve fibers, and the letter classification is used to describe motor nerve fibers. The velocity of signal transduction through the axon is directly proportional to the diameter of the axon, which is determined during development based on the structure being innervated by the axon. Therefore, it is possible to correlate the function of an axon with its cross-

sectional diameter. Only afferent type C (or IV) sensory neurons are unmyelinated. Lack of myelin, coupled with their small diameter, results in the relatively slow signal transmission speed that is associated with type C sensory neurons.

Nerve Physiology
Electrochemical Physiology of Neurons
The primary function of peripheral neurons is to rapidly conduct electrical signals through the body. Peripheral neurons are able to perform this function because of the axolemma, which is populated by specialized ion-transporting protein channels that modulate the electrical potential across the plasma membrane. Like most cells in the body, peripheral neurons contain sodium-potassium pumps that establish the resting potential of the cell. These are active-transport ion pumps that require energy to function. In the unphosphorylated state, three sodium ion (Na^+) binding sites are exposed on the intracellular domain of the pump. When these binding sites have been occupied by Na^+, the complex can react with adenosine triphosphate (ATP) to phosphorylate the sodium-potassium pump, thereby initiating a conformational change of the protein that transports the Na^+ to the extracellular surface. As a result of this conformational change, the binding affinity of the ion pump to the Na^+ drops precipitously. In its phosphorylated state, the pump contains two potassium ion (K^+) binding domains on the extracellular surface. Upon binding with K^+, the protein dephosphorylates, shifts the protein back to its original conformation, and transports the K^+ inside the cell. The Na^+ re-

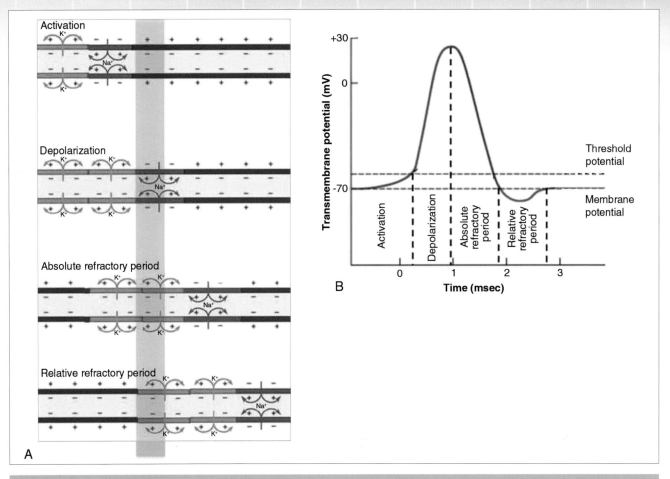

Figure 2 Schematic diagrams showing the action potential. **A,** The action potential at four time points during the propagation of the electrical current down the axon as the action of voltage-gated channels. **B,** The membrane potential of the shaded area in **(A)** is shown over time.

mains outside the cell; in contrast, the K⁺ can leak through the membrane by diffusion or specialized transmembrane proteins that serve as K⁺ leakage channels.

Resting potential is the term used to describe the electrical potential across the membrane of a cell in its inactive, unexcited state. This value is determined by the concentration of Na⁺ and K⁺ inside and outside the cell, and therefore it is highly sensitive to the number of sodium-potassium pumps on the cell membrane and the rate of K⁺ leakage back across the membrane. The resting potential of most nonneuronal cells is −10 to −30 mV. Neurons maintain a resting potential of approximately −70 mV, however, because of the high concentration of sodium-potassium pumps in the axolemma. It is estimated that the neuron expends almost two thirds of its energy output to maintain this high membrane potential, which makes the neurons a sufficiently excitable cell type to propagate signals rapidly throughout the body.

The transmission of signals along the neuron is made possible by voltage-gated channels, a specialized type of ion transporter. The voltage gated channels are transmembrane proteins containing a central channel that is designed to al-

low specific types of ions to move down their diffusion gradient, and therefore they do not require energy. However, electrochemical interactions with the transporter protein alter its conformation so that the ion channel is partially occluded when the membrane is at its resting potential. As the membrane crosses a specific threshold potential, the transporter can undergo a conformational change that opens the channel and allows ions to pass through, rapidly depolarizing the cell as the concentration on both sides of the membrane is normalized.

The Action Potential

Stimulation of neurons occurs to transmit information through the body. Motor neurons are stimulated by neurons in the spinal cord to transmit information controlling muscle contraction, and sensory neurons are stimulated by the sensory end organs to transmit information about the environment to the CNS. In response, the neuron undergoes a well-orchestrated depolarization process involving voltage-gated sodium and potassium channels, called the action potential (**Figure 2**). When the membrane potential increases to approximately −50 mV, voltage-gated sodium channels

Table 2

Sensory End Organs

End Organ	Location	Sensation
Merkel cell	Dermis	Sustained touch and pressure
Meissner corpuscle	Dermis	Light touch
Pacinian corpuscle	Dermis	Deep pressure and vibrations
Ruffini ending	Dermis	Sustained pressure
Free nerve ending	Epidermis	Pain
Nociceptor	Dermis, joints, muscles	Pain
Thermoreceptor	Dermis	Temperature
Golgi organ	Tendon	Muscle length and tension
Muscle spindle	Interfusal muscle fibers	Velocity of muscle movement

rapidly open to allow Na^+ to enter the cell, and the membrane potential spikes to more than 30 mV. However, this open-channel conformation is unstable and exists only for a fraction of a second before a second conformational change causes an inactivation gate to block the sodium channel, thereby stopping the flow of sodium ions. The rapid depolarization of the membrane also triggers the more slowly acting voltage-gated potassium channels to open and allows K^+ to exit the cell. The flow of K^+ from the cell has a longer duration than the flow of Na^+ into the cell, and the cell begins to repolarize as soon as the sodium channels close. The potassium channels do not have an inactivation gate, and they change conformation slowly after dropping back below the threshold potential. Therefore, they continue to allow K^+ out of the cell after the membrane potential exceeds the normal resting potential. As a result, the cell becomes hyperpolarized to approximately −75 mV. When the potassium channels have closed and the voltage-gated channels have been reset, the voltage across the membrane returns to the resting potential maintained by the sodium-potassium pumps.

The action potential enables the neuron to transmit a neural signal in response to a stimulus along its neuron. In motor neurons, depolarization first occurs in the dendrites, as neurotransmitters from the CNS are transmitted across a synapse in the spinal cord and trigger the opening of a sodium channel. The resulting electrical signals are graded potentials, which decrease in magnitude as the electrical potential is dissipated over the area of cell body. In sensory neurons, depolarization is initiated in the dendrites, where the dendrites interact with the sensory end organs (**Table 2**). In either case, if the magnitude of the signal is sufficient to trigger the voltage-gated channels in the axon hillock (< −55 mV) an axon potential will be propagated down the axon, and the magnitude of the axon potential will remain the same for the entire length of the axon. Thus, by triggering an action potential in the axon, the neuron generates an all-or-nothing response to the stimulus and ensures that any neural signal initiated at the beginning of an axon will be transmitted to the axon terminus.

The propagation of the action potential in one direction along the axon results from the refractory period of the axolemma. When an action potential is initiated at the axon hillock, this region of the neuron rapidly depolarizes, and the Na^+ transported into the cell begins to diffuse in both directions along the axon. As a result, the membrane potential just beyond the axon hillock exceeds the triggering potential of the voltage-gated sodium channels in that region, causing depolarization to spread further down the axon in a wavelike fashion. At every point along the axon where depolarization occurs, the Na^+ entering the cell diffuses along the axon in both directions. However, the voltage-gated sodium channels closer to the cell body are still in their inactive phase and cannot be triggered a second time until that region of the axolemma has been repolarized. The period in which the voltage-gated sodium channels cannot be reactivated, called the absolute refractory period, ensures that the action potential will propagate in only one direction along the axon toward its terminus. During the relative refractory period that follows the absolute refractory period, a larger-than-normal stimulus is required to propagate a second action potential as a result of the hyperpolarization phase of the previous action potential. The duration of these refractory periods can be determined experimentally by stimulating the neuron directly with a supermaximal electoral pulse, which will overcome the hyperpolarization of the membrane and trigger an antidromic volley characterized as an action potential transmitted in the reverse direction.[4]

The action potential can travel down along the axolemma at 5 to 20 m/s. Given the length of human extremities, these propagation rates could result in unsatisfactory delays in resultant signal transmission. The speed of the action potential is directly proportional to the diameter of the axon; larger axons allow more freedom of movement for the Na^+ along the axon to trigger the adjacent voltage-gated channels. Myelination increases the propagation speed

2: Physiology of Musculoskeletal Tissues

without increasing the diameter of the axon. Myelin is primarily made from a dielectric lipid called galactocerebroside. A myelin sheath prevents the electrical current associated with the action potential from leaking away from the axon and instead allows it to propagate through the electrically conductive axoplasm in a process called saltatory conduction. As a result, the action potential jumps along the axon to voltage-gated channels concentrated at the nodes of Ranvier, and it propagates the signal at approximately 100 m/s.

When the action potential reaches the axon terminal, the electrical signal is translated into a chemical signal for transmission across the synapse. Specialized intercellular signaling molecules called neurotransmitters are packaged into vesicles by the neurons and positioned in an organized cytoskeletal network in the presynaptic active zone. As the action potential reaches this active zone, voltage-gated calcium ion (Ca^{2+}) channels on the presynaptic membrane open and allow Ca^{2+} to enter the axon terminal. The Ca^{2+} reacts with several proteins associated with the cytoskeleton and vesicle to stimulate the vesicle to fuse with the presynaptic membrane, thereby releasing the neurotransmitters into the synapse. Neurotransmitter receptors on the postsynaptic membranes bind with these neurotransmitters and translate the chemical signal back into an electrical signal to continue the transmission.

Maintenance and Homeostasis of the Neuron

To perform their primary function, neurons have evolved into specialized structures that allow them to span large distances in the body. As a result, the intracellular functions required to maintain the metabolism of the neuron must occur over a length several times larger than that of any other cell type. Nonetheless, most intracellular functions related to gene expression and protein synthesis occur within the cell body, where they can occur in close proximity to the nucleus. The protein products then can be transported throughout the neuron to wherever they are needed. Other cellular functions, such as cellular respiration, can be effectively distributed throughout the entire length of the cell.

Neurons maintain a high level of energy expenditure to sustain their resting potential and restore membrane polarity after each action potential. As a result, the density of mitochondria is high throughout the axon for the purpose of generating ATP. The mitochondria are concentrated at the nodes of Ranvier in myelinated axons, where the energy demand is the greatest. A substantial amount of glucose must be metabolized by these mitochondria to serve as the primary source of metabolic energy for the peripheral neurons. Glucose can be transported directly from the adjacent capillaries through glucose transporters located in the nodes of Ranvier. Schwann cells also can facilitate glucose uptake by transporting glucose out of the capillaries and passing it through neuroglial contacts at the interface between the axolemma and the Schwann cell membranes. By distributing the mechanisms of metabolic energy generation, the neuron can ensure an adequate supply of ATP and maintain an excitable state.

Although neurotransmitters are released by the neurons at their axon terminals, the protein synthesis associated with these molecules occurs in the cell body. The primary neurotransmitters in the peripheral nervous system are acetylcholine and noradrenaline. These nonpeptide molecules are produced by enzymes in the axon terminus and are transported into vesicles for release into the synapse. All of the proteins and enzymes that coordinate neurotransmitter production and packaging are synthesized in the cell body and are transported into the terminus through mechanisms of slow-axonal anterograde transport (0.5 to 5 mm/day). A variety of involved neuropeptides (such as substance P and calcitonin gene-related peptide) interact with neurotransmitter-based signaling; their role in pain perception has been most extensively studied.[5] Neuropeptides are synthesized in the endoplasmic reticulum of the cell body, processed in the Golgi apparatus, and transported along the axon in vesicles to the terminus by fast-axonal anterograde transport (up to 400 mm/day).

Neuron functionality requires the neuron to maintain an active innervation with a healthy end organ. To provide a biochemical signal back to the neuron to indicate connectivity, the end organ produces neurotrophic factors. Although multiple neurotrophic factors are believed to perform various functions for this feedback mechanism, it has been studied most extensively in nerve growth factor.[6] When nerve growth factor has bound with its receptor on the presynaptic membrane, the receptors become endocytosed into a vesicle that is transported through slow-axonal retrograde transport along the axon. Upon arrival in the cell body, the vesicle-bound nerve growth factor promotes survival as well as the upregulation of various functions related to neuron function. Nerve growth factor also may initiate an intracellular signaling cascade at the axon terminus to antagonize a constitutive apoptotic signal.[7] In the absence of nerve growth factor, the mediators of apoptosis are retrogradely transported along the axis into the cell body,[8] thereby signaling that the nerve has lost its end-organ connection and should undergo apoptosis.

This mechanism is useful to ensure that the neuron is correctly innervating the appropriate target. A series of experiments by Brushart demonstrated aspects of the interaction between rat femoral nerves with mixed sensory and motor neurons; they show that motor neurons preferentially reinnervate the motor branch even when there is a situation of purposeful misalignment or gapping. The interaction or signal is independent of mechanical axon alignment.[9] Further studies demonstrated a mechanism for preferential motor reinnervation (PMR), namely selective "pruning" of sprouting regenerating nerves.[10] Thus, if the cell body receives a biochemical signal indicating that the axon has lost its end-organ connection or has become improperly reinnervated, it can undergo pruning by programmed cell death to avoid inappropriate neuronal signaling.

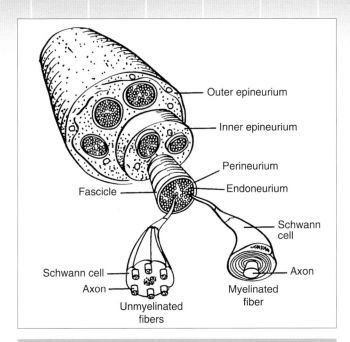

Figure 3 Schematic drawing showing the gross anatomy of a peripheral nerve. In cross section, the epineurium, perineurium, and endoneurium can be identified in relation to myelinated and unmyelinated nerve fibers. (Adapted with permission from Diao E, Vannuyen T: Techniques for primary nerve repair. *Hand Clinics* 2000;16[1]:54.)

Gross Anatomy

Nerve Organization

The nerve fibers travel from the spinal cord to their end organs inside peripheral nerves (**Figure 3**). These structures have a high content of extracellular matrix proteins, particularly collagen type I, which provides mechanical strength to protect the axons and the supporting Schwann cells. The nerve fibers also provide a framework for the delicate vascular network required to nourish these neuronal cell types. Based on their function and location relative to the axon bundles, the connective tissues of the peripheral nerve are classified as the endoneurium, perineurium, or epineurium.

Endoneurium is located directly adjacent to the nerve fibers and produced by endoneurial fibroblasts, which are derived from the neural crest and migrate into the soma with the Schwann cells during development.[11] These cells form collagen sheaths around the axons, which support the capillaries that provide nutrients to the Schwann cells. The cells of the endoneurium also produce a low-protein aqueous solution called endoneurial fluid that is similar to the cerebrospinal fluid and provides mechanical support, protection from physical insult, and metabolic stability for the cells in the peripheral neuron. Each axon, with its surrounding myelin sheath, supporting Schwann cells, and endoneurium, constitutes a nerve fiber. Perineurium surrounds the nerve fibers and forms bundles known as fascicles. Perineurium is generated by mesenchymal cells, which form concentrically around the fascicles and generate protective layers of extra-

cellular matrix. As a result, the perineurium consists of seven or eight layers of fibrous tissue in a lamellar arrangement. Myoepithelioid cells that line the perineurium are connected by tight junctions and provide a diffusion barrier for the nerve, acting as an extension of the blood-brain barrier. The myoepithelioid cells also maintain positive fluid pressure within the perineurium, and this component of the nerve provides the greatest resistance to compressive injury.

Epineurium is the outermost connective tissue component of the nerve; it has an external and an internal part. The external epineurium is an extension of the dural sleeve of the spinal cord. This tough, fibrous sheath primarily consists of collagen type I. The external layer generates most of the tensile strength of the nerve and provides an anchor for blood vessels to enter the nerve. The internal epineurium contains collagen type I but also has a high content of collagen types III and IV. As a result, the arrangement of the internal epineurium is less lamellar than that of the external epineurium. Instead, the internal epineurium generates a spongy extracellular matrix that cushions the fascicles and internal blood vessels from exterior forces.

Nerve Topography

Sunderland's classic work on the internal topography of nerve fascicles emphasized the intraneural fascicular arrangement along the nerve.[12] By examining nerve cross sections level by level and millimeter by millimeter, Sunderland constructed a three-dimensional diagram to show the arrangement of fascicles in a short, proximal segment of the musculocutaneous nerve. He found the cross sections of the fascicles to be modified continually along the entire length of the nerve because of repeated division, anastomosis, and migration of the fascicular bundles. However, this complex fiber bundling occurs only in the proximal portion of the extremity nerves. The motor and sensory fibers are progressively sorted out as they travel distally and approach the motor or sensory end organs, and there is an indirect relationship between the number of plexus formations and the distance from the brachial plexus to the end organ.[13] Moreover, interfascicular plexi are more common in nerves with mixed function, carrying both motor and sensory fibers, as well as in nerves with a wide sensory distribution or innervating multiple muscles.

The fibers within a fascicle also are organized by the anatomic locations they eventually innervate. The route of nerve fibers within individual fascicles can be followed over long distances by using the Brushart retrograde horseradish tracer technique.[3,14] Chow et al.[15] developed methods to identify distinct motor and sensory fascicles within nerves and traced them to exact anatomic points, where they were joined and became indistinguishable. These studies indicate that adjacent fascicles within the nerve fiber innervate adjacent anatomic locations. The bundles are separate and readily identifiable, and group fascicular repair has been promoted as a means of aligning the proximal and distal motor and sensory stumps during surgical repair.

2: Physiology of Musculoskeletal Tissues

Blood Supply

The peripheral nerves do not have a dedicated vasculature but instead rely on offshoots from nearby arteries and veins for blood exchange. Most nerves are located in anatomic proximity to the primary blood vessels running to the extremities or the large vessels within muscles, and branches from these vessels connect with the epineurium. These arteries typically branch one or more times before passing through the exterior epineurium, and they form a vascular plexus within the interior epineurium that surrounds the nerve fascicles. Smaller vessels branch from this network, penetrate the perineurium, and connect with the intrafascicular capillary plexus that surrounds the individual nerve fibers to provide nutrient and waste product exchange. Blood drains from the capillary plexus into the vascular plexus and leaves the nerve through veins that penetrate the epineurium in a structure that is the reverse of the arteries feeding into the nerve. These dense networks of vessels ensure a robust and redundant blood supply for nourishing the neural cells and enabling a rapid response to nerve injury.

Dorsal Root Ganglia

The dorsal root ganglia form an extension of the spinal cord outside the spinal dura and therefore are considered to be part of the peripheral nervous system. They consist of the clustered cell bodies of the pseudounipolar sensory neurons. The dorsal root ganglia do not contain Schwann cells but instead are populated by satellite cells, which are a specialized type of glial cell. These cells surround the sensory neuron bodies within the ganglia and supply neurotrophic factors to the adjacent neurons. The satellite cells are believed to serve a structural function by protectively cushioning the neurons. The neurons and satellite cells are surrounded by an extension of the endoneurium, which supports the capillary network for the dorsal root ganglia. The perineurium and epineurium of the peripheral nerve extends around the ganglion to provide mechanical strength to these structures.

Nerve Injury

Acute Response to Nerve Injury

Peripheral nerves respond to injury by undergoing a well-orchestrated sequence of pathophysiologic processes (**Figure 4**). These processes include a multitude of predictable changes that are initiated at the specific site of nerve injury and spread throughout the cell to the cell body and all points along the distal nerve segment, extending to the end organ, motor end plates, or specialized sensory receptors. Within hours of the injury, chromatolysis can be observed in the cell body as the cell rapidly depletes its intracellular stores of neurotransmitter precursors. A change in the appearance of the cell can be seen under light microscopy. Simultaneously, the nucleus begins to migrate to a peripheral location near the axon hillock, the cell body becomes

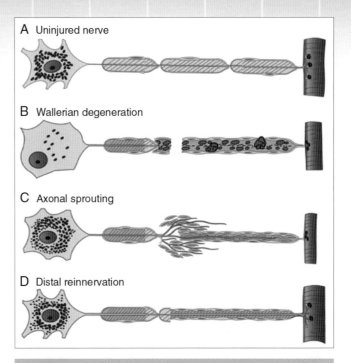

Figure 4 Schematic drawing showing four stages in peripheral nerve regeneration. After a segmentation injury to an uninjured nerve (**A**), the peripheral nerve fiber undergoes a predictable series of events to enable regeneration of the axon (**B** and **C**) and eventual reinnervation of the target organ (**D**). (Adapted with permission from Waxman SG: *Clinical Neuroanatomy*, ed 26. New York, NY, McGraw-Hill Medical, 2009.)

rounded, and RNA transcription is significantly upregulated. The cellular metabolism is altered as the neuron shifts from production of neurotransmitters to the synthesis of membrane and cytoskeletal proteins, especially tubulin, in an effort to reconstruct the axon. The biochemical changes throughout the nerve fiber include a marked increase in lipid synthesis to replenish the Schwann cell membranes.

Injury to the peripheral nerve initiates an acute immune response. Mast cells in the endoneurium may be directly stimulated by mechanical forces, as in a crush injury, and respond by rapid degranulation to release several immunomodulatory molecules, such as histamine, serotonin, and activated extracellular proteases.[16] Histamine and serotonin act on the endothelium of the adjacent capillary plexus by upregulating the surface expression of nitric oxide and P-selectin. P-selectin is a cell-to-cell adhesion protein that is critical for initiating an immune response. If the capillary network becomes compromised, circulating platelets may be activated through contact with the extracellular matrix and undergo degranulation to release inflammatory cytokines, complement factors, and surface P-selectin. Circulating neutrophils can become attached to the exposed P-selectin at the site of injury and infiltrate the wound, releasing additional extracellular proteases and reactive oxygen species to facilitate degeneration of the tissue in the region of the injury and maintain tissue sterility.

The neutrophils release proinflammatory cytokines that promote macrophage proliferation. Peripheral nerves contain a resident population of macrophages that migrate into the endoneurium through the capillary plexus and migrate through the tissue.[17] Approximately 50% of the endoneurial macrophages turn over after 12 weeks of injury by returning to the vasculature and are replaced by new macrophages. These cells normally act as dedicated antigen-presenting cells by extending cellular processes into the connective tissue, endocytosing threat antigens, and presenting the antigens to activated T cells. The resident endoneurial macrophages also provide a reservoir of macrophages that can respond to early injury signals by proliferating and initiating an inflammatory response. This response is particularly important after a crush injury, when the blood flow to the injury region may be compromised. However, the initial inflammatory response attracts circulating monocytes into the wound, and they subsequently differentiate into hematogenous macrophages. Both populations of macrophages play an important role in clearing the damaged nerve components through wallerian degeneration.

Wallerian Degeneration

In 1850, Waller described the events that occur in distal segments of peripheral nerves after injury, based on observation of severed frog glossopharyngeal and hypoglossal nerves.[18] The process of wallerian degeneration specifically refers to the events that occur in the distal nerve segments of myelinated nerves and extend proximally, usually for the distance of one node of Ranvier. Within hours of injury, damaged axons from the proximal ends of the nerve are sealed, and the distal axon remnants have significant increases in intracellular Ca^{2+} flux through ion-specific channels. Elevated intracellular Ca^{2+} concentrations in these distal axons activate calcium-dependent proteases, which autodigest the cell membrane and lead to the formation of numerous axonal membrane fragments.[19] As a result, the axon and its myelin sheath are broken down. During this time, the contents of the neural tube appear turbid and granular. The proliferating macrophages subsequently migrate into the tube to phagocytize and digest the axonal and myelin debris. Complete axoplasmic clearance along the entire length of the distal segment can require as long as 3 months. The macrophages stimulate the Schwann cells to begin proliferating and produce cytokines important in coordinating the early phases of nerve regeneration. In particular, the Schwann cells produce interleukin-1, which triggers local production of nerve growth factor as well as insulin-like growth factor–1, which promotes the growth of axons.

As the axon is autodigested, the endoneurial tube, consisting of the intact endoneurium, basement membrane, and adjacent Schwann cells, shrinks in diameter. When the axon has been completely resorbed, the Schwann cells and macrophages fill the volume of the tube. The Schwann cell–filled tubes are called the bands of Bunger. In preparation for reinnervation, the Schwann cells upregulate the expression of nerve growth factor receptors and the neural cell adhesion molecule on their surface, and they begin generating an extracellular matrix rich in the growth promoters tenascin and laminin.[20] As a result, the bands of Bunger are a highly inductive environment for axonal growth.

Nerve Regeneration

Nerve regeneration begins within 6 hours of nerve injury. As the distal segments of the neuron are being digested through wallerian degeneration, axons begin to sprout within several millimeters from the transection at the terminal nodes of Ranvier. The initial axonal sprouts typically are unstable because they are formed before the neuron has fully shifted to a regenerative metabolism, and usually they are resorbed within hours. Approximately 27 hours after the injury, permanent axonal sprouts emerge that contain a fully functional internal cytoskeleton with an actin-rich filopodia at the distal end.[21] This growth cone advances along the fibronectin- and laminin-rich regions of the bands of Bunger and preferentially directs axon growth through the inner surfaces of Schwann cell basal laminae.[22,23] Upon reaching the appropriate distal end organ or receptor, the forward movement of the axon is terminated, and the growth cone becomes a functional synaptic terminal. Eventually, axon sprouts that do not reach an end organ or a neuromuscular junction are pruned away. At first, all of the axon sprouts are unmyelinated, regardless of whether the parent nerve was myelinated. Schwann cells continue to proliferate at both the proximal and distal stumps as the axon elongates, and they initiate myelination of the appropriate nerve fibers when the axons have reached their targets.

The functional outcome of regenerating nerves depends on the rate of axon extension and the specificity with which the regenerating axons reach their end organs. The term neurotrophism refers to factors that promote fiber maturation and regeneration, and the term neurotropism refers to the selective guidance of an end organ or distal conduit. The belief that axons preferentially determine their direction of growth to extend toward an appropriate target arose as a result of experiments showing how peripheral nerves regenerate across small gaps.[24] These and other experiments suggest that the distal nerve stump generates neurotrophic factors that provide growth and guidance signals to axon sprouts.[25] Schwann cells located in the motor tubes produce a different profile of neurotrophic factors as compared to Schwann cells located in the sensory tubes of the distal stump, and the differential neurotrophic factor profiles further support specificity during nerve regeneration.[26] If a mixed nerve is transected, the regenerating motor axons preferentially reinnervate distal motor fibers, despite intentional misalignment of stumps, although a critical distance of 5 mm between the proximal and distal stumps is necessary for

2: Physiology of Musculoskeletal Tissues

optimal neurotropic effects to influence preferential motor nerve growth. There is both topographic and end-organ specificity for motor and sensory neurons. This phenomenon of end-organ specificity helps to ensure that the muscle fibers, muscle spindles, and sensory nerve endings are reinnervated by the correct type of neuron.

The rate of nerve regeneration can vary widely and has been estimated at 1 to 4.5 mm/day. This rate can be measured clinically by observing the position of the Tinel sign, in which a prickly, pins-and-needles sensation is elicited by tapping over the leading edge of a regenerating nerve. The rate of Tinel sign movement most often is 1 to 2 mm/day.[27] Axonal sprouting and growth are more vigorous when cellular debris can be rapidly cleared away from the repair site. Conversely, distal sprout progression can be delayed for several days to weeks because of scar tissue formation within the perineurium near the site of nerve transection. Exuberant proliferation of Schwann cells also can impede axonal regeneration if the nerve endings are not approximated. Failure of the position of the Tinel sign to advance over time probably indicates that nerve regeneration has been obstructed. As a result, the regenerating axons will fail to reach their end organs, and a local neuroma may form. Clinically, this process can lead to chronic pain, and functional recovery of the end organs may not be possible.

Somatic Effects of Nerve Injury

Denervation of skeletal muscle tissue is associated with several well-documented sequelae. Within one week of denervation, muscles begin to lose bulk, with marked atrophy, and splintering of muscle fibers can be observed at a microscopic level. Muscle tissue that has not been innervated after approximately 3 months will begin to develop interstitial fibrosis as fibroblasts begin to proliferate and deposit collagen around the atrophying fibers. This process begins in the perimysium. As the perimysium surrounding the muscle fibers thickens, it begins to physically separate atrophied muscle fibers. The fibroblasts eventually become pervasive in the endomysium, and the fibrosis radiates inward and throughout the muscle tissue. Poor functional recovery after a long period of denervation primarily is the result of fibrotic interference along the intramuscular nerve pathways, rather than atrophy of muscle itself. The use of passive motion and splinting may help prevent this fibrosis during denervation, but the return of muscle function after reinnervation primarily depends on the duration of denervation. The best functional outcomes can be expected if reinnervation occurs within 1 to 3 months of denervation; some functional reinnervation can be expected for as long as 1 year, and no further reinnervation can reasonably be expected after 3 years.

Unlike muscle, most sensory organs can be reinnervated for years after the initial injury. No upper limit has been defined for the time period in which restoration of useful sensation is likely to occur. However, a nerve repair more than 6 months after the injury is relatively unlikely to lead to the return of functional sensation, as characterized, for example, by an increase in the distance required for two-point discrimination. Interestingly, nerve growth factor produced by nociceptive receptors has been shown to stimulate collateral axonal sprouting by adjacent, intact nociceptive neurons and to innervate areas in which injured axons do not regenerate. As a result, the regions with nociception may continue to expand after successful reinnervation. This process apparently does not occur for axons involved in mechanoreception, however. Pacinian corpuscles become filled with fibrous tissue after denervation, and a mechanical obstruction physically prevents reinnervation. Other mechanoreceptors, including Ruffini endings, Merkel cells, and Meissner corpuscles, also can be reinnervated with some success, although reinnervation is not always correlated with clinical test results or subjective sensation.

Nerve Injury Classification

Nerve injuries were classified by Seddon et al[28,29] in 1943, with the classification expanded by Sunderland[30] in 1951 and later refined by Mackinnon and Dellon[31] (**Table 3**). The Seddon classification includes three types of injuries: neurapraxia, axonotmesis, and neurotmesis. Sunderland specified five degrees of injury, and Mackinnon and Dellon added a sixth degree of injury to indicate the simultaneous occurrence of several injury types at separate locations within a nerve.

Neurapraxia, or first-degree injury, essentially is a local conduction block resulting in paralysis but no peripheral degeneration. Despite injury at a discrete point along the nerve fibers, the nerve factors remain intact and wallerian degeneration does not occur. Full recovery can be expected; the time required varies from a few minutes to several days or weeks. The nerve may appear grossly normal, but histologic analysis may reveal demyelinated segments of the nerve fiber. Without any axonal damage, nerve regeneration will not accompany recovery. A Tinel sign will not be present at the site of injury, nor will an advancing Tinel sign be seen. Neurapraxia typically is resolved within 12 weeks.

Axonotmesis, or second-degree injury, is a nerve injury with damage to the axon leading to wallerian degeneration distally and regeneration with axonal sprouting at the proximal nerve stump. The supporting endoneurium and perineurium remain intact and are available to direct the mechanisms of regeneration along the proper path. Concomitantly, a Tinel sign is apparent at the level of injury and advances distally as the nerve regenerates. The classic rate of nerve recovery is 1 inch per month or 1.5 mm per day. Most importantly, the Schwann cell basement membrane is not damaged, and therefore full recovery of motor and sensory function to preinjury levels may occur. Diagnosis of this extent of nerve injury is made only after recovery occurs.

Sunderland's third-degree nerve injury differs from a second-degree injury (axonotmesis) in that it includes endoneurial damage and subsequent scarring. Regeneration will be incomplete, as fibrotic scar tissue becomes a barrier

Table 3

The Classification of Nerve Injuries

Seddon[28,29]	Sunderland-Mackinnon[30,31]	Injury	Recovery Potential
Neurapraxia	I	Ionic block with segmental demyelinization	Complete
Axonotmesis	II	Axon severed Intact endoneurium	Complete
	III	Axon severed Torn endoneurium	Incomplete
	IV	Severed endoneurium Epineurium intact	Neuroma
Neurotmesis	V	Loss of nerve continuity Epineurium severed	None
	VI	Combination (types I through V)	Unpredictable

that prevents the nerve fibers from reaching their end organs or receptors. The internal structure of fascicles becomes disorganized, although the fascicles remain in continuity. There is a greater risk of mismatched fibers and receptors because the Schwann cell basal lamina and endoneurial tubes were destroyed. This type of injury occurs within an intact perineurium, and fibers within the perineurium are likely to regenerate appropriately. Recovery occurs as the Tinel sign advances and at the same rate as after a second-degree injury, but it will not be complete. The extent of regeneration depends on several factors: the level of injury; whether the fascicles are mixed (as in the proximal extremity) or pure (as in the distal extremity); and the extent of the scar tissue impeding regeneration. Outcomes associated with this type of injury are variable; complete functional recovery is possible, but some loss of function is to be expected.

Sunderland describes a fourth-degree injury as involving complete disorganization of the internal structure of the nerve and loss of functionality but no damage to the epineurium. Therefore, the physical continuity of the nerve remains intact. Although the nerve trunk itself is preserved, the mechanism of functional impairment can be attributed to continuous scar tissue throughout the nerve, so that the fascicles themselves are no longer intact. Wallerian degeneration occurs distally, but proximal nerve regeneration is prevented by scar tissue. The Tinel sign is present only at the injury level and will not advance distally. Because proximal regeneration has been obstructed, there cannot be motor or sensory recovery after a fourth-degree injury. Most fourth-degree injuries are caused by significant stretch or traction of the nerve. Only surgical intervention can allow any recovery, but no surgery should be undertaken for at least 3 months after the injury to allow any possible recovery and to rule out the presence of a first-, second-, or third-degree nerve injury. If there is no evidence of recovery, a fourth-degree injury can be diagnosed, and surgical intervention is indicated.

Neurotmesis, or fifth-degree injury, is complete transaction of the nerve trunk. This most severe form of site-specific nerve disruption is characterized by significant disorganization of the nerve microarchitecture and macroarchitecture because the nerve envelope has lost all continuity. This type of injury often leads to the formation of a neuroma. Surgical intervention provides the only hope of restoring any nerve function. Early surgical exploration may be indicated because neurotmesis often occurs with an open injury leading to associated peripheral nerve deficit.

The sixth-degree injury represents the presence of all or several of Sunderland's injury classifications within the same zone of injury. Sixth-degree injury can accurately be identified in the neuroma incontinuity injury, in which the pattern of injury is mixed in the various fascicles and is followed by a varying amount of regeneration. No regeneration may occur in the areas characterized by fourth- or fifth-degree injury, but complete regeneration may be possible in adjacent sections of nerve characterized by first-, second-, or third-degree injury. The surgeon is responsible for a careful functional assessment of each nerve fascicle and group of fascicles to determine which lesions are likely to require surgical intervention.

Compression Injury

Compression nerve injuries, also called entrapment neuropathies, are caused by cumulative, chronic nerve damage rather than by acute nerve damage.[32] Generally, compression nerve injuries are caused by repetitive stress in a region where the nerves pass through a fibrous tunnel near a joint bridging two body segments, as in carpal tunnel syndrome.[33,34] The etiology of compression injuries is largely unknown, but it is assumed that repeated mechanical loading of the nerve leads to mast cell activation, degranulation, and the release of vasodilators such as histamine. The resulting edema causes the endoneurial pressure to rise because there is no lymphatic component in the endoneurium to allow the fluid to drain out of the tissue. Over time, the region becomes more susceptible to mechanically activated mast cells, and the result is escalating edema and discomfort.

Increasing edema-caused fluid pressure can eventually constrict the vasculature that allows transport of fresh blood into the endoneurium. Poor circulation in the vicinity of the nerve fibers leads to tissue ischemia and accumulation of cellular by-products, including free radicals that initiate further cell and tissue damage. Circulating immune cells respond to the tissue damage by infiltrating the region and initiating an inflammatory response. Over time, chronic inflammation can dysregulate the reparative cell types and promote the formation of fibrotic tissues and neovascularization. The formation of fibrotic lesions within the nerve causes additional discomfort and nerve dysfunction. This vicious cycle can be interrupted surgically by releasing the ligaments that are constraining the nerve, thus relieving pressure at the joint. This procedure usually is sufficient to reduce the tissue edema, allowing resolution of the inflammatory response and restoring normal function to the nerve.[35] However, the disease can become irreversible and similar to axonotmesis if fibrotic lesion formation becomes exuberant and interferes with the continuity of adjacent nerve fibers.

Summary

The orthopaedic specialist must have a thorough understanding of normal and abnormal peripheral nervous system function as well as the probable natural history of specific nerve injuries, if recovery is to be maximized. After some injuries, the body's own ability to repair and regenerate the peripheral nerves must be carefully monitored. After other injuries, however, optimal management requires acute surgical repair of severed nerves to allow the regeneration process to occur. Nerve grafts or nerve transfers may be indicated for certain injuries. For nerve injuries where little functional regeneration is expected, muscle transfers allow sufficient reinnervation to a portion of the tissue required for mobility. In other cases joint fusion may be appropriate to maximize limb function when a part of the musculature is not expected to regain function. The therapeutic options continue to expand as the understanding of neural function expands and methods are developed for enhancing nerve function and regeneration by manipulating the mechanical and biologic signaling that controls these processes.

References

1. Vogler JA, Jackson WM, Nesti LJ: Tissue engineering and regeneration, in Owens BD, Belmint PJ, eds: *Combat Orthopaedic Surgery: Lessons Learned in Iraq and Afghanistan.* Thorofare, NJ, Slack, 2011, pp 101-108.

2. Beltran MJ, Anderson RC, Hsu JR: Lower extremity limb salvage, in Owens BD, Belmint PJ, eds: *Combat Orthopaedic Surgery: Lessons Learned in Iraq and Afghanistan.* Thorofare, NJ, Slack, 2011, pp 193-204.

3. Campana WM: Schwann cells: Activated peripheral glia and their role in neuropathic pain. *Brain Behav Immun* 2007; 21(5):522-527.

4. Boërio D, Hogrel JY, Créange A, Lefaucheur JP: A reappraisal of various methods for measuring motor nerve refractory period in humans. *Clin Neurophysiol* 2005;116(4): 969-976.

5. Birklein F, Schmelz M: Neuropeptides, neurogenic inflammation and complex regional pain syndrome (CRPS). *Neurosci Lett* 2008;437(3):199-202.

6. Campenot RB, MacInnis BL: Retrograde transport of neurotrophins: Fact and function. *J Neurobiol* 2004;58(2):217-229.

7. MacInnis BL, Campenot RB: Retrograde support of neuronal survival without retrograde transport of nerve growth factor. *Science* 2002;295(5559):1536-1539.

8. Mok SA, Lund K, Campenot RB: A retrograde apoptotic signal originating in NGF-deprived distal axons of rat sympathetic neurons in compartmented cultures. *Cell Res* 2009; 19(5):546-560.

9. Brushart TM: Preferential reinnervation of motor nerves by regenerating motor axons. *J Neurosci* 1988;8(3):1026-1031.

10. Brushart TM: Motor axons preferentially reinnervate motor pathways. *J Neurosci* 1993;13(6):2730-2738.

11. Joseph NM, Mukouyama YS, Mosher JT, et al: Neural crest stem cells undergo multilineage differentiation in developing peripheral nerves to generate endoneurial fibroblasts in addition to Schwann cells. *Development* 2004;131(22):5599-5612.

12. Sunderland S: The intraneural topography of the radial, median and ulnar nerves. *Brain* 1945;68:243-299.

13. Diao E, Vannuyen T: Techniques for primary nerve repair. *Hand Clin* 2000;16(1):53-66, viii.

14. Brushart TM, Tarlov EC, Mesulam MM: Specificity of muscle reinnervation after epineurial and individual fascicular suture of the rat sciatic nerve. *J Hand Surg Am* 1983;8(3): 248-253.

15. Chow JA, Van Beek AL, Bilos ZJ, Meyer DL, Johnson MC: Anatomical basis for repair of ulnar and median nerves in the distal part of the forearm by group fascicular suture and nerve-grafting. *J Bone Joint Surg Am* 1986;68(2):273-280.

16. Olsson Y: Degranulation of mast cells in peripheral nerve injuries. *Acta Neurol Scand* 1967;43(3):365-374.

17. Müller M, Leonhard C, Krauthausen M, Wacker K, Kiefer R: On the longevity of resident endoneurial macrophages in the peripheral nervous system: A study of physiological macrophage turnover in bone marrow chimeric mice. *J Peripher Nerv Syst* 2010;15(4):357-365.

18. Waller AV: Experiments on the plossopharyngeal and hypoglossal nerves of the frog and observations produced thereby in the structure of their primitive fibres. *Philos Trans R Soc Lond B Biol Sci* 1850;140:450.

19. George EB, Glass JD, Griffin JW: Axotomy-induced axonal degeneration is mediated by calcium influx through ion-specific channels. *J Neurosci* 1995;15(10):6445-6452.

20. Gundersen RW: Response of sensory neurites and growth

cones to patterned substrata of laminin and fibronectin in vitro. *Dev Biol* 1987;121(2):423-431.

21. Yamada KM, Spooner BS, Wessells NK: Ultrastructure and function of growth cones and axons of cultured nerve cells. *J Cell Biol* 1971;49(3):614-635.

22. Letourneau PC: Cell-substratum adhesion of neurite growth cones, and its role in neurite elongation. *Exp Cell Res* 1979;124(1):127-138.

23. Ide C, Tohyama K, Yokota R, Nitatori T, Onodera S: Schwann cell basal lamina and nerve regeneration. *Brain Res* 1983;288(1-2):61-75.

24. Politis MJ, Ederle K, Spencer PS: Tropism in nerve regeneration in vivo: Attraction of regenerating axons by diffusible factors derived from cells in distal nerve stumps of transected peripheral nerves. *Brain Res* 1982;253(1-2):1-12.

25. Lundborg G, Dahlin L, Danielsen N, Zhao Q: Trophism, tropism, and specificity in nerve regeneration. *J Reconstr Microsurg* 1994;10(5):345-354.

26. Höke A, Redett R, Hameed H, et al: Schwann cells express motor and sensory phenotypes that regulate axon regeneration. *J Neurosci* 2006;26(38):9646-9655.

27. Tinel J: *Nerve Wounds.* London, England, Balliere, Tindall and Cox, 1917.

28. Seddon HJ, Medawar PB, Smith H: Rate of regeneration of peripheral nerves in man. *J Physiol* 1943;102(2):191-215.

29. Seddon HJ: Three types of nerve injury. *Brain* 1943;66(4):237-288.

30. Sunderland S: A classification of peripheral nerve injuries producing loss of function. *Brain* 1951;74(4):491-516.

31. Mackinnon SE, Dellon AL: Classification of nerve injuries as the basis for treatment, in *Surgery of the Peripheral Nerve.* New York, NY, Thieme, 1988, pp 35-63.

32. Rempel DM, Diao E: Entrapment neuropathies: Pathophysiology and pathogenesis. *J Electromyogr Kinesiol* 2004;14(1):71-75.

33. Diao E, Shao F, Liebenberg E, Rempel D, Lotz JC: Carpal tunnel pressure alters median nerve function in a dose-dependent manner: A rabbit model for carpal tunnel syndrome. *J Orthop Res* 2005;23(1):218-223.

34. Yoshii Y, Zhao C, Zhao KD, Zobitz ME, An KN, Amadio PC: The effect of wrist position on the relative motion of tendon, nerve, and subsynovial connective tissue within the carpal tunnel in a human cadaver model. *J Orthop Res* 2008;26(8):1153-1158.

35. Ablove RH, Moy OJ, Peimer CA, Wheeler DR, Diao E: Pressure changes in Guyon's canal after carpal tunnel release. *J Hand Surg Br* 1996;21(5):664-665.

2: Physiology of Musculoskeletal Tissues

Chapter 15

Form and Function of the Intervertebral Disk

Isaac L. Moss, MD, MASc, FRCSC

Howard S. An, MD

Anatomy and Development

The vertebral column is the main component of the axial spine. The 24 segments of the vertebral column traditionally are divided into the cervical, thoracic, and lumbar regions, which are composed of 7, 12, and 5 vertebrae, respectively. With the exception of the first two cervical levels, each vertebral body is separated from its adjacent vertebrae by an intervertebral disk (IVD). Collectively, the IVDs are responsible for approximately one third of the height of the spine. The IVD and the superior and inferior articular processes (the facet joints) form a three-joint complex that allows multiaxial movement and loading of the spine and is essential for maintaining upright posture and protecting the contents of the spinal canal. The facet joints are true synovial joints with features similar to those of other synovial articulations. In contrast, the IVD is a load-bearing structure with unique characteristics.

Each IVD has two components. The inner nucleus pulposus is composed of a gel-like substance with high proteoglycan content. The nucleus pulposus is surrounded by an organized fibrous, collagenous ring called the anulus fibro-

sus. The nucleus pulposus and the anulus fibrosus are bordered cranially and caudally by cartilaginous end plates. The varied composition of these tissues reflects their embryonic origins (**Figure 1**). The embryonic spine is formed from the central notochord and the surrounding mesoderm. The notochord coalesces to form the nucleus pulposus, and the mesoderm forms the remainder of the spinal column, including the anulus fibrosus.[1] This distinct origin gives rise to a well-defined border between the nucleus pulposus and the anulus fibrosus. The notochordal cells and the nucleus pulposus chondrocytes produce large amounts of negatively charged aggregating proteoglycans, which generate a significant osmotic gradient that attracts and holds water within the tissue and thereby confers compressive strength to the nucleus pulposus.

Beginning at birth, the population of notochordal cells undergoes apoptosis through a Fas-mediated mitochondrial caspase-9 pathway.[2] The population of notochordal cells is $2,000/mm^3$ at birth and $100/mm^3$ at age 1 year; by late childhood, no notochordal cells can be identified.[1] These cells are replaced by chondrocyte-like cells that have been shown to migrate from the cartilaginous end plate to the nucleus pulposus (**Figure 2**), producing matrix consisting of both proteoglycan and type II collagen.[3] Adult IVD cells are presumed to be derived from these migrated chondrocytes, and therefore the biology of the nucleus pulposus in many ways is similar to that of articular cartilage. The distinct margins of the nucleus pulposus and the anulus fibrosus become blurred with age. The result is an outer anulus fibrosus that remains fibrous and highly organized and an inner anulus fibrosus with fibrocartilaginous properties.

The mesoderm-derived anulus fibrosus is populated by fibrocyte-like cells that primarily produce type I collagen organized into concentric lamellae. The collagen fibrils in each layer run parallel to one another and are oriented

Dr. An or an immediate family member has received royalties from U & I; serves as a paid consultant for or is an employee of Smith & Nephew, Life Spine, Zimmer, Pioneer, and Advanced Biologics; has stock or stock options held in Pioneer, Spinal Kinetics, U & I, Annulex, and Articular Engineering; has received research or institutional support from Synthes, Baxter, Spinalcytes, and Globus; and is a board member, owner, officer, or committee member of the International Society for the Study of the Lumbar Spine. Neither Dr. Moss nor any immediate family member has received anything of value from or owns stock in a commercial company or institution related directly or indirectly to the subject of this chapter.

2: Physiology of Musculoskeletal Tissues

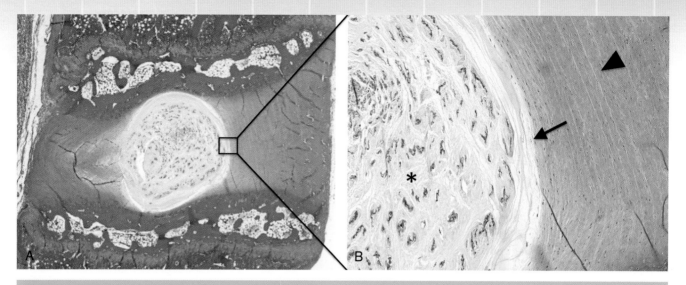

Figure 1 Hematoxylin-eosin–stained histologic section of an immature IVD at low power (**A**) and high power (**B**). In **B**, the nucleus pulposus (asterisk) is populated by clusters of cells within a gelatinous matrix. A clear border (arrow) is seen between the nucleus pulposus and the anulus fibrosus. The anulus fibrosus has organized fibrocartilage lamellae (arrowhead).

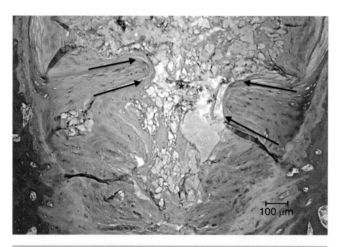

Figure 2 Photomicrograph of the rabbit IVD, showing the migration of end-plate chondrocytes toward the nucleus pulposus (arrows) and apoptosis of the notochordal cells (pyknotic nuclei surrounding the asterisk).

approximately 30° from the long axis of the spine, with alternating layers running in opposing directions. This arrangement allows the IVD to withstand tensile and shearing loads. Proteoglycans are found within the anulus fibrosus but are responsible for only a small percentage of the dry weight. Above and below each disk, mesenchymal cells form the bony vertebral bodies and cartilaginous end plates, with penetrating blood vessels providing the disk with nutrients.[4]

The blood vessels that penetrate the vertebral end plate to supply the center of the disk recede by the third decade of life. Consequently, the IVD is dependent on diffusion through the end plate and outer anulus fibrosus for nutritional support.[5] This diffusion is impeded by calcification of the end plates that occurs as a result of aging. In mature IVDs, the cells at the center of the nucleus pulposus can be several millimeters from the nearest blood supply and receive little, if any, diffusion of nutrients.[5] Furthermore, as the disk grows with age and extracellular matrix is laid down, overall cell density decreases to a level lower than that of almost any other tissue in the body.[6] The sparse cell population is concentrated near the periphery of the IVD in the regions closest to the source of nutrition.

The consequence of this developmental process is a relatively acellular, avascular tissue with little potential for self-repair. Over time, an imbalance in the production and degradation of extracellular matrix components can lead to a perturbed mechanical balance between the nucleus pulposus and the anulus fibrosus, giving the structural appearance of IVD degeneration. These changes can result in symptomatic discogenic low back pain; however, the correlation between structural degeneration and clinical symptoms is quite variable.

Pain originating from the IVD, called discogenic pain, is clinically well described and is a major source of disability. The anatomic etiology of the pain is not well understood, however. It has been shown that the central end plate and the periannular tissues have the most abundant nerve supply in the IVD.[7] The outer rim of the anulus fibrosus and the posterior longitudinal ligament contain most of the IVD nociceptive fibers. These fibers primarily arise from the sinuvertebral nerve, a meningeal branch of the spinal nerve. Pain sensation is believed to be transmitted through the sympathetic system by segmental and nonsegmental routes, through the dorsal root ganglia and the paravertebral sympathetic chain, respectively.[8] There is some evidence that with degeneration of the IVD, nociceptive fibers extend deep within the substance of the disk and may contribute to discogenic back pain.[9]

Biomechanics

The functional spinal unit consists of two adjacent vertebrae, an IVD, the facet joints, and the connecting ligaments. In a healthy functional spinal unit there is an even distribution of stress across the end plates with both axial compression and eccentric loading.[10] The hydrated nucleus pulposus acts as a relatively incompressible fluid contained by the end plates and the anulus fibrosus. In the unloaded condition, positive intradiscal pressure is generated by the ability of nucleus pulposus proteoglycans to attract and hold water (its hydrostatic pressure). With loading of the spine, the load is transmitted to the nucleus pulposus through the compact subchondral bone of the end plate. The elevated pressure in the nucleus pulposus is converted into tensile hoop stress within the organized lamellar structure of the anulus fibrosus, resulting in changes in the spatial arrangement of the collagen network and a small immediate decrease in disk height. If the applied load remains constant, the IVD exhibits the viscoelastic property of creep and continues to lose height over time, mainly as a result of the outflow of fluid through the anulus fibrosus and the end plates. In the healthy IVD, disk height slowly recovers when the load is removed, as the osmotic pressure generated within the nucleus pulposus causes an influx of fluid from the surrounding tissue.[11] This creep phenomenon leads to regular diurnal variation in IVD height.

As the IVD degenerates, the nucleus pulposus becomes fibrous, with decreased proteoglycan and increased collagen content, and its mechanical properties begin to resemble those of a solid rather than a viscous semifluid.[12] The more fibrous nucleus pulposus has a decreased overall swelling capacity and a limited ability to conform to and transmit loads. The result is an uneven stress distribution across the spinal motion segment.[13] This uneven stress distribution is particularly relevant with eccentric loading, and it can cause progressive damage to the overloaded anulus fibrosus. As the degenerative process proceeds, containment of the nucleus pulposus can be compromised, often through fissures developing in the anulus fibrosus. The creep characteristics of the degenerated IVD are altered, with larger and more rapid deformation under a load and slower recovery when the load is removed.[14] A greater portion of load bearing shifts to the posterior elements, and the overloaded facet joints may begin to manifest osteoarthritic changes similar to those found in other cartilaginous synovial articulations.

Kirkaldy-Willis and Farfan described the pathomechanics of the lumbar spine through three progressive phases of spinal motion segment degeneration.[15] In the early dysfunction stage, microscopic damage accumulates within the disk, and synovitis is present in the facet cartilage. As degeneration progresses, the spinal motion segment becomes unstable, and IVD height is diminished. This process is accompanied by capsular laxity and subluxation of the facet joints. In the final stage, disk osteophyte formation and facet enlargement allow stabilization of the segment, and spinal stenosis often develops. This observation was supported by cadaver

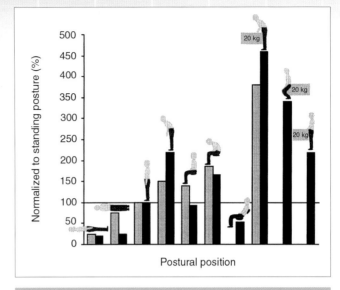

Figure 3 Schematic diagram showing intradiscal pressure in common postural positions, as measured by Nachemson and Morris[18] (gray bars) and Wilke et al[20] (black bars). (Adapted with permission from Wilke HJ, Neef P, Caimi M, Hoogland T, Claes LE: New in vivo measurements of pressures in the intervertebral disc in daily life. *Spine [Phila Pa 1976]* 1999;24(8): 755-762.)

studies of the relationship between spinal motion and disk degeneration in the lumbar and cervical spine.[16,17]

In the classic Nachemson and Morris study of in vivo intradiscal pressure in various functional positions, the highest intradiscal pressure was found in the unsupported sitting position (0.8 to 1.5 MPa), and the lowest pressure was found in a relaxed, supine position (0.1 to 0.2 MPa).[18] Pressure was observed to increase significantly with lifting and other strenuous activity. These classic measurements form the basis of traditional rehabilitation for patients with discogenic back pain. Two more recent studies generally confirmed the trends observed by Nachemson and Morris and added the finding that degenerated IVDs have significantly decreased intradiscal pressure[19,20] (**Figure 3**).

Biochemistry

The biomechanical behavior of the IVD is heavily dependent on the biochemical makeup of its components. The extracellular matrix molecules of the IVD are similar to those of hyaline cartilage. Collagen is the most abundant protein, accounting for approximately 60% of the dry weight of the anulus fibrosus and 20% of the dry weight of the nucleus pulposus. Several fibril-forming (I, II, III, V, XI) and short helical (VI, IX, XII) types of collagen are found throughout the disk.[21] In the nucleus pulposus, type II collagen is predominant; it forms a disorganized fibrillar framework for the cells and other matrix molecules. Organized type I collagen becomes more abundant where the nucleus pulposus makes its transition to the surrounding anulus fibrosus, and it accounts for approximately 80% of the collagen in the outer anulus fibrosus.

Proteoglycans are the second major group of extracellular matrix molecules in the IVD, accounting for as much as 50% of the dry weight of the nucleus pulposus and 20% of the dry weight of the anulus fibrosus. The IVD contains several different proteoglycans; these include versican, lumican, decorin, biglycan, and fibromodulin, but aggrecan is by far the most abundant.[12] The large, highly charged aggrecan molecules consist of chondroitin-6 sulfate and keratan sulfate side chains bound to a core protein. Through interaction with link protein, the aggrecan of the IVD has the ability to bind to hyaluronan to form large proteoglycan aggregates, thus further augmenting its water-binding capacity.

Remodeling and homeostasis of the IVD matrix is modulated by a variety of biochemical stimuli including growth factors, enzymes, enzyme inhibitors, and cytokines. The principal proteolytic enzymes produced by native disk cells are the matrix metalloproteinases and the ADAMTs (a disintegrin and metalloprotease with thrombospondin motifs).[22] Tissue inhibitors of metalloproteinases serve as natural antagonists to the matrix metalloproteinases. Although some turnover is necessary to clear damaged molecules, biomechanical dysfunction, genetic predisposition, and metabolic changes can disturb the balance between anabolic and catabolic processes within the IVD. The heightened catabolism can cause changes in the biochemical structure of the disk typical of degeneration (**Figure 4**).

At least three significant changes to the distribution and structure of collagen occur with degeneration of the IVD.[12] First, the ratio of type I to type II collagen increases in both the anulus fibrosus and the nucleus pulposus, resulting in a more fibrous tissue. Second, the collagens nonenzymatically cross-link, yielding advanced glycation end products. Third, collagen fibers are subject to proteolytic cleavage by collagenases produced by disk cells. These events result in an accumulation of incompetent fibrous collagen and limit the overall swelling ability of the nucleus pulposus.[23]

The aggrecan of the IVD undergoes changes in both amount and character. Less aggrecan is produced because of decreasing cell numbers and a reduced proteoglycan synthesis rate per cell. The glycosaminoglycan side chains, which predominantly consist of chondroitin sulfate at birth, with advancing age are replaced by keratan sulfate.[24] Proteolytic degradation of aggrecan and aggrecan-hyaluronan aggregates produces large molecules that are not as efficient at retaining water and, because of their size, are not easily cleared from the disk. They therefore accumulate and are subject to nonenzymatic cross-linking (as is collagen), resulting in advanced glycation end products.[23] These extracellular matrix changes together produce progressive mechanical incompetence of the IVD that limits its ability to efficiently dissipate compressive loads. Because the adult IVD relies on diffusion for the exchange of nutrients, the reduced swelling pressure in the degenerated disk results in

decreased flow of nutrients into the tissue, starving the few remaining disk cells even further. These cells are subject to increased stress in the progressively fibrous matrix, which can set off a chain of intracellular events leading to cell death and/or further upregulation of type I collagen and proteolytic enzyme expression, possibly creating a downward degenerative spiral.[25]

Biologic Therapy for Disk Degeneration

The current standard of care for IVD degeneration typically involves nonsurgical therapeutic modalities, with fusion or arthroplasty of the affected motion segment for the small number of patients with severe, unremitting symptoms. Although these mechanical approaches to the treatment of degenerative disk disease have advanced during recent decades, no perfect solution has been found. Biologic repair of the IVD for the purpose of slowing or reversing the degeneration process may be preferable to the current end-stage treatment strategies. Biologic therapy schemes generally involve the delivery of cells, the application of therapeutic molecules, or the supplementation of matrix.[4]

To achieve meaningful tissue repair, cells in the IVD must survive in the hostile degenerative environment and produce appropriate extracellular matrix molecules, including proteoglycans and collagens. For this purpose, new healthy cells can be implanted into the disk, and/or native cells can be stimulated with bioactive molecules. The harvest, ex vivo expansion, and subsequent reimplantation of autologous IVD cells has been attempted in a small clinical study.[26] However, theoretical and practical concerns related to this approach, including the time necessary between harvest and re-implantation, the local infrastructure required for ex vivo expansion, and the unpredictable nature of primary cell culture, have led investigators to explore other cell sources. Mesenchymal stem cells, a primitive cell population readily available from a variety of sources, are excellent candidates for such applications and are the subject of active investigation. Both in vitro and in vivo experiments have shown that mesenchymal stem cells can differentiate themselves into chondrocyte-like cells capable of expressing appropriate surface markers and IVD matrix proteins.[27-35] In vivo studies have shown the long-term viability of mesenchymal stem cells in IVDs, with improvement in disk height and hydration.

A second important strategy for IVD regeneration is the application of bioactive molecules to modulate the catabolic environment of the degenerating IVD. The potentially therapeutic molecules can be divided into four basic categories: anticatabolics, mitogens, chondrogenic morphogens, and intracellular regulators.[4] The chondrogenic morphogens, consisting of transforming growth factor–β and the bone morphogenetic protein (BMP) family, are among the most studied molecules for this application. In vitro experiments have shown that transforming growth factor–β can increase

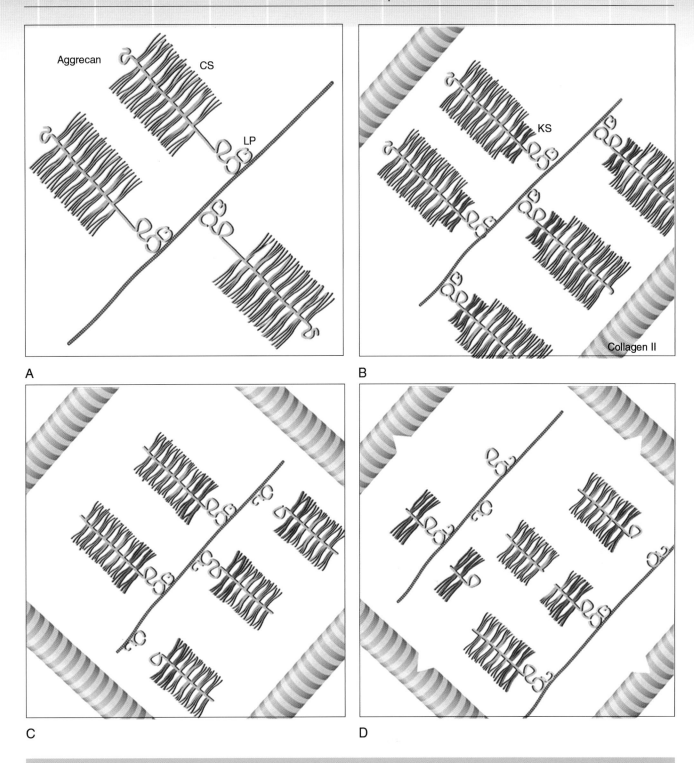

Figure 4 Schematic drawings showing changes in the nucleus pulposus extracellular matrix from fetal development through adulthood. In the fetus (**A**), the nucleus pulposus contains aggrecan rich in chondroitin sulfate (CS) that is bound to hyaluronan via link protein (LP). In the young child (**B**) and adolescent–young adult (**C**), collagen is produced, and CS is replaced by keratan sulfate (KS). In the mature adult (**D**), the nucleus pulposus has degenerated, all matrix molecules show evidence of proteolytic processing, there is greater hyaluronan content, and the proportion of aggrecan in a nonaggregated form is increased. (Adapted with permission from Roughley PJ: Biology of intervertebral disc aging and degeneration: Involvement of the extracellular matrix. *Spine [Phila Pa 1976]* 2004;29(23):2691-2699.)

the rate of proteoglycan and collagen synthesis in both healthy and degenerated IVD cells.[36-38] The members of the

BMP family of growth factors are known to be potent stimulators of osteogenesis and have been used to promote fracture healing and spinal fusion. In vitro and in vivo studies found that the application of BMP-2 and BMP-7 (osteogenic protein–1) to disk cells can increase the production of collagen type II and proteoglycans without osteogenic effects.[39-41] The direct injection of a single dose of BMP-7 into degenerating IVDs led to improved disk height, healthier functional metabolism, and restoration of viscoelastic biomechanical properties in a preclinical animal model.[42,43] Growth differentiation factor–5, another member of the BMP family, was found to improve in vitro IVD cell and extracellular matrix expression and to curb in vivo progression of degeneration.[44] Interleukin-1 receptor antagonist, platelet-derived growth factor, and insulin-like growth factor–1 are among the many other molecules whose therapeutic potential is being investigated.

Direct injection of therapeutic molecules is the simplest method of stimulating the biologic rescue of a degenerating IVD. Unfortunately, the success of this approach may be limited because of the short duration of activity of the injected factors. Gene therapy has the potential to overcome this obstacle by generating sustained expression of stimulatory molecules from cells within the IVD. The use of viral vectors for gene therapy elsewhere in the body has raised safety concerns related to immune reaction and the possible spread of disease. However, because the IVD is a relatively avascular tissue, cells of the immune system have limited access and it is considered an immune-privileged environment. Thus, there has been successful research into the use of this technique to transfect both native cells and exogenous chondrocytes with therapeutic factors. The genes of interest include both intracellular regulatory proteins and growth factors. Sox-9, a transcription factor known to drive the chondrocytic phenotype, has been delivered via a recombinant adenovirus to nucleus pulposus cells in culture and in vivo, resulting in upregulation of proteoglycan synthesis and reversal of early degeneration.[45,46] Adenoviral transfection of both animal and human nucleus pulposus cells with several growth factors including transforming growth factor–β1, BMP-2, BMP-7, and insulin-like growth factor–1 has yielded equally encouraging results, demonstrating increased cell viability and augmented production of extracellular matrix molecules.[46-48] Transfections of exogenous cells with stimulatory genes and subsequent implantation of these altered cells into the degenerating IVD represent a potentially effective strategy for delivering both cells and therapeutic molecules in a single treatment.

The final component of a successful IVD tissue-engineering strategy is the development of a scaffold to serve as a cell or drug carrier and possibly to supplement the degenerating extracellular matrix. A variety of materials are under investigation as scaffolds for IVD tissue engineering. To be successful in vivo, a scaffold must provide a microenvironment conducive to cell growth, migration, and synthesis of extracellular matrix. Constructs must be able to withstand the mechanical forces in the IVD during the acute phase of treatment, and they ideally will remodel into appropriate tissues in the long term.[49] For clinical application, spinal biocompatibility and the ability to provide initial mechanical stability also are of paramount importance. Many of the investigated scaffolds attempted to re-create the components of the IVD by combining fibrillar molecules and glycosaminoglycans.[50-54] This therapeutic approach is under active investigation.

Although techniques for IVD regeneration are becoming more sophisticated, it is important to understand that the relationship between the severity of disk degeneration and the clinical entity of back pain is not clear. Investigation into the molecular mechanism of back pain generation and biologic markers to help identify symptomatic IVDs is an active area of research. Advanced nuclear MRI techniques have been used to detect biochemical differences in IVDs in patients with discogenic back pain.[55] Exposure of human IVD cells to the proinflammatory cytokines interleukin-1β and tumor necrosis factor–α stimulates the production of nerve growth factor and may promote nociceptive nerve fiber infiltration into the disk.[56] Research in this area may lead to novel diagnostic and therapeutic approaches to painful IVDs.

Summary

The IVD is a complex organ that beautifully illustrates the intimate relationship among the biochemical composition, anatomic form, and biomechanical function of the musculoskeletal system. With aging and degeneration, the IVD can be transformed from an efficient shock absorber capable of withstanding significant loads to a mechanically incompetent fibrous tissue that ultimately can be responsible for a variety of clinically significant disorders. The understanding of the biochemical makeup and behavior of the IVD is progressing, and new therapeutic avenues for treating disk degeneration are being explored. These innovations ultimately may lead to the ability to restore normal IVD function in the large population of patients with symptomatic IVD degeneration.

References

1. Roberts S, Evans H, Trivedi J, Menage J: Histology and pathology of the human intervertebral disc. *J Bone Joint Surg Am* 2006;88(suppl 2):10-14.

2. Kim KW, Kim YS, Ha KY, et al: An autocrine or paracrine Fas-mediated counterattack: A potential mechanism for apoptosis of notochordal cells in intact rat nucleus pulposus. *Spine (Phila Pa 1976)* 2005;30(11):1247-1251.

3. Kim KW, Lim TH, Kim JG, Jeong ST, Masuda K, An HS: The origin of chondrocytes in the nucleus pulposus and histologic findings associated with the transition of a notochordal nucleus pulposus to a fibrocartilaginous nucleus pulposus in intact rabbit intervertebral discs. *Spine (Phila Pa 1976)* 2003;28(10):982-990.

4. Yoon ST: Molecular therapy of the intervertebral disc. *Spine J* 2005;5(6, suppl):280S-286S.

5. Urban JP, Smith S, Fairbank JC: Nutrition of the intervertebral disc. *Spine (Phila Pa 1976)* 2004;29(23):2700-2709.

6. Oegema TR Jr: Biochemistry of the intervertebral disc. *Clin Sports Med* 1993;12(3):419-439.

7. Fagan A, Moore R, Vernon Roberts B, Blumbergs P, Fraser R: The innervation of the intervertebral disc: A quantitative analysis. *Spine (Phila Pa 1976)* 2003;28(23):2570-2576.

8. Edgar MA: The nerve supply of the lumbar intervertebral disc. *J Bone Joint Surg Br* 2007;89(9):1135-1139.

9. Peng B, Wu W, Hou S, Li P, Zhang C, Yang Y: The pathogenesis of discogenic low back pain. *J Bone Joint Surg Br* 2005;87(1):62-67.

10. Horst M, Brinckmann P: Measurement of the distribution of axial stress on the end-plate of the vertebral body. *Spine (Phila Pa 1976)* 1981;6(3):217-232.

11. Broberg KB: Slow deformation of intervertebral discs. *J Biomech* 1993;26(4-5):501-512.

12. Roughley PJ: Biology of intervertebral disc aging and degeneration: Involvement of the extracellular matrix. *Spine (Phila Pa 1976)* 2004;29(23):2691-2699.

13. Adams MA, McNally DS, Dolan P: 'Stress' distributions inside intervertebral discs: The effects of age and degeneration. *J Bone Joint Surg Br* 1996;78(6):965-972.

14. Pollintine P, van Tunen MS, Luo J, Brown MD, Dolan P, Adams MA: Time-dependent compressive deformation of the ageing spine: Relevance to spinal stenosis. *Spine (Phila Pa 1976)* 2010;35(4):386-394.

15. Kirkaldy-Willis WH, Farfan HF: Instability of the lumbar spine. *Clin Orthop Relat Res* 1982;165:110-123.

16. Tanaka N, An HS, Lim TH, Fujiwara A, Jeon CH, Haughton VM: The relationship between disc degeneration and flexibility of the lumbar spine. *Spine J* 2001;1(1):47-56.

17. Miyazaki M, Hong SW, Yoon SH, et al: Kinematic analysis of the relationship between the grade of disc degeneration and motion unit of the cervical spine. *Spine (Phila Pa 1976)* 2008;33(2):187-193.

18. Nachemson A, Morris JM: In vivo measurements of intradiscal pressure: Discometry, a method for the determination of pressure in the lower lumbar discs. *J Bone Joint Surg Am* 1964;46:1077-1092.

19. Sato K, Kikuchi S, Yonezawa T: In vivo intradiscal pressure measurement in healthy individuals and in patients with ongoing back problems. *Spine (Phila Pa 1976)* 1999;24(23):2468-2474.

20. Wilke HJ, Neef P, Caimi M, Hoogland T, Claes LE: New in vivo measurements of pressures in the intervertebral disc in daily life. *Spine (Phila Pa 1976)* 1999;24(8):755-762.

21. Walker MH, Anderson DG: Molecular basis of intervertebral disc degeneration. *Spine J* 2004;4(6, suppl):158S-166S.

22. Le Maitre CL, Pockert A, Buttle DJ, Freemont AJ, Hoyland JA: Matrix synthesis and degradation in human intervertebral disc degeneration. *Biochem Soc Trans* 2007;35(pt 4):652-655.

23. Verzijl N, DeGroot J, Ben ZC, et al: Crosslinking by advanced glycation end products increases the stiffness of the collagen network in human articular cartilage: A possible mechanism through which age is a risk factor for osteoarthritis. *Arthritis Rheum* 2002;46(1):114-123.

24. Sztrolovics R, Alini M, Roughley PJ, Mort JS: Aggrecan degradation in human intervertebral disc and articular cartilage. *Biochem J* 1997;326(Pt 1):235-241.

25. Hutton WC, Elmer WA, Boden SD, et al: The effect of hydrostatic pressure on intervertebral disc metabolism. *Spine (Phila Pa 1976)* 1999;24(15):1507-1515.

26. Meisel HJ, Siodla V, Ganey T, Minkus Y, Hutton WC, Alasevic OJ: Clinical experience in cell-based therapeutics: Disc chondrocyte transplantation. A treatment for degenerated or damaged intervertebral disc. *Biomol Eng* 2007;24(1):5-21.

27. Hiyama A, Mochida J, Iwashina T, et al: Transplantation of mesenchymal stem cells in a canine disc degeneration model. *J Orthop Res* 2008;26(5):589-600.

28. Richardson SM, Hughes N, Hunt JA, Freemont AJ, Hoyland JA: Human mesenchymal stem cell differentiation to NP-like cells in chitosan-glycerophosphate hydrogels. *Biomaterials* 2008;29(1):85-93.

29. Risbud MV, Shapiro IM, Vaccaro AR, Albert TJ: Stem cell regeneration of the nucleus pulposus. *Spine J* 2004;4(6, suppl):348S-353S.

30. Sakai D, Mochida J, Iwashina T, et al: Regenerative effects of transplanting mesenchymal stem cells embedded in atelocollagen to the degenerated intervertebral disc. *Biomaterials* 2006;27(3):335-345.

31. Sobajima S, Vadala G, Shimer A, Kim JS, Gilbertson LG, Kang JD: Feasibility of a stem cell therapy for intervertebral disc degeneration. *Spine J* 2008;8(6):888-896.

32. Miyamoto T, Muneta T, Tabuchi T, et al: Intradiscal transplantation of synovial mesenchymal stem cells prevents intervertebral disc degeneration through suppression of matrix metalloproteinase-related genes in nucleus pulposus cells in rabbits. *Arthritis Res Ther* 2010;12(6):R206.

33. Yang F, Leung VY, Luk KD, Chan D, Cheung KM: Mesenchymal stem cells arrest intervertebral disc degeneration through chondrocytic differentiation and stimulation of endogenous cells. *Mol Ther* 2009;17(11):1959-1966.

34. Chen WH, Liu HY, Lo WC, et al: Intervertebral disc regeneration in an ex vivo culture system using mesenchymal stem cells and platelet-rich plasma. *Biomaterials* 2009;30(29):5523-5533.

35. Zhang Y, Drapeau S, Howard SA, Thonar EJ, Anderson DG: Transplantation of goat bone marrow stromal cells to the degenerating intervertebral disc in a goat disc injury model. *Spine (Phila Pa 1976)* 2011;36(5):372-377.

36. Tan Y, Hu Y, Tan J: Extracellular matrix synthesis and ultrastructural changes of degenerative disc cells transfected by Ad/CMV-hTGF-beta 1. *Chin Med J (Engl)* 2003;116(9):1399-1403.

37. Nishida K, Kang JD, Gilbertson LG, et al: Modulation of the biologic activity of the rabbit intervertebral disc by gene therapy: An in vivo study of adenovirus-mediated transfer of the human transforming growth factor beta 1 encoding gene. *Spine (Phila Pa 1976)* 1999;24(23):2419-2425.

38. Thompson JP, Oegema TR Jr, Bradford DS: Stimulation of mature canine intervertebral disc by growth factors. *Spine (Phila Pa 1976)* 1991;16(3):253-260.

2: Physiology of Musculoskeletal Tissues

39. An HS, Takegami K, Kamada H, et al: Intradiscal administration of osteogenic protein-1 increases intervertebral disc height and proteoglycan content in the nucleus pulposus in normal adolescent rabbits. *Spine (Phila Pa 1976)* 2005;30(1): 25-32.

40. Kim DJ, Moon SH, Kim H, et al: Bone morphogenetic protein-2 facilitates expression of chondrogenic, not osteogenic, phenotype of human intervertebral disc cells. *Spine (Phila Pa 1976)* 2003;28(24):2679-2684.

41. Zhang Y, Phillips FM, Thonar EJ, et al: Cell therapy using articular chondrocytes overexpressing BMP-7 or BMP-10 in a rabbit disc organ culture model. *Spine (Phila Pa 1976)* 2008;33(8):831-838.

42. Masuda K, Imai Y, Okuma M, et al: Osteogenic protein-1 injection into a degenerated disc induces the restoration of disc height and structural changes in the rabbit anular puncture model. *Spine (Phila Pa 1976)* 2006;31(7):742-754.

43. Miyamoto K, Masuda K, Kim JG, et al: Intradiscal injections of osteogenic protein-1 restore the viscoelastic properties of degenerated intervertebral discs. *Spine J* 2006;6(6):692-703.

44. Chujo T, An HS, Akeda K, et al: Effects of growth differentiation factor-5 on the intervertebral disc: In vitro bovine study and in vivo rabbit disc degeneration model study. *Spine (Phila Pa 1976)* 2006;31(25):2909-2917.

45. Paul R, Haydon RC, Cheng H, et al: Potential use of Sox9 gene therapy for intervertebral degenerative disc disease. *Spine (Phila Pa 1976)* 2003;28(8):755-763.

46. Zhang Y, An HS, Thonar EJ, Chubinskaya S, He TC, Phillips FM: Comparative effects of bone morphogenetic proteins and sox9 overexpression on extracellular matrix metabolism of bovine nucleus pulposus cells. *Spine (Phila Pa 1976)* 2006; 31(19):2173-2179.

47. Moon SH, Gilbertson LG, Nishida K, et al: Human intervertebral disc cells are genetically modifiable by adenovirus-mediated gene transfer: Implications for the clinical management of intervertebral disc disorders. *Spine (Phila Pa 1976)* 2000;25(20):2573-2579.

48. Sobajima S, Kim JS, Gilbertson LG, Kang JD: Gene therapy for degenerative disc disease. *Gene Ther* 2004;11(4):390-401.

49. Lotz JC, Staples A, Walsh A, Hsieh AH: Mechanobiology in intervertebral disc degeneration and regeneration. *Conf Proc IEEE Eng Med Biol Soc* 2004;7:5459.

50. Halloran DO, Grad S, Stoddart M, Dockery P, Alini M, Pandit AS: An injectable cross-linked scaffold for nucleus pulposus regeneration. *Biomaterials* 2008;29(4):438-447.

51. Mizuno H, Roy AK, Zaporojan V, Vacanti CA, Ueda M, Bonassar LJ: Biomechanical and biochemical characterization of composite tissue-engineered intervertebral discs. *Biomaterials* 2006;27(3):362-370.

52. Sakai D, Mochida J, Iwashina T, et al: Atelocollagen for culture of human nucleus pulposus cells forming nucleus pulposus-like tissue in vitro: Influence on the proliferation and proteoglycan production of HNPSV-1 cells. *Biomaterials* 2006;27(3):346-353.

53. Yang SH, Chen PQ, Chen YF, Lin FH: An in-vitro study on regeneration of human nucleus pulposus by using gelatin/chondroitin-6-sulfate/hyaluronan tri-copolymer scaffold. *Artif Organs* 2005;29(10):806-814.

54. Moss IL, Gordon L, Woodhouse KA, Whyne CM, Yee AJ: A novel thiol-modified hyaluronan and elastin-like polypeptide composite material for tissue engineering of the nucleus pulposus of the intervertebral disc. *Spine (Phila Pa 1976)* 2011;36(13):1022-1029.

55. Keshari KR, Lotz JC, Link TM, Hu S, Majumdar S, Kurhanewicz J: Lactic acid and proteoglycans as metabolic markers for discogenic back pain. *Spine (Phila Pa 1976)* 2008;33(3): 312-317.

56. Abe Y, Akeda K, An HS, et al: Proinflammatory cytokines stimulate the expression of nerve growth factor by human intervertebral disc cells. *Spine (Phila Pa 1976)* 2007;32(6): 635-642.

Chapter 16

Kinesiology of the Knee Joint

Jing-Sheng Li, MS
Ali Hosseini, PhD
Hemanth Reddy Gadikota, MS
Guoan Li, PhD

Introduction

The knee joint, located between the hip and ankle joints, is the largest joint in humans. The knee transmits the weight of the body from the femur to the tibia, and the two-joint structure of the knee provides the mobility needed for locomotor activities such as walking, running, climbing, descending stairs, and standing from a sitting position. In addition, the knee joint provides the necessary stability for controlling the body's alignment in a static posture.

Knee Joint Structure and Motion

The knee joint is classified as a synovial hinge joint with two component joints. The tibiofemoral joint consists of the distal femur and the proximal tibia, and the patellofemoral joint consists of the patella and the trochlear groove. The femur and tibia are two of the longest bones in the human body. In the tibiofemoral joint, the distal femur has an asymmetric shape with two convex condyles at the distal end. The tibia also is asymmetric and has a concave tibial plateau. Two C-shaped menisci are located between the femur and tibia. The menisci increase the contact area between the femur and the tibia, help transfer the load between the bones, and stabilize the joint.[1]

The patella, the largest sesamoid bone in the human body, is embedded in the quadriceps tendon. In the patellofemoral joint, this triangular bone acts as an anatomic pulley, gliding on the trochlear groove and efficiently transferring the muscle load from the quadriceps to the tib-

ial tuberosity by increasing the moment arm (defined as the perpendicular distance between the center of rotation on the femur and the line along the patellar tendon). The cartilage of the patella and femur build an environment of minimal friction for patellofemoral movement.[1]

The knee joint is surrounded by many active muscles and passive structures such as the ligaments and menisci, all of which work synergistically to maintain normal knee functions. **Figure 1** and **Table 1** identify the major muscles acting as motion generators of the knee joint.[1] The quadriceps, which is the major extensor of the knee, consists of the rectus femoris, vastus medialis, vastus lateralis, and vastus intermedius. The rectus femoris is a two-joint muscle that originates in the ilium and crosses the hip and knee joints. The vastus medialis, vastus lateralis, and vastus intermedius originate in the femur. The quadriceps tendon inserts into the proximal patella and connects to the tibial tuberosity through the patellar tendon (also called the patellar ligament). These four parts of the quadriceps function to extend the knee.[1]

The knee flexors include the semimembranosus, semitendinosus, biceps femoris, popliteus, sartorius, gracilis, and gastrocnemius muscles (**Table 1**). The semimembranosus, semitendinosus, and long and short heads of the biceps femoris muscles, known as the hamstrings, have a common origin in the ischial tuberosity, with the exception of the short head of the biceps femoris. The semitendinosus, sartorius, and gracilis muscles insert into the upper medial shaft of the tibia. Their common tendon is called the pes anserinus. These muscles both flex and rotate the knee joint.[1]

The stability of the knee joint is provided by active and passive stabilizers. The stability provided by a structure depends on its orientation.[2] **Table 2** shows the stabilizers categorized by function. The ligaments are passive stabilizers of the knee joint (**Figure 2**). One of the major characteristics of

2: Physiology of Musculoskeletal Tissues

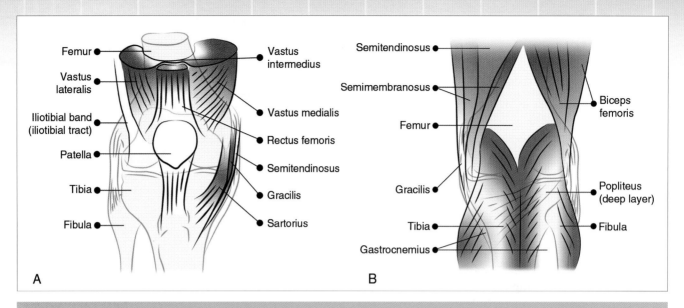

Figure 1 Schematic drawings showing the bones and major muscles of the knee joint. **A,** Anterior view. **B,** Posterior view.

ligaments is their high resistance to tensile forces. **Table 3** shows the proximal and distal attachments of the four major knee ligaments: the anterior cruciate ligament (ACL), posterior cruciate ligament (PCL), lateral collateral ligament (LCL), and medial collateral ligament (MCL). Ligamentous structures not only bear high tensile stress but also act as a position sensor, providing proprioceptive sensation and assisting in controlling and coordinating the position and movement of the knee during activity. This feedback system can help protect the knee from injury.[3]

The tibia stabilizes the knee as it externally rotates to move from slight flexion to full extension. This phenomenon is known as a screw-home mechanism and it places the knee in a locking position. The asymmetric geometry of the condyles of the femur and the restraint forces from the cruciate ligaments may contribute to the screw-home mechanism.[2,4]

All knee joint motions are based on three anatomic planes (**Figure 3,** *A*). Three-axis coordinate systems describe the relative motion of the femur, tibia, and patella in the tibiofemoral and patellofemoral joints (**Figure 3,** *B*). Each axis has one degree of freedom in rotation and one degree of freedom in translation. Therefore, the knee joint has a total of six degrees of freedom, with three rotations and three translations. The femur, tibia, and patella have their own coordinate systems that are defined by anatomic landmarks. For example, four key components of the femoral coordinate system are the long axis of the femur, the transepicondylar axis connecting the medial and lateral epicondyles, the axis perpendicular to the long and the transepicondylar axes, and the midpoint of the transepicondylar axis as the center of the femur. The tibial coordinate system is composed of the long axis of the tibia, the mediolateral axis connecting the center of the medial and lateral plateaus, the axis perpendicular to the long and mediolateral axes, and the

midpoint of the mediolateral axis as the center of the tibia. The flexion-extension, valgus-varus, and internal-external rotations are relative rotations around the mediolateral, anteroposterior, and long axes of the tibia, respectively. The tibiofemoral translations are relative, shifting between the centers of the tibia and femur along the anteroposterior, mediolateral, and long axes of the tibia. The key components of the patellar coordinate system include the proximodistal axis, the mediolateral axis connecting the medial and lateral borders, the axis perpendicular to the proximodistal and mediolateral axes, and the midpoint of the mediolateral axis as the center of the patella. Flexion-extension, mediolateral rotation, and mediolateral tilt are relative rotations around the mediolateral, anteroposterior, and long axes of the femur, respectively. The patellofemoral translations are the relative shifting between the midpoints of the transepicondylar and mediolateral axes along the anteroposterior, transepicondylar and long axes of the femur[5] (**Figure 3,** *B*). Other coordinate systems sometimes are used to describe knee motion, depending on the research methodology.

The primary motion of the tibiofemoral joint is flexion-extension in the sagittal plane, and the secondary motion is internal-external rotation in the transverse plane. **Table 4** outlines the range of tibiofemoral joint motion in the sagittal plane during common activities.[6,7]

The patellofemoral indices obtained from the skyline radiographic view are widely used in the clinical evaluation of patellofemoral joint congruence. **Figure 4** shows the patellofemoral indices, including the sulcus angle, congruence angle, lateral patellofemoral angle, lateral patellar tilt, and lateral patellar displacement.[8]

Each of the functional activities can be described as an open or a closed kinetic chain. In an open kinetic chain, the extremity is not fixed at the distal end and can move in any

Table 1

Major Muscles of the Knee Joint

Muscle	Origin	Insertion	Functions
Rectus femoris	Straight head: anteroinferior iliac spine Reflected head: ilium above acetabulum	Quadriceps tendon to patella, via patellar ligament into tibial tuberosity	Extends knee Flexes hip
Vastus medialis	Lower intertrochanteric line, spiral line, medial linea aspera, and medial intermuscular septum	Medial quadriceps tendon to patella and directly into medial patella, via patellar ligament into tibial tuberosity	Extends knee Stabilizes patella
Vastus lateralis	Upper intertrochanteric line, base of greater trochanter, lateral linea aspera, lateral supracondylar ridge, and lateral intermuscular septum	Lateral quadriceps tendon to patella, via patellar ligament into tibial tuberosity	Extends knee
Vastus intermedius	Anterolateral shaft of femur	Quadriceps tendon to patella, via patellar ligament into tibial tuberosity	Extends knee
Semimembranosus	Upper outer quadrant of posterior surface of ischial tuberosity	Medial condyle of tibia below articular margin, fascia over popliteus, and oblique popliteal ligament	Flexes and internally rotates knee Extends hip
Semitendinosus	Upper inner quadrant of posterior surface of ischial tuberosity	Upper medial shaft of tibia below gracilis	Flexes and internally rotates knee Extends hip
Biceps femoris	Long head: ischial tuberosity Short head: femoral shaft	Styloid process of head of fibula, lateral collateral ligament, and lateral tibial condyle	Flexes and laterally rotates knee Long head extends hip
Popliteus	Middle facet of lateral surface of lateral femoral condyle	Posterior tibia, inferior to tibial condyle	Internally rotates and flexes knee
Sartorius	Inferior to the anterosuperior iliac spine	Anteromedial surface of upper tibia in pes anserinus	Flexes knee Flexes, abducts, and externally rotates hip
Gracilis	Outer surface of ischiopubic ramus	Upper medial shaft of tibia below sartorius	Flexes and internally rotates knee Adducts hip
Gastrocnemius	Lateral head: posterior surface of lateral condyle of femur and highest of three facets on lateral condyle Medial head: posterior surface of femur above medial condyle	Achilles tendon to middle of three facets on posterior aspect of calcaneus	Flexes knee Plantar flexes foot
Tensor fascia lata	Iliac crest	Iliotibial tract (further attached to lateral condyle of tibia)	Stabilizes knee (works with iliotibial tract)

2: Physiology of Musculoskeletal Tissues

Table 2

Knee Stabilizers Categorized by Function

Function	Stabilizer
Prevent excessive anterior tibial translation	Anterior cruciate ligament Iliotibial band (iliotibial tract) Hamstring muscles Soleus muscle (weight bearing) Gluteus maximus muscle (weight bearing)
Prevent excessive posterior tibial translation	Posterior cruciate ligament Medial collateral ligament Meniscofemoral ligament Quadriceps muscle Popliteus muscle Gastrocnemius muscle
Prevent excessive valgus rotation	Medial collateral ligament Anterior cruciate ligament Posterior cruciate ligament Arcuate ligament Posterior oblique ligament Sartorius muscle Gracilis muscle Semitendinosus muscle Semimembranosus muscle Medial head of gastrocnemius muscle
Prevent excessive varus rotation	Lateral collateral ligament Iliotibial band (iliotibial tract) Anterior cruciate ligament Posterior cruciate ligament Arcuate ligament Posterior oblique ligament Biceps femoris muscle Lateral head of gastrocnemius muscle
Prevent excessive internal tibial rotation	Anterior cruciate ligament Posterior cruciate ligament Posteromedial capsule Meniscofemoral ligament Biceps femoris muscle
Prevent excessive external tibial rotation	Posterolateral capsule Medial collateral ligament Posterior cruciate ligament Lateral collateral ligament Popliteus muscle Sartorius muscle Gracilis muscle Semitendinosus muscle Semimembranosus muscle

Adapted with permission from Levangie PK, Norkin CC, eds: *Joint Structure and Function: A Comprehensive Analysis*, ed 4. Philadelphia, PA, FA Davis Co, 2005.

direction. In a closed kinetic chain, movement at the distal end is fixed. In the stance phase of gait, for example, the supporting limb is in contact with the ground, and the distal end of the limb is fixed; the movement, therefore, is a closed kinetic chain. In the swing phase of gait, the swing leg can move freely, and the movement is an open kinetic chain.[2,9] These motions usually are classified as weight bearing or not weight bearing. In kicking a ball, for example, the leg used for kicking is not weight bearing, and the standing leg is weight bearing.[2,9]

Kinematics of the Knee Joint

The kinematics of the knee joint describe the motion of the femur, tibia, and patella without considering forces. Knee joint kinematics are activity dependent. An understanding of the six degrees of freedom in knee kinematics is critical for analyzing physiologic knee joint motion in different pathologies and treatments. In gait (walking) and stair climbing, the most common daily activities, the lower body joints, including the knee joint, constantly adjust to maintain a smooth progression of the center of the body mass through space.

Gait

Human gait is a cyclic symmetric bipedal locomotion having two distinct phases: the stance phase (the initial 60% of the full gait cycle) and the swing phase (the subsequent 40% of the full cycle). During the stance phase, the supporting foot is in contact with the ground. During the swing phase, this foot is completely separated from the ground. A stride (one full gait cycle) consists of a consecutive stance phase and swing phase by one leg.

The stance phase can be divided by five events into four periods,[9,10] as shown in **Figure 5**. The initial contact takes place as soon as the heel contacts the ground, and it initiates the loading response at 0% of gait cycle. The contralateral (opposite) toe-off occurs when the sole of the contralateral foot is completely off the floor. The contralateral toe-off marks the end of the loading response and the beginning of the midstance (single-limb support). The heel rise corresponds to the heel lifting from the floor and starts the terminal stance. The contralateral (opposite) initial contact is the event at which the contralateral foot contacts the floor, and it marks the end of the terminal stance and the beginning of the preswing. The toe-off occurs the instant that the toe ends contact with the floor, and it begins the swing phase of the gait.

The stance phase also can be described as a double-limb support (loading-response and preswing) and single-limb support (midstance and terminal stance). The contralateral foot is in contact with the ground during the double-limb support and is in the swing phase during the single-limb support.[10]

During the double-limb support (constituting the initial approximately 10% of the gait cycle), the foot receives the body weight during a shift from the contralateral leg to the supporting leg. The first double-limb support is also called weight acceptance. The supporting leg rotates over the stationary foot during the midstance (occurring from the 10% to 30% point in the gait cycle) and the terminal stance (from the 30% to 50% point), and the body weight transfers from the heel to the forefoot (from the 10% to the 50% point). At this moment the contralateral initial contact occurs, and the body weight begins to transfer from the supporting leg to the contralateral leg; this preswing occurs approximately at the 50% to 60% point in the gait cycle. At completion of approximately 60% of the cycle, the toe breaks contact with the floor. The initially supporting leg swings about the hip joint for the remaining 40% of the gait cycle.

The swing phase is subdivided into the initial swing, midswing, and terminal swing, each of which lasts approximately one third of the entire swing phase. The initial swing phase begins with the supporting foot's toe-off and ends when the swing foot is next to the standing foot (at 60% to 73% of gait cycle). The midswing lasts until the tibia of the swing leg is vertical (at 73% to 87% of gait cycle). The terminal swing extends from the moment of the vertical tibial position to the moment of the next initial contact (at 87% to 100% of the cycle).[9,10]

Gait is analyzed in both overground and treadmill walking.[11-16] Some researchers found no differences between these two walking conditions,[17] but many other investigators reported differences in several aspects of overground and treadmill walking.[12,14,18,19] Some studies found a significant increase in cadence (number of steps per minute) and a decrease in step and stride length (as in **Table 5**) and the time of the stance phase in treadmill walking compared with overground walking.[12,14,20,21] **Table 5** presents one report of overground and treadmill gait parameters in adults.[12]

Table 3
Proximal and Distal Attachments of Knee Ligaments

Ligament	Proximal Attachment	Distal Attachment	Major Function
Anterior cruciate	Posteromedial aspect of lateral femoral condyle	Anterior tibial spine	Prevents excessive anterior tibial translation
Posterior cruciate	Lateral aspect of medial femoral condyle	Posterior tibial spine	Prevents excessive posterior tibial translation
Lateral collateral	Lateral femoral condyle	Fibular head	Prevents excessive valgus rotation
Medial collateral	Superficial: medial femoral epicondyle / Deep: inferior aspect of medial femoral condyle	Superficial: medial aspect of proximal tibia to pes anserinus / Deep: proximal aspect of tibial plateau	Prevents excessive varus rotation

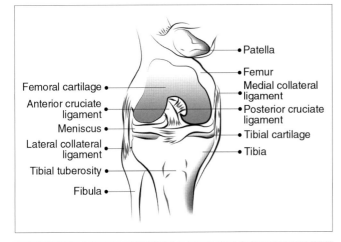

Figure 2 Schematic drawing showing the bones and major ligaments of the knee joint.

Table 4
Range of Tibiofemoral Joint Motion in the Sagittal Plane During Common Activities

Activity	Range of Motion (°)
Walking	0 to 60[a]
Ascending stairs	0 to 94[a]
Descending stairs	0 to 87[a]
Sitting down	0 to 93[b]
Tying a shoe	0 to 106[b]
Lifting an object	0 to 117[b]

[a]Mean for 20 subjects.(Data from Kaufman KR, Hughes C, Morrey BF, Morrey M, An KN: Gait characteristics of patients with knee osteoarthritis. *J Biomech* 2001;34(7):907-915.)
[b]Mean for 30 subjects.
Data from Laubenthal KN, Smidt GL, Kettlekamp DB: A quantitative analysis of knee motion during activities of daily living. *Phys Ther* 1972;52(1):34-43.

2: Physiology of Musculoskeletal Tissues

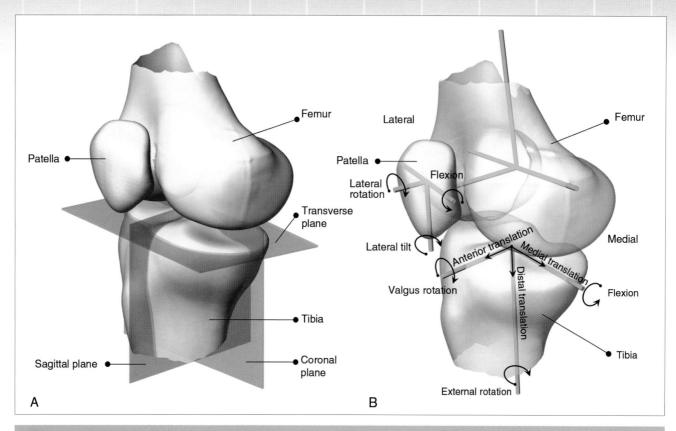

Figure 3 Schematic drawings showing the anatomic planes of the knee joint **(A)** and the motions of the tibiofemoral and patellofemoral joints **(B)**.

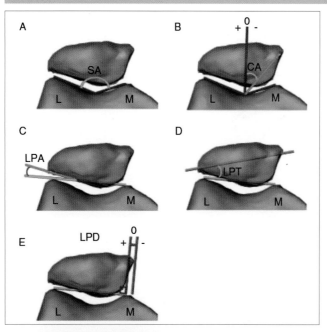

Figure 4 Schematic drawings showing the patellofemoral indices. **A,** The sulcus angle (SA). **B,** The congruence angle (CA). **C,** The lateral patellofemoral angle (LPA). **D,** The lateral patellar tilt (LPT). **E,** Lateral patellar displacement (LPD). L = lateral, M = medial. (Reproduced with permission from Nha KW, Papannagari R, Gill TJ, et al: In vivo patellar tracking: Clinical motions and patellofemoral indices. *J Orthop Res* 2008;26[8]:1067-1074.)

Gait Kinematics

The predominant motion of the knee during the stance phase of gait is in the sagittal plane. The knee is extended at initial contact, gradually flexes during the loading response, and reaches the first flexion peak (approximately 8°) during early midstance. Thereafter, the knee begins to extend until about 40% of stance phase, and it remains in slight hyperextension throughout the midstance. Approximately halfway through the terminal stance phase, the knee flexes again. The flexion continues throughout the preswing and reaches its peak at toe-off of the initially supporting leg, when the stance phase ends. The average magnitude of this second flexion peak is 35°[22] (**Figure 6**).

The pattern of axial (internal-external) knee rotation is similar to that of knee flexion-extension. At initial contact, the tibia is slightly externally rotated. The tibia then rotates internally and reaches the first peak of external rotation (5°) shortly after contralateral toe-off (in early midstance). The direction of axial rotation then reverses, and the tibia rotates internally throughout midstance. During the preswing, the tibia rotates internally until toe-off and it reaches the second maximum internal rotation (7.4°)[22] (**Figure 6**).

The average magnitude of knee motion in the coronal plane is 4°. At initial contact the knee is in an average 3° of valgus, and it rotates slightly into further valgus during the loading response. At early midstance the direction of this

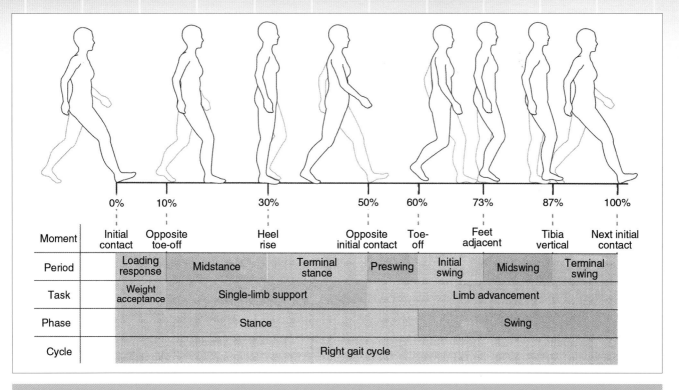

Figure 5 Schematic diagram showing the temporal sequence from the beginning to the end of the gait cycle (0% to 100%). (Reproduced with permission from Neumann DA: *Kinesiology of the Musculoskeletal System: Foundations for Physical Rehabilitation.* St. Louis, MO, Mosby, 2002.)

Table 5

Gait Parameters for Adults During Overground and Treadmill Walking

Gait Parameter	Overground Walking (mean ± SD)	Treadmill Walking (mean ± SD)
Velocity (m/s)	1.5 ± 0.2	1.5 ± 0.2
Stride length (cm)	162.6 ± 16.0	[a]155.7 ± 14.7
Step length related to leg length	0.9 ± 0.1	[a]0.8 ± 0.1
Step length related to body height	0.5 ± 0.03	[a]0.5 ± 0.03
Cadence (steps/min)	113.1 ± 11.1	[b]120.7 ± 5.2
Step width (mm)	81.2 ± 19.6	[a]104.3 ± 17.6
Foot angle (°)	9.1 ± 4.4	[a]11.3 ± 3.8
Stance phase (ms)	630.2 ± 43.6	[a]587.0 ± 29.2
Swing phase (ms)	406.6 ± 27.3	[b]426.2 ± 26.5
Double-limb support (ms)	111.7 ± 17.4	[a]81.1 ± 11.2
Cycle duration (ms)	1036.8 ± 65.6	[b]1013.2 ± 51.0

[a]$P < 0.01$; [b]$P < 0.05$.
Adapted with permission from Stolze H, Kuhtz-Buschbeck JP, Mondwurf C, et al: Gait analysis during treadmill and overground locomotion in children and adults. *Electroencephalogr Clin Neurophysiol* 1997;105(6):490-49

rotation reverses, and the knee rotates back toward varus until completion of approximately 40% of the stance phase. Thereafter, the knee remains in approximately 3° of valgus until 70% of the stance phase is complete (at terminal stance), when the knee begins to rotate into valgus again. At toe-off, the knee joint is in 6° of valgus[22] (**Figure 6**).

The pattern of anteroposterior shift of the tibia in relation to the femur also is one of flexion-extension. At initial

2: Physiology of Musculoskeletal Tissues

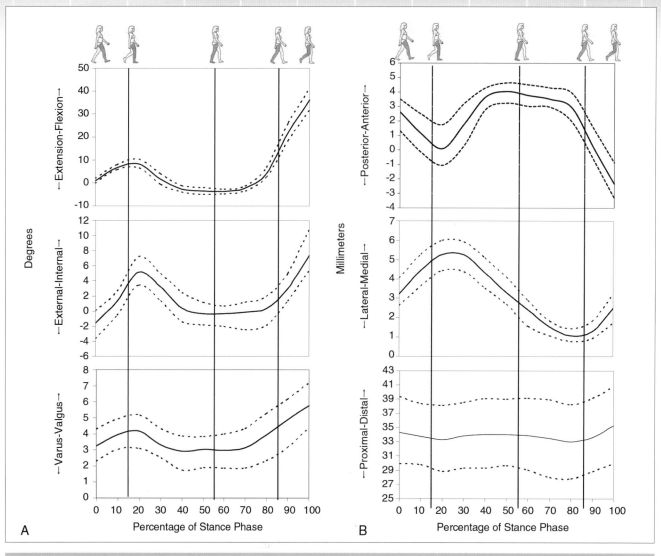

Figure 6 Schematic diagrams showing the six degrees of freedom (A and B each describe three degrees of freedom) in the tibiofemoral kinematics of the knee joint, as measured during the stance phase of treadmill gait. The figure drawings represent the motion of the tibia relative to the femur. **A,** Rotations; solid lines = contralateral toe-off, ipsilateral heel rise, and contralateral initial contact in extension-flexion, internal-external rotation, and varus-valgus, respectively. **B,** Translations; solid lines = contralateral toe-off, ipsilateral heel rise, and contralateral initial contact in posterior-anterior, lateral-medial, and proximodistal, respectively. Dashed lines = kinematic range (maximal and minimal displacement). The intervals between the solid lines represent loading response, midstance, terminal stance, and preswing, respectively. (Adapted with permission from Kozanek M, Hosseini A, Liu F, et al: Tibiofemoral kinematics and condylar motion during the stance phase of gait. *J Biomech* 2009;42[12]:1877-1884.)

contact, the tibia is 2.6 mm anterior to the femur. The tibia shifts posteriorly during the loading response and reaches the first peak of posterior shift during early midstance. At this point, the tibia is an average 0.1 mm posterior to the femur. The tibia shifts anteriorly during the midstance. Anterior motion reaches its peak at completion of 50% of the stance phase, when it is 4 mm anterior to the femur. The direction thereafter reverses, and the tibia shifts posteriorly until toe-off, when it reaches the second maximum. The average excursion in the anteroposterior direction during the stance phase is approximately 5 mm[22] (**Figure 6**).

In the coronal plane, the mediolateral motion of the knee (the tibia relative to the femur) consists of an initial medial shift of the tibia followed by a lateral motion that peaks before toe-off. At initial contact, the center of the tibia is oriented 3.2 mm medially with respect to the femoral center. Thereafter the tibia moves medially during the loading response until early midstance and reaches a maximum of 5.2 mm. The direction of the mediolateral motion is then reversed, and the tibia moves laterally until completion of 80% of the stance phase, when the center of the tibial coordinate system is 1.1 mm medial to the center of the femoral

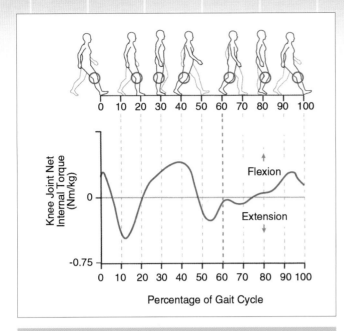

Figure 7 Schematic diagram showing sagittal plane knee joint net internal torques through a full gait cycle (normalized to body mass). (Adapted with permission from Neumann DA: *Kinesiology of the Musculoskeletal System: Foundations for Physical Rehabilitation.* St. Louis, MO, Mosby, 2002.)

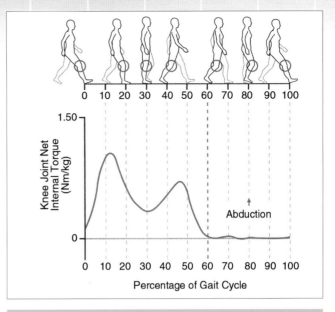

Figure 8 Schematic diagram showing frontal plane knee joint net internal torques through a full gait cycle (normalized to body mass). (Adapted with permission from Neumann DA: *Kinesiology of the Musculoskeletal System: Foundations for Physical Rehabilitation.* St. Louis, MO, Mosby, 2002.)

coordinate system. Thereafter, the tibia begins to shift medially toward its position at initial contact. The average measured mediolateral displacement is 4.1 mm. The average motion of the tibia with respect to the femur in the proximodistal direction is 2 mm, with amplitudes occurring at 20% and 80% of the stance phase[22] (**Figure 6**).

Gait Kinetics

The muscles around the knee joint actively control the motion of the knee. In addition, the ligaments inside and around the knee (the ACL, PCL, MCL, and LCL) passively control the kinematics of the knee (**Table 3**). Quadriceps and hamstrings have major roles in providing locomotion at the knee joint.[10] The quadriceps, which are the primary knee extensors, become active at the end of the swing phase in preparation for initial contact. After initial contact, the activity of the quadriceps reaches its peak around the end of the loading response to control knee flexion. The muscles elongate as they generate force to smoothly control the acceptance of body weight onto the standing leg without excessive knee flexion. Thereafter, the quadriceps begin to shorten during force generation to extend the knee and support the body weight during the midstance. The hamstrings are the primary flexors of the knee joint. Before initial contact, the hamstrings decelerate knee extension to prepare for the landing of the foot on the ground. The hamstrings stabilize the knee joint during midstance. Knee flexion during

the preswing and swing phases is provided with minor gastrocnemius activation.

Both knee flexors and extensors act during the gait cycle to maintain smooth, stable locomotion. At initial contact, a minor flexion torque is applied to ensure the knee flexes; this movement provides adequate knee alignment for shock absorption.[10] During the loading response, the quadriceps apply an extension torque to the knee to transfer the body weight to a position over the standing foot (**Figure 7**). The extension torque remains until the middle of the midstance to maintain the stability of the joint (at 20% of the gait cycle). At 20% to 50% of the gait cycle, a net flexion torque counterbalances the external torque at the foot to transfer the body weight from the heel to the toe. Before toe-off, a minor extension torque occurs for the purpose of controlling the toe-off. A flexion torque occurs during the terminal swing to decelerate knee extension before initial contact.

The moment of the ground reaction force acting about the center of the knee joint in the frontal plane determines adduction torque during the gait cycle. The total abduction torque is balanced with the abduction moments generated by active structures (such as the iliotibial tract and the tensor fascia lata) and passive structures (the lateral ligaments of the knee). Muscles provide most of the resistance during midstance and terminal stance, and the ligaments have a significant role during the loading response and midstance.[23] Both the quadriceps and hamstrings provide the abduction moment inside the knee. The abduction torques have two

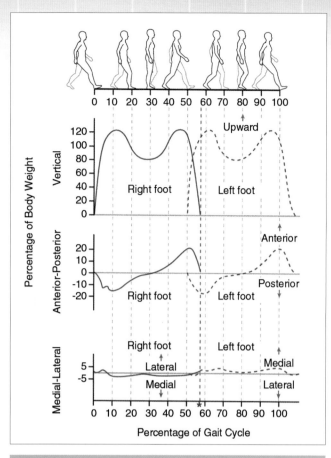

Figure 9 Schematic diagram showing ground reaction forces through a full gait cycle, in the vertical, anteroposterior, and mediolateral directions. Asterisk = toe-off is at 57%. (Adapted with permission from Neumann DA: *Kinesiology of the Musculoskeletal System: Foundations for Physical Rehabilitation.* St. Louis, MO, Mosby, 2002.)

peaks in each gait cycle (**Figure 8**). The first peak occurs at the contralateral toe-off, as the entire body weight is shifted to the supporting foot. The abduction torque then decreases during the late midstance and early terminal stance. At contralateral initial contact, the abduction torque reaches its second peak and shows that the muscles are responsible for providing significant abduction moments when both feet are in contact with the ground.

Ground Reaction Forces

The forces applied to the foot by the ground are called the ground reaction forces. The ground reaction forces are the sum of local contact forces (contact pressure) over the entire contact area of the foot and the ground. The three components of the ground reaction forces are in the vertical, anteroposterior, and mediolateral directions (**Figure 9**). The vertical ground reaction forces peak twice during a single gait cycle, with a magnitude of 120% of body weight. The peaks occur during the loading response and terminal stance. The ground reaction forces are slightly less than body weight during midstance, when the knee is extended

and the body's center of mass is higher than in the remainder of the stance phase. In other words, a relative unweighting caused by upward momentum of the center of mass means that the ground reaction forces are less than the body weight in midstance. In contrast, the body's center of mass is moving downward during the loading response and preswing; extra force, therefore, is required to decelerate the center of mass and accelerate it upward again.[10]

The ground reaction forces in the anteromedial direction are not always in the anterior direction; during the first half of the stance phase, this force is in the posterior direction. From initial contact to contralateral toe-off, the posterior component of the ground reaction forces increases to provide enough frictional resistance for the standing leg. This posterior force is necessary to keep the heel stationary (when the contralateral foot is propelling the body forward) and prepare the condition to support the body weight over the heel and during the period when the tibia is rolling forward over the heel of the standing leg.[10] The posterior force peaks at the contralateral toe-off with a magnitude equal to 20% of body weight. During midstance, this horizontal force decreases until the entire body weight is over the ankle. At this moment (50% of the stance phase), the horizontal component of the ground reaction forces does not exist. The direction of the ground reaction forces thereafter changes in the horizontal plane to create a propulsive force to move the body forward. The second peak horizontal force occurs at contralateral initial contact. The magnitude of the peak horizontal force depends on the length of the step. The longer the step, the higher the horizontal force is.[10,23]

The mediolateral component of the ground reaction forces is relatively small. Except during the loading response (double-support), these ground reaction forces are in the medial direction. The body's center of mass is to the medial (inner) side of the foot, and applying a lateral force to the ground therefore results in a medially directed ground reaction force during the midstance and terminal stance. However, the ground reaction forces are directed laterally at the beginning of the loading response and the end of the preswing. The magnitude of the mediolateral ground reaction force is less than 5% of body weight.[10]

Step-up Kinematics

Stair climbing is another major activity of daily living. In this chapter, climbing a single step is considered a step-up. The primary rotation of the knee occurs in the sagittal plane (flexion-extension), and its average range is approximately 45°. The secondary rotations in other rotational planes are much smaller (on average, less than 5°). From the beginning to the end of the step-up, the flexion angle consistently decreases from an average of 45° to full extension[24] (**Figure 10, A**). The axial plane (internal-external) rotation of the knee does not change noticeably. In the coronal plane, the knee is in an average 2° of varus at 45° of knee flexion, and it then rotates slightly into valgus. At the end of activity, when the knee is in full extension, the knee is in approximately 2° of

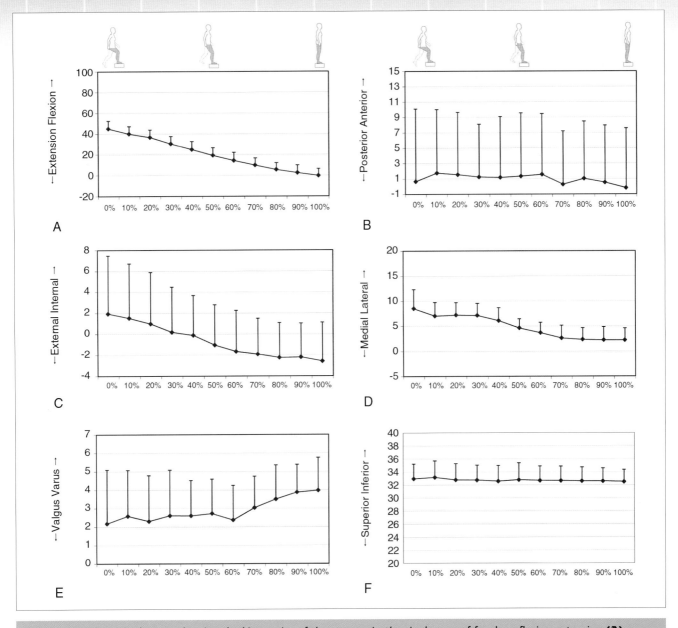

Figure 10 Schematic diagram showing the kinematics of the step-up in the six degrees of freedom: flexion-extension **(A)**, internal-external **(B)**, varus-valgus **(C)**, anteroposterior **(D)**, mediolateral **(E)**, and proximodistal **(F)**. Horizontal axis represents in 10% increments the activity from the beginning to the end of weight bearing.

valgus[24] (**Figure 10**, *B* and *C*).

In the sagittal plane, the tibia is approximately 9 mm anterior to the femur at the beginning of the activity. As the step-up progresses, the tibia translates in the posterior direction. At full extension, the tibia is 2 mm anterior to the femur. In the coronal plane, the mediolateral motion of the knee is less than in the sagittal plane. The tibia has an initial lateral shift of 2 mm at 45° of knee flexion. During step-up, the tibia moves more laterally toward its final position at full extension. At its final position, the tibia is 4 mm lateral relative to the femur[24] (**Figure 10**, *D* and *E*). The motion of the tibia with respect to the femur in the proximodistal di-

rection is less than 1 mm[24] (**Figure 10**, *F*).

Kinematics of the Patellofemoral Joint

The coordinate systems used to determine patellar tracking vary by activity and investigator.[25,26] Femur-fixed reference systems, in which patellar movement is defined with respect to a fixed femur,[27-29] as well as tibia-fixed and patella-fixed systems, have been used to describe patellar tracking.[30-33] Patellar indices based on patellofemoral joint geometry, including the femoral sulcus angle, patellofemoral congruence angle, lateral patellar displacement, lateral patellofemoral angle, and lateral patellar tilt,[34] have been clinically used to

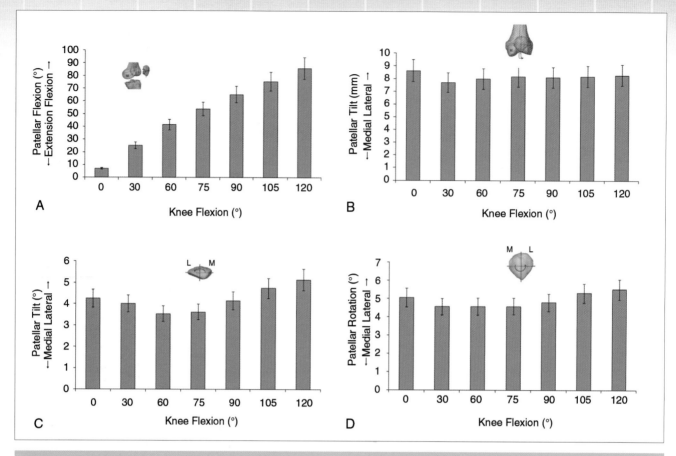

Figure 11 Schematic diagrams showing patellar kinematics with respect to knee flexion angles: patellar flexion(**A**), patellar shift (**B**), patellar tilt (**C**), patellar rotation (**D**). Bracketed lines = 95% confidence intervals. (Adapted with permission from Nha KW, Papannagari R, Gill TJ, et al: In vivo patellar tracking: Clinical motions and patellofemoral indices. *J Orthop Res* 2008;26[8]: 1067-1074.)

evaluate joint abnormalities.[8,32]

Patellofemoral tracking is clinically described in terms of flexion, tilt, rotation, and mediolateral shift[8,26] (**Figure 11**). Patellar flexion increases with knee flexion but at a lower rate. As the knee flexes from 0° to 90°, the patella flexes approximately 10° to 65°.[8,35,36] At approximately 135° of knee flexion, patellar flexion of 95° occurs.[8] During weight-bearing flexion from 0° to 120°, the patella rotates laterally less than 1°.[8] The patella tilts medially less than 1° as the knee flexes to 60°, then tilts laterally approximately 2° as knee flexion continues to 120°. The lateral shift of the patella with respect to the femur is less than 2 mm during weight-bearing flexion (from full extension to 120°). The patella shifts slightly medially at early flexion and then consistently shifts laterally as the knee flexes to 120°.[35] The femoral sulcus angle varies approximately 10° and 15°, depending on the knee flexion angle (**Figure 12**, *A*). By increasing flexion from full extension to 45°, the femoral sulcus angle decreases. From 45° to 90° of knee flexion, the femoral sulcus angle increases to its peak value (approximately 145°) and then decreases as the knee continues to flex to 120°.

The range of mean congruence angle is −20° to −30° (**Figure 12**, *B*). The lateral patellofemoral angle consistently increases less than 10° as knee flexion increases from full extension to 120° (**Figure 12**, *C*). Lateral patellar tilt decreases less than 10° as the knee flexes (**Figure 12**, *D*). Lateral patellar displacement increases less than 6 mm during weight-bearing knee flexion[8] (**Figure 12**, *E*). The kinematics of the patellofemoral joint depend on the type of loading. Studies have used different loading conditions, reference points, and coordinate systems for determining patellofemoral tracking.

Kinematics of Knee Injuries

Knee injuries account for 19% to 23% of all musculoskeletal injuries.[37] Knee injuries are classified either as direct stress injuries or repeated stress injuries. Direct stress injuries occur when knee stress in a specific direction overloads the structures that restrain the forces. The LCL, MCL, medial and lateral menisci, ACL, and PCL are commonly injured by direct stress. Often several similarly functioning structures are injured together. For example, the O'Donoghue triad is an injury to the MCL, medial meniscus, and ACL; similarly, LCL injury commonly is associated with injury to the ACL and PCL.

In contrast to direct stress injuries, repeated stress inju-

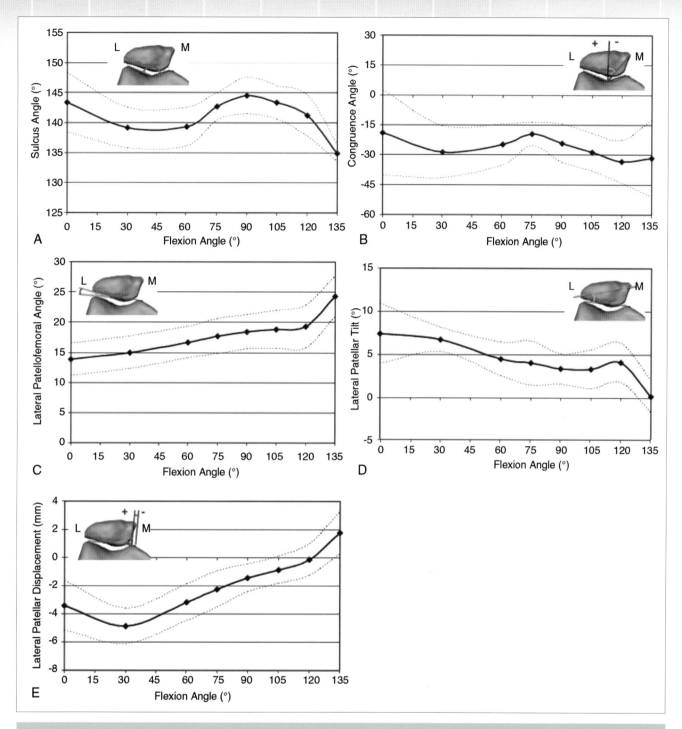

Figure 12 Schematic diagrams showing the femoral sulcus angle **(A)**, congruence angle **(B)**, lateral patellofemoral angle **(C)**, lateral patellar tilt **(D)**, and lateral patellar displacement **(E)**, all with respect to knee flexion in lunge weight bearing. L = lateral, M = medial, dotted lines = 95% confidence intervals. (Reproduced with permission from Nha KW, Papannagari R, Gill TJ, et al: In vivo patellar tracking: Clinical motions and patellofemoral indices. *J Orthop Res* 2008;26[8]:1067-1074.)

ries are caused by overuse of the joint. Iliotibial band syndrome occurs in individuals who perform repetitive activities such as long distance running and cycling. The symptoms of this syndrome include pain and swelling in the lateral aspect of the femur. Patellar tendinitis (an inflammation of the patellar tendon) is another common overuse injury. Patellar tendinitis is likely to occur in participants in long jumping, long distance running, tennis, or basketball.

2: Physiology of Musculoskeletal Tissues

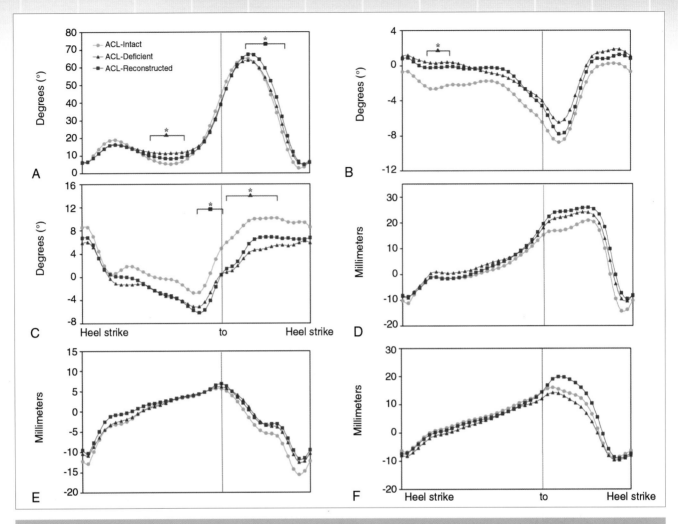

Figure 13 Schematic diagrams showing the kinematics of ACL-deficient, reconstructed, and intact knees in flexion-extension **(A)**, varus-valgus **(B)**, and external-internal **(C)** tibial rotation; and in anteroposterior **(D)**, mediolateral **(E)**, and superoinferior **(F)** translation of the femur relative to the tibia. All are shown over the full gait cycle from initial contact to toe-off. Segments with significant statistical differences ($P < 0.05$) between the patients and the control groups were marked with asterisks. (Adapted with permission from Gao B, Zheng NN: Alterations in three-dimensional joint kinematics of anterior cruciate ligament-deficient and -reconstructed knees during walking. *Clin Biomech (Bristol, Avon)* 2010;25[3]:222-229.)

Such injuries to knee joint structures alter the normal joint kinematics and performance.

ACL Injury

The ACL provides knee joint stability by preventing excessive anteromedial tibial translations, internal-external tibial rotations, and varus-valgus rotations. The exposure of the knee joint to high-stress conditions means that the ACL is one of the most commonly injured ligaments in the body. The annual incidence of injury is estimated at 80,000 to more than 250,000 in the United States.[38] Approximately 70% of ACL injuries are noncontact injuries.[39] The etiology of noncontact injuries is believed to be manifold and to involve several kinematic and kinetic factors. An abrupt change in direction, in combination with deceleration of the body, results in tibial internal or external rotation and ante-rior translation with the foot planted, and it is detrimental to the ACL. Other biomechanical, environmental, anatomic, and hormonal risk factors for noncontact injury have been identified.[38]

ACL impairment changes the kinematics of the knee. Tibiofemoral kinematics during activities such as gait (walking), quasistatic lunging, and stair climbing have been evaluated using radiostereometric techniques, optoelectronic tracking systems, fluoroscopy, and MRI.[40-42] Several studies have evaluated the kinematics of ACL-deficient knees during gait, compared with healthy knee kinematics. Patients with an ACL-deficient knee were found to have significantly less extension during the midstance phase of the gait cycle, and there was a significant increase in varus rotation (2° to 3°) during the stance phase of the gait cycle.[43] The ACL-deficient knees had significantly less external tibial rotation during the swing phase of the gait cycle. No signif-

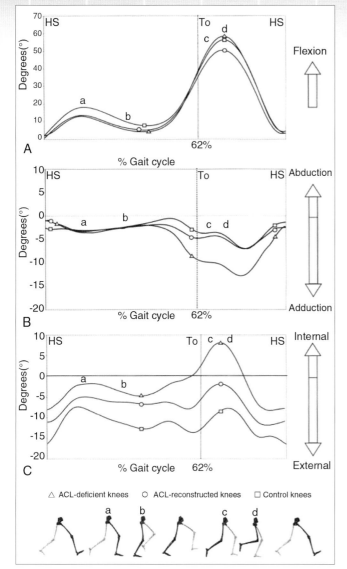

Figure 14 Schematic diagrams showing mean curves for knee flexion-extension **(A)**, tibial abduction-adduction **(B)**, and tibial internal-external rotation **(C)** in different periods of the gait cycle: loading response (a), midstance (b), initial swing (c), midswing (d). HS = heel strike (initial contact), TO = toe-off. (Reproduced with permission from Georgoulis AD, Papadonikolakis A, Papageorgiou CD Mitsou A, Stergiou: Three-dimensional tibiofemoral kinematics of the anterior cruciate ligament-deficient and reconstructed knee during walking. *Am J Sports Med* 2003;31(1):75-79.)

icant differences in translation were observed between normal and ACL-deficient knees[43] (**Figure 13**). In another study, no significant differences were found between ACL-intact and ACL-deficient knees in flexion-extension, varus-valgus, and internal-external rotations[42] (**Figure 14**). However, significant differences were observed in the maximal tibial rotations of ACL-intact and ACL-deficient knees.

ACL-deficient knees rotated internally during the initial swing phase of the gait cycle.

During quasistatic lunge activity, ACL-deficient knees were found to have increased anterior tibial translation and internal tibial rotation.[44] An increase in medial tibial translation also was observed in patients with ACL rupture. The oblique orientation of the ACL from medial on the tibia to lateral on the femur explains the increase in medial tibial translation when the ACL is injured. During stair climbing, as in other activities, ACL deficiency causes an increase in anterior tibial translation. However, the maximal anterior tibial translation was observed to occur at a lower flexion angle in ACL-injured knees than in ACL-intact knees.[44]

ACL deficiency changes the contact characteristics of the tibiofemoral joint. Abnormal stress distributions in the cartilage may predispose the knee to degenerative changes.[45] ACL deficiency causes the tibiofemoral cartilage contact points to shift both posteriorly and laterally on the surface of the tibial plateau. In the medial compartment, the contact points shift toward the medial tibial spine. Increased medial shift is of particular interest because it can lead to increased cartilage contact stress in this region. An increase in medial shift is well correlated with the observation that cartilage degeneration is likely to occur in the medial femoral condyle with chronic ACL injuries.[44,46] The observed medial shifts are minimal (approximately 2 mm) because of tibiofemoral contact congruity. Minimal alterations in tibiofemoral kinematics can profoundly alter the cartilage contact biomechanics of the tibiofemoral joint, however. The altered kinematics of the ACL-deficient knee shift the location of cartilage contact to a smaller region of thinner cartilage and increase the magnitude of cartilage contact deformation in both the medial and lateral compartments.[47]

In addition to the short-term complications associated with an ACL injury, such as functional impairment, secondary meniscal injury, and changes in knee joint loading, considerable evidence suggests that ACL injury disrupts the homeostasis of the healthy cartilage and can accelerate the development of osteoarthritis. Both mechanical and non-mechanical factors have been proposed as contributors to disease progression, but the precise mechanism for the initiation of posttraumatic osteoarthritis remains obscure.

Patients with an ACL deficiency often have altered quadriceps muscle performance, characterized by weakness and atrophy, as well as degeneration of the patellofemoral joint cartilage.[48] Because the patellofemoral and tibiofemoral joints are biomechanically related, patellofemoral kinematics are influenced by changes in the tibiofemoral kinematics. ACL injury causes an increase in the apparent elongation of the patellar tendon,[49] which could be responsible for the quadriceps muscle weakness associated with ACL injury. ACL injury can cause a decrease in the sagittal and coronal plane angles and an increased external twist of the patella.[49] This altered orientation of the patellar tendon is a coupled effect of increased anterior translation, internal rotation,

2: Physiology of Musculoskeletal Tissues

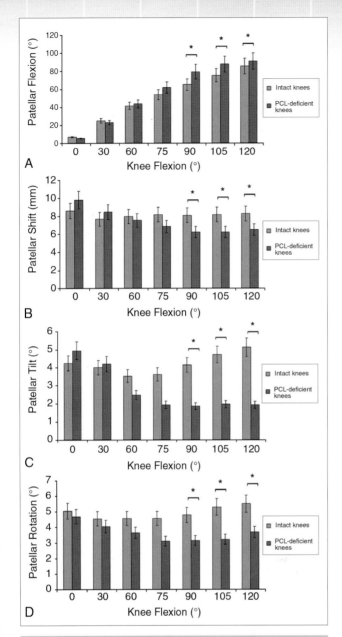

Figure 15 Schematic diagrams showing patellar flexion **(A)**, patellar shift **(B)**, patellar tilt **(C)**, and patellar rotation **(D)** as a function of knee flexion angle in intact and PCL-deficient knees. Bracketed vertical lines = mean ± standard deviation, asterisk = *P* < 0.007 between intact and PCL-deficient knees (as determined using the Wilcoxon signed-rank test). (Reproduced with permission from Van de Velde SK, Bingham JT, Gill TJ, Li G: Analysis of tibiofemoral cartilage deformation in the posterior cruciate ligament-deficient knee. *J Bone Joint Surg Am* 2009;91[1]:167-175.)

and medial translation of the tibia, as observed in ACL deficiency.

PCL Injury

PCL injury occurs much less often than ACL injury.[50] Injury to the PCL can result from high-energy motor vehicle

trauma or sports-related knee hyperflexion. The PCL is most often injured in conjunction with the posterolateral corner structures. Isolated PCL injury is relatively uncommon. PCL injuries are believed to be underdiagnosed because they are often asymptomatic; any symptoms are more subtle than those of ACL injury. Patients with a PCL injury have difficulty in ascending or descending stairs, and they report knee pain in deep knee flexion.

The primary functional role of the PCL is to restrain posterior tibial translation. In addition, the PCL provides secondary restraint to tibial varus, valgus, and external rotations. In vitro and in vivo studies found that PCL deficiency increases posterior tibial translation, lateral tibial translation, and tibial external rotation.[51,52] This finding might be explained by the structural orientation of the PCL, which is anterior with respect to the tibia to constrain posterior tibial translation and medial to constrain lateral translation and external rotation of the tibia.

The pathologic changes associated with PCL injuries were found to include posterior displacement of the tibia and degenerative osteoarthritic changes in the tibiofemoral and patellofemoral joints.[5] Joint degeneration was found in 36% to 90% of patients with a PCL injury.[52] The changes may be attributable to observed increases in the magnitude of anteromedial peak cartilage deformation in comparison with normal knees.[53] In cadaver knees, elevated patellofemoral contact pressures were found when the PCL was sectioned.[5] The observed patellofemoral kinematic alterations changed the location of the patellofemoral cartilage contact points. In vivo research found that PCL deficiency causes a distal and medial shift of cartilage contact points from 75° to 120° of flexion[35] (**Figure 15**).

Summary

The knee joint has an important role in transmitting loads, maintaining body alignment, and facilitating locomotor activities. The surrounding active and passive structures work together to achieve these functions. Knee kinesiology is a science of knee joint movements. Kinematics are commonly used to describe knee motion. The kinematics and kinetics of the knee are activity dependent. Knowledge of kinesiology is critical to understanding the etiology of disease states of the knee joint and developing effective treatment modalities.

References

1. Callaghan JJ, Rosenberg AG, Rubash HE, Simonian PT, Wickiewicz TL: *The Adult Knee*. Philadelphia, PA, Lippincott Williams & Wilkins, 2003.

2. Levangie PK, Norkin CC: *Joint Structure and Function: A Comprehensive Analysis*, ed 4. Philadelphia, PA, FA Davis, 2005.

3. Hogervorst T, Brand RA: Mechanoreceptors in joint function. *J Bone Joint Surg Am* 1998;80(9):1365-1378.

4. Welsh RP: Knee joint structure and function. *Clin Orthop Relat Res* 1980;147:7-14.

5. Gill TJ, DeFrate LE, Wang C, et al: The effect of posterior cruciate ligament reconstruction on patellofemoral contact pressures in the knee joint under simulated muscle loads. *Am J Sports Med* 2004;32(1):109-115.

6. Kaufman KR, Hughes C, Morrey BF, Morrey M, An KN: Gait characteristics of patients with knee osteoarthritis. *J Biomech* 2001;34(7):907-915.

7. Laubenthal KN, Smidt GL, Kettelkamp DB: A quantitative analysis of knee motion during activities of daily living. *Phys Ther* 1972;52(1):34-43.

8. Nha KW, Papannagari R, Gill TJ, et al: In vivo patellar tracking: Clinical motions and patellofemoral indices. *J Orthop Res* 2008;26(8):1067-1074.

9. Nordin M, Frankel VH: *Basic Biomechanics of the Musculoskeletal System*, ed 3. Philadelphia, PA, Lippincott Williams & Wilkins, 2001.

10. Neumann DA: *Kinesiology of the Musculoskeletal System: Foundations for Physical Rehabilitation*. St. Louis, MO, Mosby, 2002.

11. Larish DD, Martin PE, Mungiole M: Characteristic patterns of gait in the healthy old. *Ann N Y Acad Sci* 1988;515:18-32.

12. Stolze H, Kuhtz-Buschbeck JP, Mondwurf C, et al: Gait analysis during treadmill and overground locomotion in children and adults. *Electroencephalogr Clin Neurophysiol* 1997;105(6):490-497.

13. Wall JC, Charteris J: A kinematic study of long-term habituation to treadmill walking. *Ergonomics* 1981;24(7):531-542.

14. Murray MP, Spurr GB, Sepic SB, Gardner GM, Mollinger LA: Treadmill vs. floor walking: Kinematics, electromyogram, and heart rate. *J Appl Physiol* 1985;59(1):87-91.

15. Barbeau H: Locomotor training in neurorehabilitation: Emerging rehabilitation concepts. *Neurorehabil Neural Repair* 2003;17(1):3-11.

16. Owings TM, Grabiner MD: Step width variability, but not step length variability or step time variability, discriminates gait of healthy young and older adults during treadmill locomotion. *J Biomech* 2004;37(6):935-938.

17. van Ingen Schenau GJ: Some fundamental aspects of the biomechanics of overground versus treadmill locomotion. *Med Sci Sports Exerc* 1980;12(4):257-261.

18. Warabi T, Kato M, Kiriyama K, Yoshida T, Kobayashi N: Treadmill walking and overground walking of human subjects compared by recording sole-floor reaction force. *Neurosci Res* 2005;53(3):343-348.

19. Alton F, Baldey L, Caplan S, Morrissey MC: A kinematic comparison of overground and treadmill walking. *Clin Biomech (Bristol, Avon)* 1998;13(6):434-440.

20. Pearce ME, Cunningham DA, Donner AP, Rechnitzer PA, Fullerton GM, Howard JH: Energy cost of treadmill and floor walking at self-selected paces. *Eur J Appl Physiol Occup Physiol* 1983;52(1):115-119.

21. Strathy GM, Chao EY, Laughman RK: Changes in knee function associated with treadmill ambulation. *J Biomech* 1983;16(7):517-522.

22. Kozanek M, Hosseini A, Liu F, et al: Tibiofemoral kinematics and condylar motion during the stance phase of gait. *J Biomech* 2009;42(12):1877-1884.

23. Shelburne KB, Torry MR, Pandy MG: Contributions of muscles, ligaments, and the ground-reaction force to tibiofemoral joint loading during normal gait. *J Orthop Res* 2006;24(10):1983-1990.

24. Kozánek M, Hosseini A, de Velde SK, et al: Kinematic evaluation of the step-up exercise in anterior cruciate ligament deficiency. *Clin Biomech (Bristol, Avon)* 2011;26(9):950-954.

25. Katchburian MV, Bull AM, Shih YF, Heatley FW, Amis AA: Measurement of patellar tracking: Assessment and analysis of the literature. *Clin Orthop Relat Res* 2003;412:241-259.

26. Bull AM, Katchburian MV, Shih YF, Amis AA: Standardisation of the description of patellofemoral motion and comparison between different techniques. *Knee Surg Sports Traumatol Arthrosc* 2002;10(3):184-193.

27. Pinar H, Akseki D, Karaolan O, Genç I: Kinematic and dynamic axial computed tomography of the patello-femoral joint in patients with anterior knee pain. *Knee Surg Sports Traumatol Arthrosc* 1994;2(3):170-173.

28. Powers CM, Shellock FG, Pfaff M: Quantification of patellar tracking using kinematic MRI. *J Magn Reson Imaging* 1998;8(3):724-732.

29. Sheehan FT, Zajac FE, Drace JE: In vivo tracking of the human patella using cine phase contrast magnetic resonance imaging. *J Biomech Eng* 1999;121(6):650-656.

30. Reider B, Marshall JL, Ring B: Patellar tracking. *Clin Orthop Relat Res* 1981;157:143-148.

31. Stein LA, Endicott AN, Sampalis JS, Kaplow MA, Patel MD, Mitchell NS: Motion of the patella during walking: A video digital-fluoroscopic study in healthy volunteers. *AJR Am J Roentgenol* 1993;161(3):617-620.

32. Li G, Papannagari R, Nha KW, Defrate LE, Gill TJ, Rubash HE: The coupled motion of the femur and patella during in vivo weightbearing knee flexion. *J Biomech Eng* 2007;129(6):937-943.

33. Heegaard J, Leyvraz PF, Van Kampen A, Rakotomanana L, Rubin PJ, Blankevoort L: Influence of soft structures on patellar three-dimensional tracking. *Clin Orthop Relat Res* 1994;299:235-243.

34. Kujala UM, Osterman K, Kormano M, Komu M, Schlenzka D: Patellar motion analyzed by magnetic resonance imaging. *Acta Orthop Scand* 1989;60(1):13-16.

35. Van de Velde SK, Gill TJ, Li G: Dual fluoroscopic analysis of the posterior cruciate ligament-deficient patellofemoral joint during lunge. *Med Sci Sports Exerc* 2009;41(6):1198-1205.

36. Wilson NA, Press JM, Koh JL, Hendrix RW, Zhang LQ: In vivo noninvasive evaluation of abnormal patellar tracking during squatting in patients with patellofemoral pain. *J Bone Joint Surg Am* 2009;91(3):558-566.

37. Hootman JM, Macera CA, Ainsworth BE, Addy CL, Martin M, Blair SN: Epidemiology of musculoskeletal injuries among sedentary and physically active adults. *Med Sci Sports Exerc* 2002;34(5):838-844.

38. Griffin LY, Albohm MJ, Arendt EA, et al: Understanding and preventing noncontact anterior cruciate ligament injuries: A review of the Hunt Valley II meeting, January 2005. *Am J Sports Med* 2006;34(9):1512-1532.

2: Physiology of Musculoskeletal Tissues

39. Boden BP, Breit I, Sheehan FT: Tibiofemoral alignment: Contributing factors to noncontact anterior cruciate ligament injury. *J Bone Joint Surg Am* 2009;91(10):2381-2389.

40. Andriacchi TP, Dyrby CO: Interactions between kinematics and loading during walking for the normal and ACL deficient knee. *J Biomech* 2005;38(2):293-298.

41. Brandsson S, Karlsson J, Eriksson BI, Kärrholm J: Kinematics after tear in the anterior cruciate ligament: Dynamic bilateral radiostereometric studies in 11 patients. *Acta Orthop Scand* 2001;72(4):372-378.

42. Georgoulis AD, Papadonikolakis A, Papageorgiou CD, Mitsou A, Stergiou N: Three-dimensional tibiofemoral kinematics of the anterior cruciate ligament-deficient and reconstructed knee during walking. *Am J Sports Med* 2003; 31(1):75-79.

43. Gao B, Zheng NN: Alterations in three-dimensional joint kinematics of anterior cruciate ligament-deficient and -reconstructed knees during walking. *Clin Biomech (Bristol, Avon)* 2010;25(3):222-229.

44. Defrate LE, Papannagari R, Gill TJ, Moses JM, Pathare NP, Li G: The 6 degrees of freedom kinematics of the knee after anterior cruciate ligament deficiency: An in vivo imaging analysis. *Am J Sports Med* 2006;34(8):1240-1246.

45. Andriacchi TP, Mündermann A, Smith RL, Alexander EJ, Dyrby CO, Koo S: A framework for the in vivo pathomechanics of osteoarthritis at the knee. *Ann Biomed Eng* 2004; 32(3):447-457.

46. Li G, Papannagari R, DeFrate LE, Yoo JD, Park SE, Gill TJ: The effects of ACL deficiency on mediolateral translation and varus-valgus rotation. *Acta Orthop* 2007;78(3):355-360.

47. Van de Velde SK, Bingham JT, Hosseini A, et al: Increased tibiofemoral cartilage contact deformation in patients with anterior cruciate ligament deficiency. *Arthritis Rheum* 2009; 60(12):3693-3702.

48. Hsieh YF, Draganich LF, Ho SH, Reider B: The effects of removal and reconstruction of the anterior cruciate ligament on patellofemoral kinematics. *Am J Sports Med* 1998; 26(2):201-209.

49. Van de Velde SK, Gill TJ, DeFrate LE, Papannagari R, Li G: The effect of anterior cruciate ligament deficiency and reconstruction on the patellofemoral joint. *Am J Sports Med* 2008;36(6):1150-1159.

50. Colvin AC, Meislin RJ: Posterior cruciate ligament injuries in the athlete: Diagnosis and treatment. *Bull NYU Hosp Jt Dis* 2009;67(1):45-51.

51. Gollehon DL, Torzilli PA, Warren RF: The role of the posterolateral and cruciate ligaments in the stability of the human knee: A biomechanical study. *J Bone Joint Surg Am* 1987;69(2):233-242.

52. Li G, Papannagari R, Li M, et al: Effect of posterior cruciate ligament deficiency on in vivo translation and rotation of the knee during weightbearing flexion. *Am J Sports Med* 2008;36(3):474-479.

53. Van de Velde SK, Bingham JT, Gill TJ, Li G: Analysis of tibiofemoral cartilage deformation in the posterior cruciate ligament-deficient knee. *J Bone Joint Surg Am* 2009;91(1): 167-175.

Section 3

Basic Principles and Treatment of Musculoskeletal Disease

Section Editor

Constance R. Chu, MD

Chapter 17

Bone Biology and Engineering

Jennifer J. Westendorf, PhD

Lichun Lu, PhD

Michael J. Yaszemski, MD, PhD

3: Basic Principles and Treatment of Musculoskeletal Disease

Introduction

Bone provides both structural and physiologic functions to vertebrates. From a structural perspective, bone protects vital organs and bears loads that the body experiences, both from external forces and those that occur from muscle contraction. Bone serves as the anchor point for that muscle contraction through its specialized tendon insertion sites. The articular cartilage that covers the ends of long bones contributes to the joints, which permit locomotion via the lower extremities and the positioning of the hands in space via the upper extremities. Bone's ligament insertion sites, which have the same architecture as its tendon insertion sites, are integral to the structure and function of joints. Bone contributes to the body's physiologic functions via several mechanisms. Bone is the largest reservoir of calcium in the body, and the constant remodeling of bone mobilizes its calcium as one component of the process that tightly controls calcium homeostasis. In addition, bone retains reserve stores of phosphate and other important ions. Bone

Dr. Westendorf or an immediate family member has stock or stock options held in Amgen and serves as a board member, owner, officer, or committee member of the Orthopaedic Research Society and the American Society for Bone and Mineral Research. Dr. Yaszemski or an immediate family member has stock or stock options held in BonWrx and serves as a board member, owner, officer, or committee member of the American Academy of Orthopaedic Surgeons, the Minnesota Orthopedic Society, the Orthopaedic Research and Education Foundation, the Scoliosis Research Society, and the Society of Military Orthopaedic Surgeons. Neither Dr. Lu nor any immediate family member has received anything of value from or owns stock in a commercial company or institution related directly or indirectly to the subject of this chapter.

remodeling also serves a structural purpose. This process positions the available mineralized bone tissue in an optimum distribution to bear the loads experienced by the skeleton. The spaces between the bony struts and plates that make up trabecular bone contain the bone marrow, which produces and stores cells for several hematologic and regenerative body functions.

This chapter will discuss the normal anatomy of both trabecular and compact bone tissue, and will include a discussion of normal bone development, regeneration, and remodeling processes. Its focus will then shift to the age-related structural changes that result in osteoporosis, and will include the molecular strategies to slow or reverse this bone loss, along with an overview of the novel regenerative medicine and tissue-engineering strategies currently emerging to address bone defects.

Bone Tissue Anatomy

The mammalian skeleton consists of two types of bone tissue: compact bone and trabecular bone. Compact bone, a term that is synonymous with both the terms cortical bone and osteonal bone, contributes approximately 80% of the skeletal mass in humans. Trabecular bone, which is synonymous with both the terms cancellous bone and spongy bone, contributes approximately 20% of human skeletal mass (**Figure 1**). The external bone surface is covered with a connective tissue called periosteum, which consists of both an outer fibrous layer and a deeper cambium layer. The cambium layer of the periosteum contains osteoblast progenitor cells, which participate in fracture healing. Trabecular bone consists of an array of bony rods and plates, which form an interconnected pore space that contains the bone marrow. The age-related (or disease-related) loss of bone mass, called osteoporosis, results in a preferential loss of trabecular bone as opposed to cortical bone[1] (**Figure 2**).

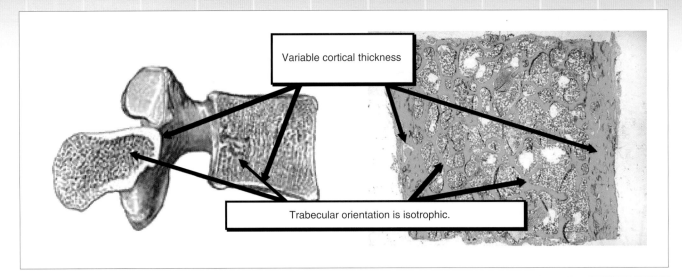

Variable cortical thickness

Trabecular orientation is isotrophic.

Figure I   Normal bone microanatomy.

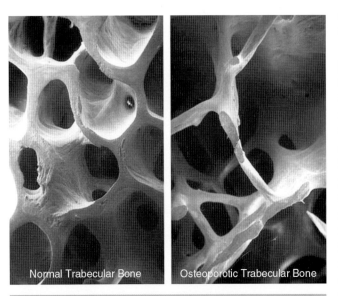

Normal Trabecular Bone   Osteoporotic Trabecular Bone

Figure 2   Trabecular bone changes in osteoporosis.

Both compact and trabecular bone are composed of an assembly of individual bone structural units (BSUs), each of which represents the structural end result of a focus of bone renewal (remodeling). Architecturally, cortical and trabecular BSUs are distinct. In cortical bone, BSUs may appear in cross section as concentric rings (lamellae), forming cylindrical-shaped structures. In cancellous bone, the lamellae are flat and appear stacked in saucer-shaped depressions. Cortical BSUs are laminated bony cylinders that have central (haversian) canals enclosing vascular structures, nerves, and a thin membranous lining (cortical endosteum) that contains flat, inactive-appearing lining cells. Cortical BSUs arise from haversian and other communicating channels called Volkmann canals, which are approximately 0.4 mm in width and are several millimeters in length. The Volkmann

canals are oriented in a branching pattern and lie perpendicular to the long axis of the bone.

All normal adult human bone undergoes renewal and repair through a process called bone remodeling. The cellular and molecular aspects of this process will be described in detail in the next section of this chapter. Groups of bone-resorbing and bone-forming cells form basic multicellular units (BMUs) that function at discrete sites throughout the skeleton in a highly coordinated sequence of cellular activity. At any given remodeling site, bone resorption always precedes bone formation, resulting in the removal and subsequent replacement of a section of bone at each site. Under normal steady-state conditions, the amount of bone removed is precisely replaced by the amount of new bone formed, and the end result consists of no net change in bone mass. Only the bone architecture is changed, to optimize the distribution of the available bone mass in a manner that optimally resists the stresses experienced in that region of the skeleton. This process usually results in anisotropic (mechanical properties differ in different loading directions) bone being formed in most parts of the skeleton. An example of a bone that has a complex loading pattern, such that its architecture is isotropic (similar in all directions), is the anterior portion of the ilium. This observation, coupled with the relatively easy surgical accessibility of the anterior ilium, has made this part of the skeleton the preferred site from which to obtain a bone biopsy to perform quantitative bone histomorphometry. This laboratory analysis technique, along with its associated tissue-staining and immunohistochemical procedures, assists clinicians in the diagnosis and treatment of many bone diseases. A thorough discussion of bone histomorphometry occurs later in this chapter.

The sequential events of the bone remodeling cycle are driven by an evolution of cellular events that occur over a time period of 3 to 6 months. The first phase, called activation, populates a quiescent bone surface with cells that have been recruited from circulating mononuclear phagocyte precursors and become preosteoclasts, which cannot be visually identified by standard microscopy. These cells are destined to become bone-resorbing osteoclasts. In the next phase, called resorption, the osteoclasts mature and remove a finite amount of mineralized bone via the following sequence: The basal surface of the osteoclast is rich in transfer organelles for both hydrochloric acid and cathepsin, and is called the ruffled border. The osteoclasts attach to the exposed mineralized bone surface to form an isolated, sealed microenvironment that becomes rich in both hydrochloric acid and lysosomal enzymes (for example, cathepsin) as the transfer organelles deliver their contents into the sealed microenvironment. Mature osteoclasts move over the bone surface, removing both the mineral and organic components of bone simultaneously, and leaving serrated footprints, or Howship lacunae, on the remaining bone surface.

Osteoclasts have variable morphology. Though often appearing as large multinuclear cells, they may be small, appear mononuclear, and, except for their characteristic location within Howship resorption lacunae, can be difficult to distinguish from fibroblasts, osteoblasts, and other cells. Positive identification may be made using acid phosphatase stains. Osteoclastic resorption of mineralized bone releases both minerals and the products of collagenous protein degradation into the circulation. The released minerals participate in the body's mineral homeostasis process. The collagen degradation product concentrations can be measured in blood or urine, and reflect the degree of bone-resorbing activity. They are considered to be markers of bone resorption. The phase that follows resorption is called reversal, during which osteoclast activity and numbers decline, and the osteoclasts are replaced by preosteoblasts (bone-forming cell precursors).

As the resorptive phase wanes and is replaced by the reversal phase, the Howship resorption lacunae become populated by mononuclear preosteoblasts (cells that are derived from recruited mesenchymal progenitors in the bone marrow, pericytes associated with capillaries, and circulating bone-forming cell precursors). Preosteoblasts are destined to become bone-forming osteoblasts. Osteoclasts ultimately undergo cell death (apoptosis). Preosteoblasts can be visually identified by their proximity to the resorption surface, clear cytoplasm, single nuclei, and positive alkaline phosphatase staining. The phase that follows reversal is called formation.

During formation, preosteoblasts become mature osteoblasts and secrete bone matrix, which subsequently undergoes mineralization. The osteoblasts, which appear as mononuclear cells with prominent nucleoli and deeply stained cytoplasm, form a cellular monolayer on the resorption surface previously abandoned by osteoclasts. Osteoblasts secrete type I collagen, called osteoid, from their basal surface, which is apposed to the remaining mineralized bone surface of the Howship lacuna. Type I collagen is composed of three peptide chains (two $\alpha1$ chains and one $\alpha2$ chain). Type I collagen is synthesized in a procollagen form, which undergoes posttranslational hydroxylation and glycosylation of selective amino acid residues. It further undergoes removal of terminal sequences before being secreted in its mature form, collagen, from the basilar surface of osteoblasts into the underlying extracellular space. This osteoid forms the organic matrix of the new bone. Under normal conditions, the collagen molecules of the newly secreted osteoid establish covalent carbon-to-nitrogen cross-links that result in both end-to-end and side-to-side alignment, forming mats of aligned and interconnected collagen molecules. These collagen mats periodically alternate their spatial orientation, resulting in the layered structure that, when mineralized, is called lamellar bone. Ten to 15 days after secretion, osteoid undergoes maturational changes that prepare it for the initial deposition of calcium phosphate crystals. This mineral deposition occurs along an interface between mineralized and unmineralized bone called the mineralization front. The mineralization front moves as mineralization proceeds, but its starting point is called the reversal line, which defines the limit of bone erosion and the original site of bone formation (**Figure 3**). Under conditions of rapid bone turnover (for example, normal skeletal growth, fracture healing, or bone-forming tumors), osteoid is deposited in a disorganized fashion, resulting in a relatively isotropic structure called woven bone (**Figure 4**). Osteoblasts secrete collagenous and noncollagenous proteins into the circulation, including alkaline phosphatase, osteocalcin, and the C- and N-terminal fragments of procollagen. The concentrations of these products in serum and urine serve as markers of bone turnover during the formation phase, just as the products of osteoclastic activity, mentioned previously, serve during the resorption phase.

Between the BMU and bone marrow is a structure called the bone remodeling compartment (BRC). The BRC is thought to be a component of the BMU that provides a local environment for regional cell signaling to coordinate the coupling of bone formation to bone resorption. Though the remodeling cycle begins with osteoclastic bone resorption and ends with osteoblastic bone formation and its subsequent mineralization, osteoclasts and osteoblasts are otherwise simultaneously present in different regions of the same BMU during most of the active remodeling cycle. Trabecular bone remodeling occurs over a trabecular surface and within a canopy of lining cells, whereas compact bone remodeling occurs in a cylinder that lies within the compact bone tissue (**Figure 5**). Bone cell function and the sequence of cell activities are otherwise similar. Trabecular bone remodeling units (synonymous with bone BMUs) occur in greater numbers than those in contact bone, causing the trabecular bone turnover rate to be approximately tenfold that of compact bone. Compact bone BMUs originate from haversian or Volkmann canals, where osteoclasts excavate a resorption cavity called a cutting cone, which extends in a linear path through the cortex and forms a resorption tunnel.

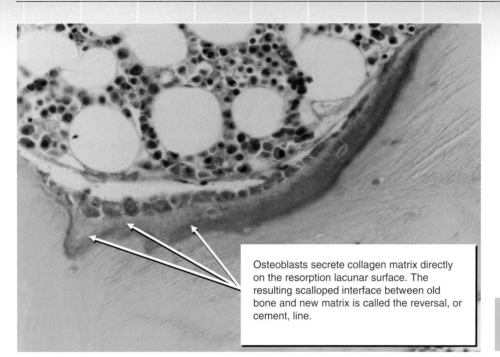

Osteoblasts secrete collagen matrix directly on the resorption lacunar surface. The resulting scalloped interface between old bone and new matrix is called the reversal, or cement, line.

Figure 3 Histology slide demonstrating the reversal (cement) line.

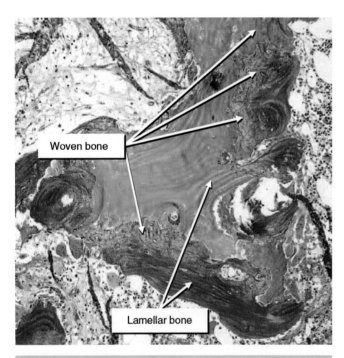

Woven bone

Lamellar bone

Figure 4 Histology slide demonstrating the difference between lamellar and woven bone.

Behind the advancing cutting cone is an irregular area somewhat devoid of active cells, the reversal zone. An elongated tapering tunnel, the closing cone, lined by osteoid and osteoblasts that circumferentially refill the resorption tunnel, follows the reversal zone. Bone formation eventually terminates, leaving a central haversian canal that contains blood vessels, lymphatic vessels, and connective tissue elements. A complete cortical remodeling cycle requires 6 to 9 months. The next section of this chapter will discuss these bone development and remodeling processes from the perspective of the detailed molecular and cellular events that simultaneously occur.

Bone Development, Remodeling (Regeneration), and Regeneration Signaling Pathways

Bone forms via two mechanisms: intramembranous or endochondral ossification. Intramembranous ossification occurs when mesenchymal progenitor cells differentiate directly into osteoblasts. This process forms many of the flat bones of the skull and most of the bones in the clavicles. In contrast, during endochondral ossification the progenitor cell condensations differentiate into chondrocytes, which form a cartilaginous scaffold that becomes vascularized, recruits osteoblasts and osteoclasts that remodel the scaffold, and then mineralizes. Long bones and vertebrae develop via endochondral ossification. These developmental processes are reactivated in response to injury or stress.[2] For example, intramembranous ossification is the primary means of bone formation during distraction osteogenesis and for fractures that are stabilized (for example, by external fixation). In contrast, endochondral ossification occurs when motion exists at a fracture site and during many conditions that produce ectopic mineralization. In all cases, progenitors are likely recruited from the periosteum, blood vessel pericytes, and potentially from marrow and circulating populations. Tissue-engineering approaches facilitate these processes through the addition of cytokines to the scaffold and variability in its structural rigidity (for example, transforming growth factor–β (TGF-β) and bone morphogenetic protein–2 (BMP-2) for endochondral ossification and fabrica-

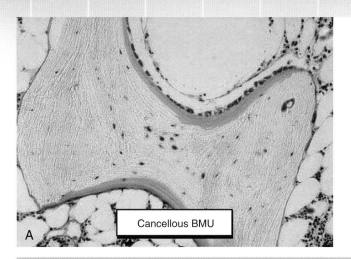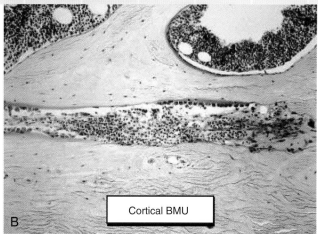

Cancellous BMU

Cortical BMU

Figure 5 Histology slides demonstrating the difference between remodeling in compact and trabecular bone. Cancellous remodelling (**A**) occurs over a trabecular surface, whereas cortical remodeling (**B**) occurs within a cylinder.

tion of a more rigid scaffold to promote osteoblast maturation).

During a person's life span, bones are constantly being remodeled and regenerated. The same processes that are involved in the healing of clinically significant fractures are active during repair of microfractures and in response to physiologic situations, such as low calcium levels. The cells that have major roles in remodeling and regeneration are osteoblasts, osteocytes, and osteoclasts. Osteocytes are derived from mesenchymal progenitor cells. They produce an extracellular matrix rich in type I collagen and mineralization-promoting factors. Runx2 (Cbfa1) is a master transcription factor for osteoblast maturation because many cellular signaling pathways converge on Runx2 in cell nuclei to regulate gene expression programs (**Figure 6**). Osteocytes are terminally differentiated osteoblastic cells that become embedded in the mineralized matrix. They constitute 90% of cells in bone and are responsible for sensing the environment (for example, loading or damage). They communicate with each other and with cells on the bone surface, including preosteoclasts and preosteoblasts, via long processes called dendrites. This communication is a factor in the regulation of bone regeneration. The osteocytes are the major producers of sclerostin, an inhibitor of bone formation. Anabolic stimuli (for example, loading and parathyroid hormone [PTH]) suppress sclerostin expression and thus promote bone formation.[3,4] Osteoclasts are myeloid-derived cells that resorb proteins and mineral in the bone matrix to remove damaged tissue or to release stored calcium and stimulate new bone formation.[5] There is extensive cross-talk (coupling) between osteoblasts and osteoclasts on the bone surface under a protective cellular canopy and within bone remodeling units (BMUs).[6,7] Osteoclasts are crucial for remodeling woven bone and initiating its replacement with the stronger lamellar bone.

Bone Morphogenetic Proteins

BMPs are secreted factors with similarity to TGF.[8] Multiple BMPs (BMPs 2 through 18) exist in humans; some are promoters of bone and cartilage formation and others act as suppressors. BMPs bind cell surface protein complexes consisting of type I and type II receptors, which are serine-threonine kinases. Through these receptors, BMPs trigger intracellular signaling cascades that involve the dimerization of SMAD proteins and activation of other kinases, such as Erk. These events culminate in cell nuclei where Runx2 is activated and gene expression programs are altered (**Figure 6**). Two BMPs, BMP-2 and BMP-7 (osteogenic protein–1), were approved by the Food and Drug Administration and are delivered from absorbable collagen scaffolds. Since that time, numerous variations of BMP delivery have been tested in a variety of models to improve bone healing.[9]

Wnts and Wnt Inhibitors, Sclerostin, and Dkk1

Wnts are secreted proteins that bind the transmembrane receptors Lrp5/6 and Frizzleds 1 through 10 on cell surfaces to promote osteoblast survival and proliferation.[10,11] Wnt pathway activation is essential for peak bone mass acquisition during development and is reactivated during fracture repair.[12] Thus, suboptimal Wnt signaling through Lrp5/6 causes severe osteopenia, whereas excessive Wnt signaling causes high bone mass. Wnts can be sequestered by other secreted factors, two being sclerostin (Scl) and dickkopf-related protein 1 (Dkk1). Neutralizing antibodies to Scl and Dkk1 stimulate fracture healing in nonhuman primates and rodents and are in clinical trials to promote bone formation in osteoporosis by enhancing Wnt/Lrp signaling.[13-15]

Parathyroid Hormone

PTH is a systemic hormone released from the thyroid gland when circulating calcium levels decrease. PTH stimulates

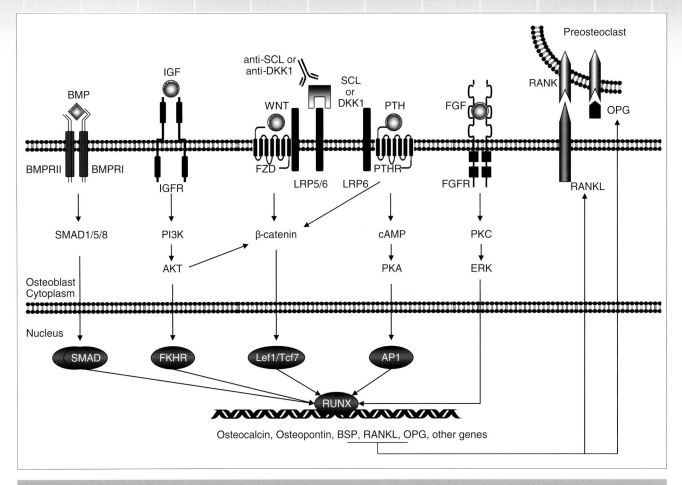

Figure 6 Osteogenic cell signaling pathways. AP, activator protein; BMP, bone morphogenetic protein; BMPR, bone morphogenetic protein receptor; cAMP, cyclic adenosine monophosphate; DKK, dickkopf; LRP, low-density lipoprotein receptor-related protein; OPG, osteoprotegerin; PTH, parathyroid hormone; PTHR, parathyroid hormone receptor; RANK, receptor activator of nuclear factor-κB; RANKL, receptor activator of nuclear factor-κB ligand; SCL, sclerostin.

bone resorption and calcium release from mineralized tissues to normalize serum calcium levels. When administered in a continuous fashion or at high concentrations, PTH stimulates bone resorption, but at lower levels and with intermittent exposure, it paradoxically stimulates bone formation. The first 34 amino acids of PTH (teriparatide) are sufficient to stimulate signaling from the PTH receptor (PTHR1).[16] PTH and PTHR1 can co-opt Lrp6 from the Wnt signaling pathway to enhance bone formation.[17] PTH also induces Wnt expression in fracture callus and suppresses sclerostin expression by osteocytes to indirectly promote Wnt signaling and bone formation.[18-23] Teriparatide is the only anabolic therapy approved in the United States for osteoporosis. The recommended treatment duration is 2 years because of the carcinogenic potential of PTH in animal models.[24,25]

RANK-RANKL-Osteoprotegerin and Denosumab

Receptor activator of nuclear factor-κB (RANK) is the transmembrane cell surface. The RANK molecule and its ligand, RANKL, mediate osteoclast activation. Within bone cells, RANK is expressed on preosteoclasts, whereas RANKL is expressed on osteoblasts. In the presence of macrophage colony-stimulating factor, the interactions between RANK and RANKL stimulate osteoclast fusion and maturation.[5] Osteoprotegerin is a natural soluble protein that interferes with RANK-RANKL associations to prevent osteoclastogenesis and subsequent bone resorption. Denosumab is a monoclonal antibody that binds RANKL and blocks its interactions with RANK, thus preventing osteoclast maturation and function. It was approved by the Food and Drug Administration in 2010 to treat postmenopausal women with osteoporosis, who are at high risk of insufficiency fractures, and to mitigate pathologic fractures in oncology patients with bone metastases. As with other antiresorptive therapies (for example, bisphosphonates), rare cases of osteonecrosis of the jaw have been documented in patients taking denosumab. However, the benefits from significant reductions in fracture incidence make it an attractive treatment option for its approved indications.

Bone Tissue Analysis: Quantitative Bone Histomorphometry

The measurement and analysis of bone structure and bone remodeling is done via a technique called bone histomorphometry.[26] Histomorphometry is usually performed on trabecular bone from transiliac biopsies. The isotropic (randomly oriented) nature of trabeculae in iliac bone is somewhat unusual in the skeleton, and reflects the complex, multidirectional loading pattern experienced by the iliac bones. Most other bones experience anisotropic loading patterns, and consequently have anisotropic trabecular (in trabecular bone) or osteonal (in compact bone) orientation. The fundamental stereologic principle used in bone histomorphometry depends on the trabecular isotropy of the iliac biopsy specimens. This principle states that two-dimensional measurements (area) can be converted to and expressed as three-dimensional (volume) measurements.[27] Isotropy also implies that the bony trabecular structures are viewed and measured at some random degree of obliquity. Therefore, a correction factor for obliquity ($4/\pi$) is used in all thickness measurements.

The transiliac biopsy is an outpatient surgical procedure that is done under monitored anesthesia care supplemented with local anesthetic infiltration. The hole-saw hand drill has an internal diameter of 7 mm, and is placed through a sheath that has been positioned onto the external cortex of the ilium via intramuscular dilation. An appropriate biopsy position is approximately 3 cm posterior to the anterior-superior iliac spine along the iliac crest, and 3 cm inferior to the iliac crest from that point. The drill is advanced sequentially through the external iliac cortex, the trabecular bone between the cortices, and the internal iliac cortex. The surgeon can sense the transitions between the cortices and the trabecular bone by the change in resistance to the drill as each junction is crossed. Once the internal cortex has been crossed, the drill is withdrawn, and the specimen is removed from the drill by pushing it out with an obturator. An acceptable specimen is an intact bone cylinder that has cortical bone on both sides of the trabecular bone from between the tables of the ilium. This intact specimen increases the likelihood that the trabecular portion of the specimen, which will be used for the analysis, has not been crushed or altered in any other way during its harvest. The specimen is passed from the surgical field to the histomorphometry technologist. The surgeon and technologist together assess the specimen for its suitability for analysis. If the specimen is not suitable, then additional passes at nearby points on the ilium are made until an appropriate specimen is harvested.

In the histomorphometry laboratory, the transiliac biopsy specimen is cut into sections and mounted on slides. **Figure 7** depicts a stained slide of a normal transiliac biopsy specimen. Using a digitizing computer graphics program, multiple fields on such a slide are selected and analyzed. Bone tissue volume is the sum of mineralized and nonmin-

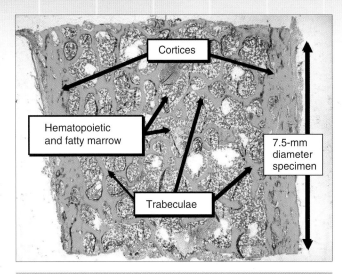

Figure 7 Histology slide demonstrating a normal transiliac bone biopsy.

eralized volumes from all the selected fields. Remember that the isotropy property of iliac trabecular bone is used to convert the area measurements from the slides into volume measurements reported as the quantitative histomorphometry output. All trabeculae within each selected field are then graphically outlined, and both the trabecular bone volume and total trabecular bone surface are calculated. The trabecular bone volume is the ratio of the trabecular bone volume to the total measured bone tissue volume. Trabecular bone volume is approximately 20% in women and 22% in men, and is related to cancellous bone mass. It declines with age and with bone loss. Trabecular bone volume is also commonly referred to as bone volume/total volume, or Tb.V/TV.

Trabecular separation is the mean distance (in millimeters) between trabeculae. Trabecular separation is a measure of trabecular connectivity. Trabecular separation increases with aging and trabecular bone loss. Mean trabecular thickness is a measure of trabecular structure, and is calculated as the reciprocal of the trabecular separation. Trabecular thickness is reduced by aging and osteoporosis. Trabecular number is the number of trabeculae present per lineal millimeter. Trabecular number is calculated as trabecular bone volume/trabecular thickness. Trabecular number is a measure of trabecular connectivity, and it decreases with bone loss. In the ilium, the average combined cortical thickness (the summation of the cortical widths of the inner and outer cortices of the ilium) in women and men is approximately 820 µm and 915 µm, respectively. The combined cortical thickness correlates with dual-energy x-ray absorptiometric (DEXA) measurements of bone density. The metrics described previously are referred to as static measurements. If the patient is injected twice with fluorescent dyes (such as tetracycline) before the iliac biopsy, dynamic measurements of bone formation can also be calculated. For example, the average distance between visible labels divided by the label-

Table 1

Normal Values for Quantitative Bone Histomorphometry Parameters

Parameter	Female Mean	Male Mean
Cortical thickness	823 µm	915 µm
Cancellous bone volume	21.8%	19.7%
Osteoid thickness	12.3 µm	11.1 µm
Osteoid surface	8.4%	6.5%
Osteoblast/osteoid interface	22.1%	14.4%
Osteoclasts/trabecular surface	3.0/100 mm	3.5/100 mm
Eroded surface	2.3%	1.5%
Single-labeled surface	2.3%	2.4%
Double-labeled Surface	6.2%	3.0%
Wall thickness	49.8 µm	49.8 µm
Mineral apposition rate	0.88 µm/day	0.89 µm/day
Bone formation rate/surface area $(mm^3/mm^2/year) = (mm/year)$	0.019	0.009
Bone formation rate/volume $(mm^3/mm^3/year) = year^{(-1)}$	0.250	0.131
Mineralization lag time	21.1 d	27.6 d
Activation frequency	0.42 y	0.42 y

ing time interval is the mineral apposition rate (MAR, in µm/day). The MAR is the average rate at which new bone mineral is being added on any actively forming bone surface. The mineral apposition rate is the basic measurement on which all dynamic estimates of bone formation are based. It is usually expressed as the adjusted appositional rate (Aj.AR). The Aj.AR is a calculated quantity, defined as the product of the mineral apposition rate and the quotient (MS/BS), where MS is the total volume of all mineralizing surfaces and BS represents the area of all bone enclosed by trabecular surfaces [Aj.AR = MAR (MS/BS)]. The total mineralizing surfaces include all double-labeled surfaces and half of all single-labeled surfaces. The total mineralizing surface area is expressed relative to the total bone surface area (MS = total labeled bone surface/BS). The total mineralizing surface is used in the calculations for bone formation rate, activation frequency, and mineralization lag time. The osteoid thickness is the mean thickness, in µm, of osteoid seams on cancellous surfaces. The osteoid thickness is normally less than 12.5 µm. An increased osteoid thickness suggests abnormal mineralization, as occurs in osteomalacia. The time interval between osteoid secretion and its subsequent mineralization, in days, is known as the mineralization lag time. The mineralization lag time is a measure of mineralization competence and is normally less than 22 days in women and 27 days in men. The average time that it takes for a new remodeling cycle to begin on any point on a cancellous surface is called the activation frequency. The activation frequency is a measure of bone turnover and is ex-

pressed in years. The wall thickness is the average thickness of the trabecular BSUs. The wall thickness is used to assess the overall balance between resorption and formation. Bone formation rates are the calculated rates at which cancellous bone surface and bone volume are being replaced annually. They are derived from estimates of the mineral apposition rate.

These measured and calculated bone histomorphometry quantities help the treating physician arrive at a diagnosis and treatment plan for people with disorders of bone metabolism. The average normal values for these quantities appear in Table 1. Novel additional techniques exist that are being evaluated for inclusion in the bone histomorphometry test battery. These include Fourier transform infrared spectroscopy and Raman spectroscopy, which are tests that provide chemical analysis of the iliac trabecular bone biopsy specimen.

Clinical Effects of Bone Changes With Aging: Osteoporosis and Its Treatment

Approximately 1.5 million fractures occur in the United States each year as a result of osteoporosis. Approximately 250,000 of these are hip fractures, and the hip fracture patients have a 20% excess mortality over that expected for their age within the first year after fracture. More than 500,000 are vertebral fractures. These patients often have kyphotic spinal deformity after fracture and are at risk for chronic back pain. Distal forearm fractures account for approximately 200,000 of these fractures, and there are approximately 550,000 other limb fractures. The fracture rates are highest in Caucasians and Asians and are lower in Hispanics and African Americans. The economic cost of these fractures is approximately $14.8 billion/year, and much of this cost is spent on long-term rehabilitation and care. Low bone mass is the single most accurate predictor of increased fracture risk: for every one standard deviation decrease below the mean, fracture risk roughly doubles at the spine and hip. The World Health Organization has stratified levels of bone mass into normal, osteopenia, and osteoporosis[28] (Table 2). The clinical evaluation of bone mass, coupled with treatment strategies for people whose bone mass places them at risk for fracture, is the cornerstone of osteoporotic fracture prevention. The clinical evaluation includes a DEXA scan and a bone metabolism laboratory test panel. This panel includes the measurement of serum calcium, phosphate, alkaline phosphatase, creatinine, liver function tests, erythrocyte sedimentation rate, thyroid-stimulating hormone, and serum protein electrophoresis. Additional tests may be needed to establish a diagnosis. These tests include serum intact PTH, 25-hydroxyvitamin D, 1,25-dihydroxyvitamin D, urine protein electrophoresis, serum or urine immunoelectrophoresis, 24-hour urine calcium, creatinine, free cortisol, histamine, and prostaglandin F2-α.

The clinical approach to the evaluation and treatment of osteoporosis depends on whether the patient is premenopausal, perimenopausal, or postmenopausal, and whether the patient has had a fracture under loading conditions that would not normally be expected to result in fracture (for example, a cough or sneeze that results in a vertebral compression fracture, or "minimal" trauma that results in an extremity or pelvic fracture). These fractures are called either fragility fractures or insufficiency fractures. The recommendations for a premenopausal patient are avoidance of lifestyle risk factors (smoking, alcohol), adequate calcium intake (1,000 mg/day), and regular weight-bearing exercise. Bone densitometry and further workup are needed only if fractures occur. The approach to the perimenopausal or postmenopausal patient depends on the bone densitometry score and the presence or absence of a fragility fracture. If the bone densitometry score is in the osteopenic range, and the patient has not had a fragility fracture, then treatment consists of calcium supplementation, weight-bearing exercise, and the administration of an anticatabolic agent, such as a bisphosphonate. The mechanism of action of the anticatabolic agents[29] is outlined in **Figure 8**. If the patient's bone densitometry is in the osteoporotic range, or if the patient has had a fragility fracture even though the bone densitometry is in the osteopenic range, then the treatment recommendations include calcium supplementation, weight-bearing exercise, and the administration of an anticatabolic agent and/or an anabolic agent. The mechanism of action of the anabolic agents[29] is outlined in **Figure 9**. Multiple clinical studies exist in the literature that assess the effect of var-

Table 2

Categories of Bone Mineral Density Test Results

Bone Mineral Density T-Score	Interpretation
+1.0 to -1.0	Normal
-1.0 to -2.5	Osteopenia
Below -2.5	Osteoporosis

ious treatment regimens of anticatabolic and anabolic drugs on specific fragility fracture rates and on improvements in bone mineral density.[30-36]

Bone Regenerative Medicine and Tissue Engineering

The molecular treatment strategies for osteoporosis that were mentioned in the previous section focus on decreasing the bone resorption rate, increasing the bone formation rate, or both. These anticatabolic and anabolic drugs address the balance between bone resorption and bone formation from a systemic perspective. Additional treatment strategies target both systemic and local bone defects. These regenerative medicine strategies are generally classified as tissue-engineering technologies.[37] They consist of some combination of a scaffold (often a polymeric analogue of the extracellular matrix), cells, and bioactive molecules to direct the cells' activity.[38-41] In addition, these tissue-engineering approaches to bone regeneration may include the sustained, controlled delivery of drugs, growth factors, and/or other signaling molecules to provide a systemic treatment effect.[40,41] The approaches that are currently under investigation address either segmental or trabecular bone defects in the axial, appendicular, or craniomaxillofacial skeleton. The segmental bone defect treatment strategies often include a scaffold that has mechanical properties appropriate for temporary stabilization of the reconstructed region during the period of bone regeneration.[39] The scaffold is designed to resorb after a time interval sufficient to allow new bone to form throughout its porous structure.[39] The polymeric scaffold walls may also serve as a reservoir and delivery vehicle for growth factors, antibiotic agents, chemotherapeutic agents, or other signaling molecules, as determined by the needs of a specific patient.[42] The second regeneration category, that of a trabecular bone defect, may occur in several clinical scenarios, such as simple bone cysts, benign bone tumors, or osteoporotic fractures (for example, vertebra and distal radius). A benign tumor example would be that of a giant cell tumor or enchondroma that has undergone curettage and left a bone void at the site of the tumor removal. The tissue-engineering strategies for trabecular defects include injectable scaffolds and particulate bone void fillers. The injectable scaffold strategy is attractive for those defects that can be approached via a minimally inva-

3: Basic Principles and Treatment of Musculoskeletal Disease

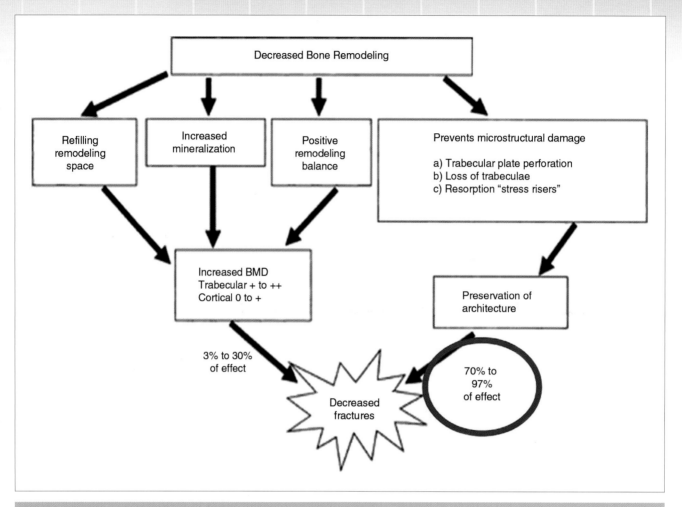

Figure 8 Mechanism of action of anticatabolic agents. BMD, bone mineral density.

sive surgical procedure.[43] An example of such a situation would be a simple bone cyst in either the humerus or the proximal femur, where the trabecular defect is contained within an intact cortical structure. The injectable scaffold conforms to the shape of the defect, and hardens in situ to provide an osteoinductive and osteoconductive environment. The particulate bone void filler strategy is appropriate for a trabecular defect that can be stabilized with instrumentation or a cast, and that may or may not be contained by an intact or fractured cortex.

A wide range of biomaterials has been explored to serve as scaffolds for bone tissue-engineering. Synthetic biodegradable polymers are among the most promising scaffold materials due to their low cost, design flexibility, ease of handling, and modulated chemical, physical, mechanical, and degradation properties. The scaffold properties can be changed by varying the polymer chemistry, molecular weight, and cross-linking conditions, and by forming copolymers or polymer blends. Calcium phosphates such as hydroxyapatite and tricalcium phosphate may be incorporated into the scaffolds as surface coatings or to produce composites to enhance the osteoconductivity of the scaffolds.[44] In addition to the composition and surface chemistry of the scaffolds, internal architecture such as porosity, pore size, pore structure, and pore interconnectivity is crucial to the bone regeneration potential of the scaffolds.[45] The common polymer processing techniques to produce porous structures are salt leaching, gas foaming, electrospinning, and solid freeform fabrication techniques, including stereolithography and ink-jet printing.

The ability of demineralized bone to induce ectopic bone formation and the discovery of the vital roles growth factors played in the process launched the promising strategy of bone tissue engineering based on bioactive molecules. Various proteins involved in bone induction have been investigated for their therapeutic potential in bone regeneration, including BMPs, TGF-β, fibroblast growth factor, insulin-like growth factor, vascular endothelial growth factor, platelet-derived growth factor, epidermal growth factor, PTH/parathyroid hormone-related protein, and interleukins.[46] A variety of delivery vehicles have been developed for localized, controlled, sustained BMP-2 release. Because natural bone healing involves the simultaneous action of multiple growth factors and cytokines, it is possible that the

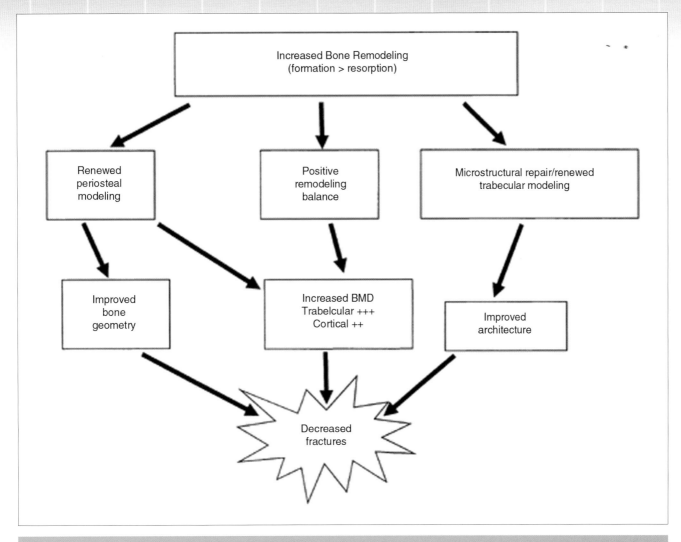

Figure 9 Mechanism of action of anabolic agents. BMD, bone mineral density.

controlled delivery of several bioactive molecules in a specific temporal fashion may be more effective in stimulating bone healing than the delivery of any single agent. Enhanced vessel and bone formation by sequential vascular endothelial growth factor and BMP-2 delivery from composite polymeric scaffolds were demonstrated in an animal model.[47]

These tissue-engineering strategies for local bone defects may be extended, via sustained, controlled delivery of anti-catabolic or anabolic agents, to become systemic treatments of generalized osteoporosis.[42] Intermittent PTH administration increases bone mass and reduces the fracture rate, making it an effective treatment of osteoporosis in humans.[36] Because PTH acts on cells committed to the osteoblastic lineage, the combined effects of PTH with osteoinductive BMPs were explored. Systemic PTH treatment increased the local BMP-2–induced bone formation and reversed the age-related decrease in osteoinductive potential of BMP-2.[46] In both an ectopic site and a critical-sized femoral defect model, the combination of intermittent systemic PTH treat-

ment and local BMP-2 delivery synergistically enhanced bone formation.[48] BMP-2 has also been combined with systemic administration of prostaglandin E_2 and 1,25-dihydroxyvitamin D_3. Systemic administration of either prostaglandin E_2 or vitamin D_3 significantly increased the alkaline phosphatase activity and the calcium content of ectopic BMP-2–loaded implants.[49,50]

Future Directions

The recent United States Bone and Joint Decade focused the nation's interest on bone health in people of all ages, and saw improved combinations of physiologic (exercise and sunlight) and pharmacologic measures to treat bone disease. The continuing advances in the understanding of bone developmental biology, remodeling, cellular and molecular bone signaling, and bone regeneration throughout the various stages of life will hopefully continue to contribute to an increasing array of these methods to maintain optimum bone health.

Regenerative medicine and tissue-engineering strategies are beginning to reach clinical use. Combinations of polymeric scaffolds, bioactive molecules, and osteogenic cells are offering new strategies to address injured and diseased bone. These novel treatment options will increase the ability to provide the affected person an opportunity to regain lost musculoskeletal function and to improve her or his performance of activities of daily living.

References

1. Dempster DW, Shane E, Horbert W, Lindsay R: A simple method for correlative light and scanning electron microscopy of human iliac crest bone biopsies: Qualitative observations in normal and osteoporotic subjects. *J Bone Miner Res* 1986;1(1):15-21.

2. Zuscik MJ, Hilton MJ, Zhang X, Chen D, O'Keefe RJ: Regulation of chondrogenesis and chondrocyte differentiation by stress. *J Clin Invest* 2008;118(2):429-438.

3. Keller H, Kneissel M: SOST is a target gene for PTH in bone. *Bone* 2005;37(2):148-158.

4. Robling AG, Bellido T, Turner CH: Mechanical stimulation in vivo reduces osteocyte expression of sclerostin. *J Musculoskelet Neuronal Interact* 2006;6(4):354.

5. Edwards JR, Mundy GR: Advances in osteoclast biology: Old findings and new insights from mouse models. *Nat Rev Rheumatol* 2011;7(4):235-243.

6. Khosla S, Westendorf JJ, Oursler MJ: Building bone to reverse osteoporosis and repair fractures. *J Clin Invest* 2008;118(2):421-428.

7. Pederson L, Ruan M, Westendorf JJ, Khosla S, Oursler MJ: Regulation of bone formation by osteoclasts involves Wnt/BMP signaling and the chemokine sphingosine-1-phosphate. *Proc Natl Acad Sci U S A* 2008;105(52):20764-20769.

8. Bessa PC, Casal M, Reis RL: Bone morphogenetic proteins in tissue engineering: The road from laboratory to clinic, part II (BMP delivery). *J Tissue Eng Regen Med* 2008;2(2-3):81-96.

9. Bessa PC, Casal M, Reis RL: Bone morphogenetic proteins in tissue engineering: The road from the laboratory to the clinic, part I (basic concepts). *J Tissue Eng Regen Med* 2008;2(1):1-13.

10. Monroe DG, McGee-Lawrence ME, Oursler MJ, Westendorf JJ: Update on Wnt signaling in bone cell biology and bone disease. *Gene* 2012;492(1):1-18.

11. Westendorf JJ, Kahler RA, Schroeder TM: Wnt signaling in osteoblasts and bone diseases. *Gene* 2004;341:19-39.

12. Secreto FJ, Hoeppner LH, Westendorf JJ: Wnt signaling during fracture repair. *Curr Osteoporos Rep* 2009;7(2):64-69.

13. Komatsu DE, Mary MN, Schroeder RJ, Robling AG, Turner CH, Warden SJ: Modulation of Wnt signaling influences fracture repair. *J Orthop Res* 2010;28(7):928-936.

14. Li X, Grisanti M, Fan W, et al: Dickkopf-1 regulates bone formation in young growing rodents and upon traumatic injury. *J Bone Miner Res* 2011;26(11):2610-2621.

15. Ominsky MS, Li C, Li X, et al: Inhibition of sclerostin by monoclonal antibody enhances bone healing and improves bone density and strength of nonfractured bones. *J Bone Miner Res* 2011;26(5):1012-1021.

16. Potts JT: Parathyroid hormone: Past and present. *J Endocrinol* 2005;187(3):311-325.

17. Wan M, Li J, Herbst K, et al: LRP6 mediates cAMP generation by G protein-coupled receptors through regulating the membrane targeting of Gα(s). *Sci Signal* 2011;4(164):ra15.

18. Andreassen TT, Willick GE, Morley P, Whitfield JF: Treatment with parathyroid hormone hPTH(1-34), hPTH(1-31), and monocyclic hPTH(1-31) enhances fracture strength and callus amount after withdrawal fracture strength and callus mechanical quality continue to increase. *Calcif Tissue Int* 2004;74(4):351-356.

19. Kakar S, Einhorn TA, Vora S, et al: Enhanced chondrogenesis and Wnt signaling in PTH-treated fractures. *J Bone Miner Res* 2007;22(12):1903-1912.

20. Komatsu DE, Brune KA, Liu H, et al: Longitudinal in vivo analysis of the region-specific efficacy of parathyroid hormone in a rat cortical defect model. *Endocrinology* 2009;150(4):1570-1579.

21. Kramer I, Loots GG, Studer A, Keller H, Kneissel M: Parathyroid hormone (PTH)-induced bone gain is blunted in SOST overexpressing and deficient mice. *J Bone Miner Res* 2010;25(2):178-189.

22. O'Brien CA, Plotkin LI, Galli C, et al: Control of bone mass and remodeling by PTH receptor signaling in osteocytes. *PLoS One* 2008;3(8):e2942.

23. Seebach C, Skripitz R, Andreassen TT, Aspenberg P: Intermittent parathyroid hormone (1-34) enhances mechanical strength and density of new bone after distraction osteogenesis in rats. *J Orthop Res* 2004;22(3):472-478.

24. Dhillon RS, Schwarz EM: Teriparatide therapy as an adjuvant for tissue engineering and integration of biomaterials. *J Mater Res* 2011;4(6):1117-1131.

25. Takahata M, Awad HA, O'Keefe RJ, Bukata SV, Schwarz EM: Endogenous tissue engineering: PTH therapy for skeletal repair. *Cell Tissue Res* 2012;347(3):545-552.

26. Hodgson S, Clarke B, Wermers R, Hefferan T, Yaszemski M: *Bone Histology and Histopathology for Clinicians.* Rochester, MN, Mayo Foundation for Medical Education and Research, 2007.

27. Recker R: *Bone Histomorphometry: Techniques and Interpretation.* Boca Raton, FL, CRC Press, 1983.

28. WHO Scientific Group: Prevention and management of osteoporosis. Geneva, Switzerland, World Health Organization, 2003. http://whqlibdoc.who.int/trs/who_trs_921.pdf.

29. Riggs BL, Parfitt AM: Drugs used to treat osteoporosis: The critical need for a uniform nomenclature based on their action on bone remodeling. *J Bone Miner Res* 2005;20(2):177-184.

30. Black DM, Cummings SR, Karpf DB, et al: Randomised trial of effect of alendronate on risk of fracture in women with existing vertebral fractures. *Lancet* 1996;348(9041):1535-1541.

31. Bone HG, Hosking D, Devogelaer JP, et al: Ten years' experience with alendronate for osteoporosis in postmenopausal women. *N Engl J Med* 2004;350(12):1189-1199.

32. Chesnut CH III, Silverman S, Andriano K, et al: A randomized trial of nasal spray salmon calcitonin in postmenopausal women with established osteoporosis: The prevent recurrence of osteoporotic fractures study. *Am J Med* 2000; 109(4):267-276.

33. Chesnut CH III, Skag A, Christiansen C, et al: Effects of oral ibandronate administered daily or intermittently on fracture risk in postmenopausal osteoporosis. *J Bone Miner Res* 2004; 19(8):1241-1249.

34. Ettinger B, Black DM, Mitlak BH, et al: Reduction of vertebral fracture risk in postmenopausal women with osteoporosis treated with raloxifene: Results from a 3-year randomized clinical trial. *JAMA* 1999;282(7):637-645.

35. Harris ST, Watts NB, Genant HK, et al: Effects of risedronate treatment on vertebral and nonvertebral fractures in women with postmenopausal osteoporosis: A randomized controlled trial. *JAMA* 1999;282(14):1344-1352.

36. Neer RM, Arnaud CD, Zanchetta JR, et al: Effect of parathyroid hormone (1-34) on fractures and bone mineral density in postmenopausal women with osteoporosis. *N Engl J Med* 2001;344(19):1434-1441.

37. Ripamonti U, Tsiridis E, Ferretti C, Kerawala CJ, Mantalaris A, Heliotis M: Perspectives in regenerative medicine and tissue engineering of bone. *Br J Oral Maxillofac Surg* 2011; 49(7):507-509.

38. Colnot C: Cell sources for bone tissue engineering: Insights from basic science. *Tissue Eng Part B Rev* 2011;17(6):449-457.

39. Hutmacher DW, Schantz JT, Lam CX, Tan KC, Lim TC: State of the art and future directions of scaffold-based bone engineering from a biomaterials perspective. *J Tissue Eng Regen Med* 2007;1(4):245-260.

40. Murphy WL: Temporal and spatial control over soluble protein signaling for musculoskeletal tissue engineering. *Conf Proc IEEE Eng Med Biol Soc* 2009;2009:2103-2105.

41. Rosen V: Harnessing the parathyroid hormone, Wnt, and bone morphogenetic protein signaling cascades for successful bone tissue engineering. *Tissue Eng Part B Rev* 2011; 17(6):475-479.

42. Mouriño V, Boccaccini AR: Bone tissue engineering therapeutics: Controlled drug delivery in three-dimensional scaffolds. *J R Soc Interface* 2010;7(43):209-227.

43. Shi X, Hudson JL, Spicer PP, Tour JM, Krishnamoorti R, Mikos AG: Injectable nanocomposites of single-walled carbon nanotubes and biodegradable polymers for bone tissue engineering. *Biomacromolecules* 2006;7(7):2237-2242.

44. Lee KW, Wang S, Yaszemski MJ, Lu L: Physical properties and cellular responses to crosslinkable poly(propylene fumarate)/hydroxyapatite nanocomposites. *Biomaterials* 2008;29(19):2839-2848.

45. Lee KW, Wang S, Fox BC, Ritman EL, Yaszemski MJ, Lu L: Poly(propylene fumarate) bone tissue engineering scaffold fabrication using stereolithography: Effects of resin formulations and laser parameters. *Biomacromolecules* 2007;8(4): 1077-1084.

46. Kempen DH, Creemers LB, Alblas J, et al: Growth factor interactions in bone regeneration. *Tissue Eng Part B Rev* 2010;16(6):551-566.

47. Kempen DH, Lu L, Heijink A, et al: Effect of local sequential VEGF and BMP-2 delivery on ectopic and orthotopic bone regeneration. *Biomaterials* 2009;30(14):2816-2825.

48. Kempen DH, Lu L, Hefferan TE, et al: Enhanced bone morphogenetic protein-2-induced ectopic and orthotopic bone formation by intermittent parathyroid hormone (1-34) administration. *Tissue Eng Part A* 2010;16(12):3769-3777.

49. Kabasawa Y, Asahina I, Gunji A, Omura K: Administration of parathyroid hormone, prostaglandin E2, or 1-alpha,25-dihydroxyvitamin D3 restores the bone inductive activity of rhBMP-2 in aged rats. *DNA Cell Biol* 2003;22(9):541-546.

50. Cui L, Ma YF, Yao W, et al: Cancellous bone of aged rats maintains its capacity to respond vigorously to the anabolic effects of prostaglandin E2 by modeling-dependent bone gain. *J Bone Miner Metab* 2001;19(1):29-37.

3: Basic Principles and Treatment of Musculoskeletal Disease

Chapter 18

Posttraumatic Osteoarthritis

Constance R. Chu, MD

Introduction

Osteoarthritis (OA) is a leading cause of disability and is the most common form of physician-diagnosed arthritis.[1] Arthritis affects more than one in five Americans and OA affects 20 times more people than rheumatoid arthritis, the second most common form of arthritis. Although the morbidity and deformity caused by end-stage rheumatoid arthritis has improved through early institution of disease-modifying agents, there are currently no proven strategies to delay or prevent the onset of OA. With increasing rates of OA due to obesity and an aging population, a massive rise in costs for treatment and disability is expected. Development of effective strategies for early diagnosis and early treatment of osteoarthritis is therefore a public health priority that has focused new attention on posttraumatic osteoarthritis (PTOA).[2]

PTOA is a subset of OA resulting from a significant joint injury such as intra-articular fracture and/or soft-tissue injury (anterior cruciate ligament [ACL], meniscal, or labral tear) that alters joint congruency, stability, and homeostasis. Although OA is typically a decades-long multifactorial disease process with variable joint involvement, joint trauma initiates accelerated OA development in both animal models and humans from a known point in time.[2] As such, joint injury cohorts provide a unique opportunity from which OA pathogenesis and intervention strategies in humans can be studied from the earliest time points. This chapter will pro-

vide a bench-to-bedside analysis of emerging research in PTOA.

Human Clinical Data

Joint injury as the precipitating event to the development of symptomatic, radiographic OA is common.[3-11] In clinical teaching, PTOA has traditionally been described following severe joint trauma such as intra-articular fractures and dislocations where the onset of radiographic OA can be observed within a few years after injury.[3-5]

More recently, lesser degrees of joint trauma have been linked to PTOA. Through extrapolation of data on patients presenting for lower extremity joint arthroplasty with PTOA, it has been estimated that 12% of symptomatic OA is attributable to hip, knee, and ankle injuries.[6] Soft-tissue injuries of the knee also frequently lead to premature OA. Meniscal and ACL tears are common knee injuries, following which approximately half of individuals develop OA 10 to 20 years later.[7-14] Twelve years after ACL tear, approximately 80% of male and female soccer players showed radiographic signs of OA, with more than half exhibiting symptoms.[8,9] Traumatic meniscal tears frequently occur with ACL injury and are important cofactors in the development of OA in these cohorts (**Figure 1**). The effect of concomitant meniscal tear on subsequent development of OA after knee injuries is high, especially when treated with meniscectomy.[4,10]

The role of meniscal tear in knee OA depends on the nature of the traumatic event, the meniscal tear pattern, and the condition of the joint. Although the lines of demarcation are not clear and deserve additional study, the traumatic meniscal tear can be thought of as a cause of PTOA, whereas the degenerative meniscal tear is likely the result of progressive joint degeneration that may be a sentinel event marking impending OA onset.[11,15] Regardless of etiology,

---

Dr. Chu or an immediate family member serves as a board member, owner, officer, or committee member of the American Orthopaedic Association, the American Orthopaedic Society for Sports Medicine, the Forum Society, the International Society of Arthroscopy, Knee Surgery, and Orthopaedic Sports Medicine, and the Orthopaedic Research Society.

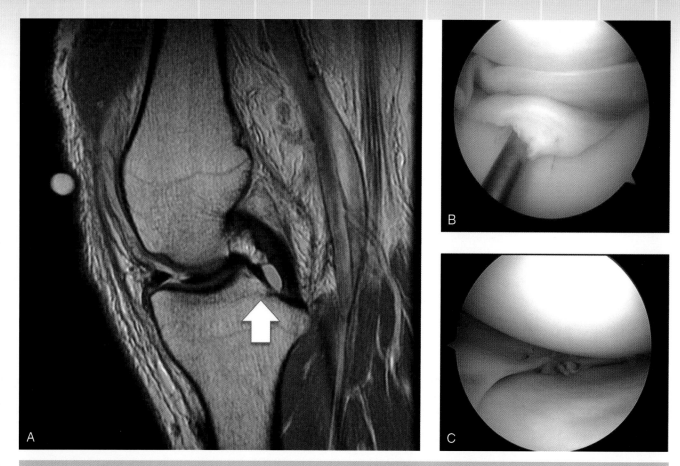

Figure 1 Traumatic meniscal tear. Traumatic meniscal tears occur after moderate- to high-energy knee injuries where the central meniscus is healthy and the meniscus tears through the periphery. This bucket-handle meniscal tear occurred in conjunction with an anterior cruciate ligament tear. **A**, MRI shows the displaced meniscal tissue within the notch (arrow). **B**, Arthroscopic view of the displaced and inverted meniscal body. **C**, Arthroscopic view after reduction and repair.

loss of meniscal function due to meniscal tear substantially increases OA risk.

Bench-to-Bedside Approaches to PTOA

As a result of the traditional clinical emphasis on PTOA associated with intra-articular fracture, animal models for fracture and impact injury have been created to assist in understanding pathogenesis and developing disease-modifying treatments. This represents a situation where the clinical need motivated development of the model.

In contrast, animal models of meniscectomy and ACL resection have long been used by basic researchers to model OA. Yet, the standard clinical diagnosis of OA has been based on factors such as age older than 50 years, pain, and radiographic changes.[16] Osteophytes and degree of joint-space narrowing are used to stage radiographic OA[17] (Table 1 and Figure 2). Additional radiographic signs of OA include subchondral cysts and sclerosis, periarticular ossicles, and alteration of bony contour such as femoral condylar flattening. These criteria define late-stage disease where cartilage loss, synovial hypertrophy, and bone and joint adap-

tations have already occurred. For this reason, subsequent clinical studies of disease-modifying treatments found to be effective in animal models of OA using ACL and meniscus injury have been conducted in elderly clinical cohorts with advanced disease (Table 2). Because of this mismatch between animal model and clinical disease, studies of chondroprotective agents in OA cohorts with advanced cartilage loss have not shown demonstrable benefits.[18]

There is increasing recognition that animal models of ACL transection and meniscectomy more closely model clinical cohorts involving patients sustaining ACL and meniscal injuries than OA cohorts.[2] Consequently, efforts are under way to perform future clinical trials of therapies shown to delay OA onset in animal models of ACL transection in human acute ACL injury cohorts.[14] In this situation, successful animal models have been more closely matched with the appropriate clinical conditions, providing new opportunities to study human OA pathogenesis. This approach will likely increase opportunity for successful bench-to-bedside translation of potential disease-modifying therapies.

Table 1

Radiographic Grading Scales for Osteoarthritis of the Tibiofemoral Joint

Kellgren-Lawrence Grading Scale		Ahlback Grading Scale	
Grade	Description	Grade	Description
0	No radiographic findings of osteoarthritis	0	No radiographic findings of osteoarthritis
1	Minute osteophytes of doubtful clinical significance		
2	Definite osteophytes with unimpaired joint space		
3	Definite osteophytes with moderate joint space narrowing	1	Joint space narrowing <3 mm
4	Definite osteophytes with severe joint space narrowing and subchondral sclerosis	2	Joint space obliterated or almost obliterated
		3	Minor bone attrition (<5 mm)
		4	Moderate bone attrition (5 to 15 mm)
		5	Severe bone attrition (>15 mm)

Pathogenesis of PTOA

To modify the course of disease, it is essential to understand pathogenesis. Human OA is typically a multifactorial, decades-long process. For these reasons, OA has eluded systematic characterization. Similarly, the pathogenesis of PTOA remains incompletely understood. However, the compressed timeline for OA development as well as the presence of common sequelae of joint injury such as biomechanical changes, articular cartilage injury, and altered soft-tissue milieu provide unique clinical opportunities to study OA pathogenesis. As such, understanding factors that contribute to the development of PTOA represent rich areas for additional study to identify new therapeutic targets.

The traditional divisions in OA research, such as the divide between mechanical and biologic factors or between cartilage and bone pathologies, are artificial. Mechanical factors related to joint loading and kinematics influence cartilage and bone biology. Biologic factors related to chondrocyte death and dysfunction affect cartilage matrix mechanical properties as well as the biochemical environment within the joint. An altered joint milieu favoring catabolism over repair processes negatively affect joint-tissue mechanics, structure, and function over time. Neuromuscular factors additionally influence joint kinematics, function, and biology. A multidisciplinary approach to the study of PTOA is critical to the development of effective clinical treatment strategies.

By definition, PTOA is preceded by a significant joint injury sustained at energy levels sufficient to disrupt the integrity of bone, cartilage, ligaments, and other joint tissues. These types of injuries typically result in impact injuries to articular cartilage, joint surface incongruity or instability, and hemarthrosis with loss of joint homeostasis. The initial trauma is followed by inflammation and repair during which the joint may be more vulnerable to degeneration

Table 2

OA Research: Animal Versus Human Studies

Laboratory Animal Study	Human Clinical Study
Young, healthy	Elderly, comorbidities
Disease onset known	Disease onset unknown
Acute inciting event	Chronic/advanced
ACL transection,	disease
meniscectomy	Idiopathic
Cartilage present	No or little cartilage
Sensitive assessments	Insensitive assessments
Histology	Radiographs
Biomechanics	Subjective patient
Biochemistry	reported outcomes
Cellular/molecular	Functional outcomes

Adapted with permission from Chu CR, Beynnon BD, Buckwalter JA, et al: Closing the gap between bench and bedside research for early arthritis therapies (EARTH): Report from the AOSSM/NIH U-13 Post-Joint Injury Osteoarthritis Conference II. *Am J Sports Med* 2011;39(7):1569-1578.

than before injury. Injury severity is an important variable, with higher energy injuries such as pilon fractures or knee dislocations generally leading to more rapid development of PTOA than lower energy injuries such as ankle fracture or isolated meniscus tear. Efforts to elucidate the relative importance of these factors in the pathogenesis of PTOA range from basic science to animal models to clinical studies involving joint injury cohorts.

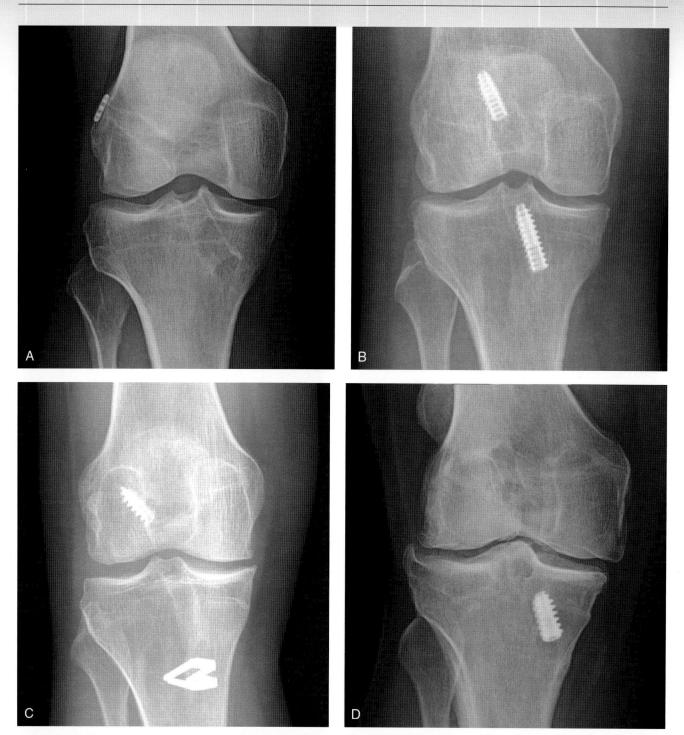

Figure 2 Radiographic knee OA. Radiographs do not directly image intra-articular soft tissues. Radiographic grading scales show variability in description of structural severity and are difficult to use in staging early OA. **A,** Radiograph of the knee of a 41-year-old asymptomatic man 1 year after ACL reconstruction showing small osteophytes with preserved joint spaces reflective of Kellgren-Lawrence (K-L) grade 1 or 2 radiographic changes with no corresponding Ahlback grade. **B,** Radiograph of the knee of a 37-year-old symptomatic woman 7 years after ACL reconstruction showing K-L 3 and Ahlback 1 radiographic OA. **C,** Radiograph of the knee of a 40-year-old asymptomatic woman 22 years after ACL reconstruction showing K-L 3 and Ahlback 1 radiographic joint space narrowing. Subchondral sclerosis is present that is difficult to account for with either grading scale. **D,** Radiograph of the knee of a 37-year-old symptomatic man 6 years after revision ACL reconstruction showing K-L 4 and Ahlback 5 radiographic OA.

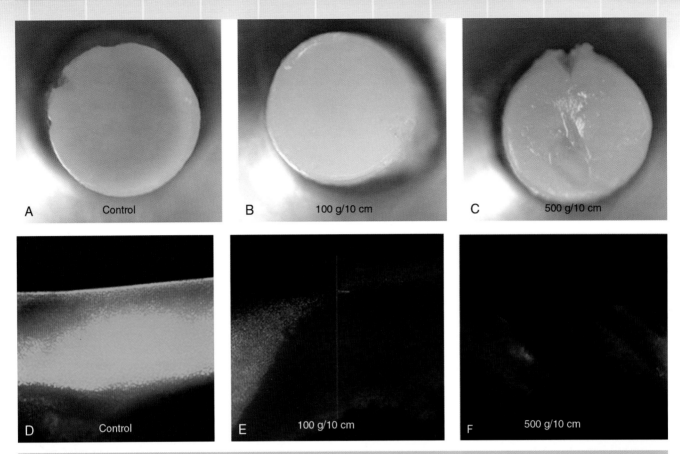

Figure 3 Subsurface injury to articular cartilage after impact. Articular cartilage-retaining intact surfaces appear undamaged to gross and arthroscopic surface evaluation. Unimpacted bovine osteochondral cores (**A**) appear similar to bovine osteochondral cores impacted using a customized drop tower at energies insufficient to fracture the articular surface (**B**). At higher energies, the articular surface is visibly disrupted (**C**). Intravital staining of fresh tissues from these cores show viable chondrocytes in the uninjured core (**D**) and substantial cell death in both impacted cores (**E** and **F**). Loss of healthy chondrocytes reduces the ability of articular cartilage to maintain the matrix and increases OA risk. These images illustrate that subsurface pathology may not be evident to visual inspection in specimens retaining intact articular surfaces (**B** and **E**).

Pathogenesis: Studies of Intra-articular Fracture

Intra-articular fracture involves disruption of the articular surface and the underlying subchondral bone. These injuries are commonly treated surgically whereby orthopaedic surgeons strive to restore joint congruity, alignment, and stability to improve functional outcomes and potentially reduce PTOA risk. The sequelae of early degeneration, PTOA, and disability, however, continue to affect a large proportion of patients with intra-articular fractures. This group includes those for whom surgical goals of anatomic fracture reduction and restoration of joint surface congruity were optimally achieved. An improved understanding of the pathogenesis and risk factors for PTOA is needed. Animal and in vitro impact models play important roles in understanding pathogenesis of PTOA from mechanical, biologic, and molecular perspectives.

In vitro impact injury models generally involve use of a drop tower to generate a short duration but high-energy load to the chondral surface of an osteochondral specimen

(**Figure 3**). Depending on the material properties of the cartilage being impacted, the tissue thickness, and the impact energy, the resulting injuries can reach three levels of severity: (1) subsurface, involving chondrocyte and matrix injury without disruption of the articular surface; (2) chondral fracture, with visible fissuring or rupture of the articular surface but intact subchondral bone; and (3) osteochondral fracture, where both bone and cartilage are disrupted. In the setting of intra-articular fracture, all three types of injuries will be present and are potential contributors to later development of PTOA. It is generally accepted that osteochondral injuries have the potential to heal with fibrocartilaginous repair tissue, whereas chondral fractures do not heal and undergo progressive degeneration. Evidence for chondroprotection in animal studies where treatment is instituted before breakdown of the articular surface suggests that articular cartilage has the capacity to heal subsurface matrix perturbations due to injury or early degeneration.[19-23] Strategies to detect and treat subsurface injuries therefore have the potential to delay or prevent the onset of PTOA.

3: Basic Principles and Treatment of Musculoskeletal Disease

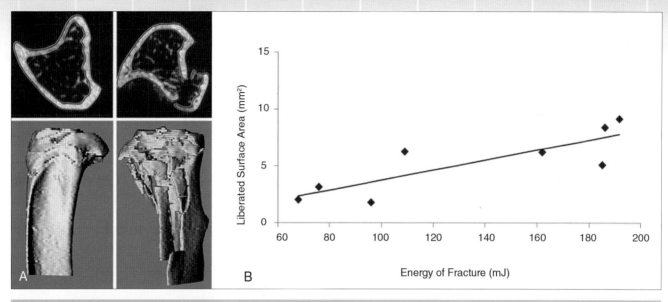

Figure 4 Quantitative measures of fracture severity correlate with energy of fracture in a mouse model. **A**, Micro-CT images were segmented using semiautomated custom software in both the intact contralateral control limb (left) and the fractured experimental limb (right). These models were then registered to each other using an interactive closest-point technique and used to calculate liberated surface area. **B**, Fracture severity, as measured from the liberated surface area, correlated to the energy of fracture as calculated from load-displacement data. (Reproduced with permission from Lewis JS, Hembree WC, Furman BD, et al: Acute joint pathology and synovial inflammation is associated with increased intra-articular fracture severity in the mouse knee. *Osteoarthritis Cartilage* 2011;19(7):864-873.)

As a soft tissue with viscoelastic properties, healthy articular cartilage appears able to withstand impact loads greater than required to fracture long bones without visible surface disruption.[24] Several groups, however, have shown chondrocyte death and subsurface matrix disruption following impact injury at energies insufficient to fracture the articular surface. Although proteoglycan synthetic activity decreased and water content increased with higher impact stresses, there appeared to be a critical threshold stress (15 to 20 MPa) that caused cell death and apparent rupture of the collagen fiber matrix at the time of impact.[25] In addition, significant and possibly irreversible articular cartilage damage was observed within 24 hours after a single high-energy impact load.[26] In cores remaining intact after impact, chondrocyte death increased with increasing impact energy ($P < 0.05$) and with greater time after impact ($P < 0.05$). Another study showed that visible fracturing of the articular surface occurred with higher energy impact loading and that thinner articular cartilage specimens were more vulnerable to surface fracturing even at lower energy levels.[27] Longitudinal studies of impacted cartilage explants show a progressive increase in both the number and extent of chondrocyte necrosis following impact injury.[27,28] Progressive chondrocyte death occurred in the hours to days after injury, revealing a potential window for chondroprotective therapies.

Animal models of impact injury and intra-articular fractures are critical to understanding joint interactions important to the pathogenesis of PTOA. Unlike a soft-tissue procedure such as ACL transection, development of impact and fracture models is more complex, requiring calibration, measuring, and testing of the applied mechanical force for ability to consistently generate the desired injury patterns. Further study is then needed to determine whether the injury pattern obtained predictably leads to accelerated joint degeneration.

To evaluate the effect of direct impact load on articular cartilage in vivo, a pendulum device was successfully used intraoperatively to deliver defined levels of impact to the medial femoral condyle of rabbit knees as measured using pressure-sensitive film and a piezoelectric load cell.[29] These investigators showed induction of chondrocyte apoptosis that was increased with higher impact loads. A subsequent in vivo study using the same pendulum impacting device showed proteoglycan loss without significant macromolecular signs of cartilage breakdown through 12 weeks after injury, leading the authors to conclude cartilage tolerates a single impact load of as much as half the joint fracture threshold.[30] Chondrocyte viability was not directly assessed in this study. A longer term study by another group using an extra-articular rabbit patellar impact model showed chondral softening at 1 year.[31] If the animal was exercised, however, pathologic changes were observed following a single impact load 3 months after injury.[32] These studies show both the difficulty in detecting early subsurface changes and that increased mechanical loading in the setting of cartilage impact injury accelerates development of degenerative changes.

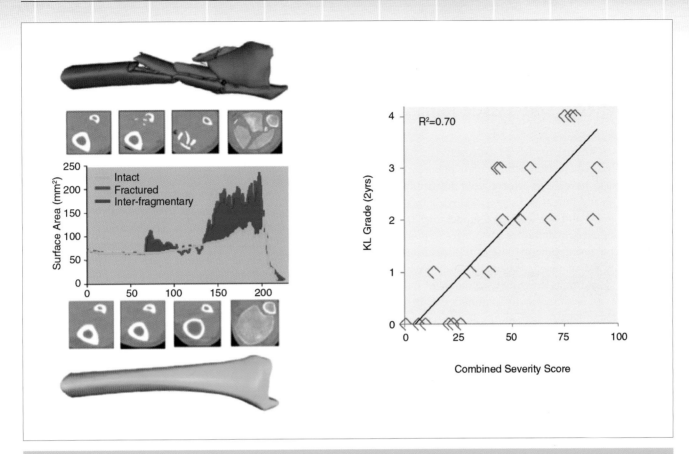

Figure 5 Fracture severity indices correlate with PTOA development in humans. **A,** Quantification of distal tibia comminution after pilon fracture is shown where the surface area for the fractured (red) and intact contralateral (green) are plotted along the length of the tibia. The total interfragmentary surface area is graphically represented by the blue area between the intact and fractured curves. The data on liberated surface area was then used to derive fracture energy. **B,** A combined fracture severity score was then formulated from measures of fracture energy and articular involvement. Linear regression showed correlation of arthrosis scores 2 years after injury with the combined fracture severity score. (Reproduced with permission from Thomas TP, Anderson DD, Mosqueda TV, et al: Objective CT-based metrics of articular fracture severity to assess risk for posttraumatic osteoarthritis. *J Orthop Trauma* 2010;24(12):764-769.)

Recently, a mouse model of closed intra-articular fracture has been developed using an externally applied indentor followed by rapid compression.[33,34] This model showed that fracture severity as measured by liberated surface area correlated with fracture energy calculated by load displacement data (**Figure 4**). Interestingly, although biomarkers for bone injury and inflammation increased with intra-articular fracture severity, chondrocyte viability decreased to the same degree acutely after the injury regardless of the degree of bone comminution in this model.[34] Although increasing bone comminution and inflammation may have long-term negative joint effects, the study substantiates that acute loss of articular chondrocytes is a likely contributor to later development of PTOA. The presence of a mouse model opens the door to the use of transgenic and knockout mice for mechanistic study of PTOA.

Animal studies have been equivocal concerning the relationships between the energy applied to create the injury as well as the degree of measured bone comminution and the extent of injury to articular cartilage, which is presumably related to PTOA risk.[34,35] Bone injury is easier to measure in situ using nondestructive techniques than cartilage injury both clinically and in animal models. As such, bony comminution measured using CT has been evaluated as a surrogate measure of joint and cartilage injury severity.[36] When the quantitative CT-based assessment was validated against clinical assessment by three experienced orthopaedic traumatologists in 20 patients with tibial plafond fractures, agreement was high for fracture energy and displacement.[37] The same patients were followed for 2 years, during which 11 of 20 (55%) developed moderate to severe OA, to determine whether the quantitative CT assessments predicted radiographic and clinical measures of OA.[38] Building on animal and ex vivo work where fragment displacement has been used to calculate fracture energy,[34] CT measures of the liberated surface area in human subjects after tibial plafond fractures were used to derive fracture energy.[38] CT measures of articular disruption combined with fracture energy successfully predicted PTOA severity 2 years after injury[38] (**Figure 5**). This bench-to-bedside series of studies provides both a quantitative method to stratify clinical cohorts for further study and serves as a model for translational research with the promise to provide the basis for new treatment strategies to combat PTOA.

Pathogenesis: Soft-Tissue Joint Injuries

Experimental animal models of osteoarthritis have classically involved ACL transection and meniscectomy.[39-41] These models have been widely used for studying both pathogenesis and potential disease-modifying treatments of OA in general,[41] and not solely as a model for PTOA. These surgically induced models offer advantages of more predictable time course and potential use of transgenic and knockout animals for in vivo mechanistic study over so-called natural models such as the guinea pig model of spontaneous OA or the study of naturally acquired OA in dogs and horses. These soft-tissue procedures do not require complex equipment, are relatively easy to perform, and yield reproducible results. Consequently, they have been widely used in general OA research. Injection models have been less popular due to concern that the resulting arthritic changes would be more similar to inflammatory arthritides than OA. It has been increasingly recognized that these existing animal models offer direct advantages for bench-to-bedside study of joint injury and PTOA.[2]

Large and small animal models of meniscectomy and ACL transection have been described.[41-44] Similar to humans, combined ACL transection and meniscectomy in rats induces more rapid development of OA than isolated ACL tear.[45] In mice, either ACL transection alone or meniscectomy alone generates rapid development of severe OA with subchondral bone erosion, raising concern that these models may be too severe for general OA studies.[41,46] As such, destabilization of the medial meniscus has emerged as a surgical method to generate slower disease progression more similar to that of aged spontaneous mouse models of OA.[46] The destabilization of the medial meniscus model has sufficient sensitivity to show disease modification, and is being increasingly used with transgenic and knockout mice for mechanistic study of OA pathogenesis.[47,48]

Reasons to use large animal models generally relate to perceived translatability to the human condition. In general, when evaluating chondroprotective strategies, there is concern that an improved cartilage repair capability may be seen in smaller animal models with greater cellularity and substantially thinner cartilage than in humans.[49] The use of skeletally mature animals has been advocated for similar reasons. Cartilage thickness may be just a few cell layers in the mouse compared to several millimeters thick in humans. Of the common large animal models (horse, sheep, goat, dog, and swine), large animal studies of OA have primarily involved osteochondral injury to the equine fetlock model, meniscectomy models in the sheep, and the canine ACL transection model. Although the equine fetlock model

is well described, the lack of comparable disease in human metacarpophalangeal joints reduces potential translatability to human disease.

Few studies of ACL injury in sheep have been performed as prior studies suggest that ACL transection alone induces relatively little cartilage degeneration in ovine and caprine fetlock joints.[50] Recently, an ovine model for ACL injury did show that synovial response biomarkers of interleukin (IL)-1β, IL-6, and matrix metalloproteinase-3 may predict early gross changes of joint tissues after arthrotomy and were likely to be involved in early osteophyte formation.[51] Meniscectomy in sheep has been more consistently shown to generate cartilage degeneration and early osteoarthritic changes.[52] Consequently, the sheep meniscectomy model has been used for large animal studies evaluating the chondroprotective effects of potential new treatments.[44,53]

Transection of the ACL to generate OA in large animal models has been best described in dogs.[39,42,54] Morphologic changes in bone, cartilage, synovial membrane, and joint capsule as well as serum and synovial fluid biomarker studies following ACL transection in dogs have been performed.[42,54-56] Although the canine ACL transection model has historically been popular, studies show this model rarely results in full-thickness cartilage loss. Rather, an active chondrocyte synthetic response has been observed, resulting in hypertrophic cartilage repair that was sustained for more than 1 year.[39] In response to altered mechanical stress following ACL transection, it has additionally been shown that canine chondrocytes synthesize proteoglycans containing more chondroitin sulfate relative to keratan sulfate than normally, as in immature articular cartilage.[57] This type of anabolic repair response to surgical instability is not known to consistently occur in humans and may therefore render canine ACL transection models less relevant to understanding human OA.

The rat ACL transection model offers several advantages for translational studies of potential disease-modifying treatments of osteoarthritis. It is a cost-effective small animal model resulting in predictable and progressive joint degeneration leading to OA measurable in the major tissues of relevance: articular cartilage, synovium, subchondral bone, osteophytes, and menisci.[20-22,45,58-60] In rats, there is sufficient cartilage to perform gene expression studies that show changes in this model mimicking that of human OA.[61] Measures of pain expressed through gait alteration are possible in this model.[60] In addition, rats can be exercised at defined levels.[62,63] Exercise has been shown to both accelerate degenerative changes and to potentially exert chondroprotective effects depending on timing and intensity following ACL transection in this model. Given these benefits, studies evaluating potential chondroprotective and other disease-modifying strategies using the rat ACL transection model are increasing.[21,22,64,65]

Translation of Early Diagnosis and Early Treatment Strategies to Human Disease

Human joint injury cohorts provide unique opportunities for bench-to-bedside translation of new therapeutic strategies to reduce acute cartilage damage or subsequent PTOA risk. Although important human clinical studies have been performed in intra-articular fracture cohorts, the injuries are relatively rare, leading to small cohorts collected over long periods, even at level I trauma centers.[5,66] In contrast, ACL and meniscal injuries are common. Similar to animal models of ACL transection, ACL tear in humans initiates events resulting in progressive joint degeneration and early OA.[7-9,67-71] ACL tear is a common knee injury occurring in approximately 80,000 to 100,000 Swedes and 1 in 3,000 Americans annually.[12,13] It is estimated that more than 250,000 ACL injuries occur annually in the United States. The injury occurs most frequently in healthy teenagers and young adults. As such, human ACL-injured cohorts provide opportunities for evaluating joint changes from the earliest time points that increase OA risk in a population less likely to have multiple joint involvement and other comorbidities than traditional cohorts of elderly individuals with advanced disease.[2,72]

Clinical studies of human ACL- and meniscus-injured cohorts are leading to new insights into the earliest structural and metabolic properties of cartilage injury and degeneration. Of significance, these patients frequently present with intact articular surfaces. This is important when evaluating promising disease-modifying treatments evaluated in ACL- and meniscus-injured animal models because those therapies are typically initiated immediately after the surgically induced injury when the articular surface is still intact. Another reason this is notable is that compromise of the articular surface results in acute structural changes that are considered progressive. This is because loss of surface integrity compromises the complex functional architecture of articular cartilage and because partial-thickness injuries to articular cartilage do not heal. Animal and laboratory studies show that the earliest changes to articular cartilage associated with progressive joint degeneration occur before breakdown of the articular surface.[20-23,27] It is at these earliest stages when the articular surface remains intact that pathologic processes are likely the most readily reversible. For these reasons, clinical methods to detect subsurface injury and degeneration in human cartilage retaining intact articular surfaces are needed to maximize opportunities for early diagnosis and early treatment strategies to reduce OA risk.

Early Diagnosis

New cross-sectional imaging techniques such as optical coherence tomography, structural MRI, and quantitative MRI that directly image articular cartilage have been translated into clinical use. These methods are beginning to show subsurface changes to the biochemistry and matrix properties of surface-intact articular cartilage and meniscus in early degeneration and acutely following ACL injury.[69,73-76] Quantitative MRI techniques such as delayed gadolinium-enhanced MRI of cartilage, T2 mapping, T1rho weighting, ultrashort echo time–enhanced T2* mapping, and sodium MRI to evaluate subsurface changes to the biochemistry and matrix properties of still-intact articular cartilage show promise in diagnosis and staging of the earliest changes that may be indicative of heightened OA risk.[72] Other nondestructive imaging modalities such as optical coherence tomography have been important in early diagnosis of subsurface cartilage damage following impact injury and in early degeneration[72,76] (**Figure 6**). This new technology has also been used clinically to assist in clinical validation of MRI T2 mapping of articular cartilage. Recently, it has also been shown that acute changes to articular cartilage and menisci after ACL tear can be detected clinically in humans using MRI T1 rho and ultrashort echo time–enhanced T2* mapping MRI (**Figure 6**), and that structural changes can be observed by conventional MRI within 5 years.[69,74,75]

Due to ease of access, relative cost-effectiveness, and clinical success in early diagnosis for diseases ranging from atherosclerosis to rheumatoid arthritis, there has been long-standing interest in identifying serum biomarkers of osteoarthritis. Animal models of ACL transection have shown promising results.[54] Biomarker validation in humans, however, has proved challenging due in part to a traditional focus on elderly cohorts with end-stage, variable disease and multiple joints involved. Additional issues for biomarker development and validation include variables of hydration and nutritional status, biorhythms, as well as difficulty evaluating sensitivity, specificity, and predictive value without concomitant sensitive structural measures of early disease.[72]

Metabolic changes in articular cartilage, synovium, and subchondral bone, however, are generally considered reversible and may represent some of the earliest metabolic changes in preosteoarthritic conditions. Evaluation of biomarkers of inflammation, cartilage turnover, and altered gene expression in the ACL-injured knee show detectable changes. Alterations in biomarkers for cartilage lubrication such as lubricin and hyaluronic acid have been shown acutely after joint injury.[66] An initial proteoglycan loss is followed by collagen loss.[77,78] Cartilage oligomeric matrix protein, a noncollagenous extracellular matrix protein surrounding chondrocytes, is additionally elevated in synovial fluid from ACL-injured knees.[77] Markers of inflammation are also elevated.[79] Several studies show transient elevation of inflammatory mediators acutely after ACL injury with levels decreasing over time.[72] These studies represent the beginning of new emphasis on evaluation and validation of biochemical biomarkers in ACL-injured cohorts. Long-term follow-up of clinical cohorts yielding carefully controlled serum, synovial fluid, and imaging data collections will be needed to identify usable serum biomarkers of pre-OA conditions and for evaluation of OA risk. Specifically,

3: Basic Principles and Treatment of Musculoskeletal Disease

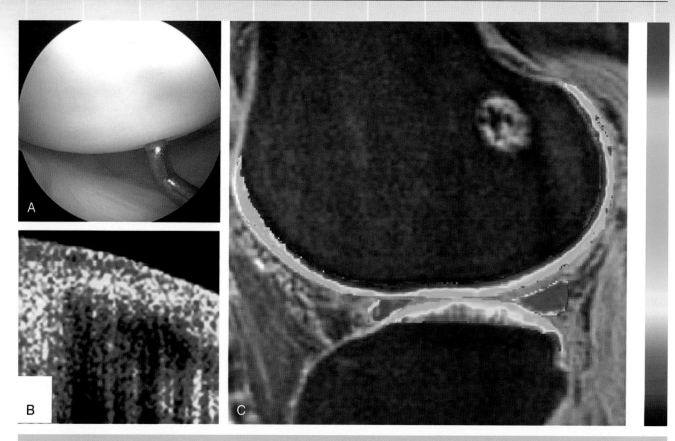

Figure 6 **A**, Arthroscopic view of an ACL injury showing intact articular surfaces. **B**, Optical coherence tomography showing subsurface changes to articular cartilage in ACL-injured knees. **C**, Novel ultrashort echo time–enhanced T2* mapping is sensitive to matrix changes to deep articular cartilage and menisci. (Courtesy of Constance R. Chu, MD, Pittsburgh, PA.)

systematic longitudinal evaluation of serum biomarkers in large human clinical cohorts that are also followed by validated structural and clinical outcome measures are needed.[72]

Emerging Treatment Strategies to Prevent PTOA

Mechanical, biologic, and genetic effects all play a role in the development of OA. Mechanical factors include body mass index, mechanical alignment, joint kinematics, joint surface congruity, joint stability, and neuromuscular fitness. Weight management can be achieved through diet and exercise. Surgical goals for treatment of joint injury include restoration of joint surface congruity and joint stability. There has been strong interest in the role of neuromuscular fitness in optimizing joint kinematics to prevent ACL injury.[13,70] These data show that neuromuscular training can improve joint function. As such, optimization of neuromuscular fitness is a promising intervention strategy for prevention of PTOA through improving joint mechanics.

Biologic treatment targets encompass at least four major therapeutic strategies: (1) optimizing chondrocyte survival and function; (2) preventing matrix breakdown; (3) enhancing matrix synthesis; and (4) reducing inflammation. Restoration of articular cartilage homeostasis can be

thought of as maintaining a balance between catabolism and anabolism. Joint trauma with accompanying impact injury, hemarthrosis, and altered biomechanics initiates a catabolic state from which recovery may be lengthy. In some instances, substantial chondrocyte death, cartilage tissue loss, and altered joint geometry and mechanics result in insurmountable changes, with clinical studies showing higher rates and more rapid development of PTOA with increasing injury severity. Host factors such as age, genetics, and sex also have biologic implications that need to be taken into consideration when designing, testing, and implementing biologic treatment strategies. Aging joints show higher incidence and more rapid development of PTOA. Although these factors complicate human clinical trials, in vitro studies as well as animal studies where PTOA is induced through surgically induced joint injuries in young animals with previously healthy joints consistently show promise for biologic early intervention strategies.

In vitro and in vivo impact studies support a role for acute and progressive loss of articular chondrocytes as a factor in the pathogenesis of PTOA.[27-29] Loss of healthy articular chondrocytes through death or disease resulting in altered metabolism likely reduces the ability of the tissue to maintain the matrix leading to reduced functional capacity with increased injury to lower levels of loading.[80,81] When

304

catabolic processes overwhelm repair processes, a vicious cycle ensues, resulting in progressive degeneration. The threshold at which this occurs remains unclear. In a small animal study evaluating the effects of a single injection of bupivacaine, 80% chondrocyte loss resulting from monoiodoacetate injection was shown to result in visible breakdown and degeneration of the articular cartilage by 6 months whereas the matrix remained intact through 6 months in the bupivacaine-injected group, showing 50% chondrocyte loss.[81] In humans, cartilage breakdown and loss is observed within a few years after transplantation of frozen osteoarticular allografts that are largely devoid of viable chondrocytes.[82] Fresh osteochondral allografts retaining viable articular chondrocytes have shown good longevity in long-term studies.[83] These data suggest efforts to rescue chondrocytes from death acutely after injury and to restore healthy chondrocyte metabolism in the long term may be important in delaying the onset of PTOA.

A final consideration for early intervention and prevention strategies includes temporal factors related to initiation and duration of therapy. Therapies to alter the acute response to injury inclusive of strategies to improve chondrocyte survival, to mitigate the effects of hemarthrosis, and to alter the early inflammatory response potentially need to be initiated within hours to days after injury and continued until resolution of the acute phase. Longitudinal follow-up would then be needed to determine whether the acute intervention impacted later development of clinically detectable joint degeneration and eventual osteoarthritis. An alternative early intervention strategy would be to identify joints "at risk" through imaging or biochemical biomarkers in high-risk populations. Because these joints will have ideally been identified before clinically detectable OA, intervention strategies would likely involve long-term treatments. For biologic agents, the intra-articular bioavailability and the potential adverse effects of orally administered medications are important considerations.

Intra-articular injection of therapeutic agents has a long history; cortisone and hyaluronic acid injections are commonly used. Compared with oral administration, biologic effects are more concentrated and localized to the joint in question. Systemic consequences from long-term use of oral medications can be severe, with 16,500 deaths attributed to nonsteroidal anti-inflammatory drugs commonly used for symptomatic relief of OA in 2004.[84] Direct intra-articular administration of bioactive agents through joint injection, however, is invasive and impractical for daily or long-term administration of small molecules with short half-lives. Several of the more promising biologic strategies, such as anti-inflammatory treatment with interleukin receptor antagonist protein, anticatabolic treatment with parathyroid hormone, or anabolic treatment with bone morphogenetic protein–7, fall into this category.[18,23,85,86]

Localized intra-articular gene therapy is one potential strategy for sustained administration of bioactive substances to joints at risk.[21] In a human clinical study involving rheumatoid arthritis patients undergoing metacarpophalangeal joint arthroplasty, intra-articular injection of the interleukin receptor antagonist gene through adenoviral vectors was shown to result in localized transgene expression.[86] Use of the smaller adenoassociated virus, a newer gene transfer vector with a greater safety profile that is not known to cause any human disease, shows strong promise for sustained delivery of small therapeutic proteins to diarthrodial joints. Following single injection of adenoassociated virus luciferase, intra-articular transgene expression was localized to the injected joint and sustained through the 1-year study period in a rat model.[87] Furthermore, introduction of a tetracycline response element permitted external control of intra-articular transgene expression through use of oral doxycycline.[87] These studies show promise for strategies such as localized gene therapy in long-term intra-articular delivery of bioactive agents to delay osteoarthritis through restoration of joint homeostasis.

Summary

Osteoarthritis is a highly prevalent and disabling disease process for which disease-modifying treatments are lacking. Similar to OA, development of PTOA is multifactorial. However, development of PTOA occurs from a known start date and over a shorter period of time than conventional OA. This situation parallels OA development in several animal models used to study OA pathogenesis and for preclinical study of new OA prevention treatments. These similarities in PTOA development to animal models of OA provide unique opportunities to study human OA pathogenesis and develop new intervention strategies using joint injury cohorts composed of young adults without preexisting OA. Identification of factors contributing to the development of PTOA from the earliest events after joint injury in select clinical cohorts will yield new therapeutic targets to prevent or delay the onset of disabling OA. Because PTOA typically still develops over periods of time measured in years if not decades, disease modification will require a multidisciplinary approach. Longitudinal follow-up will be critical to successful modification of a chronic disease process reflecting the cumulative effects of multiple factors over long periods of time. Improved understanding of PTOA is important for both comprehensive patient care as well as opportunities to transform the clinical treatment of OA from palliation to prevention.

References

1. United States Bone and Joint Initiative: *The Burden of Musculoskeletal Diseases in the United States*, ed 2. Rosemont, IL, American Academy of Orthopaedic Surgeons, 2008.

2. Chu CR, Beynnon BD, Buckwalter JA, et al: Closing the gap between bench and bedside research for early arthritis therapies (EARTH): Report from the AOSSM/NIH U-13 Post-Joint Injury Osteoarthritis Conference II. *Am J Sports Med* 2011;39(7):1569-1578.

3. Matta JM: Fractures of the acetabulum: Accuracy of reduction and clinical results in patients managed operatively

3: Basic Principles and Treatment of Musculoskeletal Disease

within three weeks after the injury. *J Bone Joint Surg Am* 1996;78(11):1632-1645.

4. Honkonen SE: Degenerative arthritis after tibial plateau fractures. *J Orthop Trauma* 1995;9(4):273-277.

5. Marsh JL, Weigel DP, Dirschl DR: Tibial plafond fractures: How do these ankles function over time? *J Bone Joint Surg Am* 2003;85-A(2):287-295.

6. Brown TD, Johnston RC, Saltzman CL, Marsh JL, Buckwalter JA: Posttraumatic osteoarthritis: A first estimate of incidence, prevalence, and burden of disease. *J Orthop Trauma* 2006;20(10):739-744.

7. Lohmander LS, Englund PM, Dahl LL, Roos EM: The long-term consequence of anterior cruciate ligament and meniscus injuries: Osteoarthritis. *Am J Sports Med* 2007;35(10):1756-1769.

8. Lohmander LS, Ostenberg A, Englund M, Roos H: High prevalence of knee osteoarthritis, pain, and functional limitations in female soccer players twelve years after anterior cruciate ligament injury. *Arthritis Rheum* 2004;50(10):3145-3152.

9. von Porat A, Roos EM, Roos H: High prevalence of osteoarthritis 14 years after an anterior cruciate ligament tear in male soccer players: A study of radiographic and patient relevant outcomes. *Ann Rheum Dis* 2004;63(3):269-273.

10. Øiestad BE, Engebretsen L, Storheim K, Risberg MA: Knee osteoarthritis after anterior cruciate ligament injury: A systematic review. *Am J Sports Med* 2009;37(7):1434-1443.

11. Englund M, Roos EM, Lohmander LS: Impact of type of meniscal tear on radiographic and symptomatic knee osteoarthritis: A sixteen-year followup of meniscectomy with matched controls. *Arthritis Rheum* 2003;48(8):2178-2187.

12. Swedish ACL Register: *Annual Report 2011.* 2011, p. 32.

13. Boden BP, Dean GS, Feagin JA Jr, Garrett WE Jr: Mechanisms of anterior cruciate ligament injury. *Orthopedics* 2000;23(6):573-578.

14. Chu CR, Beynnon BD, Dragoo JL, et al: The feasibility of randomized controlled trials for Early Arthritis Therapies (EARTH) involving acute anterior cruciate ligament tear cohorts. *Am J Sports Med* 2012;40(11):2648-2652.

15. Englund M, Guermazi A, Gale D, et al: Incidental meniscal findings on knee MRI in middle-aged and elderly persons. *N Engl J Med* 2008;359(11):1108-1115.

16. Altman R, Asch E, Bloch D, et al: Development of criteria for the classification and reporting of osteoarthritis: Classification of osteoarthritis of the knee. *Arthritis Rheum* 1986;29(8):1039-1049.

17. Kijowski R, Blankenbaker D, Stanton P, Fine J, De Smet A: Arthroscopic validation of radiographic grading scales of osteoarthritis of the tibiofemoral joint. *AJR Am J Roentgenol* 2006;187(3):794-799.

18. Malemud CJ: Anticytokine therapy for osteoarthritis: Evidence to date. *Drugs Aging* 2010;27(2):95-115.

19. Pickarski MT, Hayami T, Zhuo Y, Duong T: Molecular changes in articular cartilage and subchondral bone in the rat anterior cruciate ligament transection and meniscectomized models of osteoarthritis. *BMC Musculoskelet Disord* 2011;12:197.

20. Pascual Garrido C, Hakimiyan AA, Rappoport L, Oegema TR, Wimmer MA, Chubinskaya S: Anti-apoptotic treatments prevent cartilage degradation after acute trauma to human ankle cartilage. *Osteoarthritis Cartilage* 2009;17(9):1244-1251.

21. Hsieh JL, Shen PC, Shiau AL, et al: Intraarticular gene transfer of thrombospondin-1 suppresses the disease progression of experimental osteoarthritis. *J Orthop Res* 2010;28(10):1300-1306.

22. Jay GD, Elsaid KA, Kelly KA, et al: Prevention of cartilage degeneration and gait asymmetry by lubricin tribosupplementation in the rat following anterior cruciate ligament transection. *Arthritis Rheum* 2012;64(4):1162-1171.

23. Hurtig M, Chubinskaya S, Dickey J, Rueger D: BMP-7 protects against progression of cartilage degeneration after impact injury. *J Orthop Res* 2009;27(5):602-611.

24. Repo RU, Finlay JB: Survival of articular cartilage after controlled impact. *J Bone Joint Surg Am* 1977;59(8):1068-1076.

25. Torzilli PA, Grigiene R, Borrelli J Jr, Helfet DL: Effect of impact load on articular cartilage: Cell metabolism and viability, and matrix water content. *J Biomech Eng* 1999;121(5):433-441.

26. Torzilli PA, Grigiene R, Huang C, et al: Characterization of cartilage metabolic response to static and dynamic stress using a mechanical explant test system. *J Biomech* 1997;30(1):1-9.

27. Szczodry M, Coyle CH, Kramer SJ, Smolinski P, Chu CR: Progressive chondrocyte death after impact injury indicates a need for chondroprotective therapy. *Am J Sports Med* 2009;37(12):2318-2322.

28. Tochigi Y, Buckwalter JA, Martin JA, et al: Distribution and progression of chondrocyte damage in a whole-organ model of human ankle intra-articular fracture. *J Bone Joint Surg Am* 2011;93(6):533-539.

29. Borrelli J Jr, Tinsley K, Ricci WM, Burns M, Karl IE, Hotchkiss R: Induction of chondrocyte apoptosis following impact load. *J Orthop Trauma* 2003;17(9):635-641.

30. Borrelli J Jr, Zhu Y, Burns M, Sandell L, Silva MJ: Cartilage tolerates single impact loads of as much as half the joint fracture threshold. *Clin Orthop Relat Res* 2004;426:266-273.

31. Newberry WN, Zukosky DK, Haut RC: Subfracture insult to a knee joint causes alterations in the bone and in the functional stiffness of overlying cartilage. *J Orthop Res* 1997;15(3):450-455.

32. Newberry WN, Mackenzie CD, Haut RC: Blunt impact causes changes in bone and cartilage in a regularly exercised animal model. *J Orthop Res* 1998;16(3):348-354.

33. Furman BD, Strand J, Hembree WC, Ward BD, Guilak F, Olson SA: Joint degeneration following closed intraarticular fracture in the mouse knee: A model of posttraumatic arthritis. *J Orthop Res* 2007;25(5):578-592.

34. Lewis JS, Hembree WC, Furman BD, et al: Acute joint pathology and synovial inflammation is associated with increased intra-articular fracture severity in the mouse knee. *Osteoarthritis Cartilage* 2011;19(7):864-873.

35. Borrelli J Jr, Silva MJ, Zaegel MA, Franz C, Sandell LJ: Single high-energy impact load causes posttraumatic OA in young rabbits via a decrease in cellular metabolism. *J Orthop Res* 2009;27(3):347-352.

36. Beardsley C, Marsh JL, Brown T: Quantifying comminution as a measurement of severity of articular injury. *Clin Orthop Relat Res* 2004;423:74-78.

37. Anderson DD, Mosqueda T, Thomas T, Hermanson EL, Brown TD, Marsh JL: Quantifying tibial plafond fracture severity: Absorbed energy and fragment displacement agree with clinical rank ordering. *J Orthop Res* 2008;26(8):1046-1052.

38. Thomas TP, Anderson DD, Mosqueda TV, et al: Objective CT-based metrics of articular fracture severity to assess risk for posttraumatic osteoarthritis. *J Orthop Trauma* 2010; 24(12):764-769.

39. Adams ME, Brandt KD: Hypertrophic repair of canine articular cartilage in osteoarthritis after anterior cruciate ligament transection. *J Rheumatol* 1991;18(3):428-435.

40. Moskowitz RW, Goldberg VM, Malemud CJ: Metabolic responses of cartilage in experimentally induced osteoarthritis. *Ann Rheum Dis* 1981;40(6):584-592.

41. Bendele AM: Animal models of osteoarthritis in an era of molecular biology. *J Musculoskelet Neuronal Interact* 2002; 2(6):501-503.

42. Matyas JR, Ehlers PF, Huang D, Adams ME: The early molecular natural history of experimental osteoarthritis: I. Progressive discoordinate expression of aggrecan and type II procollagen messenger RNA in the articular cartilage of adult animals. *Arthritis Rheum* 1999;42(5):993-1002.

43. Yoshioka M, Coutts RD, Amiel D, Hacker SA: Characterization of a model of osteoarthritis in the rabbit knee. *Osteoarthritis Cartilage* 1996;4(2):87-98.

44. Young AA, McLennan S, Smith MM, et al: Proteoglycan 4 downregulation in a sheep meniscectomy model of early osteoarthritis. *Arthritis Res Ther* 2006;8(2):R41.

45. Hayami TM, Pickarski M, Zhuo Y, Wesolowski GA, Rodan GA, Duong T: Characterization of articular cartilage and subchondral bone changes in the rat anterior cruciate ligament transection and meniscectomized models of osteoarthritis. *Bone* 2006;38(2):234-243.

46. Glasson SS, Blanchet TJ, Morris EA: The surgical destabilization of the medial meniscus (DMM) model of osteoarthritis in the 129/SvEv mouse. *Osteoarthritis Cartilage* 2007; 15(9):1061-1069.

47. Malfait AM, Ritchie J, Gil AS, et al: ADAMTS-5 deficient mice do not develop mechanical allodynia associated with osteoarthritis following medial meniscal destabilization. *Osteoarthritis Cartilage* 2010;18(4):572-580.

48. Wang Q, Rozelle AL, Lepus CM, et al: Identification of a central role for complement in osteoarthritis. *Nat Med* 2011; 17(12):1674-1679.

49. Chu CR, Szczodry M, Bruno S: Animal models for cartilage regeneration and repair. *Tissue Eng Part B Rev* 2010;16(1): 105-115.

50. Mastbergen SC, Pollmeier M, Fischer L, Vianen ME, Lafeber FP: The groove model of osteoarthritis applied to the ovine fetlock joint. *Osteoarthritis Cartilage* 2008;16(8):919-928.

51. Heard BJ, Achari Y, Chung M, Shrive NG, Frank CB: Early joint tissue changes are highly correlated with a set of inflammatory and degradative synovial biomarkers after ACL autograft and its sham surgery in an ovine model. *J Orthop Res* 2011;29(8):1185-1192.

52. Little CB, Ghosh P, Bellenger CR: Topographic variation in biglycan and decorin synthesis by articular cartilage in the early stages of osteoarthritis: An experimental study in sheep. *J Orthop Res* 1996;14(3):433-444.

53. Smith MM, Cake MA, Ghosh P, Schiavinato A, Read RA, Little CB: Significant synovial pathology in a meniscectomy model of osteoarthritis: Modification by intra-articular hyaluronan therapy. *Rheumatology (Oxford)* 2008;47(8):1172-1178.

54. Matyas JR, Atley L, Ionescu M, Eyre DR, Poole AR: Analysis of cartilage biomarkers in the early phases of canine experimental osteoarthritis. *Arthritis Rheum* 2004;50(2):543-552.

55. Desrochers J, Amrein MA, Matyas JR: Structural and functional changes of the articular surface in a post-traumatic model of early osteoarthritis measured by atomic force microscopy. *J Biomech* 2010;43(16):3091-3098.

56. McDevitt C, Gilbertson E, Muir H: An experimental model of osteoarthritis; early morphological and biochemical changes. *J Bone Joint Surg Br* 1977;59(1):24-35.

57. McDevitt CA, Muir H: Biochemical changes in the cartilage of the knee in experimental and natural osteoarthritis in the dog. *J Bone Joint Surg Br* 1976;58(1):94-101.

58. McErlain DD, Appleton CT, Litchfield RB, et al: Study of subchondral bone adaptations in a rodent surgical model of OA using in vivo micro-computed tomography. *Osteoarthritis Cartilage* 2008;16(4):458-469.

59. Nielsen RH, Stoop R, Leeming DJ, et al: Evaluation of cartilage damage by measuring collagen degradation products in joint extracts in a traumatic model of osteoarthritis. *Biomarkers* 2008;13(1):79-87.

60. Wen ZH, Tang CC, Chang YC, et al: Glucosamine sulfate reduces experimental osteoarthritis and nociception in rats: Association with changes of mitogen-activated protein kinase in chondrocytes. *Osteoarthritis Cartilage* 2010;18(9): 1192-1202.

61. Appleton CT, Pitelka V, Henry J, Beier F: Global analyses of gene expression in early experimental osteoarthritis. *Arthritis Rheum* 2007;56(6):1854-1868.

62. Galois L, Etienne S, Grossin L, et al: Dose-response relationship for exercise on severity of experimental osteoarthritis in rats: A pilot study. *Osteoarthritis Cartilage* 2004;12(10): 779-786.

63. Coyle CH, Henry SE, Haleem AM, O'Malley MJ, Chu CR: Serum CTXii correlates with articular cartilage degeneration after anterior cruciate ligament transection or arthrotomy followed by standardized exercise. *Sports Health* 2012.

64. Braza-Boïls A, Alcaraz MJ, Ferrándiz ML: Regulation of the inflammatory response by tin protoporphyrin IX in the rat anterior cruciate ligament transection model of osteoarthritis. *J Orthop Res* 2011;29(9):1375-1382.

65. Elsaid KA, Zhang L, Waller K, et al: The impact of forced joint exercise on lubricin biosynthesis from articular cartilage following ACL transection and intra-articular lubricin's effect in exercised joints following ACL transection. *Osteoarthritis Cartilage* 2012;20(8):940-948.

66. Ballard BL, Antonacci JM, Temple-Wong MM, et al: Effect of tibial plateau fracture on lubrication function and composition of synovial fluid. *J Bone Joint Surg Am* 2012;94(10): e64.

67. Amin S, Guermazi A, Lavalley MP, et al: Complete anterior cruciate ligament tear and the risk for cartilage loss and progression of symptoms in men and women with knee osteoarthritis. *Osteoarthritis Cartilage* 2008;16(8):897-902.

68. Asano H, Muneta T, Ikeda H, Yagishita K, Kurihara Y, Sekiya I: Arthroscopic evaluation of the articular cartilage after anterior cruciate ligament reconstruction: A short-term prospective study of 105 patients. *Arthroscopy* 2004;20(5): 474-481.

69. Potter HG, Jain SK, Ma Y, Black BR, Fung S, Lyman S: Cartilage injury after acute, isolated anterior cruciate ligament tear: Immediate and longitudinal effect with clinical/MRI follow-up. *Am J Sports Med* 2012;40(2):276-285.

70. Chaudhari AM, Briant PL, Bevill SL, Koo S, Andriacchi TP: Knee kinematics, cartilage morphology, and osteoarthritis after ACL injury. *Med Sci Sports Exerc* 2008;40(2):215-222.

71. Neuman P, Englund M, Kostogiannis I, Fridén T, Roos H, Dahlberg LE: Prevalence of tibiofemoral osteoarthritis 15 years after nonoperative treatment of anterior cruciate ligament injury: A prospective cohort study. *Am J Sports Med* 2008;36(9):1717-1725.

72. Chu CR, Williams AA, Coyle CH, Bowers ME: Early diagnosis to enable early treatment of pre-osteoarthritis. *Arthritis Res Ther* 2012;14(3):212.

73. Brophy RH, Rai MF, Zhang Z, Torgomyan A, Sandell LJ: Molecular analysis of age and sex-related gene expression in meniscal tears with and without a concomitant anterior cruciate ligament tear. *J Bone Joint Surg Am* 2012;94(5):385-393.

74. Li X, Kuo D, Theologis A, et al: Cartilage in anterior cruciate ligament-reconstructed knees: MR imaging T1rho and T2. Initial experience with 1-year follow-up. *Radiology* 2011; 258(2):505-514.

75. Williams A, Qian Y, Golla S, Chu CR: UTE-T2* mapping detects sub-clinical meniscus injury after anterior cruciate ligament tear. *Osteoarthritis Cartilage* 2012;20(6):486-494.

76. Chu CR, Williams A, Tolliver D, Kwoh CK, Bruno S III, Irrgang JJ: Clinical optical coherence tomography of early articular cartilage degeneration in patients with degenerative meniscal tears. *Arthritis Rheum* 2010;62(5):1412-1420.

77. Catterall JB, Stabler TV, Flannery CR, Kraus VB: Changes in serum and synovial fluid biomarkers after acute injury (NCT00332254). *Arthritis Res Ther* 2010;12(6):R229.

78. Larsson S, Lohmander LS, Struglics A: Synovial fluid level of aggrecan ARGS fragments is a more sensitive marker of joint disease than glycosaminoglycan or aggrecan levels: A cross-sectional study. *Arthritis Res Ther* 2009;11(3):R92.

79. Cuellar VG, Cuellar JM, Golish SR, Yeomans DC, Scuderi GJ: Cytokine profiling in acute anterior cruciate ligament injury. *Arthroscopy* 2010;26(10):1296-1301.

80. Dye SF: An evolutionary perspective of the knee. *J Bone Joint Surg Am* 1987;69(7):976-983.

81. Chu CR, Coyle CH, Chu CT, et al: In vivo effects of single intra-articular injection of 0.5% bupivacaine on articular cartilage. *J Bone Joint Surg Am* 2010;92(3):599-608.

82. Ohlendorf C, Tomford WW, Mankin HJ: Chondrocyte survival in cryopreserved osteochondral articular cartilage. *J Orthop Res* 1996;14(3):413-416.

83. Gross AE, Shasha N, Aubin P: Long-term followup of the use of fresh osteochondral allografts for posttraumatic knee defects. *Clin Orthop Relat Res* 2005;435:79-87.

84. Singh G, Fort JG, Goldstein JL, et al: Celecoxib versus naproxen and diclofenac in osteoarthritis patients: SUCCESS-I Study. *Am J Med* 2006;119(3):255-266.

85. Sampson ER, Hilton MJ, Tian Y, et al: Teriparatide as a chondroregenerative therapy for injury-induced osteoarthritis. *Sci Transl Med* 2011;3(101):01ra93.

86. Evans CH, Gouze JN, Gouze E, Robbins PD, Ghivizzani SC: Osteoarthritis gene therapy. *Gene Ther* 2004;11(4):379-389.

87. Payne KA, Lee HH, Haleem AM, et al: Single intra-articular injection of adeno-associated virus results in stable and controllable in vivo transgene expression in normal rat knees. *Osteoarthritis Cartilage* 2011;19(8):1058-1065.

Articular Cartilage Repair and Regeneration

Rocky S. Tuan, PhD
Robert L. Mauck, PhD

Introduction

Articular cartilage ulcerations have long been considered a troublesome clinical issue.[1] Until recently, the barriers to effective cartilage repair were considered insuperable,[2] with few treatment options for most patients. The last several decades have seen a shift in this thinking, with new clinical approaches engendering repair tissues that are increasingly functional and durable in the defect site, making minimally invasive approaches to cartilage repair a new therapeutic reality. This chapter reviews the underlying biologic and mechanical barriers to effective cartilage repair and describes current clinical practice and outcomes with respect to this basic science understanding. Emerging concepts that constitute the next generation of cartilage repair strategies are outlined, namely, a regenerative medicine approach that combines cells, biomolecules, and material delivery to the defect site. Clinical and preclinical data using this regenerative medicine approach are reviewed, and future directions discussed.

Dr. Tuan or an immediate family member serves as a paid consultant to or is an employee of Alacer Technologies and serves as a board member, owner, officer, or committee member of the American Society for Matrix Biology and the Tissue Engineering and Regenerative Medicine International Society. Neither Dr. Mauck nor any immediate family member has received anything of value from or owns stock in a commercial company or institution related directly or indirectly to the subject of this chapter.

Brief Overview of Articular Cartilage
Structure, Content, and Function

Articular cartilage is the dense white connective tissue lining the bony surfaces of diarthrodial joints. Articular (or hyaline) cartilage is distinguished from elastic, nasoseptal, and other fibrocartilages by its unique structure and composition. In the adult, articular cartilage extracellular matrix (ECM) is principally composed of collagens (mostly collagen type II) and sulfated proteoglycans.[3] These elements constitute nearly three fourths and one fourth of the dry weight of the tissue and establish its unique tensile and compressive native tissue properties, respectively.[4] The tissue composition and organization of joint cartilage varies as a function of depth from the articulating surface (**Figure 1**), with the superficial zone possessing the highest tensile properties (and collagen content), and the deeper regions possessing the greatest compressive properties (and proteoglycan content).[5,6] This distribution of mechanical properties evolves with load-bearing use and development,[7] and it is critical for the tissue to function in its complex mechanical loading environment.

In addition to the solid components of the ECM, articular cartilage contains almost 75% water by wet weight. This high water content is established to balance the fixed charges and counterions associated with the high density of proteoglycans in the tissue, and it plays a critical role in cartilage mechanical operation. Specifically, this fluid is constrained from exiting the tissue too quickly when the tissue is loaded (due to the very small pore sizes created by the dense ECM). As a consequence, this interstitial water pressurizes and contributes to the load-bearing capacity of the tissue. In vitro testing of cartilage with direct measurement of fluid pressurization has shown that, under dynamic conditions, this fluid component bears more than 90% of the

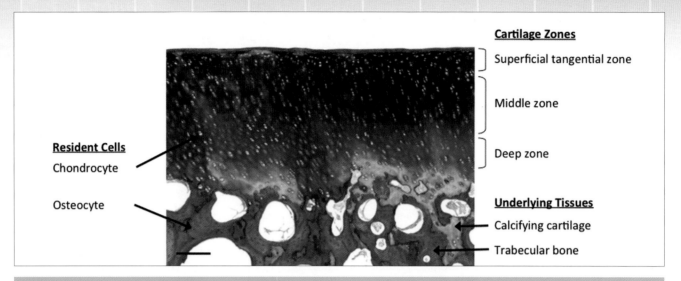

Figure 1 Articular cartilage structure and organization. Histologic image of ovine tibial plateau articular cartilage stained for sulfated proteoglycans (blue) and collagens (red), with cell types and cartilage regions identified. Scale: 100 μm.

stress applied to the native tissue, acting as a protective medium for the solid matrix.[8] Moreover, this fluid pressurization, coupled with the specialized superficial zone of the tissue containing lubricating molecules, presents an extremely slippery (low coefficient of friction) surface that limits tissue wear.[9,10] Indeed, this exquisite balance between content and structure enables cartilage load-bearing function through a lifetime of use.

That articular cartilage can operate in such a demanding environment for such a long period of time is a marvel of engineering. This is especially true given that the forces acting on the cartilage surface reach many times body weight in the major joints of the lower extremities with normal daily activities.[11] Very few synthetic materials can withstand such aggressive loading patterns, and no material can do so while also dissipating load and enabling low-friction motion between contacting surfaces. In the human adult, articular cartilage thickness can range from hundreds of microns to more than 7 mm (on the retropatellar articulating surface). The tissue attains (and sustains) these large thicknesses, despite the fact that the mature tissue is almost entirely devoid of blood supply (and also lacks both neural and lymphatic support). In synovial joints, cartilage is continuously bathed in a viscous solution of synovial fluid, which is itself a distillate of the blood supply, with supplementation from synoviocytes lining the inner synovial membranes. Nearly all nutrition of cartilage results from passive diffusion through the tissue as well as compression-induced exchange of water from within the tissue with the synovial fluid.[12]

Chondrocytes, the primary cell type of cartilage, reside within this dense matrix, occupying 1% to 10% of the tissue volume. These cells operate in a demanding load-bearing, high-stress environment with very little nutritional support. Oxygen tension in the deepest zones of cartilage is on the order of 1% (compared with 21% in air), and nutrient sup-

ply is primarily limited to that provided by the synovial fluid, as the subchondral bone presents a near-impermeable barrier to all except very small molecules. Despite this taxing environment, chondrocytes operate to first establish (in the fetus) and then maintain (in the adult) the cartilage ECM through their biosynthetic activities. Indeed, these cells act as mechanoreceptors, continually fine-tuning their operations to ensure that production of ECM matches levels of degradation, thus maintaining tissue structure and function.[13,14] This careful balance is well orchestrated through most of life, although the numeric density of chondrocytes within the tissue decreases considerably with organismal aging,[15] presenting a significant barrier to effective repair and tissue maintenance in the older adults.

Cartilage Failure and Degeneration

Although cartilage functions well over a lifetime of demanding use, acute trauma, congenital anatomic misalignment, and/or slower pathologic changes can alter tissue homeostasis and lead to degeneration.[16] Degenerative processes in cartilage (not associated with trauma) are generally referred to as osteoarthritis (OA) and are characterized by a gradual loss of cartilage matrix content, loss of structural integrity, and eventual erosion of the articulating surfaces. As noted previously, aging decreases chondrocyte numerical density while at the same time decreasing their biosynthetic capacity. For example, chondrocytes from adult mammals and humans produce fewer (or lower quality) proteoglycans and collagens than fetal and juvenile chondrocytes.[17-19] Disease processes may likewise affect chondrocyte activities; for example, collagen production by OA chondrocytes is lower than that by healthy age-matched chondrocytes.[20] These gradual reductions in cartilage health and regenerative properties represent a significant problem in the aging population.

In addition to OA associated with aging, posttraumatic OA can arise after a singular mechanical event that interrupts cartilage function at any age. High-impact loading events can radically alter the physical structure of cartilage and instigate pathologic processes within the tissue. Early traumatic events can be visualized in instances of subchondral fracture and cartilage fissuring.[21] In controlled in vitro studies, Quinn et al[22,23] showed that strain rates of 7 or 70%/s applied to 3- or 14-MPa peak stress result in cartilage damage macroscopically and microscopically (fissures and cracks), as well as progressive loss of proteoglycans and tissue changes over a 2-week time course. Chen et al[24] have likewise shown progressive catabolic and apoptotic cascades in the 48 hours following impact injury. Importantly, this latter work suggests that a very short surgical timeline exists after injury in which intervention can be palliative and/or reverse the degeneration/apoptotic cascade. In vivo models of impact have shed further light on the long-term consequences of cartilage trauma. In rabbit models developed by Borrelli et al and Haut et al,[25,26] trauma-induced changes in cartilage persist indefinitely.[27,28] Importantly, these animal models serve as a functional system in which to evaluate small molecules that may delay or reverse the immediate and long-term sequelae that follow articular trauma.[29]

Injury and Endogenous Repair

The incidence of articular cartilage injuries varies with age, anatomic location, and other associated risk factors. In the adult population, 9% of those age 30 years and older have OA of the hip or knee, costing an estimated $28.6 billion dollars with more than 200,000 knee replacements currently being performed each year in the United States alone.[30] A recent study of young adults undergoing arthroscopic procedures of the knee revealed that more than 60% had some form of cartilage damage or degeneration, with more than 10% having defects that would be appropriate for cartilage repair procedures.[31] In the fetus, cartilage heals regeneratively if the insult is created earlier in gestation.[32] However, no such healing occurs in cartilage defects in the adult. Indeed, longitudinal studies in both animals and humans have shown that focal defects in articulating surfaces rarely improve with time, and in fact most progress to larger or more serious lesions.[33,34] Although not every observed instance of cartilage damage will progress to symptomatic OA, even focal defects can impair quality of life by decreasing activity levels.[35] Furthermore, although treatment of cartilage lesions (as discussed in the following paragraphs) can improve knee function over a 5-year window, knee function will generally remain inferior to preinjury levels, and a general decline in activity levels is to be expected.[36] Indeed, the natural history of cartilage repair shows a general trend toward improvement only if the subchondral bone is broached, and then again only if the defect is of a small enough size (see the microfracture discussion in the following paragraphs).[2]

Biologic and Mechanical Barriers to Repair

Why is it, then, that cartilage in the adult cannot undergo self-repair? As detailed previously, several biologic constraints may predispose the tissue to poor healing. For instance, in the fetus, where healing does occur, a much higher density of biosynthetically active cells is present, and the ECM is considerably less dense than in the adult. Because cartilage integration requires both an active cell population at the defect site and matrix deposition,[37] the lower density of cells (most of which either are senescent or have decreased biosynthetic activities) may predispose the tissue to progressive damage accumulation. Likewise, inflammatory factors present in a damaged joint may limit tissue formation.[38] Although therapeutic delivery of factors such as parathyroid hormone–related protein may reduce injurious strain-induced initiation of inflammatory cascades,[39] such technologies have not yet proved successful in the joint environment.

In addition to the disadvantageous biologic healing environment, additional constraints are placed on the repair material via the intense loading of the normally active joint. It is not uncommon for the cartilage within the larger joints in the lower extremity to experience compressive forces on the order of multiples of body weight, translating to stresses on the order of 5 to 10 MPa. Widespread degeneration across the articular surface will result in aberrant deformations within the remaining cartilage, leading to increased catabolic events within the tissue. Likewise, local defects that reach a critical size threshold generate stress concentrations near the defect site with joint loading[40] (Figure 2). Moreover, when repair tissue does form, it is often inferior in properties compared with native tissue and so does not bear load.[41] Consequently, the surrounding regions are forced to bear additional load, and thus progressive degeneration can ensue from the precipitating focal defect. Furthermore, radially directed contact stresses about the defect site are an order of magnitude greater than that experienced by the intact cartilage.[42] This would tend to increase fracture at the defect edges, predisposing any repair tissue that does form to dehiscence at the defect edge and eventual failure.

First-Generation Cartilage Repair: Current Clinical Practice

Given the widespread prevalence of cartilage damage and degeneration and the lack of endogenous repair, several reparative strategies have been developed. For many decades, the mainstay of treatment was either masking of symptoms or an irreversible procedure, namely, the palliative treatment of the patient with anti-inflammatory agents and/or pain killers, and ultimately the replacement of the entire damaged bearing surface (in end-stage OA) with a metal and plastic (or ceramic) joint prosthesis. As treatment modalities have shifted to treating cartilage damage in the younger, more active patient population, along with the

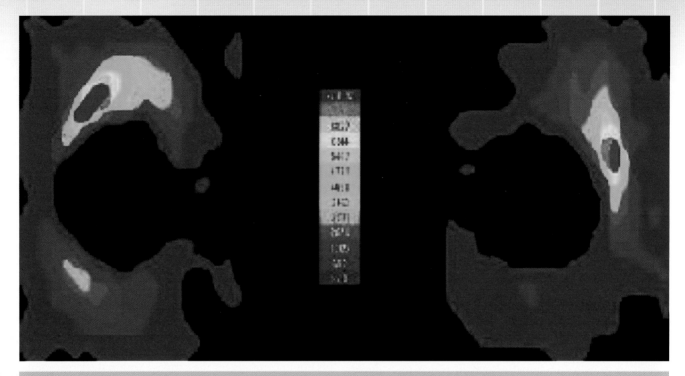

Figure 2 Cartilage defects alter load transmission and local stress profiles. Stress concentrations arising in cartilage surrounding a 12-mm-diameter articular defect on the medial (left) or lateral (right) condyle. (Adapted with permission from Guettler JH, Demetropoulos CK, Yang KH, Jurist KA: Osteochondral defects in the human knee: Influence on defect size on cartilage rim stress and load redistribution to surrounding cartilage. *Am J Sports Med* 2004;32(6):1451-1458.)

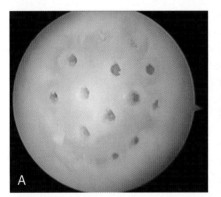
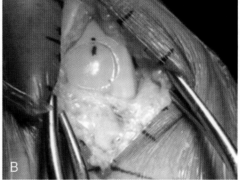
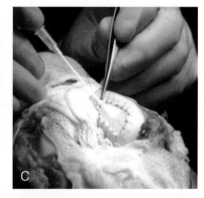

Figure 3 Current clinical approaches to the treatment of articular defects. **A,** Arthroscopic image of a prepared microfracture repair site. **B,** Press-fit osteochondral graft. **C,** Chondrocyte implantation during an autologous chondrocyte implantation procedure after suture fixation of the flap. (Adapted with permission from Gomoll AH, Farr J, Gillogly SD, Kercher J, Minas T: Surgical management of articular cartilage defects of the knee. *J Bone Joint Surg Am* 2010;92:2470-2490.)

general increases in life expectancies over this same time period, focus has shifted toward biologic and/or reconstructive measures to treat cartilage damage.[43] These methods are briefly described in the following paragraphs and depicted in **Figure 3**.

Microfracture

The most direct and straightforward of the cartilage treatments is microfracture. This approach is predicated on the finding that below a certain size, osteochondral defects (those that broach the subchondral plate) will fill with a fibrous tissue and 'heal' the defect.[44] Microfracture procedures mimic this process with the creation of small interruptions to the subchondral plate (with an awl or other device) in a regular pattern.[45-47] This enables communication between the underlying bone marrow elements and blood supply and the cartilage defect itself. Marrow elements clot and congeal within the defect, and the clot serves as a structural template to support progenitor cell migration into the defect site. Importantly, the bone marrow contains a progenitor cell population that can undergo chondrogenesis (that is, take on a chondrocyte-like phenotype).[48,49] However, absent precise control of the differentiation process, the tissue formed within microfractured defects is generally mixed (both cartilaginous and fibrous in nature). As such, the repair material does not match the native tissue properties and so is susceptible to breakdown. This approach is generally restricted to defects that are small in size, and a long and slow rehabilitation regimen is required to protect the forming tissue, with patients unable to resume full sporting activities for 12 to 18 months postsurgery. Despite these limitations, microfracture procedures are readily accomplished arthroscopically and can return patients to normal activities while forestalling (but perhaps not eliminating) the need for a more aggressive repair at a later date.

Osteochondral Grafting

A slightly more complicated repair procedure, osteochondral grafting or mosaicplasty, involves the transfer of bone-cartilage units from either autologous 'healthy' non–load-bearing regions of the same joint or from allogeneic cadaver sources to regions of full-thickness cartilage erosion.[50,51] In both instances, tissue placement restores load-bearing capacity and cartilage structure at the defect site and can provide more rapid restoration of function relative to other repair procedures. Despite its promise, there are several issues related to this procedure. First, it is technically challenging and best performed by those trained in this specialty; improper graft placement results in aberrant stresses at the graft surface and between adjacent grafts,[52] leading to rapid graft failure. If autologous tissue is used, donor site morbidity is common, whereas tissue derived from cadaver sources has diminished viability and the potential for disease transmission. In some instances, however, the patient in need of repair lacks sufficient healthy tissue for transfer, necessitating an allogeneic source. Finally, even under optimal conditions in controlled large animal models with long follow-up durations, significant gaps and clefts are observed at the defect margins, suggesting poor integration between graft and host tissues.[53] Despite the effectiveness of osteochondral grafting relative to microfracture, technical and other limitations limit its use to select patient populations.

Autologous Chondrocyte Implantation

Although the first two repair procedures take advantage of either cells that can be brought to the defect site or cartilage/bone segments that can be transferred en bloc, a newer method takes advantage of the remaining chondrocyte cell population in the surrounding healthy tissue and does so in a controlled fashion. Autologous chondrocyte implantation (ACI) was developed in the early 1990s to address focal defects in the articulating surfaces.[54-57] In this procedure, a small cartilage segment is isolated from a non–weight-bearing site, and the chondrocytes are isolated and expanded ex vivo. Upon successful expansion, these cells are returned to the defect site at a high density and secured in

place (in early versions of the procedure) using a periosteal flap. This method has shown promise, particularly in small defects in non– and low–load-bearing sites. However, as with the previously mentioned methods, significant limitations exist. For example, as with microfracture, the forming tissue is a mixture of fibrous and hyaline cartilage, although in the case of ACI a greater portion of the tissue remains cartilaginous. Another limitation is that because autologous cartilage tissue is used as a cell source, two invasive procedures are required, imposing an additional burden on the patient. ACI is a technically demanding procedure, requiring extensive training. Even with training, in some instances, periosteal flap failure can occur, leading to graft rupture,[58] and clefts and other delaminations of the repair and native tissue are not uncommon. It has recently been reported as well that the sutures used to secure the flap can cause irreparable damage in the surrounding healthy cartilage,[59] and that cells from patients with OA may be inferior in terms of matrix-forming capacity.[20] Moreover, when periosteal flaps are used, hypertrophy and tissue overgrowth have been observed. Because the graft is very fragile at early stages of regeneration, the procedure is approved only for small, nonkissing lesions, and typically in non– or low-load-bearing regions of the joint. As with microfracture, lengthy rehabilitation regimens are necessary to protect the maturing repair material. A further consideration with this procedure in particular is cost, as it involves isolation and expansion of a patient's own cells in a good manufacturing practice facility.[60] Despite these limitations, ACI remains an attractive procedure for the treatment of early-stage defects, and represents the first true 'regenerative' approach to cartilage repair in clinical use.

Each of the previously mentioned procedures has found widespread market acceptance over the past 20 years and in select instances, has provided long-term relief of symptoms to patients with cartilage lesions. Given the competitive (and high-cost) health care environment, several meta-analyses have been published comparing the relative value of each procedure over the past decade.[61] For example, early reports suggested that at 2 years postsurgery, ACI is not definitively superior to microfracture,[62-64] although further and longer term follow-ups may suggest otherwise and need to be interpreted in the context of improved technology for both procedures. Moreover, although the procedures are 'biologic,' and therefore should provide the option for repeated attempts at defect repair, recent studies suggest that ACI procedures may fail at a higher rate if performed in a lesion in which microfracture was previously attempted.[65] Each method has been fine-tuned over the years, with additional considerations and technologies brought to bear. For example, for ACI, selected chondrocyte subpopulations may have better potential than whole chondrocyte isolates,[66] and rehabilitation regimens may be tuned to improve outcomes and earlier return to activity.[67] Both microfracture and ACI procedures have likewise been modified to incorporate a variety of biomaterial implants to potentially improve formation and retention of repair tissue, as well as to obviate the need for the protective periosteal flap (in the case of ACI).[68-70] These new methods and materials, and the next-generation constructs based on this principle, are described in the following section.

Next-Generation Cartilage Repair: Emerging Regenerative Medicine Strategies

The 'first-generation' repair methods that are now established in the literature and in clinical practice have proved that some efficacy can be achieved, short of total joint arthroplasty, for the repair of cartilage defects. To further this progress, several exciting new regenerative medicine strategies have been developed that either harness endogenous healing potential (via modulation of the wound environment) or deliver cells or mature constructs to the defect site to foster a more robust or rapid repair response.[71] Several case examples are outlined in the following paragraphs, but the key concepts of this paradigm are outlined first.

The paradigm of regenerative medicine for cartilage repair was first proposed more than two decades ago. Indeed, in the early days of this new field, it was expected that cartilage repair would be one of the first 'successes' of tissue engineering/regenerative medicine, given the relative simplicity of the tissue (that is only one cell type, no vascular supply). Although the difficulties in achieving functional repair were perhaps more serious than first anticipated, marked progress has been made in achieving this goal, with several approaches now reaching the stage of clinical trial and/or acceptance in the United States and Europe. The basic components of each of these approaches arise from recognized deficits in either endogenous repair or current biologic repair strategies. Regenerative medicine attempts to foster cartilage repair through provision of a supporting structure (a scaffold) on or in which repair can occur, addition of biologic agents (growth factors or other agents) that can manipulate cellular recruitment to or activity in the repair site, and cells themselves (delivered ex vivo or recruited from within) to initiate and sustain the repair response.[72] These approaches can range from the immediate implantation of a repair construct/material to the implantation of a construct grown in the laboratory that more closely matches native tissue properties at the time of implantation.

In the following sections, experimental and commercially available agents and devices are mentioned. The authors are not advocating for the use or acceptance of any one of these devices in particular but rather use these emerging tools to discuss the field as a whole. Both clinical trials evaluating safety and efficacy and market forces will ultimately determine which product and/or approach is superior.

Direct Material Implants and In Situ Repair

The earliest of the 'next-generation' materials for cartilage regeneration arose as a direct consequence of limitations found in existing repair strategies as they became more widely adopted. In the case of both ACI and microfracture, the initial repair tissue is quite fragile, lacking a structural support on which to coalesce. Further, for ACI in particular, the laborious stitching and common observation of delamination of the periosteal flap motivated further refinements to the process.

In response to this need, biomaterial scientists have provided several scaffolding materials to foster rapid stabilization of the forming repair tissue. Scaffolds have been developed from several materials, both natural and synthetic in origin, and with varying degrees of complexity. For example, very early biodegradable nonwoven polyester meshes were shown to have in vitro and in vivo potential as a supporting structure for the formation of cartilaginous tissues.[73,74] Likewise, coupling chondrocytes with a simple collagen gel promoted osteochondral repair in a rabbit model.[75] Some of these materials have already been adopted in cartilage repair applications in humans (**Figure 4**). For example, to address limitations in ACI surgery, a collagen-based material was developed (sold commercially as Chondro-Gide) to sequester chondrocytes at the implantation site.[76] Importantly, this material is biologic in construction and so can remodel as the repair tissue matures in place. Moreover, it obviates the need for the periosteal flap, greatly reducing surgical duration and donor site morbidity. Clinical studies show good retention of the graft in the defect, and fewer complications with this 'matrix-assisted ACI' procedure compared with traditional ACI.[70] Similarly, microfracture procedures have been improved with synthetic polymer [poly(glycolic acid)] implants that are coupled with hyaluronan (a natural glycosaminoglycan constituent of articular cartilage). Fixation of these scaffolds in defects subjected to microfracture improved cartilage regeneration in early reports.[77] Another scaffold that serves as an adjuvant to cartilage repair procedures is Hyalgraft C (Fidia Advanced Biopolymers).[78,79] Hyalgraft C is an esterified hyaluronan product that can be formed into fibrous meshes and foams and is used in conjunction with both ACI and microfracture. Cell/material implants can be formed and implanted without the need for suture fixation, and the procedure can be performed arthroscopically, reducing surgical time and comorbidity. With long-term follow-up (up to 5 years), Hyalgraft C treatment appears to be more durable than microfracture alone.[80,81] Interestingly, this approach also has some efficacy in already diseased (osteoarthritic) joints.[82]

In addition to these natural and polymeric structures that have already been adopted for human clinical use, continual scaffold optimization and development has occurred in the intervening years (**Figure 5**). For example, novel processing methods have been developed for the fabrication of organized three-dimensional constructs with defined pore structures to foster cartilage tissue formation.[83-85] Weaving technologies, adopted from the textile industry, have likewise been developed to produce fibrous structures that re-

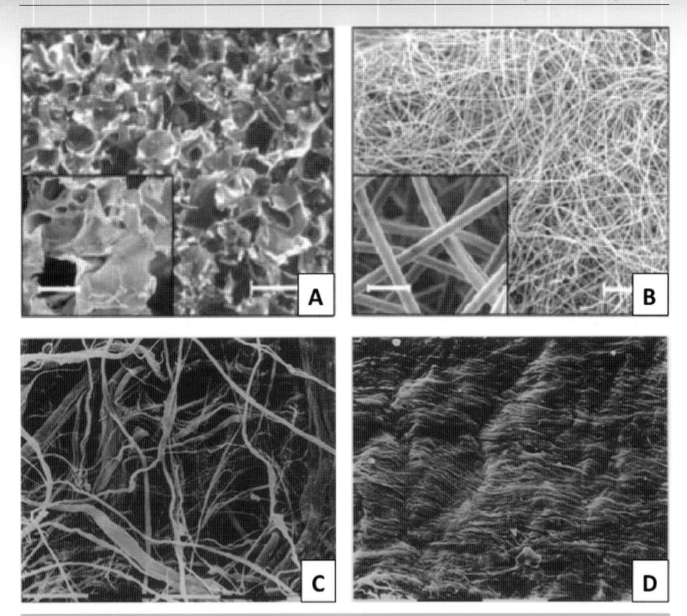

Figure 4 Scaffolding products in clinical use for the stabilization of early tissue formation during microfracture and ACI procedures. Hyaff-11 sponge (**A**) and nonwoven mesh (**B**) and a collagen type I/III membrane (sold commercially as Chondro-Gide, Geistlich Pharma) showing both porous (**C**) and less porous (**D**) surfaces for cell interaction. (Panels A and B adapted with permission from Pei M, Solchaga LA, Seidel J, et al: Bioreactors mediate the effectiveness of tissue engineering scaffolds. *Faseb J* 2002;16(12):1691-1694. Panels C and D adapted with permission from Ehlers EM, Fuss M, Rohwedel J, Russlies M, Kuhnel W, Behrens P: Development of a biocomposite to fill out articular cartilage lesions: Light, scanning and transmission electron microscopy of sheep chondrocytes cultured on a collagen I/III sponge. *Ann Anat* 1999;181(6):513-518.)

create the direction-dependent properties of the native tissue.[86] Further refinements have generated scaffolds with nanoscale topographies (comparable to the length scale of elements of the ECM) that are likewise conducive to chondrocyte growth and tissue maturation.[87,88] In vivo testing of these nanofibrous materials showed promise in a large animal defect model.[89] Still more recently, hollow microspheres with nanofibrous walls have been shown to be efficacious as cell carriers to initiate and stabilize cartilage formation both in vitro and in vivo[90] (**Figure 6**). Although most scaffolds

are evaluated in conjunction with isolated chondrocytes, cartilage fragments (morcellized) can also be combined directly with materials to serve as an immediate cell source for cartilage repair.[91]

Although most of the materials described earlier are intended to interact with cells at the time of implantation (with ACI), or capture marrow elements (with microfracture), not every material is required to do so immediately. For example, fibrin materials, into which cells can migrate, have been used to fill cartilage and osteochondral defects.

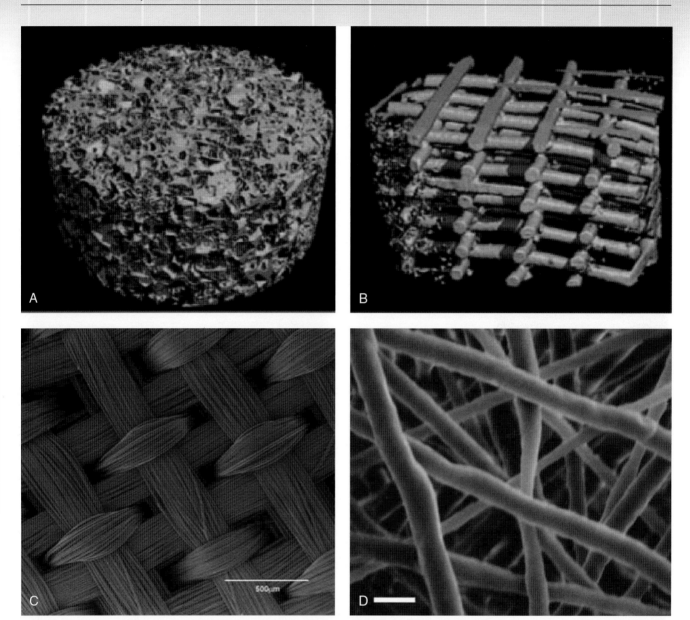

Figure 5 Advanced scaffolding technologies under development and in preclinical testing for cartilage tissue engineering and repair applications. Poly(ethyleneglycol)/polybutylene terephthalate porous scaffold (**A**) and fiber scaffold (**B**) of the same composition formed via bioplotting. **C**, Custom-woven polyglycolic acid microfiber meshes that replicate key mechanical properties of native articular cartilage. **D**, Ultrafine poly(ε-caprolactone) nanofibers (scale, 1 μm) that replicate key length scales of the cellular microenvironment and improve chondrocyte function (Panels A and B adapted with permission from Hollister SJ: Porous scaffold design for tissue engineering. *Nat Mater* 2003;64A(4):1105-1114. Panel C adapted from Moutos FT, Freed LE, Guilak F: A biomimetic three-dimensional woven composite scaffold for functional tissue engineering of cartilage. *Nat Mater* 2007;6(2):162-167. Panel D adapted with permission from Li WJ, Danielson KG, Alexander PG, Tuan RS: Biologic response of chondrocytes cultured in three-dimensional nanofibrous poly(epsilon-caprolactone) scaffolds. *J Biomed Mater Res* 2003;64A(4):1105-1114.)

These materials have been additionally modified to deliver growth factors to improve cartilage repair.[92] Other gel-based materials, formulated from polymerizable and biologically relevant elements, have also been developed to fill defects. These include gel-based versions of hyaluronan[93,94] as well as novel protein-based materials based on elastin-like subunits.[95,96] Similarly, short peptide repeats that self-assemble into a stable gel upon exposure to ions have demonstrated some efficacy in vitro and in vivo,[97,98] with and without cell delivery. In one interesting gel-based application, a two-phase approach was implemented to address both tissue formation and stable integration into the defect. In this system, the cartilage surfaces were first chemically modified, after which a photopolymerizable polymer gel was covalently coupled to the cartilage interface. These gels thus formed a contiguous and covalently integrated interface, and when

316

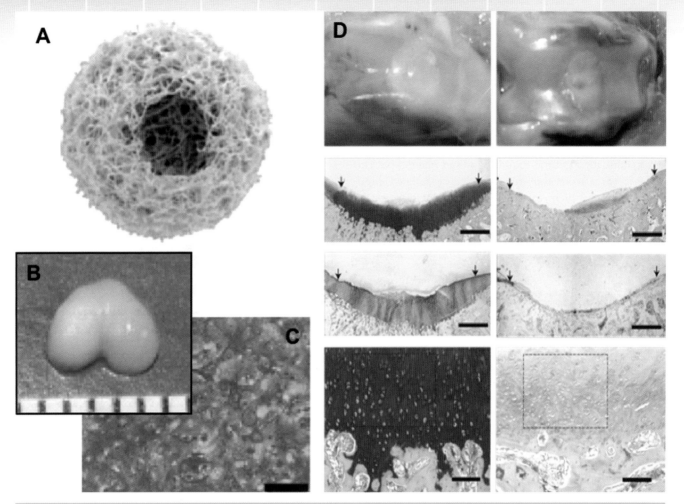

Figure 6 Novel cell delivery devices for cartilage repair. Hollow core nanofibrous shell microspheres (**A**) can be seeded with chondrocytes and packed into various shapes to generate engineered cartilage in anatomic forms (**B**) with dense ECM formation upon culture in vitro (**C**). In vivo repair of full-thickness cartilage defects (**D**) is improved with delivery of cells via these hollow nanofibrous microspheres (left) compared with empty defects (right). (Adapted with permission from Liu X, Jin X, Ma PX: Nanofibrous hollow microspheres self-assembled from star shaped polymers as injectable cell carriers for knee repair. *Nat Mater* 2011;10(5):398-406.)

coupled with microfracture performed at the time of gel polymerization, improved cartilage repair in a large animal model.[99]

Cell-Based Implants Grown in the Laboratory

Although many materials have been evaluated in vivo directly, or immediately after combination with chondrocytes, an alternative approach may be to mature the engineered construct in vitro in the laboratory for subsequent implantation.[100] This would mirror osteochondral allografting procedures described earlier where a mature and load-bearing cell-based construct could function in the defect space immediately upon implantation. Indeed, no matter what the final application intended, in vitro evaluation of construct maturation often precedes in vivo studies to demonstrate the potential of a select material. In such studies, chondrocytes are generally combined with a scaffolding ma-

terial to sequester cells and capture accumulated ECM, forming a cartilage-like replacement tissue. A variety of scaffold materials, fabrication methods, cell types, and stimulation (chemical and physical) have been used to accomplish this.[101,102]

As noted previously, porous scaffolds (foams and fibrous meshes) fabricated from poly(α-hydroxy esters), including poly(glycolic acid), poly(lactic acid), and their copolymers have been extensively investigated.[103-107] Additional work has shown that foams and meshes based on natural materials (collagen types I and II, proteoglycan/collagen composites) support cartilage growth as well.[108,109] Chondrocytes cultured on these porous scaffolds form ECM and increase in mechanical properties with culture duration. However, uniform seeding throughout the scaffold expanse is a challenge and cells may flatten and line the pore spaces, influencing phenotypic stability.

Alternatively, hydrogels are attractive biomaterials for

cartilage regeneration, and many natural (for example, collagen, hyaluronan, alginate) and synthetic (for example, Pluronics and poly[ethylene glycol]) polymers have been investigated. Specific examples in the literature include alginate,[110-112] agarose,[113,114] fibrin,[92,115] collagen types I and II,[116,117] peptide gels,[97] and photocrosslinkable hyaluronic acid[93,94] and poly(ethylene glycol).[118-120] This focus on hydrogels is motivated by the observation that in hydrogel culture, chondrocytes can be well dispersed and cells may assume their natural round shape and phenotype. This shape is particularly important, as dedifferentiated chondrocytes regain their cartilage ECM-producing capacity when seeded in even simple hydrogels.[121] Furthermore, these gels efficiently entrap the cartilage-like ECM produced by the cells[121-123] and can rapidly assemble a neocartilage-like matrix with functional properties, in a sense, recapitulating developmental cartilage formation in the embryo.[124]

Additional factors may be tuned in the in vitro setting to improve cartilage tissue formation. For example, several studies have shown that increasing the initial cell number within the construct can lead to more rapid and/or greater cartilage-ECM formation and mechanics.[107,113,114,125,126] Alterations in hydrogel density and pore size can likewise influence matrix distribution and cell activity.[127,128] Further work has shown that inclusion of anabolic growth factors normally found in the maturing and mature synovial fluid (such as insulin-like growth factor-1, transforming growth factor-β [TGF-β] family members, and fibroblast growth factor) can further improve cartilage-like tissue development in engineered constructs.[129-134] Indeed, in several recent studies, transient application of TGF-β3 in a serum-free, chemically defined medium enhanced the compressive properties and proteoglycan content of chondrocyte-laden hydrogels to match native tissue levels.[135,136] In those studies, after removal of the growth factor, constructs achieved equilibrium compressive moduli of approximately 0.8 MPa and proteoglycan levels of 6% to 7% wet weight in less than 2 months. Such mature constructs, matching native tissue properties, would enable load transmission directly upon implantation, much like an allograft, although issues of integration with the underlying bone and surrounding cartilage will have to be addressed to complete the repair process (see next paragraphs).

The Future of Cartilage Repair
Exogenous Adult Stem Cell Sources
Despite the progress made with chondrocytes for cartilage repair and tissue-engineering applications, these cells are somewhat limited in potential given their scarcity in adult tissue, potentially diseased source leading to inferior cells, and complications with tissue harvesting.[137] As a result, over the past 20 years, considerable interest has focused on the potential of adult mesenchymal stem cells (MSCs) for therapeutic applications.[138-140] Indeed, recent notable successes indicate that these cells can form native tissue struc-

tures in vitro and in vivo, including cartilage.[141] MSCs and similar progenitor cells are easily obtained from bone marrow aspirates, adipose tissue, periosteum, and several other tissue sources.[48,49,142-145] MSCs are multipotent and capable of differentiating toward several lineages of the musculoskeletal system, including bone, cartilage, and fat,[146] and are readily expandable in culture and retain their multipotential characteristics.[147] This capacity was first described more than three decades ago.[148] Since the early descriptions of chondrogenesis in pellet culture,[149-151] the ability of these cells to generate cartilage-like tissues has been widely investigated. In general, MSC chondrogenic differentiation is initiated with growth factors, including TGF-β family members,[149,152-154] ascorbate, and dexamethasone. Indeed, several studies have demonstrated that chondrogenesis can occur in most scaffolding materials used for chondrocyte-based cartilage repair and tissue engineering.[155]

With chondrogenesis, MSCs initiate expression of the master transcription factor sox9 as well as production of cartilage-specific matrix, including collagen type II and the large proteoglycan aggrecan. Although these markers are appropriate evidence that a chondrogenic event has occurred, they do not necessarily correlate with mechanical function. For clinical translation, the mechanical properties of engineered constructs will ultimately dictate in vivo success. However, few studies of MSC chondrogenesis consider this critical metric. Those studies that have been performed suggest a puzzling scenario. That is, although most markers of the 'chondrocyte' phenotype are expressed, the mechanical properties of constructs populated by these cells are typically inferior to both native tissue and tissue-engineered constructs formed by differentiated chondrocytes.[155,156] For example, **Figure 7** shows the development of mechanical and biochemical properties of constructs formed from bovine MSCs embedded within agarose, self-assembling peptide, and photocrosslinked hyaluronic acid hydrogels. These properties increase substantially over the 8 weeks of culture, with robust deposition of proteoglycan evident in histologic sections.[157] However, the values achieved with both human and bovine MSCs in these natural ECM hydrogel materials (0.1-0.2 MPa[157-161]) are far lower than those achieved with chondrocyte-based constructs cultured identically. These data support the notion that MSCs are a useful and promising tool for cartilage repair, but that their full functional capacity has yet to be realized.

Notwithstanding their clear potential for the formation of a cartilage-like tissue, a significant concern with the use of MSCs lies in their potential lack of phenotypic stability after implantation. For example, Pelttari et al[162] showed that subcutaneous implantation of chondrogenic MSC pellets resulted in mineralized deposits within the original cartilaginous matrix. In recent studies using MSC-seeded hyaluronic acid gels that were engineered to deliver TGF-β over the first week of implantation, chondrogenesis was induced when implanted subcutaneously, though hypertrophy and mineralization were observed as early as the fourth

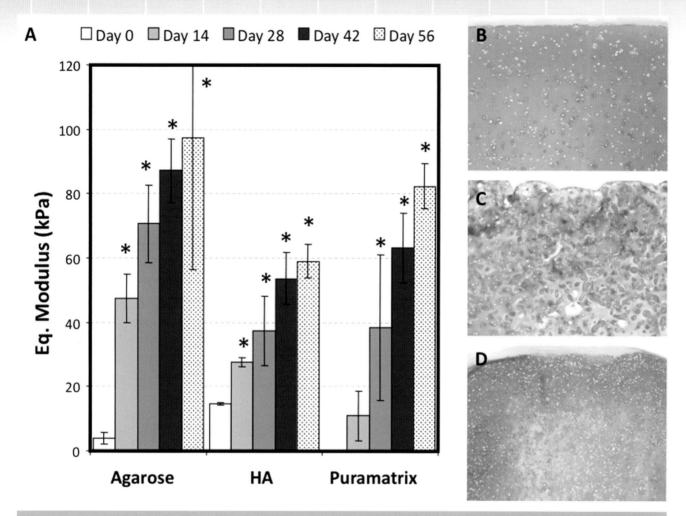

Figure 7 Mesenchymal stem cells (MSCs) can produce a cartilage-like tissue in three-dimensional culture. MSCs differentiate toward a chondrocyte-like phenotype and amass matrix with increasing mechanical properties in several three-dimensional hydrogels. Mechanical properties (**A**) and proteoglycan deposition in agarose (**B**), hyaluronic acid (**C**), and self-assembling peptide gels (**D**) with time in chondrogenic culture. The asterisks indicate difference from day 0, n = 4 to 5 per group. HA = hyaluronic acid. (Adapted with permission from Huang AH, Farrell MJ, Mauck RL: Mechanics and mechanobiology of mesenchymal stem cell-based engineered cartilage. *J Biomech* 2011;43:128-136.)

week of implantation.[160] Notably, chondrocyte control groups maintain phenotypic stability under similar in vivo conditions and form additional cartilage matrix with no evidence of mineralization. This shift toward an osteogenic phenotype can be realized in vitro as well, with modulation of the chemical environment.[163] These data suggest that the standard benchmarks of chondrogenesis as currently applied may reflect the phenotype of 'transient' chondrocytes (which reside in the growth plate and undergo hypertrophy and eventual ossification) rather than that of 'permanent' chondrocytes (which reside in the articular cartilage and maintain a fixed chondrocyte phenotype throughout life).[164] Because the permanent hyaline cartilage (and the chondrocytes within) shows a remarkable ability to first establish functional matrix and then resist progressive phenotypic conversion toward the osteogenic lineage, these cells in

particular should serve as the 'gold standard' for chondrogenesis.

Total Joint Arthroplasty With Engineered (Osteo)Chondral Anatomic Grafts

Although the advances to date in scaffold formulation and construct maturation have been striking, additional considerations remain to be addressed to achieve functional repair. As was noted previously, full repair of a cartilage defect will require not just filling with a cartilage equivalent, but that the new tissue integrates seamlessly with both the surrounding cartilage as well as with the underlying subchondral bone. To address this, in vitro models have assessed integration strength of both chondrocyte- and MSC-laden scaffolds and hydrogels within cartilage defects,[165,166] and cell-laden hydrogel formulations have been used to foster integration between native cartilage segments (as a potential

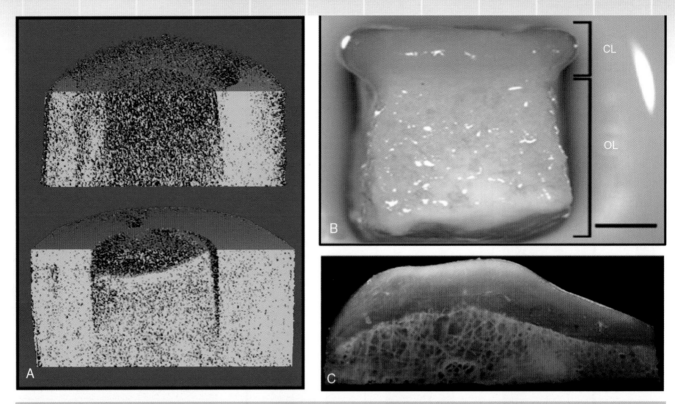

Figure 8 Formation and integration of engineered osteochondral constructs for cartilage repair. **A,** Integration of cartilage with itself (bottom) and with an engineered stem cell–seeded hydrogel (top) visualized by contrast-enhanced micro CT. (**B**) Engineered osteochondral stem cell–based constructs with cartilage layer (CL) and osteogenic layer (OL). **C,** Retropatellar osteochondral construct (image width, approximately 6 cm) formed from cell-seeded hydrogels infused into trabecular bone, with both gel and bone topographies recreating the anatomic form. (Panels A and B adapted with permission from Tuli R, Nandi S, Li WJ, et al: Human mesenchymal progenitor cell-based tissue engineering of a single-unit osteochondral construct. *Tissue Eng* 2004;10(7-8): 1169-1179. Panel C adapted with permission from Hung CT, Mauck RL, Wang CC, Lima EG, Ateshian GA: A paradigm for functional tissue engineering of articular cartilage via applied physiologic deformational loading. *Ann Biomed Eng* 2004;32:35-49.)

improvement to allografting procedures).[167] When polymerized within a defect, hydrogels can form a contiguous interface with the native cartilage boundaries (**Figure 8**) and so enhance integration strength and matrix deposition at these interfaces.

To address the issue of integration with subchondral bone, materials supportive of cartilage formation have been combined with a variety of materials that can foster bone formation and integration. This process generates an osteochondral construct, much like the native tissue structures used in allografting procedures. These composites have been formed using a variety of materials, including porous polymer layers annealed to ceramic[168] and via the creation of multiphasic constructs (with gels and foams) containing chondrogenic and osteogenic cell sources in distinct regions.[169] Gels have also been combined directly with devitalized trabecular bone,[170,171] although some recent efforts have shifted toward the use of bioglass[172] and tantalum (trabecular metal) bone regions,[173] these being more clinically applicable substrates. These formulations are particularly exciting as they combine materials that can foster cartilage formation in one region while taking advantage of the

proven potential and clinical acceptance of porous glasses and metals to achieve bony integration. These osteochondral technologies are being tested in large animal models as well; for example, one recent study showed that stem cell–based composites[174] could improve repair of osteochondral defects in a minipig model.[175]

Although these advances address cartilage-to-cartilage and cartilage-to-bone integration, in cases where cartilage damage is more severe (such as with advanced OA), replacement of the entire cartilage surface must be considered. In such circumstances, the barriers to biologic repair will be considerable: the entire joint milieu is altered in advanced OA, including degeneration of supporting structures, and the biomechanical demands placed on such an implant will be markedly higher than that placed on a repaired focal lesion. Despite these challenges, several technologies have been developed to address whole joint resurfacing. Injection molding has long been used to fabricate shaped implants,[125] and similar anatomic renderings have been used to generate molds for the formation of gel/bone composites that recreate the anatomy of large articulating surfaces[176] (**Figure 8**). Most recently, this approach has been implemented via

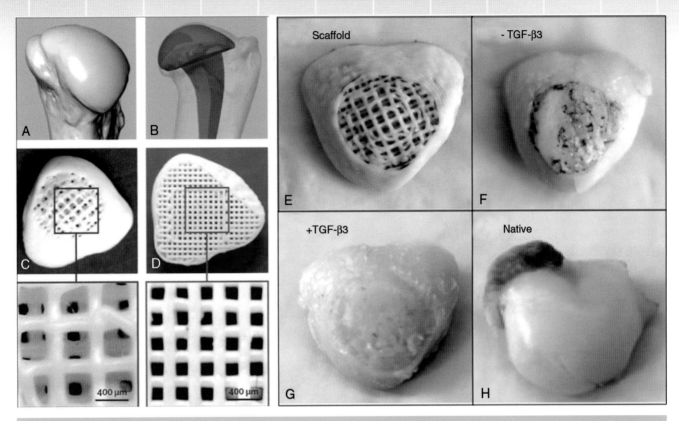

Figure 9 Construction of anatomic biodegradable prostheses for total joint arthroplasty. Rapid prototyping was used to fabricate a prosthesis for the anatomic reconstruction of the rabbit shoulder (**A** and **B**). Defined pores (**C** and **D**) engineered into the implant were filled with collagen gel (with and without TGF-β3 supplementation). After 6 weeks of implantation (**E-H**), growth factor delivery enhanced stem cell homing to the implant site and improved cartilage repair (**G**). (Adapted with permission from Lee CH, Cook JL, Mendelson A, Moioli EK, Yao H, Mao JJ: Regeneration of the articular surface of the rabbit synovial joint by cell homing: A proof of concept study. *Lancet* 2010;376:440-448.)

the formation and implantation of anatomic biodegradable constructs formed by rapid prototyping of degradable materials.[177] These anatomic 'prostheses' were designed to insert into the remaining bone stock, while presenting a porous and anatomically shaped surface in which cartilage formation could occur. When these implants were infused with collagen gels containing TGF-β and implanted into rabbit shoulders, regeneration of the complete load-bearing surface was observed (**Figure 9**). Although this technology will need to be evaluated in larger animal models, it points to the next generation of cartilage repair devices, where biologic replacement of entire articulating cartilage surfaces will be possible. This would provide a regenerative medicine/tissue engineering approach that could eliminate the need for joint arthroplasty with metal and plastic implants and could dramatically improve the health and mobility of the many individuals with OA worldwide.

Cartilage Repair: Where Do We Go From Here?

The past 20 years have witnessed an intense focus on the development of novel strategies for the treatment of chondral defects. The need for such treatments is self-evident: carti-

lage in the adult does not heal, and accumulated damage will predispose the patient to early onset of OA. Although metal and plastic prosthetics are extremely valuable as an end-stage treatment paradigm, early intervention in younger patients may forestall or even eliminate the need for these total joint arthroplasties. Since the mid-1990s, several treatment options have been developed and have seen widespread acceptance in clinical practice. Although there is certainly an ongoing debate as to which specific treatment modality is superior, there is no question that interventional therapeutic treatment is now an option and that the devices and methods are improving.

As with all new technologies, these emergent cartilage repair strategies will need to be evaluated with respect first and foremost to safety and efficacy. However, they must also be evaluated in the marketplace, where increasing medical costs may drive (and even limit) device design. Regenerative medicine/tissue-engineering efforts have culminated in laboratory-grown cartilage that recapitulates, in many important regards, the functional properties of the native tissue. Continued improvements to such engineered constructs will need to address the issue of maturation in the in vivo setting as well as integration with remaining joint structures. Moreover, technologic developments in stem cell biology will need to focus not just on the induction of a cartilage-like phenotype, but also on maintenance of that state if these cells are to become a clinical reality. Furthermore, the articular cartilage is but one part of the entire joint, and inflammatory cues present in the diseased joint 'organ' will likely have a negative effect on any implanted material. Although recent reports suggest that MSCs can be immunomodulatory,[178] considerable work remains to understand this mechanism and to optimize it for the creation of 'hardy' engineered constructs that can function in the potentially inflammatory repair environment. Some of these advances may depend on genetic modulation of implanted cells. Gene therapy approaches have already been used to induce stem cell chondrogenesis[179,180] and may be used to overcome the remaining challenges in functional and durable cartilage repair through direct molecular manipulation of cellular machinery. Although there remain considerable challenges to overcome, the future of cartilage repair is now. Next-generation products involving advanced materials, selected progenitor cell populations, and engineered constructs are steadily proving more efficacious in preclinical models. The next decade will see a wealth of new products and devices making their way into clinical trials. These products must prove themselves to be better and more cost-effective than current therapies, and to provide functional and long-term repair of cartilage defects. With these advances, the troublesome clinical issue of cartilage ulcerations, long considered insuperable, may well be on its way to becoming a thing of the past.

References

1. Hunter W: Of the structure and disease of articulating cartilages: 1743. *Clin Orthop Relat Res* 1995;317:3-6.

2. Hunziker EB: Articular cartilage repair: Are the intrinsic biological constraints undermining this process insuperable? *Osteoarthritis Cartilage* 1999;7(1):15-28.

3. Maroudas A: Physicochemical properties of articular cartilage, in Freeman MAR (ed): *Adult Articular Cartilage*. Kent, England, Pitman Medical, 1979, pp 215-290.

4. Mow VC, Ratcliffe A, Woo SL: *Biomechanics of Diarthrodial Joints*. New York, NY, Springer-Verlag, 1990.

5. Huang CY, Stankiewicz A, Ateshian GA, Mow VC: Anisotropy, inhomogeneity, and tension-compression nonlinearity of human glenohumeral cartilage in finite deformation. *J Biomech* 2005;38(4):799-809.

6. Schinagl RM, Gurskis D, Chen AC, Sah RL: Depth-dependent confined compression modulus of full-thickness bovine articular cartilage. *J Orthop Res* 1997;15(4):499-506.

7. Williamson AK, Chen AC, Sah RL: Compressive properties and function-composition relationships of developing bovine articular cartilage. *J Orthop Res* 2001;19(6):1113-1121.

8. Soltz MA, Ateshian GA: Experimental verification and theoretical prediction of cartilage interstitial fluid pressurization at an impermeable contact interface in confined compression. *J Biomech* 1998;31(10):927-934.

9. Krishnan R, Kopacz M, Ateshian GA: Experimental verification of the role of interstitial fluid pressurization in cartilage lubrication. *J Orthop Res* 2004;22(3):565-570.

10. Jones AR, Gleghorn JP, Hughes CE, et al: Binding and localization of recombinant lubricin to articular cartilage surfaces. *J Orthop Res* 2007;25(3):283-292.

11. Ateshian GA, Hung CT: Patellofemoral joint biomechanics and tissue engineering. *Clin Orthop Relat Res* 2005;436:81-90.

12. O'Hara BP, Urban JP, Maroudas A: Influence of cyclic loading on the nutrition of articular cartilage. *Ann Rheum Dis* 1990;49(7):536-539.

13. Kim YJ, Sah RL, Grodzinsky AJ, Plaas AH, Sandy JD: Mechanical regulation of cartilage biosynthetic behavior: Physical stimuli. *Arch Biochem Biophys* 1994;311(1):1-12.

14. Guilak F, Ratcliffe A, Mow VC: Chondrocyte deformation and local tissue strain in articular cartilage: A confocal microscopy study. *J Orthop Res* 1995;13(3):410-421.

15. Jadin KD, Bae WC, Schumacher BL, Sah RL: Three-dimensional (3-D) imaging of chondrocytes in articular cartilage: Growth-associated changes in cell organization. *Biomaterials* 2007;28(2):230-239.

16. Mueller MB, Tuan RS: Anabolic/catabolic balance in pathogenesis of osteoarthritis: Identifying molecular targets. *PM R* 2011;3(6, Suppl 1):S3-S11.

17. Thonar EJ, Buckwalter JA, Kuettner KE: Maturation-related differences in the structure and composition of proteoglycans synthesized by chondrocytes from bovine articular cartilage. *J Biol Chem* 1986;261(5):2467-2474.

18. Adkisson HD, Gillis MP, Davis EC, Maloney W, Hruska KA: In vitro generation of scaffold independent neocartilage. *Clin Orthop Relat Res* 2001;391(Suppl):S280-S294.

19. Erickson IE, van Veen SC, Sengupta S, Kestle SR, Mauck RL: Cartilage matrix formation by bovine mesenchymal stem cells in three-dimensional culture is age-dependent. *Clin Orthop Relat Res* 2011;469(10):2744-2753.

20. Tallheden T, Bengtsson C, Brantsing C, et al: Proliferation and differentiation potential of chondrocytes from osteoarthritic patients. *Arthritis Res Ther* 2005;7(3):R560-R568.

21. Atkinson TS, Haut RC, Altiero NJ: Impact-induced fissuring of articular cartilage: An investigation of failure criteria. *J Biomech Eng* 1998;120(2):181-187.

22. Quinn TM, Allen RG, Schalet BJ, Perumbuli P, Hunziker EB: Matrix and cell injury due to sub-impact loading of adult bovine articular cartilage explants: Effects of strain rate and peak stress. *J Orthop Res* 2001;19(2):242-249.

23. Quinn TM, Grodzinsky AJ, Hunziker EB, Sandy JD: Effects of injurious compression on matrix turnover around individual cells in calf articular cartilage explants. *J Orthop Res* 1998;16(4):490-499.

24. Chen CT, Burton-Wurster N, Borden C, Hueffer K, Bloom SE, Lust G: Chondrocyte necrosis and apoptosis in impact damaged articular cartilage. *J Orthop Res* 2001;19(4):703-711.

25. Borrelli J Jr, Burns ME, Ricci WM, Silva MJ: A method for delivering variable impact stresses to the articular cartilage of rabbit knees. *J Orthop Trauma* 2002;16(3):182-188.

26. Haut RC, Ide TM, De Camp CE: Mechanical responses of

the rabbit patello-femoral joint to blunt impact. *J Biomech Eng* 1995;117(4):402-408.

27. Isaac DI, Meyer EG, Kopke KS, Haut RC: Chronic changes in the rabbit tibial plateau following blunt trauma to the tibiofemoral joint. *J Biomech* 2010;43(9):1682-1688.

28. Ewers BJ, Weaver BT, Sevensma ET, Haut RC: Chronic changes in rabbit retro-patellar cartilage and subchondral bone after blunt impact loading of the patellofemoral joint. *J Orthop Res* 2002;20(3):545-550.

29. Isaac DI, Golenberg N, Haut RC: Acute repair of chondrocytes in the rabbit tibiofemoral joint following blunt impact using P188 surfactant and a preliminary investigation of its long-term efficacy. *J Orthop Res* 2010;28(4):553-558.

30. Frankowski JJ, Watkins-Castillo S: *Primary Total Knee and Hip Arthroplasty Projections for the U.S. Population to the Year 2030.* Rosemont, IL, American Academy of Orthopaedic Surgeons, Department of Research and Scientific Affairs, 2002, pp 1-8.

31. Arøen A, Løken S, Heir S, et al: Articular cartilage lesions in 993 consecutive knee arthroscopies. *Am J Sports Med* 2004;32(1):211-215.

32. Namba RS, Meuli M, Sullivan KM, Le AX, Adzick NS: Spontaneous repair of superficial defects in articular cartilage in a fetal lamb model. *J Bone Joint Surg Am* 1998;80(1):4-10.

33. Davies-Tuck ML, Wluka AE, Wang Y, et al: The natural history of cartilage defects in people with knee osteoarthritis. *Osteoarthritis Cartilage* 2008;16(3):337-342.

34. Wang Y, Ding C, Wluka AE, et al: Factors affecting progression of knee cartilage defects in normal subjects over 2 years. *Rheumatology (Oxford)* 2006;45(1):79-84.

35. Heir S, Nerhus TK, Røtterud JH, et al: Focal cartilage defects in the knee impair quality of life as much as severe osteoarthritis: A comparison of knee injury and osteoarthritis outcome score in 4 patient categories scheduled for knee surgery. *Am J Sports Med* 2010;38(2):231-237.

36. Løken S, Heir S, Holme I, Engebretsen L, Årøen A: 6-year follow-up of 84 patients with cartilage defects in the knee: Knee scores improved but recovery was incomplete. *Acta Orthop* 2010;81(5):611-618.

37. DiMicco MA, Sah RL: Integrative cartilage repair: Adhesive strength is correlated with collagen deposition. *J Orthop Res* 2001;19(6):1105-1112.

38. Steinert AF, Ghivizzani SC, Rethwilm A, Tuan RS, Evans CH, Nöth U: Major biological obstacles for persistent cell-based regeneration of articular cartilage. *Arthritis Res Ther* 2007;9(3):213.

39. Wang D, Taboas JM, Tuan RS: PTHrP overexpression partially inhibits a mechanical strain-induced arthritic phenotype in chondrocytes. *Osteoarthritis Cartilage* 2011;19(2):213-221.

40. Guettler JH, Demetropoulos CK, Yang KH, Jurist KA: Osteochondral defects in the human knee: Influence of defect size on cartilage rim stress and load redistribution to surrounding cartilage. *Am J Sports Med* 2004;32(6):1451-1458.

41. Nelson BH, Anderson DD, Brand RA, Brown TD: Effect of osteochondral defects on articular cartilage: Contact pressures studied in dog knees. *Acta Orthop Scand* 1988;59(5):574-579.

42. Brown TD, Pope DF, Hale JE, Buckwalter JA, Brand RA: Effects of osteochondral defect size on cartilage contact stress. *J Orthop Res* 1991;9(4):559-567.

43. Gomoll AH, Farr J, Gillogly SD, Kercher J, Minas T: Surgical management of articular cartilage defects of the knee. *J Bone Joint Surg Am* 2010;92(14):2470-2490.

44. Jackson DW, Lalor PA, Aberman HM, Simon TM: Spontaneous repair of full-thickness defects of articular cartilage in a goat model: A preliminary study. *J Bone Joint Surg Am* 2001;83(1):53-64.

45. Insall J: The Pridie debridement operation for osteoarthritis of the knee. *Clin Orthop Relat Res* 1974;101:61-67.

46. Steadman JR, Rodkey WG, Briggs KK: Microfracture to treat full-thickness chondral defects: Surgical technique, rehabilitation, and outcomes. *J Knee Surg* 2002;15(3):170-176.

47. Steadman JR, Rodkey WG, Rodrigo JJ: Microfracture: Surgical technique and rehabilitation to treat chondral defects. *Clin Orthop Relat Res* 2001;391(Suppl):S362-S369.

48. Chen FH, Tuan RS: Mesenchymal stem cells in arthritic diseases. *Arthritis Res Ther* 2008;10(5):223.

49. Chen FH, Rousche KT, Tuan RS: Technology insight: Adult stem cells in cartilage regeneration and tissue engineering. *Nat Clin Pract Rheumatol* 2006;2(7):373-382.

50. Yamashita F, Sakakida K, Suzu F, Takai S: The transplantation of an autogeneic osteochondral fragment for osteochondritis dissecans of the knee. *Clin Orthop Relat Res* 1985;201:43-50.

51. Hangody L, Kish G, Kárpáti Z, Szerb I, Udvarhelyi I: Arthroscopic autogenous osteochondral mosaicplasty for the treatment of femoral condylar articular defects: A preliminary report. *Knee Surg Sports Traumatol Arthrosc* 1997;5(4):262-267.

52. Wu JZ, Herzog W, Hasler EM: Inadequate placement of osteochondral plugs may induce abnormal stress-strain distributions in articular cartilage–finite element simulations. *Med Eng Phys* 2002;24(2):85-97.

53. Lane JG, Massie JB, Ball ST, et al: Follow-up of osteochondral plug transfers in a goat model: A 6-month study. *Am J Sports Med* 2004;32(6):1440-1450.

54. Brittberg M, Lindahl A, Nilsson A, Ohlsson C, Isaksson O, Peterson L: Treatment of deep cartilage defects in the knee with autologous chondrocyte transplantation. *N Engl J Med* 1994;331(14):889-895.

55. Brittberg M, Nilsson A, Lindahl A, Ohlsson C, Peterson L: Rabbit articular cartilage defects treated with autologous cultured chondrocytes. *Clin Orthop Relat Res* 1996;326:270-283.

56. Grande DA, Pitman MI, Peterson L, Menche D, Klein M: The repair of experimentally produced defects in rabbit articular cartilage by autologous chondrocyte transplantation. *J Orthop Res* 1989;7(2):208-218.

57. Grande DA, Singh IJ, Pugh J: Healing of experimentally produced lesions in articular cartilage following chondrocyte transplantation. *Anat Rec* 1987;218(2):142-148.

58. Nehrer S, Spector M, Minas T: Histologic analysis of tissue after failed cartilage repair procedures. *Clin Orthop Relat Res* 1999;365:149-162.

59. Hunziker EB, Stähli A: Surgical suturing of articular carti-

lage induces osteoarthritis-like changes. *Osteoarthritis Cartilage* 2008;16(9):1067-1073.

60. Clar C, Cummins E, McIntyre L, et al: Clinical and cost-effectiveness of autologous chondrocyte implantation for cartilage defects in knee joints: Systematic review and economic evaluation. *Health Technol Assess* 2005;9(47):iii-iv, ix-x, 1-82.

61. Meyerkort D, Wood D, Zheng MH: One-stage vs two-stage cartilage repair: A current review. *Orthop Res Rev* 2010;2:95-106.

62. Knutsen G, Engebretsen L, Ludvigsen TC, et al: Autologous chondrocyte implantation compared with microfracture in the knee: A randomized trial. *J Bone Joint Surg Am* 2004; 86(3):455-464.

63. Van Assche D, Staes F, Van Caspel D, et al: Autologous chondrocyte implantation versus microfracture for knee cartilage injury: A prospective randomized trial, with 2-year follow-up. *Knee Surg Sports Traumatol Arthrosc* 2010;18(4): 486-495.

64. Coleman SH, Malizia R, Macgillivray J, Warren RF: Treatment of isolated articular cartilage lesions of the medial femoral condyle: A clinical and MR comparison of autologous chondrocyte implantation vs. microfracture. *Ortop Traumatol Rehabil* 2001;3(2):224-226.

65. Minas T, Gomoll AH, Rosenberger R, Royce RO, Bryant T: Increased failure rate of autologous chondrocyte implantation after previous treatment with marrow stimulation techniques. *Am J Sports Med* 2009;37(5):902-908.

66. Gerlier L, Lamotte M, Wille M, et al: The cost utility of autologous chondrocytes implantation using ChondroCelect® in symptomatic knee cartilage lesions in Belgium. *Pharmacoeconomics* 2010;28(12):1129-1146.

67. Fazalare JA, Griesser MJ, Siston RA, Flanigan DC: The use of continuous passive motion following knee cartilage defect surgery: A systematic review. *Orthopedics* 2010;33(12): 878.

68. Wegener B, Schrimpf FM, Pietschmann MF, et al: Matrix-guided cartilage regeneration in chondral defects. *Biotechnol Appl Biochem* 2009;53(Pt 1):63-70.

69. Niemeyer P, Pestka JM, Kreuz PC, et al: Characteristic complications after autologous chondrocyte implantation for cartilage defects of the knee joint. *Am J Sports Med* 2008; 36(11):2091-2099.

70. Haddo O, Mahroof S, Higgs D, et al: The use of chondrogide membrane in autologous chondrocyte implantation. *Knee* 2004;11(1):51-55.

71. Kuo CK, Li WJ, Mauck RL, Tuan RS: Cartilage tissue engineering: Its potential and uses. *Curr Opin Rheumatol* 2006; 18(1):64-73.

72. Tuan RS: A second-generation autologous chondrocyte implantation approach to the treatment of focal articular cartilage defects. *Arthritis Res Ther* 2007;9(5):109.

73. Freed LE, Grande DA, Lingbin Z, Emmanual J, Marquis JC, Langer R: Joint resurfacing using allograft chondrocytes and synthetic biodegradable polymer scaffolds. *J Biomed Mater Res* 1994;28(8):891-899.

74. Freed LE, Marquis JC, Nohria A, Emmanual J, Mikos AG, Langer R: Neocartilage formation in vitro and in vivo using

cells cultured on synthetic biodegradable polymers. *J Biomed Mater Res* 1993;27(1):11-23.

75. Wakitani S, Kimura T, Hirooka A, et al: Repair of rabbit articular surfaces with allograft chondrocytes embedded in collagen gel. *J Bone Joint Surg Br* 1989;71(1):74-80.

76. Ehlers EM, Fuss M, Rohwedel J, Russlies M, Kühnel W, Behrens P: Development of a biocomposite to fill out articular cartilage lesions: Light, scanning and transmission electron microscopy of sheep chondrocytes cultured on a collagen I/III sponge. *Ann Anat* 1999;181(6):513-518.

77. Erggelet C, Endres M, Neumann K, et al: Formation of cartilage repair tissue in articular cartilage defects pretreated with microfracture and covered with cell-free polymer-based implants. *J Orthop Res* 2009;27(10):1353-1360.

78. Pavesio A, Abatangelo G, Borrione A, et al: Hyaluronan-based scaffolds (Hyalograft C) in the treatment of knee cartilage defects: Preliminary clinical findings. *Novartis Found Symp* 2003;249:203-217.

79. Grigolo B, Roseti L, Fiorini M, et al: Transplantation of chondrocytes seeded on a hyaluronan derivative (hyaff-11) into cartilage defects in rabbits. *Biomaterials* 2001;22(17): 2417-2424.

80. Gobbi A, Kon E, Berruto M, et al: Patellofemoral full-thickness chondral defects treated with second-generation autologous chondrocyte implantation: Results at 5 years' follow-up. *Am J Sports Med* 2009;37(6):1083-1092.

81. Kon E, Gobbi A, Filardo G, Delcogliano M, Zaffagnini S, Marcacci M: Arthroscopic second-generation autologous chondrocyte implantation compared with microfracture for chondral lesions of the knee: Prospective nonrandomized study at 5 years. *Am J Sports Med* 2009;37(1):33-41.

82. Hollander AP, Dickinson SC, Sims TJ, et al: Maturation of tissue engineered cartilage implanted in injured and osteoarthritic human knees. *Tissue Eng* 2006;12(7):1787-1798.

83. Sherwood JK, Riley SL, Palazzolo R, et al: A three-dimensional osteochondral composite scaffold for articular cartilage repair. *Biomaterials* 2002;23(24):4739-4751.

84. Schek RM, Taboas JM, Segvich SJ, Hollister SJ, Krebsbach PH: Engineered osteochondral grafts using biphasic composite solid free-form fabricated scaffolds. *Tissue Eng* 2004; 10(9-10):1376-1385.

85. Hollister SJ: Porous scaffold design for tissue engineering. *Nat Mater* 2005;4(7):518-524.

86. Moutos FT, Freed LE, Guilak F: A biomimetic three-dimensional woven composite scaffold for functional tissue engineering of cartilage. *Nat Mater* 2007;6(2):162-167.

87. Li WJ, Danielson KG, Alexander PG, Tuan RS: Biological response of chondrocytes cultured in three-dimensional nanofibrous poly(epsilon-caprolactone) scaffolds. *J Biomed Mater Res A* 2003;67(4):1105-1114.

88. Li WJ, Jiang YJ, Tuan RS: Chondrocyte phenotype in engineered fibrous matrix is regulated by fiber size. *Tissue Eng* 2006;12(7):1775-1785.

89. Li WJ, Chiang H, Kuo TF, Lee HS, Jiang CC, Tuan RS: Evaluation of articular cartilage repair using biodegradable nanofibrous scaffolds in a swine model: A pilot study. *J Tissue Eng Regen Med* 2009;3(1):1-10.

90. Liu X, Jin X, Ma PX: Nanofibrous hollow microspheres self-

assembled from star-shaped polymers as injectable cell carriers for knee repair. *Nat Mater* 2011;10(5):398-406.

91. Lu Y, Dhanaraj S, Wang Z, et al: Minced cartilage without cell culture serves as an effective intraoperative cell source for cartilage repair. *J Orthop Res* 2006;24(6):1261-1270.

92. Nixon AJ, Fortier LA, Williams J, Mohammed H: Enhanced repair of extensive articular defects by insulin-like growth factor-I-laden fibrin composites. *J Orthop Res* 1999;17(4): 475-487.

93. Smeds KA, Pfister-Serres A, Miki D, et al: Photocrosslinkable polysaccharides for in situ hydrogel formation. *J Biomed Mater Res* 2001;54(1):115-121.

94. Burdick JA, Chung C, Jia X, Randolph MA, Langer R: Controlled degradation and mechanical behavior of photopolymerized hyaluronic acid networks. *Biomacromolecules* 2005; 6(1):386-391.

95. Nettles DL, Chilkoti A, Setton LA: Applications of elastin-like polypeptides in tissue engineering. *Adv Drug Deliv Rev* 2010;62(15):1479-1485.

96. Nettles DL, Kitaoka K, Hanson NA, et al: In situ crosslinking elastin-like polypeptide gels for application to articular cartilage repair in a goat osteochondral defect model. *Tissue Eng Part A* 2008;14(7):1133-1140.

97. Kisiday J, Jin M, Kurz B, et al: Self-assembling peptide hydrogel fosters chondrocyte extracellular matrix production and cell division: Implications for cartilage tissue repair. *Proc Natl Acad Sci U S A* 2002;99(15):9996-10001.

98. Miller RE, Grodzinsky AJ, Vanderploeg EJ, et al: Effect of self-assembling peptide, chondrogenic factors, and bone marrow-derived stromal cells on osteochondral repair. *Osteoarthritis Cartilage* 2010;18(12):1608-1619.

99. Wang DA, Varghese S, Sharma B, et al: Multifunctional chondroitin sulphate for cartilage tissue-biomaterial integration. *Nat Mater* 2007;6(5):385-392.

100. Nöth U, Rackwitz L, Steinert AF, Tuan RS: Cell delivery therapeutics for musculoskeletal regeneration. *Adv Drug Deliv Rev* 2010;62(7-8):765-783.

101. Chung C, Burdick JA: Engineering cartilage tissue. *Adv Drug Deliv Rev* 2008;60(2):243-262.

102. Hung CT, Mauck RL, Wang CC, Lima EG, Ateshian GA: A paradigm for functional tissue engineering of articular cartilage via applied physiologic deformational loading. *Ann Biomed Eng* 2004;32(1):35-49.

103. Schaefer D, Martin I, Jundt G, et al: Tissue-engineered composites for the repair of large osteochondral defects. *Arthritis Rheum* 2002;46(9):2524-2534.

104. Vunjak-Novakovic G, Martin I, Obradovic B, et al: Bioreactor cultivation conditions modulate the composition and mechanical properties of tissue-engineered cartilage. *J Orthop Res* 1999;17(1):130-138.

105. Davisson T, Kunig S, Chen A, Sah R, Ratcliffe A: Static and dynamic compression modulate matrix metabolism in tissue engineered cartilage. *J Orthop Res* 2002;20(4):842-848.

106. Rotter N, Bonassar LJ, Tobias G, Lebl M, Roy AK, Vacanti CA: Age dependence of biochemical and biomechanical properties of tissue-engineered human septal cartilage. *Biomaterials* 2002;23(15):3087-3094.

107. Puelacher WC, Kim SW, Vacanti JP, Schloo B, Mooney D,

Vacanti CA: Tissue-engineered growth of cartilage: The effect of varying the concentration of chondrocytes seeded onto synthetic polymer matrices. *Int J Oral Maxillofac Surg* 1994;23(1):49-53.

108. Yates KE, Allemann F, Glowacki J: Phenotypic analysis of bovine chondrocytes cultured in 3D collagen sponges: Effect of serum substitutes. *Cell Tissue Bank* 2005;6(1):45-54.

109. Nehrer S, Breinan HA, Ramappa A, et al: Canine chondrocytes seeded in type I and type II collagen implants investigated in vitro. *J Biomed Mater Res* 1997;38(2):95-104.

110. Häuselmann HJ, Fernandes RJ, Mok SS, et al: Phenotypic stability of bovine articular chondrocytes after long-term culture in alginate beads. *J Cell Sci* 1994;107(Pt 1):17-27.

111. Paige KT, Cima LG, Yaremchuk MJ, Vacanti JP, Vacanti CA: Injectable cartilage. *Plast Reconstr Surg* 1995;96(6): 1390-1400.

112. Rowley JA, Madlambayan G, Mooney DJ: Alginate hydrogels as synthetic extracellular matrix materials. *Biomaterials* 1999;20(1):45-53.

113. Mauck RL, Seyhan SL, Ateshian GA, Hung CT: Influence of seeding density and dynamic deformational loading on the developing structure/function relationships of chondrocyte-seeded agarose hydrogels. *Ann Biomed Eng* 2002;30(8):1046-1056.

114. Mauck RL, Wang CC, Oswald ES, Ateshian GA, Hung CT: The role of cell seeding density and nutrient supply for articular cartilage tissue engineering with deformational loading. *Osteoarthritis Cartilage* 2003;11(12):879-890.

115. Brittberg M, Sjögren-Jansson E, Lindahl A, Peterson L: Influence of fibrin sealant (Tisseel) on osteochondral defect repair in the rabbit knee. *Biomaterials* 1997;18(3):235-242.

116. Hunter CJ, Imler SM, Malaviya P, Nerem RM, Levenston ME: Mechanical compression alters gene expression and extracellular matrix synthesis by chondrocytes cultured in collagen I gels. *Biomaterials* 2002;23(4):1249-1259.

117. Kawamura S, Wakitani S, Kimura T, et al: Articular cartilage repair: Rabbit experiments with a collagen gel-biomatrix and chondrocytes cultured in it. *Acta Orthop Scand* 1998;69(1):56-62.

118. Elisseeff JH, Lee A, Kleinman HK, Yamada Y: Biological response of chondrocytes to hydrogels. *Ann N Y Acad Sci* 2002;961:118-122.

119. Bryant SJ, Anseth KS: The effects of scaffold thickness on tissue engineered cartilage in photocrosslinked poly(ethylene oxide) hydrogels. *Biomaterials* 2001;22(6):619-626.

120. Burdick JA, Peterson AJ, Anseth KS: Conversion and temperature profiles during the photoinitiated polymerization of thick orthopaedic biomaterials. *Biomaterials* 2001; 22(13):1779-1786.

121. Benya PD, Shaffer JD: Dedifferentiated chondrocytes reexpress the differentiated collagen phenotype when cultured in agarose gels. *Cell* 1982;30(1):215-224.

122. Buschmann MD, Gluzband YA, Grodzinsky AJ, Kimura JH, Hunziker EB: Chondrocytes in agarose culture synthesize a mechanically functional extracellular matrix. *J Orthop Res* 1992;10(6):745-758.

123. Ragan PM, Staples AK, Hung HK, Chin V, Binette F, Grodzinsky AJ: Mechanical compression influences chon-

3: Basic Principles and Treatment of Musculoskeletal Disease

drocyte metabolism in a new alginate disk culture system. *Trans Orthop Res Soc* 1998;23:918.

124. DeLise AM, Fischer L, Tuan RS: Cellular interactions and signaling in cartilage development. *Osteoarthritis Cartilage* 2000;8(5):309-334.

125. Chang SC, Rowley JA, Tobias G, et al: Injection molding of chondrocyte/alginate constructs in the shape of facial implants. *J Biomed Mater Res* 2001;55(4):503-511.

126. Vunjak-Novakovic G, Obradovic B, Martin I, Bursac PM, Langer R, Freed LE: Dynamic cell seeding of polymer scaffolds for cartilage tissue engineering. *Biotechnol Prog* 1998;14(2):193-202.

127. Bryant SJ, Nuttelman CR, Anseth KS: The effects of cross-linking density on cartilage formation in photocrosslinkable hydrogels. *Biomed Sci Instrum* 1999;35:309-314.

128. Chung C, Mesa J, Randolph MA, Yaremchuk M, Burdick JA: Influence of gel properties on neocartilage formation by auricular chondrocytes photoencapsulated in hyaluronic acid networks. *J Biomed Mater Res A* 2006;77(3):518-525.

129. Blunk T, Sieminski AL, Gooch KJ, et al: Differential effects of growth factors on tissue-engineered cartilage. *Tissue Eng* 2002;8(1):73-84.

130. Gooch KJ, Blunk T, Courter DL, et al: IGF-I and mechanical environment interact to modulate engineered cartilage development. *Biochem Biophys Res Commun* 2001;286(5):909-915.

131. Gooch KJ, Blunk T, Courter DL, Sieminski AL, Vunjak-Novakovic G, Freed LE: Bone morphogenetic proteins-2, -12, and -13 modulate in vitro development of engineered cartilage. *Tissue Eng* 2002;8(4):591-601.

132. Mauck RL, Nicoll SB, Seyhan SL, Ateshian GA, Hung CT: Synergistic action of growth factors and dynamic loading for articular cartilage tissue engineering. *Tissue Eng* 2003;9(4):597-611.

133. Byers BA, Mauck RL, Chiang IE, Tuan RS: Transient exposure to transforming growth factor beta 3 under serum-free conditions enhances the biomechanical and biochemical maturation of tissue-engineered cartilage. *Tissue Eng Part A* 2008;14(11):1821-1834.

134. Pei M, Seidel J, Vunjak-Novakovic G, Freed LE: Growth factors for sequential cellular de- and re-differentiation in tissue engineering. *Biochem Biophys Res Commun* 2002;294(1):149-154.

135. Byers BA, Mauck RL, Chiang IE, Tuan RS: Transient exposure to transforming growth factor beta 3 under serum-free conditions enhances the biomechanical and biochemical maturation of tissue-engineered cartilage. *Tissue Eng Part A* 2008;14(11):1821-1834.

136. Lima EG, Bian L, Ng KW, et al: The beneficial effect of delayed compressive loading on tissue-engineered cartilage constructs cultured with TGF-beta3. *Osteoarthritis Cartilage* 2007;15(9):1025-1033.

137. Lee CR, Grodzinsky AJ, Hsu HP, Martin SD, Spector M: Effects of harvest and selected cartilage repair procedures on the physical and biochemical properties of articular cartilage in the canine knee. *J Orthop Res* 2000;18(5):790-799.

138. Caplan AI, Bruder SP: Mesenchymal stem cells: Building blocks for molecular medicine in the 21st century. *Trends Mol Med* 2001;7(6):259-264.

139. Dominici M, Hofmann TJ, Horwitz EM: Bone marrow mesenchymal cells: Biological properties and clinical applications. *J Biol Regul Homeost Agents* 2001;15(1):28-37.

140. Nöth U, Steinert AF, Tuan RS: Technology insight: Adult mesenchymal stem cells for osteoarthritis therapy. *Nat Clin Pract Rheumatol* 2008;4(7):371-380.

141. Macchiarini P, Jungebluth P, Go T, et al: Clinical transplantation of a tissue-engineered airway. *Lancet* 2008;372(9655):2023-2030.

142. Erickson GR, Gimble JM, Franklin DM, Rice HE, Awad H, Guilak F: Chondrogenic potential of adipose tissue-derived stromal cells in vitro and in vivo. *Biochem Biophys Res Commun* 2002;290(2):763-769.

143. Tallheden T, Dennis JE, Lennon DP, Sjögren-Jansson E, Caplan AI, Lindahl A: Phenotypic plasticity of human articular chondrocytes. *J Bone Joint Surg Am* 2003;85(Suppl 2):93-100.

144. O'Driscoll SW, Keeley FW, Salter RB: The chondrogenic potential of free autogenous periosteal grafts for biological resurfacing of major full-thickness defects in joint surfaces under the influence of continuous passive motion: An experimental investigation in the rabbit. *J Bone Joint Surg Am* 1986;68(7):1017-1035.

145. Nöth U, Osyczka AM, Tuli R, Hickok NJ, Danielson KG, Tuan RS: Multilineage mesenchymal differentiation potential of human trabecular bone-derived cells. *J Orthop Res* 2002;20(5):1060-1069.

146. Baksh D, Song L, Tuan RS: Adult mesenchymal stem cells: Characterization, differentiation, and application in cell and gene therapy. *J Cell Mol Med* 2004;8(3):301-316.

147. Kolf CM, Cho E, Tuan RS: Mesenchymal stromal cells: Biology of adult mesenchymal stem cells. Regulation of niche, self-renewal and differentiation. *Arthritis Res Ther* 2007;9(1):204.

148. Friedenstein AJ, Deriglasova UF, Kulagina NN, et al: Precursors for fibroblasts in different populations of hematopoietic cells as detected by the in vitro colony assay method. *Exp Hematol* 1974;2(2):83-92.

149. Johnstone B, Hering TM, Caplan AI, Goldberg VM, Yoo JU: In vitro chondrogenesis of bone marrow-derived mesenchymal progenitor cells. *Exp Cell Res* 1998;238(1):265-272.

150. Pittenger MF, Mackay AM, Beck SC, et al: Multilineage potential of adult human mesenchymal stem cells. *Science* 1999;284(5411):143-147.

151. Prockop DJ: Marrow stromal cells as stem cells for nonhematopoietic tissues. *Science* 1997;276(5309):71-74.

152. Awad HA, Halvorsen Y-D, Gimble JM, Guilak F: Effects of transforming growth factor beta1 and dexamethasone on the growth and chondrogenic differentiation of adipose-derived stromal cells. *Tissue Eng* 2003;9(6):1301-1312.

153. Majumdar MK, Banks V, Peluso DP, Morris EA: Isolation, characterization, and chondrogenic potential of human bone marrow-derived multipotential stromal cells. *J Cell Physiol* 2000;185(1):98-106.

154. Majumdar MK, Wang E, Morris EA: BMP-2 and BMP-9 promotes chondrogenic differentiation of human multipotential mesenchymal cells and overcomes the inhibitory effect of IL-1. *J Cell Physiol* 2001;189(3):275-284.

155. Huang AH, Farrell MJ, Mauck RL: Mechanics and mechanobiology of mesenchymal stem cell-based engineered cartilage. *J Biomech* 2010;43(1):128-136.

156. Mauck RL, Yuan X, Tuan RS: Chondrogenic differentiation and functional maturation of bovine mesenchymal stem cells in long-term agarose culture. *Osteoarthritis Cartilage* 2006;14(2):179-189.

157. Erickson IE, Huang AH, Chung C, Li RT, Burdick JA, Mauck RL: Differential maturation and structure-function relationships in mesenchymal stem cell- and chondrocyte-seeded hydrogels. *Tissue Eng Part A* 2009;15(5):1041-1052.

158. Chung C, Beecham M, Mauck RL, Burdick JA: The influence of degradation characteristics of hyaluronic acid hydrogels on in vitro neocartilage formation by mesenchymal stem cells. *Biomaterials* 2009;30(26):4287-4296.

159. Bian L, Zhai DY, Mauck RL, Burdick JA: Coculture of human mesenchymal stem cells and articular chondrocytes reduces hypertrophy and enhances functional properties of engineered cartilage. *Tissue Eng Part A* 2011;17(7-8):1137-1145.

160. Bian L, Zhai DY, Tous E, Rai R, Mauck RL, Burdick JA: Enhanced MSC chondrogenesis following delivery of TGF-β3 from alginate microspheres within hyaluronic acid hydrogels in vitro and in vivo. *Biomaterials* 2011;32(27):6425-6434.

161. Erickson IE, Huang AH, Sengupta S, Kestle S, Burdick JA, Mauck RL: Macromer density influences mesenchymal stem cell chondrogenesis and maturation in photocrosslinked hyaluronic acid hydrogels. *Osteoarthritis Cartilage* 2009;17(12):1639-1648.

162. Pelttari K, Winter A, Steck E, et al: Premature induction of hypertrophy during in vitro chondrogenesis of human mesenchymal stem cells correlates with calcification and vascular invasion after ectopic transplantation in SCID mice. *Arthritis Rheum* 2006;54(10):3254-3266.

163. Mueller MB, Tuan RS: Functional characterization of hypertrophy in chondrogenesis of human mesenchymal stem cells. *Arthritis Rheum* 2008;58(5):1377-1388.

164. Winter A, Breit S, Parsch D, et al: Cartilage-like gene expression in differentiated human stem cell spheroids: A comparison of bone marrow-derived and adipose tissue-derived stromal cells. *Arthritis Rheum* 2003;48(2):418-429.

165. Vinardell T, Thorpe SD, Buckley CT, Kelly DJ: Chondrogenesis and integration of mesenchymal stem cells within an in vitro cartilage defect repair model. *Ann Biomed Eng* 2009;37(12):2556-2565.

166. Obradovic B, Martin I, Padera RF, Treppo S, Freed LE, Vunjak-Novakovic G: Integration of engineered cartilage. *J Orthop Res* 2001;19(6):1089-1097.

167. Maher SA, Mauck RL, Rackwitz L, Tuan RS: A nanofibrous cell-seeded hydrogel promotes integration in a cartilage gap model. *J Tissue Eng Regen Med* 2010;4(1):25-29.

168. Gao J, Dennis JE, Solchaga LA, Awadallah AS, Goldberg VM, Caplan AI: Tissue-engineered fabrication of an osteochondral composite graft using rat bone marrow-derived mesenchymal stem cells. *Tissue Eng* 2001;7(4):363-371.

169. Alhadlaq A, Mao JJ: Tissue-engineered osteochondral constructs in the shape of an articular condyle. *J Bone Joint Surg Am* 2005;87(5):936-944.

170. Lima EG, Mauck RL, Han SH, et al: Functional tissue engineering of chondral and osteochondral constructs. *Biorheology* 2004;41(3-4):577-590.

171. Lima EG, Grace Chao PH, Ateshian GA, et al: The effect of devitalized trabecular bone on the formation of osteochondral tissue-engineered constructs. *Biomaterials* 2008;29(32):4292-4299.

172. Jayabalan P, Tan AR, Rahaman MN, Bal BS, Hung CT, Cook JL: Bioactive glass 13-93 as a subchondral substrate for tissue-engineered osteochondral constructs: A pilot study. *Clin Orthop Relat Res* 2011;469(10):2754-2763.

173. Bal BS, Rahaman MN, Jayabalan P, et al: In vivo outcomes of tissue-engineered osteochondral grafts. *J Biomed Mater Res B Appl Biomater* 2010;93(1):164-174.

174. Tuli R, Nandi S, Li WJ, et al: Human mesenchymal progenitor cell-based tissue engineering of a single-unit osteochondral construct. *Tissue Eng* 2004;10(7-8):1169-1179.

175. Jiang CC, Chiang H, Liao CJ, et al: Repair of porcine articular cartilage defect with a biphasic osteochondral composite. *J Orthop Res* 2007;25(10):1277-1290.

176. Hung CT, Lima EG, Mauck RL, et al: Anatomically shaped osteochondral constructs for articular cartilage repair. *J Biomech* 2003;36(12):1853-1864.

177. Lee CH, Cook JL, Mendelson A, Moioli EK, Yao H, Mao JJ: Regeneration of the articular surface of the rabbit synovial joint by cell homing: A proof of concept study. *Lancet* 2010;376(9739):440-448.

178. Petrie Aronin CE, Tuan RS: Therapeutic potential of the immunomodulatory activities of adult mesenchymal stem cells. *Birth Defects Res C Embryo Today* 2010;90(1):67-74.

179. Steinert AF, Nöth U, Tuan RS: Concepts in gene therapy for cartilage repair. *Injury* 2008;39(Suppl 1):S97-S113.

180. Palmer GD, Steinert A, Pascher A, et al: Gene-induced chondrogenesis of primary mesenchymal stem cells in vitro. *Mol Ther* 2005;12(2):219-228.

Chapter 20

Tendinopathy and Tendon Repair

Stavros Thomopoulos, PhD

Peter C. Amadio, MD

Chunfeng Zhao, MD

Richard H. Gelberman, MD

Introduction

Tendinopathies are debilitating and can lead to significant pain, disability, and lost time from work. The range of tendon disorders includes ruptures at the tendon midsubstance, the tendon-to-bone junction, and the tendon-muscle junction. These injuries can occur after an acute injury (such as laceration or sports injury) or after chronic tendon degeneration (such as tendinitis, tendinosis, or overuse). Any disruption of tendon function will result in a decreased ability to transmit forces from muscle to bone, reducing motion and debilitating joint function. This chapter will review tendinopathy and tendon repair by comparing intrasynovial with extrasynovial tendons, midsubstance with tendon-to-bone repair, and chronic tendinopathy with acute injury. To illustrate these concepts, two clinically relevant examples of tendinopathy will be examined in depth: acute flexor tendon lacerations and chronic rotator cuff tears. The unique biologic environments for each of these tendons will be discussed and the strategies necessary for successful repair will be compared.

Dr. Amadio or an immediate family member has stock or stock options held in Johnson & Johnson and Merck. Dr. Gelberman or an immediate family member has received royalties from Medartis and Wright Medical Technology and serves as a board member, owner, officer, or committee member of the American Society for Surgery of the Hand, the American Foundation for Surgery of the Hand, and the American Orthopaedic Association. Neither of the following authors nor any immediate family member has received anything of value from or owns stock in a commercial company or institution related directly or indirectly to the subject of this chapter: Dr. Thomopoulos and Dr. Zhao.

Intrasynovial Versus Extrasynovial Tendon Biology and Healing

Intrasynovial tendons are defined as the tendons or tendon portions enclosed within a synovial sheath, which contains synovial fluid as a lubricant. This unique structure effectively decreases friction, reduces abrasion, and eliminates wear. Flexor tendons in the zone II area of the hand are typical intrasynovial tendons. Extrasynovial tendons lack a synovial sheath and the lubricating mechanisms that are important for intrasynovial tendon function. Examples of extrasynovial tendons include the Achilles and patellar tendons.

Recent studies have provided a better understanding of the intrasynovial flexor tendon reparative response.[1,2] Tendon healing, as with many injured tissues, follows three healing phases: inflammation, proliferation, and remodeling. Following tendon transection and repair, a clot is formed from hemorrhage between the tendon stumps and in the space between the gliding surface and the tendon sheath. Cellular elements within the clot release growth factors that induce the recruitment of neutrophils with monocytes and macrophages to clean up necrotic material and apoptotic cells. This early inflammatory response is followed a few days after tendon suture by the proliferation phase of tendon healing; additional growth factors are involved with this phase, such as transforming growth factor–β (TGF-β), insulin-like growth factor–1 (IGF-1), platelet-derived growth factor (PDGF), vascular endothelial growth factor (VEGF), and basic fibroblast growth factor (bFGF).[3,4] Because the flexor tendon is hypovascular and hypocellular, the proliferation phase can last as long as 6 weeks. During the proliferative and early reparative stages of healing, fibroblasts migrate to the wound and synthesize type I collagen, forming an immature granulation tissue matrix. By 17 days, the first intrinsic blood vessels reach the repair site, having extended through the tendon's 3-cm avascular zone.[4] The remodeling phase, which begins at least 3 weeks after repair, is critical for functional tissue regeneration. During this phase, factors such as matrix metalloproteinases and mechanical loading promote a reduction in proliferation and an increase in collagen synthesis. Collagen is realigned along the direction of tensile muscle force and a smooth gliding surface is produced to allow tendon gliding.

Flexor tendons heal via intrinsic and extrinsic mechanisms. Intrinsic healing relies on the proliferation and migration of cells within injured tendons to bridge the lacerated tendon directly. Because these "endotenon" cells have less capability to proliferate and differentiate, the involvement of cells from the surface of the tendon (the "epitenon" cells) is critical for intrinsic healing[4] (**Figure 1**). In contrast, extrinsic healing depends on the invasion of cells from the surrounding tissues to bridge tendons together. Therefore, extrinsic healing results in adhesion formation between tendon and surrounding tissues and jeopardizes tendon gliding. For the flexor tendon, however, extrinsic healing is faster and more abundant compared with intrinsic healing because of a rich blood supply and high cellularity in the surrounding soft tissues. The strategies to eliminate extrinsic healing and enhance intrinsic healing have been investigated for several decades and will continue to be an important research topic.

The healing of extrasynovial tendons follows a wound healing course similar to that of intrasynovial tendons. However, because gliding ability is typically less important for extrasynovial tendon function in comparison with intrasynovial tendon function, extrinsic healing can augment the strength of the extrasynovial tendon repair without negative functional consequences for joint motion. The time course of healing is also accelerated in extrasynovial tendons in comparison with intrasynovial tendons. This is because of the typically higher vascularity, cellularity, and proliferation capacity of these tendons compared with those within synovial sheaths.[5] In addition, as has been described in anterior cruciate ligament healing,[6] synovial fluid may reduce the ability of the intrasynovial tendon fibroblasts to mount a healing response compared with extrasynovial tendon fibroblasts.

Midsubstance Versus Tendon-to-Bone Healing

As described in the previous section, many tendon injuries require healing of two tendon ends to each other. Functional repair of several tendinopathies (such as Achilles tendon tear, chronic rotator cuff tear, and flexor tendon avulsion), however, often requires healing of tendon to bone. Experimental studies in animal models have demonstrated that tendon-to-bone healing occurs through the generation of a fibrovascular scar rather than regeneration of a graded fibrocartilaginous transition.[7,8] Notably, the structure, com-

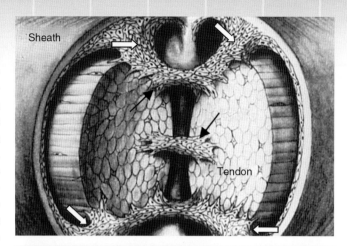

Figure 1 Intrasynovial tendons heal primarily through infiltration of fibroblasts from the outer and inner surfaces of the tendon (black arrows). Adhesions forming between the outer surface of the tendon and the sheath (white arrows) may limit tendon excursion. (Courtesy of Dr. R.H. Gelberman, Boston, MA.)

position, and mechanical properties of the healing tendon and its bony insertion do not approach normal, even by the longest time points studied.[9] In a rat rotator cuff model, it was shown that while the structural properties reached two thirds of normal after 8 weeks of healing, the material properties (indicating the "quality" of the tissue) remained an order of magnitude weaker than normal.[7] The healing tissue had a higher cross-sectional area compared with the uninjured tissue but was made up of poorly organized collagen fibers without re-creation of a fibrocartilaginous transitional zone. Experimental studies on canine flexor tendon to distal phalanx repair indicated that insertion-site healing demonstrates little improvement in repair-site failure force from the time of suture through 42 days after repair.[10] In all animal models, rather than regeneration of a graded fibrocartilaginous transition between tendon and bone, the interface is filled with fibrous scar tissue. This is in contrast to tendon midsubstance healing, which requires only the generation of well-aligned collagen fibers for return of function.

Bone loss following tendon injury further complicates tendon-to-bone repair. Reduced bone mineral density was observed in the humeri of patients 9 years after cuff rupture and repair.[11] These changes, however, were seen only in patients who did not have full return of function, suggesting that the bone loss was due in part to reduced joint loading. Significant bone loss was also demonstrated in the canine flexor tendon model.[12] Decreased bone mineral density was seen at the distal phalanx 10, 21, and 42 days after injury and repair, indicating that bone resorption may be a factor that contributes to the low values of repair-site failure force.[12] Similar results were reported in the rat rotator cuff model.[13,14] Bone mineral density was significantly decreased after tendon injury and repair. A delay between injury and repair resulted in inferior tendon-to-bone healing, in part because of decreased bone quality.

Chronic Tendinopathy Versus Acute Injury

Tendinopathies can be categorized into either chronic injuries or acute injuries. The approach for treatment of the tendinopathy depends on the pathogenesis of the injury. Acute injuries typically involve sharp lacerations (such as intrasynovial flexor tendon laceration) or sports injuries (such as Achilles tendon rupture). Chronic injuries (such as rotator cuff tear), on the other hand, typically result after years of degeneration; this degeneration may occur due to several etiologic factors, including intrinsic, extrinsic, and overuse.[15,16] Intrinsic factors include direct tendon overload, intrinsic degeneration, or other insult. Extrinsic factors include tendon damage caused by compression against surrounding structures (for example, rotator cuff degeneration due to impingement of the tendon under the coracoacromial arch). Overuse conditions can also lead to microdamage accumulation and degeneration of the tendon.

Acute injuries have a better prognosis for success than chronic injuries.[17] Treatment approaches begin with a robust suture repair, although typically not in an emergent care setting.[17] The capacity to regain strength after suture repair is high for acutely injured tendons that are repaired within a few weeks of surgery.[18,19] Chronic injuries, on the other hand, are often problematic. In the rotator cuff, prognosis for success after surgical repair depends on several factors, including the chronicity of the injury.[20]

Current and Future Treatment Strategies

The choice of treatment strategy for tendon injuries depends on the tendinopathy and local tissue environment. Repair of intrasynovial tendon lacerations, for example, must take into consideration the potential formation of adhesions between the tendon surface and the sheath within which it glides. Adhesion formation must be managed while strength accrual is promoted at the repair site. In contrast, extrasynovial repairs often require tendon-to-bone repair. Strength accrual in this case involves effective integration of two materials, tendon and bone. Current repair strategies focus on manipulation of the rehabilitation (loading) environment, optimization of surgical techniques, and augmentation with substitute materials. Future repair strategies will likely focus on biologic interventions; growth factor and cell-based treatments have shown great promise in animal models for improving the repair of both intrasynovial and extrasynovial tendon injuries.

Biologically based approaches for enhancing tendon-to-bone healing have focused on one or more aspects of the tissue engineering paradigm, that is, the use of signaling biofactors (for example, growth factors), responding cells (for example, mesenchymal stem cells), and scaffold microenvironments (for example, collagen matrices).[21] Numerous studies have attempted to enhance tendon midsubstance and tendon-to-bone healing by delivering growth factors to the repair site.

Examples of Tendinopathy and Tendon Repair

Example 1: Acute Injury and Repair of the Intrasynovial Flexor Tendon (Midsubstance)
Basic Science of Healing

Lacerations of the flexor tendons in the hand are common, both in the workplace and household settings.[22] The number of tendon injuries is difficult to quantify because epidemiologic studies have not been done, but estimates suggest that approximately 40,000 inpatient tendon repairs are done each year in the United States.[23] A much larger number of tendon surgeries are done on an outpatient basis. More importantly, these injuries occur almost exclusively in a young, working-age population, and they result in considerable disability. These injuries often necessitate reconstructive surgery to repair the tendon and extensive rehabilitation to regain finger function. Basic research and clinical practice over the past 3 decades have led to improvements in surgical repair technique and rehabilitation parameters. However, outcomes remain less than ideal. A large percentage of these injuries remain debilitating despite treatment, leading to substantial costs and loss of hand function.[23] Studies have shown that two primary factors lead to poor clinical outcomes following tendon repair: adhesion formation within the intrasynovial sheath and repair-site elongation and rupture.[24,25] These complications are likely caused by insufficient accrual of repair-site strength and stiffness in the early period after suture and are exacerbated by increases in gliding resistance within the digital sheath.[3,24,25] As described in subsequent sections, significant advances have been made in suppressing adhesion formation and improving gliding after repair. Efforts have focused on increasing repair strength by modified suture techniques, controlling the loading environment via rehabilitation, or biochemically manipulating the surface of the tendon. However, attempts have been only partially successful.[26,27] Future strategies to improve repair will likely include tissue engineering and cell-based therapies to enhance tendon healing and surface modification to decrease adhesions.[28-30]

Two healing patterns can be observed after flexor tendon repair: contact healing and gap healing. Contact healing is the ideal scenario; the lacerated tendon ends are in direct contact with each other and heal by first intention with a dominated intrinsic healing process. However, intrasynovial flexor tendons often follow a gap healing process. Because muscle forces are transmitted to bone through tendon, tensile force always exists during joint motion, especially during postoperative rehabilitation. Although lacerated tendon ends can be brought together with surgical repair, the tensile force across the repair site can result in gap formation at the repair site. This gap healing not only elongates the healing phases, but also involves extrinsic healing mechanisms. Strategies to eliminate gap healing have been studied for many decades and include improvements in surgical repair technique, suture materials, and postoperative rehabilitation protocols, but tendon gap healing still remains a problem in many cases.[31]

Treatment Approach: Rehabilitation

Rehabilitation after flexor tendon repair influences the healing process, especially with regard to adhesion formation. The role of rehabilitation variables in modulating flexor tendon healing was recently reviewed by Boyer et al.[31] Although it has been known for many years that controlling the postoperative loading regimen is critical for preventing adhesions and promoting healing,[32] it is only recently that the variables of load magnitude and tendon excursion have been critically and separately evaluated. Adhesion-free healing was demonstrated by several groups both experimentally and clinically with passive and active motion rehabilitation.[31] However, results were mostly empirical and it was unclear whether the reduction in adhesions was due to higher loads on the repair or higher tendon excursion during the rehabilitation.

In vitro and in vivo studies have demonstrated that tendon fibroblasts are responsive to mechanical load. Both static and cyclic load have been shown to stimulate fibroblast migration, fibroblast proliferation, and extracellular matrix synthesis. Hannafin et al[33] showed that load is necessary for tendon explants to maintain mechanical properties. Slack et al[34] applied load to cultured flexor tendons and demonstrated increased DNA and protein synthesis in loaded tendons. The concept that mechanical load can promote cellular activity and potentially improve flexor tendon healing was applied by several groups in experimental and clinical studies. Small et al[35] reported improvements in clinical outcomes with active motion rehabilitation. However, this study also showed a 9% rupture rate, demonstrating the risks involved with high-load rehabilitation. The high rupture rate was likely due to the difficulty in controlling the load across the repair site during active motion. In vivo forces in one clinical study ranged from 1 to 34 N for a passive digit flexion followed by an active tip pinch.[36] Therefore, although load does promote cell proliferation and matrix synthesis in a controlled environment, application of the concept to flexor tendon healing has proved difficult because of the increased risk of repair site gapping or rupture.

Passive motion rehabilitation (cyclic excursion of the tendon through the sheath at low loads) has also led to improvements in flexor tendon healing, primarily by preventing adhesion formation. To critically evaluate the role of loading versus tendon excursion, a series of studies was performed in the clinically relevant canine model.[32,37,38] For low-load rehabilitation, the wrist was held in flexion and the digit was taken through passive flexion-extension. This re-

sulted in less than 5 N of force across the repair site and 1.7 mm of tendon excursion. For high-load rehabilitation, the wrist was held in extension and the digit was taken through passive flexion-extension. This resulted in 17 N of force across the repair site and 3.5 mm of tendon excursion. The authors found that the tensile properties did not differ between low- and high-force rehabilitation. Therefore, it is preferable to rehabilitate using a low-load regimen to minimize the risk for gapping or rupture. There was also no difference between the low excursion and the high excursion groups when examining mechanical properties; both resulted in significantly fewer adhesions and improved gliding properties compared with immobilized tendons.

To further improve on the passive motion approach, a modified rehabilitation program, synergistic motion protocol was developed by Horii et al[39] in which the finger joints were passively flexed with the wrist and the finger joints in extension. This motion paradigm decreases the tension on the repaired tendon compared with active motion, and it increases tendon excursion compared with passive motion. This rehabilitation program was verified using an in vivo canine model; tendon gliding ability increased and postoperative adhesions were reduced in comparison with a passive rehabilitation.[40] More recently, Tanaka et al[41] further modified the synergistic motion protocol by grouping the wrist and metacarpophalangeal joints together synergistically with the proximal interphalangeal and distal interphalangeal joints. With this modification, both tendon tension and excursion were increased compared with the traditional synergistic motion. This could be beneficial for tendon gliding if a high-friction surgical technique is used to repair the tendon.[41]

A proper understanding of the postoperative mechanical environment, including repair strength, tendon gliding resistance, and the force applied to the repair by rehabilitation, is essential for appropriate clinical care. Manipulation of these parameters in each individual case may improve clinical outcomes. Based on the extensive literature examining rehabilitation variables for flexor tendon repair, initially a passive motion protocol should be used that emphasizes tendon excursion through the sheath rather than high force across the repair.[42] Excessive loading only increases the risk of gap and repair failure. However, this rehabilitation is only effective when the friction of the repaired tendons is lower than the force applied to the tendon during rehabilitation. Thus, an emphasis on low-friction repairs, such as the many variations of the modified Kessler suture, with the knot inside the repair site, are frequently preferred over variations that place many suture loops and knots on the tendon surface, as do the MGH or Tsuge repairs.[42] Over time, as the repair heals, active motion can be added followed by progressive resistance.[42] Unfortunately, there are not yet ways to accelerate the healing process clinically, but, as discussed in the previous paragraphs, experimental results suggest that augmentation with various growth factors may help.

Treatment Approach: Biochemical Modifications of the Tendon Surface

Lubricants within the synovial fluid or binding on the tendon surface are essential to maintain the gliding function of intrasynovial tendons. Restoration of the native tendon surface following surgical repair is critical for adhesion-free healing. Recent studies have revealed that the lubricants for flexor tendon gliding are similar to the lubricants for articular cartilage contact sliding, including hyaluronic acid (HA), proteoglycans, and phospholipids.[43] One approach to achieve adhesion-free healing has therefore involved biochemical modification of the tendon surface, which has shown a clear beneficial effect when the lubricants are chemically bound to the tendon surface with cross-linking agents, such as in the carbodiimide (cd) reaction[44-46] (Figure 2). These findings have been validated in an in vivo canine model in which HA-treated tendon grafts had gross, histologic, mechanical, and functional evidence of improved outcomes compared with the grafts that were not treated.[46]

The combination of HA and dipalmitoyl phosphatidylcholine, a phospholipid implicated in lubrication of synovial joints, was tested by Moro-oka et al.[47] These investigators found that although the HA-phospholipid combination did not decrease the coefficient of friction for tendon gliding, it did contribute to fewer adhesions in an in vivo rabbit model. It was hypothesized that the dipalmitoyl phosphatidylcholine adsorbed to tendon surfaces, acting as a boundary lubricating film. No cross-linking agents were used in this study, however.

Lubricin, one of the principal lubricants of articular cartilage, is also present in tendon. A study by Taguchi et al[48] tested lubricin's synergistic effect with HA when added to cd-gelatin and cd-HA-gelatin treatments in the repaired intrasynovial tendons. After surgical repair and 1,000 simulated flexion-extension cycles, the cd-HA-gelatin treatment, supplemented with lubricin, displayed a smaller increase in excursion resistance than cd-HA-gelatin treatments. In a recent in vivo canine model, cd-HA plus lubricin treatment after flexor tendon repair also decreased adhesion formation and improved digit function. However, these positive gliding outcomes were countered with impaired tendon healing.[49] Future strategies to enhance flexor tendon healing, such as cell or growth factor–based engineering techniques, may potentially provide methods to conquer this adverse effect of cd-HA lubricin on tendon healing while preserving its antiadhesive properties.

Treatment Approach: Modification of the Biologic Environment

Modification of the biologic environment holds great promise for improving flexor tendon healing. The growth factors bFGF, TGF-β, and PDGF-BB have been delivered to repaired tendons in an effort to increase collagen production and hence repair site strength. In vitro studies have revealed that flexor tendon fibroblasts exposed to both bFGF and PDGF-BB increased their mitogenic activity and their colla-

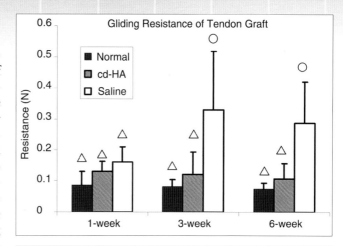

Figure 2 The gliding resistance in the cd-HA–treated tendons was similar to normal and significantly lower than in the saline-treated tendons 3 and 6 weeks after the repair. A difference in symbols denotes a significant difference between values ($P < 0.05$), with the triangle being significantly less than the circle. (Reproduced with permission from Zhao C, Sun YL, Amadio PC, Tanaka T, Ettema AM, An KN: Surface treatment of flexor tendon autografts with carbodiimide-derivatized hyaluronic acid: An in vivo canine model. *J Bone Joint Surg Am* 2006;88:2181-2191.)

gen production severalfold.[50] When combined, the growth factors displayed synergistic mitogenic effects, with further increased cell replication. PDGF-BB, when studied in vivo, has also been shown to increase cell proliferation and collagen production in a canine model.[51,52] Similarly, in situ injection of exogenous bFGF resulted in increases in cell proliferation and matrix synthesis in a rat patellar tendon injury model[53]

It is clear that the potential utility of growth factors to clinically augment tendon repair cannot be exploited through bolus administration; local concentration, timing, half-life, and growth factor synergy all play important roles in healing and must be considered in the development of therapies. Because of early inconsistent results with simple bolus administration, approaches incorporating controlled release kinetics and sustained delivery systems have recently been used. Sakiyama-Elbert et al[54] developed a fibrin/heparin-based delivery system to control the release of any heparin binding growth factor (for example, bFGF and PDGF-BB); by varying the various components of the delivery system, the growth factor release kinetics could be controlled for tendon repair.[51,54]

This fibrin/heparin delivery system was used in several in vivo canine flexor tendon studies. Delivery of PDGF-BB resulted in increased fibroblast numbers, fibroblast proliferation, collagen type I deposition, and collagen cross-links at the site of tendon repair.[51] These data suggest that the sustained delivery of PDGF-BB may be superior to bolus administration, leading to an early acceleration of the cellular processes involved in tendon healing. Although some

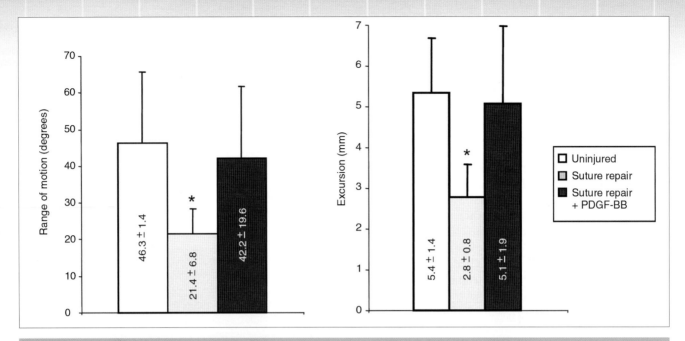

Figure 3 Range of motion and tendon excursion were significantly improved due to PDGF-BB treatment (*P < 0.05). (Reprinted with permission from Gelberman RH, Thomopoulos S, Sakiyama-Elbert SE, Das R, Silva MJ: The early effects of sustained platelet-derived growth factor administration on the functional and structural properties of repaired intrasynovial flexor tendons: An in vivo biomechanic study at 3 weeks in canines. *J Hand Surg Am* 2007;32:373-379.)

studies have shown unwanted effects because of growth factors, such as increases in adhesions with bFGF and TGF-β1,[55,56] the tendons in this study did not show evidence of early adhesion formation, and neither was there evidence of increased cell replication in the epitenon. On the contrary, tendon gliding was enhanced by PDGF-BB administration, presumably due to increased production of molecules important for gliding (such as HA and lubricin)[52,57] (**Figure 3**). Digits treated with PDGF-BB displayed significantly improved joint motion, increased total arc of motion, and greater excursion values than untreated repairs. However, although range of motion was improved, PDGF-BB did not significantly improve the strength of the repair at 3- or 6-week time points. In summary, the use of growth factors holds great promise for improving flexor tendon healing. However, additional studies are necessary to test different growth factors, alone and in combination, and to optimize growth factor dosage and release kinetics to achieve improvements in both tendon function (for example, gliding) and repair-site mechanical properties (for example, failure load).

Researchers have also used gene transfection techniques to deliver growth factors to a tendon repair site.[58] Tang et al[58] transfected tendon fibroblasts with bFGF using an adenovirus vector. Expression of bFGF at the lacerated ends of surgically repaired chicken flexor tendons led to increased tensile strength at 2 and 4 weeks. Gene delivery of growth and differentiation factor–5 (GDF-5) onto freeze-dried flexor tendon allografts led to improvements in joint flexion

compared with control samples.[59] Bone morphogenetic protein–12 (BMP-12), a growth and differentiation factor implicated in tenogenesis, has also been used to enhance tendon healing.[60] Fibroblasts transfected with BMP-12 produced more collagen compared with control samples in vitro. A flexor tendon injury model in chickens was used to test the effect of the growth factor on tendon healing. A suspension of BMP-12 adenoviral vectors was injected into repaired tendons. BMP-12–transduced tendons had similar gross appearance at 2 and 4 weeks and similar biomechanical profiles at 2 weeks compared with the control tendons. However, the BMP-12–transduced tendons displayed a significant increase in tensile strength at 4 weeks compared with the control tendons. These data suggest that increasing expression of BMP-12 can enhance flexor tendon healing.

Cell-based therapies also hold great potential for enhancing tendon healing. Adult mesenchymal stem cells (MSCs) show excellent regenerative capacity, including the ability to proliferate rapidly in culture and the capacity to differentiate into a wide range of cell types. Recent attempts have been made to apply MSC therapy to flexor tendon repair. In one study, the effects of GDF-5 and MSCs on tendon healing were investigated in vitro.[61] GDF-5 and MSCs were placed in a collagen matrix and delivered to canine flexor tendon repair sites. At 2 and 4 weeks of tissue culture, the tendons with GDF-5– and MSC-seeded matrices at the repair site were stronger than the untreated tendons. However, neither MSCs nor GDF-5 alone significantly increased the strength of healing tendons. In a similar study, the effect of

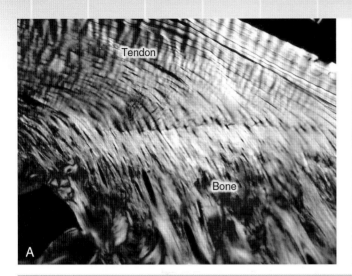
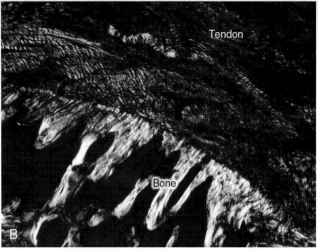

Figure 4 Histologic sections stained with hematoxylin-eosin viewed under polarized light (10× objective). **A,** Control, intact flexor tendon insertion site, illustrating a characteristic transition zone with highly aligned collagen fiber orientation. **B,** Repaired tendon at 21 days, illustrating disorganized scar tissue with little integration of tendon fibers with bone fibers.

MSCs, with and without platelet-rich plasma (PRP), was tested using the same in vitro tissue culture model. The strength and stiffness of the healing tendons with MSC-seeded PRP were higher than those of the healing tendons without a patch or with a cell-seeded patch.[62] These results suggest that the combination of MSCs with an appropriate growth factor stimulus may accelerate flexor tendon healing. These results need to be tested and verified further using in vivo animal models.

Basic Science Pearls

- Successful intrasynovial flexor tendon healing requires suppression of adhesion formation (for tendon gliding) and promotion of matrix synthesis (for accrual of strength).
- Delivering cells and growth factors at the time of surgical repair holds great promise for enhancing healing.
- Biochemical modification of the tendon surface can improve tendon gliding after repair.

Clinical Pearls

- Controlled motion after surgical repair is important to prevent adhesion formation.
- Loading above that needed for tendon motion does not improve outcomes.
- Preserving nutrition sources (vascular if present; synovial pumping via motion) is critical for healing.

Example 2: Chronic Injury and Repair of the Rotator Cuff (Tendon-to-Bone)
Basic Science of Healing
The rotator cuff muscles provide stability and motion at the glenohumeral joint. The rotator cuff is made up of four muscles and their tendons: the supraspinatus, the infraspi-

natus, the subscapularis, and the teres minor. Collagen bundles from the cuff tendons interdigitate to form a hood that inserts around the humeral head via a fibrocartilaginous transition zone. Clinically, any of the four rotator cuff tendons may be affected by injury and disease. However, the most frequently affected is the supraspinatus tendon.[63] The incidence of injury is high; approximately 30% of the population older than 60 years has a rotator cuff tear.[63] Rotator cuff repair to recover shoulder function is one of the most common orthopaedic surgical procedures, with more than 75,000 repairs performed each year in the United States.[64] It is the most common shoulder condition, with more than 17 million individuals in the United States affected. Healing after rotator cuff repair is a well-known clinical challenge. Tears occur at the tendon-to-bone insertion site, and the goal of rotator cuff repair is anatomic restoration of the tendon attachment. However, clinical studies have shown failure rates ranging from 30% to 94%.[65,66] Although pain relief can be obtained in the setting of a failed cuff repair, strength and function are not restored. Loss of strength and function results in permanent disability and leads to lost days from work, occupational challenges, and recreational limitations for patients.[23] Factors associated with failure include muscle degeneration (fatty atrophy), tear size, chronicity, patient age, and other environmental factors.[67] Tendon-to-bone healing is characterized by the formation of connective tissue with vastly inferior biomechanical properties in comparison with normal, uninjured tendon. A graded fibrocartilaginous transition between tendon and bone is not re-created[7] (**Figure 4**). Efforts to improve outcomes after rotator cuff injury have focused on surgical repair technique and rehabilitation. Future strategies may include the use of extracellular matrix scaffolds, growth factors, and cell-based therapies.

Treatment Approach: Rehabilitation

It is well established that musculoskeletal tissues, including tendon, bone, and cartilage, respond to their mechanical environment. Therefore, significant efforts have been made to enhance tendon-to-bone healing via rehabilitation protocols (via control of the mechanical loads across the healing interface). Increased force is beneficial to healing in a variety of clinical settings. Early mobilization improves healing and function after anterior cruciate ligament reconstruction in the knee.[68] Early passive range of motion decreases adhesions and improves strength after flexor tendon repair.[31] Controlled static stress is beneficial to medial collateral ligament healing in the knee.[69] On the other hand, excessive force and motion can cause microdamage and/or gapping and thus be detrimental to healing.[7] Optimizing the mechanical environment in the postoperative setting is therefore critical for improving outcomes.

To determine the effects of a variety of activity levels on tendon-to-bone healing, rotator cuff repairs were performed in rats.[7] Rat shoulders were then immobilized, allowed cage activity, or exercised. Shoulders that were immobilized demonstrated superior collagen orientation and biomechanical properties compared with those that were exercised. The exercised rats had a greater quantity of tissue, but the tissue was lower in quality. The composition of extracellular matrix generated at the immobilized insertion better resembled a normal, uninjured insertion. The immobilized group was superior to the cage activity group, and the cage activity group was superior to the exercised group. A second study using this animal model investigated the effect of short and long durations of these activity levels on the healing insertion site.[70] The activity level had no effect on the biomechanical properties of the insertion site at the early (4-week) time point. However, decreased activity (such as cast immobilization) had a positive effect on biomechanical properties at the late (16-week) time point. In these studies, decreasing the activity level by immobilizing the shoulder improved tendon-to-bone healing, as measured by collagen organization and biomechanical properties. These results demonstrate that increased activity can be detrimental to healing. The notion of negative effects due to motion at the healing rotator cuff insertion site was substantiated in a subsequent study that examined tendon biomechanics and joint range of motion in rat shoulders after rotator cuff repair.[71] Continuous immobilization was compared with two different passive range-of-motion protocols for 2 weeks followed by a 4-week remobilization period. Both passive range-of-motion groups had less joint range of motion compared with the continuous immobilization group. All joints were stiffer in comparison with preinjury levels. No differences were found in tendon collagen organization or mechanical properties in the three groups. Similar results were seen in an anterior cruciate ligament tendon-to-bone healing animal model; delayed application of cyclic axial load after reconstruction resulted in improved properties of the repair compared with immediate loading or prolonged

postoperative immobilization.[72] Recent work has demonstrated that improved healing via immobilization is due to suppression of macrophage accumulation, leading to improved tendon-bone integration.[73]

It is unclear if the improved outcomes in immobilized animals were due simply to prevention of gaps and/or ruptures or an optimal loading environment. As described for flexor tendon repair, gap healing may lead to disorganized collagen deposition and weak mechanical properties. The experimental results in the rotator cuff, however, are in sharp contrast to those in the flexor tendon. Whereas mobilization after flexor tendon repair prevents adhesion formation and improves tendon gliding function, mobilization after tendon-to-bone repair can be detrimental. Because adhesions are not an issue in short tendons and in extrasynovial tendons, there appears to be little motivation for aggressive early motion postoperatively in these situations. However, these results from animal models have not yet been substantiated with clinical data.

To further clarify the role of loading after tendon-to-bone repair, the effect of decreasing load below that seen in immobilized repairs was examined in two studies.[74,75] After surgical injury and repair, rat shoulders in two groups were immobilized. One experimental group had botulinum toxin A injected into the supraspinatus muscle to completely remove load from the healing insertion site. A second group was immobilized and had saline injections into the muscle. A third group underwent botulinum toxin A injections and rats were allowed cage activity after repair. The saline/casted group had greater scar volume and cross-sectional area of the repair tissue at the insertion site and improved structural properties in comparison with the botulinum toxin paralyzed groups, demonstrating that complete removal of load from the healing insertion site was detrimental to healing. Although reduced loading (through cast immobilization) can be beneficial to healing (presumably by eliminating excessive motion at the repair site), some load applied to the site via normal muscle contraction without causing repair site gapping or rupture may be necessary for effective healing.

Treatment Approach: Modification of the Biologic Environment

Several growth factors have been tested for enhanced tendon-to-bone repair. Two recent studies demonstrated that TGF-β3 may accelerate healing.[76,77] This growth factor has been implicated in fetal development and scarless fetal healing and, thus, exogenous addition of TGF-β3 may enhance tendon-to-bone healing. In a rat rotator cuff animal model, TGF-β3 treatment led to increases in inflammation, cellularity, vascularity, and cell proliferation at the early time points. Moreover, delivery of TGF-β3 to the healing tendon-to-bone insertion led to significant improvements in mechanical properties in comparison with control samples. However, contrary to the hypothesis that the growth factor would promote scarless healing, improvements in mechanical properties were due to increased production of disorganized matrix and not due to regeneration of the natural tendon-to-bone insertion.

Because significant bone loss has been demonstrated after tendon-to-bone injury and repair, one approach for improving healing has been to target the bony side of the insertion for treatment. The growth factor BMP-2 is well established as a potent stimulator of bone formation. One experiment showed that the healing of tendon in a bone tunnel occurred through bone ingrowth into tendon.[78] The authors demonstrated an improvement in structural properties of the tendon healing in a bone tunnel after application of exogenous BMP-2. Preventing bone resorption at the healing insertion using bisphosphonate treatment has also been effective in improving healing.[79]

Cell- and gene-transfer–based therapies have also demonstrated some success for enhancing tendon-to-bone repair. Gulotta et al[80] showed that MSCs delivered to the repair site in a rat rotator cuff model did not improve tendon-to-bone healing. However, positive results were seen when MSCs were transfected with scleraxis (Scx), a transcription factor that is necessary for tendon fibroblast differentiation.[81] Supraspinatus tendons in rats were injured and repaired to their bony insertions. One group received Scx-transfected MSCs in fibrin carriers and one group received non-transfected MSCs in fibrin carriers. The Scx-transfected MSC group had higher strength and stiffness compared with the MSC group at 2 and 4 weeks of healing. In a similar study, MSCs were transfected with membrane type 1 matrix metalloproteinase (MT1-MMP), a factor that is upregulated during embryogenesis at tendon-bone insertion sites.[28] Although there were no differences between groups at 2 weeks of healing, significant improvements due to MT1-MMP–transfected MSC treatment were seen at 4 weeks. Fibrocartilage production at the repair site and mechanical properties were increased. As with the in vitro tissue culture results for flexor tendon repair presented in the previous section, MSCs show great promise for enhanced repair provided they are stimulated with the appropriate factor. However, further studies are needed to determine if results can be applied clinically.

A recent review of scaffolds currently used clinically for rotator cuff tendon-to-bone repair revealed that further work is necessary to optimize scaffold properties.[82] Particularly lacking in the currently available scaffolds is an appropriate re-creation of the native tissue's gradation in properties between the relatively extensible tendon and the relatively stiff bone. The lack of gradation in properties may lead to stress concentrations at the interface and rupture of the scaffold and/or repair. To address this lack of complexity, in vitro work in scaffold design has focused on stratified and continuously graded approaches. Biphasic[83] and triphasic scaffolds[84] were generated and seeded with multiple cell types. These studies demonstrated the importance of signaling between the various tendon-to-bone cell types for generation of a functional insertion. Recent approaches have also attempted to create continuous gradients in properties to re-create the interface that is seen at the natural tendon-to-bone insertion. To this end, electrospun polymer nanofiber scaffolds were synthesized with gradations in mineral, mimicking the mineral gradation seen at the native insertion.[85] The gradation in mineral content resulted in a spatial variation in the stiffness of the scaffold. Similar results were reported using a cell-seeded collagen scaffold with a gradient in retrovirus encoding an osteogenic transcription factor.[86] A tissue-engineered scaffold with a gradation in properties and seeded with the appropriate cells and biofactors may ultimately provide a solution to the clinical problem of tendon-to-bone healing. A functionally graded material implanted at the time of surgical repair may provide mechanical stability and guide the repair process, leading to a successful attachment of tendon to bone.

Basic Science Pearls

- The natural tendon-to-bone insertion is a functionally graded tissue that transitions from relatively extensible tendon to relatively brittle bone.
- This graded insertion is not regenerated during tendon-to-bone healing, leaving the repair prone to rupture.
- Growth factor–, cell-, and scaffold-based approaches have shown promise in animal models for enhancing tendon-to-bone healing.

Clinical Pearls

- Rehabilitation influences healing; however, a fine balance must be reached between loads that are too low (leading to a catabolic state) and too high (leading to microdamage).
- Bone loss before and after repair must be considered in treatment plans.

Summary

Tendinopathies include a wide-ranging set of conditions that must be considered individually. Treatment approaches must bear in mind the anatomic context of the tendon and the etiology of the injury. Repair of intrasynovial tendon injuries requires addressing both the gliding requirements and the tensile strength requirements of the tendon. Repair of tendon to bone must consider the attachment of two materials (tendon and bone) with dramatically different mechanical properties. Tendons that are chronically degenerated before injury have a lower likelihood of successful healing. Manipulation and modulation of the mechanical and biologic environments of repaired tendons through surgical techniques, supplementary growth factor and cell augmentations, and postoperative rehabilitation hold promise for enhancing healing.

References

1. Gelberman RH, Khabie V, Cahill CJ: The revascularization of healing flexor tendons in the digital sheath: A vascular injection study in dogs. *J Bone Joint Surg Am* 1991;73(6): 868-881.

2. Duffy FJ Jr, Seiler JG, Gelberman RH, Hergrueter CA: Growth factors and canine flexor tendon healing: Initial studies in uninjured and repair models. *J Hand Surg Am* 1995;20(4):645-649.

3. Beredjiklian PK: Biologic aspects of flexor tendon laceration and repair. *J Bone Joint Surg Am* 2003;85(3):539-550.

4. Gelberman RH, Vandeberg JS, Manske PR, Akeson WH: The early stages of flexor tendon healing: A morphologic study of the first fourteen days. *J Hand Surg Am* 1985;10(6, pt 1): 776-784.

5. Abrahamsson SO, Gelberman RH, Lohmander SL: Variations in cellular proliferation and matrix synthesis in intrasynovial and extrasynovial tendons: An in vitro study in dogs. *J Hand Surg Am* 1994;19(2):259-265.

6. Murray MM, Martin SD, Martin TL, Spector M: Histological changes in the human anterior cruciate ligament after rupture. *J Bone Joint Surg Am* 2000;82(10):1387-1397.

7. Thomopoulos S, Williams GR, Soslowsky LJ: Tendon to bone healing: Differences in biomechanical, structural, and compositional properties due to a range of activity levels. *J Biomech Eng* 2003;125(1):106-113.

8. Fujioka H, Thakur R, Wang GJ, Mizuno K, Balian G, Hurwitz SR: Comparison of surgically attached and non-attached repair of the rat Achilles tendon-bone interface: Cellular organization and type X collagen expression. *Connect Tissue Res* 1998;37(3-4):205-218.

9. St Pierre P, Olson EJ, Elliott JJ, O'Hair KC, McKinney LA, Ryan J: Tendon-healing to cortical bone compared with healing to a cancellous trough: A biomechanical and histological evaluation in goats. *J Bone Joint Surg Am* 1995;77(12): 1858-1866.

10. Silva MJ, Boyer MI, Ditsios K, et al: The insertion site of the canine flexor digitorum profundus tendon heals slowly following injury and suture repair. *J Orthop Res* 2002;20(3): 447-453.12038617

11. Kannus P, Leppälä J, Lehto M, Sievänen H, Heinonen A, Järvinen M: A rotator cuff rupture produces permanent osteoporosis in the affected extremity, but not in those with whom shoulder function has returned to normal. *J Bone Miner Res* 1995;10(8):1263-1271.

12. Ditsios K, Boyer MI, Kusano N, Gelberman RH, Silva MJ: Bone loss following tendon laceration, repair and passive mobilization. *J Orthop Res* 2003;21(6):990-996.

13. Cadet ER, Vorys GC, Rahman R, et al: Improving bone density at the rotator cuff footprint increases supraspinatus tendon failure stress in a rat model. *J Orthop Res* 2010;28(3): 308-314.

14. Galatz LM, Rothermich SY, Zaegel M, Silva MJ, Havlioglu N, Thomopoulos S: Delayed repair of tendon to bone injuries leads to decreased biomechanical properties and bone loss. *J Orthop Res* 2005;23(6):1441-1447.

15. Soslowsky LJ, Thomopoulos S, Esmail A, et al: Rotator cuff tendinosis in an animal model: Role of extrinsic and overuse factors. *Ann Biomed Eng* 2002;30(8):1057-1063.

16. Safran O, Derwin KA, Powell K, Iannotti JP: Changes in rotator cuff muscle volume, fat content, and passive mechanics after chronic detachment in a canine model. *J Bone Joint Surg Am* 2005;87(12):2662-2670.

17. Bassett RW, Cofield RH: Acute tears of the rotator cuff: The timing of surgical repair. *Clin Orthop Relat Res* 1983;175 :18-24.

18. Iannotti JP, Bernot MP, Kuhlman JR, Kelley MJ, Williams GR: Postoperative assessment of shoulder function: A prospective study of full-thickness rotator cuff tears. *J Shoulder Elbow Surg* 1996;5(6):449-457.

19. Lähteenmäki HE, Virolainen P, Hiltunen A, Heikkilä J, Nelimarkka OI: Results of early operative treatment of rotator cuff tears with acute symptoms. *J Shoulder Elbow Surg* 2006; 15(2):148-153.

20. Lähteenmäki HE, Hiltunen A, Virolainen P, Nelimarkka O: Repair of full-thickness rotator cuff tears is recommended regardless of tear size and age: A retrospective study of 218 patients. *J Shoulder Elbow Surg* 2007;16(5):586-590.

21. Bell E: *Principles of Tissue Engineering*, ed 2. San Diego, CA, Academic Press, 2000, pp xxxv-xl.

22. Feuerstein M, Miller VL, Burrell LM, Berger R: Occupational upper extremity disorders in the federal workforce: Prevalence, health care expenditures, and patterns of work disability. *J Occup Environ Med* 1998;40(6):546-555.

23. Kelsey JL: *Frequency, Impact and Cost.* New York, NY, Churchill Livingstone, 1997.

24. Gelberman RH, Boyer MI, Brodt MD, Winters SC, Silva MJ: The effect of gap formation at the repair site on the strength and excursion of intrasynovial flexor tendons: An experimental study on the early stages of tendon-healing in dogs. *J Bone Joint Surg Am* 1999;81(7):975-982.

25. Zhao C, Amadio PC, Paillard P, et al: Digital resistance and tendon strength during the first week after flexor digitorum profundus tendon repair in a canine model in vivo. *J Bone Joint Surg Am* 2004;86(2):320-327.

26. Silva MJ, Brodt MD, Boyer MI, et al: Effects of increased in vivo excursion on digital range of motion and tendon strength following flexor tendon repair. *J Orthop Res* 1999; 17(5):777-783.

27. Boyer MI, Gelberman RH, Burns ME, Dinopoulos H, Hofem R, Silva MJ: Intrasynovial flexor tendon repair: An experimental study comparing low and high levels of in vivo force during rehabilitation in canines. *J Bone Joint Surg Am* 2001;83(6):891-899.

28. Gulotta LV, Kovacevic D, Montgomery S, Ehteshami JR, Packer JD, Rodeo SA: Stem cells genetically modified with the developmental gene MT1-MMP improve regeneration of the supraspinatus tendon-to-bone insertion site. *Am J Sports Med* 2010;38(7):1429-1437.

29. Young RG, Butler DL, Weber W, Caplan AI, Gordon SL, Fink DJ: Use of mesenchymal stem cells in a collagen matrix for Achilles tendon repair. *J Orthop Res* 1998;16(4):406-413.

30. Awad HA, Boivin GP, Dressler MR, Smith FN, Young RG, Butler DL: Repair of patellar tendon injuries using a cell-collagen composite. *J Orthop Res* 2003;21(3):420-431.

31. Boyer MI, Goldfarb CA, Gelberman RH: Recent progress in flexor tendon healing: The modulation of tendon healing with rehabilitation variables. *J Hand Ther* 2005;18(2):80-86.

32. Woo SL, Gelberman RH, Cobb NG, Amiel D, Lothringer K, Akeson WH: The importance of controlled passive mobilization on flexor tendon healing: A biomechanical study. *Acta Orthop Scand* 1981;52(6):615-622.

33. Hannafin JA, Arnoczky SP, Hoonjan A, Torzilli PA: Effect of stress deprivation and cyclic tensile loading on the material and morphologic properties of canine flexor digitorum profundus tendon: An in vitro study. *J Orthop Res* 1995;13(6): 907-914.

34. Slack C, Flint MH, Thompson BM: The effect of tensional load on isolated embryonic chick tendons in organ culture. *Connect Tissue Res* 1984;12(3-4):229-247.

35. Small JO, Brennen MD, Colville J: Early active mobilisation following flexor tendon repair in zone 2. *J Hand Surg Br* 1989;14(4):383-391.

36. Schuind F, Garcia-Elias M, Cooney WP III, An KN: Flexor tendon forces: In vivo measurements. *J Hand Surg Am* 1992; 17(2):291-298.

37. Takai S, Woo SL, Horibe S, Tung DK, Gelberman RH: The effects of frequency and duration of controlled passive mobilization on tendon healing. *J Orthop Res* 1991;9(5):705-713.

38. Lieber RL, Silva MJ, Amiel D, Gelberman RH: Wrist and digital joint motion produce unique flexor tendon force and excursion in the canine forelimb. *J Biomech* 1999;32(2):175-181.

39. Horii E, Lin GT, Cooney WP, Linscheid RL, An KN: Comparative flexor tendon excursion after passive mobilization: An in vitro study. *J Hand Surg Am* 1992;17(3):559-566.

40. Zhao C, Amadio PC, Momose T, Couvreur P, Zobitz ME, An KN: Effect of synergistic wrist motion on adhesion formation after repair of partial flexor digitorum profundus tendon lacerations in a canine model in vivo. *J Bone Joint Surg Am* 2002;84(1):78-84.

41. Tanaka T, Amadio PC, Zhao C, Zobitz ME, An KN: Flexor digitorum profundus tendon tension during finger manipulation. *J Hand Ther* 2005;18(3):330-338.

42. Amadio PC: Friction of the gliding surface: Implications for tendon surgery and rehabilitation. *J Hand Ther* 2005;18(2): 112-119.

43. Sun Y, Chen MY, Zhao C, An KN, Amadio PC: The effect of hyaluronidase, phospholipase, lipid solvent and trypsin on the lubrication of canine flexor digitorum profundus tendon. *J Orthop Res* 2008;26(9):1225-1229.

44. Ikeda J, Sun YL, An KN, Amadio PC, Zhao C: Application of carbodiimide derivatized synovial fluid to enhance extrasynovial tendon gliding ability. *J Hand Surg Am* 2011;36(3): 456-463.

45. Taguchi M, Sun YL, Zhao C, et al: Lubricin surface modification improves tendon gliding after tendon repair in a canine model in vitro. *J Orthop Res* 2009;27(2):257-263.

46. Zhao C, Sun YL, Amadio PC, Tanaka T, Ettema AM, An KN: Surface treatment of flexor tendon autografts with carbodiimide-derivatized hyaluronic acid: An in vivo canine model. *J Bone Joint Surg Am* 2006;88(10):2181-2191.

47. Moro-oka T, Miura H, Mawatari T, et al: Mixture of hyaluronic acid and phospholipid prevents adhesion formation on the injured flexor tendon in rabbits. *J Orthop Res* 2000;18(5):835-840.

48. Taguchi M, Sun YL, Zhao C, et al: Lubricin surface modification improves extrasynovial tendon gliding in a canine model in vitro. *J Bone Joint Surg Am* 2008;90(1):129-135.

49. Zhao C, Sun YL, Kirk RL, et al: Effects of a lubricin-containing compound on the results of flexor tendon repair in a canine model in vivo. *J Bone Joint Surg Am* 2010;92(6): 1453-1461.

50. Thomopoulos S, Harwood FL, Silva MJ, Amiel D, Gelberman RH: Effect of several growth factors on canine flexor tendon fibroblast proliferation and collagen synthesis in vitro. *J Hand Surg Am* 2005;30(3):441-447.

51. Thomopoulos S, Zaegel M, Das R, et al: PDGF-BB released in tendon repair using a novel delivery system promotes cell proliferation and collagen remodeling. *J Orthop Res* 2007; 25(10):1358-1368.

52. Thomopoulos S, Das R, Silva MJ, et al: Enhanced flexor tendon healing through controlled delivery of PDGF-BB. *J Orthop Res* 2009;27(9):1209-1215.

53. Chan BP, Fu S, Qin L, Lee K, Rolf CG, Chan K: Effects of basic fibroblast growth factor (bFGF) on early stages of tendon healing: A rat patellar tendon model. *Acta Orthop Scand* 2000;71(5):513-518.

54. Sakiyama-Elbert SE, Das R, Gelberman RH, Harwood F, Amiel D, Thomopoulos S: Controlled-release kinetics and biologic activity of platelet-derived growth factor-BB for use in flexor tendon repair. *J Hand Surg Am* 2008;33(9):1548-1557.

55. Chang J, Thunder R, Most D, Longaker MT, Lineaweaver WC: Studies in flexor tendon wound healing: Neutralizing antibody to TGF-beta1 increases postoperative range of motion. *Plast Reconstr Surg* 2000;105(1):148-155.

56. Thomopoulos S, Kim HM, Das R, et al: The effects of exogenous basic fibroblast growth factor on intrasynovial flexor tendon healing in a canine model. *J Bone Joint Surg Am* 2010;92(13):2285-2293.

57. Gelberman RH, Thomopoulos S, Sakiyama-Elbert SE, Das R, Silva MJ: The early effects of sustained platelet-derived growth factor administration on the functional and structural properties of repaired intrasynovial flexor tendons: An in vivo biomechanic study at 3 weeks in canines. *J Hand Surg Am* 2007;32(3):373-379.

58. Tang JB, Cao Y, Zhu B, Xin KQ, Wang XT, Liu PY: Adeno-associated virus-2-mediated bFGF gene transfer to digital flexor tendons significantly increases healing strength: An in vivo study. *J Bone Joint Surg Am* 2008;90(5):1078-1089.

59. Basile P, Dadali T, Jacobson J, et al: Freeze-dried tendon allografts as tissue-engineering scaffolds for Gdf5 gene delivery. *Mol Ther* 2008;16(3):466-473.

60. Lou J, Tu Y, Burns M, Silva MJ, Manske P: BMP-12 gene transfer augmentation of lacerated tendon repair. *J Orthop Res* 2001;19(6):1199-1202.

61. Hayashi M, Zhao C, An KN, Amadio PC: The effects of growth and differentiation factor 5 on bone marrow stromal cell transplants in an in vitro tendon healing model. *J Hand Surg Eur Vol* 2011;36(4):271-279.

62. Morizaki Y, Zhao C, An KN, Amadio PC: The effects of platelet-rich plasma on bone marrow stromal cell transplants for tendon healing in vitro. *J Hand Surg Am* 2010; 35(11):1833-1841.

63. Lehman C, Cuomo F, Kummer FJ, Zuckerman JD: The incidence of full thickness rotator cuff tears in a large cadaveric population. *Bull Hosp Jt Dis* 1995;54(1):30-31.

3: Basic Principles and Treatment of Musculoskeletal Disease

64. Vitale MA, Vitale MG, Zivin JG, Braman JP, Bigliani LU, Flatow EL: Rotator cuff repair: An analysis of utility scores and cost-effectiveness. *J Shoulder Elbow Surg* 2007;16(2):181-187.

65. Harryman DT II, Mack LA, Wang KY, Jackins SE, Richardson ML, Matsen FA III: Repairs of the rotator cuff: Correlation of functional results with integrity of the cuff. *J Bone Joint Surg Am* 1991;73(7):982-989.

66. Galatz LM, Ball CM, Teefey SA, Middleton WD, Yamaguchi K: The outcome and repair integrity of completely arthroscopically repaired large and massive rotator cuff tears. *J Bone Joint Surg Am* 2004;86(2):219-224.

67. Naranja RJ, Iannotti JP, Gartsman GM: *Orthopaedic Knowledge Update: Shoulder and Elbow.* Rosemont, IL, American Academy of Orthopaedic Surgeons, 1994, pp 157-166.

68. Beynnon BD, Johnson RJ, Fleming BC: The science of anterior cruciate ligament rehabilitation. *Clin Orthop Relat Res* 2002;402:9-20.

69. Gomez MA, Woo SL, Amiel D, Harwood F, Kitabayashi L, Matyas JR: The effects of increased tension on healing medical collateral ligaments. *Am J Sports Med* 1991;19(4):347-354.

70. Gimbel JA, Van Kleunen JP, Williams GR, Thomopoulos S, Soslowsky LJ: Long durations of immobilization in the rat result in enhanced mechanical properties of the healing supraspinatus tendon insertion site. *J Biomech Eng* 2007;129(3):400-404.

71. Peltz CD, Dourte LM, Kuntz AF, et al: The effect of postoperative passive motion on rotator cuff healing in a rat model. *J Bone Joint Surg Am* 2009;91(10):2421-2429.

72. Bedi A, Kovacevic D, Fox AJ, et al: Effect of early and delayed mechanical loading on tendon-to-bone healing after anterior cruciate ligament reconstruction. *J Bone Joint Surg Am* 2010;92(14):2387-2401.

73. Dagher E, Hays PL, Kawamura S, Godin J, Deng XH, Rodeo SA: Immobilization modulates macrophage accumulation in tendon-bone healing. *Clin Orthop Relat Res* 2009;467(1):281-287.

74. Hettrich CM, Rodeo SA, Hannafin JA, Ehteshami J, Shubin Stein BE: The effect of muscle paralysis using Botox on the healing of tendon to bone in a rat model. *J Shoulder Elbow Surg* 2011;20(5):688-697.

75. Galatz LM, Charlton N, Das R, Kim HM, Havlioglu N, Thomopoulos S: Complete removal of load is detrimental to rotator cuff healing. *J Shoulder Elbow Surg* 2009;18(5):669-675.

76. Kovacevic D, Fox AJ, Bedi A, et al: Calcium-phosphate matrix with or without TGF-β3 improves tendon-bone healing after rotator cuff repair. *Am J Sports Med* 2011;39(4):811-819.

77. Manning CN, Kim HM, Sakiyama-Elbert S, Galatz LM, Havlioglu N, Thomopoulos S: Sustained delivery of transforming growth factor beta three enhances tendon-to-bone healing in a rat model. *J Orthop Res* 2011;29(7):1099-1105.

78. Rodeo SA, Suzuki K, Deng XH, Wozney J, Warren RF: Use of recombinant human bone morphogenetic protein-2 to enhance tendon healing in a bone tunnel. *Am J Sports Med* 1999;27(4):476-488.

79. Thomopoulos S, Matsuzaki H, Zaegel M, Gelberman RH, Silva MJ: Alendronate prevents bone loss and improves tendon-to-bone repair strength in a canine model. *J Orthop Res* 2007;25(4):473-479.

80. Gulotta LV, Kovacevic D, Ehteshami JR, Dagher E, Packer JD, Rodeo SA: Application of bone marrow-derived mesenchymal stem cells in a rotator cuff repair model. *Am J Sports Med* 2009;37(11):2126-2133.

81. Gulotta LV, Kovacevic D, Packer JD, Deng XH, Rodeo SA: Bone marrow-derived mesenchymal stem cells transduced with scleraxis improve rotator cuff healing in a rat model. *Am J Sports Med* 2011;39(6):1282-1289.

82. Derwin KA, Badylak SF, Steinmann SP, Iannotti JP: Extracellular matrix scaffold devices for rotator cuff repair. *J Shoulder Elbow Surg* 2010;19(3):467-476.

83. Wang IE, Shan J, Choi R, et al: Role of osteoblast-fibroblast interactions in the formation of the ligament-to-bone interface. *J Orthop Res* 2007;25(12):1609-1620.

84. Spalazzi JP, Doty SB, Moffat KL, Levine WN, Lu HH: Development of controlled matrix heterogeneity on a triphasic scaffold for orthopedic interface tissue engineering. *Tissue Eng* 2006;12(12):3497-3508.

85. Li X, Xie J, Lipner J, Yuan X, Thomopoulos S, Xia Y: Nanofiber scaffolds with gradations in mineral content for mimicking the tendon-to-bone insertion site. *Nano Lett* 2009;9(7):2763-2768.

86. Phillips JE, Burns KL, Le Doux JM, Guldberg RE, García AJ: Engineering graded tissue interfaces. *Proc Natl Acad Sci U S A* 2008;105(34):12170-12175.

The Biologic Response to Orthopaedic Implants

Stuart B. Goodman, MD, PhD

3: Basic Principles and Treatment of Musculoskeletal Disease

Introduction

Orthopaedic implants are commonly used as internal and external fixation devices for fracture repair, for stabilization/correction of spine fractures and deformities, for joint arthroplasty procedures, and for other reconstructive purposes. Orthopaedic implants are usually made of materials and substances that normally do not reside in the body (for example, metallic, artificial polymeric, and ceramic devices) or are biologically based and manufactured or manipulated (such as hyaluronic acid for injection or musculoskeletal allografts). These materials may be permanent in nature or biodegradable. This chapter will focus on the biologic response to orthopaedic implants that are intended to remain permanently in the body or degrade slowly. Other chapters will review biologically based autograft and allograft implants and related materials.

Permanent orthopaedic biomaterials must demonstrate several fundamental properties to be successful for patient care. First, orthopaedic implants must accomplish their intended clinical function in exemplary fashion, that is to say, they must be efficacious. Second, orthopaedic implants must be safe and not lead to any major or minor local or systemic adverse effects in most patients. Finally, for the benefit of society, these implants must be cost-effective.

A related topic is the concept of biocompatibility. The term has been described as follows: "Biocompatibility refers to the ability of a biomaterial to perform its desired function with respect to a medical therapy, without eliciting any undesirable local or systemic effects in the recipient or beneficiary of that therapy, but generating the most appropriate beneficial cellular or tissue response in that specific situation, and optimizing the clinically relevant performance of that therapy."[1] These key concepts—safety, efficacy, and biocompatibility of orthopaedic implants—must be considered on a backdrop of acute and (in some cases) chronic inflammation that accompanies all surgical procedures during which an implant is placed.

Orthopaedic Implants and Inflammation: General Principles

Whenever a surgical procedure is performed (whether an implant is used or not), the inflammatory cascade of events is initiated.[2-4] The surgical insult leads to local tissue destruction and the liberation of factors such as the proinflammatory cytokines (tumor necrosis factor, interleukin-1, and others), chemotactic cytokines or chemokines (interleukin-8, macrophage chemotactic protein, macrophage inflammatory protein, and others), nitric oxide and peroxide metabolites, and other substances that initiate local tissue necrosis and the migration of leukocytes both locally and systemically. This acute inflammatory response is universal and is orchestrated by polymorphonuclear leukocytes (PMNs) and macrophages. The local hematoma becomes rich in these inflammatory factors and cells, which continue the inflammatory cascade. Acute inflammation usually resolves to reconstitute relatively normal tissue ar-

Dr. Goodman or an immediate family member serves as a paid consultant to or is an employee of Biomemetic Therapeutics and Synthes; has stock or stock options held in Accelalox, Stem-Cor, and Tibion; has received research or institutional support from Amgen, Musculoskeletal Transplant Foundation, and the National Institutes of Health (NIAMS and NICHD); and serves as a board member, owner, officer, or committee member of the AAOS Biological Implants Committee, NIH MTE Panel, and the Orthopaedic Research Society. This work was supported in part by NIH grant 2 ROIARD 5565005 and the Ellenburg Chair in Surgery, Stanford University.

chitectural and functional integrity; however, if this is not the case, either fibrosis or chronic inflammation follows.[3] Chronic inflammation occurs when active inflammation, continued tissue injury, and healing are ongoing simultaneously. Histologically, chronic inflammation is demonstrated by the persistence of inflammatory cells including PMNs, macrophages, foreign body giant cells, lymphocytes, and plasma cells, in conjunction with continued fibrosis and angiogenesis. This scenario may persist or resolve. Granulomatous inflammation is a unique type of chronic inflammation, in which activated macrophages play a prominent role histologically, assuming a squamous or epithelioid appearance. Different etiologic factors may result in granulomatous inflammation, including microorganisms (some bacteria, parasites, fungi) and organic and inorganic particulate material. Granulomatous inflammation may be divided into two types: the foreign body granuloma, which is non-antigen based and therefore nonspecific and contains few lymphocytes; and the immune granuloma, which is antigen based and contains higher numbers of lymphocytes.[4] These terms are extremely important when one considers the biologic response to different materials and their by-products. For example, sufficient numbers of polyethylene and polymethyl methacrylate (PMMA) particles elicit a foreign body granuloma, whereas in specific patients, by-products of cobalt-chromium prostheses may induce an immune granuloma, often accompanied by more widespread tissue necrosis.

Biologic Response to Implants Used In and Around Bone

Biologic Response to Implants for Joint Arthroplasty

Joint arthroplasty, particularly of the hip and knee, and, to a lesser degree, of the shoulder, elbow, finger joints, ankle, and feet, is a commonly performed surgical procedure worldwide. In the United States alone, there were 482,000 hip replacements and 542,000 knee replacements performed in 2006.[5] These operations are among the most cost-effective surgeries, improving pain, function, and psychosocial well-being. Long-term survivorship of these operations has been more than 90% at 15 years of follow-up for good prosthetic designs.[6,7]

The goal of joint arthroplasty is to perform the surgical procedure meticulously in an appropriately selected patient to optimize long-term function and prosthetic fixation. Typically, there are two general methods for fixation of joint arthroplasties to the skeleton. Joint arthroplasties can be fixed to bone with PMMA, which functions as a grout; alternatively, stable fixation to the surrounding bone can be accomplished using a cementless technique. When PMMA is used, advanced cement techniques including careful cleaning and drying of the bone, manipulation and containment of the bone cement to minimize voids and contaminating fluids such as blood that can weaken the cement, and deliv-

ery techniques to ensure proper filling of cavities and prosthetic positioning are used. When cementless methods are chosen, the surrounding bone has to be prepared for an intimate fit with the prosthetic surface. Adjunctive techniques such as increasing the roughness of the prosthetic surface, the use of porous or bioactive coatings, and screws, pegs, and other mechanical methods of fixation are also commonly used to encourage bone ingrowth, a more robust, long-lasting bone-implant interface.

Cemented Metal-on-Polyethylene Implants

Sir John Charnley and others have documented the characteristics of the interface between well-fixed cemented implants and bone from postmortem human retrievals.[8-11] Charnley reported that the interface displayed cellular damage (loss of the definition of fat and hematopoietic cells) in a 500-μm radius from the cement several weeks after the surgical procedure, due to chemical, thermal, and mechanical trauma. This interface developed into a fibrous or fibrocartilaginous zone containing circular PMMA bead impressions in some areas; elsewhere, PMMA beads directly abutted bony trabecula and cortical bone. In some localized areas, the original bone became necrotic and subsequently underwent regeneration, with or without an intervening layer of fibrous tissue or fibrocartilage; this layer then underwent metaplasia to mature cancellous or lamellar bone over many months to years. A foreign-body giant cell reaction was rarely seen at the interface of well-fixed cemented femoral hip components. Maloney et al[10] found close bone-cement apposition and little evidence of fibrous tissue at the interface surrounding well-fixed femoral implants up to 17 years postoperatively. Similar to Charnley's observations, they found that a secondary, circumferential, trabecular "neocortex" formed around the cement; this neocortex communicated with the internally expanded natural cortex via radial spicules of bone. However, Fornasier et al[11] found evidence of an evolving foreign body response even when the cemented femoral implants at autopsy were not loose. The presence of macrophages and foreign body giant cells in the tissues correlated with the time after surgery, the thickness of the periprosthetic membrane, and the density of polyethylene particles. Cemented acetabular components demonstrated a progressive centripetally developing foreign body reaction to polyethylene and cement wear particles, leading to osteolysis.[12] The linear osteolytic areas continued to grow with the generation of increasing amounts of wear particles and even ballooned into the bony supporting foundation until the prosthesis became mechanically loose.

Cementless Metal-on-Polyethylene Implants

When cementless implants are used, the bone is prepared to achieve stable fixation to minimize micromotion and facilitate bone ongrowth or ingrowth without the use of an intermediary grouting material (**Figure 1**). This goal is achieved by proper sizing of the implant and "machining" the bone for an intimate fit with the prosthesis. Surface roughening, porous coating, and bioactive coating of the implant surface (for example, with hydroxyapatite) are adjunctive methods to achieve this goal. The aim is to induce prosthetic osseointegration, a stable physical and biofunctional incorporation of the implant within bone.[13] Interfacial micromotion beyond approximately 50 µm will lead to fibrous tissue formation, rather than bone. More conventional porous coatings (such as metallic beads and wires) and newer highly porous roughened cancellous-like metallic surfaces (such as porous tantalum or titanium) have demonstrated great success in facilitating osseointegration.[14-16] For porous coatings, a pore size of approximately 100 to 400 µm is optimal.[15]

The biologic stages of bone ingrowth into stable porous coated implants parallel those of primary fracture healing. The initial hematoma that forms at the interface after cementless prosthesis implantation is composed of localized areas of tissue necrosis, proinflammatory and anti-inflammatory factors, and cells that consolidate into an amorphous gel. Mesenchymal stem cells migrate into the hematoma, and in the appropriate stable environment begin to form immature woven bone via intramembranous ossification over several weeks to months. This bone undergoes remodeling to more mature cancellous and cortical bone over subsequent months to years (**Figure 1**). However, in an unstable environment with excessive micromotion, a large gap or poor vascularity, fibrous tissue, fibrocartilage, and a synovial lining layer form, and bone ingrowth is minimal. Infection will also produce a chronic inflammatory membranous interface that inhibits bone formation.

Much information concerning the interface between stable cementless implants and bone can be learned from examining well-functioning implants retrieved at autopsy, rather than specimens gathered at revision surgery. The implants from revision surgery are usually revised because of clinical failure due to a myriad of etiologies, such as chronic dislocation, unexplained pain, excessive wear, or implant breakage.[17] Clinically successful cementless implants that have been retrieved at autopsy minimize these confounding variables.[18,19] Interestingly, these studies have substantiated the concept of bone ingrowth and ongrowth; however, the amount of bone within pores or adjacent to the metal surface has varied widely.[17-19] Studies have also shown that the location and orientation of fibrous tissue and bone around porous coated implants is determined by numerous factors including the material and design of the prosthesis, the location and extent of porous coating, the size of the pores, the addition of screws, the intimacy of the fit of the prosthesis with bone, and other variables.[18] Bone ingrowth is greater in titanium alloy stems where the porous coating ends, adjacent to screws, and in locations of compressive load where there is an intimate prosthetic fit.[18] Bone ingrowth is less around smooth as opposed to roughened surfaces, and in areas of localized infection or excessive motion. In such locations, fibrous tissue or an inflammatory membrane forms and may be associated with absorption of the adjacent bone. Unfilled screw holes containing fibrous tis-

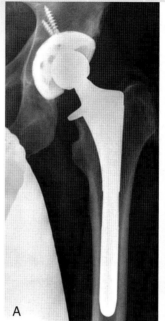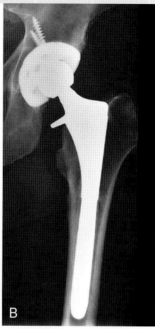

Figure 1   Osseointegrated cementless total hip replacement. **A,** 6 weeks post cementless total hip replacement. **B,** 5 years post total hip replacement. Note the rounding off of the calcar femorale underneath the collar of the femoral component. The pertrochanteric area is less radiodense than previously. There are also "spot welds" at the termination of the porous coating at the midlevel of the femoral component.

sue can provide a conduit for the migration of particles from the interface into the underlying cancellous bone. Implants that achieve intimate integration with bone (such as with porous or bioactive coatings) provide a more robust interface, preventing polyethylene particle migration compared with smooth implants.[20] Postmortem retrieval studies have also demonstrated the usefulness of hydroxyapatite coatings in facilitating bone ongrowth and preventing particle migration. This osteoconductive layer provides a scaffold for bone to form. This layer undergoes cell-mediated resorption, generally with no adverse tissue reaction. However, at least one study reported a higher incidence of loosening when hydroxyapatite coatings are used to facilitate acetabular cup fixation.[21] Recently, highly porous, corrosion-resistant metallic coatings and devices made out of tantalum, titanium, and other biocompatible materials have been introduced that mimic the structure of cancellous bone.[16] These new materials are manufactured with a higher coefficient of friction, encouraging the adhesion and proliferation of osteoprogenitor cells and other mesenchymal tissues. These materials are particularly useful in the reconstruction of areas of bone deficiency and act as a scaffold for bone formation.

Loose Metal-on-Polyethylene Implants

Loose cemented implants demonstrate radiolucent lines at the bone-cement and/or cement-prosthesis interface, and

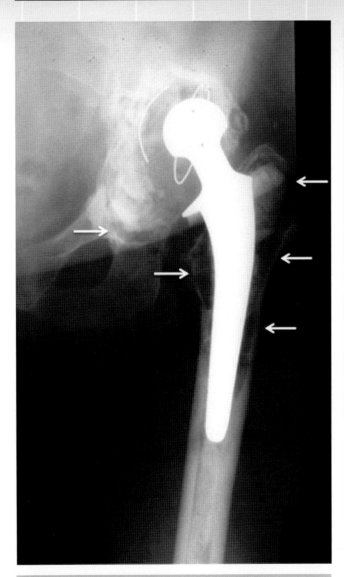

Figure 2 Loose cemented total hip replacement with osteolysis. This failed hip replacement demonstrates loosening with osteolysis (arrows) of the acetabular and femoral components secondary to cement debris.

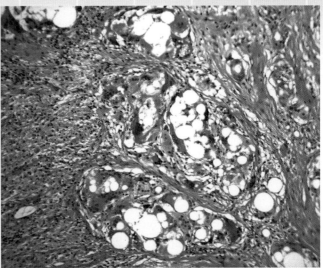

Figure 3 Granulomatous reaction to cement debris. Section from the bone-cement interface of a revised hip replacement demonstrates cement wear particles (large and small round white cement "ghosts"), surrounded by a nonspecific granulomatous reaction composed of mononucleated and multinucleated macrophages and fibrous tissue. Hematoxylin and eosin stain. (Courtesy of Patricia Campbell, PhD, Los Angeles, CA.)

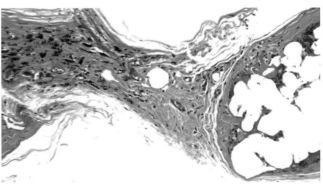

Figure 4 Histologic section from the bone-cement interface of a revised cemented hip arthroplasty. The large white circular cement "ghosts" are seen to the right of the figure, surrounded by fibrous tissue and scattered macrophages. To the left of the figure, macrophages have phagocytosed black metal debris. Hematoxylin and eosin stain. (Courtesy of Patricia Campbell, PhD, Los Angeles, CA.)

the implants often migrate from their original positions (**Figure 2**). Classically these implants are surrounded by a fibroinflammatory membrane up to several millimeters in thickness, containing particles of PMMA (when used), polyethylene, and metal (**Figures 3** and **4**). The cellular components of this chronic inflammatory and foreign body reaction include fibroblasts, macrophages, giant cells, and vascular structures, but only scant numbers of lymphocytes and polymorphonuclear leukocytes (**Figure 5**). If interfacial motion occurs, a synovium-like surface layer develops adjacent to the cement.[22,23] Large "cement lakes" in the retrieved tissue contain the remnants of PMMA (when used) because the PMMA is normally dissolved by organic solvents during processing of the tissue. Shards of polyethylene particles, which are birefringent under polarized light and stain posi-

tively with Oil Red O, are seen in the interstitium and within mononucleated and multinucleated macrophages (**Figure 5**). These particles are often needlelike and may be up to a 1 mm or longer, but most of the particulate debris is in the range of 0.3 to 5 µm in length. There is much heterogeneity throughout different locations of the tissue histologically, varying from highly oriented fibrous tissue to granulomatous inflammation, depending on the concentration of polyethylene particles. High concentrations of osteoclasts

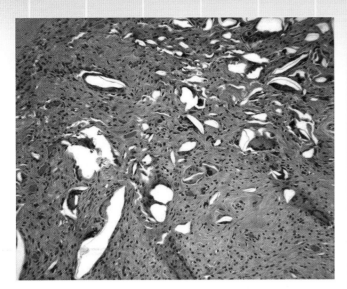

Figure 5 The biologic reaction to polyethylene wear debris. Large white shards of polyethylene are surrounded by macrophages and foreign body giant cells. Hematoxylin and eosin stain. (Courtesy of Patricia Campbell, PhD, Los Angeles, CA.)

line the membrane where bone resorption occurs; this coincides with the scalloped appearance seen around the cement mantle radiographically. Interestingly, evidence of active new bone formation is a predominant finding in the implant bone bed histologically.[24] Loose cementless implants display a similar histologic finding, except that the fibrous tissue layer is usually thinner and contains macrophages and giant cells with phagocytosed polyethylene particles.

Osteolysis

Particle-associated periprosthetic bone loss is simply designated "osteolysis," although this term is also used in other contexts when discussing more rapid bone loss associated with aggressive tumors, infections, sustained localized pressure (for example, pressure-associated remodeling of bone by a loose subsided prosthesis), and other causes. In joint arthroplasty, osteolysis refers to a radiographic phenomenon in which progressive linear, scalloped, or larger areas of bone loss are noted in conjunction with the generation of excessive wear debris (**Figures 2** and **6**). The wear debris and inflammatory fluid from chronic synovitis are pumped around the prosthesis, insinuating into the cancellous bone by waves of high pressure generated during episodic loading of the limb. In this way, the debris can be located at a great distance from where it was generated at the articulation or at other interfaces. Wear particles have been found in the local lymph nodes and in other reticuloendothelial organs such as the liver and spleen.

Osteolysis is a phenomenon in which bone degradation is accelerated and bone formation is depressed by the production of and biologic reaction to excessive wear particles. In some cases, an aggressive granulomatous lesion develops; this consists of a rapidly progressive radiographic lucent

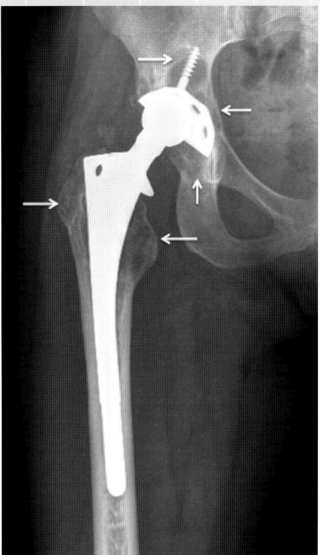

Figure 6 Cementless hip replacement with osteolysis due to polyethylene wear debris. This well-fixed cementless total hip replacement demonstrates eccentric positioning of the femoral head in the acetabulum due to polyethylene wear. Note the severe polyethylene particle–associated periprosthetic osteolysis (arrows).

area containing well-organized connective tissue, sheets of macrophages, and fibrocytic reactive zones in a highly vascularized stroma. The authors who first described aggressive granulomatosis suggest that it is due to "uncoupling of the normal sequence of monocyte-macrophage-mediated clearance of foreign material and tissue debris that is normally followed by fibroblast-mediated synthesis and remodeling of the extracellular matrix."[25] This pathologic process is quite different from that found with simple prosthetic loosening.

In vitro, in vivo, and human retrieval studies have demonstrated an association between wear particles from joint arthroplasties and periprosthetic osteolysis.[26] A plethora of biologic substances including prostaglandins (especially prostaglandin E$_2$), cytokines (such as tumor necrosis factor α (TNF-α), interleukins-1β, -6, -8, and others), chemokines (primarily macrophage chemotactic and inhibitory proteins), nitric oxide and peroxide metabolic intermediates, and other factors are liberated by particle-activated cells that initiate the inflammatory cascade.[27] This results in the degradation of bone and suppression of bone lineage cells, leading to radiographic osteolysis. Other factors may be contributory, including fluid flow-induced mechanical pressure, other mechanical factors, and previous low-grade infection.[28]

TNF-α, interleukin-1β, and many other proinflammatory and anti-inflammatory cytokines and substances are regulated primarily by the transcription factor nuclear factor kappa-B (NF-κB). This transcription factor has been shown to have great relevance to periprosthetic osteolysis associated with wear particles. RANK (receptor activator of NF-κB) activates the transcription factor NF-κB, and is a membrane-bound receptor on the surface of osteoclasts. Osteoblasts, stromal cells, and other activated cells in the inflammatory process release RANK receptor ligand (RANKL), a member of the TNF superfamily. RANKL interacts with RANK located on osteoclasts, and the cytokine macrophage colony stimulating factor (granulocyte macrophage-colony stimulating factor [GM-CSF]) to upregulate the differentiation and maturation of tissue macrophages into osteoclasts. The soluble decoy protein receptor antagonist osteoprotegerin (OPG) inhibits RANKL and is part of the homeostatic mechanism controlling bone mass. Studies have demonstrated an imbalance in the RANKL: GM-CSF:OPG axis in in vitro and in vivo experiments with wear particle challenge and in cases of periprosthetic osteolysis.[29]

Alternative Bearings

Wear and periprosthetic osteolysis associated with conventional polyethylene particles stimulated research into alternative bearing surfaces with improved wear characteristics. These new articulations include primarily newer polyethylene, ceramic-on-ceramic, and metal-on-metal (MOM) bearings. Conventional polyethylenes were originally sterilized with gamma irradiation in air and were usually stored in air-containing packaging on the shelf until used. This caused oxidative degradation of the polyethylene and suboptimal wear characteristics when implanted in vivo. More recently, the more highly cross-linked polyethylenes that are heated at or above the melting temperature and/or annealed have shown improved wear characteristics in vitro and in vivo up to 10 years postoperatively. Moreover, the particle burden is less, although the particles are slightly smaller in size and possibly induce more cellular activation, although this is controversial.[30] However, the very small number of particles generated more than compensates for the potential for increased particle-associated inflammation. Newer polyethylenes that are impregnated with the free radical scaven-

ger vitamin E, or are repetitively melted and annealed, may show even more promise.[31]

Ceramic-on-ceramic bearings are more popular in Europe and the Far East than in the United States. Although the wear particles generated are few in number secondary to extremely low volumetric wear of this bearing couple, their biologic potential is similar to that of polyethylene.[30,32] Most of the particles generated are in the nanometer size range, although damaged surfaces can generate particles of a larger size. Issues related to particle generation include surface damage during initial placement or loss of the lubricating layer, striped wear, suboptimal placement of the components with impingement or edge loading, chipping, and catastrophic fracture.

MOM bearing surfaces have been used for more than four decades, first as the McKee-Farrar and Ring prostheses in Great Britain, and more recently worldwide, as the materials, tribologic characteristics, and design of implants have improved. In addition, the resurgence of resurfacing arthroplasty of the hip (mostly in North America, Northern Europe, and Australia) has encouraged a reconsideration of MOM bearing surfaces. Hip resurfacing may have the advantage of preservation of femoral bone stock, and the use of larger femoral heads to increase stability and range of motion allows a more active lifestyle. Wear with MOM bearings is particularly low because of the smaller clearance of the components that generate thin fluid-film lubrication and the self-polishing nature of this articulation.[30,33] There is evidence (although controversial) that implants manufactured with higher carbon alloys demonstrated better wear characteristics compared with those with lower carbon alloys.[30,33] Although some MOM implants have functioned very well, new issues have arisen that have been a cause of great concern.

Metallic debris has been found in the periprosthetic tissues of metal-on-polyethylene joint arthroplasties and generally has not been a major problem, unless this debris becomes generated in large amounts (such as from corroding interfaces or particles, impingement of the femoral neck on the acetabular shell, or when the femoral head wears completely through the polyethylene liner and articulates with the metal shell). However in MOM arthroplasty, the debris that is produced is in greater quantity and the particles are very small, on the order of 10 to 50 nanometers, and have a large surface area.[30,33] Furthermore, ions of cobalt (Co) and chromium (Cr) are produced and can be found in the surrounding and remote tissues, blood, and urine. Although high levels of ions are associated with specific types of cancer in animal models, to date there is no evidence of this in humans.[30]

Retrieval and revision specimens from MOM prostheses often demonstrate different histologic findings compared with metal-on-polyethylene implants. Macrophage-laden particles are far less pervasive in MOM specimens, probably because of the lower rates of wear of MOM bearings. A subset of 19 patients with pristine-looking radiographs postoperatively, but who had early recurrence of their preoperative pain, poor function, and a joint effusion associated with a second-generation MOM articulation was studied.[34] Radiolucent lines subsequently developed in 5 of the 19 hips, and osteolysis developed in another 7 hips before revision. At surgery, the hip components were well fixed in 9 patients; "the characteristic histological features were diffuse and perivascular infiltrates of T and B lymphocytes and plasma cells, high endothelial venules, massive fibrin exudation, accumulation of macrophages with drop-like inclusions, and infiltrates of eosinophilic granulocytes and necrosis."[34] In a related publication comparing metal-on-polyethylene with MOM hip replacements, the authors found that the MOM retrievals showed pronounced ulceration superficial to the areas demonstrating perilymphocytic vascular infiltration.[35] The lymphocytic infiltration was more pronounced in specimens from MOM cases with prosthesis loosening compared with autopsy specimens or those undergoing arthrotomy. These findings suggested that degradation products from MOM implants may be associated with an allergic hypersensitivity reaction, confirmed by a positive lymphocyte transformation test in 10 of 16 patients (62%) in a subsequent report.[36]

The debris produced by metal-on-polyethylene bearings is primarily polymeric and evokes a nonspecific, nonantigenic chronic inflammatory and foreign body reaction (a nonspecific granulomatous reaction). However, MOM articulations produce metallic by-products that are soluble and can complex with serum proteins to form haptens, and subsequently, a hypersensitivity reaction mediated by the adaptive immune system involving T and B lymphocytes (immune granuloma). The most common metallic sensitizers include nickel, cobalt, and chromium. Rarely, metals such as titanium, vanadium, and tantalum function in this capacity. This allergic reaction is classified as a type IV delayed hypersensitivity immune reaction. Corrosion by-products including $CrPO_4$ may also develop from MOM bearing surfaces and other nonarticulating locations (such as the femoral head and trunnion). These by-products can elicit an immune response and act as agents in third-body wear. In addition, it is well established that patients with a MOM bearing surface had higher postoperative levels of cobalt and chromium ions in their blood, serum, erythrocytes, and urine compared with preoperative values and patients with a metal-on-polyethylene bearing.

A new adverse reaction, pseudotumor formation, has recently been described regarding MOM bearing implants. Pseudotumors are composed of large granulomatous masses of inflammatory cells (macrophages, T lymphocytes, plasma cells), fibrous tissue, and widespread tissue necrosis in conjunction with resurfacing or total hip components with MOM bearings[37,38] (Figure 7). The etiology appears to be both a cytotoxic response and delayed hypersensitivity reaction to cobalt-chromium particles and their by-products. These masses may be asymptomatic at first but often become symptomatic with time and can cause a mass effect on

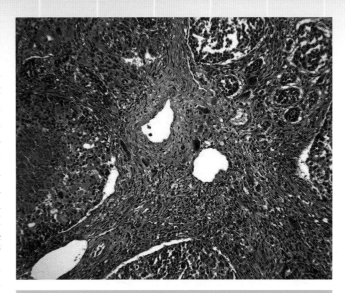

Figure 7 Metal-induced granulomatous reaction. Section from the tissue interface of a revised metal-on-metal implant demonstrating widespread infiltration of macrophages and lymphocytes in response to metal debris, in a fibrous stroma background. To the left of the photomicrograph, there are areas of tissue necrosis. Hematoxylin and eosin stain. (Courtesy of Patricia Campbell, PhD, Los Angeles, CA.)

the surrounding neurovascular structures, muscle, and bone. Risk factors for this reaction appear to be with small-sized components in younger female patients, hip dysplasia, suboptimal implant position, edge loading, and impingement of the components.[39] The incidence of pseudotumor formation is probably at least 4% of resurfacings in the Oxford series. Particularly worrisome is the high complication rate and poor outcome of revision of these cases. Surgical débridement demonstrates more widespread necrosis of muscle than was originally suspected, often compromising later function. The consensus appears to be that cases with pseudotumor formation should be revised early to a non–MOM bearing surface to avoid long-term tissue necrosis and functional loss.

Stress-Induced Bone Remodeling

In addition to affecting the biologic environment, orthopaedic implants placed within bone profoundly affect the mechanical environment. Originally, cementless femoral implants were large metallic devices made of cobalt-chromium alloy, a material that is very stiff in comparison with both cortical and cancellous bone. As load was transmitted through the intramedullary stem from proximally to distally, bypassing the proximal femur, remodeling of the proximal femur took place over time according to biomechanical principles known as Wolff's Law. The resulting radiographic findings termed "stress shielding" or "adverse bone remodeling" became apparent as marked atrophy of the proximal metaphysis of the femur near the upper end of the implant and hypertrophy of the femur adjacent to the distal end of

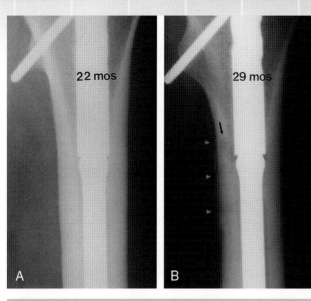

Figure 8 By-products of corrosion from the junction of a modular intramedullary nail are associated with adjacent osteolysis of the cortical bone (black arrow) and a periosteal reaction (white arrowheads). **A**, Radiograph at 22 months postoperatively. **B**, Radiograph at 29 months postoperatively showing new findings. (Reproduced with permission from Jones DM, Marsh JL, Nepola JV, et al: Focal osteolysis at the junctions of a modular stainless-steel femoral intramedullary nail. *J Bone Joint Surg Am* 2001;83[4]:537-548.)

the implant, especially at the end of the porous coating (**Figure 1**). Larger stem sizes had a more profound effect.[40] Although these radiologic events have not been associated with clinical failure of the femoral implant, the rapid disappearance of bone over time on follow-up radiographs can be daunting and might compromise the available bone stock if revision surgery should be necessary in the future. To mitigate these adverse bone-remodeling changes, modern femoral implants have been designed to provide better proximal metaphyseal fit and fill (and therefore more metaphyseal loading), and many have special features such as a tapered design that does not engage the cortex distally, metal cutouts along the length of the stem, or a compressible double-pronged distal end. Another approach has been to use materials that have a lower modulus of elasticity and are therefore less stiff than conventional stems, such as titanium alloys or composite materials.[41]

Originally, porous coating was placed over the full length of the femoral component to enhance mechanical fixation primarily by gaining a better initial "scratch fit." Fully porous coated implants would also present a more extensive surface for bone ingrowth, thereby potentially providing a more durable method for long-term prosthesis stabilization. Fully porous coated stems were thought to be another contributing factor to stress shielding; however, this point is controversial.[42] To date, there is general agreement that large diameter longer stems made of stiffer materials result in more stress shielding than shorter stems of a smaller diameter.

Carcinogenesis

There has been great interest and controversy regarding the potential for carcinogenesis due to the presence of orthopaedic implants. This is a particularly germane subject, given the fact that millions of implants are placed each year worldwide for joint arthroplasty, fracture fixation, spine fusion, and other reconstructive procedures. Furthermore, as joint arthroplasties and other implants are currently being performed in younger patients who may have the device in situ for many decades, it is good to understand the biologic implications of long-term device implantation. There is also controversy as to whether fixation devices such as intramedullary rods, plates, screws, wires, or spinal implants should be excised when their presence is no longer needed. These devices prevent normal loading of the adjacent bone and may release by-products that may have biologic sequela. For example, corrosive metallic by-products may form at modular junctions of intramedullary nails and can cause osteolysis[43] (**Figure 8**).

As discussed previously, most orthopaedic polymers and ceramics have few biologic effects in bulk form. The particulates of these materials stimulate a nonspecific chronic inflammatory and foreign body reaction. In other organ systems subjected to chronic inflammatory processes, cellular metaplasia may occur; this does seem to be the case when discussing orthopaedic implants made of polymers and ceramics. Metallic implants present a slightly different scenario because the by-products of corrosion and other processes can result in the formation of metallic-protein complexes that can function as antigenic haptens. Prolonged high levels of metallic ions and complexes containing different metals have been associated with carcinogenesis in different animal models.[44] These concerns have stimulated controversy in the use of MOM bearing surfaces in younger patients, whose blood and tissues may potentially exhibit elevated metal ion levels for many decades.

Past epidemiologic studies correlating the risk of cancer and metallic implants have been controversial and often conflicting. Perhaps the most recent and comprehensive examination of this topic has come from Visuri et al[45] in Helsinki in 2006. They reviewed a total of 46 cases of malignant tumor formation at the site of total hip replacements reported in the Western literature between 1974 and 2003. These cases included 41 sarcomas, 4 lymphomas, and 1 epidermoid carcinoma. Thirty-one of the tumors were soft-tissue carcinomas, whereas 10 were located in bone. The most common soft-tissue sarcoma was the malignant fibrous histiocytoma in 20 of the 31 cases. The mean period of latency from the first operation was 6 years (range, 0.5 to 20 years). Predisposing factors included secondary osteoarthritis, previous local complications, chronic infection, and known preconditions for cancer such as irradiation. The sarcomas were highly aggressive, with 77% of patients dying within 1 year of diagnosis. The authors concluded that particle-associated chronic inflammation does not appear to be a risk factor for the development of cancer, given the large numbers of joint arthroplasties performed each year worldwide. However, cancers associated with joint arthroplasties and other metallic fixation devices are probably underreported.

When discussing the risk of cancer around orthopaedic implants with patients, the health care team should remember that the latency for most cancers in general is many years, if not decades. Although no direct association between metal implants and cancer has been established to date, long-term follow-up and continued epidemiologic studies are warranted.

Biologic Response to Implants Used for Fracture Fixation

The biologic and biomechanical principles and the materials used in the treatment of fractures are common with those in adult reconstructive surgery and joint arthroplasty. Fracture fixation devices including intramedullary rods, plates, screws, wires, and other implants are generally manufactured from metal alloys such as stainless steel, cobalt-chromium, titanium alloy, other metallic and nonmetallic alloys and composites, and biodegradable polymeric devices. The biology and biomechanics of intramedullary nailing have been known for many years and have recently been reviewed.[46] Important factors that affect the local and systemic effects of intramedullary implants include the general condition of the patient, specific biomechanics and vascular supply of the bone involved, the type of fracture and injury characteristics, whether the canal is reamed, the type of reamer used, the design and material composition of the nail, whether it is locked with screws, and subsequent loading protocols during rehabilitation. Intramedullary reaming is superimposed on the injury to the affected bone and destroys the endosteal blood supply and the medullary contents. Reaming negatively affects cortical blood flow but increases blood flow to the surrounding muscle and soft tissues.[46] Endosteal blood supply appears to normalize within approximately 12 weeks in large animals. Reaming also facilitates the local deposition of marrow contents and proinflammatory and anti-inflammatory factors that promote osteogenesis. Whether reaming has an effect on the local rate of infection of open fractures is controversial, but at least one human study does not support this contention. Intramedullary reaming has the potential to embolize marrow contents into the systemic circulation and may affect the immune system both locally and systemically. Marrow embolization is dependent on the design of the reamer and the intramedullary pressures generated during the procedure. Reamers attached to negative pressure aspirators may potentially mitigate these embolic events. New directions include the use of new materials and bioactive coating of the nail to inhibit infection or promote fracture healing.

Traditionally, the use of full contact plates and screws with direct surgical exposure that resulted in periosteal stripping and bone devitalization led to an increased risk of nonunion and infection. These plates also dramatically altered the local stresses and interfered with local blood supply to the underlying bone. More recently, screws and plates made of newer alloys and designs have demonstrated less corrosive by-products and more limited contact with the underlying bone, minimizing local compressive forces exerted by the plate on the bone. Technical advances include preservation of the periosteum and less invasive indirect reduction and bridging osteosynthesis (instead of reduction of every single fracture fragment) in comminuted diaphyseal and metadiaphyseal fractures.[47]

Böstman and Pihlajamäki[48,49] in Finland have played a seminal role in defining the biocompatibility of bioabsorbable bone fixation devices. They report a series of 2,528 fractures and other disorders in which pins, rods, bolts, and screws were used for fixation. These devices were made of polyglycolic acid or polylactic acid. These implants were generally used around the ankle, foot, and elbow. Clinically significant foreign body reactions to the breakdown products of these polymers were seen in 4.3% of cases and manifested as a painful erythematous fluctuating papule or discharging sinus. Fifty-seven percent of these cases exhibited localized osteolytic lesions at the site of the internal fixation device. The risk of this adverse reaction was dependent on the type of polymer implanted. Polyglycolic acid implants were associated with a 5.3% incidence of significant foreign body reaction whereas only one case (0.2%) of polylactic acid implants demonstrated this reaction. Polyglycolic acid implants exhibited this reaction earlier (2 to 3 months) than polylactic acid (4.3 years). Polylactic acid is hydrophobic and has a known longer degradation time than polyglycolic acid. The presence of quinone dye additive exacerbated the inflammatory reaction. Screws and serrated bolts showed a greater propensity for this reaction compared with pins and rods, probably because of the increased surface area of screws and serrated bolts. Poorly vascularized areas were particularly susceptible. The lesions were débrided in all cases of significant reaction. Histologic specimens showed a nonspecific inflammatory foreign body mononucleated and multinucleated cell reaction to extracellular polymeric debris, approximately 25 μm in size. Important factors to consider include the molecular weight of the polymer, the thermal history, crystallinity, porosity, and presence of residual impurities and additives, as well as the methods of fabrication and sterilization. Newer polymers are being developed that may mitigate these adverse reactions. Biodegradable implants must be sufficiently strong to withstand physiologic loads during the fracture healing period and degrade at appropriate times without adverse local tissue reactions. These properties are difficult to reconcile given the great variability in fracture locations, patterns, and individual patient characteristics. If these problems could be solved, further surgery to remove biodegradable implants may be avoided.

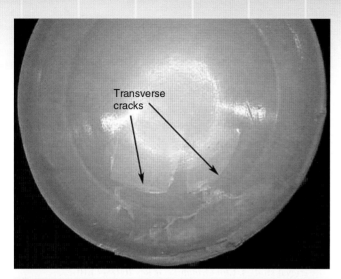

Figure 9 Transverse cracks are noted in the polyethylene component from a total disk replacement retrieved approximately 3 years postoperatively. (Reproduced with permission from Kurtz SM, Peloza J, Siskey R, Villarraga ML: Analysis of a retrieved polyethylene total disc replacement component. *Spine J* 2005;5:346-347.)

Biologic Response to Implants in Spine Surgery

Spine surgery concepts are similar to those enumerated for total joint arthroplasty and fracture fixation devices. Spinal implants generally invoke a fibrous encapsulation in the surrounding soft tissue (muscle, fascia). In some areas where there is interfacial motion, a synovial lining forms, simulating a bursa. Stable implants made of commonly used metals and alloys may osseointegrate with the surrounding bone. Implant motion within bone leads to pressure necrosis, bone resorption, and potential loosening of the implant.

Artificial spinal disks are generally made of the same materials as total joint arthroplasties and fracture fixation devices. Thus, spinal devices are subject to similar modes of failure, wear patterns, types of corrosion, and resulting biologic reactions as devices for other locations[50-52] (**Figure 9**). However, the proximity of spinal devices to the spinal cord, cauda equina, and spinal nerves, as well as major arterial and venous structures, makes adverse biologic reactions potentially very serious. Similar concerns are relevant to the use of PMMA and other materials injected into the vertebra for osteoporotic fractures.

Biologic Response to Implants in Other Orthopaedic Subspecialties

Metallic, polymeric, and biodegradable implants evoke a similar reaction as outlined previously, when placed in other locations in the musculoskeletal system. The pediatric population represents a special situation in which implants should be used judiciously because they may affect skeletal growth and development.

Biologic Response to Soft-Tissue Implants

Devices are commonly used in sports medicine, foot and ankle surgery, hand and upper extremity surgery, and other subspecialties to anchor soft tissues within bone. In general, the use of metallic, polymeric, and other implants results in biologic reactions comparable with those in other anatomic locations. In sports medicine, biodegradable implants have been used as suture anchors or arrows and are often attached to sutures made of conventional materials, which may or may not be biodegradable. The most common materials for these devices are polyglycolic acid, polylactic acid, variants/combinations of the previous two polymers, and polyglyconate.[53] In general these implants have demonstrated a high degree of success. Many of these implants are exposed to the synovial joint. By-products of these implants may cause a sterile synovitis, which is persistent until the device is explanted or overgrown by bone or fibrous tissue. A new generation of "smart polymers" that can change their shape, chemical structure, or mechanical properties when exposed to specific stimuli are also being developed. For example, temperature-sensitive metals and polymers have been developed to alter their shape and mechanical properties when exposed to certain temperatures.

The use of allograft materials, biologic scaffolds, and other devices for cartilage, bone, and soft-tissue reconstruction will be discussed in other chapters.

Summary

Implants have revolutionized the treatment of traumatic injuries and orthopaedic reconstructive procedures worldwide. These devices are tightly regulated in the United States by the Food and Drug Administration, in Canada by the Medical Devices Bureau of Health Canada, in the United Kingdom by Medicines and Healthcare Products Regulatory Agency, in the European Union by the Ministry of Health in each member state (although European Union certification is designated by the CE mark), and by other regulatory bodies in other countries around the world. These devices generally undergo exhaustive preclinical and clinical studies before use in the United States.[54] A comprehensive system is also in place for reporting of device-associated adverse events by the hospital and physician. It should be emphasized that most current devices have changed the lives of millions of patients for the better, in ways that could not have been imagined. Internal fixation of fractures, hip and knee replacement, and correction of spinal deformity are but a few examples of how our society has benefited from the use of orthopaedic implants to decrease pain, disability, functional loss, and deformity. However, with these benefits, there is risk, including perioperative complications, long-term adverse reactions, and even failure of the device.

Most implants placed within the body function well in the intermediate to long term and obtain a homeostatic level of biocompatibility with the surrounding tissues and systemic organ systems. However, some implants continue to liberate by-products that are a function of continued use, mechanical loading protocols, exposure to biologic fluids, biodegradability, and other factors. Thus, constant vigilance for continued normal function of the implant and prompt adverse event reporting are crucial to the success of these devices in the long term. In this respect, orthopaedic device registries can play an important role. One other point relates to off-label use of orthopaedic devices. This practice is very common by orthopaedic surgeons and related specialties. The surgeon should use medical devices in an off-label manner judiciously, according to his or her best knowledge and educated good medical judgment.[55] The patient's best interests are placed above all else. Further improvements and newer orthopaedic devices for expanded indications will continue to improve the quality of life for patients.

References

1. Williams DF: On the mechanisms of biocompatibility. *Biomaterials* 2008;29(20):2941-2953.

2. Anderson JA: *Inflammation, Wound Healing, and the Foreign-Body Response*. San Diego, CA, Elsevier, 2004.

3. Kumar V, Robbins SL, Cotran RS: *Robbins Basic Pathology*, ed 7. Philadelphia, PA, Saunders, 2002.

4. Majno G, Joris I: *Cells Tissues and Disease: Principles of General Pathology*, ed 2. New York, NY, Oxford University Press, 2004.

5. American Academy of Orthopaedic Surgeons: Information about Common Musculoskeletal Diseases/Disorders. 2008. http://www.aaos.org/Research/stats/patientstats.asp.

6. Vessely MB, Whaley AL, Harmsen WS, Schleck CD, Berry DJ: The Chitranjan Ranawat Award: Long-term survivorship and failure modes of 1000 cemented condylar total knee arthroplasties. *Clin Orthop Relat Res* 2006;452:28-34.

7. Callaghan JJ, Albright JC, Goetz DD, Olejniczak JP, Johnston RC: Charnley total hip arthroplasty with cement: Minimum twenty-five-year follow-up. *J Bone Joint Surg Am* 2000;82(4):487-497.

8. Charnley J: *Low Friction Arthroplasty of the Hip*. New York, NY, Springer-Verlag, 1979.

9. Charnley J: The reaction of bone to self-curing acrylic cement: A long-term histological study in man. *J Bone Joint Surg Br* 1970;52(2):340-353.

10. Maloney WJ, Jasty M, Burke DW, et al: Biomechanical and histologic investigation of cemented total hip arthroplasties: A study of autopsy-retrieved femurs after in vivo cycling. *Clin Orthop Relat Res* 1989;249:129-140.

11. Fornasier V, Wright J, Seligman J: The histomorphologic and morphometric study of asymptomatic hip arthroplasty: A postmortem study. *Clin Orthop Relat Res* 1991;271:272-282.

12. Schmalzried TP, Kwong LM, Jasty M, et al: The mechanism of loosening of cemented acetabular components in total hip arthroplasty: Analysis of specimens retrieved at autopsy. *Clin Orthop Relat Res* 1992;274:60-78.

13. Albrektsson T, Albrektsson B: Osseointegration of bone implants: A review of an alternative mode of fixation. *Acta Orthop Scand* 1987;58(5):567-577.

14. Galante J: *Bone Ingrowth in Porous Materials*. Park Ridge, IL, American Academy of Orthopaedic Surgeons, 1985.

15. Bobyn JD, Pilliar RM, Cameron HU, Weatherly GC: The optimum pore size for the fixation of porous-surfaced metal implants by the ingrowth of bone. *Clin Orthop Relat Res* 1980;150:263-270.

16. Patil N, Lee K, Goodman SB: Porous tantalum in hip and knee reconstructive surgery. *J Biomed Mater Res B Appl Biomater* 2009;89(1):242-251.

17. Cook SD, Thomas KA, Haddad RJ Jr: Histologic analysis of retrieved human porous-coated total joint components. *Clin Orthop Relat Res* 1988;234:90-101.

18. Hirakawa K, Jacobs JJ, Urban R, Saito T: Mechanisms of failure of total hip replacements: Lessons learned from retrieval studies. *Clin Orthop Relat Res* 2004;420:10-17.

19. Engh CA, Zettl-Schaffer KF, Kukita Y, Sweet D, Jasty M, Bragdon C: Histological and radiographic assessment of well functioning porous-coated acetabular components: A human postmortem retrieval study. *J Bone Joint Surg Am* 1993;75(6):814-824.

20. Bobyn JD, Jacobs JJ, Tanzer M, et al: The susceptibility of smooth implant surfaces to periimplant fibrosis and migration of polyethylene wear debris. *Clin Orthop Relat Res* 1995; 311:21-39.

21. Stilling M, Rahbek O, Søballe K: Inferior survival of hydroxyapatite versus titanium-coated cups at 15 years. *Clin Orthop Relat Res* 2009;467(11):2872-2879.

22. Goldring SR, Schiller AL, Roelke M, Rourke CM, O'Neil DA, Harris WH: The synovial-like membrane at the bone-cement interface in loose total hip replacements and its proposed role in bone lysis. *J Bone Joint Surg Am* 1983;65(5): 575-584.

23. Goodman SB, Chin RC, Chiou SS, Schurman DJ, Woolson ST, Masada MP: A clinical-pathologic-biochemical study of the membrane surrounding loosened and nonloosened total hip arthroplasties. *Clin Orthop Relat Res* 1989;244:182-187.

24. Kadoya Y, Revell PA, al-Saffar N, Kobayashi A, Scott G, Freeman MA: Bone formation and bone resorption in failed total joint arthroplasties: Histomorphometric analysis with histochemical and immunohistochemical technique. *J Orthop Res* 1996;14(3):473-482.

25. Santavirta S, Konttinen YT, Bergroth V, Eskola A, Tallroth K, Lindholm TS: Aggressive granulomatous lesions associated with hip arthroplasty: Immunopathological studies. *J Bone Joint Surg Am* 1990;72(2):252-258.

26. Bostrom M, O'Keefe R, Implant Wear Symposium 2007 Biologic Work Group: What experimental approaches (eg, in vivo, in vitro, tissue retrieval) are effective in investigating the biologic effects of particles? *J Am Acad Orthop Surg* 2008; 16(Suppl 1):S63-S67.

27. Tuan RS, Lee FY: T Konttinen Y, Wilkinson JM, Smith RL, Implant Wear Symposium 2007 Biologic Work Group: What are the local and systemic biologic reactions and mediators to wear debris, and what host factors determine or modulate the biologic response to wear particles? *J Am Acad Orthop Surg* 2008;16(Suppl 1):S42-S48.

28. Greenfield EM, Bechtold J, Implant Wear Symposium 2007 Biologic Work Group: What other biologic and mechanical factors might contribute to osteolysis? *J Am Acad Orthop Surg* 2008;16(Suppl 1):S56-S62.

29. Schwarz EM, Implant Wear Symposium 2007 Biologic Work Group: What potential biologic treatments are available for osteolysis? *J Am Acad Orthop Surg* 2008;16(Suppl 1):S72-S75.

30. Campbell P, Shen FW, McKellop H: Biologic and tribologic considerations of alternative bearing surfaces. *Clin Orthop Relat Res* 2004;418:98-111.

31. Jarrett BT, Cofske J, Rosenberg AE, Oral E, Muratoglu O, Malchau H: In vivo biological response to vitamin E and vitamin-E-doped polyethylene. *J Bone Joint Surg Am* 2010; 92(16):2672-2681.

32. D'Antonio JA, Sutton K: Ceramic materials as bearing surfaces for total hip arthroplasty. *J Am Acad Orthop Surg* 2009; 17(2):63-68.

33. Jacobs JJ, Urban RM, Hallab NJ, Skipor AK, Fischer A, Wimmer MA: Metal-on-metal bearing surfaces. *J Am Acad Orthop Surg* 2009;17(2):69-76.

34. Willert HG, Buchhorn GH, Fayyazi A, et al: Metal-on-metal bearings and hypersensitivity in patients with artificial hip joints: A clinical and histomorphological study. *J Bone Joint Surg Am* 2005;87(1):28-36.

35. Davies AP, Willert HG, Campbell PA, Learmonth ID, Case CP: An unusual lymphocytic perivascular infiltration in tissues around contemporary metal-on-metal joint replacements. *J Bone Joint Surg Am* 2005;87(1):18-27.

36. Thomas P, Braathen LR, Dörig M, et al: Increased metal allergy in patients with failed metal-on-metal hip arthroplasty and peri-implant T-lymphocytic inflammation. *Allergy* 2009;64(8):1157-1165.

37. Mahendra G, Pandit H, Kliskey K, Murray D, Gill HS, Athanasou N: Necrotic and inflammatory changes in metal-on-metal resurfacing hip arthroplasties. *Acta Orthop* 2009; 80(6):653-659.

38. Pandit H, Glyn-Jones S, McLardy-Smith P, et al: Pseudotumours associated with metal-on-metal hip resurfacings. *J Bone Joint Surg Br* 2008;90(7):847-851.

39. Glyn-Jones S, Pandit H, Kwon YM, Doll H, Gill HS, Murray DW: Risk factors for inflammatory pseudotumour formation following hip resurfacing. *J Bone Joint Surg Br* 2009; 91(12):1566-1574.

40. Engh CA, Bobyn JD: The influence of stem size and extent of porous coating on femoral bone resorption after primary cementless hip arthroplasty. *Clin Orthop Relat Res* 1988;231: 7-28.

41. Hartzband MA, Glassman AH, Goldberg VM, et al: Survivorship of a low-stiffness extensively porous-coated femoral stem at 10 years. *Clin Orthop Relat Res* 2010;468(2):433-440.

42. McAuley JP, Sychterz CJ, Engh CA Sr: Influence of porous coating level on proximal femoral remodeling: A postmortem analysis. *Clin Orthop Relat Res* 2000;371:146-153.

43. Jones DM, Marsh JL, Nepola JV, et al: Focal osteolysis at the junctions of a modular stainless-steel femoral intramedullary nail. *J Bone Joint Surg Am* 2001;83-A(4):537-548.

44. Lewis CG, Sunderman FW Jr: Metal carcinogenesis in total joint arthroplasty: Animal models. *Clin Orthop Relat Res* 1996;(329 Suppl):S264-S268.

45. Visuri T, Pulkkinen P, Paavolainen P: Malignant tumors at the site of total hip prosthesis: Analytic review of 46 cases. *J Arthroplasty* 2006;21(3):311-323.

46. Bong MR, Kummer FJ, Koval KJ, Egol KA: Intramedullary nailing of the lower extremity: Biomechanics and biology. *J Am Acad Orthop Surg* 2007;15(2):97-106.

47. Wagner M: General principles for the clinical use of the LCP. *Injury* 2003;34(Suppl 2):B31-B42.

48. Böstman O, Pihlajamäki H: Clinical biocompatibility of biodegradable orthopaedic implants for internal fixation: A review. *Biomaterials* 2000;21(24):2615-2621.

49. Böstman OM, Pihlajamäki HK: Adverse tissue reactions to bioabsorbable fixation devices. *Clin Orthop Relat Res* 2000; 371:216-227.

50. Kurtz SM, Walker PS, Implant Wear Symposium 2007 Engineering Work Group: How have new designs and new types of joint replacement influenced wear behavior? *J Am Acad Orthop Surg* 2008;16(Suppl 1):S107-S110.

51. Jacobs JJ, Hallab NJ, Urban RM, Wimmer MA: Wear particles. *J Bone Joint Surg Am* 2006;88(Suppl 2):99-102.

52. Kurtz SM, Peloza J, Siskey R, Villarraga ML: Analysis of a retrieved polyethylene total disc replacement component. *Spine J* 2005;5(3):344-350.

53. Gunja NJ, Athanasiou KA: Biodegradable materials in arthroscopy. *Sports Med Arthrosc* 2006;14(3):112-119.

54. Kirkpatrick JS, Stevens T: The FDA process for the evaluation and approval of orthopaedic devices. *J Am Acad Orthop Surg* 2008;16(5):260-267.

55. Buch B: FDA medical device approval: Things you didn't learn in medical school or residency. *Am J Orthop* 2007; 36(8):407-412.

Chapter 22

Metabolic Bone Disease

Susan V. Bukata, MD

Wakenda K. Tyler, MD, MPH

Introduction

Bone is a dynamic organ that is constantly undergoing constructive and deconstructive processes. It is one of the few major organs in the body capable of regeneration after injury. In addition to providing structural stability, the human skeleton functions as a reservoir for calcium and phosphate and allows rapid mobilization of calcium to ensure a constant state of calcium homeostasis. The skeleton also serves as the major site of hematopoiesis for both red and white blood cells. Alterations to the bony environment and cellular milieu can have a dramatic effect on these essential functions. Metabolic bone diseases are a broad spectrum of disorders that effect the normal formation, remodeling, and mineralization of bone. These diseases may be caused by genetic, environmental, medication, other disease, or a combination of factors, but the result is compromised bone that is not optimal either as an endocrine organ for mineral storage or as a support structure for the body.

Basics of Bone Biology

There are three main cell populations that regulate bone metabolism: osteoblasts, osteocytes, and osteoclasts. The os-

teoblasts originate from mesenchymal stem cells, which in turn are derived from the paraxial and lateral plate mesoderm (the skull mesenchymal cells are derived from the neural crest). Osteocytes develop from precursor osteoblast cells and are the most abundant bone cell, occurring 10 times more frequently than the osteoblast or osteoclast.[1] In contrast, the osteoclast is derived from the mononuclear cell of the hematopoietic stem cell line (similar to monocytes and macrophages). It is induced into differentiation into a large multinucleated osteoclast by a series of cell signals, many of which are derived from osteoblasts.[1] These three cell populations work in a closely coupled system to build and resorb bone in a process known as bone remodeling. Bone, more than any other tissue, remodels through a lifelong process of existing bone breakdown and removal and new bone formation and replacement. Early in life, this process is geared toward bone building and bone mass gains. During the third through fifth decades of life, the process is fairly well balanced and bone mass remains stable. At some time during the fourth decade, a shift occurs such that bone resorption begins to exceed bone formation and a net loss in bone mass results. It is the interaction of these cells with themselves and the surrounding environment that allows for this bone remodeling process to continue throughout life.

Osteoblasts

The pluripotent mesenchymal stem cells that eventually differentiate into osteoblasts also have the ability to differentiate into other cell types, including chondroblasts, adipoblasts, and fibroblasts. The mesenchymal stem cell undergoes early osteoblastic differentiation after exposure to bone morphogenetic proteins (BMPs). BMPs are a class of molecules that belong to the transforming growth factor–β (TGF-β) superfamily of proteins.[2] They were initially discovered when they were identified as the component of demineralized bone matrix that induced the formation of subcutaneous bone nodules in mice. BMP-1, -2, and -3 were the first BMPs to be fully characterized in the 1980s. Subsequently, more than 20 different BMPs have been identified, and their roles in embryogenesis, skeletal homeostasis, and tissue regulation throughout the body are still being determined through ongoing research in the area.

BMPs are first produced intracellularly as a large precursor protein that is cleaved and then secreted as a heterodimer or homeodimer.[2] In the case of osteoblastogenesis, the BMP molecule then binds to its receptor (type 1 and 2 serine/threonine receptor kinase) on the cell surface of the mesenchymal stem cell. Binding of BMP to its receptor results in phosphorylation of intracellular molecules known as Smads. The phosphorylated Smad can join with another Smad (Smad 4) and then translocate to the nucleus, where the Smad complex initiates gene transcription specific for osteoblast differentiation.[3] It appears that BMP-2 and BMP-4 are the molecules most involved in early osteoblastic differentiation from a stem cell precursor.[2] BMP-2 and BMP-4 have been shown to induce the *cbfa-1* (core-binding factor a1) and *Runx2* genes in mesenchymal stem cells.[2] These genes, in turn, have been shown to induce osteoblast-specific genes, such as osteopontin, osteocalcin, and type I collagen.

Once the preosteoblastic cell (also known as the stromal-osteoblastic cell) has developed from a mesenchymal stem cell, several other proteins interact with the cell to further its differentiation into a terminal phase osteoblast. Along with BMPs, other TGF-β proteins, platelet-derived growth factor, fibroblast growth factor (FGF), insulin-like growth factor (IGF), and interleukin-6 (IL-6) all influence the differentiation of the preosteoblast cell into a fully activated osteoblast.[4] This osteoblast is now capable of the production of fully functional type I collagen, as well as several other proteins that make up unmineralized bone matrix (osteoid). The osteoblast is also capable of regulating the mineralization of the osteoid and receives most of its signals to do this through systemic hormones and the local environment of the bone (discussed in the following paragraphs). The development of the osteoblast is negatively regulated by several proteins that have been shown to inhibit differentiation of the mesenchymal stem cell into a preosteoblast. Molecules such as noggin and chordin have been shown to directly bind and inhibit BMP-2 and BMP-4 and thereby inhibit osteoblastic differentiation.[1]

The completely differentiated osteoblast has an approximate 3-month life span, and during that time one of its main functions is to produce osteoid. Osteoblasts produce type I collagen, which is the main type of collagen present in osteoid, as well as several noncollagenous components of osteoid, including osteocalcin and osteonectin. Type I collagen, which is a three-chained triple helix molecule with a C-terminus and N-terminus domain, undergoes extracellular modulation and becomes connected to other type I collagen

molecules through pyridinoline cross-links. Once osteoid is deposited, the osteoblast then regulates the local concentrations of calcium and phosphate to allow for hydroxyapatite formation, which thereby allows for mineralization of the osteoid. Hydroxyapatite in bone is a complex biomineral that is deposited in a highly organized manner within the bone collagen structure to provide improved mechanical properties to the bone and increased bone strength. Hydroxyapatite crystal size as well as crystal orientation relative to the collagen structure both affect bone strength and are altered in many metabolic bone diseases. Aside from the very important role of bone formation and mineralization, the osteoblast and preosteoblast cells also play a critical role in the differentiation and activity of osteoclasts. Although not a precursor cell, osteoblasts influence osteoclast function. The preosteoblast cell expresses on its surface a very important membrane-bound protein, known as receptor activator of nuclear factor–κB ligand (RANKL). RANKL can bind to preosteoclasts and osteoclasts through the osteoclast membrane receptor RANK. The binding of these two proteins, along with the presence of macrophage colony-stimulating factor leads to osteoclastogenesis from the precursor monocytic stem cell.[5] Another important regulatory molecule known as osteoprotegrin (OPG) is secreted by the osteoblast as well as several other cell types, including endothelial cells, lymphoid cells, and smooth muscle cells. OPG binds to RANKL and inhibits its ability to bind to RANK, thereby exerting a negative control on osteoclastogenesis.[5,6] Several other molecules that exert both a positive and negative effect on osteoclast maturation and activity, including cytokines such as IL-6 and IL-11, are also secreted by the osteoblast and other white blood cells to modulate osteoclast activity.[4,7]

There is another important pathway of osteoblast and osteoclast differentiation (**Figure 1**). The Wnt/β-catenin pathway has recently been found to play a very important role in osteoblastic differentiation and thereby indirectly influence osteoclastic differentiation.[8] The Wnt-mediated pathway also plays an important role in various stages of embryogenesis in the skeletal system as well as several other organ systems. There are more than 19 different Wnt molecules identified, some with overlapping activities.[9] There are two main pathways for the Wnt molecule, the canonical and noncanonical. The canonical pathway uses intracellular β-catenin, whereas the noncanonical pathway acts either independently of or as an antagonist of β-catenin. It is the canonical β-catenin–dependent pathway that has been most associated with osteoblastogenesis and bone regulation. The Wnt molecules (Wnts 1, 2, 3, 3a, 7a, 7b, 8a, 8b, and 10a) associated with the canonical pathway are secreted proteins that bind to a dual complex receptor on the cell surface of the target cell (osteoblast in this case).[9,10] The receptors Frizzled (Fz) and lipoprotein-related protein 5 (LRP5) or LRP6 conjugate together after binding with Wnt. This allows β-catenin to translocate into the nucleus of the osteoblast and upregulate genes that are specifically associated with os-

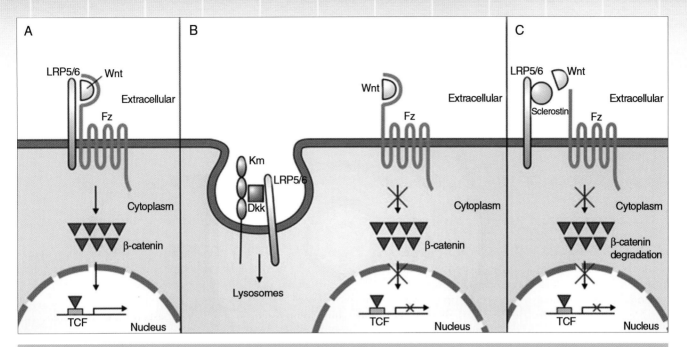

Figure I The canonical Wnt/β-catenin signaling pathway and its extracellular regulation. **A,** Extracellular binding of Wnt to the Fz–LRP5/6 receptor complex causes intracellular accumulation of β-catenin that can induce the expression of target genes after translocation to the nucleus. **B,** In the presence of Dkk and Krm, a tertiary protein complex can be made with LRP5/6 for internalization, thus inhibiting Wnt signaling as β-catenin will no longer be stabilized but will be phosphorylated and subsequently degraded. **C,** The extracellular sclerostin prevents, by binding to Fz–LRP5/6, further signaling. (Reproduced with permission from Piters E, Boudin E, Van Hol W: Wnt signaling: A win for bone. *Arch Biochem Biophysics* 2008;473:112–116.)

teoblastogenesis while at the same time β-catenin downregulates genes associated with osteoclastogenesis. It has been shown that activation of the Wnt/β-catenin pathway leads to increased OPG production and decreased RANKL production, resulting in decreased osteoclastogenesis.[8] Similarly, the Wnt/β-catenin pathway has been found to enhance mineralization by increased osteoblast activity and differentiation.

The Wnt/β-catenin pathway is a complex pathway whose components are still being studied. Like many pathways in human physiology, the Wnt/β-catenin pathway has inhibitors. There are several inhibitors that are currently under study and may prove to be important regulatory molecules. Dickkopf (DKK) is one such molecule that binds to a cell surface receptor and causes internalization of the LRP5 and LRP6 receptors.[9] This results in the inability of Wnt to bind to its receptor complex, thereby inhibiting the pathway. Similarly, sclerostin, another inhibitor of the Wnt/β-catenin pathway, is thought to directly bind to LRP5 and LRP6 receptors and block Wnt binding. Several other inhibitors of the Wnt/β-catenin pathway have been identified, such as Wnt inhibitors factor-1 (WIF1) and secreted frizzled-related protein (sFRP), and their roles in this complex pathway are still being studied.[9,11] It has been shown that these two inhibitors may even interact with each other to enhance the effects of each on osteoblast and osteoclast formation and activity.[12]

Osteocytes

A proportion of the osteoblasts eventually become embedded in the osteoid matrix and live out the rest of their lives as osteocytes. The osteocyte is not an inactive cell; there is ample evidence to support that the osteocyte may be the key regulator of mechanosensory changes in bone density that are seen as a response to loading and unloading of the bone (Wolff postulate).[9] Osteocytes have extensions of their cytoplasm that extend through the bone canaliculi to communicate and interact with other osteocytes, osteoblasts, and bone-lining cells. These extensions allow them to detect changes in the pressure that the surrounding fluid experiences and microdamage in the area. These projections allow them to sense changes in the hormonal milieu, particularly hormones such as glucocorticoids and estrogen that influence their survival. The osteocytes communicate directly with the osteoblast and bone-lining cells (also decedents of the osteoblast), which allows them to influence bone remodeling. Osteocytes function as both mechanosensors and mechanotransducers by translating mechanical force signals they experience in the bone tissue into both intracellular and intercellular biochemical signals. Gap junctions on osteocytes allow both intracellular and extracellular communication between the osteocyte and its surrounding tissue.

Osteoclasts

The mature osteoclast has a life span of only 2 weeks, but it is one of the most efficient cells in the body. These cells are

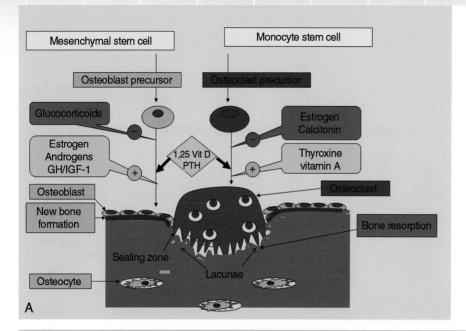

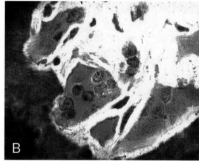

Figure 2. **A,** Factors that affect osteoblast and osteoclast activity in bone remodeling. GH = growth hormone; IGF = insulin-like growth factor; PTH = parathyroid hormone. (Adapted with permission from Valsamis HA, Arora SK: Antiepileptic drugs and bone metabolism. *Nutr Metab* 2006;3:36.) **B,** Mature osteoclasts actively resorbing bone.

responsible for the breakdown of osteoid and the release of calcium and phosphate into the bloodstream. They also break down calcium hydroxyapatite bone. Through attachments to adhesion molecules, such as integrins and cadherins, the preosteoclast cell is stimulated to migrate to an area of active bone remodeling. Once there, full differentiation occurs as a result of interactions with the osteoblasts and other environmental cytokines (released by osteoblasts or other cells in the area). In many instances, the modulation of osteoclasts is through the stimulation of osteoblasts to secrete specific proteins that directly act on the osteoclast. It is also true that osteoclasts can be influenced directly to either continue to be active or to undergo apoptosis. Molecules such as tumor necrosis factor, granulocyte-macrophage colony-stimulating factor, and several members of the TGF-β family can influence osteoclast activity both through their action on osteoblasts and directly through the osteoclast or preosteoclast itself.[7]

Once fully differentiated, the osteoclast is a very large, multinucleated cell that has a unique feature known as the ruffled border (Figure 2). The attachment of the osteoclast to surface adhesion molecules is thought to play a role in the polarization of the cell, allowing the ruffled border to face the bone surface. The ruffled border is a series of fingerlike projections in the cytoplasm of the cell that allow for increased surface area. This area is surrounded by the clear zone, which has a smooth surface and facilitates the attachment of the osteoclast to the bone. Once attached to the bone, the osteoclast produces an acidic environment through an adenosine triphosphate-fueled proton pump.[7] The mineral matrix is dissolved as a result of this acidic en-

vironment, but the protein components that make up the osteoid must be degraded by matrix metalloproteinases and cathepsins (cathepsins K, B, and L). The degraded osteoid is endocytosed by the osteoclast and transported to the cell membrane opposite the ruffled border and then secreted from the cell. Established bone in the form of calcium hydroxyapatite is broken down in a similar manner.

Hormones Influencing Bone Remodeling

There are several major systemic hormones that act to influence the development, life span, and activity of osteocytes. There are two main hormones that largely affect osteoclast and osteoblast differentiation and activity. Parathyroid hormone (PTH) and 1,25-dihydroxyvitamin D (1,25-vitamin D) both work in concert to raise serum calcium levels and as antagonists in bone remodeling and mineralization.[13,14] Other systemic hormones such as estrogens, androgens, and calcitonin also affect bone remodeling. Estrogen, androgen, and exogenous glucocorticoids influence both osteoblastic and osteoclastic development through their ability to regulate the production of cytokines by other cells. Both estrogen and androgen have been found to suppress IL-6 and IL-6 receptor production, resulting in suppression of osteoclastic function.[4] Loss of estrogen and androgen results in increased bone turnover. Estrogen has also been shown to directly initiate osteoclast apoptosis and therefore lack of it results in an increased life span of the osteoclast. Exogenous glucocorticoids, on the other hand, have been found to promote osteoblast and osteocyte apoptosis, and to inhibit osteoblastogenesis. They also have an effect on 1,25-vitamin D formation.[15] Calcitonin is known to counter the effects of

Table 1

Daily Calcium Requirements by Age

Age	Recommended Daily Calcium Intake
0-6 months	200 mg
7-12 months	260 mg
1-3 years	700 mg
4-8 years	1,000 mg
9-18 years	1,300 mg
19-50 years	1,000 mg
50 years or older	1,200 mg
Pregnant or lactating woman	1,300 mg

Source: Institute of Medicine

PTH. In the presence of high serum calcium levels, calcitonin is secreted by the parafollicular cells in the thyroid and acts to decrease serum calcium levels. It has receptors both in the kidney and on osteoclasts.

Markers of Bone Remodeling

Bone remodeling is a complex process, and several markers allow determination of the rate of bone turnover in patients. This can be very helpful in diagnosing a pathologic state as well as monitoring treatment.[16] Alkaline phosphatase is a protein produced by osteoblasts and is thought to play a role in bone mineralization. In states of increased osteoblastic activity, serum alkaline phosphatase levels can be elevated. Alkaline phosphatase is also produced by the liver and can be elevated in states of liver injury, so bone-specific forms of the protein must be studied for this to be a useful test. Osteocalcin is one of the major noncollagenous components of osteoid, and its presence at high levels in the serum suggests increased osteoclastic breakdown of mineralized bone. It is often used as a marker for patients' response to antiresorptive treatment of osteoporosis, with an anticipated decline in serum levels with a good response to treatment. N-terminal telopeptide (NTX) is another marker of increased bone turnover. It represents the cleavage product of type I collagen. It was mentioned previously that type I collagen has an N- and-C terminus domain; NTX represents the N-terminal domain of type I collagen. It is usually measured in the urine of patients (the second urination of the day) and again is frequently used to determine response to treatment, with an expected decrease in levels over time. Similar to NTX, the pyridinoline cross-links of collagen are excreted into the urine following osteoclastic activity. They can also be used as markers of increased bone turnover.

Basics of Mineral Metabolism

In addition to providing physical structure to the body, the skeleton functions as an integral part of the endocrine system. It is the principal storage center for calcium (99% of body total) and the first structure that can provide additional calcium if needed. Most calcium is actively absorbed in the duodenum through calcium-binding protein. In an average adult, this active absorption mechanism saturates at 500 to 600 mg oral intake at any one time, with the unabsorbed calcium excreted in fecal matter. In the kidney, approximately 98% of filtered calcium is reabsorbed, 85% passively in the proximal tubule and loop of Henle and the remainder actively in the distal convoluted tubule. The calcium not reabsorbed by the kidney is excreted in the urine. Calcium balance that prevents calcium from being drawn out of the skeleton occurs when daily intestinal absorption equals renal excretion. Daily dietary intake recommendations for calcium vary with age (Table 1), and a combination of food plus supplements can be used to achieve these levels. Patients with intestinal malabsorption issues, including celiac disease (wheat gluten sensitivity), gastric bypass, and diseases affecting the small bowel, may not absorb sufficient calcium from oral intake to maintain balance. In the kidney, additional calcium can be lost in the urine if calcium exchange channels responsible for passive reabsorption are faulty, or when medications (furosemide, heparin, corticosteroids, tetracycline) decrease calcium reabsorption. Thiazide diuretics (hydrochlorothiazide, chlorthalidone) increase calcium reabsorption through renal channels and can be used to help patients who have excess renal calcium loss.[17]

Vitamin D is a fat-soluble hormone that is important for calcium regulation and bone health. Vitamin D can be obtained from the diet or produced in the skin fueled by UV exposure. In the skin, 7-dehydrocholesterol is converted to cholecalciferol (vitamin D_3) after exposure to sunlight. The quantity of sunlight required to produce sufficient quantities varies due to individual characteristics such as age and skin tone, as well as external factors such as sunlight strength (which varies with latitude and season), sunblock (SPF 8 blocks 95% of vitamin D production in the skin), and protective clothing. Vitamin D can also be obtained through the diet as cholecalciferol (vitamin D_3) from animal sources, or as ergocalciferol (vitamin D_2) from plants and yeast. All forms of vitamin D are then hydroxylated at the 25th carbon in the liver to form 25-hydroxyvitamin D (25-vitamin D), which is the principal storage form for vitamin D in the body and the level that is reported with clinical vitamin D testing for most patients. This is the level that is used to describe whether the patient is vitamin D sufficient or deficient. This reservoir of 25-vitamin D is then processed by the 1α-hydroxylase in the kidney to form 1,25-dihydroxyvitamin D. This is the active form of vitamin D that provides the tissue effect of vitamin D. Only the vitamin D hydroxylated in the kidney is measured in the serum as circulating 1,25-vitamin D. However, 85% of all vitamin

D used by the body is processed by other tissues (immune cells, a variety of epithelial cells) that contain 1α-hydroxylase and used by those tissues locally. The half-life of 25-vitamin D is several weeks, whereas the half-life of 1,25-vitamin D is only a few hours. Patients with renal impairment (glomerular filtration rate < 40) or renal diseases that severely affect renal function may not be able to adequately produce 1,25-vitamin D quantities and require supplementation with this form of vitamin D (calcitriol). Patients with good renal function should not require testing of 1,25-vitamin D levels, and supplementation with precursor forms of vitamin D should correct any deficiencies.[18]

For the skeletal system, vitamin D plays several roles. In the kidney it increases calcium reabsorption in the proximal tubule. In the intestine, it regulates the production of calcium-binding protein and thus influences gut absorption of calcium. It also increases intestinal absorption of phosphorous, although the mechanism is not known. In bone, vitamin D receptors on osteoblasts stimulate RANKL production, which influences osteoclast development and activity. Vitamin D also regulates Runx2, which regulates osteoblast differentiation and appears to affect bone formation. Appropriate vitamin D levels remain highly debated, but currently vitamin D deficiency is considered to be present with serum 25-vitamin D levels of 20 ng/mL or less. At these levels rickets, osteomalacia, and hypocalcemia may be present. Although most newly formed bone is mineralized with 25-vitamin D levels over 20 ng/mL, mineralization rates do not plateau until the serum level reaches the low 40 ng/mL range.[19] In women older than 60 years, gait speed and lower extremity function tests also continue to improve until serum 25-vitamin D levels reach 40 ng/mL.[20,21] Vitamin D supplementation can be given as ergocalciferol (vitamin D_2) in 50,000 IU supplements and as cholecalciferol (vitamin D_3) in a variety of doses ranging from 400 to 50,000 IU. Physiologically, the body is able to recognize the differences between the D_2 and D_3 moieties, and 50,000 IU of vitamin D_2 is essentially functionally equivalent to 10,000 IU of vitamin D_3. Patient supplemental needs are highly variable and dependent on body fat (which sequesters vitamin D), intestinal absorption if given as supplements, and skin production efficiency (which declines with age). In general, oral supplementation of 1,000 IU daily of vitamin D_3 will raise serum 25-vitamin D levels by a maximum of 7 ng/mL, with obesity and advanced age each reducing that increase by up to 50%.[22]

PTH regulates serum calcium levels and can have both an anabolic and a catabolic effect on bone. Receptors in the parathyroid gland respond to low serum calcium levels and stimulate the chief cells in the parathyroid gland to secrete hormone. Receptors on osteoblasts respond to PTH and increase signaling to osteoclasts to increase bone resorption and release calcium into the serum. In the kidney, PTH increases calcium reabsorption, decreases phosphate reabsorption, and increases 1α-hydroxylase activity to produce more 1,25-vitamin D. This increases calcium binding pro-duction in the intestine and has the greatest quantitative effect on available serum calcium. Parathyroid hormone-related protein, which is produced by some cancers, can have a similar effect and cause hypercalcemia associated with malignancy. Elevation of PTH levels is the appropriate physiologic response to low calcium levels and can be seen transiently after large boluses of intravenous fluids (such as during surgery or with medical treatments) or can be sustained in response to low vitamin D levels (termed secondary hyperparathyroidism), certain medications and medical conditions, or renal disease. When PTH levels remain within physiologic range, PTH can have an anabolic effect on osteoblasts, increasing bone formation at a greater level than osteoclastic bone resorption and resulting in a net gain in bone mass.[23]

Calcitonin is secreted by the parafollicular cells (also known as C cells) of the thyroid gland and interacts with a G protein–coupled receptor on the osteoclast. A physical change occurs in the shape and activity of the osteoclast and bone resorption is inhibited. The physiologic significance of calcitonin in humans is not clear, and patients who undergo thyroidectomy do not have any notable deficit associated with calcitonin loss. Calcitonin has been used historically in treatment of both osteoporosis and Paget disease, but other antiresorptive medications have supplanted its use.

Metabolic Bone Diseases

Osteoporosis

Bone strength is the basic parameter that provides fracture resistance to bone. Bone strength is determined by a complex combination of bone mass, bone architecture, collagen structure and strength, bone mineralization, and bone remodeling. Osteoporosis is a disease characterized by low bone mass and a microarchitectural deterioration of bone tissue that results in enhanced bone fragility and a consequent increase in fracture risk. Essentially, osteoporosis is a disease where bone strength is reduced and bones become susceptible to fracture, even with low-energy trauma. A fragility fracture is defined as a fracture occurring from low-energy trauma such as a fall from standing height or less. Osteoporosis is the most common metabolic bone disease in US adults older than 50 years and if untreated, 50% of women and 20% of men will suffer a fragility fracture in their lifetime. One of the greatest challenges in diagnosis and treatment of osteoporosis is estimating fracture risk. Although contributors such as age, bone mineral density (as measured by dual-energy x-ray absorptiometry scan), and bone turnover rates can be measured, many of the elements that are thought to contribute to bone quality (collagen, mineral structure, mineralization rates, trabecular structure and connectivity) are difficult to measure except with an invasive bone biopsy and may vary with skeletal location. One of the best estimators of future fracture risk is a prior fragility fracture in an adult individual. Orthopaedic surgeons are in a unique position to identify these high-risk individuals

Table 2
Secondary Causes of Osteoporosis

Vitamin D deficiency

Autoimmune disease

Glucocorticoid therapy (5 mg prednisone daily for ≥3 months)

Eating disorder

Malabsorption diseases (celiac, gastric bypass, small intestine disorders)

Hormonal suppressive agents (for breast and prostate cancer treatment)

Cushing disease

Hypogonadism

Malignancy

Hypothyroidism

Hyperthyroidism

Hyperparathyroidism

HIV

Table 3
Treatment of Osteoporosis

Antiresorptive	Anabolic
Bisphosphonates	PTH
Selective estrogen receptor modulators	Antisclerostin antibody (in research development)
Denosumab (RANKL inhibitors)	Anti–DKK-1 antibody (in research development)
Estrogen	Strontium (some derivitives not available in US)
Calcitonin	
Cathepsin K inhibitors (in research development)	
Strontium (some derivatives not available in US)	

and direct them toward appropriate osteoporosis care.[24]

During growth and development, people continue to gain bone mass until approximately age 25 years, then after age 30 years, they begin a chronic phase of bone loss. Women experience bone loss at a greater rate than men, exacerbated by an almost decade-long period of accelerated bone loss around the time of menopause before settling back to the baseline loss rate associated with aging. Genetics appears to play a significant role (possibly 60% to 80%) in many of the factors that contribute to bone structure and bone strength. Except in the situation of a few rare diseases of bone fragility, the genetic contribution to osteoporosis risk appears to be multifactorial and involve interactions between multiple genes.[25] Elements such as bone size, bone shape, and bone density have strong genetic associations. This genetic predisposition combined with environmental factors contributes to an individual's fracture risk. Currently the fracture risk assessment tool, or FRAX, highlights several of the other factors that contribute to fracture risk, including age, ethnicity, personal history of fragility fracture, parental history of fragility fracture, female sex, low body mass, smoking, glucocorticoid use, autoimmune disease, and alcohol intake of three units or more daily.[26] Some of these factors are modifiable, or under the patient's control to change, whereas others are not. Several other diseases and conditions can increase bone loss and fracture risk and are considered secondary causes of osteoporosis (Table 2). One third of postmenopausal women and two thirds of men and premenopausal women have a secondary cause contributing to their osteoporosis that must be addressed to adequately control osteoporosis progression.[27]

Epidemiologic studies of osteoporosis and fracture risk have identified several genes that appear to play a significant role in bone strength. Osteogenesis imperfecta, the genetic disease of severe bone fragility and increased fracture risk, is associated with severe defects in the collagen type Ia1 gene (COL1A1). This same gene has been shown to be related to both bone mineral density and fracture risk in the general population. LRP5 is associated with a low bone mass disorder with loss of function (osteoporosis-pseudoglioma syndrome), and a disorder of increased bone mass with gain of function. Polymorphisms have also been associated with variable bone mass levels in men. A loss of function in the sclerostin gene (SOST) is associated with a high bone mass disorder and increased fracture resistance (sclerosteosis), an observation that has led to research and development of an antisclerostin antibody for possible use in the treatment of osteoporosis.[28]

Treatment of osteoporosis focuses on two strategies: antiresoptive and anabolic (Table 3). Estrogen, which was the mainstay of therapy for many years, is important in maintaining skeletal homeostasis in growth and development, and loss of estrogen at menopause causes increased bone remodeling rates and subsequent bone loss. The exact mechanism of action of estrogen is not completely understood, but the RANK/RANKL/OPG pathway appears to play a role, especially at menopause. The relative ratio of RANKL and OPG appears to change at menopause, so that more RANKL signal is available to stimulate osteoclast development and activity. After several years, this imbalance reaches a new steady state and rapid bone loss slows. Estrogen with progesterone has been associated with increased risk of breast cancer and increased cardiovascular events, including heart attack and stroke, limiting its use in the postmenopausal population. Similar studies of estrogen alone in women who have had a hysterectomy (because estrogen alone increases the risk of endometrial cancer) actually showed a significant decreased risk of breast cancer, but cardiovascular risk persisted. Both arms of the study (estrogen with progesterone and estrogen alone) showed a clear reduction in fracture risk from estrogen treatment, from 30% to 70% depending upon anatomic site.[29] Selective estrogen receptor modulators (SERMs) are not hormones themselves but work through selective activation of estrogen receptors. The SERMs used in osteoporosis treatments are agonists to bone while being antagonists to breast. They decrease rates of bone loss as well as decrease rates of breast cancer (in women in whom breast cancer has not been diagnosed). SERMs demonstrate fracture reduction in the spine, but not in the hip.[30] Both estrogen and SERMs lose their protective effect when they are stopped, returning the patient to a period of increased bone loss such as that seen at menopause. For that reason, estrogen is often tapered off in these patients slowly over several years and additional osteoporosis treatments added if necessary.

Bisphosphonates are analogs of pyrophosphate and bind to the surface of hydroxyapatite crystals in the bone. They are released during cycles of bone remodeling and inhibit osteoclast function through the mevalonate pathway. This pathway, which includes the HMG Co-A reductase pathway through which statins exert their physiologic effects in other tissues, interferes with protein prenylation and transit of cell produced vesicles through the cell membrane. For osteoclasts, this reduces the delivery of protons and lysosomal enzymes and induces cellular apoptosis. Fewer osteoclasts are active and fewer osteoclasts develop, resulting in decreased bone turnover and remodeling rates.[31] Bisphosphonates are available in both oral and intravenous forms and are effective in decreasing bone turnover rates. Currently prescribed second- and third-generation bisphosphosphonates decrease spine fracture risk, but nonvertebral fracture risk varies among the medications.[32-34] Bisphosphonates have a long half-life in the skeleton, and termination of use after a steady state is reached permits sustained efficacy for a period of time. Recent concerns about long-term use of bisphosphonates has resulted in the US Food and Drug Administration statement that safety and efficacy for these drugs is really only known for the length of their individual clinical trials. Use beyond these time periods should be done with caution and further research is certainly needed. Rare clinical events, such as osteonecrosis of the jaw and atypical femur fractures, have been associated with extended periods of bisphosphonate use, but the exact mechanism and association with bisphosphonates is not fully elucidated.[32-34]

Denosumab is the first drug developed to specifically modulate the RANK/RANKL/OPG signaling pathway that controls osteoclast development and activity. Denosumab is a human monoclonal antibody that acts as a decoy receptor for RANKL. This inhibits the development and activation of osteoclasts and decreases bone resorption rates. The anti-

body clears approximately every 6 months so that efficacy is lost unless additional doses are received. This potent antiresorptive agent has also been associated with rare cases of osteonecrosis of the jaw, although like bisphosphonates, the exact mechanism is not clear. Unlike bisphosphonates, which are cleared intact through the kidneys, drug clearance is not renal dependent, and renal function declines (glomerular filtration rate <35) are not a contraindication for use. In patients with low renal function (glomerular filtration rate <35), posttreatment hypocalcemia occurs more frequently.[35]

Calcitonin is a nonsex, nonsteroid hormone that binds to osteoclasts and causes a change in osteoclast cell shape and structure through an unknown mechanism, although effects on the osteoclast cytoskeleton are suspected to be involved. This leads to a decrease in osteoclast activity and number and a reduction in vertebral fracture, but no effect on nonvertebral fracture including hip fracture. Calcitonin is given as a nasal spray for osteoporosis, although previously injectable forms were used to treat Paget disease. Calcitonin nasal spray has been noted to have an analgesic effect for painful vertebral fractures, but its mechanism is unknown.[36]

Strontium is a divalent cation available as strontium ranelate, which attaches to the hydroxyapatite crystal. Strontium ranelate is not available in the United States for treatment of osteoporosis, but is available elsewhere. Strontium appears to have both antiresorptive and mild anabolic effects on bone. Strontium stimulates preosteoblast differentiation to osteoblasts and possible bone formation activity. It also stimulates osteoblasts to produce increased quantities of OPG, which inhibits osteoclast formation and activity through the RANKL signaling pathway.[37]

PTH hormone is the only anabolic agent that is currently available for osteoporosis treatment. It is available in the United States in the 1-34 amino acid form, with the full-length 1-84 amino acid molecule also available in other countries. The first 29 amino acids are needed for the bone anabolic function of the molecule whereas the remaining amino acids provide half-life stability to the molecule. The receptor for PTH is present on osteoblasts and preosteoblasts, and intermittent doses stimulate bone formation at a greater rate than bone resorption, resulting in a net anabolic effect on bone. Sustained dosing or secretion by the parathyroid gland results in increased osteoclast activity and bone resorption, such as seen in hyperparathyroidism. The anabolic effect of PTH leads to bone formation of the surface of cortical and trabecular bone and reconnection of disrupted trabeculae. Duration of anabolic affect is limited, and with sustained usage, osteoclastic activity reaches a new balance with osteoblastic activity and the net anabolic effect is lost. With current available forms, this net anabolic effect is sustained for several months while under treatment. The newly formed bone is indistinguishable from normal bone and is maintained after treatment cessation in the same manner that normal bone is maintained.[38]

Several agents are currently under investigation as potential treatments of osteoporosis. Cathepsin K is a lysosomal enzyme responsible for the degradation of bone collagen by osteoclasts. Cathepsin K inhibitors interfere with osteoclast resorptive function and prevent bone loss. The WNT signaling pathway is involved in bone formation through the LRP5 pathway, and both sclerostin and DKK-1 are known inhibitors of this pathway. Antibodies to sclerostin and DKK-1 have been developed as potential intermittent-dosed anabolic agents. Several other pathways remain under basic science investigation.[39]

Osteomalacia and Rickets

Undermineralized newly formed bone is the hallmark of both osteomalacia and rickets. Both diseases are present in children with open growth plates, whereas only osteomalacia occurs in adults whose growth plates are already closed. This undermineralization creates weak areas within the bones and increases susceptibility to microfractures as well as low-energy trauma fractures. In these conditions, bone biopsy shows widening of osteoid seams by the lack of mineralization and smudging of tetracycline labels from the slow mineralization rate. On radiographs, bones begin to appear osteopenic and stress fractures with radiodense lines adjacent to regions of radiolucency (called Looser lines) begin to appear on the concave sides of long bones. In growth plates, the lack of mineralization in the provisional zone of calcification leads to widening and metaphyseal flaring. This undermineralization of growing bones can lead to frontal skull bossing, enlarged costochondral junctions (the rachitic rosary), bowing of long bones, growth plate cupping and deformity, and delayed eruption of permanent teeth. In children and adults, in addition to increased fracture risk, proximal muscle weakness and gait instability can occur. Laboratory findings for osteomalacia and rickets include elevated PTH and bone-specific alkaline phosphatase, with low to low normal serum calcium and low 25-vitamin D levels.[40,41]

Most cases of osteomalacia and rickets are associated with nutritional vitamin D deficiency and are the result of inadequate intestinal calcium absorption. Treatment is correction of the vitamin D deficiency. Several genetic anomalies can also result in osteomalacia and rickets. Deficiency in 1α-hydroxylase prevents vitamin D conversion to the active 1,25-dihydroxyvitamin D. Treatment involves supplementation with calcitriol. Mutations affecting the vitamin D receptor can be treated with high doses of vitamin D or its metabolites, although this treatment does not completely resolve the problems associated with this receptor anomaly.[41] A mutation in the PHEX gene leads to X-linked hypophosphatemic rickets, and supplementation with both vitamin D and phosphate is necessary to manage the skeletal effects.[42] Both benign and malignant tumors can secrete factors that cause osteomalacia (referred to as oncogenic osteomalacia). FGF-23 has been associated with hemangiopericytoma, fibrosarcoma, and osteosarcoma, and in rare cases with fibrous dysplasia. FGF-23 inhibits phosphate re-

absorption in the kidney and reduces the production of 1,25-vitamin D. Preferred treatment is excision of the responsible tumor, but if this is not possible, then treatment with phosphate and calcitriol is used.[43] Osteomalacia associated with renal disease as a result of complex issues with calcium, phosphate, and vitamin D metabolism is discussed later in this chapter.

Primary Hyperparathyroidism

Excessive PTH production results in net calcium release from the skeleton and resulting hypercalcemia. Most of the clinical sequelae are a result of this hypercalcemia. Associated laboratory anomalies include elevated PTH, calcium, and bone alkaline phosphatase levels with a low serum phosphate level. Both calcium and phosphate levels are elevated in the urine. Demineralization of bones, mostly cortical, can be seen on radiographs, and in sustained cases, brown tumors of bone can be seen. Most cases occur from a solitary adenoma on one of the four parathyroid glands. Gene rearrangements in the PRAD-1 oncogene with overexpression of the cyclin D1 gene have been seen in these tumors. In some cases, hyperplasia of all four glands is seen. Treatment can be observation only if vitamin D levels are within the normal range and only asymptomatic hypercalcemia is present. Otherwise, surgical excision of the parathyroid gland with the adenoma or excision of part of the hyperplastic glands is used for treatment. After treatment, bone mass gradually improves, but it can take several years for maximal recovery to occur.[44]

Renal Osteodystrophy (or Chronic Kidney Disease Mineral Bone Disorder)

In the advanced stages of kidney disease, problems with renal clearance of phosphate and low 1α-hydroxylase levels leads to high serum phosphate levels and low serum calcium levels. Parathyroid glands are stimulated to increase hormone production in an attempt to raise serum calcium levels. Eventually, hyperplasia of the parathyroid glands results, and the bone develops a resistance to the ability of PTH to liberate calcium from the skeleton. Before the mid-1980s, aluminum-based phosphate binders were used in patients with renal failure. Aluminum deposited in the skeleton prevents mineralization of newly formed bone, further exacerbating the osteomalacia associated with renal disease. Iron and lanthanum can also accumulate in the skeleton of the patient with renal disease and interfere with bone mineralization.[45] FGF-23 levels rise with progressive renal disease, but it is unclear if mineralization is also impaired by FGF-23 in renal disease.[46] Secondary hyperparathyroidism and osteomalacia develop, leading to increased risk of fragility fractures, especially of the ribs and spine. β2-microglobulin amyloidosis can also occur, further weakening bone and disrupting musculoskeletal tissues. In rare advanced cases of renal-associated bone disease, a decline of osteoblast function leads to adynamic bone and minimal bone formation capacity. Treatment involves careful management of phosphate, calcium, vitamin D, and bone turnover in the early stages of renal failure with the added management of acidosis as disease progresses. Parathyroid glands many need surgical excision in cases of severe hyperparathyroidism.[47]

Osteopetrosis

Osteopetrosis describes a group of genetic disorders that result in osteoclast dysfunction and a deficiency in bone and cartilage resorption. Osteoclasts may be present in high numbers, but defective in function, or decreased or almost absent in the skeleton. Bone formation remains normal and a diffuse increase in skeletal density occurs. The newly formed bone is immature woven bone, and due to the remodeling defect, does not get remodeled into lamellar bone. Despite the dense, sclerotic appearance on radiographs, bone is fragile and susceptible to fracture. Four major phenotypes are recognized. Most patients have the autosomal dominant form (adult or tarda form) and experience a normal life span with mild anemia and increased skeletal fragility. Patients also can experience hearing loss, carpal tunnel syndrome, slipped capital femoral epiphysis, and osteomyelitis of the mandible. The most severe form is the autosomal recessive infantile (or malignant) form that results in severe anemia, thrombocytopenia, hepatosplenomegaly, immune system compromise, and cranial and optic nerve palsies. Most patients die in early childhood. An intermediate form exists with severity between adult and infantile forms. An autosomal recessive mutation in the carbonic anhydrase II gene results in osteopetrosis associated with renal tubular acidosis, cerebral calcifications, and mental retardation. More recently an X-linked form of the disease, termed OL-EDA-ID, was identified in boys having osteopetrosis, lymphedema, and an anhydrotic ectodermal dysplasia. Treatment depends upon the type of disease, with the severe infantile form sometimes responding to early bone marrow transplant and gamma interferon treatment and milder forms treated with 1,25-vitamin D supplementation and a course of PTH to stimulate bone remodeling in adulthood.[48]

Paget Disease

Paget disease, which is a localized disorder of bone remodeling, is the second most common metabolic bone disease. Little is known about the pathogenesis of Paget disease, but the clinical presentation has some common features. In the affected bone, a local increase in osteoclastic bone resorption occurs with an increase in bone formation that results in a disordered woven and lamellar bone pattern. The process tends to spread across the affected bone, causing an increase in bone size and a dense sclerotic appearance on radiographs. The newly formed bone is also hypervascular and susceptible to microfracture that can result in bowing deformity. For most patients, this process is asymptomatic, and the sequelae are seen incidentally on radiographs. Other patients experience pain from the microfracture and secondary arthritic changes from the bone expansion, not the bony deformity, or experience symptoms associated with nerve compression in nerve adjacent to the affected bones.[49]

Although a direct genetic link to Paget disease has not been found, studies of patient cohorts suggest a genetic predisposition in an autosomal dominant pattern in affected families. Paget disease is more common in persons of Anglo-Saxon decent. An association with a chronic paramyxoviral infection has been noted, with cytoplasmic inclusions that are characteristic of this family of viruses seen in osteoclasts from patients with Paget disease. Measles virus, respiratory syncytial virus, and canine distemper virus have all been suggested as candidates from the paramyxovirus family, but none has been directly associated with Paget disease. The reason for recent rapid decreases in Paget disease incidence is not known, but either vaccination or decreased exposure to the responsible virus has been proposed as a possible mechanism for this change.[50]

Bisphosphonates that control osteoclast activity and bone resorption have become the mainstay of treatment of symptomatic individuals. Diagnosis is confirmed when elevated bone alkaline phosphatase and urine N-telopeptide levels are seen, and treatment continues until these levels decline to normal levels. In most instances this provides sustained remission of the condition; however, recurrence of the increased osteoclast activity in the same bone or disease presenting in another bone can occur.

Summary

Orthopaedic surgeons need to have a fundamental understanding of the metabolic bone diseases discussed in this chapter because these diseases compromise bone strength and potentially increase fracture risk. A number of patients treated by orthopaedic surgeons, particularly in the population older than 50 years, are at risk for a metabolic bone disease, including those patients who seek elective orthopaedic care such as joint replacement and spine surgery. Knowledge of the diagnosis and treatment modalities will help orthopaedic surgeons take an active role in the diagnosis and treatment of these diseases. Identification of the at-risk patient and appropriate referral are extremely important to ensuring ongoing care of these patients.

References

1. Manolagas SC: Birth and death of bone cells: Basic regulatory mechanisms and implications for the pathogenesis and treatment of osteoporosis. *Endocr Rev* 2000;21(2):115-137.

2. Li X, Cao X: BMP signaling and skeletogenesis. *Ann N Y Acad Sci* 2006;1068:26-40.

3. Bahamonde ME, Lyons KM: BMP3: To be or not to be a BMP. *J Bone Joint Surg Am* 2001;83(pt 1, suppl 1):S56-S62.

4. Manolagas SC: The role of IL-6 type cytokines and their receptors in bone. *Ann N Y Acad Sci* 1998;840:194-204.

5. Trouvin AP, Goëb V: Receptor activator of nuclear

factor-κB ligand and osteoprotegerin: Maintaining the balance to prevent bone loss. *Clin Interv Aging* 2010;5:345-354.

6. Lacey DL, Timms E, Tan HL, et al: Osteoprotegerin ligand is a cytokine that regulates osteoclast differentiation and activation. *Cell* 1998;93(2):165-176.

7. Boyle WJ, Simonet WS, Lacey DL: Osteoclast differentiation and activation. *Nature* 2003;423(6937):337-342.

8. Tamura M, Nemoto E, Sato MM, Nakashima A, Shimauchi H: Role of the Wnt signaling pathway in bone and tooth. *Front Biosci (Elite Ed)* 2010;2:1405-1413.

9. Bonewald LF, Johnson ML: Osteocytes, mechanosensing and Wnt signaling. *Bone* 2008;42(4):606-615.

10. Boyden LM, Mao J, Belsky J, et al: High bone density due to a mutation in LDL-receptor-related protein 5. *N Engl J Med* 2002;346(20):1513-1521.

11. Ducy P, Zhang R, Geoffroy V, Ridall AL, Karsenty G: Osf2/Cbfa1: A transcriptional activator of osteoblast differentiation. *Cell* 1997;89(5):747-754.

12. Tao J, Chen S, Lee B: Alteration of Notch signaling in skeletal development and disease. *Ann N Y Acad Sci* 2010;1192:257-268.

13. Miao D, He B, Karaplis AC, Goltzman D: Parathyroid hormone is essential for normal fetal bone formation. *J Clin Invest* 2002;109(9):1173-1182.

14. Goltzman D: Emerging roles for calcium-regulating hormones beyond osteolysis. *Trends Endocrinol Metab* 2010;21(8):512-518.

15. Hansen KE, Wilson HA, Zapalowski C, Fink HA, Minisola S, Adler RA: Uncertainties in the prevention and treatment of glucocorticoid-induced osteoporosis. *J Bone Miner Res* 2011;26(9):1989-1996.

16. Brown JP, Albert C, Nassar BA, et al: Bone turnover markers in the management of postmenopausal osteoporosis. *Clin Biochem* 2009;42(10-11):929-942.

17. Emkey RD, Emkey GR: Calcium metabolism and correcting calcium deficiencies. *Endocrinol Metab Clin North Am* 2012;41(3):527-556.

18. Holick MF: Vitamin D deficiency. *N Engl J Med* 2007;357(3):266-281.

19. Priemel M, von Domarus C, Klatte TO, et al: Bone mineralization defects and vitamin D deficiency: Histomorphometric analysis of iliac crest bone biopsies and circulating 25-hydroxyvitamin D in 675 patients. *J Bone Miner Res* 2010;25(2):305-312.

20. Wicherts IS, van Schoor NM, Boeke AJ, et al: Vitamin D status predicts physical performance and its decline in older persons. *J Clin Endocrinol Metab* 2007;92(6):2058-2065.

21. Bischoff-Ferrari HA, Dawson-Hughes B, Staehelin HB, et al: Fall prevention with supplemental and active forms of vitamin D: A meta-analysis of randomised controlled trials. *BMJ* 2009;339:b3692.

22. Lee P, Greenfield JR, Seibel MJ, Eisman JA, Center JR: Adequacy of vitamin D replacement in severe deficiency is dependent on body mass index. *Am J Med* 2009;122(11):1056-1060.

23. Silva BC, Costa AG, Cusano NE, Kousteni S, Bilezikian JP: Catabolic and anabolic actions of parathyroid hormone on the skeleton. *J Endocrinol Invest* 2011;34(10):801-810.

24. Unnanuntana A, Gladnick BP, Donnelly E, Lane JM: The assessment of fracture risk. *J Bone Joint Surg Am* 2010;92(3):743-753.

25. Ralston SH, Uitterlinden AG: Genetics of osteoporosis. *Endocr Rev* 2010;31(5):629-662.

26. Kanis JA, Johnell O, Oden A, Johansson H, McCloskey E: FRAX and the assessment of fracture probability in men and women from the UK. *Osteoporos Int* 2008;19(4):385-397.

27. Painter SE, Kleerekoper M, Camacho PM: Secondary osteoporosis: A review of the recent evidence. *Endocr Pract* 2006;12(4):436-445.

28. Rachner TD, Khosla S, Hofbauer LC: Osteoporosis: Now and the future. *Lancet* 2011;377(9773):1276-1287.

29. Rossouw JE, Anderson GL, Prentice RL, et al: Risks and benefits of estrogen plus progestin in healthy postmenopausal women: Principal results from the Women's Health Initiative randomized controlled trial. *JAMA* 2002;288(3):321-333.

30. Ettinger B, Black DM, Mitlak BH, et al: Reduction of vertebral fracture risk in postmenopausal women with osteoporosis treated with raloxifene: Results from a 3-year randomized clinical trial. *JAMA* 1999;282(7):637-645.

31. Russell RG, Watts NB, Ebetino FH, Rogers MJ: Mechanisms of action of bisphosphonates: Similarities and differences and their potential influence on clinical efficacy. *Osteoporos Int* 2008;19(6):733-759.

32. Black DM, Thompson DE, Bauer DC, et al: Fracture risk reduction with alendronate in women with osteoporosis: The Fracture Intervention Trial. *J Clin Endocrinol Metab* 2000;85(11):4118-4124.

33. Harris ST, Watts NB, Genant HK, et al: Effects of risedronate treatment on vertebral and nonvertebral fractures in women with postmenopausal osteoporosis: A randomized controlled trial. *JAMA* 1999;282(14):1344-1352.

34. Lyles KW, Colón-Emeric CS, Magaziner JS, et al: Zoledronic acid and clinical fractures and mortality after hip fracture. *N Engl J Med* 2007;357(18):1799-1809.

35. Cummings SR, San Martin J, McClung MR, et al: Denosumab for prevention of fractures in postmenopausal women with osteoporosis. *N Engl J Med* 2009;361(8):756-765.

36. Knopp-Sihota JA, Newburn-Cook CV, Homik J, Cummings GG, Voaklander D: Calcitonin for treating acute and chronic pain of recent and remote osteoporotic vertebral compression fractures: A systematic review and meta-analysis. *Osteoporos Int* 2012;23(1):17-38.

37. Reginster JY, Seeman E, De Vernejoul MC, et al: Strontium ranelate reduces the risk of nonvertebral fractures in postmenopausal women with osteoporosis: Treatment of Peripheral Osteoporosis (TROPOS) study. *J Clin Endocrinol Metab* 2005;90(5):2816-2822.

38. Neer RM, Arnaud CD, Zanchetta JR, et al: Effect of parathyroid hormone (1-34) on fractures and bone mineral density in postmenopausal women with osteoporosis. *N Engl J Med* 2001;344(19):1434-1441.

39. Rachner TD, Hadji P, Hofbauer LC: Novel therapies in benign and malignant bone diseases. *Pharmacol Ther* 2012; 134(3):338-344.

40. Parfitt AM: Vitamin D and the pathogenesis of rickets and osteomalacia, in Feldman D, Pike JW, Glorieux FH, eds: *Vitamin D*, ed 2. San Diego, CA, Elsevier Academic Press, 2005, pp 1029-1048.

41. Lips P, van Schoor NM, Bravenboer N: Vitamin D-related disorders, in Rosen CF, ed: *Primer on the Metabolic Bone Diseases and Disorders of Metabolism*, ed 7. Washington, DC, American Society for Bone and Mineral Research, 2008, pp 329-335.

42. Carpenter TO: The expanding family of hypophosphatemic syndromes. *J Bone Miner Metab* 2012;30(1):1-9.

43. Chong WH, Molinolo AA, Chen CC, Collins MT: Tumor-induced osteomalacia. *Endocr Relat Cancer* 2011;18(3):R53-R77.

44. Fraser WD: Hyperparathyroidism. *Lancet* 2009;374(9684): 145-158.

45. Goodman WG: Renal osteodystrophy for nonnephrologists. *J Bone Miner Metab* 2006;24(2):161-163.

46. Manghat P, Fraser WD, Wierzbicki AS, Fogelman I, Goldsmith DJ, Hampson G: Fibroblast growth factor-23 is associated with C-reactive protein, serum phosphate and bone mineral density in chronic kidney disease. *Osteoporos Int* 2010;21(11):1853-1861.

47. Kidney Disease: Improving Global Outcomes (KDIGO) CKD-MBD Work Group: KDIGO clinical practice guideline for the diagnosis, evaluation, prevention, and treatment of Chronic Kidney Disease-Mineral and Bone Disorder (CKD-MBD). *Kidney Int Suppl* 2009;(113):S1-S130.

48. Tolar J, Teitelbaum SL, Orchard PJ: Osteopetrosis. *N Engl J Med* 2004;351(27):2839-2849.

49. Siris ES, Roodman GD: Paget's disease of bone, in Rosen CF, ed: *Primer on the Metabolic Bone Diseases and Disorders of Metabolism*, ed 7. Washington, DC, American Society for Bone and Mineral Research, 2008, pp 335-343.

50. Albagha OM, Wani SE, Visconti MR, et al: Genome-wide association identifies three new susceptibility loci for Paget's disease of bone. *Nat Genet* 2011;43(7):685-689.

Chapter 23

Neuromuscular Disorders

Mary Ann Keenan, MD

Introduction

Neuromuscular disorders can be divided into five categories: dystrophinopathies, muscular atrophies, hereditary neuropathies, neurodegenerative diseases, and acquired neurologic problems such as poliomyelitis, cerebral palsy, stroke, spinal cord injury, and traumatic brain injury (**Table 1**). These disorders commonly result in weakness, atrophy, joint contractures, and decreasing mobility with increasing disability.

Neuromuscular disorders are best classified as motor unit diseases because the primary abnormality may involve the neurons, the neuromuscular junction, or the muscle fiber. Two broad categories are considered. Myopathies are diseases of the muscle fibers. Neuropathies are disorders in which muscle degeneration is secondary to either upper or lower motor neuron disease. Most childhood-onset neuromuscular disorders are hereditary, although point mutations may result in spontaneous cases. Early diagnosis is important, not only for initiation of appropriate therapy but also for genetic counseling. Treatment programs are primarily aimed at symptomatic and supportive care. Appropriate orthopaedic intervention can significantly increase the functional capacity of patients with neuromuscular disorders.

Diagnosis
History and Physical Examination

For childhood or young adult–onset disorders, a careful genetic history is important.[1-4] The clinical history and phys-

ical examination will delineate the onset and pattern of muscle involvement. Neuropathies generally present with distal involvement. Muscle fasciculation and spasticity are common, and muscle atrophy is in excess of the weakness. The clinical features of myopathy include weakness of the proximal limb musculature, myalgia, relative preservation of muscle-stretch reflexes, and intact sensation. Muscle fasciculation and spasticity are not seen.

Muscle Enzyme Studies

The serum creatine kinase (CK) level is the most important blood value when myopathy is suspected.[5] The CK level, however, is not definitive in distinguishing myopathy from neuropathy. A greatly elevated level generally indicates muscle disease. Mild elevations can be seen in either myopathy or neuropathy. Normal CK levels are unlikely in myopathy, except in patients who have a reduced muscle mass. Because of its longer half-life in serum, the serum aldolase level is sometimes elevated in the setting of myopathy when the CK level is normal.

CK levels are the most elevated in the Duchenne type of muscular dystrophy and less elevated in the more slowly progressive disease forms. In Duchenne muscular dystrophy, the highest enzyme levels are seen at birth and during the first few years of life, before the disease is clinically apparent. As the disease progresses and the muscle mass deteriorates, the enzyme levels will decrease.

Electromyography and Nerve Conduction Velocity Studies

Electromyography (EMG) and nerve conduction velocity studies will differentiate primary muscle diseases and neuropathies. EMG is useful in differentiating between muscle diseases, peripheral nerve disorders, and anterior horn cell

Neither Dr. Keenan nor any immediate family member has received anything of value from or owns stock in a commercial company or institution related directly or indirectly to the subject of this chapter.

Table 1

The Most Common Neuromuscular Disorders

Disease by Category	Etiology	Mean Age of Onset	Cell Target
Dystrophinopathies	*Hereditary*		
Duchenne muscular dystrophy	X-linked recessive	Childhood	Lower motor neuron
Becker muscular dystrophy	X-linked recessive	Childhood	Lower motor neuron
Limb-girdle muscular dystrophies	Autosomal dominant or recessive	Childhood	Lower motor neuron
Fascioscapulohumeral muscular dystrophy	Autosomal dominant in 70% to 90%	Childhood	Lower motor neuron
Emery-Dreifuss muscular dystrophy	X-linked or autosomal	Childhood	Lower motor neuron
Muscular Atrophies	*Hereditary*		
Spinal muscular atrophy	Autosomal recessive	Childhood	Muscle
Werdnig-Hoffman disease	Autosomal recessive	Childhood	Muscle
Kugelberg-Welander syndrome	Autosomal recessive	Childhood	Muscle
Focal muscular atrophy	Autosomal recessive		Muscle
Hereditary Motor Sensory Neuropathies	*Hereditary*		
Charcot-Marie-Tooth disease (CMT)			
CMT1	Autosomal Dominant	< 10 years in 75%	Lower motor neuron
CMT2	Autosomal Dominant	Variable (2 to 40 years)	Lower motor neuron
CMT3	Autosomal Dominant	Childhood	Lower motor neuron
Dejerine-Sottas	Autosomal Dominant	Infancy	Lower motor neuron
CMTX	X-linked	Childhood	Lower motor neuron
CMT4	Autosomal Recessive	Childhood	Lower motor neuron
Neurodegenerative Diseases	*Unknown*		
Multiple sclerosis	Unknown	18 to 50 years	Lower motor neuron
Amyotrophic lateral sclerosis	Sporadic in 90% to 95% of cases; familial pattern in 5% to 10%	65 years	Lower motor meuron
Acute disseminated encephalomyelitis	Unknown	Childhood (prepubertal)	Upper motor neuron
Parkinson disease	Unknown	60 years	Lower motor neuron
Acquired Disorders	*Variable Causes*		
Poliomyelitis	Viral infection	Variable	Lower motor neuron
Stroke	Vascular abnormality	75% > 65 years	Upper motor neuron
Traumatic brain injury	Trauma	Variable	Upper motor neuron
Spinal cord injury	Trauma	Variable	Upper motor neuron
Cerebral palsy	Unknown	Birth	Upper motor neuron
Guillain-Barré syndrome			Lower motor neuron

abnormalities.[6,7] The motor unit (defined as a nerve cell and the muscle cells it innervates) is the basic functional element of skeletal muscle. A motor unit consists of the anterior horn cell or α motor neuron, its axon, and the muscle fibers it innervates.

The characteristic process in myopathies is the loss or dysfunction of muscle fibers. In most situations, such abnormality is reflected in changes in the myogenic signal. A myopathic pattern on EMG is characterized by increased frequency, decreased duration, and decreased amplitude of action potentials. In addition, increased insertional activity, short polyphasic potentials, and a retained interference pattern are evident. If significant muscle atrophy is present, the motor unit action potential amplitude is reduced. The motor unit action potential amplitude may be normal if the recording electrode is adjacent to a functioning muscle fiber, but may be increased if the muscle fiber is hypertrophied. The myogenic signal may not be altered if the process involves primarily the subsarcolemmal structures. Increased motor unit action potential complexity may be observed as a sensitive but nonspecific finding of abnormality in early or mild myopathy. Abnormalities specific for myopathy include shortened motor unit action potential duration or reduced area, particularly area-to-amplitude ratio.

In neurogenic disorders, entire motor units are lost secondary to the loss of motor neurons. The motor unit uses two basic compensatory mechanisms to regain strength and function: muscle hypertrophy and reinnervation of orphaned muscle fibers that have lost their controlling motor neurons.

A neuropathic pattern on EMG is characterized by decreased frequency, increased duration, and increased amplitude of action potentials. In addition, frequent fibrillation potentials, a group polyphasic potential, and a decreased interference pattern can be seen.

Muscle Biopsy

Advances in molecular genetics have eliminated the need for muscle biopsy in most patients with dystrophinopathies. In these patients, mutations can be demonstrated in the gene for dystrophin, located on the X chromosome (Xp21) that codes for a structural protein of skeletal muscle located on the internal surface of the muscle plasma membrane. Muscle biopsy is usually only performed in patients with clinical syndromes that differ from typical dystrophinopathies, such as adults with limb-girdle syndromes, some of whom are found to have abnormalities of dystrophin.

To gain the maximal amount of information from muscle biopsy, the clinician should choose a muscle that has mild to moderate involvement and has not been recently traumatized by electrodes during EMG. Muscle biopsy can be used to differentiate myopathy, neuropathy, and inflammatory myopathy.[2,6,8-11] The biopsy, however, cannot be used to determine prognosis. Histochemical staining will further distinguish the congenital forms of myopathy.

Histologically, myopathies are characterized by muscle fiber necrosis, fatty degeneration, proliferation of the connective tissue, and an increased number of nuclei, some of which have migrated from their normal peripheral position to the center of the muscle fiber.

Neuropathies display small, angulated muscle fibers. Bundles of atrophic fibers are intermingled with bundles of normal fibers. There is no increase in the amount of connective tissue.

Biopsy findings in polymyositis include prominent collections of inflammatory cells, edema of the tissues, perivasculitis, and segmental necrosis with a mixed pattern of fiber degeneration and regeneration.

Dystrophinopathies
Duchenne Muscular Dystrophy

Duchenne muscular dystrophy is the most common muscular dystrophy and is progressive.[1,5,12,13] It is inherited in an X-linked recessive manner and occurs in early childhood, affecting 1 in 3,500 boys. Generally, affected children have had a normal birth and developmental history. By the time these children reach age 3 to 5 years, sufficient muscle mass has been lost to impair function. The diagnostic criteria include (1) weakness with onset in the legs; (2) hyperlordosis and a wide-based gait; (3) hypertrophy of weak muscles; (4) a progressive course; (5) reduced muscle contractility on electrical stimulation in advanced stages of the disease; and (6) the absence of bladder or bowel dysfunction, sensory disturbance, or febrile illness.[14,15]

Kunkel et al[16,17] identified the Duchenne muscular dystrophy gene and provided molecular genetic confirmation of the X-linked inheritance pattern in 1986. The Duchenne muscular dystrophy gene was named *dystrophin*. It is the largest recorded human gene encoding a 427-kd protein, dystrophin. Dystrophin protein is integral to the structural stability of the myofiber. Dystrophin levels in Duchenne muscular dystrophy are less than 5% of normal. In the absence of dystrophin, muscles are susceptible to mechanical injury and undergo repeated cycles of necrosis and regeneration. Over time, the regenerative capabilities of the muscles are exhausted. Several studies have shed further light on the complex association of the dystrophin protein with several transmembrane proteins and glycoproteins, referred to as sarcoglycans and dystroglycans.[18-22]

Early signs of disease include pseudohypertrophy of the calf, which is the result of the increase in connective tissue; planovalgus deformity of the feet, which is secondary to heel cord contracture; and proximal muscle weakness. Muscle weakness in the hips may be exhibited by the Gower sign, in which the patient uses the arms to support the trunk while attempting to rise from the floor. Other signs are hesitance when climbing stairs, acceleration during the final stage of sitting, and shoulder weakness.

Weakness and contractures prevent independent ambulation in approximately 45% of patients by age 9 years and in the remainder by age 12 years. It is common for patients to have difficulty first in rising from the floor, next in ascending the stairs, and then in walking. Cardiac involvement is seen in 80% of patients. Findings generally include posterobasal fibrosis of the ventricle and electrocardiographic changes. In patients with a decreased level of activity, clinical evidence of cardiomyopathy may not be obvious. Pulmonary problems are common in the advanced stages of the disease and are found during periodic evaluations of pulmonary function. Mental retardation, which has been noted in 30% to 50% of patients, is present from birth and is not progressive.

Efforts are made to keep patients ambulating for as many years as possible to prevent the complications of obesity, osteoporosis, and scoliosis. The hip flexors, tensor fasciae latae, and triceps surae develop ambulation-limiting contractures. With progressive weakness and contractures, the base of support decreases and the patient cannot use normal mechanisms to maintain upright balance. The patient walks with a wide-based gait, hips flexed and abducted, knees flexed, and the feet in equinus and varus position. Lumbar lordosis becomes exaggerated to compensate for the hip flexion contractures and weak hip extensor musculature.

Equinus contractures of the Achilles tendon occur early and are caused by the muscle imbalance between the calf and pretibial muscles. Initially, this problem can be managed by heel cord stretching exercises and night splints. A knee-ankle-foot orthosis may be needed to control foot position and substitute for weak quadriceps muscles. Stretching exercises and pronation can be used to treat early hip flexion contractures.

Surgical intervention is directed toward the release of ambulation-limiting contractures. Early postoperative mobilization is important to prevent further muscle weakness. Anesthetic risks are increased in these patients because of their limited pulmonary reserve and because the incidence of malignant hyperthermia is higher than normal in patients with muscle disease.

The triceps surae and tibialis posterior are the strongest muscles in the lower extremity of the patient with muscular dystrophy. These muscles are responsible for equinus and varus deformities. Treatment that consists of releasing the contracted tensor fasciae latae, lengthening the Achilles tendon, and transferring the tibialis posterior muscle anteriorly is indicated and will prolong walking for approximately 3 years. Postoperative bracing is required.

Scoliosis is common in nonambulatory patients confined to a wheelchair. Adaptive seating devices that hold the pelvis level and the spine erect are useful in preventing deformity. Alternatively, a rigid plastic spinal torso orthosis may be used for support. When external support is not effective, scoliosis develops rapidly. Spinal fusion is occasionally indicated. Blood loss during surgery is high, and the incidence of pseudarthrosis is increased. Postoperative immobilization is to be avoided; therefore, segmental spinal stabilization is often the preferred technique of internal stabilization.

Fractures in patients with myopathies occur secondary to osteoporosis from inactivity and loss of muscle tension. No abnormalities of bone mineralization are present. The incidence of fracture increases with the severity of the disease. Most fractures are metaphyseal in location, show little displacement, cause minimal pain, and heal in the expected time without complication.

Becker Muscular Dystrophy

Becker muscular dystrophy is a recessive, X-linked dystrophinopathy with a male distribution pattern.[13,16,23,24] Translocations allow the possibility of Becker muscular dystrophy in girls. Affected boys in approximately 30% of cases of Becker muscular dystrophy phenotype do not have a demonstrable mutation/deletion. Abnormal but functional dystrophin may be produced. Dystrophin levels in Becker muscular dystrophy are generally 30% to 80% of normal.

The clinical picture is similar to that of Duchenne muscular dystrophy but is generally milder. The onset of symptoms occurs later with a mean age of 11 years (range, 2 to 21 years). The clinical distinction between the two conditions is comparatively easy because of the less severe muscle weakness in patients with Becker muscular dystrophy. Another distinction is that affected maternal uncles with Becker muscular dystrophy continue to be ambulatory until a mean age of 27 years. A typical developmental history may include delayed gross motor milestones. Increasing numbers of falls, toe walking, and difficulties rising from the floor are later features. Elbow contractures may be seen later in life. Death usually results from respiratory or cardiac failure at a mean age of 42 years (range, 23 to 63 years). The accuracy of diagnosis has been advanced with the recognition of the dystrophin gene defects and with dystrophin staining of muscle biopsy specimens. Dystrophin gene deletion analysis shows specific exon deletions in approximately 98% of cases. Serum CK levels show moderate to severe elevation.

Limb-Girdle Muscular Dystrophy

Limb-girdle muscular dystrophy can be expressed in either boys or girls and generally presents in the late first or second decade of life.[25-28] Limb-girdle muscular dystrophy is usually autosomal recessive but less frequently is autosomal dominant. There is involvement of shoulder or pelvic girdle muscles with variable rates of progression. Severe disability occurs within 20 to 30 years. Muscular pseudohypertrophy and contractures are uncommon, and the condition exhibits a wide range of phenotypic variability.

Limb-girdle muscular dystrophy classification has been revolutionized with the advent of molecular genetics.[29-32] The current classification system is based on both clinical and molecular characteristics.[33] It divides cases into autosomal dominant and autosomal recessive syndromes (**Tables 2 and 3**).

All patients with autosomal recessive limb-girdle muscular dystrophy have progressive, proximal muscle weakness. Limb-girdle muscular dystrophy 2A is likely the most common autosomal recessive type, accounting for up to 30% of all cases. In some geographic locations, such as northern Spain, limb-girdle muscular dystrophy 2A accounts for almost 80% of all cases of the disease. A founder mutation has been identified in this area. In other regions, it is quite rare.

Approximately two thirds of patients present at age 8 to 15 years, with a range of 2 to 40 years. The most typical presentation is of weakness due to scapulohumeropelvic weak-

Table 2

Characteristics of Autosomal Recessive Limb-Girdle Muscular Dystrophies

Subtype	Age at Presentation	Phenotype	Prevalence	Progression
LGMD 2A (calpainopathy)	8-15 years	Scapulohumeropelvic weakness	30% of LGMD	Slow
LGMD 2B (dysferlinopathy)	15-35 years	Limb-girdle or distal myopathy	20% of LGMD	Slow
LGMD 2C-2F (sarcoglycano-pathies)	6-8 years	Severe Duchenne-like weakness	20%-25% of LGMD	Rapid
LGMD 2G (telethoninopathy)	2-15 years	Highly variable	Rare	
LGMD 2H (tripartite motif–containing gene 32–related dystrophy)	8-27 years	Mild limb-girdle weakness	Rare (Hutterite people of Manitoba)	Slow
LGMD-2I (fukutin-related proteinopathy)	11-40 years	Variable	11%-38% of LGMD	Variable
LGMD-2J (titinopathy)	10-30 years	Limb-girdle myopathy	Finnish families	Slow
LGMD-2K	1-6 years	Severe proximal muscleweakness	Turkish and Italian families	Slow
LGMD-2L	11–50 years	Variable quadriceps weakness and atrophy	French-Canadian families	Slow
LGMD-2M	Hypotonia before 1 year	Proximal weakness greater than distal weakness. Affects the legs more than the arms	Very rare; described in three patients in two families with a mutation in the fukutin gene	Moderate

All patients have a history of progressive, proximal muscle weakness. LGMD = limb-girdle muscular dystrophy.

ness that may be similar to the presentation of fascioscapulohumeral dystrophy, but without facial weakness. Limb-girdle muscular dystrophy 2I may also have a similar phenotype.

Autosomal dominant limb-girdle muscular dystrophy is less common than the autosomal recessive type, accounting for approximately 10% of all cases. Patients with autosomal dominant limb-girdle muscular dystrophy have a later onset and slower course. CK elevations are not as great in the autosomal dominant type as in the recessive type.

Fascioscapulohumeral Muscular Dystrophy

Fascioscapulohumeral muscular dystrophy is the third most common muscular dystrophy.[34,35] The estimated prevalence is 1 case in 20,000 persons. Most patients have a normal life expectancy.

Fascioscapulohumeral muscular dystrophy is an autosomal dominant disease in 70% to 90% of patients and is sporadic in the remainder. One of the fascioscapulohumeral muscular dystrophy genes has been localized to chromosome band 4q35, but the affected gene or genes are still unknown.[36] Approximately 2% of patients with fascioscapulohumeral muscular dystrophy are not linked to the locus at 4q35.

Fascioscapulohumeral muscular dystrophy is caused by a deletion of D4Z4 macrosatellite repeats in the subtelomeric region of the 4qA161 haplotype of chromosome 4.[34] At least one copy of D4Z4 is required to develop the condition. Mosaic males are mostly affected, whereas mosaic females with an equal complement of affected cells are more often asymptomatic carriers. Although the genetic lesion in fascioscapulohumeral muscular dystrophy is described, the causal gene and the protein products are not known.

Fascioscapulohumeral muscular dystrophy has been established as a distinct muscular dystrophy with specific diagnostic criteria,[28] with distinct regional involvement and progression. The usual presentation is between the first and third decades. Ninety-five percent of patients show clinical features before age 20 years. Approximately one third of patients are asymptomatic.

Initial weakness is seen in facial muscles.[37] Patients may have difficulty with labial sounds, whistling, or drinking through a straw. The weakness can be asymmetric. Shoulder

Table 3

Characteristics of Autosomal Dominant Limb-Girdle Muscular Dystrophies

Subtype	Age at Presentation	Phenotype	Progression
LGMD 1A (myotilino-pathy)	Young adulthood to the mid 70s	Variable distal and proximal weakness; footdrop common; dysarthria, cardiomyopathy, or arrhythmia in 50%	Slow
LGMD 1B (laminopathy)	Childhood (<10 years) to the mid 30s	Proximal weakness; distal limb and facial weakness may be late manifestations	Slow
LGMD 1C (caveolino-pathy)	First or second decade	Usually with proximal weakness but can be with distal weakness	Slow to moderate
LGMD 1D	Adulthood	Proximal weakness Dysarthria may be present	Slow
LGMD 1E	Early adulthood	Dilated cardiomyopathy with conduction defect and muscular dystrophy	Slow
LGMD 1F	Infancy to the mid 50s	Early proximal weakness with progression to distal weakness	Rapid
LGMD 1G	30–50 years	Early proximal weakness with progression to distal weakness	Slow

Autosomal dominant limb-girdle muscular dystrophy (LGMD) is less common than autosomal recessive LGMD, accounting for approximately 10% of all cases.

weakness is the presenting symptom in more than 82% of patients. Winging of the scapula is the most characteristic sign. Weakness of foot dorsiflexion follows shoulder weakness. Tibialis anterior muscle weakness is very characteristic. Footdrop may be the presenting complaint. Posterior leg muscles are spared.

Truncal weakness occurs early. Lower abdominal muscles are weaker than upper abdominal muscles, resulting in the Beevor sign, a physical finding very specific for fascioscapulohumeral muscular dystrophy. The Beevor sign is the upward movement of the umbilicus toward the head when flexing the neck.

Extramuscular manifestations include high-frequency hearing loss, retinal telangiectasias, atrial arrhythmias, restrictive respiratory disease, mental retardation, seizures, and obstructive sleep apnea.[38] No definitive therapy is available.

Emery-Dreifuss Muscular Dystrophy

Emery-Dreifuss muscular dystrophy (EDMD) was recognized as a distinct disease in the 1960s. Dreifuss and Hogan reported a family with an X-linked form of muscular dystrophy that they considered to be a less aggressive form of Duchenne muscular dystrophy.[39] Later evaluation distinguished this type of X-linked dystrophy from the more severe Duchenne and Becker muscular dystrophies.[40,41]

Both X-linked and autosomal EDMD (EMD1 and EMD2, respectively) are caused by mutations of genes coding for proteins of the nuclear envelope. Even though these proteins are universally expressed, the disease manifestations are tissue specific. EMD1 is caused by mutations in the *EMD* gene on the X chromosome, which codes for the nuclear envelope protein emerin. Mutations occur throughout the gene and almost always result in complete absence of emerin from muscle or mislocalization of emerin. Emerin is a ubiquitous inner nuclear membrane protein, although its highest expression is in skeletal and cardiac muscle. Emerin binds to many nuclear proteins, including several gene-regulatory proteins.

EMD2 is related to mutations in the *LMNA* gene that codes for lamins A and C. Mutations in *LMNA* occur throughout the gene and can cause several different phenotypes. Lamins are intermediate filaments found in the inner nuclear membrane and nucleoplasm of almost all cells and have multiple functions, including providing mechanical strength to the nucleus, helping to determine nuclear shape, and anchoring and spacing nuclear pore complexes. Lamins are essential for DNA replication and mRNA transcription. They bind to structural components (emerin, nesprin), chromatin components (histone), signal transduction molecules (protein kinase C), and several gene regulatory molecules.

The prevalence of EMD1 or EMD2 is not known. Males are affected in X-linked EDMD. Approximately 10% to 20%

of female carriers have cardiac conduction defects, weakness, or both. In autosomal dominant EDMD, males and females are affected in equal numbers. The major cause of mortality and morbidity is cardiac disease. The most common disturbances are a result of atrial conduction defects. Sudden cardiac death has been reported in 40% of these patients.[42]

The mean age of onset is in the teenage years. Contractures, along with weakness, are common and generally occur early in the course of the disease, from the neonatal period to the third decade. This can lead to even greater functional disability than that caused by weakness. Physical therapy, bracing, and orthopaedic surgery can help prevent the formation or lessen the severity of contractures and maintain ambulation. No specific treatment exists.

Spinal Muscular Atrophies

The spinal muscular atrophies (SMAs) are the second most common autosomal recessive inherited disorders after cystic fibrosis.[43,44] The disease is characterized by degeneration and loss of anterior horn cells resulting in progressive weakness.

Several types of SMAs have been described based on the age that clinical features appear. In SMA type I (acute infantile or Werdnig-Hoffman disease), the onset is from birth to 6 months. The onset of SMA type II (chronic infantile) is between 6 and 18 months. In SMA type III (chronic juvenile or Kugelberg-Welander syndrome), onset is after 18 months; SMA type IV (adult onset) begins in the third decade. The mortality and/or morbidity rates of SMA are inversely correlated with the age at onset. Respiratory infections account for most deaths.

The genetic defects associated with SMA types I to III are located on the long arm of chromosome 5. The gene causing SMA, termed the survival motor neuron (SMN), was identified in 1995. Every person has two SMN genes, SMN1 and SMN2. More than 95% of patients with SMA have a homozygous disruption in the SMN1 gene. All patients with SMA retain a copy of SMN2. SMN2 generates only 10% of the amount of full-length SMN protein.

SMA Type I: Acute Infantile Form or Werdnig-Hoffman Disease

This severe infantile form of SMA affects 1 per 10,000 live births.[43-45] Patients present before 6 months of age and have severe progressive muscle weakness and reduced muscle tone. Bulbar dysfunction includes poor sucking ability, reduced swallowing, and respiratory failure. Facial weakness is minimal or absent. In 95% of cases, infants die of complications of the disease by age 18 months.

SMA Type II: Chronic Infantile Form

This is the most common form of SMA. Children present between age 6 and 18 months. The most common manifestation is developmental motor delay. Infants have difficulty sitting independently and are unable to stand by age 1 year.

A postural tremor of the fingers can be seen and is thought to be related to muscle fasciculations. Pseudohypertrophy of the gastrocnemius muscle, musculoskeletal deformities, and respiratory failure can occur. The life span of patients with SMA type II varies from 2 years to the third decade of life.

SMA Type III: Chronic Juvenile or Kugelberg-Welander Syndrome

SMA type III is a mild form of SMA that appears after age 18 months.[46] It is characterized by slowly progressive weakness of the proximal muscles. Most children are able to stand and walk but have trouble with stairs. Bulbar dysfunction occurs late. The overall course of SMA type III is mild. Many patients have normal life expectancies.

SMA Type IV: Adult-Onset Form

Onset of this type of SMA is typically in the mid 30s.[47-49] The overall course of the disease is benign, and patients have a normal life expectancy.

Approximately 20% of patients with SMA IV are ambulatory, and 1% are totally dependent. Fractures are common in these patients and occur secondary to decreased mobility and function. The goal of orthopaedic intervention is to prevent collapse of the spine and contractures. Orthotic support is often needed to stabilize the spine. In the nonambulatory patient, adaptive seating devices or orthotics may be used. If collapse of the spine occurs, spinal fusion is indicated.

Hereditary Motor Sensory Neuropathy: Charcot-Marie-Tooth Disease

In 1886 Charcot and Marie in France and Tooth in England independently described an inherited peripheral neuropathy characterized by slowly progressive, distal weakness and muscle atrophy, and sensory loss involving the legs and arms in a symmetric pattern.[50,51] In 1893 Dejerine and Sottas described an infant-onset inherited neuropathy with more severe symptoms.[52] Charcot-Marie-Tooth (CMT) disease is the most common inherited neuromuscular disorder. Estimates of the frequency of CMT disease vary widely.[53] A worldwide meta-analysis estimated a prevalence of 1 per 10,000 individuals. Onset is usually in childhood. The pathophysiology has been categorized into two processes: demyelination resulting in low conduction velocities (CMT1) and axonal degeneration resulting in low potential amplitudes (CMT2). The relative contribution of axonal versus demyelinative damage to the disease manifestations and progression remains controversial. Axonal degeneration is a prediction of disability.

There is significant heterogeneity in both the genetics and clinical findings of CMT neuropathy, which makes classification difficult.[54,55] The most commonly recognized forms include CMT1, CMT2, Dejerine-Sottas, CMTX, and CMT4.

CMT1 is a demyelinating form of the disease.[56] It is inherited in an autosomal dominant manner and accounts for 60% of all autosomal dominant neuropathies. This peripheral neuropathy is characterized by distal muscle weakness and atrophy, sensory loss, and slow nerve conduction velocity. Most commonly it is slowly progressive and is often associated with pes cavus foot deformity. Seventy-five percent of patients with CMT1 develop clinical signs before age 10 years. Fewer than 5% of individuals become wheelchair dependent. Life span is not shortened.

There are six subtypes of CMT1. They are clinically indistinguishable from one another and are classified only on molecular findings. CMT1A accounts for 70% to 80% of CMT1 cases. The molecular abnormality involves peripheral myelin protein 22 (PMP22). CMT1B accounts for 5% to 10% of CMT1 cases. The molecular abnormality involves myelin P0 protein (MPZ). The prevalence of CMT1C is unknown. The molecular abnormality involves lipopolysaccharide-induced tumor necrosis factor-α. The molecular abnormality of CMT1D involves early growth response protein–2. The prevalence of the CMT1D form of the disease is not known. CMT1E also has an unknown prevalence. Its molecular abnormality is in PMP22. CMT1F/2E displays an aberration in neurofilament light polypeptide. The prevalence of this disease form is also unknown.

CMT2 is a predominantly axonal, nondemyelinating form and also is dominantly inherited. It is characterized by distal muscle weakness and atrophy. Nerve conduction velocities are usually within the normal range. Peripheral nerves are not hypertrophic. CMT2 accounts for approximately 22% of CMT cases. CMT2 exhibits clinical overlap with CMT1. Individuals with CMT2 are generally less disabled and have less sensory loss than individuals with CMT1. There are 15 subtypes of CMT2. They are similar clinically and are distinguished only by molecular genetic findings.

Dejerine-Sottas is a severe form of the disease with onset in infancy. CMTX is inherited in an X-linked manner and accounts for approximately 1.6% of CMT cases. CMTX affects boys more frequently, earlier, and more severely than girls. The other forms are rarer.

CMT4 includes the various demyelinating autosomal recessive forms of CMT disease. Persons with CMT4 show the typical clinical findings of distal muscle weakness and atrophy associated with sensory loss and a cavus foot deformity.

Life expectancy is normal in patients with CMT. The degree of disability varies and is unpredictable between and within families. Characteristically, patients with hereditary neuropathy with susceptibility to pressure palsies have a good quality of life between episodes of nerve damage. Approximately 10% of patients experience incomplete recovery from episodes of nerve palsy.

EMG studies show a neuropathic pattern, and the nerve conduction velocity of the involved nerves is markedly decreased.[57] Muscle enzyme levels are normal. The peroneal muscles are affected early in the course of the disease. For this reason, CMT disease was sometimes referred to as progressive peroneal muscular atrophy. The intrinsic muscles of the feet and hands are affected later. As a rule, patients present with progressive claw toe and cavus deformities of the feet.[58] In the skeletally immature patient, release of the plantar fascia is done to correct the cavus deformity. This is often combined with transfer of the extensor digitorum longus tendon to the neck of the metatarsal and fusion of the proximal interphalangeal joints of the toes to correct the claw toe deformities. If the tibialis posterior muscle is active during the swing phase, then it can be transferred through the interosseous membrane to the lateral cuneiform bone. Triple arthrodesis is often necessary in the adult to correct the deformity.[59,60]

The "intrinsic minus" hand deformity causes difficulty in grasping objects. An orthosis with a lumbrical bar to hold the metacarpophalangeal joints in a flexed position will improve hand use. A capsulodesis of the volar portion of the metacarpophalangeal joints will accomplish the same objective. To restore active intrinsic muscle function in the hand, the flexor digitorum superficialis tendon of the ring finger can be divided into four slips and transferred through the lumbrical passages to the proximal phalanx.[61]

Neurodegenerative Diseases
Multiple Sclerosis

Multiple sclerosis (MS) is an inflammatory, demyelinating disease of the central nervous system. Clinically, MS is a dynamic, progressive, complex, and heterogeneous disease.[62-64]

MS affects females more than males; the basis for the difference and the etiology of MS are unknown. The disease appears to be exacerbated by hormonal changes, environmental agents, and infections. Genetic susceptibility may also play a role. MS is more common in Caucasian populations living in northern latitudes. In the United States, MS has a prevalence of approximately 400,000 cases, and more than 2.5 million people worldwide are estimated to be affected. MS most commonly affects people age 18 to 50 years. People with MS generally die of related complications such as recurrent urinary tract and respiratory infections, and have a mean life expectancy 5 to 7 years shorter than that of the general population.[65]

MRI is most helpful to confirm the diagnosis of MS. Characteristically, MRI shows lesions of high T2 signal intensity in the white matter that are of variable location within the brain, brain stem, optic nerves, and spinal cord.[66,67] MS lesions are characterized by perivascular infiltration of lymphocytes and monocytes, form at a steady pace, and lead to increasing physical disability. Expression of adhesion molecules on the surface seems to underlie the ability of inflammatory cells to pass through the blood-brain barrier. Molecular studies of the white matter plaque tissue have shown that interleukin (IL)-12, a potent proinflammatory substance, is present at high levels in newly formed lesions.[68,69]

Cerebrospinal fluid examination may be helpful in establishing the diagnosis of MS.[70,71] Oligoclonal band patterns can be demonstrated on electrophoresis in 85% of patients. These patterns reflect an elevation of immunoglobulin G produced by a restricted set of plasma cells. The immunoglobulin G index is frequently elevated. Myelin basic protein is a major component of myelin, and levels may be elevated.

Attacks or exacerbations of MS are characterized by new symptoms that reflect the ongoing central nervous system damage. These symptoms are normally separated in time, ranging from months to years. The clinical signs, such as limb weakness of one or more limbs and visual or sensory changes, vary. Physical and cognitive disability progression in MS often occurs in the absence of clinical exacerbations.

MS can present with different clinical phenotypes. Primary progressive, relapsing remitting, relapsing progressive, and secondary progressive forms have been described. Patients with primary progressive MS do not experience remissions; their disease progresses in a continuous manner, and they respond poorly to current therapeutic treatments. Patients with primary progressive MS have a propensity for more limb weakness and incontinence, and they become disabled at a more rapid rate.

Patients who improve after acute attacks have relapsing remitting MS. Approximately 75% to 85% of these patients then progress to secondary progressive MS. Patients who have relapsing remitting MS but continue to amass disability between and during attacks are classified as having relapsing progressive disease. MS can also present in an acute fulminant form, known as the Marburg variant of MS, that can lead to coma or death.

MS presents with a variety of clinical symptoms that may include cognitive changes, ataxia, hemiparesis or paraparesis, depression, or visual symptoms.[72,73] Bipolar disorder and dementia may occur late in the disease course. Patients also report fatigue. The fatigue is often worsened by exposure to heat.

No highly effective treatment is currently available to counteract acute exacerbations of MS attacks. The most widely used treatment is intravenous methylprednisolone, 1 g daily for 3 to 5 days. This medication may help expedite the timing of recovery but will not affect the actual extent of recovery. Considerable controversy exists regarding whether the delay in onset of new attacks by these drugs ultimately has any long-term effect on neurodegeneration.

Management of physical disability focuses on the control of spasticity, the maintenance of ambulation, and the prevention and treatment of contractures. Spasticity management includes drug therapy and intrathecal baclofen. Physical therapy, orthoses, and assistive devices help to prolong ambulation. Orthopaedic surgery is useful for both the early and late treatment of contractures.

Amyotrophic Lateral Sclerosis

Amyotrophic lateral sclerosis (ALS) is the most common neurodegenerative disease.[74,75] It affects lower motor neurons in the anterior horn of the spinal cord and brain stem; corticospinal upper motor neurons that reside in the precentral gyrus; and prefrontal motor neurons involved in motor planning. Loss of lower motor neurons leads to progressive muscle weakness and wasting (atrophy), loss of corticospinal upper motor neurons leads to spasticity, and loss of prefrontal neurons results in cognitive impairment. Death from respiratory failure occurs within a mean of 3 years.[76]

The term classic ALS is used when the disease involves both upper and lower motor neurons. Classic ALS starts as weakness and dysfunction in one location and spreads to the rest of the body. If only lower motor neurons are involved, the disease is called progressive muscular atrophy. When only upper motor neurons are involved, the disease is called primary lateral sclerosis.[77,78]

The incidence of ALS is approximately 2 per 100,000 persons per year. ALS occurs sporadically in 90% to 95% of cases and in a familial pattern in 5% to 10% of cases. Familial ALS is usually inherited in an autosomal dominant pattern and is rarely autosomal recessive.[79] Men are affected more frequently than women. The average age of onset in classic ALS is 65 years. Mean age at onset is 10 to 20 years younger in patients with familial ALS.

Nerve conduction velocity studies and needle EMG are useful for confirming the diagnosis of ALS.[80] The characteristic lower motor neuron features of ALS include decreased amplitudes of compound muscle action potentials with normal conduction velocities, little or no involvement of sensory nerves, and a mixed pattern of acute denervation and chronic reinnervation of muscles in the distribution of multiple roots at multiple levels. Electrophysiologic features compatible with upper motor neuron involvement include an increase in central motor conduction time determined by cortical magnetic stimulation and low or irregular firing rates of motor unit potentials on maximal effort during routine needle examination. MRI of the brain or spinal cord is sometimes performed to rule out structural lesions that might account for early clinical features, but imaging studies are usually not necessary in patients with advanced disease.

The signs and symptoms seen in ALS include weakness, muscle cramps, balance impairment, and bulbar problems with speech and swallowing. Clinical problems involve both upper and lower motor neuron phenomena. Upper motor neuron symptoms include spasticity, hyperreflexia, and loss of dexterity. Lower motor neuron dysfunction is characterized by muscle atrophy, weakness, and fasciculations. Respiratory difficulty, emotional lability, depression, and cognitive changes also occur.

Treatment of ALS consists of education and supportive treatment. Adaptive equipment is also important. A feeding gastrostomy tube can be considered. A tracheostomy and ventilatory support may also be considered in patients with respiratory failure.

Acute Disseminated Encephalomyelitis

Acute disseminated encephalomyelitis is a nonvasculitic inflammatory demyelinating condition that bears a striking clinical and pathologic resemblance to MS.[81-83] In most instances, acute disseminated encephalomyelitis and MS cases occurring in children are readily distinguishable on the basis of clinical features and findings on laboratory investigations. However, follow-up is important because there are instances where an initial diagnosis of acute disseminated encephalomyelitis is ultimately replaced with a diagnosis of MS.

Currently, neither condition has an identified biologic marker rendering a reliable laboratory diagnosis. MS is typically a chronic relapsing and remitting disease of young adults, whereas acute disseminated encephalomyelitis is typically a monophasic disease of prepubertal children. Abnormalities of findings on cerebrospinal fluid immunoglobulin studies are likely in MS but are much less common in acute disseminated encephalomyelitis. The onset of acute disseminated encephalomyelitis usually occurs in the wake of a clearly identifiable febrile prodromal illness or immunization and in association with prominent constitutional signs and encephalopathy of varied degree, features that are uncommon in MS.

However, the division between these processes is indistinct, which is suggestive of a clinical continuum. Moreover, other conditions along the suggested continuum include optic neuritis, transverse myelitis, and Devic syndrome, clinical entities that may occur as manifestations of either MS or acute disseminated encephalomyelitis. Other boundaries of acute disseminated encephalomyelitis merge indistinctly with a wide variety of inflammatory encephalitic and vasculitic illnesses as well as monosymptomatic postinfectious illnesses that should remain distinct from acute disseminated encephalomyelitis, such as acute cerebellar ataxia. A further indistinct boundary is shared by acute disseminated encephalomyelitis and Guillain-Barré syndrome; that entity is manifested in cases of Miller-Fisher syndrome and encephalomyeloradiculoneuropathy.

Clinically, acute disseminated encephalomyelitis is usually readily distinguishable from MS by the presence of certain clinical features, including a history of infectious illness or immunization, association with constitutional symptoms and signs such as fever, prominence of cortical signs such as mental status changes and seizures, comparative rarity of posterior column abnormalities, which are common in MS, and age younger than 11 or 12 years in acute disseminated encephalomyelitis and age older than 11 or 12 years in MS.

Parkinson Disease

Parkinson disease, one of the most common neurologic disorders, is a progressive neurodegenerative disorder associated with a loss of dopaminergic nigrostriatal neurons[84]

that affects approximately 1% of individuals older than 60 years.

No standard criteria exist for the neuropathologic diagnosis of Parkinson disease.[85-88] Major pathologic findings are a loss of pigmented dopaminergic neurons in the substantia nigra and the presence of Lewy bodies.[89] Lewy bodies are concentric, eosinophilic, cytoplasmic inclusions with peripheral halos and dense cores, whose presence within pigmented neurons of the substantia nigra is characteristic but not pathognomonic of idiopathic Parkinson disease. Approximately 60% to 80% of dopaminergic neurons are lost before the symptoms of Parkinson disease become evident.

Parkinson disease is 1.5 times more common in men than in women, with a prevalence of approximately 120 per 100,000 persons. Its incidence and prevalence increase with age, with an average age of onset of 60 years. Median survival from motor onset is approximately 15 years. Independent predictors of mortality are age of onset, chronologic age, Unified Parkinson Disease Rating Scale motor score, psychotic symptoms, and dementia.

Most cases of idiopathic Parkinson disease are thought to be due to a combination of genetic and environmental factors.[90,91] Environmental risk factors associated with Parkinson disease include exposure to herbicides or pesticides, proximity to industrial plants or quarries, and the consumption of well water. The role of genetic factors has been studied in twins. These studies suggest that genetic factors are important when the disease begins at or before age 50 years. The identification of a few large families with apparent familial Parkinson disease has sparked further interest in the genetics of the disease. One hypothesis suggests that Parkinson disease is caused by abnormalities of the proteosome system. The proteosome system is responsible for clearing abnormal proteins. Several homozygous deletions in a gene dubbed parkin (PARK2), which is located on chromosome 6, have been found to cause autosomal recessive juvenile parkinsonism. Several other gene abnormalities have been identified in families with Parkinson disease. It has been estimated that all currently known genetic causes of Parkinson disease account for less than 5% of Parkinson disease cases.[92,93] Environmental risk factors include exposure to herbicides and pesticides, living in a rural environment or in proximity to industrial plants or quarries, and consumption of well water.

Parkinson disease may have a long phase before the onset of motor dysfunction, but the signs are not specific and diagnosis is difficult at this stage. The initial symptoms of Parkinson disease may include fatigue and depression; early motor signs typically are clumsiness and a resting tremor in one hand. Over time the clinical motor features include resting tremor, rigidity, bradykinesia, postural instability, and difficulty walking.

The three fundamental signs of Parkinson disease are resting tremor, rigidity, and bradykinesia. Two of three signs are required to make the clinical diagnosis. Postural instability is the fourth cardinal sign, but it emerges late in the disease, usually after 8 years or longer. The characteristic tremor is most prominent with the limb at rest. The tremor may have the appearance of a simple oscillation of the arm or a pill-rolling motion of the hand.

Rigidity is an increase in resistance to passive movement about a joint. The resistance can be either smooth (lead pipe) or oscillating (cogwheeling). Cogwheel resistance may be related to tremor and can be present with tremors not associated with an increase in tone (essential tumor). Bradykinesia also includes a dearth of spontaneous movements and decreased amplitude of movement. Other manisfestations of bradykinesia are micrographia (small handwriting), hypomimia (decreased facial expression), decreased blink rate, and hypophonia (soft speech).

Postural instability refers to imbalance and is an important milestone because it responds poorly to treatment and is a common source of disability in late stages of the disease. Patients may freeze when starting to walk (start-hesitation), during turning, or while crossing a threshold.

No laboratory biomarkers exist for Parkinson disease. MRI and CT are unremarkable. Positron emission tomography and single-photon emission CT are useful diagnostic imaging studies but are not needed for clinical diagnosis in patients with a typical presentation.

Currently, no therapies exist to slow the loss of dopamine neurons in Parkinson disease. The goal of medical management is to provide control of signs and symptoms for as long as possible while minimizing adverse effects. Levodopa, coupled with a peripheral decarboxylase inhibitor, remains the standard of symptomatic treatment of Parkinson disease.[94-98] Levodopa and other medications usually provide good symptomatic control for 4 to 6 years. After this time, disability progresses despite best medical management, and many patients develop long-term motor complications including fluctuations and dyskinesia. Additional causes of disability in late disease include postural instability (balance difficulty) and dementia.

When medical management has been exhausted, neurosurgical interventions can be considered. Deep brain stimulation is an FDA-approved treatment of Parkinson disease that consists of a lead implanted into the targeted brain structure.[99] The thalamus, globus pallidus interna, and subthalamic nucleus may be targets of stimulation. The lead is connected to an implantable pulse generator positioned on the chest wall below the clavicle. The lead and the implantable pulse generator are connected by a subcutaneous wire. Stimulation amplitude, frequency, and pulse width can be adjusted to control symptoms and eliminate adverse events. The patient can turn the stimulator on or off using an access review therapy controller or a handheld magnet. Thalamic stimulation provides significant control of tremor but does not affect rigidity, bradykinesia, dyskinesia, or motor fluctuations. Pallidal stimulation controls tremor, rigidity, bradykinesia, and dyskinesia. Subthalamic nucleus stimulation is the most common procedure. Subthalamic nucleus deep brain stimulation controls the cardinal symptoms of Parkinson disease as well as motor fluctuations and dyskinesia and often allows for reductions in antiparkinsonian medications. The adverse effects of deep brain stimulation can include paresthesias, muscle spasms, visual disturbances, mood changes, and pain. These adverse effects are resolved with adjustments to deep brain stimulation.

Neural transplantation is a potential treatment. The site of neuronal degeneration is well defined within the striatum and is specific for dopaminergic activity. The use of stem cells is being investigated in the laboratory.

Treatment of orthopaedic conditions in patients with Parkinson disease can be problematic and result in failure of fixation or prosthetic dislocation. Despite successful pain relief, the functional results of total joint arthroplasty in these patients are poor, especially in those older than 65 years, and complications are more frequent. Success in terms of pain relief and no further need for intervention can be obtained with appropriate medical management after orthopaedic intervention.

Acquired Disorders
Poliomyelitis

Poliomyelitis is characterized by the sudden onset of paralysis and the presence of fever and acute muscle pain, often accompanied by stiff neck. Acute poliomyelitis is caused by RNA viruses of the enterovirus group of the Picornavirus family. Three distinct strains have been identified. Type I accounts for 85% of cases. Infection with one type does not protect from the other types; however, immunity to each of the three strains is lifelong.[100]

The virus infects the human intestinal tract mainly through the fecal-oral route. Only 1% to 2% of acute infections result in neurologic symptoms. The virus attacks the anterior horn cells of the spinal cord, leading to paralysis of a lower motor neuron type. Infection can lead to a variety of clinical findings, ranging from minor symptoms to paralysis. The last major epidemics in the United States occurred during the early 1950s. Because of effective immunization programs, acute poliomyelitis has now become rare. Despite the low incidence of new cases, many people continue to live with the consequences of poliomyelitis.

There are four clinical stages of poliomyelitis: acute, subacute, residual, and postpolio syndrome. The anterior horn cells are attacked during the acute stage, causing diffuse and severe paralysis. Paralysis of the respiratory muscles is life threatening in the acute stage. Treatment in the acute stage of the disease consists of providing any needed respiratory support, decreasing muscle pain, and performing regular range-of-motion exercises to prevent the formation of joint contractures.

Anterior horn cell survival, axon sprouting, and muscle hypertrophy occur in the subacute phase and provide three mechanisms for regaining strength. A variable number of anterior horn cells survive the initial infection (mean, 47%;

range, 12% to 94%). Anterior horn cell survival occurs in a random fashion. The clinical pattern of muscle weakness is therefore variable. Each anterior horn cell innervates a group of muscle cells. When a group of muscle cells is denervated by the death of the supporting anterior horn cell, an adjacent neuron can sprout additional axons and reinnervate several orphaned muscle cells. By means of this process, a motor unit can expand greatly. Muscle cells in the unit will enlarge, and this hypertrophy will provide additional strength for the patient.

Postpolio syndrome is a condition that develops in many survivors and occurs on average 30 to 40 years after the initial infection.[101-107] Increasing skeletal deformities such as scoliosis are common. Diagnosis of postpolio syndrome is based on a history of poliomyelitis, a pattern of increasing muscle weakness, and the presence of symptoms such as muscle pain, severe fatigue, muscle cramping or fasciculations, joint pain, sleep apnea, intolerance to cold, and depression. Some patients experience only minor symptoms, whereas symptoms in others are more severe. No pathognomonic tests for the syndrome are currently available. EMG can demonstrate the presence of large motor units resulting from the previous axon sprouting. This finding is supportive but not diagnostic of poliomyelitis.

Postpolio syndrome is rarely life threatening but significantly diminishes quality of life; orthopaedic surgeons continue to be called upon to treat these patients.[108]

Stroke

A stroke (cerebrovascular accident) occurs when there is acute loss of vascular perfusion to a region of the brain. This results in ischemia and the death of neurons, causing deficits in cognition, language, sensation, and motor function. Strokes are classified as either hemorrhagic or ischemic. Hemorrhagic strokes can be either intraparenchymal or subarachnoid in location. Ischemic strokes can be the result of thrombosis, embolism, or relative hypoperfusion.

In the United States, stroke is the third leading cause of death (46.6 per 100,000 in 2005) and the leading cause of disability.[109-111] The incidence of stroke is higher in men than in women. There is a higher incidence of stroke in the black population than in the white population. More than half of stroke victims survive and have an average life expectancy of 8 years. Despite a lower incidence of stroke, the mortality rate among women is higher than among men (13.2% versus 5.8%). Stroke can occur at any age, including childhood; however, the risk of stroke increases with age. Seventy-five percent of strokes occur in persons older than 64 years. Most survivors have the potential for significant function and useful lives if they receive the benefits of rehabilitation. Of stroke survivors, 50% have hemiplegia, 35% have depression, 30% have gait abnormalities requiring assistance, 26% require assistance with activities of daily living, 26% require admission to long-term care facilities, and 19% have aphasia.

Neurologic Impairment and Recovery

Infarction of the cerebral cortex in the region of the brain supplied by the middle cerebral artery or one of its branches is most commonly responsible for stroke.[112] Although the middle cerebral artery supplies the area of the cerebral cortex responsible for hand function, the anterior cerebral artery supplies the area responsible for lower extremity motion. The typical clinical picture after middle cerebral artery stroke is contralateral hemianesthesia (decreased sensation), homonymous hemianopia (visual field deficit), and spastic hemiplegia with more paralysis in the upper extremity than in the lower extremity. Because hand function requires relatively precise motor control, even for activities with assistive equipment, the prognosis for the functional use of the hand and arm is considerably worse than for the leg. Return of even gross motor control in the lower extremity may be sufficient for walking.

Infarction in the region of the anterior cerebral artery causes paralysis and sensory loss of the opposite lower limb and, to a lesser degree, the arm. The posterior cerebral artery supplies the visual cortex in the occipital region. Involvement of this artery typically results in visual impairment. Bilateral cortical involvement may lead to severe mental impairment, frontal release signs, loss of short-term memory, and inability to learn. Stroke in the vertebral basilar system is rare. Deficits in balance and coordination arise from interruption of afferent and efferent pathways between the brain and spinal cord. Balance and postural reactions are also dependent on limb control and proprioception.[113]

Patients who have cerebral arteriosclerosis and experience repeated bilateral infarctions are likely to have severe cognitive impairment that limits their general ability to function even when motor function is good.

Acute Management

The acute management of stroke has improved significantly in recent years. The brain is the most metabolically active organ in the body. When blood flow decreases, neurons stop functioning. Irreversible neuronal injury begins when blood flow is less than 18 mL/100 mg/min. Within seconds to minutes of the loss of glucose and oxygen delivery to neurons, the damage begins. The cellular processes involved are called the ischemic cascade.

The ischemic cascade process begins with loss of normal cellular electrophysiologic function. The resulting injury to both glial cells and neurons causes additional injury to the adjacent tissues. The area of the brain with significant ischemia is called the core. The cells in the core area die within minutes of stroke onset. Zones of decreased or marginal perfusion are referred to as the ischemic penumbra. Cells in the penumbra may remain viable for several hours because of marginal tissue perfusion. Acute pharmacologic interventions attempt to preserve tissue in the penumbra.

Medical intervention using thrombolytic agents has been used for acute ischemic stroke.[114] These treatments have been shown to be most effective when initiated within 3 hours from the onset of symptoms. However, pharmacologic intervention may play a role, although limited, if administered within 24 hours of onset. The efficacy of intravenous tissue plasminogen activator (tPA) was established in two randomized double-blind placebo-controlled studies published in combination by the National Institute of Neurologic Disorders and Stroke.[115,116] At 3 months after stroke, approximately 12% more patients in the tPA group experienced a cure of symptoms relative to those who did not receive it. The risk of intracerebral hemorrhage in the tPA group was 6% (50% of which were fatal), compared with 0.6% in the placebo group. Despite the differences in hemorrhage rates, there were no differences in mortality (17% in the tPA group versus 21% in the placebo group). Prourokinase is an intra-arterial therapy. The time window is 6 hours from symptom onset.

Key points about the administration of thrombolytic agents include the following: (1) an imaging study of the head (CT or MRI) must be performed before treatment to rule out hemorrhage; (2) thrombolytic agents should be administered within 3 hours of symptom onset; (3) blood pressure should be lower than 185 systolic and 110 diastolic, and the platelet count should be more than 100,000, international normalized ratio less than 1.6, prothrombin time less than 40, and glucose between 50 and 400 mg/mL.

Antiplatelet agents can be used. The Chinese Acute Stroke Trial and the International Stroke Trial are two large studies evaluating the use of aspirin (160 to 300 mg/day) within 48 hours of ischemic stroke symptom onset.[117,118] Compared with no treatment, there was approximately a 1% absolute reduction in stroke and death in the first few weeks. At further time points there was a similar absolute reduction of approximately 1% in death or dependence. Current clinical trials are under way to study the efficacy of abciximab in acute stroke. Anticoagulant use is limited. No studies have evaluated use of warfarin for the acute treatment of stroke.

The various neuroprotectants include calcium-channel antagonists, potassium channel openers, glutamate antagonists, antiadhesion molecules, N-methyl-D-aspartate receptor antagonists and modulators, α-amino-3-hydroxy-5-methyl-4-isoxazol propionic acid receptor antagonists, membrane stabilizers, growth factors, and glycine site antagonists. Currently, no neuroprotectant has shown efficacy in the treatment of acute stroke.

Subacute Management

Stroke commonly results in upper motor neuron syndrome, which is characterized by impairment of motor control, spasticity, muscle weakness, stereotypical patterns of movement (synergy), and the stimulation of distant movement by noxious stimuli (synkinesia). After stroke, motor recovery follows a fairly typical pattern. The size of the lesion and the amount of collateral circulation determine the amount of permanent damage. Most recovery occurs within 6 months, although functional improvement may continue as

the patient receives further sensorimotor reeducation and learns to cope with disability.[112,119]

Initially after a stroke, the limbs are completely flaccid. Over the next few weeks, muscle tone and spasticity gradually increase in the adductor muscles of the shoulder and in the flexor muscles of the elbow, wrist, and fingers. Spasticity also develops in the lower extremity muscles. Most commonly, there is an extensor pattern of spasticity in the leg, characterized by hip adduction, knee extension, and equinovarus deformities of the foot and ankle. In some instances, however, a flexion pattern of spasticity occurs, characterized by hip and knee flexion.

Whether the patient recovers the ability to move one joint independently of the others (selective movement) depends on the extent of the cerebral cortical damage. Dependence on the more neurologically primitive patterned movement (synergy) decreases as selective control improves. The extent to which motor impairment restricts function varies in the upper and lower extremities. Patterned movement is not functional in the upper extremity, but it may be useful in the lower extremity, where the patient uses the flexion synergy to advance the limb forward and the mass extension synergy for limb stability during standing.

The final processes in sensory perception occur in the cerebral cortex, where basic sensory information is integrated to complex sensory phenomena such as vision, proprioception, and perception of spatial relationships, shape, and texture. Patients with severe parietal dysfunction and sensory loss may lack sufficient perception of space and awareness of the involved segment of their body to ambulate. Patients with severe perceptual loss may lack balance to sit, stand, or walk. A visual field deficit further interferes with limb use and may cause patients to be unaware of their own limbs.

Treatment efforts in the subacute period are nonsurgical and are focused on minimizing spasticity, preventing contractures, and maximizing mobility and function.

Chronic Management

After 6 months the patient is usually neurologically stable. Treatment in the chronic phase involves correcting limb deformities, increasing muscle strength, maximizing motor control, training individuals to make the most effective use of residual function, and providing adaptive equipment. Definitive decisions can then be made regarding bracing or surgery to correct limb deformities and rebalance muscle forces.[120]

Traumatic Brain Injury

Traumatic brain injury from an external mechanical force causes damage to the brain and disrupts normal brain function. Traumatic brain injury often causes profound physical, psychologic, cognitive, emotional, and social effects. Annual statistics of brain injury in the United States, from the Centers for Disease Control and Prevention's National Center for Injury Prevention and Control, show that the incidence of traumatic brain injury is 1.4 million with an approximate

Table 4
Glasgow Coma Scale

Eye opening	Spontaneous = 4
	To speech = 3
	To painful stimulation = 2
	No response = 1
Motor response	Follows commands = 6
	Makes localizing movements to pain = 5
	Makes withdrawal movements to pain = 4
	Flexor (decorticate) posturing to pain = 3
	Extensor (decerebrate) posturing to pain = 2
	No response = 1
Verbal response	Oriented to person, place, and date = 5
	Converses but is disoriented = 4
	Says inappropriate words = 3
	Says incomprehensible sounds = 2
	No response = 1

Table 5
The Ranchos Los Amigos Scale of Cognitive Functioning

Level I = No response

Level II = Generalized response

Level III = Localized response

Level IV = Confused-agitated response

Level V = Confused-inappropriate response

Level VI = Confused-appropriate response

Level VII = Automatic-appropriate response

Level VIII = Purposeful-appropriate response

(Adapted from Malkmus D, et al: *Rehabilitation of the Head-Injured Adult: Comprehensive Cognitive Management.* Downey, CA, Professional Staff Association of Rancho Los Amigos Hospital, Inc., 1980.)

death rate of 50,000 people.[121] Another 80,000 to 90,000 people experience the onset of a long-term disability due to a traumatic brain injury.

Individuals at high risk for traumatic brain injury include those identified with young age, low income, substance abuse, and previous traumatic brain injury. Other high-risk groups are minorities, unmarried individuals, inner-city residents, and men. Infants and children up to 4 years and adolescents age 15 to 19 years are the two groups at highest risk for a traumatic brain injury. Males are twice as likely as females to sustain a traumatic brain injury, and polytrauma is common. Adults age 75 years or older have the highest rates of traumatic brain injury–related hospitalization and death. The leading causes of traumatic brain injury are falls (28%); motor vehicle accidents (20%); blows by or against objects (19%); and assaults (11%).[122]

The Glasgow Coma Scale is used to rate the severity of a traumatic brain injury within 48 hours of injury[123,124] (Table 4). Points are given for eye opening and response to verbal and motor stimuli. The maximum score is 15. The severity of traumatic brain injury based on the Glasgow Coma Scale score is as follows: severe = 3 to 8 points, moderate = 9 to 12 points, or mild = 13 to 15 points. Analysis of scores from patients in several countries has shed light on the chances for survival and neurologic recovery. According to the data, approximately 50% of patients with impaired consciousness survived. Six months after injury, moderate or good neurologic recovery was seen in 82% of patients with initial 24-hour Glasgow scores of 11 or higher, 68% of pa-

tients with initial scores of 8 to 10, 34% with initial scores of 5 to 7, and 7% with initial scores of 3 or 4.

Age is an important factor related to neurologic outcome. Patients younger than 20 years have moderate or good recovery in 62% of cases, whereas 46% of patients age 20 to 29 years experience moderate or good recovery. Mortality rates are higher among children up to age 4 years. The incidence of good recovery declines not only with advancing age but also with advancing duration of coma. Patients recovering from coma within the first 2 weeks of injury have a 70% chance of good recovery. The recovery rate drops to 39% in the third week and to 17% in the fourth week. Decerebrate or decorticate posturing indicates a brain stem injury and is indicative of a poor prognosis. The Ranchos Los Amigos cognition deficits scale[125] is presented in Table 5.

The two foremost mechanisms that cause primary brain injury are direct contact with object striking the head or the brain striking the inside of the skull, and acceleration-deceleration injuries. Traumatic brain injury is also divided into primary injury, which occurs at the moment of trauma, and secondary injury, which occurs directly after trauma.[126] Both can produce long-lasting consequences.

Primary injuries can manifest as focal injuries such as skull fractures, intracranial hematomas, lacerations, contusions, and penetrating wounds. Primary injuries can also result in diffuse axonal injury.[127] Diffuse axonal injury is one of the most common and important pathologic features of traumatic brain injury. Diffuse axonal injury is characterized by widespread damage to the white matter. It constitutes primarily microscopic damage, which is commonly not visible on imaging studies. The main mechanical force that causes diffuse axonal injury is rotational acceleration of the brain. Strains of the tentorium and falx during high-speed acceleration-deceleration forces to the head produce shearing and tensile forces. Axons are pulled apart at the microscopic level. Microscopic evaluation of brain tissue demonstrates numerous swollen and disconnected axons. Rapid stretching of axons is thought to damage the axonal cytoskeleton and, therefore, disrupt normal neuron function. Diffuse axonal injury can also result from ischemia.

Skull fractures can be vault fractures or basilar fractures. Hematoma, cranial nerve damage, and increased brain injury are associated with skull fractures.[128] Vault fractures tend to be linear and may extend into the sinuses. Fractures can be stellate, closed, or open, and also can be classified as depressed or nondepressed.

Several types of intracranial hemorrhages can occur. Hematomas from laceration of an artery can cause rapid neurologic deterioration. Epidural hematomas occur after impact to the skull with associated laceration of the dural arteries or veins. Subdural hematomas occur with injuries to the cortical veins or pial artery in severe traumatic brain injury. The associated mortality rate is on the order of 60% to 80%. Intracerebral hemorrhage occurs within the cerebral parenchyma. Intracerebral hemorrhage is seen from lacerations or extensive cortical contusion of the brain, with injury to the deep cerebral vessels. Intraventricular hemorrhage most commonly occurs with very severe traumatic brain injury and is associated with a poor prognosis.

Secondary Injury

Secondary types of brain injury can contribute to further damage. These injuries may develop within hours or days following the initial traumatic assault. Secondary brain injury is mediated through neurochemical mediators.[129]

Excitatory amino acids (including glutamate and aspartate, are significantly elevated after a traumatic brain injury and can cause cell swelling, vacuolization, and neuronal death.[130] They may cause an influx of chloride and sodium, leading to acute neuronal swelling. Excitatory amino acids can also cause an influx of calcium, which is linked to delayed damage, and can cause astrocytic swellings via volume-activated anion channels.

Endogenous opioid peptides also contribute to the exacerbation of neurologic damage by modulating the presynaptic release of excitatory amino acid neurotransmitters. Heightened metabolism in the injured brain is stimulated by an increase in the circulating levels of catecholamines, with associated depression in glucose utilization contributing to further brain injury.[131]

Other biochemical processes leading to a greater severity of injury include an increase in extracellular potassium, leading to edema; an increase in cytokines, contributing to inflammation; and a decrease in intracellular magnesium, contributing to calcium influx.

Increased intracerebral pressure can lead to cerebral hypoxia, ischemia, edema, hydrocephalus, and brain herniation. Brain herniation occurs from direct mechanical compression by an accumulating mass or from increased intracranial pressure.

Management

Management of traumatic brain injury comprises three distinctive phases: the acute injury period, the phase of neurologic recovery, and the residual period when neurologic recovery has largely ceased and the patient must cope with residual functional limitations. Medical complications after traumatic brain injury are common, including posttraumatic seizures (general or partial).[132] Seizures are classified according to the time elapsed after the initial injury. Immediate seizures occur within the first 24 hours of traumatic brain injury, early seizures occur in the first 2 to 7 days, and late seizures occur after 7 days. The incidence of late posttraumatic seizures is in the range of 5% to 18.9%. If a patient with traumatic brain injury has one posttraumatic seizure, the seizure recurrence rate is approximately 50%.

Another complication, hydrocephalus, exists in forms.[133] Noncommunicating hydrocephalus occurs secondary to an obstruction in the ventricular system before the point at which cerebrospinal fluid exits the fourth ventricle. Communicating hydrocephalus is the most common form and occurs when the obstruction is in the subarachnoid space. Patients with hydrocephalus can exhibit a multitude of symptoms including nausea, vomiting, headache, papilledema, obtundation, dementia, ataxia, and urinary incontinence. The diagnosis is based on clinical suspicion, diagnostic imaging, and radioisotope cisternography. Treatment usually consists of lumbar puncture or shunt placement.

Deep vein thrombosis is common in persons with traumatic brain injury, with an incidence as high as 54%.[134] Risk factors include immobility, lower extremity fracture, paralysis, and disruption in coagulation and fibrinolysis.

Upper motor neuron syndrome is common after traumatic brain injury.[129,135] It is characterized by impairment of motor control, spasticity (an overreactive response to a quick stretch stimulus), muscle weakness, stereotypic patterns of movement (synergy), and the stimulation of distant movement by noxious stimuli (synkinesia). Syndromes of restricted limb motion are the most common types of impairment. Syndromes of excessive motion are less frequent.

Heterotopic ossification is the formation of bone in nonskeletal tissue surrounding the joints.[136-138] The incidence of clinically significant heterotopic ossification is 11%. The condition causes joint pain and decreased range of motion. During the period of initial growth it is often associated with low-grade fever, periarticular swelling, warmth, and erythema and may be confused with infection. Heterotopic ossification most commonly occurs in the hips, elbows, knees, and shoulders. Risk factors include prolonged coma, male sex, young age, associated limb trauma, and spasticity. The risk of heterotopic ossification is greatest during the first 3 to 4 months after injury. Its pathophysiology remains unclear; however, inappropriate differentiation of mesenchymal cells into osteoblasts is believed to be the basic defect. Oral anti-inflammatory medications are often used during the acute and subacute phases.

3: Basic Principles and Treatment of Musculoskeletal Disease

Gastrointestinal and genitourinary complications are common after brain injury. Some of the most frequent gastrointestinal complications are stress ulcers, dysphagia, bowel incontinence, and elevated enzyme levels on liver function tests. Underlying constipation and/or impaired communication and mobility are often the causes of bowel incontinence. Genitourinary complications include urethral strictures, urinary tract infections, and urinary incontinence. An appropriate workup to evaluate genitourinary symptoms and rule out infection is indicated.

Posttraumatic agitation is common after traumatic brain injury. Aggression is commonly associated with depression or young age at the time of injury.

Brain injury is frequently the result of high-velocity accidents and associated with polytrauma. Diagnosis is problematic because multiple injuries are common, resuscitation and other lifesaving efforts make a complete examination difficult, and the patient who is comatose or disoriented cannot assist in the history or physical examination.

Under the circumstances, three important principles should be followed.[137] The first is to make an accurate diagnosis based on a thorough examination. Fractures or dislocations are missed in 11% of patients, and peripheral nerve injuries are missed in 34%. The second is to assume that the patient will make a good neurologic recovery. Basic treatment principles should not be waived on the erroneous assumption that the patient will not survive. The third principle is to anticipate uncontrolled limb motion and lack of patient cooperation. The patient often goes through a period of agitation as neurologic recovery progresses. Traction and external fixation devices are best avoided for extremity injuries. Open reduction and internal fixation of fractures and dislocations will diminish complications, require less nursing care, allow for earlier mobilization, and result in fewer residual deformities. During the subacute phase of traumatic brain injury, when the patient is generally in a rehabilitation facility, spontaneous neurologic recovery occurs.[137] During this recovery period, which may last from 12 to 18 months, spasticity is frequently present and heterotopic ossification may develop.[136-138] Management is aimed at preventing limb deformities, maintaining a functional arc of motion in the joints, and meeting both the physical and the psychological needs of the patient.[139]

Treatment in the chronic phase involves correcting limb deformities, increasing muscle strength, maximizing motor control, training individuals to make the most effective use of residual function, and providing adaptive equipment.[120,140-142] Definitive decisions can then be made regarding bracing or surgery to correct limb deformities and rebalance muscle forces.

Spinal Cord Injury

Spinal cord injury is caused by an insult to the spinal cord resulting in a change, either temporary or permanent, in its normal motor, sensory, or autonomic function. The International Standards for Neurologic and Functional Classification of Spinal Cord Injury (Table 6) is a widely accepted system describing the level and extent of injury based on a systematic motor and sensory examination of neurologic function.[143]

Approximately 400,000 people in the United States have spinal cord damage. The leading causes of spinal cord injury are motor vehicle accidents, gunshot wounds, falls, and sports and water injuries.[144,145] Patients are generally categorized into two groups: younger individuals who sustained the injury from significant trauma, and older individuals with cervical spinal stenosis caused by congenital narrowing or spondylosis often sustained from minor trauma and often no vertebral fracture spinal injury. The most common mechanisms of injury to the spinal cord are direct trauma; compression by bone fragments, hematoma, or disk material; and ischemia from damage or impingement on the spinal arteries. Edema can occur after any of these types of injury.

Terminology for the classification of spinal cord injury has been standardized.[139] Tetraplegia refers to loss or impairment of motor or sensory function in the cervical segments of the spinal cord with resulting impairment of function in the arms, trunk, legs, and pelvic organs. Paraplegia represents loss or impairment of motor or sensory function in the thoracic, lumbar, or sacral segments of the spinal cord. Arm function is intact but, depending on the level of the cord injured, impairment in the trunk, legs, and pelvic organs may be present. A complete injury is one with no spared motor or sensory function in the lowest sacral segments. Patients with complete spinal cord injury who have recovered from spinal shock have a negligible chance for any useful motor return. An incomplete injury has partial preservation of sensory or motor function below the neurologic level and includes the lowest sacral segments.

Spinal shock is a state of transient depression of cord function below the level of injury, accompanied by the loss of all sensorimotor function. An initial increase in blood pressure due to the release of catecholamines, followed by hypotension, is seen. Flaccid paralysis, including of the bowel and bladder, is observed, and sometimes sustained priapism develops. Spinal shock symptoms can last several hours to days until the reflex arcs below the level of the injury regain function. Diagnosis of complete spinal cord injury cannot be made until spinal shock has resolved, as evidenced by the return of the bulbocavernosus reflex. To elicit this reflex, the clinician digitally examines the patient's rectum, feeling for contraction of the anal sphincter while squeezing the glans penis or clitoris. If trauma to the spinal cord causes complete injury, reflex activity at the site of injury does not return because the reflex arc is permanently interrupted.

Neurogenic shock is manifested by hypotension, bradycardia, and hypothermia. Neurogenic shock occurs more frequently in injuries above T6. It results from the disruption of the sympathetic outflow from T1-L2 and to unopposed vagal tone, which leads to a decrease in vascular resistance, with associated vascular dilatation. Neurogenic shock

Table 6

ASIA Impairment Scale
(The International Standards for Neurologic and Functional Classification of Spinal Cord Injury)

Level	Injury	Description
A	Complete injury	No motor or sensory function is preserved in the sacral segments S4-S5.
B	Incomplete injury	Sensory but not motor function is preserved below the neurologic level and includes the sacral segments S4-S5.
C	Incomplete injury	Motor function is preserved below the neurologic level, and more than half of key muscles below the neurologic level have a muscle grade < 3.
D	Incomplete injury	Motor function is preserved below the neurologic level, and at least half of key muscles below the neurologic level have a muscle grade ≥ 3.
E	Normal function	Motor and sensory functions are normal.

(Adapted from American Spinal Injury Association: *International Standards for Neurologic Classifications of Spinal Cord Injury*, [rev ed]. Chicago, IL, American Spinal Injury Association, 2000, pp 1-23.)

needs to be differentiated from spinal and hypovolemic shock. Hypovolemic shock is associated with tachycardia.

International Standards for Neurologic and Functional Classification of Spinal Cord Injury, published by the American Spinal Injury Association (ASIA) and the International Medical Society of Paraplegia, represents the most reliable instrument for assessing neurologic status in the spinal cord. The extent of spinal cord injury is defined by the ASIA Impairment Scale[143] (Table 6). These standards provide a quantitative measure of sensory and motor function. The ASIA Motor Score is the sum of strength grades shown in Table 7 for each of the 10 key muscles (tested bilaterally) that represent neurologic segments from C5 to T1 and L2 to S1 (Table 8). In a neurologically intact individual, the total possible ASIA Motor Score is 100 points. The change in ASIA Motor Score is determined in successive neurologic examinations. Muscle strength always should be graded according to the maximum strength attained, no matter how briefly that strength is maintained during the examination. The muscles are tested with the patient supine. The key muscles tested and the corresponding levels of injury are listed in Table 8.

Sensory scoring is also performed for light touch and pinprick (Table 9). A score of 0 (absent sensation) is given if the patient cannot differentiate between the point of a sharp pin and the dull edge. Impaired sensation or hyperesthesia receives a score of 1. Intact sensation is scored as 2. The sensory index score is the total from adding each dermatomal score. The maximal possible total score is 112 for a neurologically intact person.

Using these criteria, the motor level is determined by the most caudal key muscles that have muscle strength of 3 or above while the segment above is normal. The sensory level is the most caudal dermatome with a normal score of 2/2 for pinprick and light touch. The neurologic level of injury

Table 7

The Medical Research Council Scale of Muscle Strength

Grade	Description
5	Normal power
4+	Submaximal movement against resistance
4	Moderate movement against resistance
4−	Slight movement against resistance
3	Movement against gravity but not against resistance
2	Movement with gravity eliminated
1	Flicker of movement
0	No movement

(Adapted from Medical Research Council: *Aids to Examination of the Peripheral Nervous System: Memorandum No. 45*. London, England, Her Majesty's Stationary Office, 1976.)

is the most caudal level at which motor and sensory levels are intact.

The lower extremities motor score uses the ASIA key muscles in both lower extremities, with a total possible score of 50. A lower extremities motor score of 20 or less indicates that the patient is likely to be a limited ambulator, and a score of 30 or more suggests that the individual is likely to become a community ambulator.

Specific spinal cord syndromes can be seen. Anterior cord syndrome results from direct contusion to the anterior cord by bone fragments or from damage to the anterior spinal artery. Depending on the extent of cord involvement, only posterior column function (proprioception and light

Table 8

The Key Muscles and the Corresponding Level of Injury in Spinal Cord Injury

Cord Level	Key Muscles
C5	Elbow flexors (biceps, brachialis)
C6	Wrist extensors (extensor carpi radialis longus and brevis)
C7	Elbow extensors (triceps)
C8	Finger flexors (flexor digitorum profundus) to the middle finger
T1	Small finger abductors (abductor digiti minimi)
L2	Hip flexors (iliopsoas)
L3	Knee extensors (quadriceps)
L4	Ankle dorsiflexors (tibialis anterior)
L5	Long toe extensors (extensor hallucis longus)
S1	Ankle plantar flexors (gastrocnemius, soleus)

(Adapted from American Spinal Injury Association: *International Standards for Neurologic Classifications of Spinal Cord Injury.* [rev ed]. Chicago, IL, American Spinal Injury Association, 2000, pp 1-23; Ditunno JF Jr, Young W, Donovan WH, et al: The international standards booklet for neurologic and functional classification of spinal cord injury: American Spinal Injury Association. *Paraplegia* 1994;32[2]:70-80.)

Table 9

Sensory Testing Levels in Spinal Cord Injury

Cord Level	Location of Sensory Testing
C2	Occipital protuberance
C3	Supraclavicular fossa
C4	Top of the acromioclavicular joint
C5	Lateral side of antecubital fossa
C6	Thumb
C7	Middle finger
C8	Little finger
T1	Medial side of antecubital fossa
T2	Apex of axilla
T3	Third intercostal space (IS)
T4	Fourth IS at nipple line
T5	Fifth IS (midway between T4 and T6)
T6	Sixth IS at the level of the xiphisternum
T7	Seventh IS (midway between T6 and T8)
T8	Eighth IS (midway between T6 and T10)
T9	Ninth IS (midway between T8 and T10)
T10	10th IS or umbilicus
T11	11th IS (midway between T10 and T12)
T12	Midpoint of inguinal ligament
L1	Half the distance between T12 and L2
L2	Midanterior thigh
L3	Medial femoral condyle
L4	Medial malleolus
L5	Dorsum of the foot at third metatarsophalangeal joint
S1	Lateral heel
S2	Popliteal fossa in the midline
S3	Ischial tuberosity
S4-5	Perianal area

One point each is given for intact pinprick and proprioception. The maximal score in a neurologically intact person is 112.

touch) may be present. The ability to respond to pain and light touch signifies that the posterior half of the cord has some intact function.

Central cord syndrome can be understood on the basis of the spinal cord anatomy. Gray matter in the spinal cord contains nerve cell bodies and is surrounded by white matter consisting primarily of ascending and descending myelinated tracts. Central gray matter has a higher metabolic requirement and is therefore more susceptible to the effects of trauma and ischemia. Central cord syndrome often results from a minor injury such as a fall in an older patient with cervical spinal canal stenosis. Most patients can walk despite severe paralysis of the upper limb.

Brown-Séquard syndrome is caused by a complete hemisection of the spinal cord, which results in a greater ipsilateral proprioceptive motor loss and greater contralateral loss of pain and temperature sensation. Affected patients have an excellent prognosis and usually will ambulate.

Mixed syndrome is characterized by diffuse involvement of the entire spinal cord. Affected patients have a good prognosis for recovery. As with all incomplete spinal cord injury syndromes, early motor recovery is the best prognostic indicator.

Conus medullaris syndrome is associated with injury to the sacral cord and lumbar nerve roots. This leads to areflexic bladder, bowel, and lower limbs. The sacral segments may occasionally show preserved reflexes, for example the bulbocavernosus and micturition reflexes.

Cauda equina syndrome is secondary to injury of the lumbosacral nerve roots in the spinal canal, leading to areflexic bladder, bowel, and lower limbs.

A complication of spinal cord injury sometimes seen is autonomic dysreflexia. This occurs from splanchnic outflow conveying sympathetic fibers to the lower body exits at the T8 region. Patients with lesions above T8 are prone to autonomic dysreflexia. Signs and symptoms include episodes of hypertension that may be heralded by dizziness, sweating, and headaches.

Heterotopic ossification occurs between the muscles and joint capsule in 20% of patients with spinal cord injury, with a higher incidence in patients 20 to 30 years old.[136,138] Heterotopic ossification is more common in cervical and thoracic level injuries than in lumbar injuries. There is a higher incidence of heterotopic ossification in patients with complete spinal cord lesions. It is most common at the hip but can occur at the knee, especially posteriorly. If the functional range of motion of a joint is limited, the heterotopic ossification should be surgically excised.

Cerebral Palsy

The term cerebral palsy loosely translates as "brain paralysis." A precise definition is not possible because cerebral palsy is not a single diagnosis. Cerebral palsy is a nonspecific term that refers to a group of disorders with nonprogressive brain lesions resulting in motor or postural abnormalities.[146,147] These abnormalities are noted during early development and are attributed to disturbances that occurred in the developing fetal or infant brain. The brain lesions of cerebral palsy occur from the fetal or neonatal period to up to age 3 years. Although the injury to the brain occurs prior to age 3 years, the diagnosis may not be made until later. Insults to the brain after age 3 years can appear clinically as similar to cerebral palsy. However, by definition, these lesions are not cerebral palsy.

Etiology and Risk Factors

Cerebral palsy is restricted to lesions of the brain only. An exact cause is not always known, but the impairment is sometimes associated with prematurity, perinatal hypoxia, cerebral trauma, or neonatal jaundice.[148,149] In the United States, more than 500,000 people are affected by cerebral palsy. The degree of neurologic impairment is severe in one third of patients and mild in approximately one sixth. The motor disorders of cerebral palsy can be accompanied by a seizure disorder and/or disturbances of sensation, cognition, communication, perception, and/or behavior.

Risk factors for cerebral palsy are multifactorial and can include preterm birth, multiple gestation, intrauterine growth restriction, male sex, low Apgar scores, intrauterine infections, maternal thyroid abnormalities, prenatal strokes, birth asphyxia, maternal methyl mercury exposure, and maternal iodine deficiency. Although preterm delivery is a well-established risk factor for cerebral palsy, a recent study suggests that postterm pregnancy at 42 weeks or later is associated with an increased risk of cerebral palsy.[149]

The immaturity of the brain and cerebral vasculature, in addition to the physical stresses experienced by premature infants, most likely explains why prematurity is a significant risk factor for cerebral palsy. The distribution of fetal circulation of the brain results in a tendency for hypoperfusion of the periventricular white matter. Hypoperfusion can result in hemorrhages within the germinal matrix and periventricular leukomalacia. Periventricular leukomalacia is usually symmetric and is thought to be due to ischemic white matter injury in premature infants. The periventricular white matter areas near the lateral ventricles are most susceptible to injury between weeks 26 and 34 of gestation. These areas of the brain carry fibers responsible for the motor control and muscle tone of the legs. Injuries here can result in spastic diplegia. With larger lesions, both the lower and upper extremities may be involved. Circulation to the brain at term resembles adult cerebral circulation. Vascular injuries at this stage most often occur in the distribution of the middle cerebral artery, resulting in a spastic hemiplegic cerebral palsy.

Classification

Given the complexity of prenatal and neonatal brain development, injury or abnormal development may occur at any time, resulting in the varied clinical presentations of cerebral palsy. Because of the diversity of neurologic findings seen in patients with cerebral palsy, a classification system is needed. Cerebral palsy can be classified by types of movement disorder and patterns of neurologic deficit.

Three types of movement disorders are seen. Spastic disorders are characterized by the presence of clonus and hyperactive deep tendon reflexes. Patients with spastic movement can be helped by orthopaedic intervention. The conditions classified as dyskinetic disorders are athetosis, ballismus, chorea, dystonia, and ataxia. For practical purposes, these conditions are grouped together because they are not amenable to surgical correction. Mixed disorders usually consist of a combination of spasticity and athetosis with total body involvement.

A variety of patterns of neurologic involvement are also seen. Monoplegia exhibits single-limb involvement, and the disorder is usually spastic in nature. Because monoplegia is rare, it is advisable to test the patient before making the diagnosis. The stress of performing an activity such as running at a fast pace will often uncover spasticity in another limb. In hemiplegia, spasticity affects the upper and lower extremities ipsilaterally. Equinovarus posturing is common in the lower extremity. The upper extremity is usually held with the elbow, wrist, and fingers flexed and the thumb adducted. The major problem interfering with upper extremity function, however, is a loss of proprioception and stereognosis. In paraplegia, neurologic deficits involve only the lower extremities. Because paraplegia is rare in patients with spastic cerebral palsy, it is important to rule out the existence of a high spinal cord lesion that could also be responsible for the neurologic findings. Bladder problems coexist with spastic paralysis that affects the lower extremities and is secondary to spinal cord damage.

Spastic diplegia is seen in 50% to 60% of patients with cerebral palsy in the United States and is the most common neurologic pattern. It is characterized by major involvement in both lower extremities with only minor incoordination in the upper extremities. Findings in the lower extremities include marked spasticity, particularly about the hips, hyperactive deep tendon reflexes, and a positive Babinski sign. The hips are commonly held in a position of flexion, adduction, and internal rotation secondary to the spasticity. The knees are in the valgus position and may have excessive external rotation of the tibia. The ankles are held in the equinus position, with the feet in valgus. Speech and intellectual functions are usually normal or only slightly impaired. Esotropia and visual perception problems are common.

Total body involvement is sometimes referred to as quadriplegia. Total body involvement is characterized by impairments affecting all four extremities, the head, and the trunk. Sensory deficits are typical, and speech and swallowing are commonly impaired. Often, the most serious deficit is the inability to communicate with others. Although mental retardation is found in approximately 45% of patients, intelligence is often masked by communication dysfunction. However, because of oromotor, fine motor, and gross motor difficulties, communication in patients with cerebral palsy may be impaired and expression of intellectual capacity may be limited. Approximately 15% to 60% of children with cerebral palsy have epilepsy. Epilepsy is more frequent in patients with spastic quadriplegia or mental retardation. Ambulation is not usually a goal because the equilibrium reactions of affected patients are severely impaired or absent. Sitting may require braces or adaptive supportive devices. Scoliosis, contractures, and dislocated hips are common orthopaedic conditions that may interfere with sitting.

Management

Physical and occupational therapy are essential in the care of patients with cerebral palsy.[139,147,150] Strengthening, joint mobility, ambulation, and training in activities of daily living all serve to maximize function and the quality of life.

Numerous medications can be used to treat movement difficulties. These drugs target spasticity, dystonia, myoclonus, chorea, and athetosis. Anticonvulsant agents may be useful in the management of myoclonus. Chorea and athetosis are difficult to manage. Seizure disorders are common in persons with cerebral palsy, and are managed with anticonvulsant medications.

Oral drug therapy can be of some assistance in controlling spasticity.[151] Drugs are used when spasticity is not severe and affects multiple large muscle groups in the body. Patients with attention deficits or memory disorders may be compromised by antispastic agents such as baclofen, diazepam, and clonidine that have sedating properties. The drug tizanidine has been reported to affect the central nervous system less than other agents and may be useful. Even a drug such as dantrolene sodium, which acts peripherally, may also cause drowsiness.

Baclofen, administered either orally or intrathecally, is also often used to treat spasticity.[152] Baclofen can inhibit both polysynaptic and monosynaptic reflexes at the spinal cord level. It does, however, depress general central nervous system function. Intrathecal baclofen is administered via an implanted pump. The pump is placed in the anterior abdominal wall and connects to a catheter inserted in the subarachnoid space overlying the conus of the spinal cord. Intrathecal baclofen can allow more local presynaptic inhibition of I-a sensory afferents and has fewer adverse effects than oral baclofen.

Neurosurgical treatment of selective dorsal rhizotomy can be considered.[153,154] Dorsal rhizotomy may be beneficial in both the short term and long term. By cutting I-a sensory fibers, selective dorsal rhizotomy decreases spasticity by decreasing reflexive motoneuron activation, which is thought to result from the lack of descending fiber input.

Chemodenervation using botulinum toxin is useful for the temporary reduction of spasticity.[155-157] Ordinarily, an action potential propagating down to a motor nerve to the neuromuscular junction triggers the release of acetylcholine into the synaptic space. The released acetylcholine causes depolarization of muscle membrane. Botulinum toxin type A is a protein produced by *Clostridium botulinum* that attaches to the presynaptic nerve terminal and inhibits the release of acetylcholine at the neuromuscular junction. Botulinum toxin is injected directly into a spastic muscle. Clinical benefit lasts 3 to 5 months. Current practice is not to administer a total of more than 400 U in a single treatment session to avoid excessive weakness or paralysis. This upper limit of 400 U may be reached rather quickly when injecting a few large muscles. A delay of 3 to 7 days between injection of botulinum toxin A and the onset of clinical effect is typical. The effect generally lasts 3 to 6 months, which can allow for improved range of motion and improved response to occupational and physical therapy, including casting to correct deformities. Effective control of spasticity can delay the need for orthopaedic surgery.

Multiple specialists are needed for optimal management of the patient with cerebral palsy.[139,150,158] Reconstructive orthopaedic surgery can restore muscle balance, release contractures, stabilize joints, and correct limb deformities and scoliosis. The severely impaired patient requires additional consultations. A gastroenterologist, nutritionist, and a feeding and swallowing team are needed for the management of feeding and swallowing difficulties, and gastroesophageal reflux. The assessment of nutritional status is also important. A pulmonologist may be needed for the management of chronic pulmonary disease due to bronchopulmonary dysplasia and frequent or recurrent aspiration.

A multidisciplinary learning disability team specializing in children with special needs should be consulted to identify specific learning disabilities, monitor cognitive progression, and guide services through early intervention and school. The child should be evaluated by a communication enhancement center to guide speech and language treatment and the use of communicative devices.

Summary

Neuromuscular disorders are classified as motor unit diseases because the primary abnormality may involve the neurons, the neuromuscular junction, or the muscle fiber. There are two broad categories. Myopathies are diseases of the muscle fibers. Neuropathies are disorders in which muscle degeneration is seen secondary to either upper or lower motor neuron disease. Neuromuscular disorders can be divided into five categories. Dystrophinopathies (muscular dystrophies) are hereditary, childhood-onset diseases that target the lower motor neuron. Muscular atrophies are autosomal recessive, childhood-onset diseases that target muscle cells directly. Hereditary neuropathies (CMT) are largely autosomal dominant disorders occurring in childhood. CMT4 is an autosomal recessive disease, and CMTX is X linked. All of the hereditary neuropathies target the lower motor neuron. Neurodegenerative diseases are diverse and include such entities as multiple sclerosis, ALS, and Parkinson disease. Their etiologies are not known. Onset is during adulthood and they target the lower motor neuron. Acute disseminated encephalomyelitis is the exception because it occurs in prepubescent children and targets the upper motor neuron. The acquired neuromuscular disorders are varied in etiology, physiology, pathology and prognosis. Poliomyelitis and Guillain-Barré syndrome are lower motor neuron disorders with flaccid paralysis. Stroke, traumatic brain injury, cerebral palsy, and spinal cord injury are upper motor neuron disorders with spastic paralysis.

References

1. Greenberg SA, Walsh RJ: Molecular diagnosis of inheritable neuromuscular disorders: Part II. Application of genetic testing in neuromuscular disease. *Muscle Nerve* 2005;31(4): 431-451.

2. Greenberg SA, Walsh RJ: Molecular diagnosis of inheritable neuromuscular disorders: Part I. Genetic determinants of inherited disease and their laboratory detection. *Muscle Nerve* 2005;31(4):418-430.

3. Rahman S, Hanna MG: Diagnosis and therapy in neuromuscular disorders: Diagnosis and new treatments in mitochondrial diseases. *J Neurol Neurosurg Psychiatry* 2009;80(9): 943-953.

4. von der Hagen M, Schallner J, Kaindl AM, et al: Facing the genetic heterogeneity in neuromuscular disorders: Linkage analysis as an economic diagnostic approach towards the molecular diagnosis. *Neuromuscul Disord* 2006;16(1):4-13.

5. Sussman M: Duchenne muscular dystrophy. *J Am Acad Orthop Surg* 2002;10(2):138-151.

6. Buchthal F: Electrophysiological signs of myopathy as related with muscle biopsy. *Acta Neurol (Napoli)* 1977;32(1): 1-29.

7. Rabie M, Jossiphov J, Nevo Y: Electromyography (EMG) accuracy compared to muscle biopsy in childhood. *J Child Neurol* 2007;22(7):803-808.

8. Chang J, Park YG, Choi YC, Choi JH, Moon JH: Correlation of electromyogram and muscle biopsy in myopathy of young age. *Arch Phys Med Rehabil* 2011;92(5):780-784.

9. Edwards R, Young A, Wiles M: Needle biopsy of skeletal muscle in the diagnosis of myopathy and the clinical study of muscle function and repair. *N Engl J Med* 1980;302(5): 261-271.

10. Lai CH, Melli G, Chang YJ, et al: Open muscle biopsy in suspected myopathy: Diagnostic yield and clinical utility. *Eur J Neurol* 2010;17(1):136-142.

11. Poulsen MB, Bojsen-Moller M, Jakobsen J, Andersen H: Percutaneous conchotome biopsy of the deltoid and quadricep muscles in the diagnosis of neuromuscular disorders. *J Clin Neuromuscul Dis* 2005;7(1):36-41.

12. Biggar WD, Klamut HJ, Demacio PC, Stevens DJ, Ray PN: Duchenne muscular dystrophy: Current knowledge, treatment, and future prospects. *Clin Orthop Relat Res* 2002;401: 88-106.

13. Holloway SM, Wilcox DE, Wilcox A, et al: Life expectancy and death from cardiomyopathy amongst carriers of Duchenne and Becker muscular dystrophy in Scotland. *Heart* 2008;94(5):633-636.

14. Duchenne GB: The pathology of paralysis with muscular degeneration (paralysie myosclerotique), or paralysis with apparent hypertrophy. *Br Med J* 1867;2(363):541-542.

15. Duchenne GB: Studies on pseudohypertrophic muscular paralysis or myosclerotic paralysis. *Arch Neurol* 1968;19(6): 629-636.

16. Kunkel LM, Hejtmancik JF, Caskey CT, et al: Analysis of deletions in DNA from patients with Becker and Duchenne muscular dystrophy. *Nature* 1986;322(6074):73-77.

17. Monaco AP, Neve RL, Colletti-Feener C, Bertelson CJ, Kurnit DM, Kunkel LM: Isolation of candidate cDNAs for portions of the Duchenne muscular dystrophy gene. *Nature* 1986;323(6089):646-650.

18. Ervasti JM: Dystrophin, its interactions with other proteins, and implications for muscular dystrophy. *Biochim Biophys Acta* 2007;1772(2):108-117.

19. Ervasti JM, Campbell KP: Dystrophin-associated glycoproteins: Their possible roles in the pathogenesis of Duchenne muscular dystrophy. *Mol Cell Biol Hum Dis Ser* 1993;3:139-166.

20. Ervasti JM, Sonnemann KJ: Biology of the striated muscle dystrophin-glycoprotein complex. *Int Rev Cytol* 2008;265: 191-225.

21. Ozawa E, Yoshida M, Suzuki A, Mizuno Y, Hagiwara Y, Noguchi S: Dystrophin-associated proteins in muscular dystrophy. *Hum Mol Genet* 1995;4(Spec No):1711-1716.

22. Yoshida M, Mizuno Y, Nonaka I, Ozawa E: A dystrophin-associated glycoprotein, A3a (one of 43DAG doublets), is retained in Duchenne muscular dystrophy muscle. *J Biochem* 1993;114(5):634-639.

23. Becker PE, Kiener F: A new x-chromosomal muscular dystrophy. *Arch Psychiatr Nervenkr Z Gesamte Neurol Psychiatr* 1955;193(4):427-448.

24. Dubowitz V: Enigmatic conflict of clinical and molecular diagnosis in Duchenne/Becker muscular dystrophy. *Neuromuscul Disord* 2006;16(12):865-866.

25. Walton JN: Research in muscular dystrophy. *Nature* 1970; 228(5270):417-418.

26. Walton JN: Muscular dystrophy: Some recent advances in knowledge. *Br Med J* 1964;1(5394):1344-1348.

27. Nattrass FJ: Recovery from muscular dystrophy. *Brain* 1954; 77(4):549-570.

28. Walton JN, Nattrass FJ: On the classification, natural history and treatment of the myopathies. *Brain* 1954;77(2):169-231.

29. Baghdiguian S, Richard I, Martin M, et al: Pathophysiology of limb girdle muscular dystrophy type 2A: Hypothesis and new insights into the IkappaBalpha/NF-kappaB survival pathway in skeletal muscle. *J Mol Med (Berl)* 2001;79(5-6): 254-261.

30. Beckmann JS, Bushby KM: Advances in the molecular genetics of the limb-girdle type of autosomal recessive progressive muscular dystrophy. *Curr Opin Neurol* 1996;9(5): 389-393.

31. Chae J, Minami N, Jin Y, et al: Calpain 3 gene mutations: Genetic and clinico-pathologic findings in limb-girdle muscular dystrophy. *Neuromuscul Disord* 2001;11(6-7):547-555.

32. Cottrell CE, Mendell J, Hart-Kothari M, et al: Maternal uniparental disomy of chromosome 4 in a patient with limb-girdle muscular dystrophy 2E confirmed by SNP array technology. *Clin Genet* 2012;81(6):578-583.

33. Teijeira-Bautista S, García-García D, Teijeiro-Ferreira A, Fernández-Hojas R, Fernández-Rodríguez JM, Navarro-Fernández-Balbuena C: Dystrophinopathies, congenital muscular dystrophy, limb-girdle dystrophies: Updated classification. *Rev Neurol* 1998;26(154):1021-1026.

34. Hawkins A: Rethinking the genetic basis and inheritance of fascioscapulohumeral muscular dystrophy. *Clin Genet* 2012; 82(3):219-220.

35. Scionti I, Greco F, Ricci G, et al: Large-scale population analysis challenges the current criteria for the molecular diagnosis of fascioscapulohumeral muscular dystrophy. *Am J Hum Genet* 2012;90(4):628-635.

36. Galluzzi G, Deidda G, Cacurri S, et al: Molecular analysis of 4q35 rearrangements in fascioscapulohumeral muscular dystrophy (FSHD): Application to family studies for a correct genetic advice and a reliable prenatal diagnosis of the disease. *Neuromuscul Disord* 1999;9(3):190-198.

37. Gilchrist JM: Other muscular dystrophies, in Gilchrist JM (ed): *Prognosis in Neurology*. Oxford, England, Butterworth-Heinemann, 1998, pp 347-349.

38. Griggs RC, Mendell JR, Miller RG: The muscular dystrophies, in *Evaluation and Treatment of Myopathies*. Philadelphia, PA, FA Davis Co, 1995, pp 122-128.

39. Dreifuss FE, Hogan GR: Survival in x-chromosomal muscular dystrophy. *Neurology* 1961;11:734-737.

40. Muntoni F, Lichtarowicz-Krynska EJ, Sewry CA, et al: Early presentation of X-linked Emery-Dreifuss muscular dystrophy resembling limb-girdle muscular dystrophy. *Neuromuscul Disord* 1998;8(2):72-76.

41. Park YE, Hayashi YK, Goto K, et al: Nuclear changes in skeletal muscle extend to satellite cells in autosomal dominant Emery-Dreifuss muscular dystrophy/limb-girdle muscular dystrophy 1B. *Neuromuscul Disord* 2009;19(1):29-36.

42. Hong JS, Ki CS, Kim JW, et al: Cardiac dysrhythmias, cardiomyopathy and muscular dystrophy in patients with Emery-Dreifuss muscular dystrophy and limb-girdle muscular dystrophy type 1B. *J Korean Med Sci* 2005;20(2):283-290.

43. Burd L, Short SK, Martsolf JT, Nelson RA: Prevalence of type I spinal muscular atrophy in North Dakota. *Am J Med Genet* 1991;41(2):212-215.

44. Pearn JH, Wilson J: Chronic generalized spinal muscular atrophy of infancy and childhood: Arrested Werdnig-Hoffman disease. *Arch Dis Child* 1973;48(10):768-774.

45. Miles JM, Gilbert-Barness E: Pathological cases of the month: Type 1 spinal muscular atrophy (Werdnig-Hoffman disease). *Am J Dis Child* 1993;147(8):907-908.

46. Tsukagoshi H, Sugita H, Furukawa T, Tsubaki T, Ono E: Kugelberg-Welander syndrome with dominant inheritance. *Arch Neurol* 1966;14(4):378-381.

47. Gdynia HJ, Sperfeld AD, Flaith L, et al: Classification of phenotype characteristics in adult-onset spinal muscular atrophy. *Eur Neurol* 2007;58(3):170-176.

48. Mazzei R, Gambardella A, Conforti FL, et al: Gene conversion events in adult-onset spinal muscular atrophy. *Acta Neurol Scand* 2004;109(2):151-154.

49. Pearn JH, Hudgson P, Walton JN: A clinical and genetic study of spinal muscular atrophy of adult onset: The autosomal recessive form as a discrete disease entity. *Brain* 1978; 101(4):591-606.

50. Charcot JM: Sur une forme particulaire d'atrophie musculaire progressive souvent familial debutant par les pieds et les jambes et atteingnant plus tard les mains. *Rev Med* 1886; 6:97-138.

51. Tooth HH: *The Peroneal Type of Progressive Muscular Atrophy*. London, England, Lewis, 1886.

52. Dejerine H, Sottas J: Sur la nevrite interstitielle, hypertrophique et progressive de l'enfance. *CR Soc Biol* 1893;45:63-96.

53. Emery AE: Population frequencies of inherited neuromuscular diseases: A world survey. *Neuromuscul Disord* 1991; 1(1):19-29.

54. Murphy SM, Laura M, Fawcett K, et al: Charcot-Marie-Tooth disease: Frequency of genetic subtypes and guidelines for genetic testing. *J Neurol Neurosurg Psychiatry* 2012;83(7): 706-710.

55. Patzko A, Shy ME: Charcot-Marie-Tooth disease and related genetic neuropathies. *Continuum (Minneap Minn)* 2012; 18(1):39-59.

56. Martini R, Berciano J, Van Broeckhoven CV: 5th Workshop of the European CMT Consortium, 69th ENMC International Workshop: Therapeutic approaches in CMT neuropathies and related disorders 23-25 April 1999, Soestduinen, The Netherlands. *Neuromuscul Disord* 2000;10(1):69-74.

57. Menotti F, Bazzucchi I, Felici F, Damiani A, Gori MC, Macaluso A: Neuromuscular function after muscle fatigue in Charcot-Marie-Tooth type 1A patients. *Muscle Nerve* 2012; 46(3):434-439.

58. Joo SY, Choi BO, Kim DY, Jung SJ, Cho SY, Hwang SJ: Foot deformity in Charcot Marie Tooth disease according to disease severity. *Ann Rehabil Med* 2011;35(4):499-506.

59. Mann DC, Hsu JD: Triple arthrodesis in the treatment of fixed cavovarus deformity in adolescent patients with Charcot-Marie-Tooth disease. *Foot Ankle* 1992;13(1):1-6.

60. Wetmore RS, Drennan JC: Long-term results of triple arthrodesis in Charcot-Marie-Tooth disease. *J Bone Joint Surg Am* 1989;71(3):417-422.

61. Brandsma JW, Ottenhoff-De Jonge MW: Flexor digitorum superficialis tendon transfer for intrinsic replacement: Long-term results and the effect on donor fingers. *J Hand Surg Br* 1992;17(6):625-628.

62. Boĭko AN, Ovcharov VV, Serkov SV, Borets OG, Gol'tsova NIu: A case of differential diagnosis between X-linked adrenomyeloneuropathy and multiple sclerosis. *Zh Nevrol Psikhiatr Im S S Korsakova* 2010;110(4):92-96.

63. Myhr KM: Diagnosis and treatment of multiple sclerosis. *Acta Neurol Scand Suppl* 2008;188:12-21.

64. Tsang BK, Macdonell R: Multiple sclerosis: Diagnosis, management and prognosis. *Aust Fam Physician* 2011;40(12):948-955.

65. Hirst C, Swingler R, Compston DA, Ben-Shlomo Y, Robertson NP: Survival and cause of death in multiple sclerosis: A prospective population-based study. *J Neurol Neurosurg Psychiatry* 2008;79(9):1016-1021.

66. Callen DJ, Shroff MM, Branson HM, et al: MRI in the diagnosis of pediatric multiple sclerosis. *Neurology* 2009;72(11):961-967.

67. Filippi M, Rocca MA: The role of magnetic resonance imaging in the study of multiple sclerosis: Diagnosis, prognosis and understanding disease pathophysiology. *Acta Neurol Belg* 2011;111(2):89-98.

68. Lucchinetti C, Brück W, Parisi J, Scheithauer B, Rodriguez M, Lassmann H: Heterogeneity of multiple sclerosis lesions: Implications for the pathogenesis of demyelination. *Ann Neurol* 2000;47(6):707-717.

69. Traboulsee AP: Magnetic resonance imaging in disease progression in multiple sclerosis, in Dangond F (ed): *Disorders of the Central and Peripheral Nervous Systems*. Boston, MA, Butterworth-Heinemann, 2002, p 170.

70. Presslauer S, Milosavljevic D, Brücke T, Bayer P, Hübl W: Elevated levels of kappa free light chains in CSF support the diagnosis of multiple sclerosis. *J Neurol* 2008;255(10):1508-1514.

71. Zipoli V, Hakiki B, Portaccio E, et al: The contribution of cerebrospinal fluid oligoclonal bands to the early diagnosis of multiple sclerosis. *Mult Scler* 2009;15(4):472-478.

72. Brück W: Clinical implications of neuropathological findings in multiple sclerosis. *J Neurol* 2005;252(suppl 3):iii10-iii14.

73. Rot U, Mesec A, Clinical MR: Clinical, MRI, CSF and electrophysiological findings in different stages of multiple sclerosis. *Clin Neurol Neurosurg* 2006;108(3):271-274.

74. Beghi E, Chiò A, Couratier P, et al: The epidemiology and treatment of ALS: Focus on the heterogeneity of the disease and critical appraisal of therapeutic trials. *Amyotroph Lateral Scler* 2011;12(1):1-10.

75. Beghi E, Logroscino G, Chiò A, et al: The epidemiology of ALS and the role of population-based registries. *Biochim Biophys Acta* 2006;1762(11-12):1150-1157.

76. Visser J, van den Berg-Vos RM, Franssen H, et al: Disease course and prognostic factors of progressive muscular atrophy. *Arch Neurol* 2007;64(4):522-528.

77. Kosaka T, Fu YJ, Shiga A, et al: Primary lateral sclerosis: Upper-motor-predominant amyotrophic lateral sclerosis with frontotemporal lobar degeneration—immunohistochemical and biochemical analyses of TDP-43. *Neuropathology* 2012;32(4):373-384.

78. Tartaglia MC, Laluz V, Rowe A, et al: Brain atrophy in primary lateral sclerosis. *Neurology* 2009;72(14):1236-1241.

79. Conte A, Lattante S, Luigetti M, et al: Classification of familial amyotrophic lateral sclerosis by family history: Effects on frequency of genes mutation. *J Neurol Neurosurg Psychiatry* 2012;83(12):1201-1203.

80. de Carvalho M, Dengler R, Eisen A, et al: Electrodiagnostic criteria for diagnosis of ALS. *Clin Neurophysiol* 2008;119(3):497-503.

81. Alper G: Acute disseminated encephalomyelitis. *J Child Neurol* 2012;27(11):1408-1425.

82. Lee YJ: Acute disseminated encephalomyelitis in children: Differential diagnosis from multiple sclerosis on the basis of clinical course. *Korean J Pediatr* 2011;54(6):234-240.

83. Tavazzi E, Ravaglia S, Franciotta D, Marchioni E: Differential diagnosis between acute disseminated encephalomyelitis and multiple sclerosis during the first episode. *Arch Neurol* 2008;65(5):676-677.

84. Parkinson J: An essay on the shaking palsy: 1817. *J Neuropsychiatry Clin Neurosci* 2002;14(2):223-236, discussion 222.

85. Abrantes AM, Friedman JH, Brown RA, et al: Physical activity and neuropsychiatric symptoms of Parkinson disease. *J Geriatr Psychiatry Neurol* 2012;25(3):138-145.

86. Bowers D, Miller K, Bosch W, et al: Faces of emotion in Parkinsons disease: Micro-expressivity and bradykinesia during voluntary facial expressions. *J Int Neuropsychol Soc* 2006;12(6):765-773.

87. Fernandez HH: Nonmotor complications of Parkinson disease. *Cleve Clin J Med* 2012;79(suppl 2):S14-S18.

88. Haller S, Badoud S, Nguyen D, et al: Differentiation between Parkinson disease and other forms of Parkinsonism using support vector machine analysis of susceptibility-weighted imaging (SWI): Initial results. *Eur Radiol* 2012: published online ahead of print July 15.

89. Del Tredici K, Rüb U, De Vos RA, Bohl JR, Braak H: Where does Parkinson disease pathology begin in the brain? *J Neuropathol Exp Neurol* 2002;61(5):413-426.

90. Kumar KR, Lohmann K, Klein C: Genetics of Parkinson disease and other movement disorders. *Curr Opin Neurol* 2012;25(4):466-474.

91. Sanyal J, Chakraborty DP, Sarkar B, et al: Environmental and familial risk factors of Parkinsons disease: Case-control study. *Can J Neurol Sci* 2010;37(5):637-642.

92. Tanner CM, Ottman R, Goldman SM, et al: Parkinson disease in twins: An etiologic study. *JAMA* 1999;281(4):341-346.

93. Polymeropoulos MH, Lavedan C, Leroy E, et al: Mutation in the alpha-synuclein gene identified in families with Parkinson's disease. *Science* 1997;276(5321):2045-2047.

3: Basic Principles and Treatment of Musculoskeletal Disease

94. Luthra PM, Kumar JS: Plausible improvements for selective targeting of dopamine receptors in therapy of Parkinson's disease. *Mini Rev Med Chem* 2012; published online ahead of print June 13.

95. Mizuno Y, Kondo T, Kuno S, Nomoto M, Yanagisawa N: Early addition of selegiline to L-Dopa treatment is beneficial for patients with Parkinson disease. *Clin Neuropharmacol* 2010;33(1):1-4.

96. Ordoñez-Librado JL, Anaya-Martinez V, Gutierrez-Valdez AL, et al: L-DOPA treatment reverses the motor alterations induced by manganese exposure as a Parkinson disease experimental model. *Neurosci Lett* 2010;471(2):79-82.

97. Stacy M, Galbreath A: Optimizing long-term therapy for Parkinson disease: Levodopa, dopamine agonists, and treatment-associated dyskinesia. *Clin Neuropharmacol* 2008; 31(1):51-56.

98. Stowe R, Ives N, Clarke CE, et al: Evaluation of the efficacy and safety of adjuvant treatment to levodopa therapy in Parkinson's disease patients with motor complications. *Cochrane Database Syst Rev* 2010;7:CD007166.

99. Sharma A, Szeto K, Desilets AR: Efficacy and safety of deep brain stimulation as an adjunct to pharmacotherapy for the treatment of Parkinson disease. *Ann Pharmacother* 2012; 46(2):248-254.

100. Baj A, Monaco S, Zanusso G, Dall'ora E, Bertolasi L, Toniolo A: The virology of the post-polio syndrome. *Future Virol* 2007;2(2):183-191.

101. Agre JC, Rodríquez AA, Tafel JA: Late effects of polio: Critical review of the literature on neuromuscular function. *Arch Phys Med Rehabil* 1991;72(11):923-931.

102. Bouza C, Muñoz A, Amate JM: Postpolio syndrome: A challenge to the health-care system. *Health Policy* 2005; 71(1):97-106.

103. Bruno RL, Frick NM, Cohen J: Polioencephalitis, stress, and the etiology of post-polio sequelae. *Orthopedics* 1991; 14(11):1269-1276.

104. Corrêa JC, Rocco CC, de Andrade DV, Peres JA, Corrêa FI: Electromyographic and neuromuscular analysis in patients with post-polio syndrome. *Electromyogr Clin Neurophysiol* 2008;48(8):329-333.

105. Klein MG, Braitman LE, Costello R, Keenan MA, Esquenazi A: Actual and perceived activity levels in polio survivors and older controls: A longitudinal study. *Arch Phys Med Rehabil* 2008;89(2):297-303.

106. Klein MG, Keenan MA, Esquenazi A, Costello R, Polansky M: Musculoskeletal pain in polio survivors and strength-matched controls. *Arch Phys Med Rehabil* 2004;85(10):1679-1683.

107. Meekins GD, So Y, Quan D: American Association of Neuromuscular & Electrodiagnostic Medicine evidenced-based review: Use of surface electromyography in the diagnosis and study of neuromuscular disorders. *Muscle Nerve* 2008; 38(4):1219-1224.

108. Sheth NP, Keenan MA: Orthopedic surgery considerations in post-polio syndrome. *Am J Orthop (Belle Mead NJ)* 2007; 36(7):348-353.

109. Wieberdink RG, Ikram MA, Hofman A, Koudstaal PJ, Breteler MM: Trends in stroke incidence rates and stroke risk factors in Rotterdam, the Netherlands from 1990 to 2008. *Eur J Epidemiol* 2012;27(4):287-295.

110. Wu SH, Ho SC, Chau PH, Goggins W, Sham A, Woo J: Sex differences in stroke incidence and survival in Hong Kong, 2000-2007. *Neuroepidemiology* 2012;38(2):69-75.

111. Zhang Y, Chapman AM, Plested M, Jackson D, Purroy F: The incidence, prevalence, and mortality of stroke in France, Germany, Italy, Spain, the UK, and the US: A literature review. *Stroke Res Treat* 2012;2012:436125.

112. Botte MJ, Waters RL, Keenan MA, Jordan C, Garland DE: Approaches to senior care #2: Orthopaedic management of the stroke patient. Part I: Pathophysiology, limb deformity, and patient evaluation. *Orthop Rev* 1988;17(6):637-647.

113. Keenan MA, Perry J, Jordan C: Factors affecting balance and ambulation following stroke. *Clin Orthop Relat Res* 1984;182:165-171.

114. Hacke WK, Kaste M, Bluhmki E, et al: Thrombolysis with alteplase 3 to 4.5 hours after acute ischemic stroke. *N Engl J Med* 2008;359(13):1317-1329.

115. Tissue plasminogen activator for acute ischemic stroke: The National Institute of Neurological Disorders and Stroke rt-PA Stroke Study Group. *N Engl J Med* 1995; 333(24):1581-1587.

116. Ingall TJ, O'Fallon WM, Asplund K, et al: Findings from the reanalysis of the NINDS tissue plasminogen activator for acute ischemic stroke treatment trial. *Stroke* 2004; 35(10):2418-2424.

117. Chen ZM, Sandercock P, Pan HC, et al: Indications for early aspirin use in acute ischemic stroke: A combined analysis of 40 000 randomized patients from the Chinese Acute Stroke Trial and the International Stroke Trial. On behalf of the CAST and IST collaborative groups. *Stroke* 2000;31(6):1240-1249.

118. CAST (Chinese Acute Stroke Trial) Collaborative Group: CAST: Randomised placebo-controlled trial of early aspirin use in 20,000 patients with acute ischaemic stroke. *Lancet* 1997;349(9066):1641-1649.

119. Botte MJ, Waters RL, Keenan MA, Jordan C, Garland DE: Approaches to senior care #3: Orthopaedic management of the stroke patient. Part II: Treating deformities of the upper and lower extremities. *Orthop Rev* 1988;17(9):891-910.

120. Hebela N, Keenan MA: Neuro-orthopedic management of the dysfunctional extremity in upper motor neuron syndromes. *Eura Medicophys* 2004;40(2):145-156.

121. Foulkes MA, Jane JA, et al: The Traumatic Coma Data Bank: Design, methods, and baseline characteristics. *J Neurosurg* 1991;75:S8-S13.

122. Kraus JF, Black MA, Hessol N, et al: The incidence of acute brain injury and serious impairment in a defined population. *Am J Epidemiol* 1984;119(2):186-201.

123. McDonald CM, Jaffe KM, Fay GC, et al: Comparison of indices of traumatic brain injury severity as predictors of neurobehavioral outcome in children. *Arch Phys Med Rehabil* 1994;75(3):328-337.

124. Teasdale G, Jennett B: Assessment of coma and impaired consciousness: A practical scale. *Lancet* 1974;2(7872):81-84.

125. Malkmus DA: *Rehabilitation of the Head-Injured Adult: Comprehensive Cognitive Management.* Downey, CA: Profes-

sional Staff Association of Rancho Los Amigos Hospital, Inc., 1980.

126. Steyerberg EW, Mushkudiani N, Perel P, et al: Predicting outcome after traumatic brain injury: Development and international validation of prognostic scores based on admission characteristics. *PLoS Med* 2008;5(8):e165.

127. Smith DH, Meaney DF, Shull WH: Diffuse axonal injury in head trauma. *J Head Trauma Rehabil* 2003;18(4):307-316.

128. Silver JM, McAllister TW, Yodofsky SC, eds: *Textbook of Traumatic Brain Injury.* Arlington, VA, American Psychiatric Publishing, 2005.

129. Zink BJ: Traumatic brain injury. *Emerg Med Clin North Am* 1996;14(1):115-150.

130. Choi DW: Ionic dependence of glutamate neurotoxicity. *J Neurosci* 1987;7(2):369-379.

131. Neary JT, Kang Y, Tran M, Feld J: Traumatic injury activates protein kinase B/Akt in cultured astrocytes: Role of extracellular ATP and P2 purinergic receptors. *J Neurotrauma* 2005;22(4):491-500.

132. Yablon SA: Posttraumatic seizures. *Arch Phys Med Rehabil* 1993;74(9):983-1001.

133. Parcell DL, Ponsford JL, Rajaratnam SM, Redman JR: Self-reported changes to nighttime sleep after traumatic brain injury. *Arch Phys Med Rehabil* 2006;87(2):278-285.

134. Cifu DX, Kaelin DL, Wall BE: Deep venous thrombosis: Incidence on admission to a brain injury rehabilitation program. *Arch Phys Med Rehabil* 1996;77(11):1182-1185.

135. Mayer NH, Esquenazi A, Childers MK: Common patterns of clinical motor dysfunction. *Muscle Nerve Suppl* 1997;6:S21-S35.

136. Cipriano CA, Pill SG, Keenan MA: Heterotopic ossification following traumatic brain injury and spinal cord injury. *J Am Acad Orthop Surg* 2009;17(11):689-697.

137. Garland DE, Keenan MA: Orthopedic strategies in the management of the adult head-injured patient. *Phys Ther* 1983;63(12):2004-2009.

138. Garland DE, Blum CE, Waters RL: Periarticular heterotopic ossification in head-injured adults: Incidence and location. *J Bone Joint Surg Am* 1980;62(7):1143-1146.

139. Keenan ME, Mehta SK: Rehabilitation, in Skinner HB, ed: *Current Diagnosis and Treatment in Orthopedics,* ed 4. New York, NY, Lange Medical Books/McGraw Hill Medical Publishers, 2006, pp 671-727.

140. Keenan MA: Surgical decision making for residual limb deformities following traumatic brain injury. *Orthop Rev* 1988;17(12):1185-1192.

141. Keenan MA: Management of the spastic upper extremity in the neurologically impaired adult. *Clin Orthop Relat Res* 1988;233:116-125.

142. Keenan MA, Esquenazi A, Mayer NH: Surgical treatment of common patterns of lower limb deformities resulting from upper motoneuron syndrome. *Adv Neurol* 2001;87:333-346.

143. American Spinal Injury Association: *International Standards for Neurological Classifications of Spinal Cord Injury* (rev ed). Chicago, IL, American Spinal Injury Association, 2000.

144. DeVivo MJ: Epidemiology of traumatic spinal cord injury, in Kirshblum S, Campagnolo DI, DeLisa JA (eds): *Spinal Cord Medicine.* Baltimore, MD, Lippincott Williams & Wilkins, 2002, pp 69-81.

145. Go BK, DeVivo MJ, Richards JS: The epidemiology of spinal cord injury, in Stover SL, DeLisa JA, Whiteneck GG (eds): *Spinal Cord Injury.* Gaithersburg, MD, Aspen, 1995 pp 21-55.

146. Bax M, Goldstein M, Rosenbaum P, et al: Proposed definition and classification of cerebral palsy, April 2005. *Dev Med Child Neurol* 2005;47(8):571-576.

147. Jones MW, Morgan E, Shelton JE, Thorogood C: Cerebral palsy: Introduction and diagnosis (part I). *J Pediatr Health Care* 2007;21(3):146-152.

148. Girard S, Kadhim H, Roy M, et al: Role of perinatal inflammation in cerebral palsy. *Pediatr Neurol* 2009;40(3):168-174.

149. Moster D, Wilcox AJ, Vollset SE, Markestad T, Lie RT: Cerebral palsy among term and postterm births. *JAMA* 2010;304(9):976-982.

150. Roberts A, Evans GA: Orthopedic aspects of neuromuscular disorders in children. *Curr Opin Pediatr* 1993;5(3):379-383.

151. Delgado MR, Hirtz D, Aisen M, et al: Practice parameter: Pharmacologic treatment of spasticity in children and adolescents with cerebral palsy (an evidence-based review). Report of the Quality Standards Subcommittee of the American Academy of Neurology and the Practice Committee of the Child Neurology Society. *Neurology* 2010;74(4):336-343.

152. Hoving MA, van Raak EP, Spincemaille GH, et al: Efficacy of intrathecal baclofen therapy in children with intractable spastic cerebral palsy: A randomised controlled trial. *Eur J Paediatr Neurol* 2009;13(3):240-246.

153. Nordmark E, Josenby AL, Lagergren J, Andersson G, Strömblad LG, Westbom L: Long-term outcomes five years after selective dorsal rhizotomy. *BMC Pediatr* 2008;8:54.

154. Trost JP, Schwartz MH, Krach LE, Dunn ME, Novacheck TF: Comprehensive short-term outcome assessment of selective dorsal rhizotomy. *Dev Med Child Neurol* 2008;50(10):765-771.

155. Elovic EP, Esquenazi A, Alter KE, Lin JL, Alfaro A, Kaelin DL: Chemodenervation and nerve blocks in the diagnosis and management of spasticity and muscle overactivity. *PM R* 2009;1(9):842-851.

156. Esquenazi AM, Mayer NH, Keenan MA: Dynamic polyelectromyography, neurolysis, and chemodenervation with botulinum toxin A for assessment and treatment of gait dysfunction. *Adv Neurol* 2001;87:321-331.

157. Simpson DM, Gracies JM, Graham HK, et al: Assessment: Botulinum neurotoxin for the treatment of spasticity (an evidence-based review): Report of the Therapeutics and Technology Assessment Subcommittee of the American Academy of Neurology. *Neurology* 2008;70(19):1691-1698.

158. Horstmann HM, Hosalkar H, Keenan MA: Orthopaedic issues in the musculoskeletal care of adults with cerebral palsy. *Dev Med Child Neurol* 2009;51(suppl 4):99-105.

3: Basic Principles and Treatment of Musculoskeletal Disease

Chapter 24

Molecular Pathophysiology of Musculoskeletal Tumors

Francis Y. Lee, MD

Sung Wook Seo, MD, PhD

Han-Soo Kim, MD, PhD

Introduction

Musculoskeletal oncology has been heavily influenced by scientific innovations and advancements in fields such as radiology, pathology, biology, and medicine. In the early 1800s, only two types of bone tumors were known. Since then, significant discoveries in science and medicine have had a major effect on the field of musculoskeletal oncology. Histologic staining using carmine dye was attempted in 1770, and hematoxylin staining was introduced in 1858. The first radiograph was obtained in 1895. Furthermore, the structure of DNA was delineated by Watson, Crick, and Collins in 1953,[1] upending the field of molecular biology. This led to the coining of molecular biology's central dogma, which describes the classic gene expression paradigm: DNA→messenger RNA (mRNA)→protein. CT became available in 1973 and MRI was introduced into the clinical arena in 1977. Beginning in 2000, the Human Genome Project accelerated the discovery of underlying molecular pathophysiologies in numerous clinical disorders and syndromes. New findings of alternative gene expression pathways or epigenetics, such as methylation or gene silencing, have initiated reassessment of the central dogmatic pathway.

During this biologic/technologic revolution, applications were used to advance many medical specialty fields. The first clinical applications of the chemotherapy agent doxorubicin for the treatment of osteosarcoma were attempted in the early 1970s.[2] Since then, combinatorial multiagent cytotoxic chemotherapy using doxorubicin, methotrexate, cisplatin, and cyclophosphamide has dramatically improved the survival rate of patients with osteosarcoma from 10% to 20% to approximately 60% to 80%. However, there has been no further increase in the cure rate for a subset of osteosarcomas in a multifocal form or in the axial skeleton for the past 20 years.[3] Current therapeutic endeavors are built upon accumulated molecular biology knowledge and tailored in the form of targeted or personalized therapy. In an era of rapidly advancing oncology fields, orthopaedic surgeons will encounter discussions of more sophisticated molecular biology jargon from patients, pathologists, and oncologists. This chapter will serve as a quick resource for orthopaedic surgeons who are interested in the clinically relevant molecular pathophysiology of cancer in a postgenomic era. Basic definitions and the clinical relevance of molecular biology as outlined in chapter 1 may be an additional reference source.

Clinically Relevant Basic Science

Hallmarks of Cancer

Cancer is characterized by uncontrolled cell growth and spread of these cells to distant sites. To cover the standard aspects of this disease, Hanahan and Weinberg proposed six hallmarks of cancer[4] (**Figure 1**).

Sustaining Proliferating Signaling

Normal cells maintain homeostasis of cell number through tight regulation of cell growth and division cycle. Cancer cells sustain their growth and proliferation signals by self-produced growth factors and receptors. In addition, cancer cells contain constitutively active signal transducers, which allow autonomous growth. For example, Ras activating mutation results in sustained activation of downstream signal transducers such as mitogen-activated protein kinase (MAPK). Another mechanism for sustained growth is a

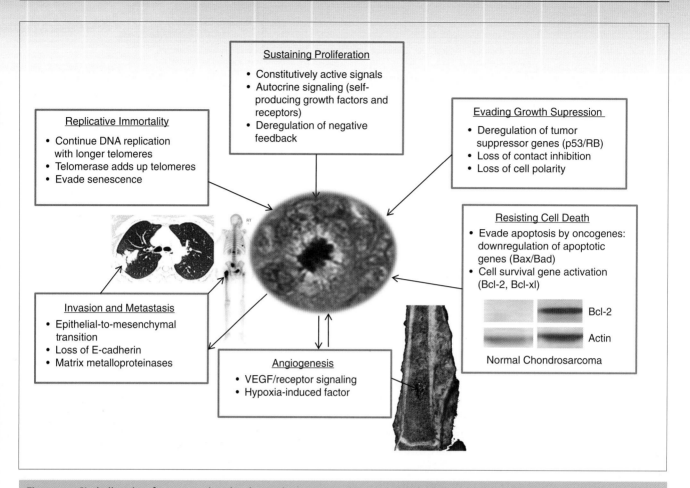

Sustaining Proliferation
- Constitutively active signals
- Autocrine signaling (self-producing growth factors and receptors)
- Deregulation of negative feedback

Replicative Immortality
- Continue DNA replication with longer telomeres
- Telomerase adds up telomeres
- Evade senescence

Evading Growth Supression
- Deregulation of tumor suppressor genes (p53/RB)
- Loss of contact inhibition
- Loss of cell polarity

Resisting Cell Death
- Evade apoptosis by oncogenes: downregulation of apoptotic genes (Bax/Bad)
- Cell survival gene activation (Bcl-2, Bcl-xl)

Bcl-2
Actin
Normal Chondrosarcoma

Invasion and Metastasis
- Epithelial-to-mesenchymal transition
- Loss of E-cadherin
- Matrix metalloproteinases

Angiogenesis
- VEGF/receptor signaling
- Hypoxia-induced factor

Figure 1 Six hallmarks of cancer and molecular explanations. VEGF = vascular endothelial growth factor.

deregulated negative feedback mechanism. As discussed in chapter 1, negative feedback mechanisms are pivotal for controlling cellular signaling pathways.

Evading Growth Suppressors

Normal cell production is disrupted by the activation of oncogenes, which results in the proliferation of renegade cells and the deactivation of tumor suppressor genes. Loss of correctly functioning tumor suppressors, inability to respond to contact inhibition, and disruption of antiproliferative cytokines (transforming growth factor–β) can result in an overgrowth of cells. Contact inhibition is a process of arresting cell growth when cells come in contact with each other (see chapter 1 for more details). Retinoblastoma (Rb)–associated and p53 proteins are well-known suppressors of the cell cycle progression. Evasion of growth suppressors can result in cancerous tumors such as retinoblastoma and osteosarcoma. Another example of a tumor suppressor is the neurofibromatosis type 2 (*NF2*) gene, which encodes for merlin. This protein is responsible for cell contact inhibition. Furthermore, loss of cell polarity via a loss-of-function mutation of *LKB1* gene in epithelial cells results in an increased activity of oncogenes.

Resisting Cell Death

Cell death is a way of maintaining homeostasis and responding to external stimuli. Necrosis is a form of death caused by chemical or physical injuries and results in an inflammatory reaction in the surrounding tissue. Apoptosis is a sequential programmed cell death involving proteins and machinery such as mitochondria, cytochrome C, Bad, Bid, and Bax. This cell death process is counterbalanced by cell survival proteins such as Bcl-2, Bcl-xL, and X-linked inhibitor of apoptosis protein. Unlike in necrosis, apoptotic cells and fragments are covered with a cellular membrane and do not cause an inflammatory response. Cancer cells escape apoptotic signals due to gene mutations in apoptosis-regulating tumor suppressors or from overactivating cell survival genes. For example, chondrosarcoma cells produce more cell-survival proteins, such as Bcl-2, when exposed to radiation or doxorubicin.

Activating Invasion and Metastasis

Cancer cells are mobile and capable of detaching from their original site, enabling them to invade local tissues and spread to distant sites. Cell-to-cell adhesion becomes loose as the cancer cells lose E-cadherin. Loss of E-cadherin is also seen in epithelial-to-mesenchymal cell transition, which is characterized by acquisition of mesenchymal cell pheno-types, loosening of intercellular connection, motility, inva-sion, and distant spread. Prostate cancer cells show epithelial-to-mesenchymal cell transition and have a predi-lection to spread to bone by assimilating to bone microen-vironments.

Replicating Immortality

Normal cells have limited capabilities of DNA replication. Telomeres ensure replication of chromosomes to their most distal ends. When telomeres are absent or dysfunctional, cells may not replicate the entire DNA sequences and lose viability. In general, longer telomeres allow more replication potential. If telomeres are used up or short, cells become se-nescent. Cancer cells have longer telomere sequences and can lengthen telomeres by a specific type of DNA poly-merase known as the telomerase, which adds telomere seg-ments to the telomeric DNA.

Inducing Angiogenesis

Cancer cells survive and increase in dimension by making their own blood vessels, which are connected to the host cir-culation. This angiogenic switch is accomplished by an an-giogenic factor called vascular endothelial growth factor (VEGF) proteins. In a response to activated oncogenes and hypoxia, VEGF signaling could be turned on, leading to the activation of tyrosine kinase receptors and subsequent downstream signaling targets. Naturally occurring inhibi-tors of VEGF are thrombospondin-1, plasmin (angiostatin), and type 18 collagen (endostatin). Cancer cells continue to survive and grow by making more blood vessels or by acti-vating cell survival machinery (antiapoptotic pathways) in relatively hypoxic conditions.

Mitosis and Cell Death in Cancer

A neoplasm is an abnormal growth of tissues resulting from an imbalance between cell proliferation and cell death. In neoplastic tissues, cell proliferation dramatically exceeds cell death, and cancer is defined as a malignant neoplasm.[4] Cell proliferation, perpetual in cancerous cells, occurs through a process known as mitosis, which comes from the Greek word meaning thread. In mitosis, DNA, a threadlike struc-ture in the nucleus, is copied and separated into two groups. The cell division process is conventionally divided into four phases: initial growth (G1: first gap), DNA synthesis/replication (S), second growth (G2: second gap), and mito-sis (M). Cells in the G0 phase are stable and do not undergo mitosis.[5] Interphase consists of the G1, G2, and S phases.[5] Organelles are replicated in the G1 and G2 phases, whereas DNA is replicated in the S phase. Cells divide during the M phase. Mitosis is a commonly used diagnostic criterion for cancers. Cyclin proteins activate many cyclin-dependent ki-nases, which promote cell division. There are also noncyclin-dependent kinases. Microtubules are involved in rearranging dividing chromosomes. Anticancer drugs target many different aspects of cell proliferation.[4]

Cell death is a very hot scientific topic. Since the first de-scription of apoptosis in 1972,[6] there has been growing in-terest in the morphologic features and molecular pathways leading to cell death. The original observation on apoptosis included nuclear condensation and shrunken morphologic features of cells, as opposed to swollen appearance, and dis-rupted cellular organelles typically seen in necrosis. Cellular and DNA fragments undergoing apoptosis are bound by double membranes and do not cause inflammatory reac-tions.[6] Necrotic cell fragments do not have protective mem-branes, and disintegrated cellular contents cause inflamma-tion. In a similar sense, oncosis refers to a cell death morphology consisting of swelling and subsequent mechan-ical rupture of the plasma membrane with dilatation of cy-toplasmic membranes. With advances in molecular biology, cell death mechanisms are better understood. There can be more than two types of cell deaths (apoptosis versus necro-sis) when the mechanisms are considered. Apoptosis can oc-cur through an intrinsic mitochondrial cytochrome C re-lease pathway or without mitochondria (extrinsic pathway). Caspases (cysteine proteases) mediate apoptosis. Caspase 3 is involved in the DNA fragmentation process.[7] Studies have shown that apoptosis can also occur without caspases.[7] Au-tophagy is based on morphologic features of massive au-tophagic vacuolization of the cytoplasm without nuclear condensation. These phagosomes contain cytoplasmic or-ganelles and are bound by two layers of membrane. Necrosis or oncosis is characterized by the swollen appearance of cells without signs of apoptosis or autophagy. There are other descriptions of cell death such as mitotic catastrophe (death after deregulated mitosis), anoikis (death after de-tachment), excitotoxicity (neuronal cell death in response to chemicals), wallerian degeneration (neuronal death after disruption of axonal flow), and cornification (skin surface death).[8] The importance of the cell death mechanism lies in the fact that different chemotherapeutic agents and radia-tion activate various cell death pathways (**Figure 2**).

Cytokines and Growth Factor

Cancers accomplish rapid localized cell growth by the pro-duction and utilization of growth-inducing cytokines. Cytokines are released by cancer cells, immune cells, bone cells, and the cells that surround the cancer cells. These sur-rounding cells are ultimately destroyed by the cancer cells. Cytokines are a group of proteins that mediate cell-to-cell communication and modulate the behavior of cells. Cytok-ines can stimulate cell growth, protein synthesis, prolifera-tion, and motility by activating specific cytokine receptors and signaling pathways.[9] Examples of cytokines are interleukin-1 (IL-1), IL-6, tumor necrosis factor (TNF), in-terferon (IFN), macrophage colony-stimulating factor (M-CSF), and receptor activator of nuclear factor κB ligand (RANKL). These cytokines promote cancer cell growth, host inflammatory response initiation, collagen degradation, and bone destruction. Chemokines (chemoattractive cytokines) are small proteins involved in recruiting or homing the cells

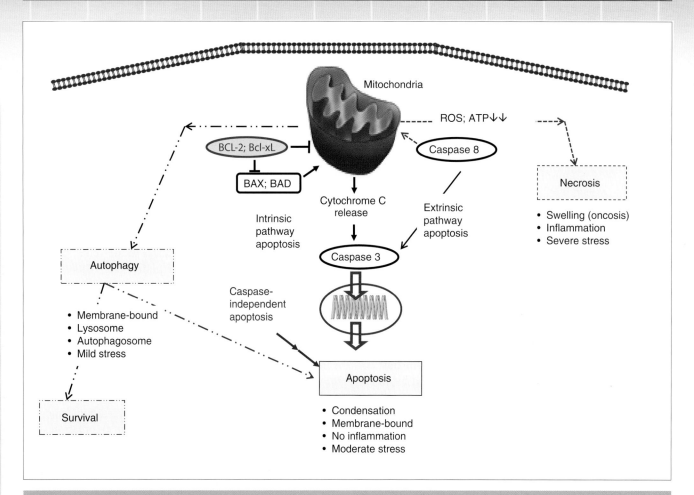

Figure 2 Cell death signals, TNF, radiation, anticancer drugs, nutritional deprivation.

by activating specific chemokine receptors.[9] Examples of chemokines are stromal cell-derived factor–1 (SDF-1), macrophage chemotactic protein–1 (MCP-1), and macrophage inflammatory protein–1 (MIP-1). Growth factors are a group of polypeptides that act as hormones and promote local cancer growth. Examples of growth factors are insulin-like growth factors (IGFs), transforming growth factors (TGFs), bone morphogenetic proteins (BMPs), VEGF, and platelet-derived growth factors (PDGFs). These biologically active cytokines, chemokines, and growth factors activate signaling pathways. Among the signal transducers, kinases relay signals to the nucleus. Some examples of these kinases are phosphoinositide 3-kinase (PI3K), tyrosine kinase, and MAPK.[5] Elucidation of growth factors, cytokines, and chemokines involved with cancers has opened many new avenues for treatment. For example, imatinib is a tyrosine kinase inhibitor that is widely used for the treatment of gastrointestinal stromal tumors and leukemias.[10] Kinase inhibitors can target many converging signals from different cytokines.

Inflammation and Cancers

The hallmarks of inflammation are pain (dolor), swelling (turgor), redness (rubor), heat (calor), and functional impairment (functio laesa).[11] More recently, the cardinal signs of inflammation have been defined as angiogenesis, increased blood flow, cytokine presence, cell proliferation, and tissue destruction. In inflammation, the response is rapid and transient. However, cancers share features similar to infection and take advantage of sustained growth. Behind uncontrolled growth of cancer cells, these cells take advantage of the inflammatory machinery, avoid cell death, and promote cell proliferation.[4] Cytokines, growth factors, and inflammatory signaling pathways are actively involved in the pathophysiology of cancer. Many cancer types, such as colon, stomach, and hepatobiliary cancer, arise from preexisting chronic inflammatory lesions. Chronic skin ulceration, secondary to osteomyelitis, is associated with squamous cell carcinoma (Majolin ulcer). The current trend is to define aberrantly activated inflammatory pathways and target them. One good example of a component in inflammatory pathways is the *Ras* oncogene. The abnormal activation of the Ras oncogene activates Raf and MAPK, which leads to cell proliferation, prolonged cell survival, and metastasis.[12]

Table 1

Important Genes Associated With Cancer

Gene	Function	Cancer
Proto-oncogenes		
Ras	G-protein, which activates multiple cell signaling pathways for survival, cell cycle progression, and motility	Colon, pancreas, lung, blood, thyroid, liver, and squamous cell cancers
c-myc	Transcription factor, which promotes cell differentiation and angiogenesis	Bone, breast, stomach, lung, cervical, and blood cancers; neuroblastoma, glioblastoma
c-Fos	In conjunction with c-Jun, promote transcription of genes involved in cell differentiation and growth	Bone, lung, colon, and breast cancers
Tumor suppressor genes		
Rb	Arrest cell cycle progression by binding to E2F protein	Eye, breast, bladder, lung, bone, and esophageal cancers
p53	Promote p21 expression to halt cell cycle progression and DNA repair	Breast, lung, brain, bone, blood, and cervical cancers

Specific inhibitors targeting Ras/Raf/MAPK currently are in clinical trials.

Oncogenes and Tumor Suppressor Genes

Genetic alterations that affect the cell cycle are key requirements for tumor development. Most of these genetic changes have been shown to occur in genes, which belong to either one of the two distinct groups known as proto-oncogenes and tumor suppressor genes. Most proto-oncogenes, the regulated forms of oncogenes, encode for proteins that stimulate cell division while inhibiting cell death and cell cycle regulation. Conversely, tumor suppressor genes play a protective role in keeping normal cells from becoming tumorigenic by repairing genetic alterations and halting cell division. It has been noted that most of these cancer-causing genetic alterations occur sporadically from somatic mutations, more so than inherited germline mutations. Regardless of the mechanisms of genetic alterations, activated oncogene and/or inactivated tumor suppressor genes are vital to the manifestation of cancerous effects. A summary of these key cancer-related genes is shown in Table 1.

Oncogenes

Under normal conditions, proto-oncogenes play a fundamental role in carrying out multiple cellular processes such as cell signaling, growth, and differentiation. However, the conversion of proto-oncogenes to hyperactive oncogenes leads to continuous cell growth and differentiation, which are key processes in tumorigenesis.[12] This functional conversion could be achieved by two different ways, which are quantitative (overproduction of the unaltered protein) or qualitative (expression of a modified protein). The quantitative conversion occurs from either gene amplification or chromosomal translocation, whereas qualitative conversion occurs from point mutations in the gene sequence.[12] Currently, more than 100 oncogenes have been identified, and the three key oncogenes are described in further detail in the following paragraphs.

Ras

Ras was the first type of proto-oncogene detected in a human tumor.[13] Once mutated, these guanosine triphosphatases (GTPase) become hyperactive and lead to the activation of multiple cellular signaling pathways, including those that contribute to the activation of apoptosis, survival, motility, and cell cycle. The activity of *Ras* is regulated by proteins known as GTPase-activating proteins (GAPs), which assist in converting *Ras* from an active GTP-bound form to an inactive GDP-bound form.[13] Furthermore, the clinical significance of this oncogene has been noted in several cancers, including colon, pancreas, lung, thyroid, liver, squamous cell, and leukemia.

Myc

Myc is an oncogene initially identified from a retrovirus.[14] Following the discovery of viral myc (*v-myc*), a homolog in humans was found and named cellular myc (*c-myc*). The activation of *c-myc* could occur by several mechanisms including chromosomal translocation, insertional mutagenesis, and amplification.[14] Several decades of research have revealed that the c-myc protein associates with a wide variety of genes and proteins, leading to numerous cellular effects that promote tumorigenesis.[14] For instance, this protein was shown to be essential for the progression of the cell cycle from G0/G1 to S phase, and upon activation, c-myc abrogates genes that are involved in cell cycle checkpoints.[15] The c-myc protein also promotes angiogenesis, cellular migration, and proliferation. However, at the same time, this protein activates *p53* tumor suppressor genes and promotes apoptosis of the cells, a process that may be used to destroy *myc*-deregulated tumors in the future.[16]

Myc has been implicated in numerous cancer types including leukemia, neuroblastoma, glioblastoma, lung, breast, stomach, cervical cancers, osteosarcoma, and Burkitt lymphoma.[14] In many cases of osteosarcoma, this protein is overexpressed, leading to tumorigenic effects.

Fos

Another well-known proto-oncogene is *c-Fos*. This protein dimerizes with another proto-oncogenic protein, c-Jun, to form a transcriptional complex known as AP-1.[17] AP-1 binds to gene promoters to cause the expression of genes involved in cellular proliferation, differentiation, and transformation. In addition, stimulation of cells with growth factors has been shown to increase the transcription of *c-fos*, demonstrating the role of this protein in cellular proliferation. Several years of research has revealed the activity of c-Fos in the formation of osteosarcoma[3] and breast cancer.[18]

Tumor Suppressor Genes

As stated previously, functional loss of tumor suppressors predisposes one to cancer, and in order for this to occur, both alleles of the gene must be in an inactivated or in a functionally weak (recessive) form.[19] In many cases of familial cancers, inactivation of these genes commonly occurs due to germline mutation of one of the two alleles followed by somatic mutation of the other allele. Alternatively, dominant alleles could be inactivated by somatic mutations or epigenetic mechanisms, such as hypermethylation of CpG, or sequential cytosine-guanine nucleotide pair regions, leading to functional loss of the gene and cancer formation.[19]

Retinoblastoma

Retinoblastoma is an eye tumor that occurs in early childhood due to germline or sporadic mutation.[3] The familial form of retinoblastoma is commonly seen in children whose parents had this disease in their childhood. In a case of familial retinoblastoma, tumors are commonly seen in both eyes (bilateral retinoblastoma), whereas in sporadic retinoblastoma, a child who has no family history presents with a tumor in a single eye (unilateral retinoblastoma).[3] These types of tumors are caused by a defect in a tumor suppressor gene known as *Rb*, which plays a vital role in controlling the progression from the G1 dormant phase to the S phase. Under normal circumstances, cyclin-dependent kinase (CDK) complexes tightly regulate Rb proteins by hyperphosphorylating (inactivating) this tumor suppressor in the late dormant G1 phase.[3] If a cell has DNA damage before entering the S phase, *Rb* is hypophosphorylated (activated) and binds to E2F protein to halt the cell cycle progression.[3] This inhibition allows the cell to correct any DNA damage and defects in the cell before proceeding into cell division.

Although *Rb* has been strongly linked to retinoblastoma, this tumor suppressor, which is found in all cells of the body, has been shown to be associated with other types of cancers including breast, bladder, lung, and esophageal cancers. Above all, sporadic osteosarcoma is commonly associated with the functional loss of *Rb*, and the incidence of this bone cancer for those who are affected by retinoblastoma is 500 times higher compared with the normal population.[3]

p53

p53 is a well-known tumor suppressor whose activity is affected by sporadic and familial mutations. Similar to *Rb*, *p53* is a gatekeeper involved in arresting the cell cycle for the maintenance of DNA integrity before cell cycle progression.[20] *p53* is a tetrameric protein regulated by MDM2 protein and activated in two distinct ways.[20] One way is by mitogenic signal-induced ARF (Alternate Reading Frame of the INK4a/ARF locus) expression and the other is by DNA damage-induced kinases (ataxia-telangiectasia mutated[ATM], checkpoint homolog CHK2, and Rad3-related). Activation of p53 induces the transcription of *p21*, which arrests the cell cycle progression in the G1 phase allowing DNA damage to be repaired.[20] If the damage is too great to repair, this protein promotes the apoptosis of the cell.

Mutations of this tumor suppressor are correlated with several different cancers including breast and lung carcinomas, brain tumors, osteosarcoma, leukemia, and virus-associated cervical cancers. Familial mutations are associated with Li-Fraumeni syndrome, which is a rare disorder that greatly increases the risk of acquiring multiple types of cancer from early age.[20] Osteosarcoma is the second most common cancer in patients with Li-Fraumeni syndrome, and inactivated p53 in osteosarcoma is commonly due to the allelic loss of this protein.[3]

Epigenetics and Cancers

Although the central dogma describes linear connections between DNA-mRNA-protein synthesis (transcription and translation), epigenetics describe modifications of gene expression by multiple factors other than genetic codes in DNA. These epigenetic factors include posttranscriptional modification, X chromosome effects, carcinogens, lifestyle factors, infection, physical factors, and chemical factors[21] (**Figure 3**). Epigenetic mechanisms include DNA methylation, histone modification, and RNA-mediated gene silencing.[21] DNA methylation and histone modification are mechanisms that silence a gene before transcription, whereas RNA-associated silencing is a mechanism of posttranscriptional silencing. DNA methylation, which is one of the well-known silencing mechanisms, occurs with the methylation of cytosine residues in the DNA by an enzyme

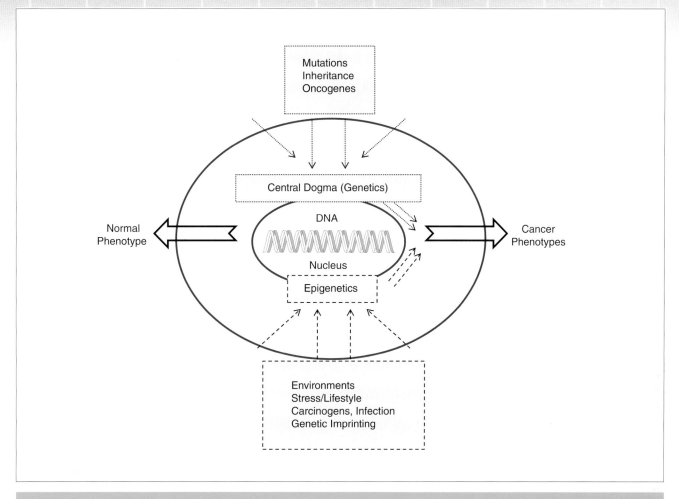

Figure 3   Genetics, epigenetics, and cancers.

known as DNA methyltransferase.[21] In histone modification, histones, which are nuclear proteins associated with DNA, are subjected to numerous modifications. These proteins could be acetylated, methylated, phosphorylated, or ubiquitinated.[21] Modifications of histones lead to inactivation of the DNA regions associated with these proteins. In RNA-associated silencing, small RNA molecules are used to inhibit gene expression.[22]

Tumor-Induced Osteolysis and Bone Formation

Changes of bone architecture in the tumor microenvironments dictate symptoms, such as pain and pathologic fractures. Radiographic changes become evident when mineral density in the bone is altered by the host-tumor interactions. Tumor cells do not directly destroy bones. Instead, these tumor cells recruit and stimulate monocytes to make osteoclasts, which destroy host bones by releasing growth factors for increased tumor growth. Tumor cells stimulate host cells with parathyroid hormone-related protein (PTHrP) to make bone-active cytokines, such as RANKL, M-CSF, TNF, IL-1, and IL-6.[23] RANKL and M-CSF are two essential cytokines necessary for the production of osteo-

clasts. Furthermore, cross-talk between cytokines (TNF, IL-1, and IL-6) and RANKL/M-CSF pathways augment the osteoclastogenic pathways.[24] Subsequently, host osteoclasts destroy the bone, leading to the release of growth factors, such as TGF-β, from the bone matrix. These growth factors then nourish the cancer cells for further growth and stimulate the cells to make more PTHrP. Multiple myeloma cells stimulate host cells to make RANKL, resulting in predominant osteolysis. Osteolytic breast cancer metastatic cells secrete PTHrP, which in turn stimulate bone marrow stromal cells and osteoblasts to make RANKL,[25] a critical osteoclastogenic cytokine.

Osteoblastic metastasis results from interaction between cancer cells and host cells. Genetic repression of noggin, one of the BMP antagonists, by prostate cancer cells results in moderate osteoblastic metastatic lesions.[26] As a result, there are more signals in favor of BMPs and bone formation. Another mechanism of osteoblastic metastasis is epithelial-mesenchymal transition, which is the acquisition of osteoblastic (mesenchymal cells) phenotypes by prostate cancer cells (epithelial cells). These prostate cancer cells secrete BMPs and promote bone formation in the tumor microenvironment[26] (**Figure 4**).

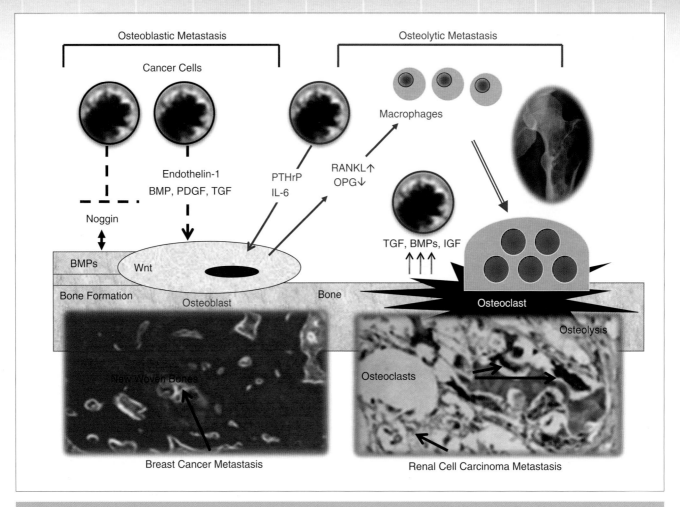

Figure 4 Cancer-induced bone destruction and bone formation.

Molecular Pathophysiology of Common Musculoskeletal Tumors

Giant Cell Tumor

The term giant cell tumor was coined on the microscopic observation that an excessive number of multinucleated osteoclast-like cells were contained within the lesion.[27] The modern interpretation of giant cell tumor is an excessive osteoclastogenesis by neoplastic stromal cells, which make pro-osteoclastogenic cytokines such as RANKL, IL-6, and TNF.[28] Osteoclast precursors, monocytes, are actively recruited by chemokines such as SDF-1 and MCP, which are also produced by giant cell tumor stromal cells. Monocytes have RANK, which is a receptor for RANKL. Monocytes have CXCR4, which is a receptor for SDF-1. TNF and IL-6 augment RANKL-induced osteoclastogenesis. This paradigm represents a self-sufficient osteoclastogenic paracrine loop in a localized area (**Figure 5**). Consistent with this paradigm, a recombinant RANK-Fc protein is currently being investigated for treatment of giant cell tumors.

Cartilaginous Tumors (Enchondroma, Enchondromatosis, Osteochondroma, Exostosis, Chondrosarcomas)

Tumoral chondrocytes in enchondromas look similar to chondrocytes in the growth plate or secondary ossification centers during skeletal development.[29] In the growth plates, chondrocytes are located in the reserve zone, proliferating zone, hypertrophic (prehypertrophic and hypertrophic) zone, and provisional calcification zone.[30] Chondrocytes in the growth plate are under a tight regulation of the Indian hedgehog (Ihh)/PTHrP negative feedback loop. The *Ihh* gene was first described in *Drosophila*.[31] A group of *Ihh* mutant *Drosophila* larvae were observed and characterized as being spiky, thus the gene was designated Indian hedgehog. Ihh is a signaling molecule that delivers a message from cell to cell. PTH-related peptides or PTH-like hormones not only have PTH-like function, but also act on endochondral ossification. Prehypertrophic chondrocytes express Ihh proteins that promote chondrocyte proliferation.[32] Ihh proteins also deliver signals to the perichondrial cells for PTHrP production, which causes the inhibition of growth plate differentiation and the repression of the *Ihh* gene in prehypertro-

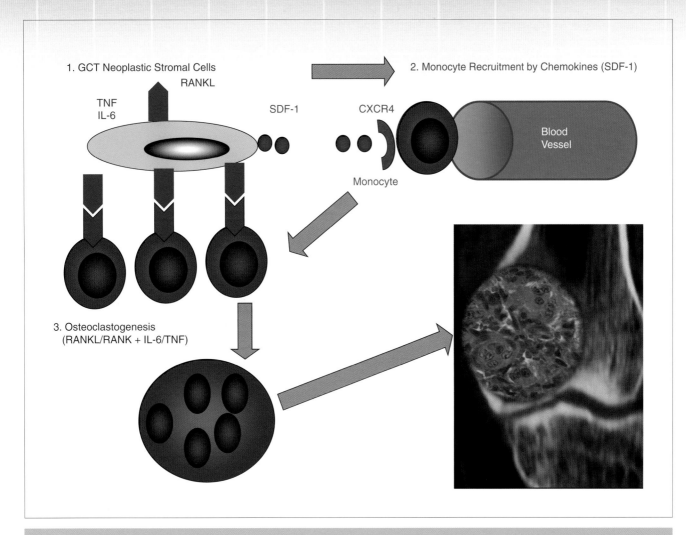

Figure 5 Osteoclastogenesis in giant cell tumor.

phic chondrocytes. As a result of this feedback loop, the growth plate maintains a pool of well-controlled proliferating hypertrophic chondrocytes. In enchodromatosis, the *Ihh* gene is abnormally active due to the absence of PTHrP receptor (loss of negative feedback).[29]

Exostosis is caused by the mutations in exostosin-1 (*EXT1*), *EXT2*, and *EXT3* genes.[33] Pathophysiology of exostosis highlights the importance of cell matrix-to-cell interactions. *EXT* genes encode for glucuronyl transferases, which are present in the matrix. Mutations in the *EXT* gene result in defective heparan sulfate proteoglycan, which is a matrix protein involved in Ihh signaling.[33] As a result of the defective Ihh signaling (communication), the peripheral component of the growth plate loses polarity of chondrocytes, which causes the sustained aberrant growth of the cartilage.[33]

Chondrosarcoma occurs when there is overactivation of tumor-related genes such as *p53*, *IGF*, cytochrome C oxidase subunit 2 (*COX2*), *AKT*, *SRC*, hypoxia-induced factor (*HIF*) and matrix metalloproteinases (*MMPs*).[32] Chondrosarco-

mas are notorious for their resistance to radiation and chemotherapy. There are several molecular mechanisms underlying chemoresistance and radioresistance. Chondrosarcomas express p-glycoprotein, which is an adenosine triphosphate-dependent membrane bound pump encoded on the multiple drug resistance–1 (*MDR-1*) gene. The p-glycoprotein expels chemotherapeutic drugs from these cancerous cells. Chondrosarcomas also use cell survival proteins such as Bcl-2, Bcl-xL, and XIAP when these cells become neoplastic.[34] When these tumoral cells are exposed to radiation and chemotherapeutic drugs, they avoid cell death. Other features of chondrosarcoma cells are high telomerase activities, VEGF expression, HIF-1α, and genetic changes of tumor suppressor gene *p16*.[34]

Fibrous Dysplasia and McCune-Albright Syndrome

Fibrous dysplasia is characterized by the proliferation of stromal cells, which leads to the production of disorganized bones.[35] McCune-Albright syndrome is associated with polyostotic fibrous dysplasia, café-au-lait skin lesions, and multiple endocrine abnormalities such as sexual precocity, hyperthyroidism, and adrenal hyperplasia.[35] Mutation of the *GNAS1* gene, which is located in chromosomal region 20q13, encoding the α subunit of Gs protein, results in the sustained activation of cyclic adenosine 3', 5'-monophosphate (cAMP).[35] This activating mutation (gain-of-function) results in abnormal cellular proliferation, differentiation, and function of osteoblastic progenitors and endocrine cells. Disorganized woven bones in fibrous dysplasia are not mechanically sufficient and fibrous dysplasia cells make redundant IL-6, which favors osteoclastogenesis and bone resorption. As a result, bone is weakened and undergoes insufficiency fractures and progressive deformity. Aberrant activation of osteoclastic activity may explain the anecdotal description of bone graft resorption in fibrous dysplasia. Café-au-lait spots are from the accumulation of melanin pigments, which are overproduced by melanocytes. These melanocytes have elevated cAMP activity, an increased number of melanosomes, and increased tyrosinase activity, which is a rate limiting step of melanin synthesis.[35] Signs of sexual precocity, such as premature menstruation and testicular enlargement, occur as a result of gonadotropin-independent activation of ovaries or seminiferous tubules, respectively.[35]

Ewing Sarcoma

Ewing sarcoma is a malignant small round cell tumor that affects adolescents and younger adults. This rare form of cancer belongs to the Ewing sarcoma family of tumors, which includes Askin tumor and primitive neuroectodermal tumor.[36] In most cases, the tumor arises from the bone, but several cases of tumor originating from the soft tissues have been reported.[37]

Ever since the 1960s and 1970s, new treatments and therapy regimens have improved the patient survival outcome of those affected with Ewing sarcoma from 10% to 20% to approximately 60%.[16] Despite the improvement in patient outcomes in the past few decades, the survival rate of Ewing sarcoma patients has plateaued due to the recurrence of the tumor and secondary malignancies.[38] To further improve the health of those affected with Ewing sarcoma, much attention has been given to molecular research, which focuses on investigating the pathophysiology of the disease.

Pathophysiology

In many circumstances, cancers are caused by deregulation or structural alteration of genes and cellular components, and Ewing sarcoma is no exception to this phenomenon. In approximately 85% of patients, Ewing sarcoma has been shown to be caused by t(11;22)(q24;q12) chromosomal translocation.[39] As a result of this chromosomal translocation, the N-terminal portion of the *EWS* gene encoded on chromosome 22 fuses with the carboxyl terminal DNA binding domain of the *FLI1* gene.[40] Although the function of EWS protein is currently unknown, it has been proposed

that this protein is most likely involved in translational control due to its ability to interact with RNA and DNA molecules.[41] *FLI1* is a proto-oncogene that encodes for a transcriptional activator of the E-twenty six (ETS) family of transcriptional factors.[42]

The fusion protein, essential for the cellular transformation of Ewing sarcoma tumor cells,[43] acts as both a potent transcription activator and a deviant transcriptional repressor.[44,45] Several studies have highlighted the regulating power of this protein in controlling more than 1,000 genes.[46,47] These regulated genes include genes involved in the cell cycle (p21,[45]CREB2,[47] CDK2, SKP2, MCM10, and CDC6), cytokines (TGF-β,[44] IL-8, VEGF[46]), transcription factors (TAF6, EP300[46]), and metastasis (MTA1[47]). Furthermore, the fusion protein was shown to cause the downregulation of tumor suppressor genes and genes involved in apoptosis while it induces upregulation of oncogenes.[47] Studies have also revealed the presence of EWS protein fusing with other transcription factors other than FLI1, which indicates that EWS is a pro-oncoprotein.[48]

Therapeutic/Prognostic Value

Before the 1960s, Ewing sarcoma was treated by radiation therapy, but patients often died due to pulmonary metastasis.[36] After the 1960s, new drugs and drug regimens, such as VAcCD (vincristine, actinomycin-D, cyclophosphamide, doxorubicin),[49] were developed to improve patient health and survival. In addition to these four drugs, ifosfamide and etoposide have also been used to treat patients with Ewing sarcoma. Currently, Ewing sarcoma is generally treated by combined chemotherapy and surgical removal of the tumor. In some cases where the patients have an inoperable tumor, radiation therapy is used.[50] In addition to these treatment routines, novel drugs such as figitumumab[51] and NVP-BEZ235,[52] which target the tumors at the molecular level, are currently being evaluated in clinical trials.

Synovial Sarcoma

Synovial sarcoma is one of the common soft-tissue tumors that frequently occurs in close vicinity to the bone and joints of children and young adults.[53] In most cases, the tumor arises from joint spaces; however, synovial sarcoma originating from bone has been reported.[54] Studies of synovial sarcoma using electron microscopy revealed the presence of two different types of histologic patterns, monophasic and biphasic. Monophasic synovial sarcoma entails spindle cells, whereas biphasic synovial sarcoma is composed of spindle cells and epithelial cells.

Pathophysiology

Synovial sarcoma is typically caused by a chromosomal translocation, which leads to the production of a chimeric protein. In most synovial sarcoma cases, chromosomal translocation t(X;18)(p11.2;q11.2) was identified to be a common abnormality.[55] The translocation of chromosomal elements leads to the fusion of the 5' portion of *SYT* gene from chromosome 18 and the 3' portion of one of the three *SSX* genes from chromosome X (*SSX1, SSX2,* or rarely *SSX4*). Under normal conditions, *SYT* is expressed ubiquitously in several human cell lines and functions as a transcriptional activator. *SSX* genes are a family of transcriptional repressors, which were shown to be expressed in certain cancers and testes.[56]

Like many proto-oncoproteins, the SYT-SSX fusion protein was shown to influence gene expression, particularly those that are involved in cell cycle checkpoints (cyclin A and D1,[57] COM1[58]) and DNA repair (XRCC4 and MSH2[59]). The powerful effect of the SYT-SSX protein in cellular normalcy was revealed by microarray analysis, which unveiled that the presence of this chimeric protein in a cell leads to alteration in the gene expression of over 700 genes.[60]

Therapeutic/Prognostic Value

Although several prognostic factors that affect patient outcome and the treatment plan have been identified (tumor size, invasiveness, practicability of surgical resection),[61] the optimal treatment regimen for synovial sarcoma still remains to be determined. In general, synovial sarcoma tumors are commonly cleared by surgery with or without adjuvant therapy such as chemotherapy and radiation therapy.[61] For chemotherapy, multidrug regimens, which include the combination of drugs such as cyclophosphamide, ifosfamide, doxorubicin, epirubicin, actinomycin D, vincristine, dacarbazine, and cisplatin, are used.[61,62] Although some of these adjuvant therapies have been implicated for tumor treatment, some studies have shown the use of chemotherapy does not significantly affect the rate of recurrences in patients with synovial sarcoma, whereas other studies support the use of such drugs.[62] These studies indicate that the best treatment option for eliminating the possibility of recurrences is adequate surgery.

Neurofibromatosis

Neurofibromatosis is a genetic syndrome in which tumors grow on nerves, leading to deformities of the skin and bone.[63] Three major forms of neurofibromatosis have been documented: neurofibromatosis type 1 (also known as von Recklinghausen disease), neurofibromatosis type 2, and schwannomatosis.[63] Neurofibromatosis type 1 is typically characterized by numerous café-au-lait macules on the skin, bone lesions/abnormalities, family history, and optic glioma[63] whereas the characteristics of neurofibromatosis type 2 include vestibular schwannomas, ophthalmologic lesions, and possibly cutaneous lesions. Schwannomatosis, which occurs in adulthood, is characterized by pain in the peripheral nerves.[64] Although the pathophysiologies of neurofibromatosis types 1 and 2 have been revealed, the genetic basis of schwannomatosis remains unknown. This section will discuss the pathophysiology and therapeutic/prognostic approaches to neurofibromatosis types 1 and 2.

Pathophysiology

Neurofibromatosis type 1 and type 2 occur due to mutations and chromosomal translocations within the *NF1* and *NF2* tumor suppressor genes.[65,66] *NF1*, which is located on 17q11.2 of chromosome 17, encodes for neurofibromin,[66] whereas *NF2* of chromosome 22 encodes for a smaller product known as merlin or schwannomin.[65] In the case of neurofibromatosis type 1, neurofibromin tightly regulates Ras, which is a protein involved in the cell cycle. Consequently, mutations that inactivate NF1 protein lead to activation of Ras and uncontrolled proliferation of neuronal cells. Merlin, which is a membrane-cytoskeleton scaffolding protein, interacts with several proteins including Ras.[63] Studies have indicated that this protein prevents tumorigenesis by repressing Ras-ERK and PI-3K-Akt pathways as well as suppressing E3 ubiquitin ligase CRL4.[67]

Therapeutic/Prognostic Value

Treatment options for neurofibromatosis are limited, and tumors commonly recur due to the difficulty of removal and the slow-growing nature of these tumors. In many cases, several surgeries for tumor removal and bone deformities must be conducted even with chemotherapy and radiation therapy.

Advances in molecular research and technology have enabled an increasing number of scientists and doctors to gain a better understanding of the molecular mechanisms behind neurofibromatosis faster than ever. This knowledge has led and is still leading to the identification of novel drug targets. In the case of neurofibromatosis type 1, tranilast, an antiallergy drug, was shown to have therapeutic effects against neurofibromatosis type 1 cells in vitro by preventing the release of chemical mediators from mast cells present in neurofibromas.[68] In addition, several studies of neurofibromatosis type 1 showed lovastatin (HMG-CoA reductase inhibitor) and farnesyl transferase inhibitors induce apoptosis of malignant cells in vitro,[69] and lovastatin improves the learning of mice with this disease in vivo.[70] For neurofibromatosis type 2, numerous therapeutic targets were identified based on molecular findings, such as those that target platelet-derived growth factor receptor–β (PDGF-β), insulin-like growth factor–1 receptor (IGF-1), and VEGF receptor.[71] A study that used bevacizumab (an anti-VEGF antibody) for the treatment of patients with neurofibromatosis type 2 showed that this drug lessens hearing loss, which commonly occurs in affected patients.[72]

Radiation

Radiation instigates cytotoxicity within the exposed cells by direct and indirect interactions. Direct interaction refers to ionizing radiation, which directly interacts with a cell's proteins and DNA, whereas indirect interaction refers to cellular damage through the transfer of radiation energy to the intracellular fluid. This transfer of energy leads to the hydrolysis of water, resulting in the formation of reactive

Table 2

DNA-Related Terminology and Definitions

DNA	A double-stranded polymer formed from multiple pairs of deoxyribonucleotides, which are connected by hydrogen bonds. Deoxyribonucleotides consist of deoxyribose, a phosphate group, and one of the four nucleobases (adenine, guanine, cytosine, or thymine). DNA contains biologic information vital for replication and regulation of gene expression. The nucleotide sequence of DNA determines the specific biologic information.
Chromosome	A nuclear structure that contains linear strands of DNA. Humans have 46 chromosomes (23 pairs).
Gene Promoter	Regulatory portion of DNA that controls initiation of transcription adjacent to the transcription start site of a gene.
Chromatin	Genetic material composed of DNA and proteins. It is located within the nucleus of the cell and becomes condensed to form chromosomes.
Gene	A specific DNA segment that contains all the information required for synthesis of a protein, including both coding and noncoding sequences.
Genome	The complete genetic information of an organism.
Mitochondrial DNA (mtDNA)	Circular DNA that is found in the mitochondria. mtDNA encodes proteins, which are essential for the function of the organelle. Mammalian mtDNAs are 16 kb in length, contains no introns, and had very little noncoding DNA.
DNA Polymerase	An enzyme that synthesizes new strands of DNA by polymerizing deoxyribonucleotides.
Exon	Portion of a gene that encodes for mRNA.
Intron	Portion of a gene that does not encode for mRNA.
Gene enhancer	Short regions of a gene that enhance the level of transcription.
Recombinant DNA	DNA that is artificially made by recombining DNA segments, which are usually not found together from splicing.
Transgene	Gene that is artificially placed into a single-celled embryo. An organism that develops from the embryo will have this gene present in all of its cells.
Single Nucleotide Polymorphism (SNP)	Difference in DNA sequence due to a single nucleotide change. SNPs are found among members of same biologic species.
Central Dogma of Molecular Biology	A framework, that shows how information is passed sequentially in a cell. It is commonly depicted as: DNA→RNA→Protein.
Epigenetics	Study of how environmental factors affect gene expression without changing the DNA sequence itself.
Genomics	Study of genomes as well as gene function.

oxygen species. Furthermore, although not as significant as DNA damage caused by radiation, damage to the cell membrane from radiation does also occur, leading to activation of signaling pathways, which lead to cell death.[73]

Radiation is known to affect dividing cells more than nondividing cells and causes cell division delays, incompletetion of mitosis, and cell death during interphase. Multiple sites of DNA damage caused by radiation increase the difficulty of distributing the DNA equally to the dividing cells, leading to insufficient cellular physiologic functions and cell death. Furthermore, radiation increases the activity of the nuclear signal transducer ATM. Although the precise mech-

Table 3

Basic Genetics

Genomic DNA	1) Human chromosomes contain 6 billion base pairs, which encode approximately 50,000 to 100,000 individual genes. All the genetic information present in a single haploid set of chromosomes constitutes the genome for a human being. A variety of orthopaedic disorders are secondary to genetic mutation. 2) Only 5% to 10% of genomic DNA in humans is transcribed. Genes in DNA are organized into introns, or noncoding sequences, and exons, which contain the code for the mRNA to produce the proteins as a gene product. 3) The noncoding sequences contain promoter regions, regulatory elements, and enhancers. About half of the coding genes in human genomic DNA are solitary genes, and their sequences occur only once in the haploid genome. 4) Directionality—Single-strand nucleic acid is synthesized in vivo in a 5' to 3' direction, meaning from the fifth to the third carbon in the nucleotide sugar ring. 5) Simple-sequence repeated DNA in long tandem array is located in centromeres, telomeres, and specific locations within the arms of particular chromosomes. Because a particular simple-sequence tandem array is variable between individuals, these differences form the basis for DNA fingerprinting for identifying individuals. 6) Mitochondrial DNA (mtDNA) encodes rRNA, tRNA, and proteins for electron transport and ATP synthesis. mtDNA originates from egg cells. Mutations in mtDNA can cause neuromuscular disorders.
Control of gene expression	1) Transcription—Transcriptional control is the primary step for gene regulation. A transcription process means the synthesis of complementary RNA by RNA polymerase from a strand of DNA molecule. Transcription is controlled by a regulatory sequence in DNA called the *cis*-acting sequence, which includes enhancer and promoter sites. *Trans*-acting factors bind to the *cis*-acting sequence and regulate gene expression. The *trans*-acting factor is usually a protein such as a transcriptional factor. Promoter regions include the binding site for various transcriptional factors, including the TATA box, and a binding site for RNA polymerase II. The TATA-binding protein, together with other transcriptional proteins, initiates transcription, followed by binding of RNA polymerase. RNA polymerase II generates mRNA template. 2) Translation—The ribosome binds to the translation start sites of the mRNA and initiates protein synthesis. tRNA interprets the code on the mRNA and delivers amino acids to the peptide chain. Each amino acid is encoded by a three-nucleotide sequence (codon). For example, UUC is a codon for lysine, and GGG or GGU is a codon for glycine. UGA, UUA, and UAG are codons that stop translation.
Inheritance patterns of genetic disease	1) Autosomal mutation—A gene mutation that is located on a chromosome other than the X or Y chromosome. 2) Sex-linked mutation—A gene mutation that is located on the X or Y chromosome. 3) Dominant mutation—A mutation of one allele is sufficient to cause an abnormal phenotype. 4) Recessive mutation—A mutation of both alleles is necessary to cause an abnormal phenotype.

3: Basic Principles and Treatment of Musculoskeletal Disease

anism of how ATM is activated by the presence of damaged DNA[74] is unknown, it has been acknowledged that this protein activates numerous downstream targets, leading to DNA repair processes, cell cycle arrest, and cell death.[73] An example of a protein that is activated by ATM is p53. p53 regulates numerous components of the cell death pathway and is considered an activator of cell death. In addition to ATM, another kinase, Rad3-related, is activated by radiation and initiates the DNA damage responses. Irreparable DNA damage initiates the cell death process. DNA damage can also arise from a bystander effect, which results from the activation of inflammatory response in the surrounding normal tissues. Radiation can be delivered by external methods and internal beams. External methods include a cyclotron (a charged particle accelerator), a synchrotron (a particle circular accelerator), a linear accelerator that uses high-energy electrons and photons, a microtron (a cyclotron that uses an electron linear accelerator and oscillating electric fields), intensity modulated radiation therapy (three-dimensional radiation therapy using CT), and a cyberknife (a radiosurgery device with a linear accelerator on a robotic arm and a three-dimensional imaging system).[75] Internal methods include an implantable radiation source, antibody-directed targeted radiation, and brachytherapy using a catheter.[75]

Terminology

DNA-related terminology and definitions are presented in **Table 2**, and a description of basic genetics is presented in **Table 3**.

Summary

The field of musculoskeletal oncology has evolved dramatically over the past few centuries, but never more rapidly than in the past three or four decades. With the advent of new and effective molecular biology research techniques, such as rapid genomic sequencing, as well as improved musculoskeletal imaging modalities such as CT and MRI, the understanding of the molecular basis of musculoskeletal tumors as well as treatment principles and subsequent outcomes have improved substantially. It is critical that practicing orthopaedic surgeons remain up to date on the latest theory and terminology in clinical musculoskeletal oncology in order to have meaningful discussions with fellow practitioners as well as an ever-increasingly educated patient population. This chapter serves as a concise, broadly applicable summary of the currently accepted theory and terminology used in the field, as well as the pathophysiology and treatment strategies of several musculoskeletal tumors that are commonly encountered in the clinical setting.

References

1. Watson JD, Crick FH: Molecular structure of nucleic acids: A structure for deoxyribose nucleic acid. *Nature* 1953; 171(4356):737-738.

2. Blum RH, Carter SK: Adriamycin: A new anticancer drug with significant clinical activity. *Ann Intern Med* 1974;80(2): 249-259.

3. Kansara M, Thomas DM: Molecular pathogenesis of osteosarcoma. *DNA Cell Biol* 2007;26(1):1-18.

4. Hanahan D, Weinberg RA: Hallmarks of cancer: The next generation. *Cell* 2011;144(5):646-674.

5. Alberts B, Johnson A, Lewis J, Raff M, Roberts K, Walter P: *Molecular Biology of the Cell*, ed 4. New York, NY, Garland Publishing, 2001.

6. Kerr JF, Wyllie AH, Currie AR: Apoptosis: A basic biological phenomenon with wide-ranging implications in tissue kinetics. *Br J Cancer* 1972;26(4):239-257.

7. Porter AG, Jänicke RU: Emerging roles of caspase-3 in apoptosis. *Cell Death Differ* 1999;6(2):99-104.

8. Zhivotovsky B, Orrenius S: Cell death mechanisms: Crosstalk and role in disease. *Exp Cell Res* 2010;316(8):1374-1383.

9. Borish LC, Steinke JW: 2: Cytokines and chemokines. *J Allergy Clin Immunol* 2003;111(2, suppl):S460-S475.

10. Gambacorti-Passerini C: Part I: Milestones in personalised medicine. Imatinib. *Lancet Oncol* 2008;9(6):600.

11. Gallazzi MB, Chiapparino R, Garbagna PG: Early radiological diagnosis and differential diagnosis of infection in orthopaedic surgery, in Meani E, Romanò C, Crosby L, Hofmann G, Calonego G, eds: *Infection and Local Treatment in Orthopedic Surgery*. Springer Berlin Heidelberg; 2007, pp 21-32.

12. Croce CM: Oncogenes and cancer. *N Engl J Med* 2008; 358(5):502-511.

13. Karnoub AE, Weinberg RA: Ras oncogenes: Split personalities. *Nat Rev Mol Cell Biol* 2008;9(7):517-531.

14. Meyer N, Penn LZ: Reflecting on 25 years with MYC. *Nat Rev Cancer* 2008;8(12):976-990.

15. Hydbring P, Larsson LG: Tipping the balance: Cdk2 enables Myc to suppress senescence. *Cancer Res* 2010;70(17):6687-6691.

16. Arai Y, Kun LE, Brooks MT, et al: Ewing's sarcoma: Local tumor control and patterns of failure following limited-volume radiation therapy. *Int J Radiat Oncol Biol Phys* 1991; 21(6):1501-1508.

17. Takayanagi H: The role of NFAT in osteoclast formation. *Ann N Y Acad Sci* 2007;1116:227-237.

18. Lu C, Shen Q, DuPré E, Kim H, Hilsenbeck S, Brown PH: cFos is critical for MCF-7 breast cancer cell growth. *Oncogene* 2005;24(43):6516-6524.

19. Weinberg RA: Tumor suppressor genes, in Weinberg RA, ed: *The Biology of Cancers*. New York, NY, Garland Publishing, 2006, pp 209-256.

20. Levine AJ: p53, the cellular gatekeeper for growth and division. *Cell* 1997;88(3):323-331.

21. Weber WW: Epigenetics, in John BT, David JT, eds: *Comprehensive Medicinal Chemistry II*. Oxford, England, Elsevier, 2007, pp 251-278.

22. Egger, G, Liang G, Aparicio A, Jones PA: Epigenetics in human disease and prospects for epigenetic therapy. *Nature* 2004; 429:457-463.

23. Wittrant Y, Théoleyre S, Chipoy C, et al: RANKL/RANK/OPG: New therapeutic targets in bone tumours and associated osteolysis. *Biochim Biophys Acta* 2004;1704(2):49-57.

24. Lee SK, Lorenzo J: Cytokines regulating osteoclast formation and function. *Curr Opin Rheumatol* 2006;18(4):411-418.

25. Käkönen S-M, Mundy GR: Mechanisms of osteolytic bone metastases in breast carcinoma. *Cancer* 2003;97(3, suppl): 834-839.

26. Secondini C, Wetterwald A, Schwaninger R, Thalmann GN, Cecchini MG: The role of the BMP signaling antagonist noggin in the development of prostate cancer osteolytic bone metastasis. *PLoS One* 2011;6(1):e16078.

27. Eckardt JJ, Grogan TJ: Giant cell tumor of bone. *Clin Orthop Relat Res* 1986;204(204):45-58.

28. Roux S, Amazit L, Meduri G, Guiochon-Mantel A, Milgrom E, Mariette X: RANK (receptor activator of nuclear factor kappa B) and RANK ligand are expressed in giant cell tumors of bone. *Am J Clin Pathol* 2002;117(2):210-216.

29. Schipani E, Provot S: PTHrP, PTH, and the PTH/PTHrP receptor in endochondral bone development. *Birth Defects Res C Embryo Today* 2003;69(4):352-362.

30. Karsenty G: Transcriptional control of skeletogenesis. *Annu Rev Genomics Hum Genet* 2008;9(1):183-196.

31. Nüsslein-Volhard C, Wieschaus E: Mutations affecting segment number and polarity in Drosophila. *Nature* 1980;287(5785):795-801.

32. Kronenberg HM: PTHrP and skeletal development. *Ann N Y Acad Sci* 2006;1068:1-13.

33. Pannier S, Legeai-Mallet L: Hereditary multiple exostoses and enchondromatosis. *Best Pract Res Clin Rheumatol* 2008;22(1):45-54.

34. Jamil N, Howie S, Salter DM: Therapeutic molecular targets in human chondrosarcoma. *Int J Exp Pathol* 2010;91(5):387-393.

35. Chapurlat RD, Orcel P: Fibrous dysplasia of bone and McCune-Albright syndrome. *Best Pract Res Clin Rheumatol* 2008;22(1):55-69.

36. Subbiah V, Anderson P, Lazar AJ, Burdett E, Raymond K, Ludwig JA: Ewing's sarcoma: Standard and experimental treatment options. *Curr Treat Options Oncol* 2009;10(1-2):126-140.

37. Horowitz ME, et al: Ewing's sarcoma family of tumors: Ewing's sarcoma of bone and soft tissue and the peripheral primitive neuroectodermal tumors, in Pizzo PA, ed: *Principles and Practice of Pediatric Oncology*. Philadelphia, PA, Lippincott-Raven, 1997, pp 831-863.

38. Bacci G, Toni A, Avella M, et al: Long-term results in 144 localized Ewing's sarcoma patients treated with combined therapy. *Cancer* 1989;63(8):1477-1486.

39. Aurias A: Chromosomal translocations in Ewing's sarcoma. *N Engl J Med* 1983;309(8):496-498.

40. Delattre O, Zucman J, Plougastel B, et al: Gene fusion with an ETS DNA-binding domain caused by chromosome translocation in human tumours. *Nature* 1992;359(6391):162-165.

41. Takahama K, Kino K, Arai S, Kurokawa R, Oyoshi T: Identification of Ewing's sarcoma protein as a G-quadruplex DNA- and RNA-binding protein. *FEBS J* 2011;278(6):988-998.

42. Prasad DD, Rao VN, Reddy ES: Structure and expression of human Fli-1 gene. *Cancer Res* 1992;52(20):5833-5837.

43. Tanaka K, Iwakuma T, Harimaya K, Sato H, Iwamoto Y: EWS-Fli1 antisense oligodeoxynucleotide inhibits proliferation of human Ewing's sarcoma and primitive neuroectodermal tumor cells. *J Clin Invest* 1997;99(2):239-247.

44. Hahm KB, Cho K, Lee C, et al: Repression of the gene encoding the TGF-beta type II receptor is a major target of the EWS-FLI1 oncoprotein. *Nat Genet* 1999;23(2):222-227.

45. Nakatani F, Tanaka K, Sakimura R, et al: Identification of p21WAF1/CIP1 as a direct target of EWS-Fli1 oncogenic fusion protein. *J Biol Chem* 2003;278(17):15105-15115.

46. Smith R, Owen LA, Trem DJ, et al: Expression profiling of EWS/FLI identifies NKX2.2 as a critical target gene in Ewing's sarcoma. *Cancer Cell* 2006;9(5):405-416.

47. Ohali A, Avigad S, Zaizov R, et al: Prediction of high risk Ewing's sarcoma by gene expression profiling. *Oncogene* 2004;23(55):8997-9006.

48. Sorensen PH, Lessnick SL, Lopez-Terrada D, Liu XF, Triche TJ, Denny CT: A second Ewing's sarcoma translocation, t(21;22), fuses the EWS gene to another ETS-family transcription factor, ERG. *Nat Genet* 1994;6(2):146-151.

49. Rosen G, Wollner N, Tan C, et al: Disease-free survival in children with Ewing's sarcoma treated with radiation therapy and adjuvant four-drug sequential chemotherapy. *Cancer* 1974;33(2):384-393.

50. Paulussen M, Bielack S, Jürgens H, Casali PG; ESMO Guidelines Working Group: Ewing's sarcoma of the bone: ESMO clinical recommendations for diagnosis, treatment and follow-up. *Ann Oncol* 2009;20 (suppl 4):140-142.

51. Olmos D, Postel-Vinay S, Molife LR, et al: Safety, pharmacokinetics, and preliminary activity of the anti-IGF-1R antibody figitumumab (CP-751,871) in patients with sarcoma and Ewing's sarcoma: A phase 1 expansion cohort study. *Lancet Oncol* 2010;11(2):129-135.

52. Manara MC, Nicoletti G, Zambelli D, et al: NVP-BEZ235 as a new therapeutic option for sarcomas. *Clin Cancer Res* 2010;16(2):530-540.

53. Sandberg AA, Bridge JA: Updates on the cytogenetics and molecular genetics of bone and soft tissue tumors: Synovial sarcoma. *Cancer Genet Cytogenet* 2002;133(1):1-23.

54. Jung SC, Choi JA, Chung JH, Oh JH, Lee JW, Kang HS: Synovial sarcoma of primary bone origin: A rare case in a rare site with atypical features. *Skeletal Radiol* 2007;36(1):67-71.

55. Turc-Carel C, Dal Cin P, Limon J, et al: Involvement of chromosome X in primary cytogenetic change in human neoplasia: Nonrandom translocation in synovial sarcoma. *Proc Natl Acad Sci U S A* 1987;84(7):1981-1985.

56. Güre AO, Wei IJ, Old LJ, Chen YT: The SSX gene family: Characterization of 9 complete genes. *Int J Cancer* 2002;101(5):448-453.

57. Xie Y, Skytting B, Nilsson G, et al: SYT-SSX is critical for cyclin D1 expression in synovial sarcoma cells: A gain of function of the t(X;18)(p11.2;q11.2) translocation. *Cancer Res* 2002;62(13):3861-3867.

58. Ishida M, Miyamoto M, Naitoh S, et al: The SYT-SSX fusion protein down-regulates the cell proliferation regulator COM1 in t(x;18) synovial sarcoma. *Mol Cell Biol* 2007;27(4):1348-1355.

59. Xie Y, Törnkvist M, Aalto Y, et al: Gene expression profile by blocking the SYT-SSX fusion gene in synovial sarcoma cells: Identification of XRCC4 as a putative SYT-SSX target gene. *Oncogene* 2003;22(48):7628-7631.

60. Cai W, Sun Y, Wang W, et al: The effect of SYT-SSX and extracellular signal-regulated kinase (ERK) on cell proliferation in synovial sarcoma. *Pathol Oncol Res* 2011;17(2):357-367.

61. Lewis JJ, Antonescu CR, Leung DH, et al: Synovial sarcoma: A multivariate analysis of prognostic factors in 112 patients with primary localized tumors of the extremity. *J Clin Oncol* 2000;18(10):2087-2094.

62. Rosen G, Forscher C, Lowenbraun S, et al: Synovial sarcoma: Uniform response of metastases to high dose ifosamide. *Cancer* 1994;73(10):2506-2511.

3: Basic Principles and Treatment of Musculoskeletal Disease

63. McClatchey AI: Neurofibromatosis. *Ann Rev Pathol* 2007;2: 191-216.

64. Delucia TA, Yohay K, Widmann RF: Orthopaedic aspects of neurofibromatosis: Update. *Curr Opin Pediatr* 2011;23(1): 46-52.

65. Jacoby LB, Jones D, Davis K, et al: Molecular analysis of the NF2 tumor-suppressor gene in schwannomatosis. *Am J Hum Genet* 1997;61(6):1293-1302.

66. Wallace MR, Marchuk DA, Andersen LB, et al: Type 1 neurofibromatosis gene: Identification of a large transcript disrupted in three NF1 patients. *Science* 1990;249(4965):181-186.

67. Li W, You L, Cooper J, et al: Merlin/NF2 suppresses tumorigenesis by inhibiting the E3 ubiquitin ligase CRL4(DCAF1) in the nucleus. *Cell* 2010;140(4):477-490.

68. Yamamoto M, Yamauchi T, Okano K, Takahashi M, Watabe S, Yamamoto Y: Tranilast, an anti-allergic drug, down-regulates the growth of cultured neurofibroma cells derived from neurofibromatosis type 1. *Tohoku J Exp Med* 2009; 217(3):193-201.

69. Wojtkowiak JW, Fouad F, LaLonde DT, et al: Induction of apoptosis in neurofibromatosis type 1 malignant peripheral nerve sheath tumor cell lines by a combination of novel farnesyl transferase inhibitors and lovastatin. *J Pharmacol Exp Ther* 2008;326(1):1-11.

70. Li W, Cui Y, Kushner SA, et al: The HMG-CoA reductase inhibitor lovastatin reverses the learning and attention deficits in a mouse model of neurofibromatosis type 1. *Curr Biol* 2005;15(21):1961-1967.

71. Ammoun S, Hanemann CO: Emerging therapeutic targets in schwannomas and other merlin-deficient tumors. *Nat Rev Neurol* 2011;7(7):392-399.

72. Plotkin SR, Stemmer-Rachamimov AO, Barker FG II, et al: Hearing improvement after bevacizumab in patients with neurofibromatosis type 2. *N Engl J Med* 2009;361(4):358-367.

73. Pawlik TM, Keyomarsi K: Role of cell cycle in mediating sensitivity to radiotherapy. *Int J Radiat Oncol Biol Phys* 2004; 59(4):928-942.

74. Kurz EU, Lees-Miller SP: DNA damage-induced activation of ATM and ATM-dependent signaling pathways. *DNA Repair (Amst)* 2004;3(8-9):889-900.

75. Sadeghi M, Enferadi M, Shirazi A: External and internal radiation therapy: Past and future directions. *J Cancer Res Ther* 2010;6(3):239-248.

Chapter 25

Orthopaedic Infection

James Cashman, MD
Javad Parvizi, MD, FRCS

General Considerations

Epidemiology

The most common complication affecting hospitalized patients is nosocomial infection, with a reported incidence of 5% to 10%.[1] Infections developing after orthopaedic procedures are also common, with 33% of surgical site infections occurring in patients undergoing orthopaedic procedures. Twenty-two percent of health care–associated infections are surgical site infections. Drug-resistant organisms, which include methicillin-resistant *Staphylococcus aureus* (MRSA) and vancomycin-resistant enterococci, colonize the skin and are spread by contact; they are of increasing concern. The death rate from MRSA is 2.5 times greater than that from nonresistant *Staphylococcus*. Orthopaedic surgical site infections prolong hospital stays by a median of 2 weeks per patient, double the rehospitalization rates, and more than triple overall health care costs.[2] Amelioration of these issues

Dr. Parvizi or an immediate family member serves as a paid consultant to or is an employee of Biomet, Covidien, National Institutes of Health (NIAMS and NICHD), Salient Surgical, Smith & Nephew, Stryker, TissueGene, and Zimmer; has received research or institutional support from 3M, Musculoskeletal Transplant Foundation, National Institutes of Health (NIAMS and NICHD), Stryker, and Zimmer; and serves as a board member, owner, officer, or committee member of the American Association of Hip and Knee Surgeons, the American Board of Orthopaedic Surgery, the British Orthopaedic Association, CD Diagnostics, the Hip Society, the Orthopaedic Research and Education Foundation, the Orthopaedic Research Society, SmartTech, and United Healthcare. Neither Dr. Cashman nor any immediate family member has received anything of value from or owns stock in a commercial company or institution related directly or indirectly to the subject of this chapter.

depends on assessment of the risk factors and incorporation of appropriate interventions. Some surgeries have much higher incidences of early postoperative infection, and this risk can be devastating in spine surgery. One survey of spine surgery found a 10% incidence of surgical site infection, and occurrence was highly correlated with older age, increased blood loss, longer surgical time, and multiple levels of arthrodesis.[3] Another study found that the rate of wound infection occurring within 90 days was 0.2% after primary total hip replacement and 0.95% after revisions.[4] Total knee replacement has been associated with similar rates: 0.25% infection after primary and 0.45% after revision arthroplasty.[5] Because the number of primary arthroplasties seems to be increasing nationwide and the proportion of primary and revision arthroplasties has remained the same during the past decade, it is predicted that the incidence of revision surgeries also will increase.

Etiology

Microorganisms that can cause infection include bacteria, viruses, parasites, and fungi. Of these, bacteria are the most common source of infection in bones and joints. Bacteria are prokaryotic cells, as they do not have a nucleus. The genetic material is aggregated in an area of the cytoplasm called the nucleoid. Bacteria do not possess a cytoplasmic compartment containing mitochondria and lysosomes. A consistent feature of all prokaryotes, but not eukaryotes, is the presence of a cell wall, which allows bacteria to resist osmotic stress. This cell wall differs in complexity between species, and bacteria are usually divided into two major groups–gram positive and gram negative–which reflect their cell wall structure. Bacteria are designated gram positive or negative depending on whether the cell membrane of the bacterium retains crystal violet indium dye after an alcohol rinse. Gram-positive bacteria retain the dye and appear blue under light microscopy. Gram-negative bacteria do not retain the dye but do retain the safranin O counterstain and appear pink under light microscopy. Bacteria can be further classified into cocci or bacilli depending on their shape. Cocci are round and bacilli are rod shaped.

Microbial resistance to antibiotic therapies is a major challenge in the treatment of orthopaedic infection. There are two types of microbiologic resistance: innate (or intrinsic) and extrinsic. Innate implies that the bacterial cell inherently has properties that do not allow the antibiotic to act on it. Examples of innate or intrinsic resistance include enzyme production that destroys the antibiotic; changes in cell wall permeability; alterations in structural target; mutations in efflux mechanisms; bypass of metabolic pathway; and resistance via a combination of the above or multiple mechanisms.

Extrinsic antibiotic resistance implies that an organism acquires resistance to an antibiotic to which it was previously sensitive. This can take place due to a chance mutation in the genetic material of the cell or the acquisition of drug-resistant genes from other drug-resistant cells. This resistance is usually mediated via plasmids, small circles of double-stranded DNA. Plasmids carry genes for specialized functions and also carry one or more genes for antimicrobial resistance.

Biomaterials and Bacterial Adherence

Bacteria in the normal environment are predominantly found in biofilms.[6] A biofilm is a highly structured community of bacterial cells that adopts a distinct phenotype, communicates through cell-cell signals, and adheres to an inert nonliving surface. A biofilm is a protected form of bacterial growth that allows survival in a hostile environment. Bacterial signaling, or quorum sensing, is a key event within biofilm.[7] This signaling is responsible for the release of bacteria from biofilm. Compared with planktonic bacterial cells, bacteria in biofilm are less susceptible to antibiotic agents and host immune responses. They are slow growing and do not react to environmental stressors such as changes in pH, osmolarity, or temperature.

The initial phase of biofilm development is adherence of the bacteria to a surface and the formation of microcolonies. The bacteria then undergo differentiation into biofilm through the production of extracellular polysaccharides. Bacterial cells thus become embedded within the biofilm matrix. This polysaccharide matrix is termed a glycocalyx. Microorganisms are attracted to the surface of the substratum by physical forces including van der Waal forces, hydrophobic interactions, and gravitational forces. Chemical interactions such as ionic, hydrogen, and covalent bonding also have a role to play in bacterial adherence.

Bacterial adherence is influenced by the chemical composition of the biomaterial. In vitro studies have identified a higher rate of bacterial adherence in titanium alloys than in stainless steel, and higher in steel than pure titanium. Tantalum appears to be more resistant to *S aureus* adherence.[8]

When a biomaterial is implanted, its surface becomes coated with a film of plasma and extracellular matrix molecules such as fibrinogen, laminin, fibronectin, and collagen. These adhesive molecules facilitate bacterial adhesion via bacterial surface receptors. Bacterial pili and flagellae facilitate adhesion, particularly in gram-negative organisms.[9]

Principles of Antimicrobial Agents

Success in treating musculoskeletal infection often requires appropriate application of surgical modalities in concert with targeted antimicrobial therapy. It is important to consider microbial factors including the type of infection, susceptibility, and virulence; patient factors such as general health and nutritional status; and drug factors such as adverse effects. Antibiotics are used for prophylaxis, to eradicate infections, and for initial care in open fractures and wounds. They can be delivered orally, intramuscularly, intravenously, locally via antibiotic beads or spaces, or via an osmotic pump. An antimicrobial agent is any substance of natural, semisynthetic, or synthetic origin that kills or inhibits the growth of a microorganism but causes little or no host damage.

There are at least five basic principles on which successful antimicrobial therapy must be based. These principles require knowledge of an antimicrobial agent's spectrum of activity, distribution and pharmacokinetics, toxicity, synergy and antagonism with other antimicrobial agents, and cost. Spectrum of activity is important in choosing an antimicrobial directed against a specific pathogen. First, the physician must determine the particular pathogen that is causing infection. Once the agent has been identified, an antimicrobial agent with particular activity against the organism causing disease can be chosen. It is important to consider antibiotic distribution and pharmacokinetics. An antimicrobial agent may have excellent activity against a particular bacterium, but treatment will not be successful unless it reaches the site of infection in adequate concentrations. The benefits of an antimicrobial agent must outweigh the risks. Some medications can have unacceptable toxicity that can obviate their therapeutic use in a given situation. When one antimicrobial agent enhances the other with more than just an additive effect, the interaction is called synergy. When an antimicrobial agent interferes with the activity of a second one, the effect is called antagonism. A bacteriostatic antimicrobial agent, for example, frequently slows the killing rate of a bactericidal antimicrobial agent. In life-threatening infections, cost will not play a major role in choosing antimicrobial therapy; however, for mild infections such as cystitis or for antimicrobial prophylaxis, regimens may vary tenfold in cost. Therefore, the clinician must have some understanding of the cost of various antimicrobial agents.

Host Factors and Immune Response

Many patients have increased risks that make them more susceptible to developing infections. Several of those infections may be preventable through the identification and

3: Basic Principles and Treatment of Musculoskeletal Disease

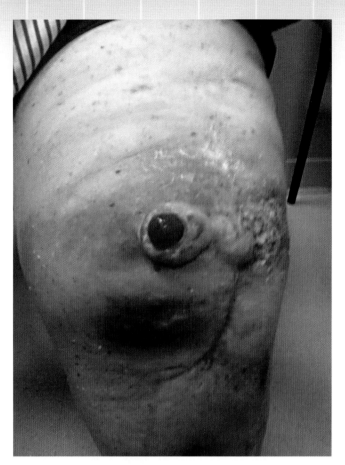

Figure 1 Total knee replacement with postoperative wound infection. Patient risk factors such as obesity, peripheral vascular disease, and poor soft tissue increase infection risk.

tion for the patient. In response to these data, several efficient and quick-acting antiseptic alcohol solutions that require no scrubbing have been produced. All these solutions are as effective as chlorhexidine solutions.[13] Preoperative hair removal also is important in postoperative infection control. Shaving immediately before a procedure decreases the infection rate compared with shaving within 24 hours, which is probably the result of microscopic abrasions that house bacteria. Furthermore, there was strong evidence that when hair removal is considered necessary, it should not be accomplished by shaving. Instead, a depilatory or electric clipping immediately before surgery should be used.

In implant surgery, air and surface contamination are important factors in postoperative wound infection. Infection rates have been shown to correlate with the number of airborne bacteria within 30 cm of the wound. This infection rate is influenced by intraoperative factors such as the number of operating room personnel, their clothing, and the type of ventilation system used.[14] In one study, it was estimated that a high contamination rate of gowns can be due to the gown packs having been left open for too long. Therefore, it was hypothesized that some infections could have been avoided if single-gown packs had been used; multiple-gown packs result in delay and traffic around the table, providing additional sources of infection.[15] Although appropriate use of drapes during invasive procedures is recommended widely as an aid in minimizing contamination of the surgical field, the efficacy of this practice in reducing surgical site infection has not been assessed by scientific studies. It has been found that bacteria easily penetrated all the woven reusable fabrics within 30 minutes.[16] Disposable, nonwoven drapes have been proved to be impermeable. Therefore, the use of nonwoven disposable drapes or woven drapes with an impermeable operating tray in all surgical cases is recommended.

One source of the environmental bacteria in the operating room has been shown to be the operating room personnel, and the quantity of environmental bacteria is related directly to the amount of bacteria the personnel shed and the number of people present. Thirty percent of people are colonized by S $aureus$, and people shed approximately 10^6 skin scales loaded with bacteria per day.[17] Another study found that when the number of operating room personnel rose from 8 to 16, the rate of surgical site infections increased from 1.5% to 3.8%.[18]

Several factors can significantly affect bacterial counts in the operating room. One such factor is the position of the door. The average colony-forming units per square foot per hour with closed doors was 13.3, that with open doors was 24.8, and that with swinging doors was 19.4.[19] Horizontal laminar airflow systems reduced bacterial counts by 92% at the wound and back table and by 60% at the periphery of the room. However, laminar airflow must be used properly because, as reported by Salvati et al,[20] any impedance of the course of the air increases the amount of bacterial contam-

treatment of modifiable risk factors. Some of these risk factors include disease states such as HIV, rheumatoid arthritis, diabetes, and other local or distant infection such as urinary tract infections. Other modifiable patient risk factors include obesity, malnutrition, smoking, and poor oral health (**Figure 1**).

Procedure-Related Risk Reduction

Preoperative skin preparation is an important factor in the prevention of infection, but it removes only up to 80% of skin flora.[10] Standard surgical antisepsis involves scrubbing the skin with antiseptic solutions. In one study, it has been found that patients who showered with chlorhexidine had the least amount of growth on cultures of the incision site compared with patients who used povidone-iodine or water.[11] Scrubbing with chlorhexidine significantly reduced hand bacterial counts compared with povidone-iodine. In addition, at 6 hours after scrubbing, chlorhexidine-scrubbed hands had significantly lower bacterial counts compared with baseline levels, whereas hands scrubbed only with povidone-iodine had higher bacterial counts.[12] Scrubbing can damage the skin, with a subsequent risk of infec-

ination downwind about the wound. The type of airflow also affects instrument contamination. In one study, half of the instruments in a conventional operating room were contaminated when the scrub nurse took the instruments and 30% were contaminated without being touched, whereas fewer than 1% were contaminated in an operating room with laminar airflow. Surgical facemasks worn in the hallway or the operating room had no effect on the bacterial counts in the hallway or the operating room. In an operating room, there were 447.3 colony-forming units per foot per hour when a facemask was worn and 449.7 colony-forming units per foot per hour when it was not worn.[19]

With regard to clean spinal procedures, risk factors that have been associated with increased surgical site infection include estimated blood loss of greater than 1 L, previous surgical site infection at the same site, diabetes, obesity, longer procedure times (more than 5 hours), current smoking, American Society of Anesthesiologists' score of 3 or higher, weight loss, dependent functional status, preoperative hematocrit less than 36, disseminated cancer, elevated preoperative or postoperative serum glucose level, suboptimal timing of antibiotic prophylaxis, and two or more surgical residents participating in the surgical procedure. Additionally, posterior approach or combined anterior-posterior approaches were associated with higher rates of infection.[21,22] For knee replacement procedures, factors associated with increased risk of postoperative wound infection include male sex, rheumatoid arthritis or fracture as the indication for arthroplasty, low volume of cases performed by the surgeon, morbid obesity, and diabetes.[23,24] Risk factors associated with higher rates of infection following clean hip procedures include arthroplasty surgery performed in a hospital with low volumes of arthroplasty procedures and prolonged wound drainage following the procedure.[25]

Diagnostic Modalities
Clinical and Laboratory Evaluation
The cardinal signs of inflammation are color, dolor, tumor, rubor or temperature, pain, swelling and erythema. Bacteria at a site of infection release a specific set of antigens that are recognized by local immune cells. The characteristic response of the immune cells leads to local and systemic changes including increased local blood flow and vascular permeability, which generate the cardinal signs of inflammation. This reaction may elicit local signs in addition to inflammation such as joint effusion or wound drainage. When determining the cause of an infection, it is important to consider systemic distant locations as the source. A thorough clinical examination of the pulmonary, urinary, gastrointestinal, and cardiovascular systems is required. The optimal medical therapy for a patient with infection requires the identification of causative microorganisms and their in vitro antimicrobial susceptibility. If possible, antimicrobial agents should be withheld until specimens are collected for culturing.

In a patient with osteomyelitis or septic arthritis, the erythrocyte sedimentation rate and C-reactive protein level may be elevated. The white cell count may be close to normal levels or elevated. In suspected osteomyelitis, definitive diagnosis can be obtained from bone biopsy. Tissue can be obtained by punch biopsy, needle biopsy, or curettage of deep tissue. Accurate tissue diagnosis can allow for prompt rationalization of antibiotics, particularly in the context of resistant organisms. Blood cultures are generally useful only in the context of systemic sepsis.

Synovial fluid aspiration is necessary for definitive diagnosis of septic arthritis. This fluid should be analyzed for white cell count, Gram stain, and culture. Fluid should also be analyzed for the presence of crystals, because crystal arthropathies can mimic septic arthritis. A white cell count of higher than 18 to 50 x 10³/uL is significant for the diagnosis of sepsis.[26] A neutrophil differential of greater than 90% is highly suggestive of infection. Values for the diagnosis of infection in arthroplasty differ from these and are discussed later.

Synovial fluid cultures can yield a definitive diagnosis and are useful for determining antimicrobial susceptibility. The sensitivity for diagnosis of nongonococcal septic arthritis is 75% to 90%, whereas the sensitivity for Gram staining is 50% to 75%.[27] Specific culture media are needed for the growth of certain fastidious microorganisms, such as *Mycobacterium tuberculosis* or fungi. Polymerase chain reaction can be used for the diagnosis of *Borrelia burgdorferi* or *Neisseria gonorrhoeae*. The diagnostic yield for gonococcal synovial fluid cultures tends to be lower, particularly in disseminated infection. In this instance, it is imperative to isolate cultures from the primary mucosal site of infection.

Imaging Studies
Plain radiography is the initial modality for imaging in musculoskeletal infections. AP and lateral radiographs should be taken to evaluate the site in question. In periprosthetic joint infection, radiographs can reveal periosteal reaction, bone cysts, and focal resorption indicative of periprosthetic joint infection (**Figure 2**). Although radiographs rarely detect osteomyelitis during the early stages, they may identify adjacent soft-tissue swelling, joint effusion, and erosion related to adjacent septic arthritis. Radiographs may show subluxation or dislocation of the joint and soft-tissue swelling around the affected joint. In the later stages of osteomyelitis, frank bone destruction and sequestered bone necrosis may be evident.

Radionuclide imaging is a sensitive but nonspecific imaging modality for infection. There are three main methods available: the technetium Tc 99m bone scan, the gallium 67 scan, and the labeled white blood cell scan. Bone scans may show a decreased uptake (a cold scan), early in the disease process and an increased uptake (hot scan) later (**Figure 3**). Nuclear medicine techniques, notably combined leukocyte–bone marrow imaging, are especially useful in the setting of infection. Although leukocytes do not usually accumulate at

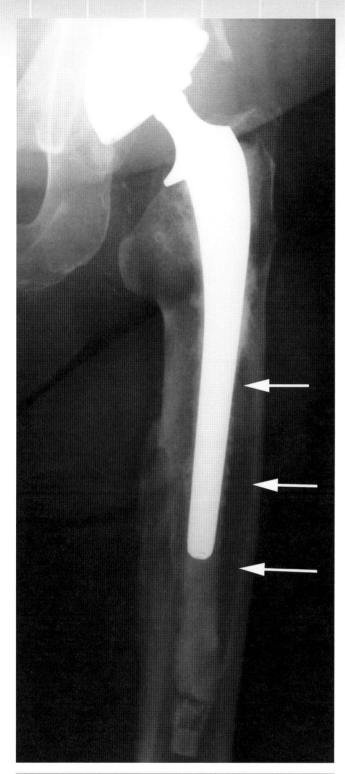

Figure 2 Plain radiograph demonstrating periprosthetic joint infection in a cemented total hip. Note the osteolysis (arrows) at the tip of the stem with expansion of the cortex.

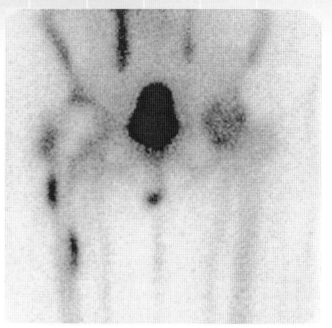

Figure 3 Technetium bone scan demonstrating increased uptake associated with periprosthetic joint infection.

sites of increased bone mineral turnover in the absence of infection, they do accumulate in the bone marrow. The implantation of orthopaedic hardware can alter the normal distribution of hematopoietically active marrow, making it

difficult to distinguish uptake of labeled leukocytes in infection from uptake in marrow. This problem can be overcome by performing complementary bone marrow scintigraphy with Tc 99m sulfur colloid. Both labeled leukocytes and sulfur colloid accumulate in the marrow, whereas only leukocytes accumulate in infection. Hence, images on which the distribution of the two radiotracers is the same indicate that the leukocyte uptake involves the marrow. Activity on the leukocyte image without corresponding activity on the bone marrow image indicates that the leukocyte uptake is due to infection. The accuracy of this dual radiotracer technique exceeds 90%.[28]

Cross-sectional imaging can be used to detect or localize a source of infection. CT findings in osteomyelitis include cortical bone destruction, periosteal new bone formation, intraosseous gas, increased attenuation of the marrow, narrowing of the medullary cavity, serpentine drainage tracts, and the presence of an involucrum or sequestrum.[29] The presence of a punctate area of increased attenuation, with a region of focal cortical destruction, suggests a sequestrum and is very specific for an infective process.[30]

MRI is also very sensitive in detecting osteomyelitis.[31] The marrow space of the involved bone demonstrates decreased signal on T1-weighted images and increased signal on T2-weighted images.[32] Cortical destruction or thickening and edema or abscess formation in the soft tissues can also be demonstrated on MRI. Although both an abscess and edema will have low signal on T1-weighted images and high signal on T2-weighted images, a well-demarcated border and a rim of decreased intensity are more characteristic of an abscess.[33] The penumbra sign is a characteristic magnetic resonance feature of subacute osteomyelitis. It can be

3: Basic Principles and Treatment of Musculoskeletal Disease

identified on unenhanced T1-weighted spin-echo images as a discrete peripheral zone of marginally higher signal intensity than the central bony abscess cavity and the surrounding lower signal intensity of the reactive new bone and edema.[34] In chronic osteomyelitis, T2-weighted images can localize areas of active infection with high signal intensity. Findings that favor chronic infection include thickening of the cortex, a relatively sharp interface between diseased and normal marrow, and a well-defined soft-tissue abnormality.[35]

Ultrasound of a septic joint, especially the hip, can detect an effusion and can be an aid in aspiration. The use of ultrasound has been described in the emergency department setting to rapidly evaluate the patient with suspected septic arthritis.[36] Ultrasound also can be used in the detection of osteomyelitis. Many of the ultrasonic features of osteomyelitis, such as deep soft-tissue swelling, periosteal thickening, and early subperiosteal fluid collection, can precede radiologic changes.[37]

Fluorine-18 fluorodeoxyglucose–positron emission tomography (^{18}F FDG-PET) is a promising modality for imaging musculoskeletal infection and might play an important role in the evaluation of chronic osteomyelitis and spinal infection. FDG-PET has shown promising results for diagnosing both acute and chronic infection of the axial and appendicular skeletons. PET imaging will have increased importance in patients with metallic implants because FDG uptake, in contrast to MRI and CT, is not hampered by metallic artifacts. PET/CT with the combination of PET and a low-dose or full-dose diagnostic CT provides exact anatomic correlation of bone and joint lesions and increases the accuracy of the test compared with PET alone. The question of the situations in which PET/CT becomes the preferred imaging method in suspected musculoskeletal infection depends on several factors, including cost and availability.[38]

Culture and Tissue Biopsy

Joint aspiration with immediate Gram stain and microscopy followed by culture and sensitivity remains the mainstay for diagnosis of septic arthritis. On direct examination, the aspirate may demonstrate gross pus. A white cell count of more than 50,000/mm³ with 75% polymorphonuclear leukocytes is usually seen.[39] Gram stains are only positive in 30% to 50% of cases, and cultures of the aspirate are positive in about 50% to 80% of cases.[40] Synovial protein levels that are more than 40 mg/dL and are less than serum protein levels are consistent with septic arthritis. The glucose level in the aspirate is lower than that in serum.

The diagnosis of osteomyelitis is usually made by a combination of clinical findings, radiography, bone scanning, and MRI, along with the aspiration of pus from the involved area and positive blood cultures. In chronic osteomyelitis, radiographic signs of necrotic bone (sequestrum) and periosteal new bone formation (involucrum) are evident.

Antimicrobial Agents
Application in Orthopaedics

Success in treating musculoskeletal infection requires an aggressive surgical approach and optimized antimicrobial therapy. The type of infection, the virulence and antimicrobial susceptibilities of the involved micro-organism, the adverse effects of the proposed antimicrobial therapy, alternative antimicrobial therapies, and the patients' general health should be considered before initiation of treatment. Antimicrobial agents have a wide variety of uses in orthopaedics. They are used in both prophylaxis and treatment of infections. The method of delivery depends on the infection involved. Antimicrobial agents can be delivered systemically, in the form of oral or parenteral dosing, or locally, in the form of topical solutions or local delivery devices such as antibiotic beads or spacers. The local delivery of antimicrobial agents to the site of orthopaedic infection is based on the need for high concentrations of these drugs to kill planktonic and biofilm-based bacteria. Many musculoskeletal infections require prolonged systemic antimicrobial therapy, often administered on an outpatient basis under the guidance of an infectious disease specialist in close collaboration with an orthopaedic surgeon.

Bioavailability

An intravenous route of administration has the greatest quantitative potential, as it permits a mass balance approach to be applied to distribution, clearance, and the body processes associated with excretion and metabolic elimination (for example, renal, hepatic). The administration of a drug by other routes, notably oral, introduces an uncertainty that reflects the unknown fraction that is actually absorbed.

The most important property of any nonintravenous dosage mode intended to treat a systemic condition is the ability to deliver the active ingredient to the bloodstream in an amount sufficient to cause the desired response. This property of a dosage form has historically been identified as physiologic availability, biologic availability, or bioavailability. Bioavailability captures two essential features: how fast the drug enters the systemic circulation (rate of absorption) and how much of the nominal strength enters the body (extent of absorption). Given that the therapeutic effect is a function of the drug concentration in a patient's blood, these two properties of nonintravenous dosage forms are, in principle, important in identifying the response to a drug dose.

Bioavailability after receipt of oral doses may vary because of either patient-related or dosage form–related factors. Patient factors can include the nature and timing of meals, age, disease, genetic traits, and gastrointestinal physiology. The dosage form factors include the chemical form of the drug (salt versus acid), its physical properties (crystal structure, particle size), and an array of formulation (nonactive ingredients) and manufacturing (tablet hardness) variables.

Elution Characteristics

The current standard of care for infected joint arthroplasty is considered to be two-stage revision arthroplasty including removal of the prosthesis and cement, thorough débridement, placement of an antibiotic-impregnated cement spacer, a course of intravenous antibiotics, and a delayed second-stage revision arthroplasty. The choice of the spacer, either articulating or nonarticulating, is based on many factors, including the amount of bone loss, the condition of the soft tissues, the need for joint motion, the availability of prefabricated spacers or molding methods, and antibiotic selection. Additionally, in nonarthroplasty infections, bone cement beads are used to deliver antibiotics to the local area after surgical débridement.

The elution of antibiotics from bone cement depends on several factors. The type of antibiotic, the amount and number of antibiotics, the porosity and type of cement, and the surface area of the spacer all play a role in the release.[41-43] Stevens et al[44] studied the in vitro elution of antibiotics from Simplex and Palacos bone cements and found Palacos to be a more effective vehicle for local drug delivery. In a study of the long-term elution of antibiotics from polymethylmethacrylate (PMMA) bone cement in vivo in 40 patients, Masri et al[43] found that effective levels of antibiotics remained 4 months after the operation. This observation is consistent with the suggestion that at least 3.6 g of tobramycin per 40 g of bone cement, with the addition of 1 g of vancomycin, is an effective antibiotic regimen in this setting. With effective levels of vancomycin not present 4 months after the operation, Masri et al[43] determined that the two antibiotics acted synergistically with one another to increase the elution rates but vancomycin should not be used alone. This finding was consistent with the results of an in vitro study that showed that combining tobramycin and vancomycin in PMMA bone cement improved the elution rates of both antibiotics.[45]

Compared with commercially available antibiotic-loaded cement, hand-mixed cement is associated with a decreased release of antibiotics, whereas vacuum mixing has been shown to result in only a minor reduction in antibiotic release.[46] Unlike antibiotics that are commercially mixed in cement, hand-mixed antibiotics do not have a homogeneous distribution in the cement, which decreases their rate of elution from a given surface area.[47] Vacuum mixing decreases the porosity of the cement, which also decreases the rate of elution of the antibiotics.[48] The elution of antibiotics from PMMA bone cement is determined by a combination of surface area and porosity.[48] One study showed that increasing the surface area of PMMA bone cement by 40% resulted in a 20% higher rate of elution of vancomycin.[49] Dextran has been added to cement to enhance porosity and increase antibiotic elution rates. Kuechle et al[50] found that the addition of 25% dextran to cement increased the release of antibiotics in the first 48 hours approximately four times compared with that associated with routine preparation and increased the duration of the elution to up to 10 days compared with only 6 days with routine preparation.

Approach to Treatment

The most important determinant of successful outcomes of acute or chronic orthopaedic infections is the quality of the surgical débridement. An aggressive débridement with a wide margin (more than 5 mm) has been found to eradicate infection in almost all cases.[51] The goal of débridement is to achieve a clean, viable wound with minimal trauma to the remaining soft tissue. For an acute infection, the most straightforward method of débridement is incision and drainage, coupled with copious lavage. In chronic infection, a more aggressive approach is required due to a compromised host and tissues, the presence of foreign bodies, and adherent biofilms.[52]

Incisions should be made either through the old scar or, if the old scar cannot be used, perpendicular to the scar so as to avoid wound edge necrosis. An extensile exposure should be used permitting lengthening of the incision to permit thorough débridement based on intraoperative findings.[53] In the context of osteomyelitis, all necrotic bony tissue must be excised to leave only viable bone. It is important not to devascularize remaining bone so as not to give rise to a new sequestrum. If 70% or more of the original cortical bone at the level of débridement is intact, the risk of fracture is low. If a more extensive débridement is required, it may be necessary to stabilize the bone with an external fixator.[52]

Specific Infections
Osteomyelitis and Septic Arthritis

Septic arthritis is a condition characterized by infection of the synovium and the joint space. The infection causes an intense inflammatory reaction and release of proteolytic enzymes, leading to the rapid destruction of the articular cartilage. Osteomyelitis is an acute or chronic inflammatory process of the bone and its structures secondary to infection. Septic arthritis in combination with osteomyelitis is common in children. Because of their unique anatomy, neonates and young children often have coexisting septic arthritis and osteomyelitis.[54] The bony cortex is thin, and the periosteum is loose. Blood vessels that connect the metaphysis and epiphysis serve as a conduit by which bone infection may easily reach the joint space. Septic arthritis can also occur in adults, usually secondary to an immunocompromised state or an underlying medical condition, such as diabetes. In the shoulder, elbow, hip, and ankle joints, the capsule overlaps a portion of the adjoining metaphyses. If the focus of osteomyelitis breaks through the metaphyseal bone, it can directly infect the joint and lead to concurrent septic arthritis.

Destruction of the articular cartilage begins quickly and is secondary to proteolytic enzymes released from synovial cells.[55] Interleukin-1 (IL-1) triggers the release of proteases from chondrocytes and synoviocytes in response to polymorphonuclear leukocytes and bacteria. Smith et al[56] showed that cartilage destruction starts to occur as early as 8 hours after infection. Early administration of antibiotics helps to slow down the process, but even if intravenous antibiotic therapy is started within the first 24 hours of infection, significant glycosaminoglycan destruction and collagen disruption occurs. Degradation results in the loss of proteoglycans from the articular cartilage by 5 days and loss of collagen by 9 days.[57] Impairment of the intracapsular vascular supply secondary to elevation of the intracapsular pressure and thrombosis of the vessels also play a role in the destruction of the articular cartilage.[58] The common sites of involvement in children are the hip and knee, but in the adult approximately 85% of cases are monoarticular, with the knee being the most commonly affected.

Acute hematogenous osteomyelitis occurs predominantly in children, with the metaphysis of long bones the most common location. Patients usually present within several days to 1 week after the onset of symptoms. In addition to local signs of inflammation and infection, patients have signs of systemic illness, including fever, irritability, and lethargy. Typical clinical findings include tenderness over the involved bone and decreased range of motion in adjacent joints.

The subacute and chronic forms of osteomyelitis usually occur in adults. Generally, these bone infections are secondary to an open wound, most often an open injury to bone and surrounding soft tissue. Localized bone pain, erythema, and drainage around the affected area are frequently present. The cardinal signs of subacute and chronic osteomyelitis include draining sinus tracts, deformity, instability and local signs of impaired vascularity, range of motion, and neurologic status. The incidence of deep musculoskeletal infection from open fractures has been reported to be approximately 23%, with a 6% osteomyelitis rate.[59] A further study divided patients into subgroups according to comorbidities and reported a range of infection rates from 4% to 30% depending on host factors.[60] Patient factors, such as altered neutrophil defense, humoral immunity, and cell-mediated immunity, can increase the risk of osteomyelitis.

Treatment

After the initial evaluation, staging, and establishment of microbial etiology and susceptibilities, treatment includes antimicrobial therapy, débridement with management of resultant dead space and, if necessary, stabilization of bone. In most patients with osteomyelitis, early antibiotic therapy produces the best results. Antimicrobial agents must be administered for a minimum of 4 weeks (ideally, 6 weeks) to achieve an acceptable rate of cure. To reduce costs, parenteral antibiotic administration on an outpatient basis or the use of oral antibiotics can be considered. In many cases, osteomyelitis can be effectively treated with antibiotics and pain medications. If a biopsy is obtained, this can help guide the choice of the best antibiotic. In some cases, the affected

area will be immobilized with a brace to reduce the pain and speed the treatment.

Osteomyelitis often requires prolonged antibiotic therapy, with a course lasting a matter of weeks or months. A peripherally inserted central catheter line or central venous catheter is often placed for this purpose. Osteomyelitis also may require surgical débridement. Severe cases may lead to the loss of a limb. Initial first-line antibiotic choice is determined by the patient's history and regional differences in common infective organisms. Treatment lasting 42 days is practiced in several facilities. Local and sustained availability of drugs has proved to be more effective in achieving prophylactic and therapeutic outcomes.

Sometimes, surgery may be necessary. If there is an area of localized bacteria (abscess), this may need to be opened, washed out, and drained. Damaged soft tissue or bone may need to be removed. If bone needs to be removed, it may need to be replaced with bone graft or stabilized during surgery.

For the treatment of septic arthritis, several surgical methods have been proposed. Needle aspiration has been historically advocated for the drainage of a septic joint.[61] Shaw and Kasser[62] in a major review of acute septic arthritis described open surgical drainage as the "gold standard." Bertone et al,[63] in a study on septic arthritis in horses, showed that arthrotomy eradicated joint infection more completely than arthroscopy, but that secondary wound infection was a problem. More recent publications have demonstrated effective use of arthroscopic techniques, particularly in conjunction with continuous irrigation, for the management of septic arthritis.[64,65]

Outcome

Acute hematogenous osteomyelitis is best managed with careful evaluation of microbial etiology and susceptibilities and a 4- to 6-week course of appropriate antibiotic therapy. Surgical débridement is not necessary when the diagnosis of hematogenous osteomyelitis is made early. Current treatment recommendations rarely require surgical débridement. However, if antibiotic therapy fails, débridement (or repeated débridement) and another 4- to 6-week course of parenteral antibiotic therapy are essential.[66]

After cultures have been obtained, an empiric parenteral antibiotic regimen (nafcillin plus either cefotaxime or ceftriaxone) is initiated to cover clinically suspected organisms. When the culture results are known, the antibiotic regimen is revised. Children with acute osteomyelitis should receive 2 weeks of initial parenteral antibiotic therapy before they are given an oral agent.[67]

Chronic osteomyelitis in adults is more refractory to therapy and is generally treated with antibiotics and surgical débridement. Empiric antibiotic therapy is not usually recommended. Depending on the type of chronic osteomyelitis, patients may be treated with parenteral antibiotics for 2 to 6 weeks. However, without adequate débridement, chronic osteomyelitis does not respond to most antibiotic regimens, no matter what the duration of therapy is. Outpatient intravenous therapy using long-term intravenous access catheters (Hickman catheters) decreases the length of hospital stays.[68] Oral therapy using fluoroquinolone antibiotics for gram-negative organisms is currently being used in adults with osteomyelitis.[69] None of the currently available fluoroquinolones provides optimal antistaphylococcal coverage, an important disadvantage in view of the rising incidence of nosocomially acquired staphylococcal resistance.[70] Furthermore, the current quinolones provide essentially no coverage of anaerobic pathogens.

Débridement

Surgical débridement in patients with chronic osteomyelitis can be technically demanding.[52] The quality of the débridement is the most critical factor in successful management. After débridement with excision of bone, it is necessary to obliterate the dead space created by the removal of tissue. Dead-space management includes local myoplasty, free-tissue transfers, and the use of antibiotic-impregnated beads. Soft-tissue procedures have been developed to improve local blood flow and antibiotic delivery

Periprosthetic Joint Infection

Periprosthetic joint infection, one of the most dreaded complications in orthopaedics, often results in repeat surgeries, patient distress and disability, increased cost, and utilization of medical resources.[71] Infection, despite being less prevalent than aseptic loosening, can lead to chronic systemic spread, osteomyelitis, possible tissue necrosis or amputation, and, in particularly difficult cases, death.[72] It is important to realize that, at the end of the day, periprosthetic infections do not affect just the patient, but this dreadful complication impinges on society at large. As far back as 1989, the annual cost of infection exceeded $200 million. More recent data show that joint revisions due to infection cost more than $50,000 per case; revision due to aseptic loosening is approximately $16,000 and primary arthroplasty is approximately $8,500. Financial analysis estimates that as little as 1% decrease in revision rate for total joint arthroplasty would save as much as $211 million in US health care costs.[73]

Diagnosis

Clinical history and physical examination are critical for determining the risk of periprosthetic infection. A good history identifying the specific presentation, duration, and localization of symptoms, predisposing factors, and response to treatments may allow an early diagnosis (**Table 1**). A diagnosis can be almost always confirmed in patients presenting with severe joint pain, fever, poor wound healing, erythema, drainage, sinus formation, and early implant failure.[74] Radiographs can provide some nonspecific information about the local environment around the prosthesis; in cases of overt infection, periosteal reaction, bone cysts, and resorption may be visible. Another aid to diagnosis is

Table 1
Risk Factors for Surgical Site Infection

Patient	Surgical
Diabetes mellitus	Blood transfusion
Urinary tract infection	Hypothermia
Chronic renal failure	Surgical technique
Rheumatoid disease	Preoperative skin preparation
Immunocompromise Obesity	Intraoperative issues: Operating room traffic/laminar flow/space suits
Nutritional status Smoking	Postoperative issues: Antibiotics/length of stay

serologic testing that is often easy to perform and provides preoperative information to aid in the diagnostic algorithm. Specifically, blood leukocyte count and differential are not sensitive or specific to periprosthetic joint infection, whereas synovial fluid leukocyte count and differential is a rapid and accurate assay for predicting periprosthetic infection.[75] A knee synovial fluid leukocyte count of more than 1,700/μL (range, 1,100-3,000/μL) and a differential of more than 65% neutrophils produced sensitivities of 94% and 97%, with specificities of 88% and 98%, for detecting periprosthetic infection, respectively.[76] Although they are generally nonspecific markers of inflammation, erythrocyte sedimentation rate and C-reactive protein level are very useful as initial screening tests of infection due to their high negative predictive values.[77] Both of these markers normally rise after surgery, with C-reactive protein level returning to normal within 3 weeks. Erythrocyte sedimentation rate, however, takes up to 6 weeks to reach normal values with some diurnal variation present even at that time.[74] Elevation of these markers after 3 months is considered abnormal and may indicate the development of periprosthetic infection. Erythrocyte sedimentation rate values of more than 30 mm/h in some studies produced 82% sensitivity and 85% specificity.[78]

C-reactive protein level is generally a better predictor of infection, with levels of 10 mg/L considered more than 96% sensitive and 92% specific for periprosthetic infection. More recently, serum levels of IL-6 have been shown to correlate with infection.[79] IL-6 is produced by monocytes and macrophages, and serum levels above 10 pg/mL have consistently predicted infection with a sensitivity of 100%, specificity of 95%, positive predictive value of 89%, negative predictive value of 100%, and accuracy of 97% against positive histopathology and culture.[80]

Imaging

Radionuclide studies have been used for diagnosis of periprosthetic joint infection; these include bone scintigra-

Table 2

Criteria for Device Salvage in Periprosthetic Infection

Acute infection for longer than 14 to 28 days

Stable implant

Clear diagnosis

Susceptible organism

Effective antimicrobial agent, preferably bacteriocidal

Compliant patient

phy with technetium 99m or indium-111 scanning, or ^{18}F-FDG imaging. Three-phase bone imaging alone showed only 33% sensitivity and 86% specificity, with poor predictive value.[81] When using more specific antigranulocyte scintigraphy with monoclonal antibodies, a meta-analysis of more than 522 implants showed a sensitivity as high as 90% and specificity of 80%. Technetium 99m sulfur colloid indium-111–labeled leukocyte bone scintigraphy had a sensitivity of more than 50% and specificity of 95% in diagnosing infection.[82] By comparison, FDG-PET showed 95% sensitivity and 93% specificity for hip prosthesis–associated infection.[83] Yet another study showed 91% sensitivity and 72% specificity for diagnosing infection around the knee and 90% sensitivity and 89% specificity around the hip.[84] Areas of infection involve inflammation and increased metabolism, especially relevant to glucose consumption. Immune system cells uptake the FDG, which gets phosphorylated to deoxyglucose-6-phosphate and trapped in the cell long enough to be imaged by PET. However, PET is generally nonspecific, and inflammatory conditions have to be ruled out to have any predictive value in the diagnosis of infection. Overall, radionuclide imaging is an exciting test but requires extensive resource utilization that is not easily available at most centers.

Intraoperative tests and frozen sections represent a much more important component in the operating room.

Treatment

Successful treatment of periprosthetic joint infection can often prove to be a difficult undertaking. Revision surgery is often indicated, although prosthesis retention with débridement and antibiotic therapy is a viable alternative in uncomplicated cases where acute presentation is within 4 weeks of initial surgery. During the management of infection, both the identity and susceptibility of the infectious organisms should be determined soon after empiric therapy is initiated. Despite availability of new antibiotics, such as linezolids or the monobactams, a basic algorithm suggests use of vancomycin for gram-positive organisms in acute or chronic infections, while cephazolin and gentamycin are recommended for hematogenous contamination.[85] Furthermore, third- or fourth-generation cephalosporin alone or in combination with vancomycin is recommended for gram-negative and mixed flora. Clindamycin or a combination of ampicillin with sulbactam is efficient against anaerobes.[86] Treatment should be continued for a minimum of 4 to 6 weeks, which coincides with the typical period of revascularization.[87] Surgical intervention allows direct removal of the biofilm, further excision of contaminated tissue, and washing with antibiotic solutions in high local concentrations. During the early postoperative period, superficial infection without joint capsule involvement can be managed with soft-tissue resection and débridement, which allows implant salvage (**Table 2**). Antibiotic-laden cement beads containing tobramycin or vancomycin are often used within the wound for up to 2 weeks.[87] Such cement beads maintain a high local antibiotic concentration inhibitory to bacterial growth while allowing the immune system to eliminate any residual bacteria. Intravenous antibiotics are continued for a duration of 4 to 6 weeks. This approach can yield very good results, with eradication reported in 26% to 71% of patients.[88] Delay in treatment, however, converts the early acute infection to a chronic status, with surgery and aggressive management necessary if symptoms persist for more than 2 weeks.

Implant removal is always involved in more severe infections where the joint capsule is involved or symptoms have a late chronic presentation. Depending on the severity of infection, risk factors, and the surgeon's ability to cleanly excise the surrounding tissue, a one-stage or two-stage revision is performed. If the infection is relatively mild, without sinus tracts or induration, and the cultured organisms show simple flora susceptible to typical antibiotics, which is currently rare, then a one-stage procedure is possible with relatively good success.[89] The rate of reinfection after one-stage procedures varies from 8% to more than 12%, allowing more than 80% survival of the implant.[90] One-stage procedures are less involved and provide faster recuperation for the patient. However, with the high risk and costs of reinfection and the very limited indications for a one-stage procedure, two-stage exchange revision is currently the standard for many physicians in the United States. After removal of the infected prosthesis with extensive débridement and soft-tissue excision, an antibiotic cement spacer is used to help eradicate the remaining bacteria. A second surgery is used to remove the spacer and implant a new joint prosthesis. The specific timing for the procedures is not clearly defined and ranges from 3 to 6 months.[91] Because biofilms are difficult to eradicate, intraoperative aspiration and culture are recommended during the extraction of the spacer.

Comparison studies of two-stage versus one-stage procedures suggest an advantage to the two-stage revision with reinfection rates of 3% to 6%, even though another study documented up to 22% infection with delayed surgery.[92,93] Despite improved treatment, the rate of infection is higher after revision surgery than after primary joint arthroplasty. Such a conclusion emphasizes the critical role of a successful primary surgery, with maximum precautions taken to eliminate infection. The consequences of an aggressive infection are further amplified by additional complications associated with revision surgery. Extensive bone loss can take place, which precludes additional revisions, leaving no choice but arthrodesis or even amputation. However, considering that two-stage procedures are the management step just before amputation, antibiotic-laden cements are currently considered the gold standard for local antibiotic delivery in cases of periprosthetic infection[93] (**Table 3**).

Cement Spacers

Use of antibiotic-impregnated PMMA bone-cement spacers is now considered to be the standard of care for patients with a chronic infection at the site of a total joint arthroplasty. These spacers provide direct local delivery of antibiotics while preserving patient mobility and facilitating reimplantation surgery.[94] This treatment decreases cost and improves patient outcomes as well as addresses some of the disadvantages of two-stage revision procedures in which spacers are not used. There are two types of antibiotic-impregnated cement spacers that are typically used in two-stage revisions of total hip and knee arthroplasties: nonarticulating (block or static) and articulating.

Nonarticulating spacers allow local delivery of a high concentration of antibiotics and at the same time function to maintain joint space for future revision procedures. Disadvantages of nonarticulating spacers include limited range of motion of the joint after the operation, possibly resulting in quadriceps or abductor shortening. In contrast, articulating spacers permit more joint motion and can improve function before the second-stage reimplantation. From a technical perspective, improved joint function and decreased scar formation after resection arthroplasty can facilitate exposure during reimplantation.[95] Although the distinction between articulating and nonarticulating spacers is somewhat controversial, use of a well-molded, well-fitted articulating spacer that restores soft-tissue tension and allows a greater degree of joint motion has been reported to have better outcomes than use of a nonarticulating spacer, specifically in terms of improved range of motion and functional knee scores without concomitant increases in infection rate and bone loss.[96,97]

Spine Infection

Spine infections can result in significant morbidity and even mortality. Smoking, obesity, malnutrition, diabetes, immunodeficiency, or local radiation treatment can predispose to infection. Pyogenic infections are most commonly caused by *S aureus*, although *Staphylococcus epidermidis*, *Streptococcus* spp, and *Escherichia coli* infections may also occur. Granulomatous infections may be caused by *Mycobacterium tuberculosis* and, rarely, fungi. Symptoms include back pain, possibly in combination with radicular pain. Less common symptoms include neurologic disability with sensory disturbance and motor weakness. Systemic manifestations of spine infection include malaise, weight loss, and altered

Table 3
Treatment Options for Periprosthetic Infection

Débridement with retention of implants

Excision arthroplasty

One-stage revision arthroplasty

Two-stage revision arthtoplasty

Arthrodesis

Amputation

mental status. The mainstay of treatment is antimicrobial therapy typically for 6 weeks; however, response to therapy can be monitored using serial erythrocyte sedimentation rate and C-reactive protein level.[98] Surgery is indicated if the infection is refractory to appropriate nonsurgical treatment. Spinal cord decompression should be performed promptly in the context of an emerging neurologic deficit. Factors associated with favorable outcome include age younger than 60 years, normal immune status, infection with *S aureus* as well as a prompt response to treatment as demonstrated by decreasing erythrocyte sedimentation rate.[99]

Infected Nonunion

Although definitions vary, infected nonunion has been defined as a state of failure of union and persistence of infection at the fracture site for 6 to 8 months. Infected nonunions are mostly due to a severe open fracture with extensive comminution and segmental bone loss or after internal fixation of a comminuted closed fracture. Factors associated with an infected nonunion include exposed bone devoid of vascularized periosteal coverage for more than 6 weeks, purulent discharge, a positive bacteriologic culture from the depth of the wound, and histologic evidence of necrotic bone containing empty lacunae.[100] Treatment and long-term recovery can be complicated by soft-tissue loss with multiple sinuses, osteomyelitis, osteopenia, complex deformities with limb-length inequality, stiffness of the adjacent joint, and polybacterial multidrug-resistant infection. These patients have been categorized into two groups. Type A is infected nonunion of long bones with nondraining (quiescent) infection, with or without implant in situ; type B is infected nonunion of long bones with draining (active) infection. Both are classified further into two subtypes: nonunion with a bone gap smaller than 4 cm or nonunion with a bone gap larger than 4 cm. Single-stage débridement and bone grafting with fracture stabilization are the methods of choice for type A1 infected nonunions. Adequate débridement, fracture stabilization, and second-stage bone grafting give desirable results in type B1 infected nonunions. Distraction histiogenesis is the preferred procedure for types A2 and B2. The autogenous infected nonvascularized fibular graft, posterolateral bone grafting for the tibia, and centralization of the ulna over distal radial remnant (single bone forearm) may be good treatment options in selected cases.[101] Although uncommon, infected nonunion of a long bone presents a great challenge to the orthopaedic surgeon in providing optimal treatment.

Summary

As the burden of orthopaedic infection increases, the orthopaedic and medical communities should become more familiar with these diseases. Periprosthetic joint infection is a significant and costly challenge to the orthopaedic community. Molecular markers in the serum and joint fluid aspirate hold immense promise and in combination with improving radiologic measures will lead to enhanced development of firm diagnostic criterion. It is hoped that the tools currently under investigation will aid clinicians in diagnosing orthopaedic infections in an accurate and timely fashion to allow prompt and appropriate treatment. Given the current knowledge and planned future research, the medical community should be prepared to effectively manage these increasingly prevalent diseases.

References

1. Burke JP: Infection control: A problem for patient safety. *N Engl J Med* 2003;348(7):651-656.

2. Whitehouse JD, Friedman ND, Kirkland KB, Richardson WJ, Sexton DJ: The impact of surgical-site infections following orthopedic surgery at a community hospital and a university hospital: Adverse quality of life, excess length of stay, and extra cost. *Infect Control Hosp Epidemiol* 2002;23(4):183-189.

3. Carreon LY, Puno RM, Dimar JR II, Glassman SD, Johnson JR: Perioperative complications of posterior lumbar decompression and arthrodesis in older adults. *J Bone Joint Surg Am* 2003;85(11):2089-2092.

4. Mahomed NN, Barrett JA, Katz JN, et al: Rates and outcomes of primary and revision total hip replacement in the United States Medicare population. *J Bone Joint Surg Am* 2003;85(1):27-32.

5. Hervey SL, Purves HR, Guller U, Toth AP, Vail TP, Pietrobon R: Provider volume of total knee arthroplasties and patient outcomes in the HCUP-Nationwide Inpatient Sample. *J Bone Joint Surg Am* 2003;85(9):1775-1783.

6. Costerton JW: Overview of microbial biofilms. *J Ind Microbiol* 1995;15(3):137-140.

7. Davies DG, Parsek MR, Pearson JP, Iglewski BH, Costerton JW, Greenberg EP: The involvement of cell-to-cell signals in the development of a bacterial biofilm. *Science* 1998;280(5361):295-298.

8. Schildhauer TA, Robie B, Muhr G, Köller M: Bacterial adherence to tantalum versus commonly used orthopedic metallic implant materials. *J Orthop Trauma* 2006;20(7):476-484.

9. O'Toole GA, Kolter R: Flagellar and twitching motility are necessary for Pseudomonas aeruginosa biofilm development. *Mol Microbiol* 1998;30(2):295-304.

10. Selwyn S, Ellis H: Skin bacteria and skin disinfection reconsidered. *Br Med J* 1972;1(5793):136-140.

11. Murray MR, Saltzman MD, Gryzlo SM, Terry MA, Woodward CC, Nuber GW: Efficacy of preoperative home use of 2% chlorhexidine gluconate cloth before shoulder surgery. *J Shoulder Elbow Surg* 2011;20(6):928-933.

12. Kaul AF, Jewett JF: Agents and techniques for disinfection of the skin. *Surg Gynecol Obstet* 1981;152(5):677-685.

13. Mulberrry G, Snyder AT, Heilman J, Pyrek J, Stahl J: Evaluation of a waterless, scrubless chlorhexidine gluconate/ethanol surgical scrub for antimicrobial efficacy. *Am J Infect Control* 2001;29(6):377-382.

14. Gosden PE, MacGowan AP, Bannister GC: Importance of air quality and related factors in the prevention of infection in orthopaedic implant surgery. *J Hosp Infect* 1998;39(3):173-180.

15. Kong KC, Sheppard M, Serne G: Dispensing surgical gloves onto the open surgical gown pack does not increase the bacterial contamination rate. *J Hosp Infect* 1994;26(4):293-296.

16. Blom A, Estela C, Bowker K, MacGowan A, Hardy JR: The passage of bacteria through surgical drapes. *Ann R Coll Surg Engl* 2000;82(6):405-407.

17. Bethune DW, Blowers R, Parker M, Pask EA: Dispersal of *Staphylococcus aureus* by patients and surgical staff. *Lancet* 1965;1(7383):480-483.

18. Pryor F, Messmer PR: The effect of traffic patterns in the OR on surgical site infections. *AORN J* 1998;68(4):649-660.

19. Ritter MA: Operating room environment. *Clin Orthop Relat Res* 1999;369:103-109.

20. Salvati EA, Robinson RP, Zeno SM, Koslin BL, Brause BD, Wilson PD Jr: Infection rates after 3175 total hip and total knee replacements performed with and without a horizontal unidirectional filtered air-flow system. *J Bone Joint Surg Am* 1982;64(4):525-535.

21. Pull ter Gunne AF, Cohen DB: Incidence, prevalence, and analysis of risk factors for surgical site infection following adult spinal surgery. *Spine (Phila Pa 1976)* 2009;34(13):1422-1428.

22. Olsen MA, Nepple JJ, Riew KD, et al: Risk factors for surgical site infection following orthopaedic spinal operations. *J Bone Joint Surg Am* 2008;90(1):62-69.

23. Dowsey MM, Choong PF: Obese diabetic patients are at substantial risk for deep infection after primary TKA. *Clin Orthop Relat Res* 2009;467(6):1577-1581.

24. Jämsen E, Huhtala H, Puolakka T, Moilanen T: Risk factors for infection after knee arthroplasty: A register-based analysis of 43,149 cases. *J Bone Joint Surg Am* 2009;91(1):38-47.

25. Patel VP, Walsh M, Sehgal B, Preston C, DeWal H, Di Cesare PE: Factors associated with prolonged wound drainage after primary total hip and knee arthroplasty. *J Bone Joint Surg Am* 2007;89(1):33-38.

26. Li SF, Cassidy C, Chang C, Gharib S, Torres J: Diagnostic utility of laboratory tests in septic arthritis. *Emerg Med J* 2007;24(2):75-77.

27. Swan A, Amer H, Dieppe P: The value of synovial fluid assays in the diagnosis of joint disease: A literature survey. *Ann Rheum Dis* 2002;61(6):493-498.

28. Palestro CJ, Torres MA: Radionuclide imaging in orthopedic infections. *Semin Nucl Med* 1997;27(4):334-345.

29. Azouz EM: Computed tomography in bone and joint infections. *J Can Assoc Radiol* 1981;32(2):102-106.

30. Hernandez RJ: Visualization of small sequestra by computerized tomography: Report of 6 cases. *Pediatr Radiol* 1985; 15(4):238-241.

31. Jaramillo D: Infection: Musculoskeletal. *Pediatr Radiol* 2011; 41(Suppl 1):S127-S134.

32. Unger E, Moldofsky P, Gatenby R, Hartz W, Broder G: Diagnosis of osteomyelitis by MR imaging. *AJR Am J Roentgenol* 1988;150(3):605-610.

33. Beltran J, Noto AM, McGhee RB, Freedy RM, McCalla MS: Infections of the musculoskeletal system: High-field-strength MR imaging. *Radiology* 1987;164(2):449-454.

34. Davies AM, Grimer R: The penumbra sign in subacute osteomyelitis. *Eur Radiol* 2005;15(6):1268-1270.

35. Cohen MD, Cory DA, Kleiman M, Smith JA, Broderick NJ: Magnetic resonance differentiation of acute and chronic osteomyelitis in children. *Clin Radiol* 1990;41(1):53-56.

36. Shavit I, Eidelman M, Galbraith R: Sonography of the hip joint by the emergency physician: Its role in the evaluation of children presenting with acute limp. *Pediatr Emerg Care* 2006;22(8):570-573.

37. Mah ET, LeQuesne GW, Gent RJ, Paterson DC: Ultrasonic features of acute osteomyelitis in children. *J Bone Joint Surg Br* 1994;76(6):969-974.

38. Strobel K, Stumpe KD: PET/CT in musculoskeletal infection. *Semin Musculoskelet Radiol* 2007;11(4):353-364.

39. Margaretten ME, Kohlwes J, Moore D, Bent S: Does this adult patient have septic arthritis? *JAMA* 2007;297(13):1478-1488.

40. Weston VC, Jones AC, Bradbury N, Fawthrop F, Doherty M: Clinical features and outcome of septic arthritis in a single UK Health District 1982-1991. *Ann Rheum Dis* 1999;58(4):214-219.

41. Durbhakula SM, Czajka J, Fuchs MD, Uhl RL: Spacer endoprosthesis for the treatment of infected total hip arthroplasty. *J Arthroplasty* 2004;19(6):760-767.

42. Hanssen AD, Spangehl MJ: Treatment of the infected hip replacement. *Clin Orthop Relat Res* 2004;420:63-71.

43. Masri BA, Duncan CP, Beauchamp CP: Long-term elution of antibiotics from bone-cement: An in vivo study using the prosthesis of antibiotic-loaded acrylic cement (PROSTALAC) system. *J Arthroplasty* 1998;13(3):331-338.

44. Stevens CM, Tetsworth KD, Calhoun JH, Mader JT: An articulated antibiotic spacer used for infected total knee arthroplasty: A comparative in vitro elution study of Simplex and Palacos bone cements. *J Orthop Res* 2005;23(1):27-33.

45. Penner MJ, Masri BA, Duncan CP: Elution characteristics of vancomycin and tobramycin combined in acrylic bone-cement. *J Arthroplasty* 1996;11(8):939-944.

46. Kuehn KD, Ege W, Gopp U: Acrylic bone cements: Mechanical and physical properties. *Orthop Clin North Am* 2005; 36(1):29-39.

47. Nelson CL, Griffin FM, Harrison BH, Cooper RE: In vitro elution characteristics of commercially and noncommercially prepared antibiotic PMMA beads. *Clin Orthop Relat Res* 1992;284:303-309.

48. Neut D, van de Belt H, van Horn JR, van der Mei HC, Busscher HJ: The effect of mixing on gentamicin release from polymethylmethacrylate bone cements. *Acta Orthop Scand* 2003;74(6):670-676.

49. Greene N, Holtom PD, Warren CA, et al: In vitro elution of tobramycin and vancomycin polymethylmethacrylate beads and spacers from Simplex and Palacos. *Am J Orthop (Belle Mead NJ)* 1998;27(3):201-205.

50. Kuechle DK, Landon GC, Musher DM, Noble PC: Elution of vancomycin, daptomycin, and amikacin from acrylic bone cement. *Clin Orthop Relat Res* 1991;264:302-308.

51. Simpson AH, Deakin M, Latham JM: Chronic osteomyelitis: The effect of the extent of surgical resection on infection-free survival. *J Bone Joint Surg Br* 2001;83(3):403-407.

52. Tetsworth K, Cierny G III: Osteomyelitis debridement techniques. *Clin Orthop Relat Res* 1999;360:87-96.

53. Heitmann C, Patzakis MJ, Tetsworth KD, Levin LS: Musculoskeletal sepsis: Principles of treatment. *Instr Course Lect* 2003;52:733-743.

54. Nade S: Acute septic arthritis in infancy and childhood. *J Bone Joint Surg Br* 1983;65(3):234-241.

55. Dingle JT: The role of lysosomal enzymes in skeletal tissues. *J Bone Joint Surg Br* 1973;55(1):87-95.

56. Smith RL, Schurman DJ, Kajiyama G, Mell M, Gilkerson E: The effect of antibiotics on the destruction of cartilage in experimental infectious arthritis. *J Bone Joint Surg Am* 1987; 69(7):1063-1068.

57. McCarthy JJ, Dormans JP, Kozin SH, Pizzutillo PD: Musculoskeletal infections in children: Basic treatment principles and recent advancements. *Instr Course Lect* 2005;54:515-528.

58. Morrey BF, Bianco AJ, Rhodes KH: Suppurative arthritis of the hip in children. *J Bone Joint Surg Am* 1976;58(3):388-392.

59. Khatod M, Botte MJ, Hoyt DB, Meyer RS, Smith JM, Akeson WH: Outcomes in open tibia fractures: Relationship between delay in treatment and infection. *J Trauma* 2003; 55(5):949-954.

60. Bowen TR, Widmaier JC: Host classification predicts infection after open fracture. *Clin Orthop Relat Res* 2005;433:205-211.

61. Goldenberg DL, Brandt KD, Cohen AS, Cathcart ES: Treatment of septic arthritis: Comparison of needle aspiration and surgery as initial modes of joint drainage. *Arthritis Rheum* 1975;18(1):83-90.

62. Shaw BA, Kasser JR: Acute septic arthritis in infancy and childhood. *Clin Orthop Relat Res* 1990;257:212-225.

63. Bertone AL, Davis DM, Cox HU, et al: Arthrotomy versus arthroscopy and partial synovectomy for treatment of experimentally induced infectious arthritis in horses. *Am J Vet Res* 1992;53(4):585-591.

64. Kuo CL, Chang JH, Wu CC, et al: Treatment of septic knee arthritis: comparison of arthroscopic debridement alone or combined with continuous closed irrigation-suction system. *J Trauma* 2011;71(2):454-459.

65. Ateschrang A, Albrecht D, Schröter S, Hirt B, Weise K, Dolderer JH: Septic arthritis of the knee: Presentation of a novel irrigation-suction system tested in a cadaver study. *BMC Musculoskelet Disord* 2011;12:180.

66. Mader JT, Mohan D, Calhoun J: A practical guide to the diagnosis and management of bone and joint infections. *Drugs* 1997;54(2):253-264.

67. Tetzlaff TR, McCracken GH Jr, Nelson JD: Oral antibiotic therapy for skeletal infections of children: II. Therapy of osteomyelitis and suppurative arthritis. *J Pediatr* 1978;92(3):485-490.

68. Couch L, Cierny G, Mader JT: Inpatient and outpatient use of the Hickman catheter for adults with osteomyelitis. *Clin Orthop Relat Res* 1987;219:226-235.

69. Mader JT, Cantrell JS, Calhoun J: Oral ciprofloxacin compared with standard parenteral antibiotic therapy for chronic osteomyelitis in adults. *J Bone Joint Surg Am* 1990;72(1):104-110.

70. Carek PJ, Dickerson LM, Sack JL: Diagnosis and management of osteomyelitis. *Am Fam Physician* 2001;63(12):2413-2420.

71. Barrack RL: Economics of revision total hip arthroplasty. *Clin Orthop Relat Res* 1995;319:209-214.

72. Bozic KJ, Ries MD: The impact of infection after total hip arthroplasty on hospital and surgeon resource utilization. *J Bone Joint Surg Am* 2005;87(8):1746-1751.

73. Kurtz S, Mowat F, Ong K, Chan N, Lau E, Halpern M: Prevalence of primary and revision total hip and knee arthroplasty in the United States from 1990 through 2002. *J Bone Joint Surg Am* 2005;87(7):1487-1497.

74. Bauer TW, Parvizi J, Kobayashi N, Krebs V: Diagnosis of periprosthetic infection. *J Bone Joint Surg Am* 2006;88(4):869-882.

75. Zimmerli W: Infection and musculoskeletal conditions: Prosthetic-joint-associated infections. *Best Pract Res Clin Rheumatol* 2006;20(6):1045-1063.

76. Trampuz A, Hanssen AD, Osmon DR, Mandrekar J, Steckelberg JM, Patel R: Synovial fluid leukocyte count and differential for the diagnosis of prosthetic knee infection. *Am J Med* 2004;117(8):556-562.

77. Parvizi J, Ghanem E, Menashe S, Barrack RL, Bauer TW: Periprosthetic infection: What are the diagnostic challenges? *J Bone Joint Surg Am* 2006;88(Suppl 4):138-147.

78. Spangehl MJ, Masri BA, O'Connell JX, Duncan CP: Prospective analysis of preoperative and intraoperative investigations for the diagnosis of infection at the sites of two hundred and two revision total hip arthroplasties. *J Bone Joint Surg Am* 1999;81(5):672-683.

79. Berbari E, Mabry T, Tsaras G, et al: Inflammatory blood laboratory levels as markers of prosthetic joint infection: A systematic review and meta-analysis. *J Bone Joint Surg Am* 2010;92(11):2102-2109.

80. Di Cesare PE, Chang E, Preston CF, Liu CJ: Serum interleukin-6 as a marker of periprosthetic infection following total hip and knee arthroplasty. *J Bone Joint Surg Am* 2005;87(9):1921-1927.

81. Levitsky KA, Hozack WJ, Balderston RA, et al: Evaluation of the painful prosthetic joint: Relative value of bone scan, sedimentation rate, and joint aspiration. *J Arthroplasty* 1991;6(3):237-244.

82. Pill SG, Parvizi J, Tang PH, et al: Comparison of fluorodeoxyglucose positron emission tomography and (111)

indium-white blood cell imaging in the diagnosis of periprosthetic infection of the hip. *J Arthroplasty* 2006;21(6, Suppl 2):91-97.

83. Schiesser M, Stumpe KD, Trentz O, Kossmann T, Von Schulthess GK: Detection of metallic implant-associated infections with FDG PET in patients with trauma: Correlation with microbiologic results. *Radiology* 2003;226(2):391-398.

84. Zhuang H, Chacko TK, Hickeson M, et al: Persistent nonspecific FDG uptake on PET imaging following hip arthroplasty. *Eur J Nucl Med Mol Imaging* 2002;29(10):1328-1333.

85. Fulkerson E, Valle CJ, Wise B, Walsh M, Preston C, Di Cesare PE: Antibiotic susceptibility of bacteria infecting total joint arthroplasty sites. *J Bone Joint Surg Am* 2006;88(6):1231-1237.

86. Frommelt L: Principles of systemic antimicrobial therapy in foreign material associated infection in bone tissue, with special focus on periprosthetic infection. *Injury* 2006;37(Suppl 2):S87-S94.

87. Tsukayama DT, Estrada R, Gustilo RB: Infection after total hip arthroplasty: A study of the treatment of one hundred and six infections. *J Bone Joint Surg Am* 1996;78(4):512-523.

88. Crockarell JR, Hanssen AD, Osmon DR, Morrey BF: Treatment of infection with débridement and retention of the components following hip arthroplasty. *J Bone Joint Surg Am* 1998;80(9):1306-1313.

89. Toms AD, Davidson D, Masri BA, Duncan CP: The management of peri-prosthetic infection in total joint arthroplasty. *J Bone Joint Surg Br* 2006;88(2):149-155.

90. Callaghan JJ, Katz RP, Johnston RC: One-stage revision surgery of the infected hip: A minimum 10-year followup study. *Clin Orthop Relat Res* 1999;369:139-143.

91. Durbhakula SM, Czajka J, Fuchs MD, Uhl RL: Antibiotic-loaded articulating cement spacer in the 2-stage exchange of infected total knee arthroplasty. *J Arthroplasty* 2004;19(6):768-774.

92. Colyer RA, Capello WN: Surgical treatment of the infected hip implant: Two-stage reimplantation with a one-month interval. *Clin Orthop Relat Res* 1994;298:75-79.

93. Garvin KL, Fitzgerald RH Jr, Salvati EA, et al: Reconstruction of the infected total hip and knee arthroplasty with gentamicin-impregnated Palacos bone cement. *Instr Course Lect* 1993;42:293-302.

94. Hanssen AD, Rand JA: Evaluation and treatment of infection at the site of a total hip or knee arthroplasty. *Instr Course Lect* 1999;48:111-122.

95. Meek RM, Masri BA, Dunlop D, et al: Patient satisfaction and functional status after treatment of infection at the site of a total knee arthroplasty with use of the PROSTALAC articulating spacer. *J Bone Joint Surg Am* 2003;85(10):1888-1892.

96. Barrack RL: Rush pin technique for temporary antibiotic-impregnated cement prosthesis for infected total hip arthroplasty. *J Arthroplasty* 2002;17(5):600-603.

97. Park SJ, Song EK, Seon JK, Yoon TR, Park GH: Comparison of static and mobile antibiotic-impregnated cement spacers for the treatment of infected total knee arthroplasty. *Int Orthop* 2010;34(8):1181-1186.

98. Chelsom J, Solberg CO: Vertebral osteomyelitis at a Norwegian university hospital 1987-97: Clinical features, laboratory findings and outcome. *Scand J Infect Dis* 1998;30(2): 147-151.

99. Carragee EJ: Pyogenic vertebral osteomyelitis. *J Bone Joint Surg Am* 1997;79(6):874-880.

100. Struijs PA, Poolman RW, Bhandari M: Infected nonunion of the long bones. *J Orthop Trauma* 2007;21(7):507-511.

101. Jain AK, Sinha S: Infected nonunion of the long bones. *Clin Orthop Relat Res* 2005;431:57-65.

3: Basic Principles and Treatment of Musculoskeletal Disease

Section 4

Clinical Science

Section Editor

Thomas A. Einhorn, MD

Chapter 26

Evidence-Based Medicine: A Practical Guide for Orthopaedic Surgeons

Suneel B. Bhat, MD, MPhil

Mohit Bhandari, MD, MSc

Richard C. Mather III, MD

Samir Mehta, MD

Introduction

Surgery has long been described as an art. For several decades, learning in orthopaedics was limited to apprenticeship, and progress was drawn solely from case studies and individual experience. Anecdotal evidence proves to be a rough measure that only unearths the broadest of changes and benefits — after initial leaps such as joint arthroplasty and open reduction/internal fixation, new methods to shape development in the field were needed.[1] In the 1980s and early 1990s a paradigm shift in medicine emerged that reduced the emphasis on observation and expert opinion and instead focused on systematic clinical research.[2] This new perspective was heralded as "evidence-based medicine" (EBM) and by promising a more objective approach to medical practice, has become increasingly incorporated into both orthopaedic practice and all of medicine.[3-5] Applying EBM to the field of orthopaedics is a multipart process, involving generating clinical research, evaluating the studies,

and incorporating data into clinical decision making. Understanding each of these steps is crucial to successfully using EBM in modern practice. Furthermore, understanding different aspects of EBM such as comparative effectiveness analysis, systematic review, and decision analysis, and their role in the research to operating room/clinic modality will provide surgeons with better tools to improve outcomes. This is not to diminish the value of clinical experience and surgeon intuition, but to facilitate translation of knowledge to practice. By rigorous use of EBM, the orthopaedic surgeon can take his or her craft from being not only an art but also a science.

Defining the Concept of Evidence-Based Orthopaedics

What does EBM actually constitute? EBM is the conscientious and explicit use of current best evidence to guide management and clinical decision making for individual patients, achieved by identifying and appraising the academic literature.[6] This is not to say by using evidence in daily patient management that clinical judgment or patient preferences are precluded; indeed, clinical experience can augment or drive the integration of data into patient care.[7,8] Orthopaedic surgeons have a strong tradition of training and an established literature. However, much of existing surgical practice is based on lower levels of evidence with only a fraction being based on randomized controlled trials, among which the quality is variable.[9-11] Decisions are often appropriately made on the best available evidence, which when adequate quality research is unavailable, may be clinician experience. What EBM brings to the field is a structured approach that most importantly necessitates critical evaluation of the strength of evidence to gauge its role in decision making between the surgeon and the patient.

Dr. Bhandari or an immediate family member serves as a paid consultant for or is an employee of Amgen, Eli Lilly, Stryker, and Smith & Nephew. Dr. Mather or an immediate family member has received research or institutional support from Forest Pharmaceuticals. Dr. Mehta or an immediate family member is a member of a speakers' bureau or has made paid presentations on behalf of Zimmer, Smith & Nephew, and AO North America; serves as a paid consultant for or is an employee of Smith & Nephew and Synthes; has received research or institutional support from Amgen, Medtronic, and Smith & Nephew; and serves as a board member, owner, officer, or committee member of the Pennsylvania Orthopaedic Society. Neither Dr. Bhat nor any immediate family member has received anything of value from or owns stock in a commercial company or institution related directly or indirectly to the subject of this chapter.

Basics of Evidence-Based Medical Practice

Although EBM as a general concept may be applied to orthopaedics variably, following a defined algorithm allows for both case-based consistency and increased efficiency in practice. The Sicily statement outlines five discrete steps to help structure EBM practice and is supported by evidence regarding its own use.[12] When presented with the need for guidance surrounding decisions in clinical practice, this approach allows for identification of a question specific to the patient in concern, a focused search to identify relevant literature, critical evaluation of identified literature, integration of the discovered knowledge into decision making in the clinical situation, and self-evaluation of the process.

Generating a Focused Question

When making a management decision or when clinical uncertainty exists, translating this uncertainty into a defined, answerable question is the first step in an evidence-based approach. A medical question may be roughly characterized as a "who?" (a patient with a given problem) a "what?" (the possible management options for the problem), and a "why?" (the desired clinical outcome). This can be formally remembered with the mnemonic PICO (patient/population/problem, intervention, comparison, outcome),[13] in which

"**P**" describes the patient/population with a problem ("In 70-year-old patients with odontoid fractures")

"**I**" describes the intervention ("would operative management")

"**C**" describes the comparison ("compared with nonsurgical management")

"**O**" describes the outcome ("reduce mortality?").

The focused question serves as the foundation of applying EBM at the patient level. By generating a question that is patient specific, incorporates feasible and accessible intervention options, and addresses the outcomes that are important to both the surgeon and the patient, identifying the best evidence-based management may subsequently be pursued.

Finding and Retrieving the Evidence

Surgical knowledge has traditionally been disseminated through textbooks, direct mentorship, or peer-reviewed journal articles. Although books and personal dissemination indeed have some value, they are also constrained by their common basis in anecdote or opinion. Furthermore, the shelf life of this knowledge is limited, as many textbooks contain clinical information that is out of date by the time the book has gone to press. Current medical journals, however, contain the most up-to-date information from clinical and basic science studies. Using modern information technology and electronic databases, these may be efficiently surveyed to retrieve the best evidence. One database commonly used in the medical field is Medline/PubMed, a project of the National Library of Medicine, which can be accessed using the Internet. Whatever means are used, a thorough and systematic review of the literature to identify relevant studies is a necessary first step for the objective research-driven aspect of EBM.

Critical Appraisal of Evidence

A rigorous critical appraisal of evidence is what truly sets EBM apart from heuristic limited approaches. To help characterize studies, the level of evidence system was developed by the Oxford Centre for Evidence-based Medicine, which ranks study designs for their strength, ranging from randomized controlled studies to expert opinion.[14] Randomized controlled trials represent the strongest type of study, followed in order by cohort studies, case-control studies, case series, and finally expert opinion. In general, systematic reviews in each category are stronger than individual studies. Each study type carries different weight and should have a graded influence when comparing management decisions. Despite level of evidence playing an influential role in manuscript acceptance in orthopaedic journals, understanding of level of evidence classifications by practitioners is not optimal.[15-17] The orthopaedic surgeon must take responsibility to be educated about the implications of these classifications when appraising evidence. Although it cannot be expected of all surgeons to become fully qualified epidemiologists or biostatisticians, it is very important for all medical practitioners to be at least well versed in basic scientific and statistical methodology, which would allow them to discriminatingly read, synthesize, and apply the literature.

Bias

Systematic error inherent in the design of a study that results in deviation from the truth is called bias. All studies have some degree of bias; however, minimizing sources of bias is an important aspect of robust research. Examples of bias include selection bias (unrepresentative study population or dissimilar study groups), determination bias (detection/recall/interviewer bias, for example, imprecise data collection), survivorship bias (patients with lower morbidity have greater associated costs and morbidity), follow-up bias (nonresponder and transfer bias), and, on a broader level, publication bias (selective publication of either positive or negative studies on a subject).

Confounding

A remote variable that is independently associated with both the dependent (effect) and independent (cause) variables and inaccurately amplifies or minimizes the apparent relationship between variables is called confounding. Confounding can be adjusted for statistical significance in data analysis.

Conflict of Interest

A conflict of interest occurs when, from the perspective of an independent observer, an individual's (or his or her family's) financial/social/academic/philosophical goals or interests may influence the individual's professional actions, decisions, judgment, or published work.

Randomized Controlled Trial

Randomized controlled trials (RCTs) are considered the gold standard of research designs for clinical evidence because they provide the most internal validity and are best at reducing the influence of bias and confounding. The basis of an RCT is random allocation of sampled patients to either a treatment or controlled group, which theoretically reduces the sources of bias and confounding found in observational studies. Well-designed RCTs are often blinded so that one or more types of individuals involved in the study – patients, investigators, data collectors, and analysts – do not know if the patient is receiving a given treatment. Well-designed RCTs also use intention-to-treat analysis, where all patients are analyzed within the treatment group to which they were initially randomized, despite any changes in treatment group. Although RCTs have excellent internal validity, they are often limited by expense, logistics, and time involved and may in some cases have reduced generalizability due to constrained patient sampling. In particular for surgical fields such as orthopaedics, RCTs may be unfeasible, fail to capture surgeon-specific differences, pose supraideal conditions, and not reflect patient motivations that are crucial in candidacy for surgery.

Cohort Study

Prospective or retrospective studies that follow a population group or compare study groups over time without randomization are called cohort studies. Cohort studies are considered the next level of study design after RCTs and allow for good controlled comparisons between study groups across time, although their unrandomized nature can result in more sources of bias than RCTs. However, there is a growing perspective that pragmatic comparative trials may more accurately reflect therapeutic realities, and thereby be more generalizable and applicable in EBM than constrained RCTs.

Case-Control Study

In case-control studies, patients of interest are identified (cases) and are matched with a set of normal control patients for comparison. Because there is no means of estimating the population in which cases occur, case-control studies are limited to calculating odds ratios instead of risk ratios, which although appropriate in instances when the outcome is rare in a population are a less intuitive result. Furthermore, case-control studies are inherently more susceptible to more sources of bias and confounding than cohort studies or RCTs.

Cross-sectional Study

Point-in-time cross-population analyses are called cross-sectional studies. Although these do allow comparison of cases and normal patients, they generally are more useful to characterize epidemiologic parameters such as the preva-

Table 1

Standard Two-Way Table Construct

	Event	No Event	
Treatment/ intervention	a	b	a+b
Control	c	d	c+d
	a+c	b+d	

lence of a condition. Although uniquely useful for baseline information, these studies are limited by their inability to provide longitudinal data.

Case Series

Descriptive studies without a control group that present a series of cases are useful for hypothesis generation but have limited applicability for making comparisons or hypothesis testing. Case series serve as a starting point to identify future research topics that subsequently provide information for evidence-based decision making.

Case Report

Case reports are descriptive presentations of single cases. Although they may make interesting reading material, they are inappropriate for utilization in evidence-based approaches because of their limited internal and external validity.

Two-Way Table

The two-way table is the fundamental way of representing binary outcomes and serves as the basis for many statistical analyses. Constructing a two-way table is often the first step in either analyzing data primarily for study analysis, or when evaluating and understanding a study already published in the literature (**Table 1**).

Risk Ratio

The risk of an event is simply the probability of the event occurring. The risk ratio, or relative risk, is the ratio of the risk of an event between two groups. This is calculated by dividing the risk of the exposed group by the risk of the unexposed group, and is expressed as

$$\frac{a/(a+b)}{c/(c+d)}$$

Risk ratios are often the preferred means of expressing relative likelihoods because they are stable across event probabilities and are more intuitive than odds ratios for clinical applications.

4: Clinical Science

Table 2

Sensitivity Analysis

	Test Positive	Test Negative	
Exposed	True Positive (TP)	False Negative (FN)	TP+FN
Unexposed	False Positive (FP)	True Negative (TN)	FP+TN
	TP+FP	FN+TN	

Odds Ratio

The odds of an event is the ratio between the number of events and the number of nonevents, which more formally is the risk of having an event divided by the risk of not having an event. The odds ratio is an expression of the likelihood of an event between groups, or the odds of an event in the treatment group relative to the odds of an event in the control group. This is calculated by the function

$$\frac{(a/b)}{(c/d)}$$

or, more simply,

$$\frac{(a \times d)}{(b \times c)}$$

Odds ratios are the only likelihood measure possible for case-control studies, but in other study designs they have the added benefit of allowing for adjustment for other variables in regression analysis. However, odds ratios become distorted as event probability increases, and are not as intuitive for clinical application as relative risk ratios.

Absolute Risk Reduction

Although ratios are useful for expressing likelihood factor differences, often an absolute difference in risks between two management approaches provides a straightforward, useful reference for clinical decision making. The absolute risk reduction, or risk difference, is expressed as

$$\frac{a}{(a+b)} - \frac{c}{(c+d)} \times 100\%$$

Number Needed to Treat

Another measure that is easy to conceptualize and directly applicable to clinical practice is the number of patients needed to treat to avoid a single event. The number needed to treat is the inverse of the risk difference, and is expressed as

$$\frac{1}{\dfrac{a}{(a+b)} - \dfrac{c}{(c+d)}}$$

Expressing outcomes as the number needed to treat is valuable for broader policy decision, individual clinical decisions, and patient communication.

Sensitivity

For a given clinical test, the ability of the test to accurately capture positive cases, or the proportion of true-positive cases that actually test positive, is called the sensitivity. A simple two-way table can be constructed to characterize all test possibilities (**Table 2**). Sensitivity is expressed as

$$\frac{TP}{(TP+FN)}$$

Specificity

For a given clinical test, the ability of the test to accurately capture negative cases, or the proportion of true-negative cases that actually test negative, is called the specificity. Using the two-way table above, sensitivity can be expressed as

$$\frac{TN}{(TN+FP)}$$

Positive Predictive Value

The proportion of patients with positive test results who are actually accurately diagnosed is the positive predictive value or precision rate. This is expressed by the ratio of true positives to test positives, or

$$\frac{TP}{(TP+FP)}$$

Negative Predictive Value

The proportion of patients with negative test results who are actually accurately diagnosed is the negative predictive value. This is expressed by the ratio of true negatives to test negatives, or

$$\frac{TN}{(TN+FN)}$$

Table 3

Checklist of Study Questions Regarding Methods and Results

Population	Is the study population representative of my patients? How homogenous is the study population?
Cohorts (in non-RCTs)	Are patient groups similar or significantly different?
Randomization (in RCTs)	Was randomization sufficient? Are patient groups similar or significantly different? Was there intention-to-treat analysis? What were the impacts of randomization on generalizability?
Bias	Is there evident bias?
Confounding	Are there evident confounding factors?
Intervention/Treatment	Is the intervention studied relevant to my question? Was the treatment adequately performed?
Blinding	Was the treatment blinded? Was the data analysis blinded?
Follow-up	Was there adequate length of follow-up? How many patients were lost to follow-up? How were patients lost to follow-up analyzed?
Outcome Measures	Are outcome measures relevant to my question? Are outcome measures biased between study groups? Were costs assessed?
Analysis	Was the statistical analysis appropriate for the data? Was statistical analysis adequately performed?
Results	How large was the effect size? How significant was the effect? How precise were the outcomes?
Implications/Practice	Are the results applicable to my question and patient? Are treatment benefits worth possible harm and costs in the context of my patient? Are treatment options feasible?

Type I Error

In hypothesis testing, a type I error, or α error, occurs when a significant association is found when there is no true association, and results in the inappropriate rejection of a true null hypothesis.

Type II Error

In hypothesis testing, a type II error, or β error, occurs when no association is found in the presence of a true significant association, and results in the inappropriate failure to reject a false null hypothesis.

Power

The probability of finding a significant association in a study if one truly exists is influenced by the probability of type II error and is called power, which is represented by $1-p(\beta)$. Acceptable power of a study is conventionally set at 80%, or a 20% probability of incorrectly failing to reject the null hypothesis. When a study does not demonstrate a significant association, it may be that the study is underpowered (not large enough a sample size), or outcome measurements are too imprecise to uncover differences.

P values

The P value represents the strength of evidence provided by data relative to the null hypothesis. This value is compared against a preset acceptable threshold for type I error (α), which often is set to 0.05 or 0.01. If the P value is less than α of 0.05, this suggests that there is less than a 5% probability that a true null hypothesis is being rejected. P values are flawed in that they represent a fixed threshold, and the actual relative strength of association is unclear. Confidence intervals (CIs) are a more precise and appropriate means of presenting significance than P values when possible.

Confidence Intervals

CIs constructed around a value also represent the strength of an association. A 95% CI suggests that given multiple samples, 95% of the time the outcome value will fall within the CI. When the CI of one outcome includes the value for the other outcome, the result is not significant and the null hypothesis cannot be rejected. The smaller the CI, the greater the confidence around an outcome estimate; looking at CIs and outcome values, the analyst or reader can evaluate the strength of the outcomes.

Causality

A set of minimal conditions necessary to provide evidence that a correlation is driven by a causal relationship is characterized by the nine Bradford-Hill criteria: statistical strength of association; consistency; specificity; temporality; dose dependency; plausibility; coherence; reversibility; and analogy. Although each criterion need not be necessarily met in every situation to suggest causality, the more criteria met the stronger the suggestion of causality.

Clinical Significance

Clinical significance exists when the difference between two approaches is appreciable to either the patient or the surgeon. Although a result may be statistically significant, the practical clinical implications of a numeric difference maybe unappreciable.

Not all data sources are created equal, and the onus of critical and rigorous appraisal of each study falls on the orthopaedic surgeon. With an understanding of basic statistics and research design, surgeons may themselves critically evaluate studies regarding quality and applicability. There are several questions about the methods and results of each study that are important to consider when weighing their relative value (Table 3).

After critically appraising the systematically identified relevant studies, the surgeon can weigh the relative strengths and weakness of the studies and their applicability toward the focused question.

Evidence-Based Clinical Decision Making

Once evidence has been collected, reviewed, analyzed, and adjusted to the clinical question at hand, a clinical decision can be made. Although patient preferences, intangible factors, and situational factors may play a role in influencing, the decision can be made with the knowledge that it is consistent with the best current practice and knowledge.

Performance Evaluation

Simply changing practice based on evidence is not sufficient. Effort must be made to audit and follow up on the effects of the change. Evidence-based medicine is a dynamic process, and as clinical decisions are made based on evidence, this should lead to the generation of more data that help further define best practice. The onus of critical evaluation of practices falls both on the orthopaedic surgeon developing the knowledge and recommendations, as well as the orthopaedic surgeon implementing changes in their own practice. By fostering and pursuing an ongoing cycle of data generation, analysis, implementation, evaluation, and new data generation, the field of orthopaedics can progress toward continually better care for patients.

Defining the Concept of Comparative Effectiveness

Over the past 3 to 4 years, the term "comparative effectiveness" has become increasingly important in the worlds of both clinical science and policy, heralded by a tremendous presence of opinions in the media, increasing legislative interest, and the significant investment of $1.1 billion by the US government.[18-22] Despite the attention, confusion remains as to what comparative effectiveness research actually entails and there is controversy regarding its implications and effect on health care.[23] The concept of comparative effectiveness research has been around for some time, and it falls within the overall umbrella of evidence-based medicine.[24] It represents a paradigm shift from a comparative study analyzing a treatment group compared with a control group to a comparative study analyzing differences in treatment groups against each other. By doing this, indirect comparisons of management options against placebo are unnecessary, and instead direct comparisons can be made against other potential treatment options, and thereby facilitate clinical decision making.

Efficacy Versus Effectiveness

The basis of what separates comparative effectiveness research from other approaches used in EBM is the focus of the study. Traditionally, clinical research has aimed to identify efficacy, which is a relationship between a treatment or management option and an outcome in a highly structured, population-regulated, and patient-homogenous setting, compared with a placebo control. This is an excellent way of showing whether a treatment biologically "works" in a specific patient population. However, trials of efficacy do not provide much insight into the performance of a treatment in the general population, or effectiveness. Comparative effectiveness research aims to evaluate the effectiveness of a treatment in a broader, more generalizable population, against other treatment options, not against a placebo control. By doing this, comparative effectiveness produces results that are directly clinically applicable, and can more easily be used for clinical decision making at the patient and population levels.

Bayesian Statistics

Comparative effectiveness analysis is particularly amenable to both Bayesian study design and Bayesian statistics.[25,26] Bayesian statistical inference relies on preexisting information to shape further data sampling or analysis. The traditional frequentist approach (often assuming a gaussian or normal distribution of trials) measures the likelihood of an observed result having occurred by chance, and is framed in terms of repeated sampling and trials; that is, given significance at 95%, if the trial was repeated 100 times, the null hypothesis would fail to be rejected only 5 times or less. The multiple sampling basis of frequentist statistics is not intuitive, and a significance of 95% is often misunderstood as a 95% probability that the conclusion is true as opposed to a 95% probability that the conclusion is not due to chance. Bayesian inference is what aims to achieve the likelihood of a true hypothesis, as opposed to rejection of a null hypothesis not due to chance. Bayesian approaches use dynamic sampling and hypothesis, where the probability of outcomes can change as data are collected, as can the hypothesis. Furthermore, by establishing multiple prior hypotheses, as data collection progresses and dynamically adapts, one may quickly be favored. As comparative effectiveness analysis is inherently comparing possible management approaches in diverse, more generalizable populations with the aim of identifying clinical truth, Bayesian statistical approaches can help generate useful data for evidence-based decision making where traditional statistics may be underpowered or too inflexible to be useful.

Cost-Benefit Analysis

With the introduction of comparative effectiveness analysis into the public and political domain in part as a means to help increase the efficiency of expenditures in health care – although legislation does not specify costs – there has been criticism that comparative effectiveness will lead to rationing, should not include cost-benefit analysis, and should not be used for health policy decisions.[18,21,27,28] This is absolutely inappropriate. Cost-effectiveness analysis, the use of cost outcomes in comparative effective analysis, although not a replacement for clinical outcomes, is an important adjunct for decision making. Although it may be unethical to purely make decisions based on cost, it is similarly unethical to ignore costs in the context of unclear clinical benefits. In particular, because it is unclear that increased intervention and increased health care expenditure actually lead to improved health outcomes, failing to include costs in the evidence base for decision making is a disservice to patients, payers, and society at large.[29] In cases of clinical equivalence between management approaches, cost can be an important deciding factor. Furthermore, comparative effectiveness can identify redundant, ineffective, and harmful medical practice, whose elimination could potentially reduce costs. Ignoring or failing to include cost as an outcome measure thereby precludes the full implications of studies and thereby limits or slows their utilization in clinical decision making.[27,28,30,31] It is important to further recognize that costs are not necessarily simply charges or reimbursement – they include distribution of economic and incentive burdens across parties involved in health care and can be multidimensional on both the supply and demand aspects of medicine. In light of the rapidly evolving and resource-reliant nature of the field, orthopaedic surgeons need to take a mature and progressive approach by incorporating costs into comparative effectiveness analysis and evidence-based decision making, and work toward not only improving the clinical outcomes and management of their patients, but simultaneously improving the efficiency and societal utility of the field.

Systematic Reviews, Meta-analysis, and Consolidating the Evidence

The Need for Systematic Reviews

One of the difficulties of EBM is that for appropriate decision making, reliable, current information is needed, and sometimes there is just too much information. With modern research and communication the turnover of research can be quite rapid, and it can be difficult for the orthopae-

dic surgeon to keep up with current information. In such circumstances, reviews are important adjunctive tools for the retrieval and appraisal steps of EBM. Systematic reviews are structured studies with strict defined a priori criteria for collecting and appraising studies – in part like the initial steps of EBM – and eliminate some of the bias that might emerge in other reviews.[32-34] Systematic reviews of a given type of study are generally considered a higher level of evidence than a single study of the same type – that is, a systematic review of RCTs of a given subject is a higher level of evidence than one of the RCTs in that systematic review independently considered.[14]

The Need for Meta-analysis

Although some systematic reviews simply present and appraise the existing evidence on a topic in a structured way, some systematic reviews also include a meta-analysis. Meta-analyses extract the data from individual studies, express the data in terms of an adjusted point estimate with CIs, and generate a pooled, weighted average across the studies. Analyses that include a broader range of studies and have gradient rating rather than simple dichotomous weighting likely more accurately capture reality. This essentially is a step forward in evidence-based decision making, takes the information derived from a systematic review, and instead of having the orthopaedic surgeon shoulder the burden of appraising individual studies, conglomerates results using set criteria. Both systematic reviews and meta-analysis facilitate the practice of EBM and are important steps to make EBM more accessible and feasible for the orthopaedic surgeon.

Decision Analysis and the Evolution of Evidence-Based Approaches

Introduction to Decision Analysis

The underlying goal of EBM is the ultimate appropriate clinical decision. Decision analysis studies attempt to supplement and facilitate decision making by applying explicit quantitative measures to analyze potential management options when uncertainty exists. These represent the actual step of evidence-based decision making in EBM, and essentially provide a preanalyzed decision set for the orthopaedic surgeon and help augment and formulate the actual clinical decision-making process, a step beyond descriptive collection and appraisal of data. Initially introduced as an aspect of game theory, decision analysis is heavily used in economics, management, and operations research, but is increasingly being applied to medicine to simultaneously weigh risks, benefits, and costs in the context of decision making at the level of both the population and the patient.[35-39] Understanding and using decision analysis is an important step toward actively and efficiently incorporating EBM into practice.

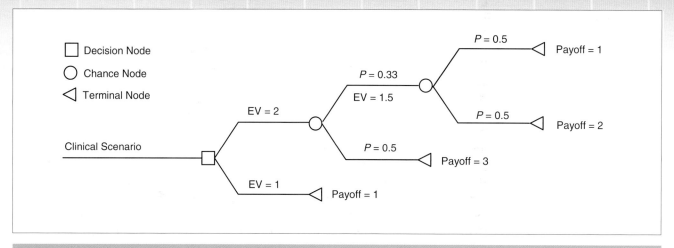

Figure 1 Theoretical rollback analysis EV = expected value. (Reproduced with permission from Phillips B, Ball C, Saukett D, et al: Oxford Center for Evidence Based Medicine Levels of Evidence. March 2009. http://cebm.net/index.aspx?o=1025.)

The Decision Model: Probabilities and Utilities

The foundation of a decision analysises[40-42] is the conceptual decision model with its graphic counterpart, the decision tree. Conceptually the decision model mirrors the EBM process, by framing a clinical question with possible management options, deriving evidence-based probabilities for events, and comparing subsequent outcomes of different management approaches. At the root of the decision tree is a decision node, which represents the choices for the orthopaedic surgeon, usually denoted by a square. Each emanating branch is a decision pathway, and is defined by a series of mutually exclusive and exhaustive probability nodes and branches, which represent downstream outcomes of a decision. Probability nodes are usually denoted by a circle. Every decision pathway has a terminal point, which is a final outcome associated with a "payoff," and is called the terminal node, usually represented by a triangle.

Probabilities may be derived from several sources, including data collection directly from patients, or from the literature. Every estimate has some degree of uncertainty, which should be reflected in the model, preferably incorporated at each probability node. As with the critical appraisal of any evidence, both the type and number of sources behind an estimate affect its uncertainty. Estimates from higher level evidence sources and multiple sources can be derived with higher certainty, and contribute to the validity of the model.

Outcome payoffs can take the form of any measure, including but not limited to dollars, deaths, complications, outcome scores, and relative measures such as quality-adjusted life-years or disability-adjusted life-years. Estimates for outcomes by definition will also have some degree of uncertainty, which should be reflected in the model. Selected outcomes should be expressed as simply as possible, allowing the flexible application to clinical decision making in practice, that is, direct costs, events, and mortality are preferable to the more abstract relative measures.

Deterministic Analysis

The most basic analysis used in decision modeling is a deterministic approach,[43] such as rollback analysis (**Figure 1**). In practice, rollback analysis takes place on the decision tree from terminal nodes across each probability node toward the decision node. At each step, the expected value (EV) of the branch is calculated by combining payoffs and probabilities. At the decision node, the total EVs of each of the pathways representing a management decision are compared, and the optimal approach identified.

$$\text{Decision node} \rightarrow \text{terminal node} - EV = \text{Payoff}$$

$$\text{Chance node} \rightarrow \text{terminal node} - EV$$

$$= \text{Payoff} \times \text{Probability}$$

$$\text{Chance node} \rightarrow \text{chance node} - EV$$

$$= [EV_{branch1} + EV_{branch2} + EV_{branchN}]$$

$$\text{Terminal node} \rightarrow \text{chance node} - EV_{decision}$$

$$= [EV_{branch1} + EV_{branch2} + EV_{branchN}]$$

Stochastic Simulation Analysis

A more elegant method than rollback analysis to analyze decision models that incorporate probability and outcome uncertainties are stochastic approaches[43] that introduce randomness into the model, such as Monte Carlo simulation (**Figure 2**). Monte Carlo methods use repeated sampling of probabilities with random numbers to generate outcomes, and are applied to a decision tree with repeated, independent trials, directly representing frequentist or Bayesian hypothesis testing. With each trial, only a single outcome is reached through the decision model, and trials are repeated, usually thousands of times, mimicking a large cohort of individual patients. A Monte Carlo simulation produces outcomes of a series of discrete, independent trials, which has particular benefit to evidence-based decision making. If

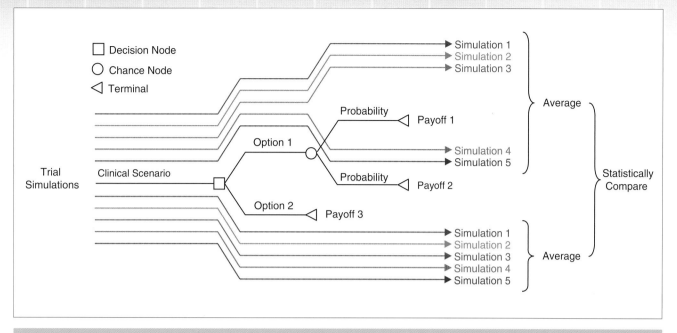

Figure 2 Theoretical Monte Carlo simulation. (Reproduced with permission from Phillips B, Ball C, Saukett D, et al: Oxford Center for Evidence Based Medicine Levels of Evidence. March 2009. http://cebm.net/index.aspx?o=1025.)

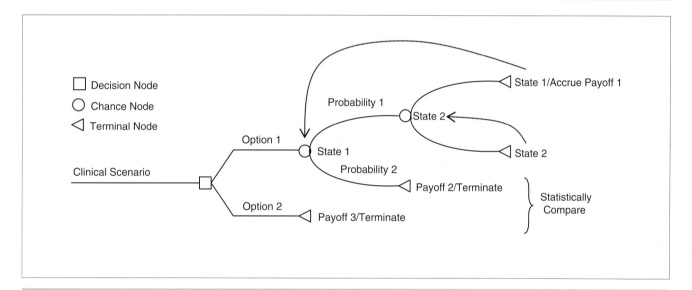

Figure 3 Theoretical Markov chain decision tree. (Reproduced with permission from Phillips B, Ball C, Saukett D, et al: Oxford Center for Evidence Based Medicine Levels of Evidence. March 2009. http://cebm.net/index.aspx?o=1025.)

probability estimates are demographically specific, the analysis can be made directly representative of the population modeled. This increases the generalizability of the study, and specific decision management approaches may be identified for very specific patient populations, enhancing the effect on practical decision making.

Markov Chain Analysis

A Markov chain Monte Carlo analysis[44] allows for analysis of a decision model in which multiple health states exist, where future states only depend on the current state and

probabilities in different health states can vary (**Figure 3**). Markov chain decision trees differ from other decision trees in three major ways. (1) Progress is not unidirectional; recursive movements from a probability node to a previous probability node are allowed. (2) At set intervals, an independent trial may transition health states where probabilities at even a previously encountered probability node may be different. (3) Payoffs and utilities are not exclusively calculated at terminal nodes, and may accrue over the duration of the simulation; outcomes and payoffs may be encountered multiple times within the same trial.

One of the benefits of Markov chain Monte Carlo simulations is that theoretical patients may be aged over time, accruing different risks and outcomes based on their age category over time. However, Markov chain models are significantly more complicated than non–Markov chain Monte Carlo simulations, which can often adequately model decision options if age categories are incorporated without state transitions.

Point-of-Care Active Decision Analysis

As orthopaedic surgeons become increasingly better versed in the literature and statistical methods, and the mechanisms for decision analysis become more user-friendly and accessible, we would like to introduce point-of-care active decision analysis (PADA) in the evolution of EBM. When faced with a difficult clinical decision, after applying the principals of EBM by formulating a specific question and finding and critically appraising the current best data, the progressive orthopaedic surgeon can generate an ad hoc decision model specifically tailored for the patient and clinical situation at hand and use quantitative methods to come to a decision. Instead of attempting to understand and apply all the data discovered in an unstructured manner, by using PADA, outcomes, risks, benefits, and costs can be simultaneously synthesized. This allows the orthopaedic surgeon to present the patient with the probabilities of combined outcomes specific to their situation, and make the most informed decision possible for that precise clinical scenario. PADA may represent the next step in optimizing EBM. With PADA, all aspects of evidence-based decision making become structured, from the initial formulation of the clinical question, to data retrieval and critical appraisal, and finally actual decision making and follow-up.

Summary

As there is increasing demand from patients, payers, and the health care industry for increased quality and efficiency of care, evidence-based decision making will become an important tool for orthopaedic surgeons. This is not a futile exercise, as strong clinical evidence is known to change the practice and clinical behavior of orthopaedic surgeons.[45] The responsibility for generating a valid clinical evidence base with research to promote decision making falls on the field of orthopaedics as a whole; using this evidence base in the care of patients is the responsibility of individual practitioners. Although generating high-quality evidence can be challenging, the principles of EBM outlined in this chapter are not particularly difficult, and are readily applied by all physicians and surgeons. By using rigorous evidence-based decision making in everyday practice and actively evolving this concept, orthopaedic surgeons will be able to help maximize the outcomes for their patients, as well as optimize the efficiency of their care.

References

1. Hayashi AC: A case for evidence-based orthopaedic clinical research. *J Orthop Res* 2011;29(6):I-III.

2. Hoppe DJ, Bhandari M: Evidence-based orthopaedics: A brief history. *Indian J Orthop* 2008;42(2):104-110.

3. Evidence-Based Medicine Working Group: Evidence-based medicine: A new approach to teaching the practice of medicine. *JAMA* 1992;268(17):2420-2425.

4. Sackett DL, Rosenberg WM: On the need for evidence-based medicine. *Health Econ* 1995;4(4):249-254.

5. Sackett DL, Rosenberg WM: The need for evidence-based medicine. *J R Soc Med* 1995;88(11):620-624.

6. Sackett DL, Rosenberg WM, Gray JA, Haynes RB, Richardson WS: Evidence based medicine: What it is and what it isn't. *BMJ* 1996;312(7023):71-72.

7. Stuebe AM: Level IV evidence: Adverse anecdote and clinical practice. *N Engl J Med* 2011;365(1):8-9.

8. Karthikeyan G, Pais P: Clinical judgement & evidence-based medicine: Time for reconciliation. *Indian J Med Res* 2010; 132(5):623-626.

9. Jones RS, Richards K: Office of evidence-based surgery charts course for improved systems of care. *Bull Am Coll Surg* 2003;88(3):11-21.

10. Panesar SS, Thakrar R, Athanasiou T, Sheikh A: Comparison of reports of randomized controlled trials and systematic reviews in surgical journals: Literature review. *J R Soc Med* 2006;99(9):470-472.

11. Chan S, Bhandari M: The quality of reporting of orthopaedic randomized trials with use of a checklist for nonpharmacological therapies. *J Bone Joint Surg Am* 2007;89(9):1970-1978.

12. Dawes M, Summerskill W, Glasziou P, et al: Sicily statement on evidence-based practice. *BMC Med Educ* 2005;5(1):1.

13. Poolman RW, Kerkhoffs GM, Struijs PA, Bhandari M; International Evidence-Based Orthopedic Surgery Working Group: Don't be misled by the orthopedic literature: Tips for critical appraisal. *Acta Orthop* 2007;78(2):162-171.

14. Phillps B, Chris B, Sackett D, et al: Oxford Centre for Evidence-based Medicine: Levels of Evidence (March 2009). http://www.cebm.net/index.aspx?o=1025. Accessed August 1, 2011.

15. Wolf JM, Athwal GS, Hoang BH, Mehta S, Williams AE, Owens BD: Knowledge of levels of evidence criteria in orthopedic residents. *Orthopedics* 2009;32(7):494.

16. Obremskey WT, Pappas N, Attallah-Wasif E, Tornetta P III, Bhandari M: Level of evidence in orthopaedic journals. *J Bone Joint Surg Am* 2005;87(12):2632-2638.

17. Kumar M, Gopalakrishna C, Swaminath PV, Mysore SS: Evidence-based surgery: Evidence from survey and citation analysis in orthopaedic surgery. *Ann R Coll Surg Engl* 2010; 93(2):133-138.

18. H.R. 1 - 111th Congress. *American Recovery and Reinvestment Act of 2009.*

19. H.R. 3163 - 110th Congress. *Enhanced Health Care Value For All Act of 2007.*

20. Steinbrook R: Health care and the American Recovery and Reinvestment Act. *N Engl J Med* 2009;360(11):1057-1060.

21. S. 3048 - 110th Congress. *Comparative Effectiveness Research Act of 2008.*

22. Sipkoff M: Comparative effectiveness: An idea whose time has finally come. *Manag Care* 2009;18(4):14-16, 19-21.

23. Saha S, Coffman DD, Smits AK: Giving teeth to comparative-effectiveness research: The Oregon experience. *N Engl J Med* 2010;362(7):e18.

24. Comparative effectiveness: Its origin, evolution, and influence on health care. *J Oncol Prac* 2009;5(2):80-82.

25. Gurrin LC, Kurinczuk JJ, Burton PR: Bayesian statistics in medical research: An intuitive alternative to conventional data analysis. *J Eval Clin Pract* 2000;6(2):193-204.

26. Bowalekar S: Adaptive designs in clinical trials. *Perspect Clin Res* 2011;2(1):23-27.

27. Weinstein MC, Skinner JA: Comparative effectiveness and health care spending: Implications for reform. *N Engl J Med* 2010;362(5):460-465.

28. Martin DF, Maguire MG, Fine SL: Identifying and eliminating the roadblocks to comparative-effectiveness research. *N Engl J Med* 2010;363(2):105-107.

29. Fisher ES, Wennberg DE, Stukel TA, Gottlieb DJ, Lucas FL, Pinder EL: The implications of regional variations in Medicare spending: Part 2. Health outcomes and satisfaction with care. *Ann Intern Med* 2003;138(4):288-298.

30. Elshaug AG, Garber AM: How CER could pay for itself: Insights from vertebral fracture treatments. *N Engl J Med* 2011;364(15):1390-1393.

31. Carroll J: Payers step in with 'real-world' comparative effectiveness research. *Manag Care* 2011;20(6):23-26.

32. Higgins JPT, Green S, eds: *Cochrane Handbook for Systematic Reviews of Interventions: Version 5.1.0 [updated March 2011].* London, England, The Cochrane Collaboration, 2011. http://www.cochrane-handbook.org.

33. Mulrow CD: Rationale for systematic reviews. *BMJ* 1994;309(6954):597-599.

34. Furlan AD, Pennick V, Bombardier C, van Tulder M; Editorial Board, Cochrane Back Review Group: 2009 updated method guidelines for systematic reviews in the Cochrane Back Review Group. *Spine (Phila Pa 1976)* 2009;34(18):1929-1941.

35. Birkmeyer JD, Welch HG: A reader's guide to surgical decision analysis. *J Am Coll Surg* 1997;184(6):589-595.

36. Lilford RJ, Thornton JD: Decision logic in medical practice. *J R Coll Physicians Lond* 1992;26(4):400-412.

37. Thornton JG, Lilford RJ, Johnson N: Decision analysis in medicine. *BMJ* 1992;304(6834):1099-1103.

38. Lilford RJ, Pauker SG, Braunholtz DA, Chard J: Decision analysis and the implementation of research findings. *BMJ* 1998;317(7155):405-409.

39. Kocher MS, Zurakowski D: Clinical epidemiology and biostatistics: A primer for orthopaedic surgeons. *J Bone Joint Surg Am* 2004;86(3):607-620.

40. Detsky AS, Naglie G, Krahn MD, Naimark D, Redelmeier DA: Primer on medical decision analysis: Part 1. Getting started. *Med Decis Making* 1997;17(2):123-125.

41. Detsky AS, Naglie G, Krahn MD, Redelmeier DA, Naimark D: Primer on medical decision analysis: Part 2. Building a tree. *Med Decis Making* 1997;17(2):126-135.

42. Naglie G, Krahn MD, Naimark D, Redelmeier DA, Detsky AS: Primer on medical decision analysis: Part 3. Estimating probabilities and utilities. *Med Decis Making* 1997;17(2):136-141.

43. Krahn MD, Naglie G, Naimark D, Redelmeier DA, Detsky AS: Primer on medical decision analysis: Part 4. Analyzing the model and interpreting the results. *Med Decis Making* 1997;17(2):142-151.

44. Naimark D, Krahn MD, Naglie G, Redelmeier DA, Detsky AS: Primer on medical decision analysis: Part 5. Working with Markov processes. *Med Decis Making* 1997;17(2):152-159.

45. Dijkman BG, Kooistra BW, Pemberton J, Sprague S, Hanson BP, Bhandari M: Can orthopedic trials change practice? *Acta Orthop* 2010;81(1):122-125.

Chapter 27

The Design of Clinical Investigations: Randomized, Cohort, and Case Studies

Charles L. Cox, MD, MPH
Kurt P. Spindler, MD

Introduction

Every aspect of the patient care process must be evaluated with a questioning mind in this era of cost minimization and rapid technologic advances. Basic science and clinical research investigators as well as practicing clinicians must find time to read and critically evaluate published literature on subjects ranging from diagnostic testing to medication use, surgical procedures, and cost-effectiveness. The best available evidence must be analyzed, and a decision-making process must be followed before clinical practice is changed.

In the past, medical training resembled an apprenticeship in which a mentor imparted knowledge based on personal experience or expert opinion (level V evidence). Published studies were lacking or unavailable for review. The Internet has made an abundance of information available, and the clinician now has the burden of critically evaluating the literature and making clinical decisions as to the validity of relevant findings. Research design and implementation serve as the foundation of scientific advancement.

Evidence-based medicine has been described as the "conscientious, explicit, and judicious use of the best evidence in making decisions about the care of individual patients."[1] Many orthopaedic journals promote the use of an evidence-based medicine pyramid for determining the overall quality of a research publication[2] (Table 1). In this method, authors and reviewers analyze a study manuscript based on factors including its design, implementation, sources of bias, and statistical analysis, and they assign a level-of-evidence rating from I to V (levels I and V representing the apex and base of

the pyramid, respectively). The level of evidence allows a reader to categorize the study for the purpose of evaluating its scientific validity and possibly incorporating the findings into clinical practice.

General Principles

Three questions must be answered before a clinical practice can be changed. The first of these questions asks whether scientific truth has been established. In other words, what is the quality of the evidence supporting the treatment in question? Do the findings of any relevant studies endure after scrutiny of the reported scientific methods? This question applies both to new findings and traditional methods of clinical care. Study results usually are presented after careful statistical analysis; the findings may be determined to be statistically significant or insignificant, as shown by a P value or confidence interval comparing the strength of the findings to the likelihood of a relationship by chance alone.

The second question asks whether the findings of the study represent a clinically relevant difference. A well-performed study may reveal a statistical difference in outcomes, but it must be decided whether this difference is actually important to patients and physicians. If the study's sample size is large enough, even a small absolute difference in outcome scores can be statistically significant. Many validated patient-reported outcome scales specify the minimal change representing a relevant difference in average scores among treatment groups. As a result, patients can detect a change that is beneficial, which may justify a change in practice.

The third question asks whether implementing the change in practice is worth the cost to society. For example, an expensive new treatment might allow professional athletes to recover from a specific injury 2 to 4 days earlier than the traditional treatment and also could be used for the gen-

Dr. Cox or an immediate family member serves as a paid consultant to or is an employee of Smith & Nephew. Dr. Spindler serves as a board member, owner, officer, or committee member of the American Orthopaedic Society for Sports Medicine.

4: Clinical Science

Table 1
Levels of Evidence for the Primary Research Question

Level of Evidence[a]	Type of Study	
	Therapeutic (Investigating the Results of Treatment)	**Prognostic (Investigating the Effect of a Patient Characteristic on Disease Outcome)**
I	High-quality randomized controlled study with statistically significant difference or no statistically significant difference but narrow confidence intervals	High-quality prospective study[d] with all patients enrolled at the same point in the disease and at least 80% follow-up of enrolled patients
	Systematic review[b] of level I randomized controlled studies with homogeneous results[c]	Systematic review[b] of level I studies
II	Lower-quality randomized controlled study (for example, less than 80% follow-up, no blinding, improper randomization)	Retrospective[f] study
	Prospective[d] comparative[e] study	Untreated control subjects from a randomized controlled study
	Systematic review[b] of level II studies or level I studies with inconsistent results	Lower-quality prospective study (for example, enrollment at different points in the disease, less than 80% follow-up)
		Systematic review[b] of level II studies
III	Case-control study[g]	Case-control study[g]
	Retrospective[f] comparative[e] study	
	Systematic review[b] of level III studies	
IV	Case series[h]	Case series[h]
V	Expert opinion	Expert opinion

[a] A complete assessment of the quality of individual studies requires critical appraisal of all aspects of the study design.
[b] A combination of results from two or more earlier studies.
[c] The studies had consistent results.
[d] The study was started before the first patient was enrolled.
[e] A comparison of patients receiving two different treatments (for example, cemented hip arthroplasty and cementless hip arthroplasty) at the same institution.
[f] The study was started after the first patient was enrolled.
[g] A comparison of patients identified on the basis of their outcome (for example, unsuccessful total hip arthroplasty) with those who did not have the outcome (for example, successful total hip arthroplasty).
[h] Patients received one treatment, without a comparison group of patients receiving another treatment.
Adapted with permission from *Journal of Bone and Joint Surgery Am*: Levels of evidence for primary research question, in Instructions for Authors, 2012. http://www.jbjs.org/public/instructionsauthors.aspx#LevelsofEvidence.

eral population, including high school and recreational athletes, if the cost-to-benefit ratio is acceptable.

The Research Question

The research question is the first and arguably the most important aspect of study design because it defines the objective of the project. The research question should be clearly defined before the study begins. The characteristics of a good research question can be evaluated using the criteria represented by the mnemonic FINER (feasible, interesting, novel, ethical, and relevant)[3] (**Table 2**). A good research question should satisfy all of the FINER criteria. It is important to review the existing literature to maximize knowledge about the area of interest; often this is an important first step in applying the FINER criteria when analyzing a proposed research question.

Study Parameters

After the research question is constructed and refined, it is important to define several additional study design parameters, including exposure (a risk factor, diagnostic test, or intervention), outcome, patient population, study design,

Table 1 *(continued)*

Levels of Evidence for the Primary Research Question

Type of Study	
Diagnostic (Investigating a Diagnostic Test)	**Economic and Decision Analysis (Developing an Economic or Decision Model)**
Testing of previously developed diagnostic criteria in consecutive patients, with a universally applied gold standard reference	Sensible costs and alternatives, values obtained from many studies; multiway sensitivity analyses
Systematic review[b] of level I studies	Systematic review[b] of level I studies
Development of diagnostic criteria based on consecutive patients, with a universally applied gold standard reference	Sensible costs and alternatives; values obtained from limited studies; multiway sensitivity analyses
Systematic review[b] of level II studies	Systematic review[b] of level II studies
Study of nonconsecutive patients, without a consistently applied gold standard reference	Analyses based on limited alternatives and costs; poor estimates
Systematic review[b] of level III studies	Systematic review[b] of level III studies
Case-control study	
No sensitivity analyses	
Poor reference standard	
Expert opinion	Expert opinion

and sample size. These parameters establish the foundation for study validity. A good prospective study exposure or outcome should be specifically defined in advance, be available for assessment in all participants, generally represent the end of participation in the study, and be amenable to unbiased measurement.[4] The study population represents a subset of the general population defined in advance by clearly stated inclusion and exclusion criteria that ultimately determine the generalizability of the study's findings to the population at large. If a study population is limited to a small subset of eligible people, it will be difficult to broadly apply any valid findings to clinical practice. The type of study design probably will have been established by this point in the process. The sample size is calculated before the study begins to ensure sufficient statistical power for detecting between-group differences. The levels of significance and power must be defined so the study results can be evaluated by others. In general, a level of significance (an α level) lower than 0.05 is considered acceptable; at this level, the likelihood that the study findings occurred by chance alone is less than 1 in 20. This level of significance serves to decrease the risk of type I error, which is defined as rejection of the null hypothesis although it is true. In other words, a type I error occurs when a researcher erroneously concludes there is a between-group difference. In contrast, a type II error occurs if the null hypothesis is not rejected even though it is false. In other words, a type II error occurs when a researcher erroneously concludes there is no between-group difference. The probability of a type II error is directly related to the power of the study, with power defined as 1 minus the maximum probability of making a type II error. By convention, power is usually considered adequate if it is at least 0.8.

Types of Study Designs
Randomized Studies

The randomized study or systematic review of randomized studies represents the apex of the evidence-based medicine pyramid. A randomized study is designed to compare study participants in two or more treatment groups and their associated outcomes in an attempt to determine the efficacy of

Table 2

The FINER Criteria for Evaluating a Research Question

Criterion	Description
Feasible	Is it possible to perform the study? Are the available expertise, resources, time, money, and access to patients sufficient for answering the question?
Interesting	Does the answer to the question have meaning to you and others?
Novel	Has similar research been done previously? Will the study results represent a meaningful contribution to existing literature?
Ethical	What are the risks to participating patients? Will an institutional review board allow the study to proceed?
Relevant	Will the findings have the potential to influence patient care strategies?

Data from Cummings SR, Browner WS, Hulley SB: Conceiving the research question, in Hulley SB; Cummings SR, Browner WS, Grady DG, Newman TB, eds: *Designing Clinical Research*, ed 3. Philadelphia, PA, Lippincott Williams & Wilkins, 2007, pp 20-22.

a clinical intervention. From an ethical standpoint, all involved researchers should have clinical equipoise regarding the study intervention, and genuine uncertainty should exist as to the benefit of the intervention. The purpose of randomization is to minimize bias. In an ideal setting, the treatment groups are statistically similar in every way except for the presence or absence of the clinical intervention of interest. With effective randomization, a study participant should have an equal likelihood of being assigned to the control or intervention group at the time of enrollment. The clinical question generally must be fairly specific to limit the topic of the study to a clinical intervention. For purposes of statistical analysis, the hypothesis compares the effect of the intervention on patients in different groups in a statistically significant manner, in terms of superiority, inferiority, or equivalency. An appropriate sample of eligible patients is identified, and patients are randomized to a treatment group after consenting to the intervention. The process of randomization can be done in many ways, but the pervasive goal is to assign the clinical intervention using a predefined system that is unpredictable to patients and investigators. This process serves to decrease bias in patient selection, minimize possible confounding variables, and allow for blinding of patients and/or investigators as to the assigned intervention groups. In general, concealing knowledge of the intervention groups from patients and investigators is desirable in an attempt to eliminate bias when determining outcomes with a subjective component.

After the study is conducted, the outcomes are recorded, data are analyzed using predetermined statistical techniques, and the results are reported. The Consolidated Standards of Reporting Trials (CONSORT) statement is a valuable reference tool for reporting randomized study results; the CONSORT checklist can be used to ensure high-quality data reporting.[5]

Although randomized studies represent the pinnacle of scientific evidence, they have several disadvantages. A randomized study normally is more expensive to conduct than other types of studies. In addition, a relatively long time period is required for achieving full enrollment, carrying out the intervention, and determining the outcome. The outcome of interest must occur with relative frequency to justify the use of this type of study design. The technology in some industries is advancing so rapidly that a study might be obsolete before it is completed and thus might not justify the cost. Patients must be followed over time to record their outcome. An adequate percentage of the originally enrolled patients must be followed to the follow-up date to determine the outcome; if too many patients are lost to follow-up, the study findings can be called into question. Some patients may decide to move from the originally assigned intervention group to another group during the course of a study. To deal with this difficulty, study results often incorporate an intention-to-treat analysis that reports the final outcome of patients by their originally assigned group, even if some have crossed over into another intervention group. This conservative technique adds value to any statistically significant findings. Finally, external validity (the extent to which the study's findings can be applied to a general population) may be limited based on the criteria for enrollment. External validity is affected by the location of the study (such as a country, city, academic center, or private hospital), the characteristics of patients (such as comorbidities, age, or smoking status), intervention factors (such as the cost of the surgery, cost of medication, experience of surgeons), and type of outcome measure (such as an objective measure or patient-reported outcome). Physicians must take all of these factors into account before incorporating the results of a study into clinical practice.

Numerous randomized studies can be found in the published orthopaedic literature. One important example is an international multicenter randomized, double-blind study of zoledronic acid administration and the subsequent risk of clinical fracture and mortality in patients undergoing surgical hip fracture repair.[6] In this study, 1,054 patients received intravenous zoledronic acid and 1,057 received intravenous placebo within 90 days of the surgical hip fracture repair. Patients who received zoledronic acid had a lower risk of a new clinical fracture and less mortality at a median 1.9-year follow-up compared with patients receiving the placebo. Another example is a randomized study that compared arthroscopic débridement, arthroscopic lavage, and placebo surgery in 180 patients with knee osteoarthritis who were being treated at a Veterans Affairs hospital.[7] Patient-reported outcomes at 24-month follow-up after surgery revealed that the arthroscopic options did not lead to a better outcome than the placebo surgery.

Cohort Studies

A cohort study follows a group of patients over time for the primary purpose of analyzing outcomes based on the presence or absence of defined risk factors. Like all types of studies, a cohort study begins with one or more clinical questions. In a prospective cohort study, the question is generated before the collection of data, the patients in the sample are followed over time, and measurements are used to assess the outcomes of interest. Such a study is at level II on the evidence-based medicine pyramid. The study is at level I if the question is one of risk factors (predictors) that significantly influence the prognosis. A cohort study is retrospective and represents level III on the evidence-based medicine pyramid if the question is posed after data collection and patient follow-up. Both prospective and retrospective cohort studies begin with a definition of the sample population. The exposure of interest is represented by the presence or absence of risk factors, and the outcome is represented by a defined clinical entity. This type of study attempts to associate the presence or absence of risk factors with the development of a specific outcome or the absence of such development.

Cohort studies are observational in nature. A prospective study generally is more expensive to perform than a retrospective study. It may be necessary to study an outcome that occurs with relative frequency to avoid the need for larger sample sizes or longer study duration, both of which can add to the cost of the study. Cohort studies are best suited for a common clinical entity in which risk factors and predictors are not well known. Because of the observational nature of the study, causation is relatively difficult to demonstrate, and confounding variables must be accounted for in the statistical design. However, multiple risk factors and outcomes can be studied at the same time, and descriptive statistics such as incidence and relative risk can be determined. A systematic review comparing prospective cohort studies with randomized controlled studies conducted during the preceding 25 years found that the results of the cohort studies did not consistently overestimate or demonstrate a qualitative difference when compared with the results obtained in randomized controlled studies.[8,9]

Cohort studies are relatively common, and cohort studies related to many topics are readily available. The Framingham Heart Study is one of the most important historical cohort studies. Prompted by dramatically rising rates of death from cardiovascular disease, researchers in 1948 recruited 5,209 middle-aged individuals from Framingham, MA.[10] Extensive information was recorded on the research subjects' lifestyle, examination findings, and laboratory tests. The subjects were followed prospectively, with the evaluation repeated every 2 years. Major risk factors for cardiovascular disease were described based on differences the study found between subjects who developed cardiovascular disease and those who did not. One good example of a recently published orthopaedic cohort study analyzed predictors of sports function and activity after unilateral anterior cruciate ligament reconstruction surgery. In this multicenter study, 84% of original patients (378 of 448 patients) completed validated outcome measures at a minimum 6-year follow-up. Through multivariable analysis of numerous risk factors documented at the time of enrollment, the authors found that the use of allograft, a positive smoking status, and an elevated body mass index were risk factors leading to lower outcome scores.[11]

Case Studies

The types of case studies include case reports, case series, and case-control studies. Case studies begin by identifying individuals who have the outcome of interest, in contrast with the cohort and randomized study designs, which begin by identifying patients who do or do not have defined risk factors before onset of outcome. Although case studies are relatively low in the hierarchy of the evidence-based medicine pyramid, valuable scientific information can be gleaned from these studies. For example, a rarely occurring disease or medical condition generally cannot be studied in a prospective fashion because a scientifically valid study would require many individuals to be followed over time to identify a sufficient number with the outcome of interest. The cost of such an undertaking cannot be justified. It is more feasible to identify individuals having the outcome of interest, then retrospectively examine the presence or absence of certain risk factors.

The case report is the simplest form of a case study. In a case report, one patient with the outcome of interest is identified, and the treatment and associated risk factors related to that one patient are described. A case series is similar to a case report except that it involves two or more patients having the outcome of interest. These studies, representing level IV on the evidence-based medicine pyramid, are valuable for studying an extremely rare condition and can serve as a foundation for the hypothesis in future studies. Case reports and case series generally are low in cost and relatively easy to perform. Their greatest weakness is the lack of a control group. Causation therefore cannot be determined. It has been suggested that one should "take them seriously and then ignore them."[12] Although it is difficult for a clinician to change practice based on the results of case studies, they can provide guidance in the setting of a rare clinical condition. By definition, case studies are descriptive: they summarize the presentation, treatment, and outcome of a previously encountered patient.

The case-control study is the best case study design and is classified as level III on the evidence-based medicine pyramid. Like other case studies, the case-control study begins with the identification of patients with the outcome of interest. Individuals from a similar population who do not have the disease are then identified to serve as control sub-

4: Clinical Science

jects. The researchers retrospectively identify the prevalence of risk factors in both the patients and control subjects with the goal of identifying risk factors that could explain the presence of the disease in the patients but not the control subjects. The researchers calculate the odds of exposure to a risk factor among the patients compared with the odds of exposure among the control subjects. The calculations are expressed as an odds ratio. Case-control studies generally are inexpensive to perform and require little time; they can serve as an exploratory study before a possible cohort or randomized clinical study. However, if the outcome is too rare to justify a cohort or randomized study, the case-control study will provide the highest available level of evidence for use in clinical decision making. The weaknesses inherent in this study design include the inability to study multiple outcomes at once and a susceptibility to bias. A case-control study begins with the identification of individuals who have the outcome of interest, and by definition it is limited to the study of that single outcome. In contrast, a prospective study retains the ability to identify outcomes other than the primary outcome of interest. In a case-control study, the control subjects are chosen independently of the case subjects. The population from which the control subjects are chosen is important to the study design. For example, if the control subjects are chosen from a population of hospital inpatients, the presence of risk factors may be affected by the general poor health of many hospital inpatients, and this factor could limit the validity of the study's findings. The presence or absence of risk factors in a case-control study is determined retrospectively from previously collected data; this factor further exposes the study to a potential for error. Descriptive findings such as prevalence and incidence cannot be calculated because the study subjects are selected based on the presence or absence of a defined outcome.

Case studies are abundant in the published literature because of the relative ease with which they can be performed. In an early orthopaedic case study, Sir John Charnley described his technique for hip arthroplasty, as justified by his past experience, laboratory experiments, and a loose description of initial outcomes in 97 patients.[13] Although the description of outcomes is lacking by current standards, this case study served as a foundation for future research into the treatment of arthritic conditions of the hip. A classic case study by James Ewing described a tumor of bone he called "a diffuse endothelioma of bone" in seven patients.[14] The first-described patient, a 14-year-old girl with a presumed osteosarcoma of the forearm, had a tumor that proved initially sensitive to radiation; subsequent analysis revealed a typical radiographic and histologic appearance. Ewing's description of this new type of tumor, now known as Ewing sarcoma, forever altered the field of orthopaedic oncology.

Summary

The foundation of clinical decision making in medicine rests on the proper design and conduct of clinical investigations to answer specific questions. The process includes generating the study question, establishing inclusion and exclusion criteria, choosing the patient population, choosing the study design, and estimating the sample size. It is easy to assume that the responsibility for adhering to these principles rests on researchers and others actively involved in studies. However, practicing clinicians remain accountable for evaluating the published literature, and they must have the ability to scrutinize study results before implementing them in patient care. In an era of rapidly advancing technology and escalating costs, the importance of these skills cannot be overstated.

References

1. Sackett DL, Rosenberg WM, Gray JA, Haynes RB, Richardson WS: Evidence based medicine: What it is and what it isn't. *BMJ* 1996;312(7023):71-72.

2. *Journal of Bone and Joint Surgery:* Levels of evidence for primary research question, in Instructions for Authors. http://www.jbjs.org/public/instructionsauthors.aspx#Levels Evidence. Accessed January 10, 2012.

3. Cummings SR, Browner WS, Hulley SB: Conceiving the research question, in Hulley SB, Cummings SR, Browner WS, Grady DG, Newman TB, eds: *Designing Clinical Research*, ed 3. Philadelphia, PA, Lippincott Williams & Wilkins, 2007, pp 20-22.

4. Friedman LM, Furberg CD, DeMets DL: What is the question, in *Fundamentals of Clinical Trials*, ed 3. New York, NY, Springer, 1998, pp 16-29.

5. Begg C, Cho M, Eastwood S, et al: Improving the quality of reporting of randomized controlled trials: The CONSORT statement. *JAMA* 1996;276(8):637-639.

6. Lyles KW, Colón-Emeric CS, Magaziner JS, et al: Zoledronic acid and clinical fractures and mortality after hip fracture. *N Engl J Med* 2007;357(18):1799-1809.

7. Moseley JB, O'Malley K, Petersen NJ, et al: A controlled trial of arthroscopic surgery for osteoarthritis of the knee. *N Engl J Med* 2002;347(2):81-88.

8. Benson K, Hartz AJ: A comparison of observational studies and randomized, controlled trials. *N Engl J Med* 2000;342(25):1878-1886.

9. Concato J, Shah N, Horwitz RI: Randomized, controlled trials, observational studies, and the hierarchy of research designs. *N Engl J Med* 2000;342(25):1887-1892.

10. Dawber TR, Meadors GF, Moore FE Jr: Epidemiological approaches to heart disease: The Framingham Study. *Am J Public Health Nations Health* 1951;41(3):279-281.

11. Spindler KP, Huston LJ, Wright RW, et al: The prognosis and predictors of sports function and activity at minimum 6 years after anterior cruciate ligament reconstruction: A population cohort study. *Am J Sports Med* 2011;39(2):348-359.

12. Mayer D: Study design and strength of evidence, in *Essential Evidence-Based Medicine*. Cambridge, England, Cambridge University Press, 2004, pp 52-61.

13. Charnley J: Arthroplasty of the hip: A new operation. *Lancet* 1961;1(7187):1129-1132.

14. Ewing J: Diffuse endothelioma of bone [*Proceedings of the New York Pathological Society*, 1921]. *Clin Orthop Relat Res* 2006;450:25-27.

4: Clinical Science

Chapter 28

Systematic Reviews and Meta-analyses

Reza Firoozabadi, MD

Saam Morshed, MD, PhD, MPH

Introduction

The number of scientific publications directed toward practicing physicians is markedly increasing every year. Reports of an estimated 25,000 randomized clinical studies are published annually, and that number continues to rise. More than 19 million publications are currently indexed in the MEDLINE database.[1] Published reviews have come to serve an important role in summarizing the ever-growing body of information, but they are of varying quality and usefulness. Distilling relevant information on a chosen clinical topic requires skillful navigation of the literature.

Evidence-based medicine has been defined as the process of "integrating individual clinical expertise with the best available external clinical evidence from systematic research."[2] The term was coined in 1991 to present a paradigm that places less emphasis on expert opinion and clinical observation than on randomized clinical studies.[3] The medical community has embraced this methodology. The initial emphasis was on treatment effect using discrete clinical end points, but evidence-based medicine increasingly has focused on patient quality of life.[4]

The scientific evidence on a particular clinical question can be summarized from a review of the relevant research. Clinicians can use these reviews as sources of evidence for practice. Reviews are presented in many forms, of which the most common are the narrative review, the systematic review, meta-analysis of published data, and pooled reanalysis

(Figure 1). However, these commonly used terms are not clearly defined in the literature.

Types of Reviews

Narrative Reviews

Although a narrative review summarizes studies from which conclusions can be drawn and interpreted, it is based on the reviewer's own experience and opinion. The study results typically are qualitatively summarized. Narrative reviews tend to deal with a broad range of issues related to a given topic, rather than to discuss a particular question in depth.[5]

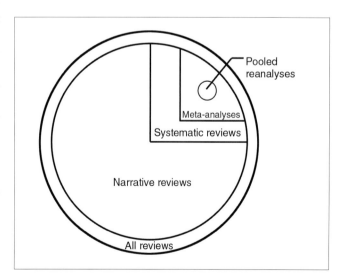

Figure 1 Schematic diagram showing the types of review summarizing medical research. Note that although narrative reviews and systematic reviews are exclusive of one another given their methodology, systematic reviews include those with and without quantitative meta-analysis or pooled reanalysis.

Dr. Morshed or an immediate family member has received research or institutional support from Stryker and Synthes. Neither Dr. Firoozabadi nor any immediate family member has received anything of value from or owns stock in a commercial company or institution related directly or indirectly to the subject of this chapter.

A narrative review on clavicle fractures, for example, might include sections on anatomy, types of clavicle fractures, forms of nonsurgical and surgical fixation, and different techniques for fixation. Narrative reviews are useful for obtaining a broad perspective on a given topic but are less likely than other types of reviews to provide a quantitative answer to a specific question. A textbook chapter typically is a narrative review.

A narrative review may have multiple deficiencies, including an inability to answer a specific question, an absence of research systematically sought from the literature, the presence of research reports that were selected by the author, and a qualitative summary of research without relative weighting based on study sample or critical appraisal. Clinical recommendations from narrative reviews are strongly based on the author's opinion.[6] The result may be a difference in the recommendations found in a narrative review compared with those of a systematic review. Many narrative reviews lag 10 or more years behind current research; the recommendations might not include a relatively new treatment of proven efficacy but instead might include a therapy that has since been proven harmful or useless.[7]

A narrative review is useful for providing background information or the historical context of a clinical topic but is no longer an appropriate means of summarizing the best or most current evidence for answering a specific question.

Systematic Reviews

A systematic review is a multistage process in which all available publications relevant to a specific question are obtained and data are assembled in a quantitative or qualitative manner.[8] In a systematic review, all available evidence is considered to assess the association between treatment and outcome, prognostic strength, or diagnostic accuracy. The key feature distinguishing a systematic review from a narrative review is that a reproducible search algorithm is used to identify and select studies for inclusion. The search strategy typically is designed with the assistance of a research librarian, with investigators blinded to authorship of candidate works. The emphasis of a systematic review is on analyzing the methodologic quality of the studies and the reasons for any discrepancies in the results of different studies. The results of each study are presented in a variety of formats and are evaluated based on defined criteria.[9]

Systematic reviews commonly are used to generate consensus on the prevention or management of common conditions. For example, the American Academy of Orthopaedic Surgeons conducts systematic reviews as the basis for developing clinical practice guidelines.[10] If the studies are sufficiently similar to allow quantitative merging of statistical estimates, the result can be called a meta-analysis.[6]

Meta-analyses

Meta-analysis has been an important component of clinical epidemiology and health-related research ever since its development.[6,11] The first medical researcher to use formal techniques to combine data from different studies probably was Karl Pearson, who assessed the efficacy of typhoid vaccination in 1904. Pearson's rationale for pooling data was that "many of the groups... are far too small to allow any definite opinion being formed at all, having regard to the size of the probable error involved."[12] By merging data, a meta-analysis can provide the power that is lacking in individual small studies.[13] The terms meta-analysis and systematic review are not interchangeable. It is important to be able to determine when a systematic review should include a meta-analysis. To conduct a meta-analysis, one must first conduct a systematic review to determine whether the available data support meta-analysis.

A meta-analysis begins with an unbiased systematic review using predetermined inclusion criteria to select specific published studies that answer a clinical question.[12] The data from these studies are analyzed to determine whether the required high level of consistency of effect measures exists across studies. If the study conditions (the inclusion criteria and details of treatment) or measures of disease or outcome vary widely, the data usually should be presented as a systematic review.[14] The effect measures should be common to all studies. For example, a clinical study might use an effect measure such as the relative risk of an undesirable outcome after an experimental treatment versus no treatment.[15] Risk reduction and odds ratio are other common effect measures used to summarize the data. Many measures of effect share components such as incident cases and number of subjects at risk; meta-analysis can be performed as long as data on the measures of disease or outcome are provided or can be obtained from the author of the original study.

Pooled Reanalyses

Investigators performing a review may need to request unpublished raw data from the authors of individual studies. These data are compiled and assessed using predetermined criteria. Such an analysis is called a pooled reanalysis, an individual patient data meta-analysis, or a meta-analysis of individual data.[9,14] Although pooled reanalysis has not been common in orthopaedic research, it can be helpful if there is a need to reformulate outcome measures across studies for the purpose of examining specific subgroups or alternative outcomes. The reanalysis process can provide the uniformity necessary for a proper meta-analysis.

The History of Reviews in Orthopaedic Surgery

For most of its history, the practice of orthopaedic surgery has been guided by expert opinion. Most published literature recounted the experience of a single surgeon or institution treating a particular condition. More recently, clinical studies that compare treatments have advanced the push for evidence-based medicine. The number of randomized controlled studies has increased over the course of the past two decades the findings of these studies often contradict conventional or expert opinion. This has led clinicians to increasingly acknowledge a hierarchy of study design that correlates with the validity of conclusions that can be drawn.[3] Meta-analysis and systematic reviews became more widely used during the 1980s, as the benefit of pooling the results of many randomized controlled studies became increasingly clear.[4] The Cochrane Collaboration became a leading source of reviews of health care interventions tested in randomized controlled studies. Researchers in orthopaedic surgery have attempted to keep up with the significant advances in evidence-based medicine in other health care fields.

Bhandari et al[16] studied the prevalence of meta-analyses in the orthopaedic literature over a 20-year period and found no meta-analyses before 1984. There was a fivefold increase in the number of meta-analyses in orthopaedic surgery from 1999 to 2008.[17] Although significant flaws in the methodology of orthopaedic research continue to be found, the methodologic quality appears to be improving. Rigorous processes for conducting and reporting are needed to ensure continued progress.

Steps in a Systematic Review

Investigators must take five key steps to ensure a proper systematic review: define the question by formulating a focused review question; conduct a comprehensive, exhaustive literature search that includes primary studies; assess the quality of the included studies and extract data by means of inclusion and exclusion criteria; analyze the data; and interpret the results and write the report[6,14,18] (Table 1).

Formulating the Question

The research question must be specific and relevant to clinical practice. A literature search should be performed to determine whether a systematic review of the topic already has been conducted. A properly formulated question should use the so-called patient-intervention-comparison-outcome (PICO) format.[19] The essential characteristics of the patient population must be identified, such as primary symptom, health status, racial identity, sex, and previous medical condition, and the investigator must determine which of these characteristics should be considered during the search for evidence. The intervention identifies the treatment or exposure the patient will undergo, such as a specific procedure, diagnostic test, adjunctive therapy, or medication. The comparison is the primary alternative (control) intervention or placebo being considered; the choice of only one alternative treatment will expedite a productive computerized search. The definition of the outcome is the final component of the PICO process. The definition of outcome identifies what end point the study intends to measure. Orthopaedic surgical outcomes typically involve improvement or maintenance of form or function, relief of symptoms, or prevention of future symptoms.[20]

Table 1

The Five Key Steps in a Systematic Review

Define the question.
Specify inclusion and exclusion criteria: population, intervention or exposure, outcome, methodology. Establish a priori hypotheses to explain heterogeneity.

Conduct a literature search.
Decide on information sources: databases, experts, funding agencies, pharmaceutical companies, manual literature search, personal files, registries, reference lists from retrieved articles.
Determine restrictions: time period, unpublished data, language.
Identify article titles and abstracts.

Apply inclusion and exclusion criteria.
Apply inclusion and exclusion criteria to article titles and abstracts.
Obtain full text of eligible articles and abstracts.
Apply inclusion and exclusion criteria.
Select final eligible articles.
Assess agreement on study selection.

Abstract data.
Data abstraction: participants, interventions, comparison interventions, study design, results, methodologic quality, agreement on validity assessment.

Conduct the analysis.
Determine method of pooling results.
Pool results (if appropriate).
Decide how to handle missing data.
Explore heterogeneity.
Perform sensitivity and subgroup analysis.
Explore the possibility of publication bias.

(Adapted with permission from American Medical Association: *User's Guides to the Medical Literature: A Manual for Evidence-Based Clinical Practice.* Chicago, IL, American Medical Association, 2002.)

Conducting a Literature Search

A well-formulated clinical question defines the criteria for including or excluding primary studies. The search for primary studies should be comprehensive and should include multiple databases so that relevant studies are not missed.[21] Most systematic reviews find most of the relevant studies and data on general databases including MEDLINE, EMBASE, the Cochrane Controlled Trials Register, and DARE. MEDLINE (PubMed) is a database compiled and maintained by the US National Library of Medicine and predominantly includes studies published in the United

4: Clinical Science

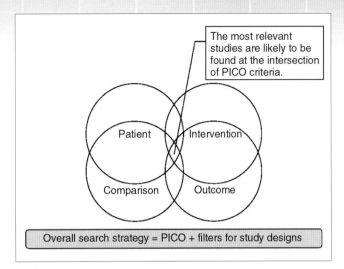

The most relevant studies are likely to be found at the intersection of PICO criteria.

Patient

Intervention

Comparison

Outcome

Overall search strategy = PICO + filters for study designs

Figure 2 The strategy for a literature search using the PICO study design filters. The most relevant studies are likely to be those that intersect all four PICO criteria. (Adapted with permission from Pai M, McCulloch M, Gorman JD, et al: Systematic reviews and meta-analyses: An illustrated, step-by-step guide. *Natl Med J India* 2004;17(2):86-95.)

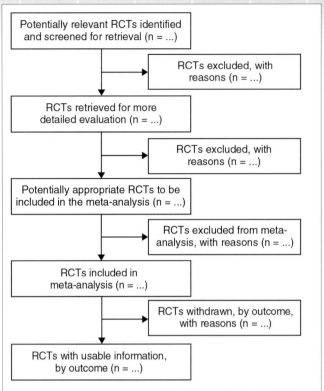

Potentially relevant RCTs identified and screened for retrieval (n = ...)

RCTs excluded, with reasons (n = ...)

RCTs retrieved for more detailed evaluation (n = ...)

RCTs excluded, with reasons (n = ...)

Potentially appropriate RCTs to be included in the meta-analysis (n = ...)

RCTs excluded from meta-analysis, with reasons (n = ...)

RCTs included in meta-analysis (n = ...)

RCTs withdrawn, by outcome, with reasons (n = ...)

RCTs with usable information, by outcome (n = ...)

Figure 3 The Quality of Reporting of Meta-Analyses (QUOROM) flowchart for recording reasons for study inclusion or exclusion. RCT = randomized controlled trial. (Adapted with permission from Moher D, Cook DJ, Eastwood S, Olkin I, Rennie D, Stroup DF: Improving the quality of reports of meta-analyses of randomized controlled trials: The QUOROM statement. *Lancet* 1999;354:1896-1900.)

States. EMBASE contains many more European citations as well as disciplines outside of medicine;[6] a MEDLINE search may not include important European studies that are available through EMBASE. The Cochrane Collaboration mainly focuses on registering and reviewing randomized controlled studies. DARE is prepared by the Centre for Reviews and Dissemination sponsored by the UK National Health Service and includes systematic reviews as well as a rich database of economic analyses and health technology assessments. Additional data can be located in subject-specific databases such as CANCERLIT (from the National Cancer Institute). Ongoing research and unpublished data can be discovered by searching references cited in relevant articles and contacting their authors as well as other experts in the field.[14,22] The authors of conference presentation abstracts can provide additional data.

Pai et al[14] described an effective strategy for searching databases, beginning with separate sensitive searches for each of the components of the PICO set. Multiple alternative terms can be combined with the Boolean operator 'OR.' The use of 'OR' expands the search results and can yield a large number of citations. The results of these separate searches can be combined using the operator 'AND' to narrow the search to studies containing all of the PICO terms (**Figure 2**). Filters also can be set to narrow the search.[14] All relevant reports found using these and other methods should be organized using reference management software, such as EndNote (Thomson Reuters, Carlsbad, CA) or RefWorks (RefWorks, Bethesda, MD). These products may be available in a Web-based platform useful for managing references, retrieving bibliographic information, and organizing reports based on specific questions. A subscriber can store references online, access them from any computer, share data with other subscribers, and use the software for personal learning.

Reference management software can allow easy access to all studies by all reviewers. To limit investigator bias, all reference citations should be screened for validity by at least two independent reviewers. Involving multiple independent reviewers can decrease the risk of selection subjectivity. If the reviewers disagree on inclusion or exclusion, an additional reviewer can become involved.[23] The selection process should be transparent. Publishers increasingly are requesting that authors submit a flowchart describing the steps used in deciding on study inclusion or exclusion[14] (**Figure 3**).

Assessing the Quality of Included Studies and Extracting the Data

After the literature search is conducted and organized, the quality of the studies is assessed to determine their credibility. Quality is a relative term used to describe the validity of a study and its lack of bias. The assessment should be done by at least two independent reviewers, with blinding of jour-

4: Clinical Science

nal and author names to preclude reviewer bias. The method of appraisal depends on the type of research design. The appraisal can be based on structured scales and questionnaires designed for specific study designs. For example, the Jadad scale is used for assessing the quality of randomized clinical studies.[14] This scale considers the presence and method of randomization, the method of blinding, and the number of patients lost to follow-up. If these criteria are in question, the reviewers may contact the study authors for clarification or consider the criteria to be not reported.[8] Numerous other composite scales and programs deal with possible bias by assessing allocation concealment, blinding, follow-up details, and intention-to-treat analysis.[8,14] If a scale appropriate for assessing a particular study cannot be found, the study characteristics are summarized, including the study design, the methods of patient selection, the loss–to–follow-up ratio, and the presence of identified bias.

The use of quality scales and scores can introduce inconsistencies into the data assessment because a study may achieve a high quality score despite a fatal flaw in its methods.[23] For example, a study could score 5 out of a possible 5 points on the Jadad scale although it lacks an explanation of the baseline demographics or clinical characteristics of the patients in each treatment group. Most study scales are not validated, and assessments of the same study using different scales can yield dramatically different quality scores.[12]

Some researchers use checklists of the elements that make up a quality study. The CONSORT Statement is commonly used in evaluating randomized controlled studies[24] (Table 2).The use of a checklist of specific study components is an objective approach that can provide a more transparent interpretation of quality assessment. In 2011, Guyatt et al[25-29] published the Grading of Recommendations Assessment, Development, and Evaluation (GRADE) system for rating the quality of evidence. This series of guidelines provides specific criteria for study design, risk of bias, imprecision, inconsistency, indirectness, and magnitude of effect; study recommendations are classified as

Table 2

Checklist of Items Used to Validate a Report of a Randomized Controlled Study

Section or Topic	Item Number	Descriptor	Locator (Page Number)
Title and abstract	1	How participants were allocated to interventions (eg, random allocation, randomized, randomly assigned)	
Introduction Background	2	Scientific background, explanation of rationale	
Methods			
Participants	3	Eligibility criteria Settings in which data were collected	
Interventions	4	Precise interventions intended for each group How and when interventions were administered	
Objectives	5	Specific objectives and hypotheses	
Outcomes	6	Clearly defined primary and secondary outcome measures and (if applicable) methods used to enhance the quality of measurements (eg, multiple observations, training of assessors)	
Sample size	7	How sample size was determined and (if applicable) explanation of interim analyses and stopping rules	
Randomization (sequence generation)	8	Method used to generate the random allocation sequence, including any restriction (eg, blocking, stratification)	
Allocation, concealment	9	Method used to implement the random allocation sequence (eg, numbered containers, central telephone), including whether the sequence was concealed until interventions were assigned	
Implementation	10	Identification of the person who generated the allocation sequence, enrolled participants, and assigned participants to a group	

Continued on next page

4: Clinical Science

Table 2 continued

Checklist of Items Used to Validate a Report of a Randomized Controlled Study

Section or Topic	Item Number	Descriptor	Locator (Page Number)
Blinding (masking)	11	Whether participants, those administering the interventions, and those assessing the outcomes were blinded to group assignment. If blinding was used, how its success was evaluated	
Statistical methods	12	Statistical methods used to compare groups for the primary outcome(s) Methods for additional analyses, such as subgroup and adjusted analyses	
Results			
Participant flow	13	Flow of participants through each stage, (a diagram is strongly recommended). For each group, the number of randomly assigned participants, participants receiving the intended treatment, participants completing the study protocol, and participants analyzed for the primary outcome Deviations of the protocol from the study as planned, with reasons	
Recruitment	14	Dates defining the periods of recruitment and follow-up	
Baseline data	15	Baseline demographic and clinical characteristics of each group	
Numbers analyzed	16	Number of participants (denominator) in each group included in each analysis and whether the analysis was by intention to treat. Results stated in absolute numbers rather than percentages (eg, 10 of 20, not 50%), if possible.	
Outcomes and estimation	17	For each primary and secondary outcome, a summary of results for each group and the estimated effect size and its precision (eg, 95% confidence interval).	
Ancillary analyses	18	Address multiplicity by reporting any other analyses performed, including subgroup analyses and adjusted analyses, indicating those prespecified or exploratory.	
Adverse events	19	All important adverse effects in each intervention group	
Discussion			
Interpretation	20	Interpretation of the results, taking into account study hypotheses, sources of potential bias or imprecision, and the dangers associated with multiplicity of analyses and outcomes	
Generalizability	21	Generalizability (external validity) of the study findings	
Overall evidence	22	General interpretation of the results in the context of current evidence	

(Adapted with permission from Moher D, Schulz KF, Altman DG, CONSORT: The CONSORT statement: Revised recommendations for improving the quality of reports of parallel group randomized trials. *BMC Med Res Methodol* 2001;11(2):3.)

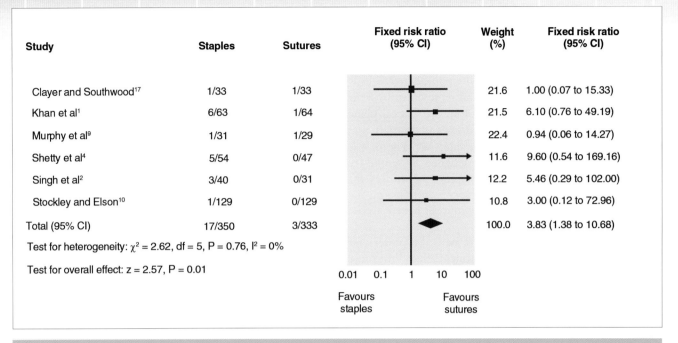

Study	Staples	Sutures	Fixed risk ratio (95% CI)	Weight (%)	Fixed risk ratio (95% CI)
Clayer and Southwood[17]	1/33	1/33		21.6	1.00 (0.07 to 15.33)
Khan et al[1]	6/63	1/64		21.5	6.10 (0.76 to 49.19)
Murphy et al[9]	1/31	1/29		22.4	0.94 (0.06 to 14.27)
Shetty et al[4]	5/54	0/47		11.6	9.60 (0.54 to 169.16)
Singh et al[2]	3/40	0/31		12.2	5.46 (0.29 to 102.00)
Stockley and Elson[10]	1/129	0/129		10.8	3.00 (0.12 to 72.96)
Total (95% CI)	17/350	3/333		100.0	3.83 (1.38 to 10.68)

Test for heterogeneity: $\chi^2 = 2.62$, df = 5, P = 0.76, $I^2 = 0\%$

Test for overall effect: z = 2.57, P = 0.01

0.01 0.1 1 10 100

Favours staples   Favours sutures

Figure 4 A sample forest plot, displaying the incidence of infection in orthopaedic wounds closed with sutures or staples. CI = confidence interval, df = degrees of freedom. (Adapted with permission from Smith TO, Sexton D, Mann C, Donell S: Sutures versus staples for skin closure in orthopaedic surgery: Meta-analysis. *BMJ* 2010;340:c1199.)

strong or weak based on these criteria. Strong recommendations have strong methods, a large and precise effect, and few disadvantages of therapy. Weak recommendations have weak methods, imprecise estimates, a small effect, and substantial adverse effects of therapy. The GRADE system allows physicians to interpret specific recommendations and determine the best treatment for their patients.

After the investigator has selected and stratified appropriate studies on the basis of their quality, the relevant data are extracted. The process of data extraction is demanding and time consuming. Meticulous recording is needed by at least two observers. Study blinding should include author, institution, and journal names as well as funding sources and acknowledgments.[12] The types of data to be extracted should be determined before investigation, and a review-specific data extraction form should be used. Information on study dynamics, methods, populations, interventions, and outcomes should be listed on the form.[12] The same data must be extracted from each study, and any missing data should be noted. Differences among patients in the control and intervention groups must be recorded as a statistical parameter. These parameters are reported differently for different types of study designs. For example, in a randomized controlled study an outcome typically is expressed as a relative risk, an odds ratio, or a difference between means if the outcome is continuous. Final exclusion decisions should be made and recorded after data extraction. The reason for the exclusion should be documented in detail for the benefit of future reviewers and readers.[23]

Analyzing the Data

The results of the selected studies must be presented in a way that answers the formulated question. The steps in data analysis are to tabulate the summary data; graph the data; check for heterogeneity; perform a meta-analysis, if heterogeneity is not a substantial concern, or identify factors that can explain the heterogeneity; evaluate the impact of study quality on results; and explore the potential for publication bias.[14] The study characteristics should be described and presented in a tabulated format.[30,31] The study population, time frame, study design, interventions, and outcomes should be included in the tables.[14,23]

The final decision to perform a meta-analysis or a systematic review depends only on the variability of the data. Data typically are pooled if the individual studies had comparable conditions and the treatment effects were similarly reported. The analytic goal of a meta-analysis is to generate a homogenous summary. Homogeneity primarily signifies the presence of narrow confidence intervals that overlap among the included studies, supporting the notion of a single population mean.[6]

Forest Plot

Forest plots are routinely used in systematic reviews and meta-analyses to visually summarize the results of the individual reviewed studies (**Figure 4**). A forest plot typically has two main components: data that identify the individual studies and the plot itself. A vertical line is drawn through the center of the plot to represent the null hypothesis (no difference between patients in the treatment and control

4: Clinical Science

groups). A square and a horizontal line correspond to each study's estimate of effect (the odds ratio, risk ratio, or risk difference) and confidence interval, respectively. The size of the square reflects the weight given to the study in the analysis.[12] At the bottom of the plot is the pooled overall estimate, with its 95% confidence interval represented by a diamond.[32] The center of the diamond on the vertical plane represents the average treatment effect, and the left and right apices represent the confidence intervals.[8] **Figure 4** is the forest plot for a meta-analysis designed to synthesize study data comparing the use of staples and sutures for wound closure after orthopaedic surgery.[33] In this plot, the pooled effect showed a statistically significant benefit to using sutures rather than staples.

Pooled results are used to increase statistical power and lead to more precise estimates of treatment effect.[34] In some analyses, all studies are considered equal for purposes of pooling, and an unweighted average value is calculated. Invalid conclusions can be drawn from this method because it fails to account for study sample size. Unfortunately, simple addition averaging is the most common traditional method of pooling in orthopaedic meta-analyses.[16] In weighted pooling, each study is assigned a weight based on the precision of its results. Precision is related to the narrow confidence intervals that arise from a larger sample size. Precise estimates are assigned more weight in the computation of averages.[12,14,34]

Heterogeneity Assessment

The consistency of the treatment effect among the studies must be assessed. Data pooling ideally would use multicenter randomized studies with identical protocols used on similar patients. These studies would describe the same target population and therefore could be validly combined, with homogeneity of effect assumed. However, most studies have their own protocol, and their variations in patient demographics, clinical situations, and methods of intervention can alter the treatment effect. The result is variability in the outcomes. Some dissimilarity of outcomes is expected secondary to chance, but the outcomes also can vary secondary to study characteristics.[12]

Excessive variability among the studies can be determined by visually assessing the forest plot or performing a statistical analysis. The forest plot can be scanned to determine the overall layout of the data. If some studies sit on the right side of the vertical null line and some studies sit on the left side, and the confidence intervals do not overlap, the variation among studies probably is more than chance and can be attributed to heterogeneity of effects. If the forest plot includes a large number of studies, this variation may be due to chance and not heterogeneity.[35] To calculate pooled estimates, a random-effects model or a fixed-effects model is used, depending on the assumption made about variance in the data. Variance can be intrastudy (within an individual study) or interstudy (between studies). When no interstudy variance is assumed, a fixed-effects model is used,

and observed differences among studies are considered to represent random error.[12,14,34] The random-effects model takes into account both intrastudy and interstudy variance when the pooled mean of the random effects is calculated.[34] The random-effects model typically is used when the data are heterogeneous, to account for both intrastudy and interstudy variability. When significant interstudy variability necessitates the use of the random-effects models, a more conservative estimate of effect with wider confidence intervals is generated. Numerous software programs are available to calculate heterogeneity and estimates using both the fixed-effects and random-effects models.

The χ^2 and the I^2 tests are the tools most commonly used to quantify heterogeneity. The results of these two tests routinely appear at the bottom of a forest plot. The χ^2 is computed by adding the squared deviation of each study's estimate from the overall meta-analysis estimate and calculating a P value using a χ^2 distribution with k-1 degrees of freedom (k = the number of studies). Smaller P values imply greater heterogeneity.[35] A cutoff of 0.10 typically is used to indicate heterogeneity. In the example in **Figure 4**, the P value of 0.76 suggests relative homogeneity among the studies. The shortcoming of the χ^2 test is that it has low power to detect true heterogeneity for a meta-analysis with a small number of studies and excessive power to detect negligible variability in meta-analyses with a large number of studies.[36]

Higgins et al[36] developed the I^2 statistic as an alternative method for quantifying the extent of true heterogeneity by measuring inconsistency in the study results. Unlike χ^2 analysis, this method is not dependent on the number of studies. The I^2 values range from 0% to 100%, with 0% indicating no observed heterogeneity and values greater than 20% indicating heterogeneity. If significant heterogeneity is present, the investigators may decide to present the data as a qualitative summary, or they may decide to pool the data and attempt to identify potential sources of variability by conducting subgroup analysis.

Figure 5 is an example of subgroup analysis using graphic methods. In this analysis, the relative reduction of the risk of mortality was studied in patients treated with fondaparinux compared with patients receiving low-molecular-weight heparin or placebo.[37] The authors wanted to determine whether comparison with placebo or low-molecular-weight heparin accounted for variability in the comparison, and therefore they divided the data into two major groups. One subgroup was composed of studies that compared fondaparinux to placebo. Studies in the other subgroup compared fondaparinux to low-molecular-weight heparin. The subgroups were further divided by type of treatment (medical, abdominal, or orthopaedic) to determine whether the procedure could account for variability. The overall summary estimate was found to approach statistical significance ($P = 0.058$), and no significant heterogeneity was noted (P for heterogeneity was greater than 0.1). As a

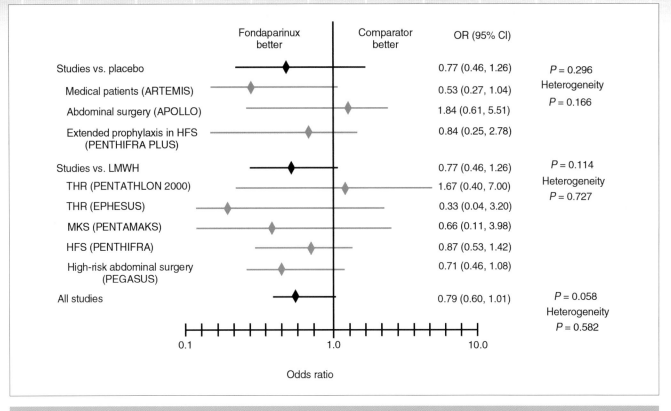

Figure 5 Subgroup analysis of the effect of fondaparinux on mortality. CI = confidence interval, HFS = hip fracture surgery, LMWH = low molecular weight heparin, MKS = major knee surgery, THR = total hip replacement. (Adapted with permission from Eikelboom JW: Effect of fondaparinux 2.5mg once daily on mortality: A meta-analysis of phase III randomized trials of venous thromboembolism prevention. *Eur Heart J* 2008;10:8-13.)

result of this analysis, the authors were able to pool the data appropriately.

Bias Assessment

Assessing for bias is crucial to any meta-analysis. The main types of bias in meta-analyses are related to reporting, publication, language, time-lag, and citations.[12,14,30] Failure to find all studies pertaining to a question can result from a combination of these biases. Reporting and publication bias tends to occur when only reports with significant positive findings are submitted or accepted for publication. Language bias occurs when studies in English are expedited during the publication process. Time-lag bias can occur if a study is published more rapidly than other studies, and citation bias can occur if a study is cited more frequently than other studies.[23] Because studies with negative results are less likely to be published than those with positive results, publication bias can significantly skew the results of a meta-analysis.[38]

An inverted funnel plot can be used to explore for the possibility of publication bias. Funnel plots are scatter plots of study results from individual studies. The study sample is marked on the y-axis, and the effect size is marked on the x-axis. This orientation relies on precise estimation of the underlying treatment effect. Larger studies should have less

variance secondary to chance and therefore should not have much scatter. Smaller studies will form the base of the plot because they have more variance and therefore more peripheral locations on the x-axis.[6] In the absence of bias, a funnel shape is produced from small studies scattered widely at the bottom of the graph, with the spread narrowing among the larger studies at the apex. If bias is present, an asymmetric funnel plot will be produced. In **Figure 6**, the upper plot represents the expected shape in the absence of bias, and the lower plot suggests publication bias against smaller, negative studies. An alternative method of determining publication bias is to use statistical methods. The most common is the Egger test, which is most useful when there is significant variation in study sizes.[12,39]

Interpreting the Results and Writing the Report

The proper reporting and discussion of the results of a systematic review, with or without meta-analysis, is necessary to allow valid interpretation by the reader. Even if all the components of a review have been properly executed, the limitations of the review must be discussed, including constraints imposed by the primary studies.[12] Any bias noted during the design process must be reported and discussed. It is important to reiterate the meaning, purpose, and relevance of the findings in the conclusion of the review. The

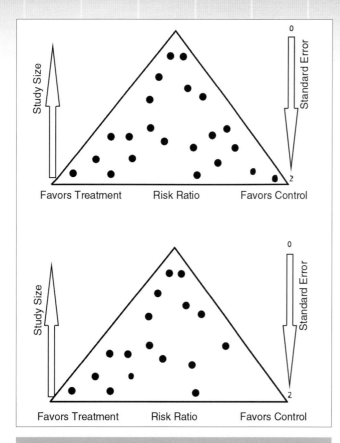

Figure 6 Inverted funnel plots. **A,** The plot reveals no publication bias. **B,** The plot suggests publication bias because small studies are not evenly distributed around the pooled risk ratio. This may occur due to lack of publication of studies that failed to show treatment effect.

answer to the clinical question should be clearly stated, with a succinct statement of the review's most important findings. These statements should focus on enhancing the reader's understanding of the study results and limitations. However, the interpretation should not extend beyond the scope of the data or the target populations of the included studies.[40] The review can be related to other studies, and the relationships of the findings can be explained. If a question related to the study findings remains unanswered or can be made more focused, further studies can be suggested. Less commonly, the evidence is sufficiently substantial that the author recommends no further studies on the specific clinical question.[12]

The format of the review should follow the guidelines for the specific study type. For a meta-analysis of randomized controlled studies, the Quality of Reporting of Meta-Analyses (QUOROM) consensus guidelines should be used. The Meta-analyses of Observational Studies in Epidemiology (MOOSE) consensus should be used for a meta-analysis of observational studies.[41,42] These guidelines provide a means for clearly presenting and organizing the information necessary for study verification and reproduction.[43]

Summary

Systematic reviews and meta-analyses summarize data from multiple studies to answer a specific clinical question. With the increased emphasis on evidence-based medicine, systematic reviews have become an important tool for guiding clinical practice. It is important to realize that an analysis is only as good as the data drawn from individual primary studies. A concerted effort toward high quality in primary studies should be the focus of future orthopaedic research.

References

1. Sackett DL, Rosenberg WM: The need for evidence-based medicine. *J R Soc Med* 1995;88(11):620-624.

2. Sackett DL, Rosenberg WM, Gray JA, Haynes RB, Richardson WS: Evidence based medicine: What it is and what it isn't. *BMJ* 1996;312(7023):71-72.

3. Guyatt GH: Evidence based medicine: Past, present, and future. *McMaster Univ Med J* 2003;1:27-32.

4. Hoppe DJ, Bhandari M: Evidence-based orthopaedics: A brief history. *Indian J Orthop* 2008;42(2):104-110.

5. Cook DJ, Mulrow CD, Haynes RB: Systematic reviews: Synthesis of best evidence for clinical decisions. *Ann Intern Med* 1997;126(5):376-380.

6. Montori VM, Swiontkowski MF, Cook DJ: Methodologic issues in systematic reviews and meta-analyses. *Clin Orthop Relat Res* 2003;413:43-54.

7. Antman EM, Lau J, Kupelnick B, Mosteller F, Chalmers TC: A comparison of results of meta-analyses of randomized control trials and recommendations of clinical experts: Treatments for myocardial infarction. *JAMA* 1992;268(2):240-248.

8. Ryś P, Władysiuk M, Skrzekowska-Baran I, Małecki MT: Review articles, systematic reviews and meta-analyses: Which can be trusted? *Pol Arch Med Wewn* 2009;119(3):148-156.

9. Ressing M, Blettner M, Klug SJ: Systematic literature reviews and meta-analyses: Part 6 of a series on evaluation of scientific publications. *Dtsch Arztebl Int* 2009;106(27):456-463.

10. American Academy of Orthopaedic Surgeons: Clinical practice guidelines. Rosemont, IL, American Academy of Orthopaedic Surgeons, http://www.aaos.org/research/guidelines/guide.asp. Accessed October 28, 2011.

11. Placket RL: Studies in the history of probability and statistics: VII. The principles of the arithmetic mean. *Biometrika* 1958;45:130-135.

12. Egger M, Smith GD, Altman D: *Systemic Reviews in Health Care: Meta-Analysis in Context*, ed 2. Hoboken, NJ, John Wiley and Sons, 2001.

13. Ioannidis JP, Lau J: Pooling research results: Benefits and limitations of meta-analysis. *Jt Comm J Qual Improv* 1999;25(9):462-469.

14. Pai M, McCulloch M, Gorman JD, et al: Systematic reviews and meta-analyses: An illustrated, step-by-step guide. *Natl Med J India* 2004;17(2):86-95.

15. Walter SD: Choice of effect measure for epidemiological data. *J Clin Epidemiol* 2000;53(9):931-939.

16. Bhandari M, Morrow F, Kulkarni AV, Tornetta P III: Meta-analyses in orthopaedic surgery: A systematic review of their methodologies. *J Bone Joint Surg Am* 2001;83(1):15-24.

17. Dijkman BG, Abouali JA, Kooistra BW, et al: Twenty years of meta-analyses in orthopaedic surgery: Has quality kept up with quantity? *J Bone Joint Surg Am* 2010;92(1):48-57.

18. American Medical Association: *User's Guide to the Medical Literature: A Manual for Evidence-Based Clinical Practice.* Chicago, IL, American Medical Association, 2002.

19. Richardson WS, Wilson MC, Nishikawa J, Hayward RS: The well-built clinical question: A key to evidence-based decisions. *ACP J Club* 1995;123(3):A12-A13.

20. Sackett D: *Evidence-Based Medicine: How to Practice and Teach EBM.* Philadelphia, PA, Churchill Livingstone, 1997.

21. Suarez-Almazor ME, Belseck E, Homik J, Dorgan M, Ramos-Remus C: Identifying clinical trials in the medical literature with electronic databases: MEDLINE alone is not enough. *Control Clin Trials* 2000;21(5):476-487.

22. Information Service Centre for Reviews and Dissemination: Finding studies for systematic reviews: A resource list for researchers. Heslington, York, England, University of York, 2002. http://www.york.ac.uk/inst/crd/finding_studies_systematic_reviews.htm. Accessed October 28, 2011.

23. Wright RW, Brand RA, Dunn W, Spindler KP: How to write a systematic review. *Clin Orthop Relat Res* 2007;455:23-29.

24. Moher D, Schulz KF, Altman DG, CONSORT: The CONSORT statement: Revised recommendations for improving the quality of reports of parallel group randomized trials. *BMC Med Res Methodol* 2001;1:2.

25. Balshem H, Helfand M, Schünemann HJ, et al: GRADE guidelines: 3. Rating the quality of evidence. *J Clin Epidemiol* 2011;64(4):401-406.

26. Guyatt G, Oxman AD, Akl EA, et al: GRADE guidelines: 1. GRADE evidence profiles and summary of findings tables. *J Clin Epidemiol* 2011;64(4):383-394.

27. Guyatt GH, Oxman AD, Kunz R, et al: GRADE guidelines: 2. Framing the question and deciding on important outcomes. *J Clin Epidemiol* 2011;64(4):395-400.

28. Guyatt GH, Oxman AD, Schünemann HJ, Tugwell P, Knottnerus A: GRADE guidelines: A new series of articles in the *Journal of Clinical Epidemiology. J Clin Epidemiol* 2011;64(4):380-382.

29. Guyatt GH, Oxman AD, Vist G, et al: GRADE guidelines: 4. Rating the quality of evidence: Study limitations (risk of bias). *J Clin Epidemiol* 2011;64(4):407-415.

30. Torgerson C: *Systematic Reviews.* London, England, Continuum, 2003.

31. Khan KS: *Systematic Reviews to Support Evidence-Based Medicine: How to Review and Apply Findings of Healthcare Research.* London, England, Royal Society of Medicine Press, 2003.

32. Lewis S, Clarke M: Forest plots: Trying to see the wood and the trees. *BMJ* 2001;322(7300):1479-1480.

33. Smith TO, Sexton D, Mann C, Donell S: Sutures versus staples for skin closure in orthopaedic surgery: Meta-analysis. *BMJ* 2010;340:c1199.

34. Lau J, Ioannidis JP, Schmid CH: Quantitative synthesis in systematic reviews. *Ann Intern Med* 1997;127(9):820-826.

35. Hardy RJ, Thompson SG: Detecting and describing heterogeneity in meta-analysis. *Stat Med* 1998;17(8):841-856.

36. Higgins JP, Thompson SG, Deeks JJ, Altman DG: Measuring inconsistency in meta-analyses. *BMJ* 2003;327(7414):557-560.

37. Eikelboom JW: Effect of fondaparinux 2.5mg once daily on mortality: A meta-analysis of phase III randomized trials of venous thromboembolism prevention. *Eur Heart J* 2008;10:8-13.

38. Dickersin K: The existence of publication bias and risk factors for its occurrence. *JAMA* 1990;263(10):1385-1389.

39. Egger M, Davey Smith G, Schneider M, Minder C: Bias in meta-analysis detected by a simple, graphical test. *BMJ* 1997;315(7109):629-634.

40. Hess DR: How to write an effective discussion. *Respir Care* 2004;49(10):1238-1241.

41. Stroup DF, Berlin JA, Morton SC, et al: Meta-analysis of observational studies in epidemiology: A proposal for reporting. Meta-analysis of Observational Studies in Epidemiology (MOOSE) Group. *JAMA* 2000;283(15):2008-2012.

42. Moher D, Cook DJ, Eastwood S, Olkin I, Rennie D, Stroup DF: Mejora de la calidad de los informes de los metaanálisis de ensayos clínicos controlados: El acuerdo QUOROM. *Rev Esp Salud Publica* 2000;74(2):107-118.

43. Margaliot Z, Chung KC: Systematic reviews: A primer for plastic surgery research. *Plast Reconstr Surg* 2007;120(7):1834-1841.

4: Clinical Science

Chapter 29

Fundamentals of Cost-Effectiveness Research

David Shearer, MD, MPH

Kevin J. Bozic, MD, MBA

Introduction

The "value" of elective healthcare interventions such as orthopaedic surgical procedures has recently come under increased scrutiny by policy makers, payers, and healthcare purchasers, such as the federal government and large employers. As such, research evaluating the cost-effectiveness of these procedures has become increasingly important in both clinical and healthcare policy decision making. Clinical decision making in orthopaedic surgery historically has been informed primarily by anecdotal surgeon experience, expert opinion, and small uncontrolled case series. This has evolved with greater emphasis on evidence-based medicine toward larger, multicenter clinical trials using randomization, blinding, and patient-centered outcome measures. However, implicit in both of these approaches is the idea that the more effective intervention is always preferred, regardless of its cost. Economic analysis is an alternative approach that incorporates the monetary cost of an intervention into the clinical and policy decision-making framework. Two underlying assumptions that are important for acceptance of this methodology are (1) resources are

constrained (for example, there is not an unlimited budget) and (2) a more effective intervention may not always be preferred if the incremental benefit is small relative to the monetary cost.[1]

The first assumption is more widely accepted. Although healthcare spending is not fixed in the United States, the steady rise in healthcare costs as a fraction of the gross domestic product over the past several decades has been labeled a healthcare crisis.[2] There is no absolute threshold, but the idea that resources are not unlimited is not debated. The second assumption, that certain high-cost interventions with small incremental benefit may be too expensive, is more politically and ethically troublesome.[3] An attempt to factor cost into a ranking system to determine Medicaid coverage in Oregon in the 1990s led to widespread public outcry due to concerns over rationing and government control of health care.[4]

To date in the United States, the Centers for Medicare & Medicaid Services has accepted comparative effectiveness research but has declined to use cost-effectiveness analysis for coverage decisions.[5,6] In other countries, economic analysis has seen greater acceptance by governments seeking to control costs of health care and maximize scarce resources. Many countries have dedicated government agencies, such as the National Institute for Clinical Excellence in the United Kingdom, that perform economic analysis, the results of which weigh heavily in coverage decisions in the frequently nationalized healthcare systems.[7]

Despite the absence of an explicit use of economic analysis by the Centers for Medicare & Medicaid Services in the United States, there are a growing number of studies published both in the orthopaedic and other medical literature.[8,9] The results are incorporated into decision-making by private insurers, professional societies, and, to some degree, individual surgeons. It is therefore important for or-

4: Clinical Science

Table 1

Summary of Recommendations of the US Panel on Cost-Effectiveness in Health and Medicine

Components of Numerator (Costs):
- Direct and indirect costs
- Exclude costs associated with added years of life

Components of Denominator (Effects):
- Quality-adjusted life-years
- Utility estimates from standard gamble/time tradeoff (TTO) or preference-weighted survey instruments (for example, EQ-5D, Health Utilities Index)

Perspective

Societal

Time Horizon

Lifetime

Discount

3%, explore with sensitivity analysis

Data Sources

Primary or secondary, best available evidence preferred

Sensitivity Analysis
- Univariate sensitivity analysis for key assumptions at a minimum
- Multivariate sensitivity analysis recommended

thopaedic surgeons to have a basic understanding of the principles of economic analysis and familiarity with the interpretation of study results.

To date, the standard for cost-effectiveness analysis (CEA) methodology in the United States is based on the recommendations of the US Panel on Cost-Effectiveness in Health and Medicine, published in 1996.[10] A summary of these recommendations is presented in **Table 1**. The panel emerged due to the lack of standardization in CEA methods and aimed to put forth a set of recommendations for each component of a CEA that would form a base case that should be performed in all studies. Although the authors recognized that no single method applies to all circumstances, the goal of the reference case is to allow greater comparability across economic analyses. Furthermore, it provides a framework for the reader to evaluate the methodologic quality of studies being interpreted. The recommendations of the panel are incorporated throughout the chapter.

Types of Economic Analysis

Although there is variability in the nomenclature used to describe types of economic analysis, the terminology described in this chapter is generally accepted.[11,12] Each approach shares the inclusion of cost but varies in the method and degree to which other data are incorporated. **Table 2** summarizes each type of economic analysis and lists the strengths and limitations.

Cost-Effectiveness Analysis

CEA is an umbrella term that seeks to identify the cost for a unit of health benefit from an intervention. It is usually expressed quantitatively in terms of the cost-effectiveness ratio. The numerator always contains cost, whereas the denominator can be any desired outcome of interest. Examples could include cost per life saved, cost per complication averted, or cost per unit of utility (for example, quality-adjusted life-years [QALYs]) gained. Although using an outcome specific to an intervention may simplify an analysis, it may limit the ability to make comparisons across studies or interventions.

Cost-Utility Analysis

Cost utility is a specific case of cost-effectiveness in which the denominator of the cost-effectiveness ratio is the preference-based measure of utility. Utility in the context of health is a measure ranging from 0 to 1 that quantifies an individual's preference for a given health state relative to perfect health (equal to 1) and death (equal to 0). The product of utility and duration of a health state yields QALYs, which are frequently used in the denominator of a cost-utility analysis. In the medical literature the term CEA is often synonymous with cost-utility analysis and the two terms may be used interchangeably, but it should be recognized in the current taxonomy that although every cost-utility analysis is a CEA, not every CEA is a cost-utility analysis.

Cost-Benefit Analysis

In cost-benefit analysis, both the cost and effect of an intervention are expressed in monetary terms. Because all terms have the same units, the result is expressed as net monetary benefit (NMB) rather than a ratio. Alolabi et al[13] used this technique to estimate the net benefit of internal fixation compared to hemiarthroplasty for displaced femoral neck fractures. The authors found a higher cost associated with internal fixation, but surveyed individuals were willing to pay more for internal fixation than hemiarthroplasty. When multiplied by the expected number of femoral neck fractures in Ontario, a total NMB of $224,000,000 was found for internal fixation. The advantage of this approach is that it allows comparisons across broad categories of intervention that could include education, environment, criminal justice, or any other societal interest competing for scarce funds. Its use is limited in medicine, however, because assigning a monetary value to health outcomes is difficult and ethically troublesome.

Table 2

Types of Economic Analysis

Analysis	Measure of Cost	Measure of Health Effect	Output	Strengths	Limitations
CEA	$	Any measure of health benefit	Incremental cost-effectiveness ratio	Can choose health effect most relevant to intervention	Difficult to make comparisons across different diseases or interventions
Cost-utility analysis	$	Utility (for example, QALYs)	Incremental cost-effectiveness ratio	Allows comparisons across diseases and interventions within health care	Need estimate of utility for each relevant outcome
Cost-benefit analysis	$	$	Net monetary benefit	Policy makers can make comparisons across healthcare and non–healthcare programs	Difficult to assign monetary value to health benefits
Cost minimization	$	None (assumed equal)	Cost difference	Simple to conduct	Effectiveness of two treatments usually not equal

Cost Minimization

The final major category of economic analysis is cost minimization, which is used when the effectiveness of two or more interventions is considered equivalent. In this case the denominator is equal to zero and only the cost differentiates the two treatments. Cost data for both treatments are collected and the intervention with lower total cost is preferred. A simple example would be comparing the costs associated with arthroscopic versus miniopen rotator cuff repair. Collecting outcome data is unnecessary because the results have been shown to be equivalent, and therefore an appropriate comparison can be made with cost data only. A study by Adla et al[14] demonstrated equivalent outcomes but an $1,850 excess cost associated with arthroscopic rotator cuff repair compared with open repair, which was attributed primarily to increased costs of instrumentation. This type of economic analysis is often simpler, and the information derived from a cost-minimization analysis can be used in future cost-effectiveness research. However, there are few cases where two interventions are exactly equivalent.

Recommendations of the US Panel on Cost-Effectiveness in Health and Medicine

The numerator of the cost-effectiveness ratio should contain the net cost of an intervention, while the denominator should be QALYs.

Study Design

There are two major categories for CEA study design: clinical trial-based and model-based studies. With trial-based studies, cost data are collected in the context of a clinical trial through empiric observation. Model-based studies rely on simulations, typically computer-generated, that make assumptions regarding the costs and effects of an intervention based on data from other sources. Each category has specific advantages and disadvantages, and the two are frequently combined to achieve the best possible result.

Clinical Trial–Based

A cost-effectiveness analysis can be conducted alongside a clinical trial by collecting economic data in addition to measuring clinical outcomes.[15] This is sometimes referred to as a CEA "piggybacked" onto a clinical trial. These studies generally require a prospective cohort design with the intention to collect all relevant cost data, which may include procedures, hospitalization, and outpatient visits.

The primary advantage of a clinical trial–based CEA is that data are generated through empiric observation, which eliminates many of the assumptions necessary for modeling. However, they are often limited by the time frame of observation, which may not include important outcomes that affect health and incur cost over a longer period of time than a trial is feasible to conduct. Furthermore, all of the same limitations that apply to a typical clinical trial such as a selection bias or confounding apply with the inclusion of cost. Generalizability is problematic because strict inclusion and exclusion criteria are frequently used in trials, and efficacy observed in a trial may not reflect the effectiveness observed with more widespread use.

An example of a trial-based cost-utility analysis in orthopaedics is the SPORT study, which assessed surgical versus nonsurgical care for disk herniation, spinal stenosis, and degenerative spondylolisthesis.[16,17] In addition to reporting clinical outcomes, Tosteson et al[18] separately published the results of the cost-effectiveness of surgical decompression compared with nonsurgical care for the management of spinal stenosis with and without spondylolisthesis. The EQ-5D, a survey instrument for estimating utility, was administered to all participants and demonstrated a difference in utility of 0.17 between the surgical and nonsurgical cohorts over the 2-year follow-up period. Cost data were determined using a combination of Medicare payment data for procedure and inpatient charges, while remaining costs incurred, such as nonsurgical care and missed work, were self-reported by the subjects in the trial. Using these data, the incremental cost-effectiveness ratio (ICER) of surgical decompression for the management of spinal stenosis was estimated to be $77,600/QALY.

Modeling

Cost-effectiveness models are typically generated after an extensive review of the available literature on the topic or in conjunction with a trial-based CEA. These models allow projection of the observed costs and benefits of an intervention over time, making lifetime estimates of the ICER more feasible.[19] Modeling is appropriate when empiric observation is not possible, typically due to practical or ethical considerations. Practical considerations include the high cost and time associated with clinical trials, particularly those considered of highest quality, using randomization, blinding, and control groups. Ethical considerations include equipoise, when one treatment is known to be superior or when there is potential for harm to trial participants.

The disadvantage is that CEA models are subject to bias and often are difficult to validate. Furthermore, many of the inputs required for a CEA model, including treatment costs, clinical outcome probabilities, and clinical effectiveness, may be unknown or not previously reported in the literature. It is important that the assumptions used in formulating the model are explicitly stated. Computer-generated models can become highly complex, leading to a lack of transparency, particularly to those unfamiliar with the methodology.

An example of a model-based CEA in orthopaedic surgery is a study by Slover et al[20] evaluating the cost-effectiveness of total hip arthroplasty after femoral neck fracture. The authors use a Markov model to estimate the projected cost and utility gain of total hip arthroplasty compared with hemiarthroplasty for active elderly patients over a 10-year period. There were several important assumptions including an equal failure rate for both interventions and a higher postoperative utility for total hip arthroplasty. One- and two-way sensitivity analysis, which will be described in detail later in the chapter, was used to explore the effect of uncertainty in those assumptions on the output of the model. The study concluded that total hip arthroplasty may

be highly cost-effective in management of femoral neck fracture with an ICER of $1,960/QALY.

Combined

It is important to recognize that modeling and clinical trial–based designs can be used in combination. This is typically done to extend the results of the trial beyond the available follow-up period. There are important assumptions regarding the degree to which the effect of treatment is maintained over time, and this should be explicitly stated.

Recommendations of the US Panel on Cost-Effectiveness in Health and Medicine

Researchers should use the best available data for determining the cost and effectiveness of a treatment strategy, whether from randomized controlled trials, observational studies, or descriptive series. Models should be used to supplement but not replace data directly observed in empirical study.

Expressing and Interpreting Cost-Effectiveness

The degree of cost-effectiveness in economic studies is commonly expressed in terms of ICER, net health benefit (NHB), or NMB. These three terms are related conceptually and mathematically by the willingness-to-pay threshold (WTP or λ).

Incremental Cost-Effectiveness Ratio

The ICER is a ratio of the difference in cost to the difference in effectiveness of an intervention in relation to a baseline comparator. It is expressed in the following formula:

$$\text{ICER} = (\text{Cost}_{\text{intervention}} - \text{Cost}_{\text{baseline}}) / (\text{Effect}_{\text{intervention}} - \text{Effect}_{\text{baseline}}).$$

Defining a baseline comparator is one of the most critical and frequently neglected elements of a cost-effectiveness study. There is seldom a true "do-nothing" approach that is without cost or effect on the patient. For example, a patient treated conservatively for a rotator cuff tear may accrue significant costs in pain medications, physical therapy, and steroid injections. He or she may also have significant improvement in pain and quality of life as a result of these treatments over time. It is important that a study of the cost-effectiveness of surgical repair of the rotator cuff over a given time frame includes the change in cost and utility of nonsurgical care as a comparator.

The cost-effectiveness plane is a graphic representation of the ICER that aids in its interpretation (**Figure 1**). There are four quadrants defined by whether the difference in cost and effect is positive or negative between the new intervention and the comparator. In quadrant II the cost of the intervention is higher but the effectiveness is lower, which results in the intervention being "dominated" by the comparator. In this case the comparator is always preferred. In quadrant IV the intervention is more effective and less costly, and therefore results in cost savings. It is therefore

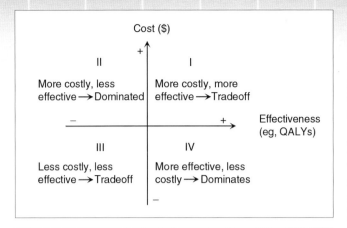

Figure I The cost-effectiveness plane.

said to "dominate" the comparator and is always preferred. In quadrant I, the cost and effect are both higher for the intervention, which is the most common scenario. In this case the choice is dependent upon the decision maker's willingness to pay for a given effect. Quadrant III is the case in which the new intervention is less costly and less effective than the established baseline. Interpretation of this scenario is controversial; the concept of willingness to pay in quadrant I can again be applied, but in this case to the comparator rather than the new intervention.

The WTP concept attempts to identify a threshold of acceptability for the incremental cost-effectiveness ratio.[21] Stated differently, it is the cost-effectiveness threshold, below which an intervention is considered to be cost-effective. Although $50,000/QALY is a frequently reported WTP threshold, it is somewhat arbitrary and is rarely used in healthcare policy decision making.

The NHB and NMB are alternative means of expressing the results of an economic analysis. The NHB is the net gain in effectiveness (eg, QALYs) from an intervention based on a given willingness to pay. It is calculated using the following formula:

$$NHB = \Delta Effect - \Delta Cost / \lambda$$

where $\Delta Effect$ is the difference in effectiveness, $\Delta Cost$ is the difference in cost, and λ is WTP. Using the same definitions, the NMB is calculated using the following formula:

$$NMB = \Delta Effect \times \lambda - \Delta Cost$$

Net monetary benefit is similar to the cost-benefit study design and has the advantage of allowing comparisons with strategies unrelated to health. It is important to recognize that assumptions regarding WTP are built into the calculations of NHB and NMB. If the ICER is greater than the WTP, the NHB and NMB will be negative, whereas if the ICER is less than the WTP, and therefore favorable, the NHB and NMB will be positive. Because the WTP is difficult to define absolutely and at the discretion of the decision maker, the ICER is often preferred.

In a hypothetical example, suppose rotator cuff repair for

a 60-year-old patient with a full-thickness supraspinatus tear costs $11,000 and results in an expected utility of 20 QALYs over the remainder of the patient's lifetime, and nonsurgical management costs $1,000 and results in an expected utility of 19 QALYs. Payer A is only willing to pay $5,000/QALY whereas Payor B is willing to pay $100,000/QALY. The ICER would be ($11,000 − $1000)/(20 QALYs − 19 QALYs) = $10,000/QALY. Using the ICER calculated, Payer A would not be willing to pay for rotator cuff repair (WTP < ICER) whereas Payer B would be willing to pay for rotator cuff repair (WTP > ICER). The NMB and NHB in contrast to the ICER would be unique for each payer and allows further quantification of the magnitude of gain or loss associated with selecting rotator cuff repair as a treatment strategy. For payer A, NMB = (20 QALYs − 19 QALYs) × $5,000/QALY − ($11,000 − $1,000) = (-$5,000), indicating a net monetary loss. For payor B, NMB = (20 QALYs − 19 QALYs) × $100,000/QALY − ($11,000 − $1,000) = $90,000, indicating a net monetary gain. The NHB would be calculated similarly but would give a result in QALYs. In practice, the WTP is rarely explicitly defined; as a result, the ICER is generally preferred to the NHB or NMB.

Recommendations of the US Panel on Cost-Effectiveness in Health and Medicine

Economic analyses should report the total cost and effectiveness, incremental cost and effectiveness, and incremental cost-effectiveness ratios.

Valuing Effectiveness
Quality-Adjusted Life-Years

The most common health outcome measure used in economic analyses is the QALY, which is a year of life spent in a health state weighted by the utility of that health state. For example, if it is assumed that the utility of hip osteoarthritis is 0.6, 10 years with the condition would yield 6 QALYs. An intervention that restores perfect hip function for 10 years would result in a net gain of 4 QALYs.

There are several significant assumptions underlying the QALY, not the least of which is that the preference for a health state remains constant regardless of the duration of the health state. For example, in the QALY model, 10 years with hip osteoarthritis results in exactly twice the number of QALYs as 5 years. This assumption is not supported by empirical evidence, which demonstrates that quality of life often declines over time in a chronic health state such as osteoarthritis.[22] Healthy-years equivalents were developed as an alternative to QALYs to avoid this assumption[23,24] and are assigned using a time tradeoff (TTO) approach specific to the expected duration of the disease. This is theoretically beneficial to more accurately reflect individual preference but has not been widely applied due to the time-consuming nature of collecting healthy-years equivalents for all relevant health states and durations. Therefore, QALYs remain the gold standard for conducting a cost-utility analysis.

Disability-adjusted life-years (DALYs) were developed and are used primarily by the World Health Organization for estimation of global disease burden, but can also be used for economic analysis.[25] The DALY is similar to the QALY but the scale is inverse; that is, a disease with high morbidity results in more DALYs. Unlike the QALY, the values assigned to a given disease are determined by an expert panel rather than using an empirically derived estimate of utility.

Recommendations of the US Panel on Cost-Effectiveness in Health and Medicine

QALYs should be used to quantify health benefits in the denominator of the incremental cost-effectiveness ratio.

Deriving Utility

There are two broad categories of methods used to estimate the utility of a health state for a CEA. The first category, the empiric method, is obtained from the general population to elicit preferences for various disease states. The standard gamble technique is the gold standard for determining the utility of a health state.[10] It involves a choice between remaining in an undesirable health state or accepting a gamble between perfect health and death. The lowest probability of perfect health that is acceptable in the gamble is the utility of the health state. For example, to determine the utility of hip osteoarthritis, healthy individuals could be asked to choose between having hip arthritis or taking a gamble in which there is a 99% chance of perfect health with no hip arthritis and a 1% chance of death. If this choice is deemed acceptable, the probability of perfect health would be lowered until reaching the threshold where the individual prefers to accept hip arthritis rather than take the gamble. If this threshold occurred when the probability of perfect health is 60% and death is 40%, the estimated utility of hip osteoarthritis would be 0.6.

An alternative method for determining utility empirically is the TTO method.[26] Subjects are asked to make a choice between a given time with the undesirable health state in question and a shorter duration with perfect health. The ratio of the two time intervals is an estimate of the utility of the health state. In the above example of hip osteoarthritis, an individual could be asked to trade 10 years of osteoarthrities to have 9 years of perfect health. If this scenario were acceptable, the number of years of perfect health would be lowered until reaching the threshold where 10 years of arthritis is preferred. If the threshold of acceptability was 6 years of perfect health versus 10 years of arthritis, the estimated utility would be 0.6.

Preference-Weighted Generic Measures

Because the standard gamble and TTO can be impractical to administer for all possible health states, the second method for estimating utility includes survey instruments that have been developed and correlated with the empiric instruments. These surveys seek to capture relevant domains of quality of life that underlie the preference for a particular health state. Unlike the empiric instruments, most can be completed quickly either in person or by mail. This is generally much more practical in the setting of most trial-based CEAs. A few of the more common preference-weighted survey instruments are the EQ-5D, Medical Outcome Survey Short Form–6(SF-6D), and Health Utilities Index.

EQ-5D

The Euroqol group developed the EQ-5D to assess health outcomes in a practical, standardized manner. The questionnaire uses five distinct domains: mobility, self-care, usual activities, pain/discomfort, and anxiety/depression. There are five questions, the results of which have been correlated to results of the standardized gamble to calculate a utility value.[27]

SF-6D

The SF-36 is a well-known and commonly used survey instrument to assess quality of life. It is not, however, designed to determine utility. The SF-6D has more recently been developed to allow calculation of utility using a subset of six SF-36 domains. It is reduced to 11 items and has been correlated with the standard gamble.

Health Utilities Index

The Health Utilities Index is a preference-based questionnaire designed to generate a utility score from 0 to 1. Three versions were developed chronologically: Mark 1, Mark 2, and Mark 3. The latter two are more commonly used and can be used together because they are complementary. Responses are then translated into a utility score using a multiplicative function that was derived from correlation with a combination of a visual analog score (the Feeling Thermometer) and the standard gamble.

Recommendations of the US Panel on Cost-Effectiveness in Health and Medicine

Utilities should reflect community preferences rather than those of patients, providers, or investigators. Empiric measures, such as the standard gamble or TTO, and preference-weighted generic measures, such as the EQ-5D or Health Utilities Index, are considered acceptable methods for estimating utility.

Estimating Costs
Perspective

Determination of the relevant costs associated with a healthcare intervention is highly dependent on the perspective of the decision maker. Perspectives commonly considered are those of government or private payers, hospitals, and society. The societal perspective is recommended by the US Panel on Cost Effectiveness Analysis and includes not only the direct costs of medical care, but economic effects of the intervention on employment, school, and other societal interests.[10] These additional effects may be less relevant to other decision-makers with a more narrow focus. This may result in the inclusion or exclusion of certain costs from the numerator of the ICER, which could result in different conclusions.

Direct and Indirect Costs

Costs included in economic analyses are divided into direct and indirect sources. The direct costs of an intervention are the more readily apparent expenses stemming from medical treatment such as hospitalization, surgery, and outpatient visits. Indirect costs, which accrue from missed work, travel time, child care, and other sources of monetary loss that may be affected by an intervention, are often more difficult to quantify but nevertheless important, especially when performing a CEA from a societal perspective. In modeling studies, missed time is frequently estimated by using the average time of missed work multiplied by the average wage nationally.

Obtaining Cost Data

There are two approaches to collecting cost data: microcosting and gross costing.[23] Microcosting is an item-by-item estimation of the costs of an intervention that could include supplies, nursing care, and other aspects of surgical care or hospitalization. This technique is more frequently used in the trial setting, where individual-level data on each resource used in the course of a treatment are recorded and tallied. In contrast, gross costing typically uses diagnostic or procedural codes to obtain the aggregate cost of a disease or intervention from large state- or national-level databases. Gross costing is often used in modeling studies in which individual level data are unavailable. It has the benefit of being relatively generalizable and easy to obtain but has less flexibility in assessing less common diseases or subpopulations that may not have a specific code to distinguish them.

Discounting

Discounting is an important economic concept that stems from the principle that there is a preference for present rather than future benefits (for example, the time-value of money). Using a monetary example, an individual would rather receive a $10,000 reward now than in 10 years. An exact discount rate could be determined empirically by surveying individuals to determine the monetary value in 10 years that would be equivalent to a current value of $10,000. The idea of discounting medical outcomes and costs is more controversial but has been empirically studied. The US Panel on Cost Effectiveness Analysis recommends using a 3% annual discount on both future health benefits and costs.[10] This has the effect of favoring interventions that improve health in the present rather than the future.

It is important to distinguish discounting and time preference from inflation. Inflation is the rise in prices of goods and services over time. Economic analyses should adjust all prices to current value based on the inflation rate, typically determined by the Consumer Price Index. For example, in a

study of total hip arthroplasty, if costs of surgery were obtained from a database generated in the year 2000 whereas other costs were from 2010, the surgical costs would have to be adjusted to 2010 dollars. This is independent of the discount rate, which would remain 3%.

Recommendations of the US Panel on Cost-Effectiveness in Health and Medicine

Costs should be estimated from the societal perspective and include both direct and indirect costs of treatment. Both costs and health effects should be estimated over a lifetime time horizon, but non–health-related costs from additional years of life added by the intervention should not be included. Costs and health effects should be discounted at 3% per year, but 5% should be tested in sensitivity analysis for comparison with older studies.

Modeling

There are a variety of modeling methods that can be used to simulate health outcomes and costs associated with an intervention ranging in complexity from the simple decision tree to dynamic models. In general, the simplest model that can effectively address the question is preferred. Most models rely on categorizing a health problem and its subsequent outcomes into discrete health states. The expected progression of disease is estimated from the best available evidence, whether from a trial, database, or published literature.[23]

Simple Decision Tree

There are several important considerations in selecting a model. One of the first is whether outcomes evolve over time or are known within a short time frame after the intervention and remain stable over time; for the the latter case, a simple decision tree is well suited, and many surgical interventions fall in this category. An example would be a patient with a tibial shaft fracture considering surgical or nonsurgical intervention. Consequences of surgery could include successful union, nonunion, or infection, whereas nonsurgical outcomes could be successful union, malunion, or nonunion. By 1 year after surgery, these outcomes are usually known and are unlikely to change significantly over the remainder of a patient's life. A proposed model is shown in **Figure 2**.

The blue square represents the decision node, which is the branch point for all possible choices. The green circles are chance nodes, reflecting potential outcomes of each possible strategy. Listed below each outcome is its probability of occurring. It is important to note that at each node the sum of the probabilities is always 100%. At the far right, next to the red triangles, are the "rewards", which can be any outcome, cost, or both. In a cost-utility analysis, cost and QALYs are the two rewards. Through a process called folding back, which involves a weighted sum of the rewards at each node, the expected value of each strategy can be calculated and compared or used to calculate the ICER. In the tibial fracture example, the expected value of intramedullary nailing is 9.65

4: Clinical Science

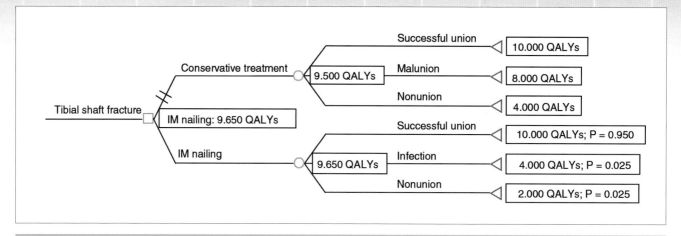

Figure 2 Simple decision tree comparing surgical and nonsurgical care for tibial shaft fracture.

whereas the expected value of nonsurgical care is 9.5, indicating that surgical treatment is expected to result in an additional 0.15 QALY compared with nonsurgical treatment.

Markov Modeling

In contrast to simple decision trees, Markov models incorporate cycling through health states over time. This facilitates a more realistic representation of the time course of diseases that progress through stages. Total joint arthroplasty procedures are commonly modeled using Markov models, because failure occurs steadily over time and is difficult to model accurately with a simple decision tree. The model output can be calculated by hand using matrix algebra but is more commonly obtained using computer-generated models. For each cycle of every health state there is a transition probability of moving to a new health state or remaining in the same health state. The model cycles over a fixed cycle length (for example, 1 year) for the time horizon of the model, which could be a specified duration relevant to the decision maker or the remainder of the lifetime. In a lifetime model there is usually a dead state (referred to as an absorbing state), meaning that transitions can occur into but not out of the state. In a lifetime model, the Markov model cycles until the entire cohort is in the dead state. If an assumption is made that the intervention does not influence mortality, as is often the case with orthopaedic interventions, the transition to the dead state is set equivalent to the national average death rate based on published life tables.

A Markov model is demonstrated comparing total hip arthroplasty to nonsurgical care in **Figure 3**. With each cycle of the model, the cohort progresses through each branch of the tree. At the terminal end of each branch (red triangle) is the starting health state for the subsequent cycle. This continues until all members of the cohort are in the dead state. Important assumptions of the Markov model include a fixed cycle length and constant transition probabilities over time. Commonly used software to generate these models allows the latter assumption of constant transition probabili-

ties to be overcome by varying the model inputs with each cycle, but classically this is not the case.

Monte Carlo Simulation

In cases where individual histories are important in predicting future events within the model, standard Markov modeling techniques, which assume a cohort of individuals progressing through the model simultaneously, are limited. For example, in a model evaluating the cost-effectiveness of total hip arthroplasty, a patient who undergoes a second or third revision may face a higher rate of failure than a patient who undergoes the first revision procedure. To account for this in a Markovian model structure, it is necessary to create a health state, called a tunnel state, for each revision, which can create a large, cumbersome Markov tree. Monte Carlo simulation addresses this problem by performing individual simulations repeatedly rather than assuming an entire cohort passes through the model simultaneously. The advantage of individual-level simulations is that events that predict future risks can be tracked and used to modify transition probabilities. In the arthroplasty example, the number of revisions could be tracked and incorporated into the risk of failure. The downside of these models is that to achieve stable estimates, hundreds of thousands or even millions of simulations must be performed, which requires significant computer power. In addition, there is a lack of transparency due to the complexity and greater difficulty in identifying and debugging errors in the model.

Other Modeling Techniques

Other types of models include dynamic models and discrete event simulation. Dynamic models incorporate interaction between individuals in the model. It is therefore most commonly applied in models of infectious disease where transmission is important for accurate simulation of the progression of a disease within a population. As musculoskeletal disease is rarely transmissible, the technique is infrequently applied in the field of orthopaedics.

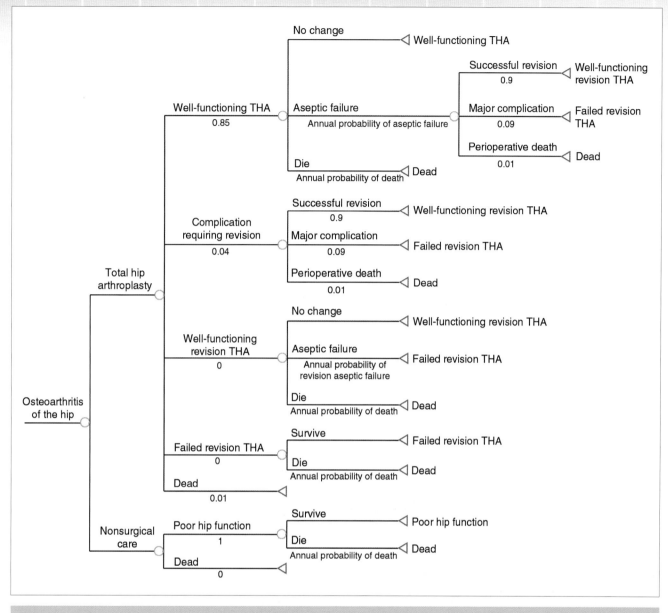

Figure 3 Markov model comparing total joint arthroplasty and nonsurgical care.

Discrete event simulation is another more complex modeling technique that allows uncoupling from several assumptions of the Markov model, notably the assumption of a constant cycle length and limited ability to track individual patient histories. Although this technique has advantages, its use has been limited in orthopaedic surgery, and further discussion is beyond the scope of this chapter.

Handling Uncertainty

Uncertainty exists in every aspect of a cost-effectiveness study, particularly when modeling is used. This includes the type of model selected (model uncertainty) and the inputs to the model such as costs, utilities, and probabilities of each health state (parameter uncertainty).

Parameter Uncertainty

Point estimates of each model variable are used, but often there is a range of plausible inputs either because of insufficient empirical data or chance error. This is referred to as parameter uncertainty. For any given model, there can be uncertainty in the estimates of cost, utilities, or the probability of events occurring within the model. The simplest method to address this is sensitivity analysis, which explores the output of the model across a range of a model input. For example, in the prior study of tibial fracture treatment, the cost-effectiveness could be calculated and plotted across a range of infection rates for surgical treatment. A sample is shown in **Figure 4**. This figure suggests that tibial fracture treatment is cost-effective for low infection rates, but if the infection rate is greater than 5%, nonsurgical treatment is

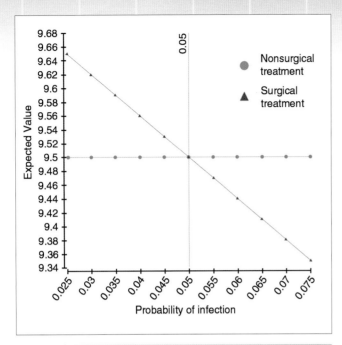

Figure 4 One-way sensitivity analysis.

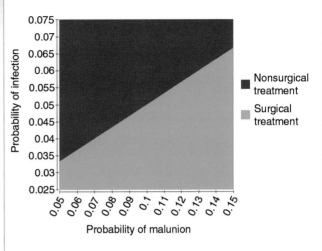

Figure 5 Two-way sensitivity analysis.

preferred. Identifying thresholds in an unknown variable is an important outcome of CEAs that informs clinicians and future research.

Two-way sensitivity analysis can be used to explore the impact of a plausible range of two variables. The value of each variable is plotted on each axis, and the plot is coded to indicate which strategy is preferred based on the value of the two variables. **Figure 5** shows a sample graph for the tibial fracture example using the probability of infection after surgical treatment and the probability of malunion after nonsurgical treatment. In the green area surgical treatment is preferred, whereas in the blue nonsurgical treatment is preferred.

Sensitivity analysis becomes more difficult if there is uncertainty in more than two variables. This is not uncommon, as there is typically a degree of uncertainty in every variable included in the model. To accomplish multivariate sensitivity analysis, probabilistic sensitivity analysis (PSA) is commonly employed. The PSA technique assigns a distribution rather than a point estimate for each variable in the model. There are different types of distributions depending on the type of data. Although a normal distribution could be used if the data supported the assumptions of normally distributed data, more commonly distributions that match the data inputs, such as the gamma distribution (ranges from 0 to infinite) and the beta distribution (ranges from 0 to 1), are used for costs and probabilities, respectively.

To conduct the PSA, the model is run using computer software thousands or even millions of iterations. In each iteration, a number is drawn for each model input from the assigned distributions. The results can then be plotted and

interpreted. Two common plots used are the 95% confidence ellipse and the cost-effectiveness acceptability curve, which are shown in **Figure 6**.

The 95% confidence ellipse is a plot on the cost-effectiveness plane of all the PSA trials with an ellipse encircling the 95% of simulations nearest the point estimate. It is analogous to a 95% confidence interval, and gives an idea of the upper and lower bounds of the ICER.

The cost-effectiveness acceptability curve can be one of the most informative methods of reporting results of a cost-effectiveness model. Along the x-axis is the WTP and on the y-axis is the proportion of trials that are acceptable based on the WTP. In the above example, using low WTP of $10,000/QALY, nonsurgical treatment is preferred in 87% of cases. In contrast, if the WTP is $50,000/QALY or $100,000/QALY, intramedullary nailing is preferred in 65% and 83% of cases, respectively.

Uncertainty also exists in estimates of the ICER from trial-based cost-effectiveness analyses. In these cases, standard statistical methods for estimating the 95% confidence interval are difficult to perform because of the calculation of the ICER. Bootstrapping is frequently used in these situations. Bootstrapping is a resampling of the data to explore the range of possible outcomes. For example, in a study of 1,000 patients, random samples of 100 could be drawn repeatedly and the ICER could be calculated for each sample. This creates a distribution of results that can then be expressed in terms of a 95% confidence interval.

Model Uncertainty

When uncertainty exists in choice of model structure or processes, it is referred to as modeling uncertainty.[28] Although there are logical reasons to choose a more or less complex model structure, it is difficult to have a high degree of confidence that the model ultimately chosen most accurately reflects the real world process being modeled. This

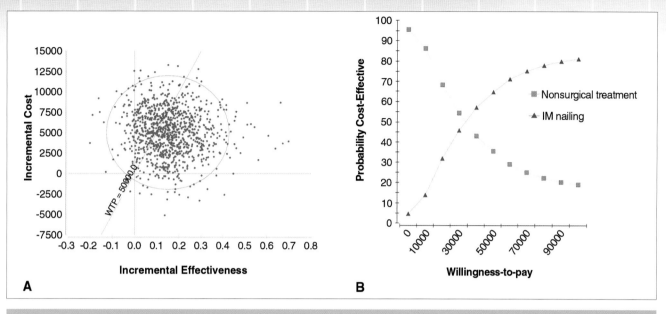

Figure 6 The 95% confidence ellipse (**A**) and cost-effectiveness acceptability curve (**B**).

can be addressed by performing the analysis using several possible modeling methods to explore the impact of the model choice. This is limited, however, by the time and resources needed to develop one model, let alone multiple models. An alternative approach uses validation of the model by comparing model predictions to real-world data or models generated by other researchers.

Recommendations of the US Panel on Cost-Effectiveness in Health and Medicine

Investigators should perform both univariate and multivariate sensitivity analysis.

Summary

As pressure to control healthcare costs increases, it will be important for orthopaedic surgeons to understand the principles of economic analysis. The US Panel on Cost-Effectiveness in Health and Medicine published a set of guidelines that are useful to understand the methods to properly conduct and report cost-effectiveness studies. The panel-recommended studies report the cost per QALY, which incorporates both the quality and quantity of life affected by an intervention. Strategies with lower cost per QALY may be preferred, but the conclusion is dependent on the willingness-to-pay threshold of the decision maker.

References

1. Weinstein MC, Stason WB: Foundations of cost-effectiveness analysis for health and medical practices. *N Engl J Med* 1977;296(13):716-721.

2. Bodenheimer T: High and rising health care costs: Part 1. Seeking an explanation. *Ann Intern Med* 2005;142(10):847-854.

3. Ubel PA, DeKay ML, Baron J, Asch DA: Cost-effectiveness analysis in a setting of budget constraints: Is it equitable? *N Engl J Med* 1996;334(18):1174-1177.

4. Firshein J: U.S. turns down Oregon plan to rank, ration Medicaid services. *J Am Health Policy* 1992;2(5):51-52.

5. Chambers JD, Neumann PJ, Buxton MJ: Does Medicare have an implicit cost-effectiveness threshold? *Med Decis Making* 2010;30(4):E14-E27.

6. Gold MR, Sofaer S, Siegelberg T: Medicare and cost-effectiveness analysis: Time to ask the taxpayers. *Health Aff (Millwood)* 2007;26(5):1399-1406.

7. Claxton K, Sculpher M, Drummond M: A rational framework for decision making by the National Institute For Clinical Excellence (NICE). *Lancet* 2002;360(9334):711-715.

8. Brauer CA, Neumann PJ, Rosen AB: Trends in cost effectiveness analyses in orthopaedic surgery. *Clin Orthop Relat Res* 2007;457:42-48.

9. Neumann PJ, Greenberg D, Olchanski NV, Stone PW, Rosen AB: Growth and quality of the cost-utility literature, 1976-2001. *Value Health* 2005;8(1):3-9.

10. Gold MR: *Cost-Effectiveness in Health and Medicine.* New York, NY, Oxford University Press, 1996.

11. Muennig P, EBooks Corporation: *Cost-Effectiveness Analyses in Health: A Practical Approach,* ed 2. San Francisco, CA, Jossey-Bass, 2008.

12. Drummond MF, McGuire A: *Economic Evaluation in Health Care: Merging Theory with Practice.* Oxford, NY, Oxford University Press, 2001.

13. Alolabi B, Bajammal S, Shirali J, Karanicolas PJ, Gafni A, Bhandari M: Treatment of displaced femoral neck fractures in the elderly: A cost-benefit analysis. *J Orthop Trauma* 2009;23(6):442-446.

14. Adla DN, Rowsell M, Pandey R: Cost-effectiveness of open versus arthroscopic rotator cuff repair. *J Shoulder Elbow Surg*

4: Clinical Science

2010;19(2):258-261.

15. Drummond M: Economic analysis alongside clinical trials: Problems and potential. *J Rheumatol* 1995;22(7):1403-1407.

16. Weinstein JN, Lurie JD, Tosteson TD, et al: Surgical versus nonoperative treatment for lumbar disc herniation: Four-year results for the Spine Patient Outcomes Research Trial (SPORT). *Spine (Phila Pa 1976)* 2008;33(25):2789-2800.

17. Weinstein JN, Lurie JD, Tosteson TD, et al: Surgical compared with nonoperative treatment for lumbar degenerative spondylolisthesis: Four-year results in the Spine Patient Outcomes Research Trial (SPORT) randomized and observational cohorts. *J Bone Joint Surg Am* 2009;91(6):1295-1304.

18. Tosteson AN, Lurie JD, Tosteson TD, et al: Surgical treatment of spinal stenosis with and without degenerative spondylolisthesis: Cost-effectiveness after 2 years. *Ann Intern Med* 2008;149(12):845-853.

19. Stahl JE: Modelling methods for pharmacoeconomics and health technology assessment: An overview and guide. *Pharmacoeconomics* 2008;26(2):131-148.

20. Slover J, Hoffman MV, Malchau H, Tosteson AN, Koval KJ: A cost-effectiveness analysis of the arthroplasty options for displaced femoral neck fractures in the active, healthy, elderly population. *J Arthroplasty* 2009;24(6):854-860.

21. Olsen JA, Smith RD: Theory versus practice: A review of 'willingness-to-pay' in health and health care. *Health Econ* 2001;10(1):39-52.

22. Bala MV, Wood LL, Zarkin GA, Norton EC, Gafni A, O'Brien BJ: Are health states "timeless"? The case of the standard gamble method. *J Clin Epidemiol* 1999;52(11):1047-1053.

23. Muennig P, Khan K: *Designing and Conducting Cost-Effectiveness Analyses in Medicine and Health Care.* San Francisco, CA, Jossey-Bass, 2002.

24. Mehrez A, Gafni A: Quality-adjusted life years, utility theory, and healthy-years equivalents. *Med Decis Making* 1989;9(2):142-149.

25. Murray CJ, Acharya AK: Understanding DALYs (disability-adjusted life years). *J Health Econ* 1997;16(6):703-730.

26. Bleichrodt H, Johannesson M: Standard gamble, time trade-off and rating scale: Experimental results on the ranking properties of QALYs. *J Health Econ* 1997;16(2):155-175.

27. Shaw JW, Johnson JA, Coons SJ: US valuation of the EQ-5D health states: Development and testing of the D1 valuation model. *Med Care* 2005;43(3):203-220.

28. Kim SY, Goldie SJ, Salomon JA: Exploring model uncertainty in economic evaluation of health interventions: The example of rotavirus vaccination in Vietnam. *Med Decis Making* 2010;30(5):E1-E28.

Chapter 30

The Scientific Foundations of Clinical Practice Guidelines

Charles M. Turkelson, PhD

Kristy Weber, MD

Introduction

The development of clinical practice guidelines began in earnest during the 1980s, and the National Guidelines Clearinghouse (http://www.guideline.gov) now houses more than 2,600 guidelines. All of these guidelines are new or updated (every 5 years). Although many of the guidelines are related to musculoskeletal conditions, some orthopaedic surgeons are unfamiliar with guidelines in general or with why and how they are developed. The American College of Surgeons described the apparent discrepancy as follows: "Thoughtful surgeons seek 'proof' to support their actions [despite] a pervasive lack of understanding and appreciation of the scientific method among clinicians." It is likely that orthopaedic surgeons increasingly will be expected by patients and payers to base their treatment decisions on the available evidence.

The orthopaedic surgery medical specialty, as represented by the American Academy of Orthopaedic Surgeons (AAOS), played a key role in the development of several sophisticated outcomes instruments such as the Disabilities of the Arm, Shoulder and Hand Questionnaire and databases such as the Musculoskeletal Outcomes Data Evaluation and Management System during the early and mid 1990s. Several years later, the AAOS produced clinical guidelines in the format of consensus algorithms developed by physician volunteers. The process was criticized because it lacked a strict

Dr. Weber or an immediate family member serves as a board member, owner, officer, or committee member of the Musculoskeletal Tumor Society and the Ruth Jackson Orthopaedic Society. Neither Dr. Turkelson nor any immediate family member has received anything of value from or owns stock in a commercial company or institution related directly or indirectly to the subject of this chapter.

methodology to combat bias, and the initiative was abandoned. In 2005 the AAOS Board of Directors made a commitment to develop evidence-based clinical practice guidelines based on accepted methodology, with a focus on maximizing transparency and minimizing bias. Between 2007 and 2011, the AAOS approved 14 evidence-based guidelines on topics including the treatment of osteoarthritis of the knee, the treatment of osteoporotic spinal compression fractures, and venous thromboembolic disease prophylaxis after total hip and knee replacements (available at http://www.aaos.org/research/research.asp).

Clinical practice guidelines have been described as "systematically developed statements to assist practitioner and patient decisions about appropriate health care for specific clinical circumstances."[1] This characterization implies both a patient-centered and a scientific focus. The reason for the emphasis on patients should be obvious. The emphasis on science arises from the ability of the scientific method to bring to bear a series of steps designed to eliminate bias. This emphasis does not always come easily to medicine because of the strength of the mentor-trainee tradition. It is important to consider whether the most convincing rationale for a procedure is "this is what I was taught by Dr. Smith" or "the evidence shows this is the best way to treat the patient's condition." (These are known as the eminence and evidence rationales, respectively.) Antman et al[2] found that the opinion of experts, as documented in textbooks and traditional review articles, lagged behind the evidence by as much as 13 years and that most experts continued to recommend some treatments even after they were shown to be ineffective or even harmful.

Although clinical practice guidelines have been criticized for promoting so-called cookbook medicine, a rigorously developed guideline is constructed to invite critical reading and transparency. A thorough guideline includes the infor-

Table 1

Guideline Developers' Possible Sources of Bias

Financial

Stock ownership or another financial interest related to the guideline topic

Professional income derived from treating a disease or condition related to the guideline topic

Long service on a health care–related government committee or with a private insurer

Intellectual

Authorship of published research on a guideline-related topic

Personal clinical experience related to the topic

Adapted with permission from Detsky AS: Sources of bias for authors of clinical practice guidelines. *CMAJ* 2006;175(9):1033-1035.

Table 2

Clinical Practice Guidelines in the National Guideline Clearinghouse, by Type of Sponsor (as of March 16, 2009)

Type of Sponsor	Number of Guidelines
Medical specialty society (US or other)	959
Professional association (US or other; mostly nonphysician or physician-nonphysician groups)	408
Government agency (non-US)	214
Federal, state, or local government agency	165
Nonprofit organization	142
Independent expert panel	97
Academic institution (US or other)	98
Disease-specific society (US or other)	202
Hospital or medical center (US or other)	26
For-profit organization	21
Managed care organization	11
Total	**2,343**

Adapted with permission from Lo B, Field MJ, eds: *Conflict of Interest in Medical Research, Education, and Practice.* Washington, DC, National Academies Press, 2009, chapter 7, pp 189-215.

mation used to construct each of its recommendations and describes how this information was identified and evaluated. Critical readers can then decide for themselves whether the guideline's recommendations are sound.[3] Authors of a scientific guideline welcome critical evaluation and modify the guideline as new evidence becomes available. This cycle of quality improvement occurs when new information informs the revision of an evidence-based guideline on a regular basis. The guideline development process, as described in this chapter and followed at the AAOS, sets a high standard for transparency, methodology, and minimization of bias. This chapter describes guideline development for the benefit of a critical reader who wishes to determine whether the recommendations are fully supported by objectively collected evidence.

Bias in Guideline Development

Not all clinical practice guidelines are truly scientific or evidence based. The development process often is subject to bias. Many current guidelines are not what the Institute of Medicine originally intended and amount merely to consensus reports.[1,4] Some of the biases that can affect a guideline are listed in **Table 1**.

A financial conflict of interest arises when an individual receives money from or owns stock in a company with a financial interest in the outcome of the guideline. Most of the published literature on bias is related to this type of financial conflict of interest.[5] However, financial conflicts of interest are not the primary source of bias in guideline development. A clinical guideline is more likely to include a favorable conclusion about a procedure or other service if the guideline was developed by individuals who receive income from performing the procedure or service. A guideline developer's service on a government committee or with a

private insurer might create a bias in favor of recommending against certain procedures to decrease costs. An investigator in a key clinical study relevant to the topic is likely to prefer that the guideline confirm the study's conclusion. A guideline developer's personal experience can become a hindrance as well as a help. For example, Antman et al[2] found that experts, on the basis of their experience, were convinced that thrombolytic agents are ineffective because they cause bleeding. This belief is understandable because bleeding is immediately seen and is likely to be remembered. Nonetheless, the accrual of information from thousands of patients enrolled in published studies showed that the lifesaving benefit of using thrombolytic agents outweighs the morbidity caused by bleeding. Individuals are not the only source of bias; hospitals and academic medical centers can introduce an institutional bias,[6] and the organization sponsoring the development of a guideline also may have a set of biases (**Table 2**).

Those with the greatest expertise on the guideline topic have the greatest potential for introducing bias into the guideline development process. One method of minimizing this risk is to structure the process so that such individuals serve as content advisors, but the analysis of the published litera-

Table 3
Clinician and Methodologist Roles in AAOS Guideline Development

Clinicians

Develop initial guideline questions

Prepare recommendations and rationales based on the evidence report

Methodologists

Are free of possible conflicts of interest

Conduct an evidence analysis and report the results

Review the draft guideline to ensure that its recommendations and rationales conform to the evidence

Both

Assemble the evidence report, rationales, and recommendations into a draft guideline

Table 4
Questions for Evaluating the Risk of Bias in Guideline Questions

Did the guideline authors begin by formulating questions instead of answers?

Are the questions specific?

Did the guideline authors seek to answer only the original questions?

Did the final guideline answer all of the original questions?

ture is performed by conflict-free methodologists.[7] The AAOS is one of the few organizations that develops guidelines in this manner (**Table 3**).

A reader should begin evaluating a final guideline by determining whether bias influenced its recommendations. If so, the guideline may not be appropriate to guide clinical care. Rigorously developed guidelines use the scientific method to combat bias.

Guideline Questions

The goal of developing a clinical practice guideline is to arrive at practice recommendations. Guideline development should avoid looking for evidence to support suggested recommendations. Like a scientific study, a scientific guideline begins with questions, not answers. The guideline questions, sometimes framed as strawman recommendations, are hypotheses to be empirically tested during the course of guideline development. The data used to test the guideline hypotheses typically arise from published literature.

A well-framed question specifies the patient groups, interventions, comparisons, and outcomes of interest (the so-called PICO format). A good question does not include appropriateness (for example, "Which treatment is most appropriate for a patient with disease X?") because this factor is subjective and may vary among patients. Similarly, a well-framed question does not ask whether an intervention is medically necessary, and neither does it attempt to determine whether an intervention is "experimental" or is a "standard of care." Questions that use such terms are subjective and lead to an opinion-based rather than a scientific (data-driven) answer.

A well-designed guideline process will adhere to questions that follow the PICO format and ensure that all questions are answered in the final guideline. Considering only these initial questions combats the development of bias by preventing work group members from asking new questions as a means of seeking data to support a predetermined conclusion. Clinicians participating in a guideline development group probably will understand the most relevant clinical questions, and they are likely to ask those questions from the beginning of the process. If data are not available to answer the questions, the guideline developers can choose to abandon further development of the guideline or to acknowledge the lack of evidence.

Requiring that all questions are answered in the final guideline ensures that no data are hidden. Ideally, guideline developers should make the initial questions publicly available before they are answered. The AAOS clinical practice guideline process follows these strict rules to minimize the risk of introducing bias. The questions that should be asked about bias prevention in guideline questions are summarized in **Table 4**.

Rules of Evidence

A well-designed clinical study contains criteria for determining whether a patient is eligible for enrollment. Similarly, a scientific guideline uses criteria for determining whether a published study should be included. These criteria constitute the guideline's rules of evidence, and studies that do not meet the criteria are not considered. The guideline should include only studies relevant to the initial questions. The guideline's rules of evidence may be even more restrictive. Sometimes a relatively old study is not considered because it does not reflect current medical practice. Traditional review articles are almost never included because they are not a source of primary data and often are written to support a particular point of view. Meeting abstracts often are not considered because they are too brief to allow the quality of the described study to be fully evaluated.

Finally, guidelines typically include only the best available evidence. Because the focus of a guideline is patient-oriented outcomes, many guidelines include only studies of humans. Animal, in vitro, and biomechanical studies are excluded or deemphasized because they can only determine whether an intervention might be of use in patients, not

4: Clinical Science

Table 5

Questions for Evaluating the Risk of Bias in Article Inclusion Criteria Used for Guidelines

Did the guideline list the inclusion criteria for published research studies?

Were the criteria developed before any studies were examined?

Did the criteria consider factors in addition to the relevance of a study?

Did the criteria ensure that studies of humans would be emphasized?

Did the criteria ensure that only the best available evidence was included?

Did the criteria establish a quality threshold below which studies would not be included?

Did the guideline authors adhere to the inclusion criteria?

---

whether it actually was successful. Study design also is a basis for inclusion. Data from randomized controlled studies are the best possible evidence, but other data can be used if they constitute the best evidence that is actually available. For example, if data from controlled nonrandomized studies are available, data from uncontrolled studies should not be included. Including only the best available evidence avoids the risk that the results of the most credible studies will be diluted by the results of less credible studies.

Guidelines should exclude low-level evidence, even if it is the best available evidence. At a minimum, a guideline should not include retrospective uncontrolled studies, such as retrospective case series. These studies have almost no components of a true scientific study, such as a hypothesis, complete data collection, and safeguards to ensure that changes in patient outcome resulted from the intervention being studied. The inclusion of such nonscientific evidence may represent an attempt to justify a predetermined opinion.

The inclusion criteria should be adopted before any literature searches are conducted to prevent the selection of studies supporting a particular point of view. If research studies are examined before the criteria are developed or if no criteria are developed, there is a risk that a study may be preferred if it supports a particular point of view. Every well-designed guideline lists the study inclusion criteria used in developing its evidence report, but presence of such a list is no guarantee that the authors of a guideline adhered to the inclusion criteria. Determining the quality of a guideline's underlying data may require checking whether the listed studies (or a representative sample) meet the inclusion criteria. It is also helpful to determine whether studies published by a guideline author were given priority over studies of equal quality, particularly if the other studies reached a different conclusion.

A rigorous guideline should include a list of excluded studies, with the reasons they were excluded. Such a list serves to inform a critical reader that studies were not excluded because of their results. AAOS guidelines often exclude published studies written by members of the guideline work group. **Table 5** summarizes the questions a reader should ask about a guideline's inclusion criteria.

The Data Search

To avoid bias, the data collection process should include an attempt to locate all literature relevant to a guideline question. A published study in which only a part of the collected data were analyzed is suspect, particularly if the authors appear to have considered only data that agreed with preconceived opinions. A clinical practice guideline is held to the same standard. Thus, guideline authors should not rely solely on readily accessible studies from their files, and work on a guideline should not begin with authors exchanging published studies they wrote. An author's files may not be complete, and a study exchange may be an author's way of informing the other authors of what he or she thinks the guideline should ultimately recommend.

A guideline literature search should be extensive and should include databases other than MEDLINE. Suarez-Almazor et al[8] found that MEDLINE searches identified only 73% of the controlled studies related to rheumatoid arthritis, osteoporosis, and low back pain but that EMBASE searches identified 85% of such studies. Wilkins et al[9] found that MEDLINE identified only 40% of the unique citations in osteoarthritis but that EMBASE identified the remaining 60%. Because an incomplete data set might represent bias, a well-designed guideline is based on searches of both MEDLINE and EMBASE, at a minimum. Ten or more databases (such as CINAHL and the Cochrane Database of Systematic Reviews) may need to be searched. Bibliographies should be examined to ensure that no published research is overlooked. A guideline typically reports the search terms used in MEDLINE and sometimes in other databases. The absence of such a list could mean that the search was not systematic and introduces the possibility that the studies represented in the guideline are not completely representative of the literature.

The most thorough way for a reader to determine whether all appropriate studies were considered is to repeat the search process using the guideline authors' stated inclusion and exclusion criteria. Doing so requires a great deal of effort but allows the reader to determine whether the guideline contains sufficient information for replicating the search process; if it does not, there is reason for concern. The questions to ask about the methods for obtaining information for a guideline are provided in **Table 6**.

Study Quality Evaluation

It is critical for guideline developers to evaluate the quality of the available evidence. The Cochrane Collaboration and

Table 6

Questions for Evaluating the Risk of Bias in a Literature Search Used for Guidelines

Did the authors search multiple databases to locate published research studies?

Are the electronic database search strategies described in the guideline?

Were the electronic database searches supplemented by hand searches of published bibliographies?

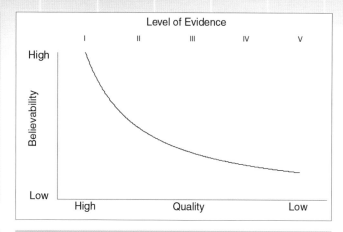

Figure 1 The relationship between study quality and the believability of its results.

some other groups prefer to evaluate studies in terms of the risk of bias.[10] "Quality" and "risk of bias" are measured in the same way, and these terms are used interchangeably in this chapter. Poor-quality evidence is common in the medical literature and is difficult to trust. The challenges posed by suboptimal evidence are particularly keen in orthopaedics, where uncontrolled studies are common.[11] Uncontrolled studies do not account for the possibility that patients' symptoms wax and wane as part of the natural course of the disease or condition. Thus, any improvements found in such a study may be the result of the disease course rather than the treatment. Randomized controlled studies on orthopaedic topics often are of relatively low quality,[12] and the validity of the results of many studies reported in orthopaedic journals is questionable.[13,14]

The believability of the study's evidence is related to its quality: results from a high-quality study are believable, and results from a low-quality study are not believable (**Figure 1**). Level of evidence is one of the methods professional societies most commonly use to index the quality of a study, and it also serves as an indicator of believability. A simplified version of the system used by *The Journal of Bone and Joint Surgery* is shown in **Table 7**. More than 50 systems for evaluating the quality of a study are available. Authors do not apply the rules consistently, however, and many of the currently available systems are not used by methodologists.[15] In addition, level I studies do not always report whether adequate safeguards were used to prevent bias.[16]

The use of a level of evidence system does not guarantee the absence of bias. Guideline developers can minimize the risk of bias by asking several individuals to independently determine a study's level of evidence, with any disagreements resolved through discussion. This approach does not ensure that all important aspects of study quality are considered, however. Another option is for guideline developers to evaluate study quality using a system other than or in addition to level of evidence. Both simple and complex methods are available for evaluating randomized controlled studies and case studies,[17-19] and it can be difficult to choose among them. The AAOS has adopted a comprehensive approach to evaluating different aspects of study quality; the

checklist in **Table 8** is used to evaluate studies with parallel control groups.

Guideline developers must follow a clear set of rules that will ensure the same standards are consistently applied to all evidence. The rules must establish the consequences of the answer to every question before the quality evaluation is begun, and they should be included in the final guideline. Otherwise, the guideline developers could be tempted to more heavily weigh a flaw in a study that contains uncomfortable data, compared with a study that has a favorable conclusion. Consider, for example, two studies designed in exactly the same manner except that only the second study used stochastic randomization. Now imagine that the first study found a procedure used by physicians in the guideline-developing organization to be ineffective and the second study found it to be effective. Without a rule that clearly defines the consequences of a negative answer to a randomization question on the quality evaluation checklist, a work group might be tempted to conclude that the studies were of equal quality, that the literature was contradictory, and that further research was needed. With a rule in place, the work group is led to conclude that the procedure is ineffective. The AAOS uses a comprehensive quality evaluation checklist and has clear-cut rules as to the consequences of the answer to every question asked during the evaluation.

A quality evaluation checklist should be composed of properly worded questions. For example, a potential for bias is created if a question asks whether the assignment of patients to groups was appropriate rather than whether randomization was stochastic. Detailed instructions for answering each checklist question enhance the accuracy of the answers, combat bias, and facilitate reproducibility. The checklist questions should be directed toward study quality rather than reporting. For example, a question that asks whether the study described how patients were assigned to groups is a question about reporting. A high score might be assigned even if the study described the use of a suboptimal method for patient assignment. The checklist should not be

4: Clinical Science

Table 7

Journal of Bone and Joint Surgery Levels of Evidence System

Level of Evidence	Type of Study			
	Therapeutic	**Prognostic**	**Diagnostic**	**Economic and Decision Analysis**
I	High-quality RCT Systematic review of Level I RCTs	High-quality prospective study Systematic review of Level I studies	Test of previously developed diagnostic criteria on consecutive patients (with universally applied reference "gold" standard) Systematic review of Level I studies	Sensible costs and alternatives; values obtained from many studies; with sensitivity analyses Systematic review of Level I studies
II	Lesser quality RCT Prospective comparative study Systematic review of Level II studies or Level I studies with inconsistent results	Retrospective study Untreated controls from an RCT Lesser quality prospective study Systematic review of Level II studies	Development of diagnostic criteria on consecutive patients (with universally applied reference "gold" standard) Systematic review of Level II studies	Sensible costs and alternatives; values obtained from limited studies; with multiway sensitivity analyses Systematic review of Level II studies
III	Case-control study Retrospective comparative study Systematic review of Level III studies	Case-control study	Study of nonconsecutive patients; without consistently applied reference "gold" standard Systematic review of Level III studies	Analyses based on limited alternatives and costs; and poor estimates Systematic review of Level III studies
IV	Case series	Case series	Case-control study Poor reference standard	Analyses with no sensitivity analyses
V	Expert opinion	Expert Opinion	Expert opinion	Expert opinion

RCT = randomized controlled trial.

used to evaluate the quality of a study as a whole but should evaluate the quality of the evidence for each of the outcomes reported across all studies.[20,21] A randomized controlled study design that was perfect for evaluating a study's primary outcome may not be well designed for evaluating other reported outcomes. The quality of evidence for some outcomes is likely to be overestimated if the reviewer assigns a level of quality to the entire study rather than to each of its outcomes.

A quality checklist must consider the number of patients enrolled in the study (its statistical power) and the number of patients at follow-up for every outcome. Most studies that report negative findings did not enroll enough patients to find a statistically significant effect.[22,23] Readers of such a study might incorrectly conclude that the study found no effect; instead, such a study is uninformative. However, a meta-analysis of small studies that found statistically nonsignificant effects might find a statistically significant effect by combining the results. Statistical power becomes lower as

the follow-up time is extended; the number of patients at long-term follow-up may be insufficient to confirm a statistically significant early effect.

The key features for determining whether a guideline used unbiased methods for quality evaluation are summarized in Table 9. A scientifically developed guideline will provide extensive documentation (in the form of tables) that provides the answers to every question about every outcome in every study considered in the guideline and allows the reader to unequivocally determine the answers to each question.

Outcomes Selection

The recommendations of clinical practice guidelines should focus on patient-oriented outcomes rather than on surrogate outcomes. Examples of patient-oriented outcomes include pain, quality of life, and death. Patient-oriented outcomes tell "what our patients want to know and would like us to fulfill as a diagnostic or treatment goal,"[24] and they let

Table 8

AAOS Checklist for Evaluating Studies With Parallel Control Groups

Did the study use stochastic randomization?

Was the study prospective?

Was blinding used for control group patients?

Was blinding used for those who assessed outcomes?

Was there empiric verification that the blinding achieved its objective?

Was the allocation to groups concealed?

Was patient follow-up greater than 80%?

Did patients in the study groups have similar baseline outcome values?

Did patients in the study groups have comparable characteristics?

Were patients in the study groups treated at the same centers?

Was the treatment duration the same in and across all groups?

Was the same concomitant treatment given to all groups?

Were the same instruments used to measure outcomes in all patient groups?

Were valid instruments used to measure outcomes?

Were the study authors free of relevant conflicts of interest?

Do the conclusions presented in the abstract agree with those presented in the full study?

Did the study report results for all outcomes mentioned in its methods section?

Were the statistical comparisons determined a priori?

Table 9

Questions for Evaluating the Risk of Bias in Guideline Quality Evaluation

Was the quality evaluation performed using a system other than or in addition to the assignment of levels of evidence?

Did the quality evaluation involve a priori rules describing the consequences of each answer to every question concerning quality?

Were the quality criteria consistently applied to all outcomes at all time points reported by all studies included in the guideline?

Were specific questions asked about quality (for example, did the study questions follow the PICO format)?

Were the questions truly about the quality of the study rather than about how well the study reported certain items related to quality?

Did the questions consider the number of patients being studied?

Did the questions determine the quality of evidence for each relevant outcome, rather than the entire study?

A scientifically developed guideline incorporates studies that used scientific measuring instruments to determine specific outcomes. Measuring quality of life and similar outcomes, such as pain, requires clinical investigators to use valid, reliable instruments. Instruments with unproven validity and reliability can be difficult to trust, especially if their use is limited to one group of investigators.

In the preferred development process for a clinical practice guideline, only the methods section of a study report is initially examined. If the study results are determined to be valid, the data presented in the results section are evaluated. Little weight is given to the discussion section and the authors' conclusions.[27] The discussion section often includes author bias, possibly stemming from manufacturer funding of the study.[28,29] A good guideline includes tables that report all outcomes from the included studies, as well as the times at which measurements were made.

A scientifically developed guideline evaluates both the benefits of a given medical treatment or diagnostic test and its adverse effects. Ignoring even a rare adverse effect, particularly if it is severe, is a form of bias that can have serious consequences for patients. Unfortunately, harms are not well reported in the medical literature,[30] and this factor affects how rigorously they can be evaluated in a guideline.

Guideline authors should specify which outcomes are critical to determining whether a medical service is effective. For example, it would be impossible to know whether total knee arthroplasty is effective without knowing whether it relieves pain; pain is therefore a critical outcome for deter-

us know "directly and without the need for extrapolation that a diagnostic, therapeutic, or preventive procedure helps patients live longer or live better".[25]

In contrast, a surrogate outcome is a substitute for a clinical event of true importance[26] and is of "uncertain clinical utility."[24] Radiographic findings, bone mineral density, laboratory results, and nerve conduction velocity are examples of surrogate outcomes. The concept is straightforward: if you want to know if you made something better, measure the thing itself rather than a substitute for it. Using a surrogate outcome can make an ineffective or harmful treatment look effective.[26] Surrogate outcomes may be measurable more quickly or less expensively than patient-oriented outcomes, but that factor does not make them superior. Surrogate outcomes may appear to be more objective than patient-oriented outcomes, but subjective outcomes usually are the outcomes that patients care about.

Table 10

Questions for Evaluating the Risk of Bias in Outcome Selection

Did the guideline give preference to patient-oriented outcomes over surrogate outcomes?

If a recommendation was made using surrogate outcome data, was the recommendation tempered accordingly?

Did the guideline give preference to measurements made using valid, reliable instruments?

Did the guideline contain evidence tables to demonstrate that the developers examined all relevant data?

Did the guideline developers consider both the benefits and the harms of the medical intervention of interest?

Did the guideline developers specify the critical outcomes?

Did the critical outcomes include both benefits and harms?

Were the critical outcomes specified before any studies were examined?

Were recommendations tempered (or not made) if critical outcomes data were lacking?

mining the effectiveness of total knee arthroplasty. Similarly, it is critical to know the mortality rate associated with total knee arthroplasty. To combat bias, the critical outcomes should be specified before work on the guideline begins. These outcomes should include both benefits and harms. If no data are available for a critical outcome, the relevant guideline recommendation should be tempered, or no recommendation should be made. The questions to be used in determining whether a guideline has examined outcomes in an unbiased fashion are summarized in **Table 10**.

Synthesis of Study Results

With rare exceptions, neither a randomized controlled study nor any other study should be interpreted in isolation.[31] The results of a single study could have been influenced by the skill and experience of the participating physicians, unique institutional practices, a patient group not representative of patients usually seen in clinical practice, the use of unique diagnostic methods, or other factors. The first randomized controlled studies published on a topic tend to find larger effects than later studies,[32,33] even when several hundred patients were enrolled, and caution is required regarding the reliability of the reported treatment effects. More than 10,000 patients must be randomized to resolve uncertainty about the first decimal point of the odds ratio derived from a meta-analysis of treatment effectiveness.[34] Guideline developers cannot control how many studies exist

on a topic but can modify the strength of their recommendations accordingly. A scientifically rigorous guideline usually is more cautious in recommending a medical device, drug, or procedure backed by sparse literature than in recommending one backed by substantial literature.

A rigorously developed scientific guideline synthesizes the results of all relevant studies. The synthesis can be qualitative (narrative) or quantitative, as in a meta-analysis, which statistically combines study results. A quantitative synthesis not only provides a numeric estimate of the size of the effect (for example, an odds ratio of 3.31) but also, if enough studies are available, explains any differences in the study results. A qualitative synthesis is performed if, as is often the case, the number of studies is too small for a quantitative synthesis.

A clinically relevant synthesis considers clinical importance as well as statistical significance. Statistically significant study results may not be clinically important, and clinical significance matters more to patients than statistical significance. The measures of clinical significance include the minimum clinically important difference and the minimum clinically important improvement (the smallest difference and the smallest improvement, respectively, that are considered acceptable by patients).[35] These two measures are related to many outcomes that are known and can be reported in the guideline, even if they were not reported in the original study.

An appropriate qualitative synthesis is not performed by tallying the number of studies that found (or did not find) statistically significant results. Instead, all outcomes are examined at all of the times they were measured. Data for a hypothetical example are presented in **Table 11.** In this example, five equal-quality studies of a treatment found at least one statistically significant result, and a study-by-study narrative description focused on statistical significance might conclude that the treatment is effective. However, these five studies reported a total of 56 measurements using 17 different outcomes instruments at 10 time points, and they reported clinical importance as well as statistical power (the number of patients measured at each time point). Of the eight statistically significant findings in favor of the treatment (in Table 11, A and B), only one is clinically important (outcome 13 at day 1). Most other statistically significant findings (A) tended to occur within the first 2 weeks after treatment and were not clinically important. One statistically significant finding suggested that the treatment led to a clinically important harm (outcome 14 at 1 week). Forty-seven observations (C) had nonsignificant results, despite a sufficiently large number of patients for finding a statistically significant effect. This data synthesis, in contrast to a narrative review, probably would lead to the conclusion that the treatment is not effective. Similar tables drawn from actual studies can be found in many AAOS guidelines.

The studies examined in a synthesis may have reached different conclusions. For example, two results for one out-

Table 11

A Sample Qualitative Synthesis of Study Outcomes

Treatment Outcome	Follow-up Point									
	1 Day	3 Days	7 Days	14 Days	1 Month	1.5 Month	3 Months	6 Months	6-12 Months	24 Months
1					C					
2							C	C		
3	A			A	C					
4			C		C		C	C		
5	A					A			C	C
6							F			
7			C		D		C	C		
8										C
9			C		C		C	C		
10					C					
11					C					
12			C		C		C	C		
13	A,B	C	C	C,F	D		C,F	C	C	C
14			E	A	C		C	C		
15		C	C	A,C	D		C	C		
16					C		F			
17					C		F			

A = statistically significant, clinically unimportant benefit.
B = statistically significant, clinically important benefit.
C = statistically insignificant (and, therefore, clinically unimportant) benefit in an adequately powered study.
D = statistically significant, clinically unimportant harm.
E = statistically significant, clinically important harm.
F = number of enrolled patients was too small for detecting a statistically significant effect; the results are uninformative.

come at one time point might differ in that one showed the treatment to have a statistically significant benefit and the other found a statistically significant harm. Accordingly, it is important that guideline authors discuss the articles that agree with their recommendations, as well as the articles that disagree with them, and explain why one set of findings was chosen over another. Guideline users should evaluate these reasons to ensure they are free from bias.

One study's statistically nonsignificant result does not necessarily disagree with another study's significant result,[36] particularly if one study was large and the other was small. Two studies that found statistically significant results may disagree with each other. Meta-analytic statistics can be used to determine whether the study results are truly different (heterogeneity testing). A crude method of determining whether two or more results are significantly different is to examine their 95% confidence intervals; if they do not overlap, the results are different. The important questions used to determine whether a guideline considered study results in a scientific manner are summarized in **Table 12**.

The Role of Expert Opinion

Effectiveness has been demonstrated for fewer than half of current medical treatments[37] (**Table 13**). Most guidelines contain some recommendations based on expert opinion, but to avoid bias a guideline must be judicious in the use of expert opinion. The US Preventive Services Task Force has proposed a useful set of guides to consider in evaluating the suitability of a recommendation based on expert opinion, including costs, potential preventable disease burden, harms, and current medical practice associated with the service.[38] AAOS guidelines may incorporate expert opinion to recommend the use of services such as a patient history and physical examination, which are of low cost, have virtually no associated harms, and can be used with all patients. However, AAOS guidelines do not use expert opinion to rec-

Table 12

Questions for Evaluating the Risk of Bias in a Research Synthesis

Was the strength of the guideline recommendations influenced by the amount of available evidence?

Did the guideline authors consider clinical importance?

Did the guideline authors synthesize all relevant results across all reported time periods, rather than conducting a study-by-study narrative review?

If the guideline's recommendations do not agree with all study findings, did the guideline authors explain their decision?

If the guideline's recommendations do not agree with all study findings, did the guideline authors always prefer higher quality evidence to lower quality evidence?

Did the synthesis determine that results of different studies were significantly different?

Table 14

Questions for Evaluating the Risk of Bias in Use of Expert Opinion

Did the guideline use a formal, a priori system for incorporating expert opinion?

Did this system preclude the use of expert opinion in some circumstances?

Did the guideline distinguish between recommendations based on data and recommendations based on expert opinion?

Table 13

The Effectiveness of Specified Medical Treatments, as Reported in Randomized Controlled Studies

Description of Effectiveness	Percentage of Treatments (N = 3,000)
Beneficial	11
Likely to be beneficial	23
Trade-off between benefits and harms	7
Unknown effectiveness	51
Unlikely to be beneficial	5
Likely to be harmful or ineffective	3

Adapted with permission from British Medical Journal Evidence Center: What conclusions has Clinical Evidence drawn about what works, what doesn't, and what we cannot draw conclusions about based on randomized controlled trial evidence? *Clinical Evidence*, 2010. http://www.clinicalevidence.org/x/set/static/cms/efficacy-categorisations.html. Accessed January 30, 2012.

ommend a costly procedure for treating a condition that is not debilitating.

A guideline should describe its specific rules for constructing a recommendation based on expert opinion and should state that the rules were determined before work on the guideline began. Furthermore, a guideline must clearly distinguish between recommendations based on evidence and those based on expert opinion. The AAOS guidelines designate a recommendation based on expert opinion as a "consensus recommendation." The important questions to ask about use of expert opinion in a guideline are summarized in Table 14.

Strength of Recommendations

A guideline may recommend some medical services without reservation and others only with caution, depending on the likelihood that future research will lead to the recommendation being modified or overturned. These concepts are re-

flected in recommendation strength. An opinion-based recommendation usually is not characterized by its strength. Designating a recommendation as strong or weak is useful for avoiding bias because guideline authors are prevented from overemphasizing their own studies or implying equal confidence in all of their recommendations.

Formal systems are available for determining a recommendation's strength as well as the strength of the underlying evidence.[1,39] The quantity of evidence is one factor in determining the strength of a recommendation, but more evidence leads to more confidence only if the evidence is of relatively high quality. Confidence is not increased if there are a large number of studies whose results are not credible. The strength of a guideline's recommendations varies with the quality of the evidence.

The definition of "sufficient evidence" should be determined before guideline development begins. One study is only rarely sufficient (as in a population-based study). The AAOS uses the system described in *The Journal of Bone and Joint Surgery*,[40] and other systems also are available. Adopting such a system before work on the guideline begins can combat the possibility of bias from overemphasis of a guideline author's own research.

The consistency of the literature also is a factor in the strength of a recommendation. If all studies relevant to a recommendation found the same result, there can be more confidence in the recommendation than if the study findings differed (with consideration of their quality). The definition of "consistent" should be established beforehand. The generalizability of the evidence is the final factor influencing the strength of a recommendation. Although randomized

Table 15

Questions for Evaluating the Risk of Bias in Applicability Evaluations

Did the evaluation of generalizability involve a priori rules that detailed the consequences of each answer to every question asked about applicability?

Were the criteria for determining generalizability consistently applied to all outcomes at all time points reported by all studies included in the guideline?

Were the questions truly about generalizability rather than about how well the study reported certain items related to generalizability?

Did the generalizability appraisal consist of determining the quality of evidence for each relevant outcome, rather than the entire study?

Table 16

Questions for Evaluating the Risk of Bias in Characterizing the Strength of Recommendations

Was the strength of each guideline recommendation characterized?

Did the characterization of strength involve the quality, quantity, consistency, and generalizability of the evidence?

Was the system for determining the strength of the recommendations determined a priori?

Table 17

Questions for Evaluating the Risk of Bias in Peer Review

Was the guideline peer reviewed?

Were individuals and/or organizations likely to disagree with the guideline's recommendations included among the peer reviewers?

Did the guideline authors document their responses to the peer review?

Were the responses to the peer review in keeping with the scientific nature of guideline development?

controlled studies typically provide the most convincing evidence that a treatment is effective, such studies may enroll carefully selected patients and treat them according to a stringent protocol. There is a substantial difference between finding a treatment effective under ideal conditions and in actual clinical practice. The results of studies conducted by a preeminent surgeon are likely to be less generalizable than those conducted by a wide array of surgeons. Formal tools for assessing a study's generalizability are still being refined, and it cannot be known whether some of the relevant factors are more important than others in actual clinical practice. Therefore, it may be wise to be conservative in reassessing a recommendation's strength based on the generalizability of the underlying evidence. As in almost every aspect of guideline development, there should be a formal, a priori system for judging generalizability. Such a system also should meet the criteria for judging study generalizability, as summarized in Table 15. The PRECIS instrument[41] is useful for this purpose.

Treadwell et al[20] list many other factors that can affect a reader's confidence in the evidence for and strength of a guideline's recommendations.[21] A rigorously developed guideline uses all of the factors discussed in this chapter, at a minimum, to determine the strength of its recommendations. The key questions to ask in evaluating whether the strength of evidence in a guideline was scientifically determined are summarized in Table 16.

Peer Review

Guidelines, like studies submitted to a journal for publication, should undergo peer review. Peer review by itself does not guarantee an unbiased guideline because guideline developers could seek out reviewers who are likely to agree with the guideline's recommendations. Instead, guideline developers should seek reviewers and reviewing organizations that may disagree with the recommendations. The

guideline should include the identity of the reviewers so that readers can verify the integrity of the process. Peer review does not imply that the developers adequately responded to the reviewers' comments, however. The AAOS publishes its responses to reviewers in the guideline and on the AAOS website. The key questions to ask about the peer review of a guideline are summarized in Table 17.

Summary

This chapter describes the development of high-quality clinical practice guidelines related to medical treatments, with an emphasis on the methodology used to develop AAOS guidelines. Evidence is the foundation of the quality focus in health care, and orthopaedic surgeons are expected to understand the tenets of evidence-based medicine. Orthopaedic residents and young practicing surgeons need to learn methodology that will improve the quality of clinical research studies. Clinical guidelines will play an increasingly greater role in patient care, and therefore it is imperative for a reader to be able to determine a guideline's quality. An inadequate guideline may be biased, rely too heavily on expert opinion, be out of date, or serve to market a drug or procedure. An ideal guideline discusses a topic with significant practice variability, for which a valid evidence base can guide recommendations. Developing a trustworthy guide-

4: Clinical Science

line, like conducting a trustworthy clinical study, requires the use of the scientific method, which is detailed and arduous. The scientific method extends far beyond citing the conclusions of authors of published papers, relying on the opinions of guideline developers, or searching for studies that support those opinions.

Physicians should not use guidelines unquestioningly; flexibility is necessary to allow for patient comorbidities. The physician should exercise sound clinical judgment by consulting high-quality clinical practice guidelines, assessing ongoing evidence, and making a decision on the care of each individual patient. Online continuing medical education courses related to evidence-based orthopaedics and clinical guideline development are available through Orthopaedic Knowledge Online (http://www.orthoportal.org) and the AAOS website (http://www.aaos.org/research/research.asp).

References

1. Field MJ, Lohr KN, Ioannidis J; Institute of Medicine Committee on Clinical Practice Guidelines: *Guidelines for Clinical Practice: From Development to Use.* Washington, DC, National Academies Press, 1992.

2. Antman EM, Lau J, Kupelnick B, Mosteller F, Chalmers TC: A comparison of results of meta-analyses of randomized control trials and recommendations of clinical experts: Treatments for myocardial infarction. *JAMA* 1992;268(2): 240-248.

3. Jones RS, Richards K: Office of Evidence-Based Surgery charts course for improved system of care. *Bull Am Coll Surg* 2003;88:11-21.

4. Shaneyfelt TM, Centor RM: Reassessment of clinical practice guidelines: Go gently into that good night. *JAMA* 2009; 301(8):868-869.

5. Detsky AS: Sources of bias for authors of clinical practice guidelines. *CMAJ* 2006;175(9):1033-1035.

6. Lo B, Field MJ, eds: *Conflict of Interest in Medical Research, Education, and Practice.* Washington, DC, National Academies Press, 2009.

7. Hirsh J, Guyatt G: Clinical experts or methodologists to write clinical guidelines? *Lancet* 2009;374(9686):273-275.

8. Suarez-Almazor ME, Belseck E, Homik J, Dorgan M, Ramos-Remus C: Identifying clinical trials in the medical literature with electronic databases: MEDLINE alone is not enough. *Control Clin Trials* 2000;21(5):476-487.

9. Wilkins T, Gillies RA, Davies K: EMBASE versus MEDLINE for family medicine searches: Can MEDLINE searches find the forest or a tree? *Can Fam Physician* 2005;51:848-849.

10. Higgins JP, Green S: *Cochrane Handbook for Systematic Reviews of Interventions.* Oxford, England, Wiley-Blackwell, 2008.

11. Obremskey WT, Pappas N, Attallah-Wasif E, Tornetta P III, Bhandari M: Level of evidence in orthopaedic journals. *J Bone Joint Surg Am* 2005;87(12):2632-2638.

12. Boutron I, Tubach F, Giraudeau B, Ravaud P: Methodological differences in clinical trials evaluating nonpharmacological and pharmacological treatments of hip and knee osteoarthritis. *JAMA* 2003;290(8):1062-1070.

13. Gartland JJ: Orthopaedic clinical research: Deficiencies in experimental design and determinations of outcome. *J Bone Joint Surg Am* 1988;70(9):1357-1364.

14. Kiter E, Karatosun V, Günal I: Do orthopaedic journals provide high-quality evidence for clinical practice? *Arch Orthop Trauma Surg* 2003;123(2-3):82-85.

15. Atkins D, Eccles M, Flottorp S, et al; GRADE Working Group: Systems for grading the quality of evidence and the strength of recommendations: I. Critical appraisal of existing approaches. *BMC Health Serv Res* 2004;4(1):38.

16. Poolman RW, Struijs PA, Krips R, Sierevelt IN, Lutz KH, Bhandari M: Does a "Level I Evidence" rating imply high quality of reporting in orthopaedic randomised controlled trials? *BMC Med Res Methodol* 2006;6:44.

17. Jadad AR, Moore RA, Carroll D, et al: Assessing the quality of reports of randomized clinical trials: Is blinding necessary? *Control Clin Trials* 1996;17(1):1-12.

18. Chalmers TC, Smith H Jr, Blackburn B, et al: A method for assessing the quality of a randomized control trial. *Control Clin Trials* 1981;2(1):31-49.

19. Carey TS, Boden SD: A critical guide to case series reports. *Spine (Phila Pa 1976)* 2003;28(15):1631-1634.

20. Treadwell JR, Tregear SJ, Reston JT, Turkelson CM: A system for rating the stability and strength of medical evidence. *BMC Med Res Methodol* 2006;6:52.

21. Schunemann H, Brozek JL, Oxman AD, eds: GRADE Working Group: *GRADE Handbook for Grading Quality of Evidence and Strength of Recommendation,* version 3.2. 2009. http://ims.cochrane.org/revman/gradepro. Accessed January 5, 2012.

22. Moher D, Dulberg CS, Wells GA: Statistical power, sample size, and their reporting in randomized controlled trials. *JAMA* 1994;272(2):122-124.

23. Bailey CS, Fisher CG, Dvorak MF: Type II error in the spine surgical literature. *Spine (Phila Pa 1976)* 2004;29(10):1146-1149.

24. Hurwitz SR, Slawson D, Shaughnessy A: Orthopaedic information mastery: Applying evidence-based information tools to improve patient outcomes while saving orthopaedists' time. *J Bone Joint Surg Am* 2000;82(6):888-894.

25. Shaughnessy AF, Slawson DC: What happened to the valid POEMs? A survey of review articles on the treatment of type 2 diabetes. *BMJ* 2003;327(7409):266.

26. Grimes DA, Schulz KF: Surrogate end points in clinical research: Hazardous to your health. *Obstet Gynecol* 2005; 105(5, pt 1):1114-1118.

27. Montori VM, Jaeschke R, Schünemann HJ, et al: Users' guide to detecting misleading claims in clinical research reports. *BMJ* 2004;329(7474):1093-1096.

28. Leopold SS, Warme WJ, Fritz Braunlich E, Shott S: Association between funding source and study outcome in orthopaedic research. *Clin Orthop Relat Res* 2003;415:293-301.

29. Ezzet KA: The prevalence of corporate funding in adult lower extremity research and its correlation with reported results. *J Arthroplasty* 2003;18(7, suppl 1):138-145.

30. Ioannidis JP, Lau J: Completeness of safety reporting in randomized trials: An evaluation of 7 medical areas. *JAMA* 2001;285(4):437-443.

31. Glasziou P, Vandenbroucke JP, Chalmers I: Assessing the quality of research. *BMJ* 2004;328(7430):39-41.

32. Gehr BT, Weiss C, Porzsolt F: The fading of reported effectiveness: A meta-analysis of randomised controlled trials. *BMC Med Res Methodol* 2006;6:25.

33. Trikalinos TA, Churchill R, Ferri M, et al: Effect sizes in cumulative meta-analyses of mental health randomized trials evolved over time. *J Clin Epidemiol* 2004;57(11):1124-1130.

34. Ioannidis J, Lau J: Evolution of treatment effects over time: Empirical insight from recursive cumulative metaanalyses. *Proc Natl Acad Sci U S A* 2001;98(3):831-836.

35. Kvien TK, Heiberg T, Hagen KB: Minimal clinically important improvement/difference (MCII/MCID) and patient acceptable symptom state (PASS): What do these concepts mean? *Ann Rheum Dis* 2007;66(suppl 3):iii40-iii41.

36. Hedges LV, Olkin I: *Statistical Methods for Meta-analysis.* Orlando, FL, Academic Press, 1985.

37. British Medical Journal Evidence Center: What conclusions has *Clinical Evidence* drawn about what works, what doesn't, and what we cannot draw conclusions about based on randomized controlled trial evidence? *Clinical Evidence*, 2010. http://clinicalevidence.bmj.com/ceweb/aboutus/knowledge.jsp. Accessed December 14, 2011.

38. Petitti DB, Teutsch SM, Barton MB, et al: Update on the methods of the U.S. Preventive Services Task Force: Insufficient evidence. *Ann Intern Med* 2009;150(3):199-205.

39. Atkins D, Best D, Briss PA, et al: Grading quality of evidence and strength of recommendations. *BMJ* 2004;328(7454):1490.

40. Wright JG, Einhorn TA, Heckman JD: Grades of recommendation. *J Bone Joint Surg Am* 2005;87(9):1909-1910.

41. Thorpe KE, Zwarenstein M, Oxman AD, et al: A pragmatic-explanatory continuum indicator summary (PRECIS): A tool to help trial designers. *J Clin Epidemiol* 2009;62(5):464-475.

4: Clinical Science

Chapter 31

Detection of Bias in Clinical Research

Andrew H. Schmidt, MD
Seth S. Leopold, MD
Steven D. Stovitz, MD, MS

Introduction

The concept of evidence-based medicine (EBM) has gained significant support during the past decade among researchers, journals, academic faculties, health policy makers, clinicians, and third-party payers.[1-3] An example of EBM in practice is the development of clinical practice guidelines; these are typically developed by a team of researchers who perform a rigorous review of the available literature using specific and well-defined search strategies applied to a defined clinical question, followed by critical assessment of the scientific methodology of each article using specific checklists that rate methodologic quality, statistical summation and comparison of the data, and finally the development of the guideline with specific mention of the weight of the evidence behind each recommended practice.[4]

However, EBM is not just for experts. Clinicians must also read and evaluate the medical literature for their own purposes, whether for patient care, continuing medical education, or licensing, credentialing, and certification.[3] In these instances, a large part of the process is the individual clinician's own assessment of the literature. One of the most important factors to take into account in evaluating published research is the identification of potential sources of bias in a given study. Recent surveys have shown disparity in the familiarity of clinicians with the fundamentals of EBM.[5] The purpose of this chapter is to review the concept of bias in clinical research, describe how bias affects the reported results of clinical trials, and provide the clinician with some tools to evaluate the literature critically.

What Is Bias, and Why Is Bias an Important Consideration in Clinical Research?

In the context of science, bias represents nonrandom error in the conduct, measurement, analysis, or reporting of data. Such errors create false differences between observed and true values and misrepresent one outcome with respect to another. Bias is therefore different from random errors or lack of precision. Although bias is often considered to be caused by human factors, nonhuman systematic errors that consistently affect one study group differently than others also introduce bias and may, in fact, be the largest cause of bias in clinical research. Unlike random error, bias is difficult or impossible to control for statistically and causes estimates of treatment effect to be either exaggerated or attenuated, leading to inaccurate conclusions. Bias can be introduced at any step in the conduct of a clinical trial. Although there are many types of bias,[6] within clinical research bias is generally categorized according to the stage of research in which the particular element of bias is introduced. Although the divisions are somewhat artificial, for this chapter four important forms of bias will be discussed: selection bias, intervention/exposure bias, measurement bias, and transfer bias. Such biases are generally a function

Dr. Schmidt or an immediate family member has received royalties from Smith & Nephew; is a member of a speakers' bureau or has made paid presentations on behalf of Synthes; serves as a paid consultant for or an employee of Medtronic, DGIMed Orthopedics, and AGA; serves as an unpaid consultant to Twin Star Medical; owns stock or stock options in Twin Star Medical, Anthem Orthopedics, and Conventus Orthopaedics; and has received research or institutional support from Twin Star Medical. Neither of the following authors nor any immediate family member has received anything of value from or owns stock in a commercial company or institution related directly or indirectly to the subject of this chapter: Dr. Leopold and Dr. Stovitz.

4: Clinical Science

of study design, and their presence and potential influence can be discerned by assessing the methodology of a given study. Other forms of bias (for example, publication bias and positive-outcome bias) create nonrandom influences affecting study reporting and publication and therefore can cause an entire body of literature on a given topic to misrepresent true research findings. These kinds of bias often are not discernible and require analysis of larger denominators – such as manuscripts submitted to institutional review boards, specialty societies, or journals[7] – or explicit experiments to be performed on the peer review process itself,[8] to identify their presence.

Bias in its many forms is very common.[9,10] Gøtzsche[10] examined 196 articles comparing nonsteroidal anti-inflammatory drugs, finding evidence of bias in the abstract or conclusion in 42% of the studies and invalid statements in 76% of the conclusions. Bias can be difficult to detect,[11] but with rigorous application of EBM methods, insight often can be gained into its most common and most important forms. Furthermore, the influence of systematic errors (bias), as opposed to random error, is not corrected simply by increasing sample size. For the same amount of error, P-values generated by statistical tests will appear smaller with increased sample size. A large sample size coupled with a small P value can result in the mistaken belief that a real difference in outcomes between treatment groups exists when, in fact, the treatment has no effect. Because bias can result in incorrect answers to clinical questions, clinicians must have a working framework to assess clinical research studies and be wary of bias.

Types of Bias

For the purposes of discussion, bias will be considered in its two broad forms: bias affecting the design and conduct of individual studies (those that often can be discerned by the careful reader), and forms of publication bias that instead influence a body of knowledge on particular topics (and typically cannot be identified even by the most critical reader of an individual study). With an understanding that experts disagree on subtleties regarding specific categories of bias, the following explanation is proposed as a guide that will serve as a useful framework when reviewing the orthopaedic literature.

Bias in Study Design
Selection Bias: Are the Subjects Who Were Analyzed (in All Groups) Representative of the Population Targeted?
The internal validity of clinical studies is diminished if there are differences among subjects in the treatment groups, aside from the intervention provided, that may influence the outcomes. Such differences constitute selection bias; when selection bias is present it cannot be known whether the outcome was the result of the treatment itself or these underlying differences. For the purposes of this discussion, se-

lection bias will be considered to involve events leading up to subject enrollment; later events (primarily differential loss to follow-up) that change the composition of study groups will be considered in the section on transfer bias.

In the context of a clinical study, selection bias can increase the likelihood of concluding that there is a difference in the outcome of interest between treatment groups when no difference actually exists. For example, imagine that a new technique for anterior cruciate ligament reconstruction is advertised with the claim that it will allow patients to compete in sports sooner after surgery. Certain patients sign up and are then followed. Their results are then compared with those of patients who had standard reconstruction. The new treatment appears better because the patients return to sport sooner. However, the new technique may have had no effect on the outcome. The difference between the groups may have been solely the result of selection of the new technique by those seeking a faster return to sport.

In an ideal study, participants are allocated into treatment groups in a manner that neither participants nor study investigators can predict or influence, and if done in a random manner, all known and unknown confounding factors will, on average, be distributed evenly in the various groups. Selection bias is caused by differential assignment of subjects by clinical investigators or use of randomization schemes that are not in fact truly random (such as those based on the day of the week or medical record number). All of these factors can cause unequal distribution of confounders among treatment groups, in turn resulting in outcome differences not related to the study intervention. The process of assigning a subject to a treatment group is concealed when the investigator has no influence or insight into the assignment process and therefore cannot predict to which group a given patient will be assigned. Some methods of randomization, such as alternating group assignment, assignment by day of the week or medical record number, or even the use of nonopaque envelopes, potentially allow the investigator to predict what group a given subject may be assigned to and perhaps use inclusion and exclusion criteria inconsistently. When selection bias occurs, it compromises the ability of the trial to demonstrate causal relationships (internal validity) and its generalizability (external validity).

Lack of adequate randomization tends to result in exaggerated estimates of treatment effect.[11] The effect of selection bias on study outcomes has been quantified by comparing the results of observational studies with randomized trials.[12,13] One such study found considerable differences in more than half the comparisons, with the differences ranging from an underestimation of the treatment effect by 76% to overestimation of effect by 160%.[13] Observational studies typically generate larger group differences, suggesting a more beneficial effect of the study intervention, than corresponding randomized trials.[13] However, both Benson and Hartz[14] and Concato et al[15] compared several published observational studies with randomized controlled trials and found that the average results were similar, concluding that in practice, well-designed cohort or case-control studies do not necessarily overestimate treatment effects. Thus, study quality is very important, and critical reviewers of the literature should be aware that the conclusions of well-designed and executed nonrandomized studies may be more valid than the results of poorly done randomized trials.[2]

In summary, it is crucial for readers judging the internal validity of a given study to consider selection bias as a major component of it. Although many studies present tables comparing the distribution of demographic and other potential confounding variables among the treatment groups, simple demonstration that these groups appear to be the same is not sufficient to rule out the possibility of bias.[16] Furthermore, the mere fact that a given study was randomized does not by itself guarantee that the study is of high quality and the results can be considered valid. High-quality studies will use fair (and explicitly stated) approaches to patient recruitment, good-quality random allocation of patients into treatment groups, and adequate concealment. When all of these factors coexist in a study, the impact of selection bias is minimized.

Exposure/Intervention Bias: How Was the Intervention Provided, and Who Received It?

By definition, studies of orthopaedic surgical interventions compare one surgical procedure to another intervention, often a different procedure. Systematic differences in how a treatment or intervention is performed, or how subjects are exposed to the study intervention, result in what is referred to as intervention or exposure bias. There are many different types of exposure bias, each reflecting a given manner in which different groups within a study may be systematically exposed to different interventions.

An important form of exposure bias that commonly affects orthopaedic studies is so-called performance bias. Clearly, surgical technique differs among surgeons. A surgeon who has taken the time and energy to design a study on a specific technique for an orthopaedic problem likely has more experience than most at treating that problem (although that surgeon may also have a vested interest in the study drawing certain conclusions). More generally, there is considerable evidence that volume and experience with a particular procedure may result in a lower likelihood of complications; if high- and low-volume surgeons contribute cases differentially to the treatment and control arms of a surgical study, one might reasonably suspect performance bias to have an impact on the outcome.

So-called cotreatment bias is a common form of performance bias. Cotreatments are therapeutic maneuvers used in addition to the main intervention being studied; they can introduce bias when applied differentially to the intervention and control groups. For example, some studies about surgical versus nonsurgical management of Achilles tendon rupture use different physical therapy protocols and immobilization approaches between the surgically and nonsurgically treated groups; both immobilization and therapy have

been separately demonstrated as having an impact on outcomes in other studies. Another common example of cotreatment bias in the orthopaedic literature is differential use of nonsteroidal anti-inflammatory drugs or analgesics between the control and intervention groups. Cotreatment bias should be suspected in particular when historical control groups are used in a study because other adjuvants to treatment (such as use of intraoperative imaging in the trauma and spine literature) have changed significantly over time.

Measurement Bias: How Is the Outcome of Interest Measured?

Research involves the collection of data, and the measurement of any parameter is associated with some degree of uncertainty in the measurement itself. As in other aspects of study design, nonrandom systematic errors can occur during collection of study data; this is referred to as measurement bias. Common sources of measurement bias are systematic errors in the instrument used to measure outcomes (instrument bias), lack of tools to demonstrate important differences among groups (insensitive measure bias), observation error during the recording of data because of lack of blinding (expectation bias), errors in the recall of past events (recall or memory bias), and differences in reported results because of the awareness of a subject that he or she is being studied (attention bias).

Measurement bias can be very subtle. For example, it is common to measure and report disease status before and after an intervention, yet doing so alters the observed effect of the treatment.[17] Diseases or health status are determined on the basis of some test, which has an inherent uncertainty. When these test values vary continuously, single determinations of their results are likely not to represent the actual state of disease because of this measurement error. If the first test result happens to be at the extreme end of the range of uncertainty, subsequent measurements of this same test (for example, after an intervention is completed) are themselves likely to be less extreme than the first. This is due in part to the regression to the mean effect.[18]

A logical outcome for a study, such as pain or time to fracture healing, is often subjective. For example, recent reports have highlighted the difficulties in defining when a fracture is considered healed.[19] In some studies, reoperation rates are used as an outcome.[9,20] However, even the decision to reoperate is somewhat subjective and may vary between investigators and sites,[9] and such differences introduce measurement bias.

A very important source of potential bias in a study is the process of ascertaining outcome. Study investigators often have some interest in the outcome of the study, whether it is as simple as generating a positive outcome that guarantees publication or as complex as a personal financial interest in whatever is being studied. When someone who has the ability to influence the determination of any outcome parameter has knowledge of the treatment group to which a given subject is assigned, there is an opportunity for differential misclassification, whereby one of the treatment groups is assessed differently than the others. To minimize this form of bias, outcomes of any study should be determined by an independent observer who is not aware of what treatment a given study subject received and who is completely disinterested in the outcome of the study. Blinding is readily accomplished in pharmaceutical trials, but is much harder to achieve in surgical studies. However, even in surgical trials, outcomes often include assessment of function or review of imaging studies; both can be done by blinded observers simply by using an independent assessor, by hiding incisions, and by masking radiographs.[21] Poolman et al[22] reviewed 32 randomized clinical trials published in a prominent orthopaedic journal and found that half of them did not report blinding of outcome assessors when blinding was possible. Of interest, this article noted that unblinded outcomes assessment was associated with a dramatically larger treatment effect for both continuous and dichotomous outcome variables.[22] Although blinding should be done whenever possible, it may not completely eliminate differential misclassification when a study outcome has multiple components.[23]

Assessment of outcomes often is done using self-reported scores on surveys that can be taken either by interview or by mail. Readers should be aware of the numerous opportunities for bias in the use of such questionnaires, which collectively can be termed response bias. One form of response bias relates to survey nonresponders, who have been shown to have worse outcomes than those who do respond to mail surveys.[24,25] This latter form of response bias is very similar to transfer bias in a cohort or randomized trial and is caused by patients being lost to follow-up, as discussed in the following section. In an attempt to evaluate whether bias occurs with the use of outcome surveys, researchers should compare variables (for example, age, sex, and preoperative pain level) of those who responded and those who did not.

Whenever possible, as with other types of outcomes, surveys done by interview should be administered by independent assessors who are blinded to the treatment provided to a patient.[26] Steps should be taken to ensure that interviewers administer the surveys as originally designed[22] and that they do not "lead" or otherwise influence the response of the patient. Finally, there can be cultural and/or language barriers that bias responses to an outcome instrument; ideally every instrument should be specifically validated for use in the language in which it is given. Many commonly used instruments have been translated and validated in several languages.[26]

Assessment of outcomes can be done at several hierarchical levels,[27] beginning with measurement of objective biologic variables associated with disease status (such as a hemoglobin A1c level in a patient with diabetes), and progressing through measures of symptom severity, functional status, general health perceptions, and overall quality of life.[27] With each higher level of assessment, there is more

opportunity for bias, often outside the control of the investigator.[26] This is because at each higher level, there are increasing inputs that are related to patient factors such as motivation, secondary gain/symptom amplification, and social support. These factors may not be adequately explained or controlled for, leading to potential bias in data. To provide a comprehensive assessment of outcome status, many researchers use multiple outcome scores, such as both a disease-specific and a general health status questionnaire. However, the use of multiple scales increases the likelihood of differences being found by chance alone, analogous to the situation when multiple statistical tests are performed.[26] When multiple outcome assessments are done, it is recommended that they be chosen to cover all five levels of outcome defined by Wilson and Cleary[27] and that the most important outcome be defined a priori, with statistical correction done for multiple comparisons.[26]

Transfer Bias: Is Subject Follow-up the Same in All Groups?

An important factor to consider in clinical studies is differential loss to follow-up between arms of a clinical series;[28] this phenomenon is referred to as transfer bias. Patients are lost to follow-up in nearly all clinical studies, and this can often introduce bias because the outcome for these patients is unknown and the investigators are forced to make assumptions about them that may not be valid. The magnitude of this problem becomes greater with studies reporting longer term outcome, as more and more patients are lost to follow-up. Thus, although long-term follow-up studies are necessary to truly understand the benefits of an intervention, these studies have to be the most carefully scrutinized for transfer bias. Loss to follow-up is a particular problem for studies of patients suffering orthopaedic trauma, who as a group may be less likely to follow up than other demographic groups. If patients who do not complete follow-up differ in any systematic way from those who do complete a clinical trial, the results of the study will not be valid. If the proportion of such patients is large (greater than 20% is a commonly accepted threshold), or if there are differences in the proportion of missing patients between study groups, the likelihood of bias is large.

Patients who are lost to follow-up often have worse outcomes than those who remain in a study,[24,25,28,29] and erroneous conclusions could be drawn about the effect of the study intervention.[29] Kim et al[24] performed a mail survey of patients who had undergone total knee arthroplasty and identified a group of nonresponders, defined as those who did not respond to two questionnaires. All of the nonresponders were contacted directly by the investigators, and this group was found to report notably worse satisfaction and outcome scores than did the responders.[24] Murray et al[28] performed a survivorship analysis of 2,268 patients who had total hip arthroplasty. During 16 years of follow-up, 142 patients were lost; these patients were reviewed and were found to have significantly worse pain, range of motion, and opinion of their progress than patients who continued to be seen. These authors concluded that unless these patients are accounted for, the results of the survival analysis will be overly optimistic and that authors should make vigorous attempts to avoid losses to follow-up.[28]

There are ways to ascertain whether transfer bias is present. Investigators can compare the outcomes at the patient's last intermediate follow-up point with that of patients who were not lost and see if there are differences. Extraordinary efforts can be made to contact patients who were lost to determine how they were doing and whether they experienced any adverse events.[30] When there are study participants who do not complete a study, their characteristics and last-known outcome should be carefully reported.[31]

Other circumstances aside from incomplete follow-up can distort the effects of randomization. Examples include the presence of crossover patients, who change from one treatment group to another, and enrolled patients, who do not meet the inclusion or exclusion criteria. These sorts of events can be best clarified for the reader in a flow diagram, as recommended by the CONSORT group (http://www.consort-statement.org).[32]

Publication Bias and Other Influences on the Literature as a Whole

So far, this chapter has examined bias in the design and execution of individual studies that can be detected by a critical review of a given study's methodology. There are other biases that affect a body of knowledge; for example, biases that affect how data are reported, published, and then, in turn, interpreted. These biases are not evident when reading one paper on a topic; instead, they can only be inferred when looking at an entire cross-section of literature on a given topic.

Publication Bias

Publication bias refers to the possibility that the medical literature may favor the publication of studies with certain characteristics, such as those that report the beneficial effects of treatment, over studies showing no difference or negative outcomes. This bias exists at several levels: researchers are less likely to submit research for publication when a difference is not found, and peer reviews or editors view studies that do not report a beneficial finding as less desirable for a particular journal. In one study, only 14% of unpublished randomized trials demonstrated benefit for a new therapy, compared with 55% of published studies.[33] Emerson et al[8] recently found strong evidence of positive-outcome bias among more than 200 reviews performed for two highly regarded orthopaedic journals. In this study, actual peer reviewers of two orthopaedic journals randomly reviewed one of two versions of a fabricated manuscript; one of the versions reported a positive outcome and the other version reported a no-difference result for the primary study end point. Importantly, the methods sections of both manuscript versions were identical, and both versions included the same pur-

posely placed errors. Reviewers of these two manuscripts strongly favored the version showing the positive outcome; they were more likely to recommend it for publication, less likely to find the purposely placed errors, and graded the quality of the (identical) methods sections more favorably.[8]

Funding Bias

Several studies have found an association between commercial funding sources and proindustry outcomes.[34,35] Leopold et al[34] reviewed all articles published in three major orthopaedic journals (one general and two specialty) and found that commercial funding was significantly associated with a beneficial outcome for the new treatment; 78.9% of industry-funded studies reported a beneficial outcome compared to 63.3% of nonindustry-funded studies. In contrast, in these same studies, the presence of a statistician or epidemiologist as a coinvestigator and the country of origin of the study were not associated with beneficial outcomes. Similar findings have been reported regarding presentations at the annual meeting of the American Academy of Orthopaedic Surgeons.[35] Another report examined not just published papers but all submissions to one high-impact orthopaedic journal and also controlled for study quality to determine whether funding source or outcome had an impact on the likelihood of a manuscript being accepted for publication.[7] When these important methodologic improvements were made (looking at the denominator of manuscripts submitted and controlling for study quality), the impact of publication bias was somewhat more subtle but was still present. Commercial funding was not found to be associated with a positive study outcome, and studies with a positive outcome were no more likely to be published than those with a negative outcome. However, commercially funded and US-based studies were more likely to be published, even though those studies were not associated with higher quality, larger sample sizes, or more rigorous levels of evidence. Even more importantly, the no-difference studies were found to be of better methodologic quality and larger sample size than the positive studies, yet the no-difference studies were not published more frequently.[7] Taking this in the context of the results cited previously by Emerson et al,[8] there does appear to be strong evidence that positive-outcome bias does affect orthopaedic peer review.

Publication bias severely affects the potential value of meta-analysis, a technique wherein the results of numerous trials are combined to increase the number of subjects and the likelihood of obtaining a realistic estimate of the true treatment effect of a given intervention. Meta-analyses are often done when large clinical trials that address specific questions are lacking. Such analyses are dependent on the assumption that all of the composite studies are themselves a random collection of possible studies. If studies are only selectively reviewed, then this basic condition of meta-analysis is not met.[33]

Importantly, if a body of literature has positive-outcome bias, then meta-analysis of that literature will systematically

4: Clinical Science

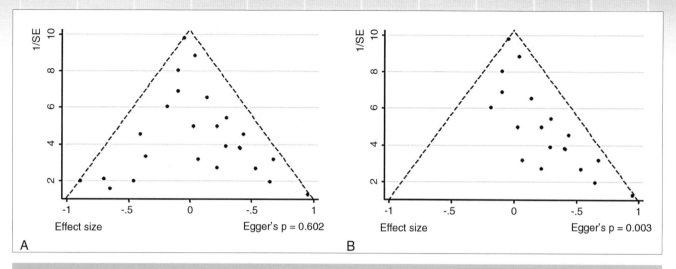

Figure 1 Examples of funnel plots. The funnel plot on the left (A) is symmetric, whereas the one on the right (B) is skewed. The lack of symmetry in plot (B) is suggestive of publication bias.(Reproduced with permission from Vauken P, Dorotka R: The prevalence and effect of publication bias in orthopaedic meta-analyses. *J Orthop Sci* 2011;16:238-244.)

result in a false inflation of the treatment effect size of the interventions being studied, making newer interventions seem more effective than they actually are. Funnel plots are a statistical tool that can be helpful in determining whether the literature surveyed in a meta-analysis has publication bias.[36] Funnel plots are graphic representations of effect estimates versus sample size (often represented as the standard error of the estimate). Larger studies should yield more precise estimates of effect and therefore cluster together at the top, whereas smaller studies with less precise results will scatter more at the bottom (**Figure 1**). The relative degree of asymmetry of a funnel plot has been associated with evidence of bias within the meta-analysis.[37, 38] However, funnel plots are not a panacea; there is good evidence that this approach is less effective than was once thought.[39, 40] Asymmetry in funnel plots — indicating lack of homogeneity in the individual studies represented in the plot — can have several explanations other than publication bias.[41]

Because meta-analysis combines data from many studies, bias in the component studies must be carefully assessed and controlled.[42] Bhandari et al[42] carefully evaluated 40 meta-analyses related to orthopaedic surgery that were published between 1969 and 1999. Eighty-eight percent were found to have methodologic flaws that could limit their validity. A critical step in meta-analysis is the selection of studies to include; this is often done by using one of many available methodologic quality scores. However, even this seemingly straightforward task can introduce bias. Jüni et al[43] have shown that the results of meta-analyses may be different depending on which quality scales are used. It has also been shown that there is a subjective component when interpreting the results of meta-analyses that can lead to discordance among different reviewers.[44]

One way to validate the concept of meta-analysis is to compare the results of single large randomized controlled trials to meta-analyses of smaller trials that address the same research question. The results of such comparisons have been inconclusive, similar to the findings when observational studies were compared to randomized studies as discussed earlier. Egger and Smith[45] report on a "misleading meta-analysis" of the effect of magnesium supplementation on improving mortality after myocardial infarction, a finding based on small studies with large treatment effects that was eventually refuted by a later megatrial. Ioannidis et al[46] point out that the different conclusions among sets of comparison studies can be explained by discrepancies in how trials and meta-analyses are selected for comparison.

Methods to Minimize Bias When Designing a Study

The key to preventing bias is first to understand the multiple ways that bias can creep into nearly every aspect of a study. More than 25 quality scales have been developed to assess the methodologic rigor of a study, which in turn reflects the likelihood of bias being present.[11] The guidelines proposed by the CONSORT group[32] seem to be most accepted by medical journals; careful integration of all of the items into the design of a proposed study will help to avoid the introduction of bias.

Selection bias can be minimized by using a prospective and truly randomized study design. When prospective randomized trials are not possible for a given research question, using a concurrent case-control design is generally better than using historical control groups. Systematic differences might exist among groups of patients treated or studied at different times; there may be unknown changes in demographic and/or clinical characteristics of the patients in each group if they were treated at different times.

Exposure bias is diminished by avoiding historical control groups and by using protocols that eliminate the poten-

Table 1
How to Review a Therapeutic Study

1. Are the Results of the Study Valid?
Primary Questions:
- Was the assignment of patients to treatment randomized?
- Were all patients who entered the trial properly accounted for and attributed at its conclusion?
- Was follow-up complete?
- Were patients analyzed in the groups to which they were randomized?

Secondary Questions:
- Were patients, health workers, and study personnel "blind" to treatment?
- Were the groups similar at the start of the trial?
- Aside from the experimental intervention, were the groups treated equally?

2. What Are the Results?
- How large was the treatment effect?
- How precise was the estimate of the treatment effect?

3. Will the Results Help Me in Caring for My Patients?
- Can the results be applied to my patient care?
- Were all clinically important outcomes considered?
- Are the likely treatment benefits worth the potential harms and costs?

Adapted with permission from Sackett DL, Straus SE, Richardson WS, et al: *Evidence-Based Medicine: How to Practice and Teach EBM*, ed 2. New York, NY, Churchill Livingstone, 2000.

tial for performance bias and cotreatment bias. Sites considered for participation in a surgical study should demonstrate competence for the study procedures; this can be done by selecting experienced investigators who have performed at a specified number of cases, and have the appropriate experience and research infrastructure to successfully carry out the study and all associated functions, such as accurately documenting and maintaining study data records. When an outcome is subjective and determined by different individuals, assessment of that outcome by a consensus committee might remove individual bias. Similarly, when reoperations are part of a given study's outcomes, the indications for that operation could be reviewed and approved by consensus, or at least very specific guidelines should be provided regarding when reoperation is appropriate. However, even use of specifically defined and agreed-upon criteria for reoperation is not sufficient to ensure comparability of results among different sites, because of differences in clinical decision making.[9]

Measurement bias is most effectively mitigated by ensuring adequately long and complete follow-up, by using validated outcome instruments, or, if doing a study on a diag-

nostic test, by ensuring that the gold standard is applied to all patients regardless of the result of the diagnostic test being studied.

Several means to minimize loss to follow-up have been reported.[47] These methods include carefully considering exclusion criteria so that patients not likely to follow up are not enrolled, such as patients who are incarcerated, live out of state, or are homeless. Of course, the exclusion of such groups will affect the generalizability of the results.

During the interim analysis of a study, reviewers should be skeptical of apparently large treatment effects, especially when they do not seem plausible or are explained by other things, such as differences in patient groups.[48] Such differences may be caused by random fluctuations in outcome, which may serve to exaggerate differences early in a study.[49]

Critical Analysis of the Scientific Literature

When reviewing any scientific study, the reader should have a critical mind and ask several questions in a systematic fashion.[50] A framework for interested readers is presented in the series of articles by Guyatt and Drummond[51] published in the *Journal of the American Medical Association* and available in compendium form, as well as a series of reviews in the *Journal of Bone and Joint Surgery*.[52-55] Much of the information contained in these articles is summarized in **Tables 1 through 4**. Several other concepts important to the critical assessment of research are reviewed in the following sections.

Common Statistical Misperceptions

As discussed, bias can be introduced at several points during the process of data analysis and reporting, but other errors are often made in the statistical tests used to analyze a study and in how those tests are used to make conclusions. Statistical errors are frequent; common pitfalls are for researchers to simply perform too many statistical comparisons, to overemphasize arbitrary levels of statistical significance as indicated by so-called *P* values, and to violate assumptions of statistical independence or repeated measures.

One example relates to how bilateral cases are handled in a study. Statistical tests often assume that measures are independent (not correlated with each other). However, if both limbs of a given patient are entered into a study, the outcomes of each limb might in fact be correlated, violating the assumption of independence.[56] Park et al[57] examined all of the articles published in the *Journal of Bone and Joint Surgery*, American volume, during 2007 and 2008. One hundred fifty-one of 486 articles (31%) included bilateral cases. One hundred twenty articles (25% of the total; 79% of the articles that had bilateral cases) were found to have possibly violated statistical independence. In the same article, Park et al[57] provide examples of how failure to account for statistical dependence leads to falsely narrow confidence intervals, thus suggesting with more certainty that a difference be-

Table 2

Evaluating and Applying the Results of Studies of Diagnostic Tests

1. Are the Results of the Study Valid?
Primary Questions:
- Was there an independent, blind comparison with a reference standard?
- Did the patient sample include an appropriate spectrum of patients to whom the diagnostic test will be applied in clinical practice?

Secondary Questions:
- Did the results of the test being evaluated influence the decision to perform the reference standard?
- Were the methods for performing the test described in sufficient detail to permit replication?

2. What Are the Results?
- Are likelihood ratios for the test results presented or is data necessary for their calculation provided?

3. Will the Results Help Me in Caring for My Patients?
- Will the reproducibility of the test result and its interpretation be satisfactory in my setting?
- Are the results applicable to my patient?
- Will the results change my management?
- Will patients be better off as a result of the test?

(Adapted with permission from Sackett DL, Straus SE, Richardson WS, et al: *Evidence-Based Medicine: How to Practice and Teach EBM*, ed 2. New York, NY, Churchill Livingstone, 2000.)

Table 3

How to Review a Study About Harm

1. Are the Results of the Study Valid?
Primary Questions:
- Were there clearly identified comparison groups that were similar with respect to important determinants of outcome, other than the one of interest?
- Were the outcomes and exposures measured in the same way in the groups being compared?
- Was follow-up sufficiently long and complete?

Secondary Questions:
- Is the temporal relationship correct?
- Is there a dose response gradient?

2. What Are the Results?
- How strong is the association between exposure and outcome?
- How precise is the estimate of the risk?

3. Will the Results Help Me in Caring for My Patients?
- Are the results applicable to my practice?
- What is the magnitude of the risk?
- Should I attempt to stop the exposure?

(Adapted with permission from Sackett DL, Straus SE, Richardson WS, et al: *Evidence-Based Medicine: How to Practice and Teach EBM*, ed 2. New York, NY, Churchill Livingstone, 2000.)

tween study groups exists (a type I statistical error). Similarly, Bryant et al[58] found that 42% of clinical studies in high-impact orthopaedic journals inappropriately used multiple observations from single individuals, leading to potential bias in their results. When reporting a study that contains some patients with bilateral data, Morris[59] recommends using the patient as the variable and, when possible, condensing bilateral data into single measurements.

Many randomized clinical trials incorporate data safety–monitoring boards and specify interim analyses of data; this is done for ethical purposes to avoid continuing a study when there is either no benefit or potential harm to one group, or a dramatic benefit realized by one group such that it seems unethical to continue the study. Interestingly, studies stopped for benefit are often published in high-impact journals (typically with great fanfare), are industry funded, and are becoming more common.[60] However, because of chance effects, early in a study the effect sizes seen between groups are typically greater than what is seen when the planned number of patients have been enrolled.[48,60] This was recently demonstrated in a comparison of 91 truncated trials whose results were compared to 424 nontruncated matching clinical trials.[49] Many published studies that are stopped early for benefit appear to suffer from significant methodologic issues that should make readers skeptical, including implausibly large treatment effects, failure to explain why the study was stopped, and no statistical accounting for interim comparisons or truncated enrollment.[60]

Many observational studies evaluate the potential influence of various factors by performing logistic regression analysis. Deeks et al[61] resampled participants from two large randomized trials to examine potential bias in nonrandomized studies. Logistic regression, a common method to examine potential prognostic factors, was actually found to increase bias because of classification and measurement errors related to confounding variables.[59]

Confidence Intervals Versus *P* Values

Many studies reported in the medical literature simply report the *P* value as a measure of the statistical likelihood that a given study outcome differs between two groups as a result of chance. The *P* value is often misinterpreted as symbolizing solely the magnitude of average difference between the two groups (and subsequently as the difference caused by the intervention). Many factors influence the calculated *P* value. Even if two groups are identical in all ways except for the intervention, the *P* value still is a measure of more than just the average difference. Variation and sample size also contribute to the *P* value. Dorey et al[62] point out that confidence intervals are a much more appropriate measure of the difference between groups. Statistically significant confi-

Table 4
How to Review a Study of Prognosis

1. Are the Results of the Study Valid?
Primary Questions:
• Was there a representative and well-defined sample of patients at a similar point in the course of the disease?
• Was follow-up sufficiently long and complete?
Secondary Questions:
• Were objective and unbiased outcome criteria used?
• Was there adjustment for important prognostic factors?

2. What Are the Results?
• How large is the likelihood of the outcome event(s) in a specified period of time?
• How precise are the estimates of likelihood?

3. Will the Results Help Me in Caring for My Patients?
• Were the study patients similar to my own?
• Will the results lead directly to selecting or avoiding therapy?
• Are the results useful for reassuring or counseling patients?

(Adapted with permission from Sackett DL, Straus SE, Richardson WS, et al: *Evidence-Based Medicine: How to Practice and Teach EBM*, ed 2. New York, NY, Churchill Livingstone, 2000.)

dence intervals allow the reader to assess the magnitude of differences between groups.[62]

Subgroup Analyses

Subgroup analysis refers to the common practice of researchers to address questions of whether the results of a specific treatment are better in subgroups of the overall study population — in other words, in patients with specific characteristics.[63] These may represent primary hypotheses (when specified a priori), although more often the research question that is addressed by subgroup analysis is generated post hoc after an initial review of the results of a study.[64] Whether a given treatment has better efficacy or different complications in specific groups of patients in comparison with the general population are important questions that provide the impetus for these sorts of analyses.[63]

Analyses of subgroups within a larger clinical trial are reported in more than one third of surgical trials.[20] Analysis of subgroups may also be the focus of follow-up reports. For example, Swiontkowski et al[65] reported a subgroup analysis of patients who were enrolled in two similar trials of bone morphogenetic protein in open tibial fractures (one published and one not published) and examined two specific subgroups: those with Gustilo type IIIA or IIIB open injuries and those treated with reamed intramedullary nails. In this report, differences in outcome were noted among the first group, but not the second. These findings were not part

of the analysis of the larger published study, in which the effect of reamed nails was not considered.

Readers need to be aware of the problems associated with subgroup analysis because the results may not be as robust as they appear. There are several well-known examples of conclusions drawn from subgroup analyses that were later shown to be false when directly examined as a primary research hypothesis.[66] To analyze subgroups, multiple statistical tests are required, which increases the likelihood of a difference being found due to chance alone. Ideally, when multiple statistical comparisons are done within a single study, the P value that is considered to be the measure of statistical significance is lowered. A common way to do this is with the Bonferroni correction, in which the adjusted level of significance for the P value for n comparisons is P/n, where P is the original level of significance (typically 0.05).[67]

Although the reader should be wary of claims based on subgroup analyses, inferences may be credible if they are based on a small number of hypotheses generated a priori, demonstrate large treatment effects, are based on within- rather than between-study comparisons, and when there is other indirect evidence that supports the hypothesis and the finding. Oxman and Guyatt[66] have presented guidelines for assessing the believability of a given subgroup analysis.[66]

Type II Error

A type II error refers to the probability of concluding that no difference between treatment groups exists in a comparative trial when, in reality, there is a difference. A type II error occurs primarily as a result of insufficient study power, generally caused by an inadequate number of subjects.

Type II errors are common in orthopaedic trials. Lochner et al[68] evaluated 117 randomized trials of fracture care and found a wide range of sample sizes from as small as 10 subjects to as large as 662. The mean study power was just under 25%, whereas the mean type II error rate for primary outcomes was just over 90%.[68] Too often, absence of proof (for example, because of type II errors) is misinterpreted as proof of absence of effect. The lack of statistical significance for a primary research hypothesis is not proof of the absence of effect, especially if the study was underpowered.

Type II errors can be avoided by performing power and sample size calculations based on previous research, or if that is not available, data based on a small pilot study.

Effect Size and Sample Size

In contrast to the situation described in the preceding paragraph, some small orthopaedic trials report large differences in effect size.[69] Readers of such studies need to be aware that these results are likely exaggerated; large clinical trials routinely demonstrate more modest treatment effects than small trials.[69] The situation in these small trials is analogous to the situation encountered when studies are stopped early for benefit. Because of chance fluctuations in data sampling,

4: Clinical Science

the treatment effect in smaller studies is likely larger than the true value.

Conversely, large trials, by virtue of their increased power, often report statistically significant differences that may be of little clinical difference. That said, small differences (effect sizes) may be of real clinical importance, and it is necessary for the reader to carefully consider this for every end point reported. For example, researchers comparing single-dose to 24 hours (three doses) of prophylactic antibiotic therapy with cefazolin documented infection rates of 2.3% and 2.8%, respectively, in orthopaedic surgeries, concluding that the 0.5% absolute risk difference was statistically insignificant.[70] However, in the scenario presented (surgical site infection), such a small effect (if indeed real) would be of clinical significance, because the inverse of the absolute risk difference represents the number-needed-to-treat, which in this case is 200. In other words, treating 200 patients with three doses of antibiotics instead of one dose (400 extra doses of antibiotics, at a few dollars per dose, or a total cost for the group of just over $1,000) would prevent one infection, which would cost tens of thousands of dollars to treat.

Summary

Bias takes numerous forms, and a careful reader of the medical literature should be aware of, at minimum, the most common and most important forms of bias and how they may influence the conclusions of a given study. Bias in the context of a study's design may result in false conclusions about differences or similarities between study groups. Even when bias is not obvious, one should be wary of large treatment effects that are demonstrated in small-size trials and of the conclusions of studies stopped early for benefit. It is also important to have at least an awareness of how publication bias and other related methodologic issues can affect an entire body of knowledge, and how results of meta-analyses may be affected by these more broadly based phenomena, specifically that if positive-outcome bias affects publication of material, this will result in inflation of apparent treatment effect sizes. Appropriate analysis of specific studies and bodies of literature on a given topic requires a skeptical frame of mind; one should remember that even meta-analyses and randomized clinical trials may not present the truth, and some well-designed studies of lower grade may in fact be quite useful. Only a reader with reasonable sophistication in the detection of bias will be able to discern these very important differences.

References

1. Brophy RH, Gardner MJ, Saleem O, Marx RG: An assessment of the methodological quality of research published in *The American Journal of Sports Medicine. Am J Sports Med* 2005;33(12):1812-1815.

2. Cowan J, Lozano-Calderón S, Ring D: Quality of prospective controlled randomized trials: Analysis of trials of treatment for lateral epicondylitis as an example. *J Bone Joint Surg Am* 2007;89(8):1693-1699.

3. Poolman RW, Sierevelt IN, Farrokhyar F, Mazel JA, Blankevoort L, Bhandari M: Perceptions and competence in evidence-based medicine: Are surgeons getting better? A questionnaire survey of members of the Dutch Orthopaedic Association. *J Bone Joint Surg Am* 2007;89(1):206-215.

4. Atkins D, Best D, Briss PA, et al: Grading quality of evidence and strength of recommendations. *BMJ* 2004; 328(7454):1490-1497.

5. Hanson BP, Bhandari M, Audige L, Helfet D: The need for education in evidence-based orthopedics: An international survey of AO course participants. *Acta Orthop Scand* 2004; 75(3):328-332.

6. Sackett DL: Bias in analytic research. *J Chronic Dis* 1979; 32(1-2):51-63.

7. Lynch JR, Cunningham MR, Warme WJ, Schaad DC, Wolf FM, Leopold SS: Commercially funded and United States-based research is more likely to be published: Good-quality studies with negative outcomes are not. *J Bone Joint Surg Am* 2007;89(5):1010-1018.

8. Emerson GB, Warme WJ, Wolf FM, Heckman JD, Brand RA, Leopold SS: Testing for the presence of positive-outcome bias in peer review: A randomized controlled trial. *Arch Intern Med* 2010;170(21):1934-1939.

9. Alho A, Austdal S, Benterud JG, Blikra G, Lerud P, Raugstad TS: Biases in a randomized comparison of three types of screw fixation in displaced femoral neck fractures. *Acta Orthop Scand* 1998;69(5):463-468.

10. Gøtzsche PC: Methodology and overt and hidden bias in reports of 196 double-blind trials of nonsteroidal anti-inflammatory drugs in rheumatoid arthritis. *Control Clin Trials* 1989;10(1):31-56.

11. Gluud LL: Bias in clinical intervention research. *Am J Epidemiol* 2006;163(6):493-501.

12. Ioannidis JP, Haidich A-B, Pappa M, et al: Comparison of evidence of treatment effects in randomized and nonrandomized studies. *JAMA* 2001;286(7):821-830.

13. Kunz R, Vist GE, Oxman AD: Randomisation to protect against selection bias in healthcare trials. *Cochrane Database Syst Rev* 2007;(2)MR000012.

14. Benson K, Hartz AJ: A comparison of observational studies and randomized, controlled trials. *N Engl J Med* 2000; 342(25):1878-1886.

15. Concato J, Shah N, Horwitz RI: Randomized, controlled trials, observational studies, and the hierarchy of research designs. *N Engl J Med* 2000;342(25):1887-1892.

16. Berger VW, Exner DV: Detecting selection bias in randomized clinical trials. *Control Clin Trials* 1999;20(4):319-327.

17. Lin H-M, Lyles RH, Williamson JM: Bias in a placebo-controlled study due to mismeasurement of disease status and the regression effect. *Control Clin Trials* 2002;23(5):497-501.

18. Barnett AG, van der Pols JC, Dobson AJ: Regression to the mean: What it is and how to deal with it. *Int J Epidemiol* 2005;34(1):215-220.

19. Corrales LA, Morshed S, Bhandari M, Miclau T III: Variability in the assessment of fracture-healing in orthopaedic trauma studies. *J Bone Joint Surg Am* 2008;90(9):1862-1868.

20. Study to Prospectively Evaluate Reamed Intramedullary

Nails in Tibial Fractures (SPRINT) Investigators, Sun X, Heels-Ansell D, et al: Is a subgroup claim believable? A user's guide to subgroup analyses in the surgical literature. *J Bone Joint Surg Am* 2011;93:(3):e8.

21. Karanicolas PJ, Bhandari M, Taromi B, et al: Blinding of outcomes in trials of orthopaedic trauma: An opportunity to enhance the validity of clinical trials. *J Bone Joint Surg Am* 2008;90(5):1026-1033.

22. Poolman RW, Struijs PA, Krips R, et al: Reporting of outcomes in orthopaedic randomized trials: Docs blinding of outcome assessors matter? *J Bone Joint Surg Am* 2007;89(3):550-558.

23. Wacholder S, Lubin JH, Dosemeci M, Gail MH: Bias despite masked assessment of clinical outcomes when an outcome is defined as one of several component events. *Control Clin Trials* 1991;12(4):457-461.

24. Kim J, Lonner JH, Nelson CL, Lotke PA: Response bias: Effect on outcomes evaluation by mail surveys after total knee arthroplasty. *J Bone Joint Surg Am* 2004;86(1):15-21.

25. Ludemann R, Watson DI, Jamieson GG: Influence of follow-up methodology and completeness on apparent clinical outcome of fundoplication. *Am J Surg* 2003;186(2):143-147.

26. Poolman RW, Swiontkowski MF, Fairbank JC, Schemitsch EH, Sprague S, de Vet HC: Outcome instruments: Rationale for their use. *J Bone Joint Surg Am* 2009;91(Suppl 3):41-49.

27. Wilson IB, Cleary PD: Linking clinical variables with health-related quality of life: A conceptual model of patient outcomes. *JAMA* 1995;273(1):59-65.

28. Murray DW, Britton AR, Bulstrode CJ: Loss to follow-up matters. *J Bone Joint Surg Br* 1997;79(2):254-257.

29. Norquist BM, Goldberg BA, Matsen FA III : Challenges in evaluating patients lost to follow-up in clinical studies of rotator cuff tears. *J Bone Joint Surg Am* 2000;82(6):838-842.

30. Smith JS, Watts HG: Methods for locating missing patients for the purpose of long-term clinical studies. *J Bone Joint Surg Am* 1998;80(3):431-438.

31. Herman A, Botser IB, Tenenbaum S, Chechick A: Intention-to-treat analysis and accounting for missing data in orthopaedic randomized clinical trials. *J Bone Joint Surg Am* 2009;91(9):2137-2143.

32. Altman DG, Schulz KF, Moher D, et al: The revised CONSORT statement for reporting randomized trials: Explanation and elaboration. *Ann Intern Med* 2001;134(8):663-694.

33. Dickersin K, Chan S, Chalmers TC, Sacks HS, Smith H Jr: Publication bias and clinical trials. *Control Clin Trials* 1987;8(4):343-353.

34. Leopold SS, Warme WJ, Fritz Braunlich E, Shott S: Association between funding source and study outcome in orthopaedic research. *Clin Orthop Relat Res* 2003;415(415):293-301.

35. Okike K, Kocher MS, Mehlman CT, Bhandari M: Conflict of interest in orthopaedic research: An association between findings and funding in scientific presentations. *J Bone Joint Surg Am* 2007;89(3):608-613.

36. Song F, Khan KS, Dinnes J, Sutton AJ: Asymmetric funnel plots and publication bias in meta-analyses of diagnostic accuracy. *Int J Epidemiol* 2002;31(1):88-95.

37. Egger M, Davey Smith G, Schneider M, Minder C: Bias in meta-analysis detected by a simple, graphical test. *BMJ* 1997;315(7109):629-634.

38. Smith TO, Sexton D, Mann C, Donell S: Sutures versus staples for skin closure in orthopaedic surgery: Meta-analysis. *BMJ* 2010;340:c1199

39. The Cochrane Collaboration: Publication bias: Interpreting funnel plots. Published 2002. http://www.cochrane-net.org/openlearning/HTML/mod15-3.htm.

40. Lau J, Ioannidis JP, Terrin N, Schmid CH, Olkin I: The case of the misleading funnel plot. *BMJ* 2006;333(7568):597-600.

41. Nüesch E, Trelle S, Reichenbach S, et al: Small study effects in meta-analyses of osteoarthritis trials: Meta-epidemiological study. *BMJ* 2010;341:c3515.

42. Bhandari M, Morrow F, Kulkarni AV, Tornetta P III: Meta-analyses in orthopaedic surgery: A systematic review of their methodologies. *J Bone Joint Surg Am* 2001;83(1):15-24.

43. Jüni P, Witschi A, Bloch R, Egger M: The hazards of scoring the quality of clinical trials for meta-analysis. *JAMA* 1999;282(11):1054-1060.

44. Shrier I, Boivin JF, Platt RW, et al: The interpretation of systematic reviews with meta-analyses: An objective or subjective process? *BMC Med Inform Decis Mak* 2008;8:19.

45. Egger M, Smith GD: Misleading meta-analysis. *BMJ* 1995;310(6982):752-754.

46. Ioannidis JP, Cappelleri JC, Lau J: Issues in comparisons between meta-analyses and large trials. *JAMA* 1998;279(14):1089-1093.

47. Sprague S, Leece P, Bhandari M, et al: Limiting loss to follow-up in a multicenter randomized trial in orthopedic surgery. *Control Clin Trials* 2003;24(6):719-725.

48. Wheatley K, Clayton D: Be skeptical about unexpected large apparent treatment effects: The case of an MRC AML12 randomization. *Control Clin Trials* 2003;24(1):66-70.

49. Bassler D, Briel M, Montori VM, et al: Stopping randomized trials early for benefit and estimation of treatment effects: Systematic review and meta-regression analysis. *JAMA* 2010;303(12):1180-1187.

50. Sackett DL, Straus SE, Richardson WS, et al: *Evidence-based Medicine: How to Practice and Teach EBM*, ed 2. Edinburgh, United Kingdom, Churchill Livingstone, 2000.

51. Guyatt G, Drummond R: *Users' Guides to the Medical Literature: A Manual for Evidence-Based Clinical Practice*. Chicago, IL, American Medical Association, 2002.

52. Bhandari M, Guyatt GH, Swiontkowski MF: User's guide to the orthopaedic literature: How to use an article about a surgical therapy. *J Bone Joint Surg Am* 2001;83(6):916-926.

53. Bhandari M, Guyatt GH, Swiontkowski MF: User's guide to the orthopaedic literature: How to use an article about prognosis. *J Bone Joint Surg Am* 2001;83(10):1555-1564.

54. Bhandari M, Guyatt GH, Montori V, Devereaux PJ, Swiontkowski MF: User's guide to the orthopaedic literature: How to use a systematic literature review. *J Bone Joint Surg Am* 2002;84-A(9):1672-1682.

55. Bhandari M, Montori VM, Swiontkowski MF, Guyatt GH: User's guide to the surgical literature: How to use an article

4: Clinical Science

about a diagnostic test. *J Bone Joint Surg Am* 2003;85(6): 1133-1140.

56. Ranstam J: Problems in orthopedic research: Dependent observations. *Acta Orthop Scand* 2002;73(4):447-450.

57. Park MS, Kim SJ, Chung CY, Choi IH, Lee SH, Lee KM: Statistical consideration for bilateral cases in orthopaedic research. *J Bone Joint Surg Am* 2010;92(8):1732-1737.

58. Bryant D, Havey TC, Roberts R, Guyatt G: How many patients? How many limbs? Analysis of patients or limbs in the orthopaedic literature: A systematic review. *J Bone Joint Surg Am* 2006;88(1):41-45.

59. Morris RW: Bilateral procedures in randomised controlled trials. *J Bone Joint Surg Br* 1993;75(5):675-676.

60. Montori VM, Devereaux PJ, Adhikari NK, et al: Randomized trials stopped early for benefit: A systematic review. *JAMA* 2005;294(17):2203-2209.

61. Deeks JJ, Dinnes J, D'Amico R, et al: Evaluating non-randomised intervention studies. *Health Technol Assess* 2003; 7(27):1-173.

62. Dorey F, Nasser S, Amstutz H: The need for confidence intervals in the presentation of orthopaedic data. *J Bone Joint Surg Am* 1993;75(12):1844-1852.

63. Wang R, Lagakos SW, Ware JH, Hunter DJ, Drazen JM: Statistics in medicine: Reporting of subgroup analyses in clinical trials. *N Engl J Med* 2007;357(21):2189-2194.

64. Bhandari M, Devereaux PJ, Li P, et al: Misuse of baseline comparison tests and subgroup analyses in surgical trials. *Clin Orthop Relat Res* 2006;447:247-251.

65. Swiontkowski MF, Aro HT, Donell S, et al: Recombinant human bone morphogenetic protein-2 in open tibial fractures: A subgroup analysis of data combined from two prospective randomized studies. *J Bone Joint Surg Am* 2006; 88(6):1258-1265.

66. Oxman AD, Guyatt GH: A consumer's guide to subgroup analyses. *Ann Intern Med* 1992;116(1):78-84.

67. Dunn OJ: Multiple comparisons among means. *Am Stat Assoc J* 1961;56:52-64.

68. Lochner HV, Bhandari M, Tornetta P III: Type-II error rates (beta errors) of randomized trials in orthopaedic trauma. *J Bone Joint Surg Am* 2001;83(11):1650-1655.

69. Sung J, Siegel J, Tornetta P, Bhandari M: The orthopaedic trauma literature: An evaluation of statistically significant findings in orthopaedic trauma randomized trials. *BMC Musculoskelet Disord* 2008;9:14.

70. Fonseca SN, Kunzle SR, Junqueira MJ, Nascimento RT, de Andrade JI, Levin AS: Implementing 1-dose antibiotic prophylaxis for prevention of surgical site infection. *Arch Surg* 2006;141(11):1109-1114.

4: Clinical Science

Chapter 32

Decision Analysis

Julius Bishop, MD

Mininder S. Kocher, MD, MPH

Introduction

What Is Decision Analysis?

Decision analysis is a methodologic tool based in gaming theory that allows for the quantitative analysis of decision making under conditions of uncertainty. Although frequently unaware of it, human decision makers routinely weigh the risks and benefits of the alternative strategies available to them before attempting to act in their own best interest. This is frequently done without explicitly identifying the scope of possible outcomes or the value that the individual might assign to each. Decision analysis facilitates a formal mathematical decision-making process in which a decision-making scenario is identified, various decision-making strategies are itemized, and the potential outcomes of each strategy are quantified. The probability of each potential outcome as well as the preferences of the decision maker are precisely defined. This then allows a rigorous evaluation of the most logical plan of action. All of the implicit variables that are routinely considered when making an important clinical decision are made explicit and available for formal analysis. These variables can then be manipulated so that the effects of different outcome probabilities as well as different sets of values among decision makers can be assessed. In this way, decision analysis can be used to examine how the optimal decision-making strategy may change under different sets of circumstances or among different types of decision makers.

History of Decision Analysis

The term "decision analysis" was first used in 1966, and many of the early applications involved helping business and industry identify the most profitable strategy among several options.[1] This methodology is attractive to health care researchers because it allows for the quantitative analysis of clinical decision making in the setting of uncertainty without requiring the same formidable commitment of time, energy, and financial resources as a randomized controlled trial (RCT). Decision analysis was first used in health care research in 1967 when a model was created to explore the role of radical neck dissection in patients with oral cancer.[2] Since that time, there has been a proliferation of decision analysis research in medicine in general, with a recently increased enthusiasm in orthopaedics in particular.[3-7]

Relevance to Orthopaedic Surgery

Many clinical questions in orthopaedics are well suited to decision analysis modeling. Throughout orthopaedics, there remain many diagnoses for which the optimal treatment remains controversial. In some instances, the uncertainty involves a decision between surgical and nonsurgical treatment whereas in others it involves choosing between distinct surgical procedures or nonsurgical treatment protocols. Although the gold standard for answering many of these questions remains the RCT, these trials can be difficult to perform in surgical disciplines for logistical, economic,

Dr. Kocher or an immediate family member has received royalties from Biomet; serves as a paid consultant to or is an employee of Biomet, OrthoPediatric, PediPed, and Smith & Nephew; has stock or stock options held in Fixes 4 Kids and Pivot Medical; and is a board member, owner, officer, or committee member of the American Academy of Orthopaedic Surgeons, the ACL Study Group, the American Orthopaedic Society for Sports Medicine, the Herodicus Society, the Pediatric Orthopaedic Society of North America, and the Steadman Hawkins Research Foundation. Neither Dr. Bishop nor any immediate family member has received anything of value from or owns stock in a commercial company or institution related directly or indirectly to the subject of this chapter.

Table 1

Summary of Orthopaedic Decision Analyses Published Through April 2011

Study	Decision Analysis
Bernstein[24]	Early versus delayed reconstruction of the anterior cruciate ligament
Bishop and Ring[9]	Exploration versus observation of radial nerve palsy associated with humeral shaft fracture
Brauer and Graham[14]	Optimal surgical technique for cubital tunnel syndrome
Cavaliere and Chung[15]	Wrist arthroplasty versus arthrodesis in rheumatoid arthritis
Chung et al[12]	Amputation versus limb salvage in open tibial fractures
Davis[16]	Posterior spinal fusion versus anterior/posterior spinal fusion for adolescent idiopathic scoliosis
Graham and Detsky[17]	Surgical technique for wrist osteoarthritis
Hernandez et al[18]	Ultrasound screening for developmental dysplasia of the hip
Kailes and Richmond[19]	Open versus arthroscopic Bankart reconstruction
Kocher et al[8]	Surgical versus nonsurgical management of Achilles tendon rupture
Kocher et al[10]	Prophylactic pinning versus watchful waiting of the contralateral hip after unilateral slipped capital femoral epiphysis
Koenig et al[11]	Internal fixation versus cast treatment of well-reduced unstable distal radius fractures
Mahan et al[20]	Ultrasound screening for developmental dysplasia of the hip
Schultz et al[13]	Prophylactic pinning versus watchful waiting of the contralateral hip after unilateral slipped capital femoral epiphysis
Seng et al[21]	Surgical versus nonsurgical treatment of anterior cruciate ligament rupture
Van der Velde et al[22]	Optimal nonsurgical treatment of neck pain
Wolf et al[25]	Comparison of one- and two-stage revision of total hip arthroplasty complicated by infection
Zangger and Detsky[23]	Resurfacing or not resurfacing the patella in total knee arthroplasty

and ethical reasons. Decision analysis provides a viable alternative that is efficient, relatively inexpensive, and does not generally involve any risk to participants. Furthermore, differing treatment strategies in orthopaedics generally fit the decision analysis model well as they are well defined and distinct, with discrete treatments and clinical outcomes. **Table 1** summarizes the orthopaedic decision analysis studies conducted to date.[8-25]

Methodologic Overview

There are several discrete steps in the decision analysis process. The first involves identifying a clinical problem, defining alternative treatment strategies, and itemizing the possible outcomes of these strategies. The decision-making scenario can then be structured as a tree.[26,27] Next, a determination of outcome probabilities and utilities is made.[28] Then a "foldback" analysis is performed to determine the optimal decision-making strategy.[29] Finally, sensitivity analysis is performed to model the effects of varying outcome probabilities and utilities on decision making and identify the factors that are most influential in the decision-making process.[29]

Creating a Decision Tree

Decision analysis begins with the creation of a decision tree. The tree is created to model the decision-making scenario and provides the foundation for all subsequent data collection and analysis.

Before the tree can be constructed, the decision to be analyzed must be clearly outlined. For instance, an investigator might ask, "In the setting of Diagnosis A, does Treatment B, Treatment C, or Treatment D optimize outcome?" Once the problem has been concisely stated in this manner, all of the relevant treatment alternatives must be identified. Finally, the possible outcomes of each of these treatment alternatives need to be itemized and defined.

The clinical problem must then be structured graphically as a decision tree. The decision tree is constructed from left to right and begins with the clinical problem. The tree then comes to a decision node, which by convention is represented by a square. The decision node represents the point at which the decision maker must choose between alternative management strategies. From here, as many branches as necessary are added to reflect the various treatment options. Each of these treatment options then leads to a chance node

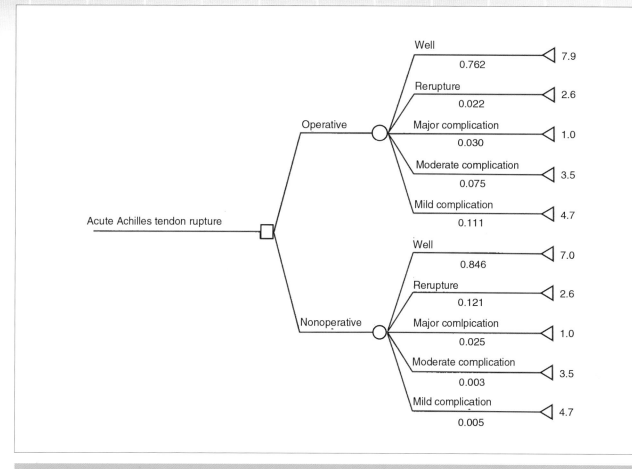

Figure 1 A decision tree to evaluate surgical versus nonsurgical treatment of acute Achilles tendon rupture. The tree starts on the left with the clinical condition in question, then reaches a choice node (square) where it branches into the alternatives of surgical and nonsurgical treatment options. At this point chance nodes are encountered (circle) and the tree branches again reflect the possible outcomes of each management strategy. Each of these outcomes is represented by a terminal node (triangle). (Adapted from Kocher MS, Bishop J, Marshall R, Briggs KK, Hawkins RJ: Operative versus nonoperative management of acute Achilles tendon rupture: Expected-value decision analysis. *Am J Sports Med* 2002;30[6]:783-790.)

or series of chance nodes, which by convention are represented by circles. The chance node is the point at which a given treatment strategy may lead to several defined clinical outcomes. At each of these chance nodes, the tree branches represent all of the possible outcomes of each treatment alternative. An assumption implicit in the decision tree is that each of these outcomes is mutually exclusive. Ultimately, each branch of the tree terminates in a terminal or outcome node, represented by a triangle. In orthopaedic decision analyses, these outcomes typically include uneventful recovery and various disability states or complications.

Example

Kocher et al[8] created a decision analysis model to identify the optimal treatment after Achilles tendon rupture. The treatment options were surgical and nonsurgical care. After both treatments, possible outcomes were identified as uneventful recovery (well), rerupture, major complication, moderate complication, and minor complication. The initial decision tree from this study is shown in **Figure 1**.

Estimating Outcome Probabilities

Once a decision tree has been created, the probability of each clinical scenario displayed in the tree must be estimated. Although obtaining valid estimates of outcome probability is important, it should be emphasized that these probabilities serve only as estimates upon which further sensitivity analysis can be performed. There are two primary approaches to selecting appropriate estimates.

Using the Medical Literature

The medical literature is the preferred source of outcome probability estimates. Generally, the most robust estimates are derived from meta-analytic synthesis of RCTs. Often in orthopaedics, this highest level of clinical evidence is not available, in which case a systematic review of the existing literature can be undertaken. Frequently, identified areas of controversy in orthopaedics have been subjected to formal meta-analysis. In these circumstances, the meta-analysis

4: Clinical Science

data can be updated and incorporated into a decision analysis model.

Example

Bishop and Ring[9] created a decision analysis model to compare early exploration versus observation for radial nerve palsy associated with humeral shaft fracture. A rigorous and contemporary meta-analysis of this question had previously been published so the authors were able to use these data to establish outcome probabilities.[30]

Expert Opinion

Sometimes, outcome probabilities for a particular condition or intervention cannot be found in the medical literature. In these cases, expert opinion may be solicited to estimate these values. It is recommended that this elicitation be structured, as with the Delphi method.[31] The Delphi method involves convening a panel of experts on a particular outcome and initially soliciting their estimates of outcome probability by questionnaire. A facilitator who provides feedback to the panel analyzes these initial responses, and the estimates of outcome probability are then discussed and modified until consensus can be reached. As the breadth and depth of the published orthopaedic literature continues to expand, expert opinion should be resorted to less frequently as a means of estimating outcome probability.

Example

Graham and Detsky[17] created a decision analysis model to compare wrist fusion, proximal row carpectomy, and excision of the scaphoid combined with midcarpal arthrodesis for the treatment of wrist osteoarthritis. Citing the lack of reliable data in the literature, these authors used their clinical experience to estimate some of the relevant outcome probabilities.

Establishing Outcome Utilities
Measuring Utility: Assessing Preferences for Health States

As noted previously, each branch of a decision tree ends in a discrete and mutually exclusive terminal node. The next step in the decision analysis is to measure the relative preference of the decision maker for each of these outcomes. The desirability of each outcome is termed the utility.

Accurately measuring utility can be complex. Because orthopaedic interventions more commonly affect pain and disability rather than life or death, life expectancy typically should not be used as a tool to quantify the benefits of these interventions. Therefore, various alternative techniques for assessing health status have been developed.[32-34] Direct rating scales allow a decision maker to rank all the possible outcomes from most to least desirable. Alternatively, reference-based rating scales analyze the tradeoffs between morbidity and mortality. In an effort to combine both a

measure of quality of life and life expectancy, the quality-adjusted life year (QALY) has also been introduced.

By convention, subjects used for utility assessment are those who potentially face the decision being studied. Those who have already experienced the clinical scenario are generally excluded because their assessments may be altered by their experiences. Therefore, the demographics of the subjects surveyed for utility measurement will vary significantly between analyses, based on the decision-making scenario being evaluated.

Direct Measures of Utility

Methods of directly measuring utility include the use of a Likert or visual analog scale. These scales allow subjects to rank various health outcomes relative to one another. This methodology is appealing because developing the scale is relatively simple for the investigator, and completing the scale is usually similarly intuitive for the subject.[35,36] These scales can be distributed in the form of a paper or online survey and have demonstrated good intrarater and interrater reliability. It has been shown in pilot studies using orthopaedic residents and attending surgeons as subjects that their utility outcomes do not differ drastically from those obtained from lay subjects.

Example

Kocher et al[10] created a decision analysis model to compare prophylactic pinning with observation of the contralateral hip after unilateral slipped capital femoral epiphysis (SCFE). Because adolescent boys are at greatest risk for SCFE, a group of boys ages 12 through 14 years without a history of hip injury were surveyed. The authors used a survey in which all possible outcomes after either prophylactic pinning or watchful waiting were described. Subjects were then asked to rate each outcome on a visual analog scale of 0 to 10 points, with 0 representing the worst possible outcome and 10 the best possible outcome. The outcome of observation followed by late contralateral SCFE leading to osteonecrosis was preselected by the authors as the worst possible outcome and assigned a score of 0, whereas the outcome of observation without contralateral slip was preselected as the best outcome and assigned a value of 10. These "anchor" values served as points of reference for subjects completing the survey.

Time Trade-off

The time trade-off is a method for measuring utilities that presents the rater with a choice between two alternative health states.[34] The rater must determine how many years of life he or she would give up to be in the healthier state compared with the less healthy state. A trained interviewer systematically varies the number of years spent in the healthy state until the rater finds it too difficult to choose between the two. Using this method, each outcome can be assigned a utility value relative to normal function and good health. The disadvantages of this technique include the large number of health states to which the rater must respond and the increased conceptual complexity.

Example

Koenig et al[11] created a decision analysis model to compare internal fixation with cast treatment of well-reduced unstable distal radius fractures. To estimate outcome utilities, a time trade-off questionnaire was constructed and administered to a group of volunteers without a history of wrist fracture. The average age of these volunteers (58 years) was noted to approximate that of individuals previously demonstrated to be at risk for distal radius fracture. The authors evaluated the outcomes of painless malunion, painless functional deficit, painful malunion, and complex regional pain. A portion of their questionnaire is included in **Figure 2**.

Standard Reference Gamble

The standard reference gamble is another method for measuring utility.[28,33,34] It involves raters choosing between two health states in which one has a certain outcome and the other is a gamble. The gamble generally involves the possibility of complete health (the best health state) with a probability of P and the possibility of death (the worst health state) with a probability of $1 - P$. Similar to the time trade-off technique, the probability P is then systematically varied until the rater finds it too difficult to choose between the certain outcome and the gamble. This method also requires the rater to respond to a large number of scenarios, is somewhat less intuitive than the time trade-off method, and generally requires that the rater reference death, which is an extreme outcome in the setting of most orthopaedic conditions. A schematic of a hypothetical standard reference gamble is represented in **Figure 3**.

Example

Chung et al[12] created a decision analysis model to examine limb salvage versus amputation in the setting of severe open tibia fracture. The authors created a standard reference gamble survey to determine outcome utilities. The survey was administered to physicians with an interest in limb salvage and amputation as well as patients who had experienced significant lower extremity trauma. The survey was administered online, and the gamble was characterized as a "magic pill," offering the possibility of complete cure but also death. Based on data from the Lower Extremity Assessment Project (LEAP), the outcomes evaluated were early amputation followed by no complications, secondary revision, or osteomyelitis; and limb salvage followed by no complications, secondary amputation, osteomyelitis, nonunion, or flap failure. A sampling from the survey created by the authors complete with theoretic responses from what the authors consider a patient with low risk tolerance is included in **Figure 4**.

Foldback Analysis: Determining the Optimal Management Strategy

Foldback analysis is the process by which the tree is analyzed and values assigned to each of the alternative choice branches.[29] Simple arithmetic is all that is required in this analysis. As decision trees get large and complex, this arithmetic can become cumbersome, so commercial software packages are often used. The required mathematics involves multiplying the outcome probability by the utility for each branch of the tree. These values are then summed for each decision strategy, creating a total value. Values can then be compared and the optimal strategy identified. This initial analysis using initial outcome probability and utility measures is termed the base case analysis.

Example

The decision analysis by Kocher et al[8] of surgical versus nonsurgical treatment of Achilles tendon rupture will be used to illustrate the process of foldback analysis. The corresponding decision tree is shown in **Figure 1**. Surgical treatment is revealed to be the optimal decision-making strategy given the probabilities and utilities studied. The calculations involved in foldback analysis are displayed in **Table 2**.

Sensitivity Analysis: Accounting for Uncertainty in the Decision Model
What Is Sensitivity Analysis?

Sensitivity analysis is performed to evaluate how variation of outcome probabilities and utilities changes the optimal decision-making strategy. The process involves varying one or several outcome probabilities or utilities within a clinically plausible range. If the optimal decision-making strategy changes as a result of manipulating a variable within this plausible range, the model is said to be "sensitive" to this variable. Conversely, if a variable does not change decision-making within a clinically plausible range, it has less effect on the decision-making process. In general, the less sensitive a decision-making model is in sensitivity analysis, the more robust the conclusions of the model.

The methodology requires identifying clinically plausible ranges for all variables. Evaluating whatever survey instrument was administered to subjects can reveal the appropriate range for each utility value. The lowest and highest utilities assigned to each outcome should be recorded and used to establish the range to be evaluated in sensitivity analysis. The appropriate range of outcome probabilities should come from review of the medical literature. The lowest and highest probabilities of a particular outcome reported in the literature should be used to direct sensitivity analysis.

Next, a sensitivity analysis of each variable should be performed. This means that each variable in the decision-making model is individually varied within the previously determined clinically plausible range while all others are

4: Clinical Science

Appendix E-1 Time Trade-Off Questionnaire

Health State Time Trade-Off

Age:

Sex: Male/Female

Do you consider yourself right-handed or left-handed? Right/Left/Both

Instructions: You will be asked to complete a questionnaire called the "Time Trade-Off" in which you imagine what it would be like to live in four different situations following a wrist fracture. You will then be asked to determine how that condition compares to living with a normal wrist.

Description of Health States

Health State 1. Painless Malunion
You have broken the wrist of your dominant arm. After treatment, it has healed. Compared to using your other wrist, you notice no difference when performing everyday tasks like opening doors, writing, or typing. You have slightly decreased grip strength and range of motion such that you notice mild difficulty when playing sports like golf or tennis. You have no pain on the affected side, but you have a noticeable bump on the back of your wrist.

Health State 2. Painless Functional Deficit
You have broken the wrist of your dominant arm. After treatment, it has healed. Compared to using your other wrist, you have minor difficulty when performing everyday tasks like opening doors, writing, or typing. You have moderately decreased grip strength and range of motion such that you have trouble playing sports like golf or tennis. You have no pain in the affected wrist.

Health State 3. Painful Malunion
You have broken the wrist of your dominant arm. After treatment, it has healed. Compared to using your other wrist, you have difficulty and pain when performing everyday tasks like opening doors, writing, or typing. You have decreased grip strength and range of motion such that you are unable to open jars with the affected hand, and have trouble with fine motor activities like threading a needle or winding your watch. You have pain when using the affected hand and sometimes at rest. There is also a noticeable bump on the back of your wrist.

Health State 4. Reflex Sympathetic Dystrophy
You have broken the wrist of your dominant arm. After treatment, it has healed. However, you have developed a syndrome in your wrist that causes frequent pain, swelling, discoloration, sweating, and weakness. You have significantly impaired function of your wrist and hand such that you cannot work. Frequent physician and physical therapy visits are required for treatment.

Figure 2 Sample time trade-off questionnaire. (Adapted from Koenig KM, Davis GC, Grove MR, Tosteson AN, Koval KJ: Is early internal fixation preferred to cast treatment for well-reduced unstable distal radial fractures? *J Bone Joint Surg Am* 2009;91[9]: 2086-2093.)

SAMPLE OF TIME TRADE-OFF QUESTION: HEALTH STATE 2
(each respondent will complete the time trade-off for each of the 4 health states)

Painless Functional Deficit	**No Wrist Fracture and Normal Function**
You have broken the wrist of your dominant arm. After treatment, it has healed. Compared to using your other wrist, you have minor difficulty when performing everyday tasks like opening doors, writing, or typing. You have moderately decreased grip strength and range of motion such that you have trouble playing sports like golf or tennis. You have no pain in the affected wrist.	You never sustained a wrist fracture and have your normal function.

Now imagine you can choose among the following options. Please indicate which option you prefer.

Live for **20 years** with *painless functional deficit* and then die (give up no time).	Live for **XX years** with *no wrist fracture and normal function* and then die (give up 20-XX years).

It is too hard to choose.

The interviewer administering the survey determines the respondents' utilities for the four health states using the template above. The only change in the template for each health state is the title of the health state and health state descriptor (above). The respondent is initially asked to choose between 20 years in the affected health state and 10 years in the "no wrist fracture and normal function" health state. The amount of time in the "no wrist fracture and normal function health state" (indicated by **XX** in the above template) is then varied systematically until the respondent reaches a state of indifference and chooses "It is too hard to choose."

Figure 2 continued

held constant. The effect on decision making is then observed. Two-way, three-way, and *n*-way sensitivity analysis can also be performed, which involves varying an increasing number of variables simultaneously and observing the effect on decision making. Simultaneous sensitivity analyses on more than three variables is infrequent because they are increasingly difficult to perform, report, and interpret.

Example

Sensitivity analyses are traditionally represented graphically. The decision analysis study conducted by Kocher et al[10] compared prophylactic pinning with observation of the contralateral hip after unilateral SCFE. In this study, the authors reported the results of one-way sensitivity analyses of

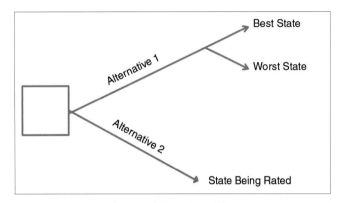

Figure 3 A schematic representation of a hypothetical standard reference gamble. Alternative strategy 1 involves entering the gamble, and alternative 2 involves the certain outcome of the state being rated.

several variables including the probability of a late contralateral SCFE (**Figure 5**). This analysis confirms in a quantifiable way the intuitive notion that as the probability of late contralateral SCFE increases, prophylactic pinning becomes an increasingly favorable treatment strategy. Specifically, the analysis reveals that when the probability of a late contralateral slip exceeds 27%, the expected value of prophylactic pinning exceeds that of watchful waiting.

Importance of Sensitivity Analysis

It is important to acknowledge that the probabilities and utilities used in a decision analysis model are merely estimates and might vary significantly based on the characteristics and preferences of an individual patient or distinct patient population. Therefore, sensitivity analysis plays a critical role in evaluating whether a decision made under one set of circumstances is equally effective under a different set of circumstances. Although one goal of a decision analysis model is to identify an optimal decision-making strategy, sensitivity analysis broadens the scope of the model and gives greater insight into how and why decisions are made. The model can then be tailored to individual patients or distinct groups of patients who may not share the same outcome utilities and probabilities used in the base case analysis.

Example

The previous example introduced the sensitivity analysis performed by Kocher et al[10] to evaluate the influence of the rate of late contralateral SCFE on a model evaluating observation versus prophylactic pinning of the contralateral hip after unilateral SCFE. This analysis revealed that when the

Table 2

A Demonstration of the Arithmetic Involved in Foldback Analysis[a]

Treatment	Outcome	Value (probability × utility)
Surgical	Well	0.762 × 7.9 = **6.02**
	Rerupture	0.022 × 2.6 = **0.06**
	Major complication	0.030 × 1.0 = **0.03**
	Moderate complication	0.075 × 3.5 = **0.26**
	Mild complication	0.111 × 4.7 = **0.52**
		Total Value: 6.9
Nonsurgical	Well	0.846 × 7.0 = **5.92**
	Rerupture	0.121 × 2.6 = **0.31**
	Major complication	0.025 × 1.0 = **0.03**
	Moderate complication	0.003 × 3.5 = **0.01**
	Mild complication	0.005 × 4.7 = **0.02**
		Total Value: 6.3

[a]Corresponds to the decision tree shown in Figure 1.

Primary Amputation with osteomyelitis as least-preferred complication

Scenario 1

Participant with low risk tolerance

The following scenarios will ask you how you feel about different possible treatments for your injury. As you consider the options. imagine that there will be no financial cost to you or your family for the treatments. If you miss work because of these treatments, you will not lose income for the time off work. However, please consider all other ways these treatments might affect your life.

Imagine that you have suffered a severe (type IIIB or IIIC) open tibial fracture.

Your surgeon offers to perform **A PRIMARY AMPUTATION** on your leg and it is guaranteed that you will develop **osteomyelitis (a bone infection)** as described here. However, your surgeon also has a MAGIC PILL that you can take INSTEAD of having Amputation with Osteomyelitis. If you take the pill, there is a chance of complete cure, but there is also a chance of death. If you refuse the pill, you will get Amputation with Osteomyelitis with complete certainty.

For each of the scenarios that follow state whether you would prefer the magic pill (with its associated probabilities) or Amputation with Osteomyelitis.

1.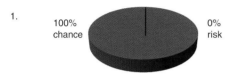

The pill has **100%** chance of cure and **0%** risk of death.

- ✓ Prefer magic Pill
- ❑ Prefer Amputation with Osteomyelitis
- ❑ Too hard to choose between the two

2.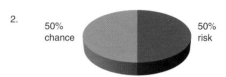

The pill has **50%** chance of cure and **50%** risk of death.

- ❑ Prefer magic Pill
- ✓ Prefer Amputation with Osteomyelitis
- ❑ Too hard to choose between the two

3.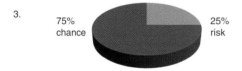

The pill has **75%** chance of cure and **25%** risk of death.

- ❑ Prefer magic Pill
- ✓ Prefer Amputation with Osteomyelitis
- ❑ Too hard to choose between the two

4.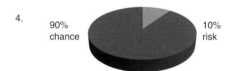

The pill has **90%** chance of cure and **10%** risk of death.

- ❑ Prefer magic Pill
- ✓ Prefer Amputation with Osteomyelitis
- ❑ Too hard to choose between the two

5.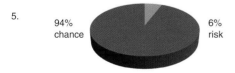

The pill has **94%** chance of cure and **6%** risk of death.

- ❑ Prefer magic Pill
- ✓ Prefer Amputation with Osteomyelitis
- ❑ Too hard to choose between the two

6.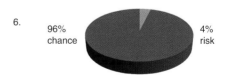

The pill has **96%** chance of cure and **4%** risk of death.

- ❑ Prefer magic Pill
- ✓ Prefer Amputation with Osteomyelitis
- ❑ Too hard to choose between the two

Figure 4 Sample standard reference gamble questionnaire. (Adapted from Chung KC, Saddawi-Konefka D, Haase SC, Kaul G: A cost-utility analysis of amputation versus salvage for Gustilo type IIIB and IIIC open tibial fractures. *Plast Reconstr Surg* 2009; 124[6]:1965-1973.)

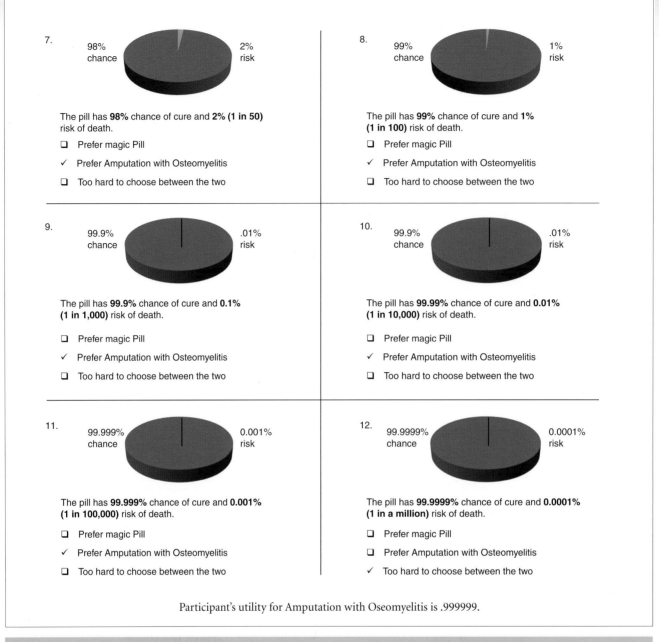

7. 98% chance — 2% risk

The pill has **98%** chance of cure and **2% (1 in 50)** risk of death.

☐ Prefer magic Pill

✓ Prefer Amputation with Osteomyelitis

☐ Too hard to choose between the two

8. 99% chance — 1% risk

The pill has **99%** chance of cure and **1% (1 in 100)** risk of death.

☐ Prefer magic Pill

✓ Prefer Amputation with Osteomyelitis

☐ Too hard to choose between the two

9. 99.9% chance — .01% risk

The pill has **99.9%** chance of cure and **0.1% (1 in 1,000)** risk of death.

☐ Prefer magic Pill

✓ Prefer Amputation with Osteomyelitis

☐ Too hard to choose between the two

10. 99.9% chance — .01% risk

The pill has **99.99%** chance of cure and **0.01% (1 in 10,000)** risk of death.

☐ Prefer magic Pill

✓ Prefer Amputation with Osteomyelitis

☐ Too hard to choose between the two

11. 99.999% chance — 0.001% risk

The pill has **99.999%** chance of cure and **0.001% (1 in 100,000)** risk of death.

☐ Prefer magic Pill

✓ Prefer Amputation with Osteomyelitis

☐ Too hard to choose between the two

12. 99.9999% chance — 0.0001% risk

The pill has **99.9999%** chance of cure and **0.0001% (1 in a million)** risk of death.

☐ Prefer magic Pill

☐ Prefer Amputation with Osteomyelitis

✓ Too hard to choose between the two

Participant's utility for Amputation with Oseomyelitis is .999999.

Figure 4 continued

rate of late contralateral SCFE exceeded 27%, prophylactic pinning is favored. A 27% incidence of late contralateral SCFE is clinically plausible, as in patients with endocrinopathy or renal failure. Therefore, the model is sensitive to this variable and suggests that prophylactic pinning may be optimal in these patient populations. This illustrates the ability of sensitivity analysis to account for patients who may have different characteristics than those used to establish baseline values. Even though data from these patients were not used to establish baseline values, decision making in their unique situations can be modeled.

Reporting and Interpreting Results
Identifying the Optimal Management Strategy
One of the primary goals of a decision analysis study is to identify the optimal management strategy for a given clinical problem. Through foldback analysis, the expected value of each of the alternative management strategies under evaluation has been determined. The strategy with the greatest expected value is then reported as the preferred strategy, although it is important to note that this conclusion is valid only for the outcome utilities and probabilities used in the model. Based on the difference between the expected values, a decision analysis model may clearly identify a superior

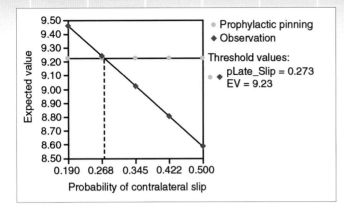

Figure 5 An example of a one-way sensitivity analysis for probability of contralateral SCFE in a model comparing observation with prophylactic pinning of the contralateral hip after unilateral SCFE. As the probability of late contralateral slip (pLate_Slip) increases, the expected value of observation (EV) decreases. The dashed line represents the threshold point (27% probability of contralateral SCFE) above which prophylactic pinning is favored. (Adapted from Kocher MS, Bishop JA, Hresko MT, Millis MB, Kim YJ, Kasser JR: Prophylactic pinning of the contralateral hip after unilateral slipped capital femoral epiphysis. *J Bone Joint Surg Am* 2004;86[12]: 2658-2665.)

strategy or reveal that the expected values after alternative strategies are very similar, making the base case analysis less conclusive.

Evaluating the Stability of the Model

As discussed previously, sensitivity analysis is employed to evaluate the stability of the model. If the optimal management strategy does not change when sensitivity analysis is performed on all variables within their plausible ranges, the findings of the model are robust and the conclusions strong. If the optimal management does change with sensitivity analysis, the conclusions of the model hold only for the particular patient population used to derive outcome utilities and probabilities. When stating the conclusions of such a model, appropriate qualifiers must be included. Outcomes in patient populations with different values and different outcome probabilities may be optimized with the alternative management strategy. Sensitivity analysis also can be used to provide insight into optimal decision making in these unique populations.

Identifying Important Variables

A decision analysis model can be helpful in identifying fruitful targets for future research. As previously noted, when a particular variable influences the optimal management strategy within a plausible range, it is highlighted as an important factor in the decision-making process. In the case of the SCFE decision analysis performed by Kocher et al[10] the model was shown to be sensitive to the probability of

Table 3

Guidelines for the Verbal Presentation of Decision Analysis Research

1.	Start with a title slide.
2.	Give appropriate background:
	Motivation, current beliefs, and main controversies.
3.	Articulate the study question:
	Losing the audience here is a disaster.
4.	Show the tree structure:
	–Clearly indicate the available strategies
	–Show the details in consecutive layers
	–Emphasize the important trade-offs
5.	List the important assumptions and data:
	Found by meta-analysis, literature review, new data, or best guess?
6.	Offer the main results:
	Base case results first, the table of one-way analysis, then a few two- or three-way sensitivity analyses.
7.	State the conclusion:
	One strategy dominates, a toss-up, or inconclusive?
8.	Discuss limitations and directions for future research.
9.	Deal with audience questions:
	Brief, simple, and nonconfrontational.

Reproduced with permission from Redelmeier DA, Detsky AS, Krahn MD, Naimark D, Naglie G: Guidelines for verbal presentations of medical decision analyses. *Med Decis Making* 1997;17(2):228-230.

late contralateral SCFE as illustrated in **Figure 5**. This highlights the importance of understanding the risk factors of late contralateral SCFE, and research efforts have been appropriately focused on this issue.[37,38]

Verbal Presentation of Decision Analysis

Because decision analysis remains a novel concept to many orthopaedic audiences, a clear presentation of such research is important. Therefore, guidelines for verbal presentations of decision analysis studies have been published.[39] Primary recommendations from these studies are summarized in Table 3.

Limitations

Modeling Complex Decisions

Depicting complex medical decision-making scenarios as a decision tree has limitations. Many tree designs assume that patients can only experience a single complication and that each of these complications is mutually exclusive. Experienced clinicians recognize that the variety of treatment algorithms and potential outcomes for a particular clinical problem are frequently more complex and nuanced than can be expressed in a decision tree. Therefore, clinical scenarios must sometimes be simplified to be modeled.[10]

Estimates of Probability and Utility

The quality of a decision analysis model is closely linked to the accuracy of estimates of outcome probability. In general, the most accurate and reliable estimates of outcome probability come from RCTs. Decision analyses are frequently performed to address questions for which RCTs are ethically, financially, or logistically nonviable, and therefore level I evidence is often unavailable for use in these models.

Reasonable outcome utility estimates can be similarly difficult to establish. Subjects with no background in medicine in general or orthopaedics in particular are often asked to assign values to outcomes to which they are introduced on only a most superficial level. A decision analysis model by Chung et al[12] comparing limb salvage with amputation for treatment of the mangled lower extremity illustrates the challenge of obtaining reliable outcome utility estimates. Outcome utilities were established using a standard reference gamble survey administered both to patients who had sustained a limb-threatening lower extremity injury and physicians from several disciples with an interest in limb salvage. As has been the case with several previous orthopaedic investigations, the physicians and patients assigned significantly different values to the various outcomes.

An additional challenge to the methodology of measuring patient preference comes from the psychology literature and the discovery of framing effects, which refers to the way in which formulation of a choice problem affects patient preferences. Ongoing psychology research has demonstrated that subjects are often risk averse in choices involving potential gains and risk taking in choices involving potential losses. A classic experiment from Tversky and Kahneman demonstrates that principle.[40] A group of students was asked to choose between two treatment programs for a hypothetical group of 600 people at risk for contracting a fatal disease. In program A, 200 people will be saved from death, whereas in program B there is a one-third probability that 600 people will be saved and a two-thirds probability that none will be saved. A separate group of students was asked to make a similar choice, but with distinct treatment programs. In program C, 400 people will die, whereas in program D there is a one-third probability that nobody will die and a two-thirds probability that everyone will die. Students strongly preferred program A to program B and program D

to program C. The two sets of programs are actually identical except that programs A and B frame the decision in terms of number of lives saved, whereas programs C and D frame the decision in terms of lives lost. The change in frame caused a significant change in preferences. If preferences are not fixed and stable, the entire decision analysis methodology is in question.[41]

Validation Studies

A formal evaluation of the quality and reproducibility of medical decision analysis studies has not been conducted. This lack of validation is an inherent limitation of the decision analysis. The orthopaedic literature provides an example of two distinct decision analyses that modeled the same clinical question and came to distinct conclusions. Two decision analysis models comparing prophylactic pinning to observation of the contralateral hip after unilateral slipped capital femoral epiphysis have been created.[10,13] The Kocher model defined outcome utilities by surveying patients to determine their preferences for various outcomes, whereas the Schultz model used Iowa hip scores obtained from a long-term study of SCFE. The definition of a late second slip also differed significantly between these studies. Kocher et al[10] estimated a 19% incidence based on a quantitative synthesis performed by Castro et al.[42] Schultz et al[13] estimated a 14% incidence of a late second slip based on a series by Hägglund[43] but also asserted that there is a 51% incidence of a late "silent" slip and incorporated this into the model. As a result, the Kocher model found that watchful waiting was the optimal management strategy, whereas the Schultz model suggested that prophylactic pinning would optimize outcome. Disparate results such as these challenge the credibility of the decision analysis method.

Summary

Decision analysis is a useful tool for quantitatively evaluating areas of uncertainty in orthopaedics, particularly when an RCT is not a viable option. The number of orthopaedic decision analyses has increased significantly over the past decade as surgeons have become increasingly familiar with the technique and applied it to many of the controversies that arise in practice. This chapter has focused on the rationale, methodology, and limitations of decision analysis as specifically applicable to orthopaedic problems. Refining the process of modeling complex decisions, accurately estimating outcome probabilities, and assigning valid and reproducible utilities should be among the objectives of ongoing decision analysis research.

References

1. Howard RA: Applied decision theory. *International Conference on Operations Research: Interscience.* Boston, MA, 1966, pp 55-71.

2. Henschke UK, Flehinger BJ: Decision theory in cancer therapy. *Cancer* 1967;20(11):1819-1826.

3. Bernstein J: Decision analysis. *J Bone Joint Surg Am* 1997; 79(9):1404-1414.

4. Kocher MS, Zurakowski D: Clinical epidemiology and biostatistics: A primer for orthopaedic surgeons. *J Bone Joint Surg Am* 2004;86(3):607-620.

5. Chen NC, Shauver MJ, Chung KC: A primer on use of decision analysis methodology in hand surgery. *J Hand Surg Am* 2009;34(6):983-990.

6. Kucey DS: Decision analysis for the surgeon. *World J Surg* 1999;23(12):1227-1231.

7. Sporer SM, Rosenberg AG: Decision analysis in orthopaedics. *Clin Orthop Relat Res* 2005;431:250-256.

8. Kocher MS, Bishop J, Marshall R, Briggs KK, Hawkins RJ: Operative versus nonoperative management of acute Achilles tendon rupture: Expected-value decision analysis. *Am J Sports Med* 2002;30(6):783-790.

9. Bishop J, Ring D: Management of radial nerve palsy associated with humeral shaft fracture: A decision analysis model. *J Hand Surg Am* 2009;34(6):991-996, e1.

10. Kocher MS, Bishop JA, Hresko MT, Millis MB, Kim YJ, Kasser JR: Prophylactic pinning of the contralateral hip after unilateral slipped capital femoral epiphysis. *J Bone Joint Surg Am* 2004;86(12):2658-2665.

11. Koenig KM, Davis GC, Grove MR, Tosteson AN, Koval KJ: Is early internal fixation preferred to cast treatment for well-reduced unstable distal radial fractures? *J Bone Joint Surg Am* 2009;91(9):2086-2093.

12. Chung KC, Saddawi-Konefka D, Haase SC, Kaul G: A cost-utility analysis of amputation versus salvage for Gustilo type IIIB and IIIC open tibial fractures. *Plast Reconstr Surg* 2009; 124(6):1965-1973.

13. Schultz WR, Weinstein JN, Weinstein SL, Smith BG: Prophylactic pinning of the contralateral hip in slipped capital femoral epiphysis: Evaluation of long-term outcome for the contralateral hip with use of decision analysis. *J Bone Joint Surg Am* 2002;84(8):1305-1314.

14. Brauer CA, Graham B: The surgical treatment of cubital tunnel syndrome: A decision analysis. *J Hand Surg Eur Vol* 2007;32(6):654-662.

15. Cavaliere CM, Chung KC: Total wrist arthroplasty and total wrist arthrodesis in rheumatoid arthritis: A decision analysis from the hand surgeons' perspective. *J Hand Surg Am* 2008; 33(10):1744-1755, e1-e2.

16. Davis MA: Posterior spinal fusion versus anterior/posterior spinal fusion for adolescent idiopathic scoliosis: A decision analysis. *Spine (Phila Pa 1976)* 2009;34(21):2318-2323.

17. Graham B, Detsky AS: The application of decision analysis to the surgical treatment of early osteoarthritis of the wrist. *J Bone Joint Surg Br* 2001;83(5):650-654.

18. Hernandez RJ, Cornell RG, Hensinger RN: Ultrasound diagnosis of neonatal congenital dislocation of the hip: A decision analysis assessment. *J Bone Joint Surg Br* 1994;76(4): 539-543.

19. Kailes SB, Richmond JC: Arthroscopic vs. open Bankart reconstruction: A comparison using expected value decision analysis. *Knee Surg Sports Traumatol Arthrosc* 2001;9(6):379-385.

20. Mahan ST, Katz JN, Kim YJ: To screen or not to screen? A decision analysis of the utility of screening for developmental dysplasia of the hip. *J Bone Joint Surg Am* 2009;91(7): 1705-1719.

21. Seng K, Appleby D, Lubowitz JH: Operative versus nonoperative treatment of anterior cruciate ligament rupture in patients aged 40 years or older: An expected-value decision analysis. *Arthroscopy* 2008;24(8):914-920.

22. van der Velde G, Hogg-Johnson S, Bayoumi AM, et al: Identifying the best treatment among common nonsurgical neck pain treatments: A decision analysis. *Spine (Phila Pa 1976)* 2008;33(4, suppl)S184-S191.

23. Zangger P, Detsky A: Computer-assisted decision analysis in orthopedics: Resurfacing the patella in total knee arthroplasty as an example. *J Arthroplasty* 2000;15(3):283-288.

24. Bernstein J: Early versus delayed reconstruction of the anterior cruciate ligament: a decision analysis approach. *J Bone Joint Surg Am* 2011;93(9):e48.

25. Wolf CF, Gu NY, Doctor JN, Manner PA, Leopold SS: Comparison of one and two-stage revision of total hip arthroplasty complicated by infection: A Markov expected-utility decision analysis. *J Bone Joint Surg Am* 2011;93(7):631-639.

26. Detsky AS, Naglie G, Krahn MD, Redelmeier DA, Naimark D: Primer on medical decision analysis: Part 2. Building a tree. *Med Decis Making* 1997;17(2):126-135.

27. Detsky AS, Naglie G, Krahn MD, Naimark D, Redelmeier DA: Primer on medical decision analysis: Part 1. Getting started. *Med Decis Making* 1997;17(2):123-125.

28. Naglie G, Krahn MD, Naimark D, Redelmeier DA, Detsky AS: Primer on medical decision analysis: Part 3. Estimating probabilities and utilities. *Med Decis Making* 1997;17(2):136-141.

29. Krahn MD, Naglie G, Naimark D, Redelmeier DA, Detsky AS: Primer on medical decision analysis: Part 4. Analyzing the model and interpreting the results. *Med Decis Making* 1997;17(2):142-151.

30. Shao YC, Harwood P, Grotz MR, Limb D, Giannoudis PV: Radial nerve palsy associated with fractures of the shaft of the humerus: A systematic review. *J Bone Joint Surg Br* 2005; 87(12):1647-1652.

31. Linstone HA, Turoff M: *The Delphi Method: Techniques and Applications.* Boston, MA, Addison-Wesley, 1975.

32. Brauer CA, Rosen AB, Greenberg D, Neumann PJ: Trends in the measurement of health utilities in published cost-utility analyses. *Value Health* 2006;9(4):213-218.

33. Morimoto T, Fukui T: Utilities measured by rating scale, time trade-off, and standard gamble: Review and reference for health care professionals. *J Epidemiol* 2002;12(2):160-178.

34. Torrance GW: Measurement of health state utilities for economic appraisal. *J Health Econ* 1986;5(1):1-30.

35. Parkin D, Devlin N: Is there a case for using visual analogue scale valuations in cost-utility analysis? *Health Econ* 2006; 15(7):653-664.

36. Stiggelbout AM, Eijkemans MJ, Kiebert GM, Kievit J, Leer JW, De Haes HJ: The 'utility' of the visual analog scale in medical decision making and technology assessment: Is it an alternative to the time trade-off? *Int J Technol Assess Health Care* 1996;12(2):291-298.

37. Park S, Hsu JE, Rendon N, Wolfgruber H, Wells L: The utility of posterior sloping angle in predicting contralateral slipped capital femoral epiphysis. *J Pediatr Orthop* 2010; 30(7):683-689.

38. Riad J, Bajelidze G, Gabos PG: Bilateral slipped capital femoral epiphysis: predictive factors for contralateral slip. *J Pediatr Orthop* 2007;27(4):411-414.

39. Redelmeier DA, Detsky AS, Krahn MD, Naimark D, Naglie G: Guidelines for verbal presentations of medical decision analyses. *Med Decis Making* 1997;17(2):228-230.

40. Tversky A, Kahneman D: The framing of decisions and the psychology of choice. *Science* 1981;211(4481):453-458.

41. Petitti DB: *Meta-Analysis, Decision Analysis, and Cost-Effectiveness Analysis: Methods for Quantitative Synthesis in Medicine*, ed 2. New York, NY, Oxford University Press USA, 2000.

42. Castro FP Jr, Bennett JT, Doulens K: Epidemiological perspective on prophylactic pinning in patients with unilateral slipped capital femoral epiphysis. *J Pediatr Orthop* 2000; 20(6):745-748.

43. Hägglund G: The contralateral hip in slipped capital femoral epiphysis. *J Pediatr Orthop B* 1996;5(3):158-161.

4: Clinical Science

Chapter 33

Biostatistics in Clinical Research

Elena Losina, PhD, MSc
William Reichmann, MA
Jeffrey N. Katz, MD, MSc

Biostatistics is the study of the collection, organization, analysis, and interpretation of numeric data applied to biologic and health sciences, including medical research. Biostatistics is used to "tell stories" with numbers, because numbers may communicate ideas more precisely than words. The use of biostatistical methods coupled with epidemiologic concepts of study design and outcome measurement is essential for the development of evidence-based medicine.[1]

Motivational Example

An orthopaedic surgeon who has spent decades performing total hip replacement on elderly individuals has noticed over the years that patients with great preoperative functional limitations are more likely to experience great functional limitations after recovering from surgery. The surgeon would like to know whether his or her observations can be summarized and compared with the experiences of other surgeons. Consequently, the surgeon decides to gather evidence that may confirm the association between preoperative and postoperative functional limitations. How should the surgeon proceed?

Dr. Katz or an immediate family member serves as a board member, owner, officer, or committee member of the OsteoArthritis Research Society International. Neither of the following authors nor any immediate family member has received anything of value from or owns stock in a commercial company or institution related directly or indirectly to the subject of this article: Dr. Losina and Dr. Reichmann.

Characteristics of a Statistical Problem

To understand how statistics can be helpful in framing and addressing scientific hypotheses related to medical questions, it is important to understand key characteristics of the statistical problem. In general, there is a large group of patients about whom clinicians and researchers would like to make some statements. This group is called the population; certain characteristics of the members of the population are of particular interest. The value of these characteristics may change from subject to subject within the population. These characteristics are called random variables. Studying the population in its entirety often is impractical. The science of biostatistics develops methods that help to make inferences about the population based on what is observed in a portion of the population, which is called the sample[1] (Figure 1).

Properties of a Good Sample

Figure 1 represents the use of statistics to address questions related to the population. Features of populations are termed parameters. Because entire populations cannot be studied, parameters cannot be calculated directly. Instead, a sample is gathered from the population, and statistics are calculated. These statistics serve to estimate parameters in the population. The sample will not have exactly the same properties as the population. Deviation of the sample statistics from the parameter is called sampling error. A smaller sample, on average, will have more sampling error than a larger sample. A good sample, from the statistical point of view, has three key properties. First, each member of the population has an equal chance of being selected into the sample. This results in a random sample. Second, members of the sample should be fair representations of the popula-

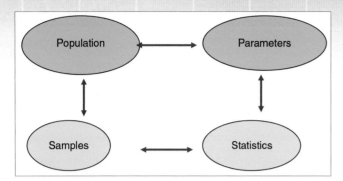

Figure 1 Overview of statistical inference from study samples.

tion. This ensures that conclusions arising from the sample are generalizable to the population. And, third, inclusion of one individual should not change the probability of choosing another individual. Members of the sample should be independent of one another.[2]

Branches of Statistical Methodology

Statistical methodology can be divided into two main branches: descriptive statistics and inferential statistics. Descriptive statistics include summary statistics such as frequencies, percentages, means, and ranges. These statistics can be presented in graphs and tables. Inferential statistics provides methodology for arriving at conclusions about the population from evidence derived from the sample. The main focus of inferential statistics is on hypothesis testing.[3]

Descriptive Statistics

Descriptive statistics comprise measures of central tendency. These include the mode, median, and mean.

Mode is defined as the value that occurs most often. The mode is best for describing nominal data because it is simple to compute, can be used for all levels of measurement, and is not affected by extreme values. Disadvantages of using the mode include that it is usually not very descriptive of the data, does not use all values, is not necessarily unique (multimodal distributions occur often), and is sensitive to how categories are defined.[1]

Median is defined as the value corresponding to the middle of all values of the variable. Half of observations are greater than the median and half are less. The median is not affected by extreme values, always exists, is easy to compute, and is good for all levels of measurement except nominal data. The median is especially useful for description of skewed distributions. It is important to note that the median does not use all the data values and categories must be properly ordered for the median to be estimated accurately.[1]

Mean is defined as an arithmetic average. The mean is the most frequently used measure of central tendency. Calculation of the mean uses all of the data and is particularly useful for describing the center of a distribution. The mean is highly sensitive to extreme values and may be misleading

if used for highly skewed distributions.[1]

Measures of central tendency do not capture the variability of the distribution. Typical measures of variability include range, which is defined by the difference between the highest and lowest value of the distribution, interquartile range, standard deviation, and variance.[1]

Types of Random Variables

A continuous variable can take any value within a specified interval and is described by mean, median, standard deviation, and range.[4] This type of categorization is sometimes useful to improve transparency of interpretation. Examples of continuous variables include weight, height, age, range of motion, and outcome scores, such as the Western Ontario and McMaster Universities Osteoarthritis Index[5] or Oswestry Disability Index.[5,6] Continuous variables are often described by using the normal distribution. In the normal distribution the mean, median, and mode all have the same value; which curves symmetrically around the mean. If a continuous random variable follows a normal distribution, 68% of its values fall within one standard deviation of the mean and 95% of values fall within two standard deviations of the mean.[4]

Continuous variables are not the only variables that can describe data arising in clinical practice. Discrete or categorical variables use a finite, countable number of possible values. Categorical variables can be further classified as nominal or ordinal. Nominal variables have categories that do not have an inherent ordering. Examples of nominal variables include sex, incision approach for total hip replacement (for example, posterolateral, lateral, anterior), side, and type of prosthesis. Nominal variables are usually described by percentages. Ordinal variables have categories that can be ordered. Examples of ordinal variables include Likert scales for satisfaction with surgery (very satisfied, somewhat satisfied, somewhat dissatisfied, very dissatisfied) and self-reported health (excellent, very good, good, fair, or poor), number of comorbidities, number of revisions, and American Society of Anesthesiologists criteria. Ordinal variables are usually described by percentages, cumulative frequencies, and medians.[4]

Inferential Statistics

In addition to describing the sample, the next step is to frame and test the hypothesis about population parameters using sample statistics. Statistical inference offers methods that facilitate making a statement about a population based on the results of a sample.

Hypothesis Testing

Testing of statistical hypotheses is a capstone of inferential statistics. The test uses the sample data to decide between two competing hypotheses or claims about a population parameter. The hypothesis is always formulated in relation to population parameters. In formulating a statistical hypothesis, the two types are the null and alternative hypothesis.

Table 1

Types of Errors in Statistical Hypothesis Testing

	Truth	
Decision	Null hypothesis is true	Alternative hypothesis is true
Do not reject the null hypothesis.	Correct decision	Wrong decision—Type II error
Reject null hypothesis.	Wrong decision—Type I error	Correct decision

The null hypothesis is often a statement of no difference between parameters with respect to levels of another factor.[1] The alternative hypothesis claims the opposite. In statistical hypothesis testing, the null hypothesis is tested most of the time. The essence of hypothesis testing is the determination of whether the sample carries sufficient evidence to state that the null hypothesis is false. If the sample does offer enough evidence, then the null hypothesis is rejected in favor of the alternative hypothesis. Often a statistical hypothesis is set up in hopes of being able to reject the null hypothesis. In most of the methods of statistical hypothesis testing, the goal is not to prove the null hypothesis but rather to have enough evidence to reject the null hypothesis. If the null hypothesis is not rejected, the null hypothesis is not supported, but rather there is insufficient evidence to reject it.[2]

Type I and Type II Errors

Every time the null hypothesis is rejected, there is the risk of being wrong. Every time a physician fails to reject the null hypothesis, there is the risk of being wrong. Table 1 describes the consequences of being wrong and acceptable levels of errors. A type I error occurs when the null hypothesis is rejected when the null hypothesis is true. It is often noted as the level of statistical significance or α. A type II error occurs when the physician fails to reject the null hypothesis when the null hypothesis is false.[2] It is often noted as β or 1 minus the power of the study (discussed later).

The level of statistical significance is determined before the test and is defined as the criterion used to reject a null hypothesis. When hypothesis testing is done, the physician formulates the hypothesis, assumes that the null hypothesis is true, collects the data, and calculates the appropriate test statistic. The p-value is defined as probability that observed or even more extreme results would be obtained assuming that the null hypothesis is true. If the p-value is lower than the chosen level of statistical significance (for example, less than 0.05), the null hypothesis is rejected.[2]

Reaching statistical significance depends on the magnitude of the effect and sample size. Values must be defined that are statistically significant and clinically important. If the sample is too large, statistically significant results may be seen in situations that are not clinically important. If the sample is too small, statistically significant results may not be seen in situations where the differences appear to be clin-

ically important.[3] In these situations the investigator can note that, although the differences could be attributed to chance alone, they may also be clinically important and merit further study. However, the use of terms such as borderline statistical significance or trend toward statistical significance is discouraged.

Power

Power of the test is defined as the probability of rejecting the null hypothesis given that the null hypothesis is false. Factors influencing power include significance level, the magnitude of the effect, and sample size.[2] A sample with more subjects allows the null hypothesis to be rejected when there is a smaller difference. More subjects will also yield narrower confidence levels for parameter estimates. Additional subjects are likely to be costly to enroll in the study. Greater numbers of subjects may also increase the complexity of the study.

To obtain a meaningful sample size estimation, prior knowledge is needed of the prevalence of risk factors, prevalence of the outcome, efficacy or effectiveness of intervention, and desired power, as well as recruitment and dropout rates.[2] Calculation of sample size estimates is critical for investigators to understand whether the study is feasible as planned and the duration of recruitment to obtain the desired sample size. For example, if desirable sample size is estimated at 1,050, and it is known that the capacity of the clinic is approximately 300 patients per month, assuming that 50% will be eligible and 50% of those eligible will be willing to participate will result in an estimated recruitment of 75 subjects per month. Therefore, such a study would require an enrollment stage of approximately 14 months.

Statistical Analysis

The appropriate statistical analysis depends on the type of data and hypothesis of interest. For examining linear associations, the Pearson correlation or linear regression are appropriate analytic tools. When means between several groups are compared, the independent sample Student *t* test (two groups) or analysis of variance (more than two groups) is appropriate. To compare risks of an event among several groups, the chi-square test or logistic regression is the most appropriate analytic tool. To compare time to an event such as death or prosthesis failure among several

Table 2

Properties and Conditions Under Which Certain Statistical Analyses Are Performed

Statistical Analysis	Outcome	Independent Variable(s)	Purpose
Correlation	Continuous	Continuous	Examine the linear association between two variables. No distinction is made between the outcome and independent variables.
Linear regression	Continuous	Continuous or categorical	Examine the linear association between two or more variables.
Independent samples (Student t test)	Continuous	Categorical—two groups	Compare the means between two independent groups.
Analysis of variance (ANOVA)	Continuous	Categorical—two or more groups	Compare the means between two or more independent groups. ANOVA is a special case of linear regression.
Chi-square test of independence	Categorical—two or more groups	Categorical—two or more groups	Compare two categorical variables to see if they are associated with each other. Similar to the correlation in that no distinction between the outcome and independent variable needs to be made.
Logistic regression	Categorical—typically two groups, but other methods of logistic regression can use more than two groups	Continuous or categorical	Examine the association with a categorical outcome and a set of predictors.

groups, survival analysis techniques should be considered.[2] A summary of statistical analyses in relationship to types of variables of interest is presented in **Table 2.**

Summary

Statistical analysis uses both descriptive and inferential statistics. In addressing a scientific question, the first and most important step is to define a clinically important scientific question. A study is then designed to address the question. An outcome measure must be identified that captures the key end point and has been validated. The sample size is calculated. The data are collected and statistical methods used to test the prespecified hypothesis. Typically either the null hypothesis is rejected on the basis of the observed data or the null hypothesis is not rejected. In this manner, the data are ultimately used to tell the clinical story.

Acknowledgment

Supported by NIH/NIAMS K24 AR057827, P60 AR 47782, T32 AR 055885.

References

1. D'Agostino RB, Sullivan LM, Beiser AS: *Introductory Applied Biostatistics.* Florence, KY, Brooks/Cole, 2006.

2. Armitage P, Colton T: *Encyclopedia of Biostatistics.* Hoboken, NJ, Wiley, 2005, 8 vols.

3. Gerstman BB: *Basic Biostatistics: Statistics for Public Health Practice.* Sudbury, MA, Jones & Bartlett Publishers, 2008.

4. Glantz SA: *Primer of Biostatistics.* New York, NY, McGraw-Hill Medical, 2005.

5. Bellamy N, Buchanan WW, Goldsmith CH, Campbell J, Stitt LW: Validation study of WOMAC: A health status instrument for measuring clinically important patient relevant outcomes to antirheumatic drug therapy in patients with osteoarthritis of the hip or knee. *J Rheumatol* 1988;15(12):1833-1840.

6. Fairbank JC, Pynsent PB: The Oswestry Disability Index. *Spine (Phila Pa 1976)* 2000;25(22):2940-2952.

4: Clinical Science

Chapter 34

Ethical Considerations in Clinical Research

James D. Capozzi, MD
Rosamond Rhodes, PhD

A Historical Perspective

Several years ago a patient came to the office of one of this chapter's authors (JC) for a consultation regarding hip and back pain. He was in his early 70s and walked with a slight limp. The patient revealed that he wore a prosthesis for an above-knee amputation on his left side that was performed during World War II. As a Jewish teenager living in Germany, he had been imprisoned in a Nazi concentration camp. The physicians there, in an attempt to assess human pain thresholds, proceeded to perform surgery on his leg without the use of anesthesia. The patient was strapped to a table where, fully conscious, doctors operated on his thigh. At some point during the procedure, restrained and screaming, he lost consciousness. When he awoke, his thigh was bandaged. His leg had been amputated.

Prior to World War II, ethical standards for conducting medical experimentation were not in place. Although a few statements on research ethics had been produced, they were not commonly known nor widely promulgated. In preparation for the trial of Nazi physicians accused of atrocities, the Nuremberg Military Tribunal requested that a panel of expert witnesses "articulate the universal standards of ethical research."[1] American physicians Andrew Ivy and Leo Alexander proposed six standards of ethical research practices. The Tribunal accepted the six standards and added an additional four. The result of their work, the Nuremberg Code, thus became the first broadly shared standard of conduct

for studies of human subjects, and it established some of the basic principles governing the ethical practice of that research.[2]

The Nuremberg Code articulated the core principle that "the voluntary consent of the human subject is absolutely essential." It continued with nine additional principles of ethical conduct in human research, which are presented in **Table 1**.

In 1964 the World Medical Association proposed its own significantly different standards for doctors conducting research on human subjects, the Declaration of Helsinki. In 1966, the United States Public Health Service, the parent body of the National Institutes of Health, issued its Policies for the Protection of Human Subjects. The policies governed research funded by the National Institutes of Health and required institutional prospective assurance review of the rights and welfare of the individuals involved, the appropriateness of informed consent methods used, and the risks and potential benefits of the investigation. In short, these policies established Institutional Review Boards (IRBs). In 1974, those policies were elevated to regulatory status by the Department of Health, Education, and Welfare.

That same year, the National Research Act was passed, establishing the National Commission for the Protection of Human Subjects of Biomedical and Behavioral Research. The Commission, comprising physicians, scientists, theologians, and attorneys, met over a 4-year period, reporting and recommending guidelines regarding the conduct of biomedical and behavioral research on human subjects. In 1979, the Commission issued its Belmont Report elucidating basic ethical principles for conducting biomedical research.

In 1981, the Department of Health and Human Services (formerly the Department of Health, Education, and Welfare) and the Food and Drug Administration, in response to the Commission's reports and recommendations, revised

Dr. Capozzi or an immediate family member has received royalties from BodyworksMD and has stock or stock options held in Pfizer. Neither Dr. Rhodes nor any immediate family member has received anything of value from or owns stock in a commercial company or institution related directly or indirectly to the subject of this chapter.

4: Clinical Science

Table 1

The Nuremberg Code: Nine Principles of Ethical Conduct in Human Research

The experiment should be such as to yield fruitful results for the good of society, unprocurable by other methods or means of study, and not random and unnecessary in nature.

The experiment should be so designed and based on the results of animal experimentation and knowledge of the natural history of the disease or other problem under study that the anticipated results will justify the performance of the experiment.

The experiment should be so conducted as to avoid all unnecessary physical and mental suffering and injury.

No experiment should be conducted where there is an a priori reason to believe that death or disabling injury will occur; except, perhaps, in those experiments where the experimental physicians also serve as subjects.

The degree of risk to be taken should never exceed that determined by the humanitarian importance of the problem to be solved by the experiment.

Proper preparations should be made and adequate facilities provided to protect the experimental subject against even remote possibilities of injury, disability, or death.

The experiment should be conducted only by scientifically qualified persons. The highest degree of skill and care of those who conduct or engage in the experiment should be required through all stages of the experiment.

During the course of the experiment the human subject should be at liberty to bring the experiment to an end if he or she has reached the physical or mental state where continuation of the experiment seems to him or her to be impossible.

During the course of the experiment the scientist in charge must be prepared to terminate the experiment at any stage, if he or she has probable cause to believe, in the exercise of the good faith, superior skill, and careful judgment required of him or her that a continuation of the experiment is likely to result in injury, disability, or death to the experimental subject.

Adapted from Appelbaum PS, Lidz CW, Meisel A: *Informed Consent: Legal Theory and Clinical Practice.* New York, NY, Oxford University Press, 1987.

their human subject regulations in what is now referred to as The Common Rule. As its name implies, the policy was designed to codify the protection of human subjects for all relevant federal agencies and departments. The Common Rule requires that consent for human research occur "only under circumstances that provide the prospective subject sufficient opportunity to consider whether or not to participate and that minimizes the possibility of coercion or undue influence."[3]

Some of the most notorious examples of ethical abuses in medical studies in the United States before the establishment of the Common Rule include the Tuskegee syphilis studies, the Willowbrook studies, and the human radiation studies.[4,5] In the Tuskegee syphilis studies, impoverished African-American men were never told that they were participants in research on syphilis and were never offered treatment with penicillin when it became available. Similarly disturbing studies were conducted at the Willowbrook State Hospital in Staten Island, NY. There, live hepatitis virus was injected into severely developmentally disabled children. Equally as disturbing, in a series of human radiation studies performed after World War II, civilians were never informed that they were deliberately exposed to radiation so that its effects could be studied. Such vivid examples demonstrate the importance of establishing and enforcing standards for the ethical conduct of human-subject research and

implementing mandatory institutional review procedures for the systematic oversight of studies.

At the same time, it is critical to remember that medicine is science applied to the moral goal of acting for the good of patients and society. When patients seek the help of a medical doctor, the patient relies on the physician to make decisions based on established biomedical science. Medical professionals are, therefore, committed to guiding their practice by science. Although the phrase evidence-based medicine is relatively new to the medical literature, patients have long believed that doctors always use evidence to guide their practice, and they turn to doctors because they expect their decisions to be based on proven scientific results.

Orthopaedic surgeons' professional responsibility to guide their practice with evidence entails a commitment to "using modern quality assurance strategies" in furthering the clinical community's knowledge.[6] Two points in The Code of Ethics and Professionalism for Orthopaedic Surgeons, articulated by the American Academy of Orthopaedic Surgeons, are particularly germane to this issue.[7] The Academy's public declaration of its ethical responsibilities asserts the following:

IV, A. The orthopaedic surgeon continually should strive to maintain and improve medical knowledge and skill and should make available to patients and colleagues the benefits of his or her professional attainments.

IX, A. The honored ideals of the medical profession imply that the responsibility of the orthopaedic surgeon extends not only to the individual but also to society as a whole. Activities that have the purpose of improving the health and well being of the patient and/or the community in a cost-effective way deserve the interest, support, and participation of the orthopaedic surgeon.

Reading these statements with a knowledge of harms resulting from a lack of data, they clearly suggest what Gruen et al[6] conclude, that "we surgeons have a professional responsibility to ensure that our interventions are more effective than alternatives and, for this reason, outcomes-based research must be supported." In other words, orthopaedic surgeons' acknowledged professional responsibility to "improve medical knowledge" and to improve the "well being of the patient" requires them to engage in research, to cooperate with research, to support research, and to advocate for the creation of national registries for follow-up of new treatments and devices.[8]

The Ethical Conduct of Clinical Research

Once the importance of clinical research is acknowledged as a central element in the professional commitments of orthopaedic surgeons, it is important to consider how orthopaedic research can be conducted in accordance with the highest ethical standards. Seven ethical requirements for evaluating human subject studies have been delineated,[9] drawing on various codes, principles, agency recommendations, and reports that had been articulated over the previous decades, to refine and synthesize key points. Together, these requirements comprise a framework for understanding the ethics of research involving human subjects. These seven requirements are explained in the following paragraphs by providing an example of each provision related to orthopaedics and elaborating on its significance and importance.

For research to be valuable it must be possible for the study design to advance knowledge. The study must be focused on trying to answer a question that will forward understanding of physiologic function or help to advance clinical treatment. The study design must be capable of providing an answer to the study question. When orthopaedic surgeons did not know whether arthroscopic débridement and lavage was an effective treatment of knee arthritis, a study to answer that question was well justified. According to one study in 2002, more than 650,000 such procedures were performed each year, at a cost of approximately $5,000 each.[10] Although arthroscopic lavage became the standard of care, it had never been proven effective. The study found that this "treatment" was in fact no more effective in relieving pain than placebo surgery. Thousands of patients had undergone seemingly unnecessary surgery, along with its risks, costs, and the burdens of pain and discomfort over a long recovery period, simply because this intervention had become the accepted practice. Data from that study showed the intervention to be ineffective. The randomized controlled prospective study by Moseley et al[10] was the basis for abandoning that particular intervention as a treatment of that specific condition.

Because cemented total knee arthroplasty has already been proven an effective treatment, and because arthroscopic débridement and lavage has already been shown to be ineffective, the study design will not contribute any new knowledge. The answer to the question, "Which of these two interventions is more effective?" is already known. In this circumstance, imposing the risks and inconveniences on subjects of the proposed study of an intervention that has already been shown to be useless cannot be justified. The human and financial resources devoted to such a project could be allocated in other more productive ways.

When the data produced by a study are inadequate to transform professional opinion, another study could be well justified. In addition, when a study seems to answer one question about a treatment while raising other questions, for example, about long-term outcomes, further study is in order. The study described above, however, suggests none of these sorts of justifications.

For a study design to be valid it must be adequate for answering the study question with a reasonable degree of certainty. Fatal pulmonary embolism is a relatively rare complication of hip replacement surgery, occurring in

Value

Case Scenario:

An orthopaedic surgeon and colleagues are planning to undertake a randomized, prospective study of two treatment modalities for severe knee arthritis. They have randomly assigned patients with advanced degenerative arthritis of the knee into two surgical groups. One group is to be treated with a standard, cemented total knee arthroplasty. The second group is to be treated with arthroscopic débridement and lavage. Both groups are followed for 2 years after the surgical procedure.

Scientific Validity

Case Scenario:

An orthopaedic surgeon who wants to study two different treatments of fatal pulmonary embolism prophylaxis following hip replacement randomly assigns patients to the two different protocol groups. The surgeon performs approximately 50 joint arthroplasties per year.

4: Clinical Science

approximately 1 in 500 patients.[11] Thus, it is not likely that any of this surgeon's patients in either arm of the study will suffer this complication. If any do, the numbers will be too small to support a statistically valid conclusion and inadequate to support anyone's confidence in choosing one treatment over the other.

A clinical trial of alternative treatment modalities is supposed to provide evidence for altering clinical practice. Thus, the study design must be sufficiently powered to provide an answer to the study question that statistically demonstrates to the community of surgeons that the results could not have occurred by mere chance. In circumstances where each of the alternative modalities has a committed following, the study design must be sufficiently robust to convince those who are skeptical and reluctant to alter their practice that a change will actually serve the interests of their patients.[12]

These proof requirements translate into the necessity for designing studies that can show what they claim to demonstrate and that will involve an adequate number of subjects to support valid conclusions. The demands of clinical research also require researchers to avoid stopping studies prematurely and to continue the studies beyond the minimal statistical standards. When a study is discontinued before the amassed evidence is sufficient for convincing the community of professionals, the study has not achieved its purpose of advancing clinical care. In addition, when the evidence provided by the data leaves uncertainty or raises new questions (for example, does the treatment that is more effective for pulmonary embolism prophylaxis increase the risk of developing some other organ system disease?), further study is in order.

Revision surgery accounts for approximately 17% to 18% of total hip replacement procedures.[13] At least some of these revisions are related to issues with the implant device. The need for these replacement procedures could be minimized

Fair Subject Selection

Case Scenario:

Several hospitals located within a geographic region elect to begin a voluntary joint arthroplasty registry program. They believe that by pooling information from several hospitals they can develop data that will allow them to follow their patients and identify unanticipated complications and potentially dangerous problems early in the course of using a new device. Several surgeons elect not to participate in the registry. Several surgeons submit some but not all of their patient information.

with ongoing data collection and prompt reporting. Joint arthroplasty surgeons will undoubtedly remember the failures of threaded acetabular shells, metal-backed patella components, titanium bearing surfaces, and first-generation

ceramic implants. The clinical impact of these failures could have been minimized with comprehensive data collection and prompt reporting. In addition, complications arising from surgical techniques, perioperative care practices, or other factors not specifically related to the device could be brought to light more quickly and lead to rapid responses and changes.[14]

Delays in reporting implant failures (for example, the Durom acetabular shell [Zimmer Holding, Warsaw, IN]) largely because of sporadic experiences and noncentralization of data, had crippling consequences for some of the thousands of patients who received that defective device. Other countries, including Australia, Britain, Norway, and Sweden, had national databases that tracked outcomes after joint arthroplasty surgery. Thus, registries in Australia and Sweden alerted surgeons in those countries to stop using flawed devices before American surgeons stopped using them.

It is very difficult for individual surgeons, whose experience is necessarily limited by the relatively small number of clinical patients they encounter, to recognize a pattern of success or failure related to a particular treatment or device. Without systematic data collection, no one can identify the small statistical differences that make one treatment choice better or worse than another. Such examples constitute an argument for the implementation of registries by the American Academy of Orthopaedic Surgeons. A joint registry is the classic example pointing to the pressing need for ongoing data collection to be a standard companion to treatment so that orthopaedic surgeons can be provided with the information that they need to avoid harming patients.

This view has profound implications for fair subject selection regarding clinical research. It suggests that just as every patient should be willing to participate in the education of future doctors, everyone should also be willing to help advance medical knowledge by participating in biomedical research. Although patients are not forced to accept the participation of trainees (such as medical students, residents, and fellows) in their care, general cooperation in the educational effort is important and patients should be encouraged to participate. Although no one should be compelled to enroll in research, patients should be encouraged to participate in studies and in registries as a feature of fair subject selection. Both principled arguments and a practical argument for this position are presented in the following paragraphs.[15,16]

The Argument From Justice

Everyone is vulnerable to death, pain, disability, and the loss of pleasure and freedom that may be consequent to disease. These are conditions that are preferably avoided, and everyone would like a remedy to be available. Almost everyone has medical needs at some point in their lives. Yet, the need to improve on the standard of care for numerous acute and chronic conditions must be acknowledged. Physicians need to learn about the causes and natural development of diseases and the effectiveness of treatments. The desired advance in treatment can only be achieved by studying the body. Study involves some sacrifice of flesh, privacy, safety, comfort, and time. Because these basic goods are precious to everyone, noninstrumental basic principles of justice, such as equality and the anti–free-rider principle, require everyone to do his or her fair share to advance the common good. Because it is expected that everyone share in the benefits of future medical advances, at least to some degree, all must participate.

The Argument From Beneficence
The obligation characterized by the phrase "do unto others as you would have them do unto you" leads to the same conclusion. Because anyone would want effective treatment for a medical need, and because such medical advances require the cooperation of many in the research enterprise, the principle of mutual love dictates that people should give of themselves to help advance medical science. Emotional and genetic interrelatedness, the lack of an adequate alternative, and the commonality of the desire to benefit from medical knowledge create this participatory duty.

A Practical Argument
Looking toward the future of personalized medicine makes the case to participate in medical research even more strongly. The expectation is that researchers will learn a great deal more about the human genome and the human microbiome, and that this new knowledge will allow medicine to tailor treatments specific to individuals. These advances promise to make medicine more effective and possibly even more affordable. The studies to advance this science will require the development of biobank and sample bank repositories with the participation of a large number of subjects. To reap the rewards of advancing the practice of medicine, broad public participation will be required. Furthermore, to the extent that any group abstains from participation, its members will be less able to share in the rewards precisely because their genetic and microbiome samples will be absent from the studied pool. When those with chronic conditions (such as osteoarthritis) or heritable medical problems (such as Gaucher disease) abstain from participating in research, it is less likely that advances to benefit people with these conditions or their genetic susceptibilities will be developed.

It would be unfair to choose a particular social group to serve as research subjects so that others could benefit at their expense. Likewise, it would also be unfair to impose research burdens on those who would have no prospects of sharing in the medical advances that biomedical research could bring. It is fair, however, to ask all of those who hope to benefit from research to contribute some modicum of effort in the communal effort to improve health care. When the orthopaedic community needs to determine what alternative treatment is most effective, it is fair to ask patients to participate in a study. When the orthopaedic community

creates a registry to track the unanticipated problems of a new device, it is fair to ask every patient who receives the device to participate.

It is always difficult to compare the risks and benefits of medical interventions because typically the advantages and disadvantages cannot be measured in the same terms. Physicians, nevertheless, are regularly called upon to make cal-

Favorable Risk-Benefit Ratio
Case Scenario:
An orthopaedic surgeon is discouraged by the high incidence of postoperative anteromedial knee pain in her patients following total knee arthroplasty. She randomizes her patients who experience pain following knee replacement surgery into two groups. One group is treated with modalities including oral NSAIDs, analgesic dermal patches, and ice. The second group receives a series of cortisone injections into the affected area over the proximal anteromedial tibia.

culations that involve balancing incommensurable factors. Surgeons, in particular, must make risk-benefit comparative assessments before every surgery: Do the significance and likelihood of promised benefits justify subjecting the patient to the risks and harms associated with surgery?

The same type of comparative assessment must be made before undertaking any study that involves human subjects. The balance, however, is somewhat different in research because the risks accrue to individual study participants whereas the possible benefits will be advantageous to future patients, a group that may or may not include the research participants.

In this case, cortisone injections into the area of a knee replacement are associated with a high likelihood of sepsis of the knee joint. Because the two alternative pain treatments may be similar in effectiveness, a situation of clinical equipoise apparently exists. Yet, the risk of harm associated with the injection arm is far too high to justify undertaking this study. No patient should be subjected to such a risky experimental intervention when there is a far less risky alternative and where the potentially devastating complication of a prosthetic joint infection far outweighs the benefit of pain relief.

It is easier to justify studies when the potential harms involved are unlikely. For the most part, in clinical research studies, as the risks increase so should the potential benefits to subjects. There may be extreme circumstances, however, in which people have very little to lose by participating. Sometimes people with little to lose may possibly have more to gain by participating in a study, as when imminent death with the intervention is certain, even if the investigational therapy offers only a slim lifesaving possibility. In other circumstances, there may be no possibility of benefit, but the possibility of contributing to knowledge and the brief duration of the investigational procedure could justify enrolling subjects in the study.

Policy makers are especially reluctant to allow research involving "vulnerable" populations, so as to protect them from risks and harms. According to the Office for Human Research Protection policies, and those of IRBs that introduce additional policies inspired by the regulations, vulnerable groups include mentally ill or mentally handicapped people, pregnant women, fetuses, products of in vitro fertilization, children, prisoners, elderly people, people who are in the midst of a medical emergency, and educationally or economically disadvantaged people. Sometimes, classifying individuals as part of a vulnerable group that requires special protections (for example, elderly or educationally or economically disadvantaged people) may be inaccurate. For example, it is disrespectful to presume that an elderly person without a high school diploma cannot make his or her own decisions. In any circumstance other than research, the presumption would be ageist and discriminatory.

Some vulnerable groups include only individuals who lack decisional capacity (for example, young children or profoundly retarded, demented, or unconscious individuals). Individuals in such groups are vulnerable to being treated thoughtlessly and carelessly. Others need to be concerned with their interests and protect them from unreasonable harm. When it comes to research, however, it may be especially important to involve these individuals. In some circumstances, it may be important to learn about their underlying debilitating condition; in other cases, it may be important to learn about how an intervention affects a particular group.

For example, it is accepted that children should be protected from avoidable risks and harms, including those associated with research. Because their bodies are small and still developing, children may be especially susceptible to harm that may have an especially dramatic effect. Although these are all legitimate concerns, the paternalistic protectionist tenor of the current research environment leaves researchers reluctant to undertake studies involving children. Without study, however, the health care of children cannot be improved upon. Studies of adults may not be applicable to children because their bodies are smaller and still developing, their metabolism is different, they are far more active than adults, and their activities are different. Without data to support the treatment of children, every treatment with an unstudied intervention is an experiment with a single subject. Thus, "treatment" with interventions that have not been studied specifically in children exposes each child to risks without providing information that might be useful in the treatment of future patients. It makes no sense to expose every child to the risks of unstudied "treatment" when the alternative of enrolling a few in carefully thought-out studies with vigilant oversight would expose those few to no greater risks than that of the unstudied "treatment." In effect, the current approach protects no children from risks and harms and prevents every child from receiving the benefits of scientific advance.

Human-subject research imposes some risk of harm on subjects. Independent review by a panel of experts and community members assures participants and society that the

Independent Review

Case Scenario:

An orthopaedic surgeon read several studies that indicated that postoperative pain medication use was decreased in patients treated preoperatively with NSAIDs. He asks all of his knee arthroscopy patients to take 200 mg of a well-established cyclooxygenase-2 inhibitor NSAID beginning 2 days prior to surgery. He notices a significant decrease in the amount of postoperative pain medications used by his patients. He wishes to publish his finding in an orthopaedic journal.

study conforms to the highest ethical standards. In the United States, granting agencies, data and safety monitoring boards, and institutional, regional, and private IRBs review and oversee the conduct of human-subject research. Reviewers have the responsibility for approving or withholding approval from proposed studies, amending them, and terminating them when appropriate.

Independent review of proposed studies requires scientists to disclose what will be done, to whom, how, when, where, and why. This disclosure allows reviewers to consider all aspects of a proposed study and to evaluate its merits to reach a decision about whether or not it conforms with ethical standards. Furthermore, although a study may appear very reasonable to a researcher, independent review allows another group of eyes to serve as a check on possible researcher bias. By giving reviewers the responsibility to assess the risk-benefit ratio of a study, independent judgment serves to confirm the reasonableness of the risks and burdens involved in study participation so that unreasonable studies are not undertaken.

Independent review and oversight of the conduct of hazardous studies ensures the trust and trustworthiness of biomedical research by promoting confidence that nothing about the project is being concealed, that informed and reasonable people find that the study design is valid, that the promised results will be valuable, that subjects are fairly selected and treated with respect, and that the risks involved have been minimized and are justified and proportional with the anticipated benefits.

Physicians are legally allowed to treat patients with any approved and available medications and to prescribe or administer medications for off-label uses. If this surgeon takes on the responsibility to improve clinical practice seriously and chooses to undertake a formal study and systematically evaluate the results, IRB approval is required by most institutions and most academic journals. The radical distinction between the totally unregulated status of "innovation" and the highly regulated bureaucratic regulation of "research" certainly seems arbitrary and conceptually incoherent because both activities involve the scientific methods of formulating and testing a hypothesis. Also, the regulatory burdens associated with IRB review of research seem to inhibit research. Nevertheless, these requirements do provide the assurance that the research question has value, that the study is well designed, that subjects are selected fairly, and that the research is conducted according to the highest ethical standards.[17,18]

To enroll any patient in this study, the surgeon will first be required to obtain the patient's informed consent for study participation. Informed consent has become en-

Informed Consent

Case Scenario:

An implant device representative explains a new, highly innovative hip prosthesis to a local orthopaedic surgeon. The device is currently under investigation for Food and Drug Administration approval. Early laboratory data and animal studies look promising. In animal studies and preliminary trials, the new high-density, microporous synthetic coating appears to result in rapid bone ingrowth and component stabilization. The surgeon wishes to participate in the early clinical trials. He signs all of the necessary paperwork to register as a clinical investigator and wants to begin immediately enrolling patients in the study.

sconced as the cornerstone principle of research ethics. According to bioethicists, the concept of autonomy explains the centrality of informed consent in the ethical practice of research.[19,20] Because knowing and understanding the relevant facts is a critical element in autonomous choices, people with the capacity to take responsibility for their actions need to have critical information when they are making important choices. When researchers ask people capable of making their own decisions to participate in a study, they must provide the information that participants will need to make participation decisions that reflect their own values and priorities. In effect, when autonomous individuals are well informed about the goals of a study and the burdens and risks involved in participation and they consent to participation, they take on a responsibility to do what they agree to do, and they can be held responsible for their choice. If they had been inadequately informed, either deliberately or carelessly, or were even deceived about critical details of the study, their agreement to participate would not be autonomous and, ethically, they would not be held responsible for their enrollment decision.

Obtaining informed consent is, therefore, important for the ethical conduct of research because it demonstrates the

researchers' respect for patients' moral capacity. Informed consent also allows participant assessment to serve as a check on the researcher and even on IRB bias by allowing participants to exercise their own judgment as to the reasonableness of the risks and burdens involved in study participation so that unreasonable studies are not undertaken. Informed consent is the principal mechanism for permitting people liberty and ensuring respect for participant autonomy. It also plays an important role in the ethical conduct of human subject research by underscoring other important goals of the research enterprise: maintaining public trust in science and research through honest and transparent practice, ensuring that avoidable harms and burdens are not imposed on participants, and treating others with the respect and dignity that they deserve.

In this case, very little is known about the risks and benefits of the new material. It could be a great boon for patients, it could be no better than the existing implants, or it could be a total short-term or long-term disaster. Although

Respect for Enrolled Subjects

Case Scenario:

An orthopaedic surgeon is approached regarding a new osteoporosis medication. Early trials seem very promising. The surgeon is asked to participate in a large, multicenter clinical trial. She enrolls hundreds of her female patients in the study over a 2-year period. Bone density is significantly increased in almost all patients. One year after the study period ends, several reports begin to surface about diminished renal function in patients who had been taking the investigational medication.

the researcher cannot provide information on the actual risks and benefits of a brand-new, highly experimental device, the researcher could explain what is known thus far and be sure to convey the uncertainty about the proposed intervention. Informed consent requires a sincere effort to accurately communicate what is known about the intervention, the results of previous studies, estimates of the risks and benefits identified as possible consequences, and the likelihood of their occurrence.

People who enroll in biomedical research often accept some burdens and some risks. By enrolling, they also express their willingness to promote the social good of producing biomedical knowledge to be shared with others. Regardless of the participants' actual motives, participation in research should always be seen as a noble choice that expresses concern and sympathy for the plight of others and solidarity with the community of humanity. People who volunteer to serve as research participants should not be seen as merely subjects being used for the purposes of others. Instead, they should be acknowledged as collaborators in important social projects, as courageous citizens who ac-

4: Clinical Science

cept their responsibility to do what they can to further biomedical research. Research participants are entitled to feel proud of doing their part, and that they have earned respect from others for their sacrifice.

Research participants should, obviously, be treated very well. They deserve careful treatment and monitoring during the course of a study to ensure that risks are minimized and that their well-being is maintained. Also, because the burdens of a study may turn out to be more significant than a subject had anticipated, thereby changing the risk-benefit ratio, subjects must be allowed to withdraw from a study without penalty. Additionally, as new information becomes available during the study period, this information should be shared with the study participants. Information regarding the intervention's effectiveness or the subject's condition should be carefully monitored and shared as the study progresses. Beyond that, as Emanuel et al[9] note, information that participants disclose to further the research project should be safeguarded according to standards of medical confidentiality.

Because research participants are collaborators in the research enterprise, they deserve to be informed of study findings so that they can partake in the pleasure of having helped to produce valuable knowledge. Once this study is completed and the data analyzed, the researchers should share their findings with the study participants. This communication expresses respect for what the participants have done to advance medical knowledge and to benefit others.

Later, if evidence of potential harm seems to be associated with the investigational drug, implant device, or other intervention, study participants should be informed of the problem. In addition, corrective treatment should be made available to the participants if so required. Excellent treatment of research subjects throughout the study period, even after the completion of the study, helps to promote and maintain society's trust in the research enterprise.

Summary

Beginning with the guidelines established after World War II for the ethical treatment of human research subjects, and progressing historically through the subsequent codes of behavior, respect for human research subjects remains the central tenet of research ethics. Recently, seven requirements for evaluating the ethical validity of human research studies have been proposed: value, scientific validity, fair subject selection, favorable risk-benefit ratio, independent review, informed consent, and respect for enrolled subjects. It behooves all medical researchers involved in human subject studies to evaluate their research designs in light of these ethical requirements to ensure the safety and respect of their subjects and to affirm that the risks assumed by the study participants are warranted, justified, and appreciated.

References

1. Appelbaum PS, Lidz CW, Meisel A: *Informed Consent: Legal Theory and Clinical Practice*. New York, NY, Oxford University Press, 1987.

2. Penslar RL, ed: *Office for Human Research Protections (OHRP): IRB Guidebook*. Washington, DC, US Department of Health & Human Services, 1987. http://www.hhs.gov/ohrp/archive/irb/irb_guidebook.htm.

3. National Science Foundation: 45 CFR Part 690: Federal Policy for the Protection of Human Subjects. Subpart A: The Common Rule for the Protection of Human Subjects. http://www.nsf.gov/bfa/dias/policy/docs/45cfr690.pdf.

4. Rothman DJ: *Strangers at the Bedside: A History of How Law and Bioethics Transformed Medical Decision Making*. New York, NY, Basic Books, 1991.

5. Rothman DJ: Ethics and human experimentation: Henry Beecher revisited. *N Engl J Med* 1987;317(19):1195-1199.

6. Gruen RL, Arya J, Cosgrove EM, et al: Professionalism in surgery. *J Am Coll Surg* 2003;197(4):605-608.

7. Code of medical ethics and professionalism in orthopaedic surgery, in *Guide to Professionalism and Ethics in the Practice of Orthopaedic Surgery*. Rosemont, IL, American Academy of Orthopaedic Surgeons, 2009, pp 3-7.

8. Rhodes R, Gligorov N, Schwab A, eds: Research ethics, in *The Human Microbiome Research: Ethical, Legal, and Social Concerns*. New York, Oxford University Press, 2013.

9. Emanuel EJ, Wendler D, Grady C: What makes clinical research ethical? *JAMA* 2000;283(20):2701-2711.

10. Moseley JB, O'Malley K, Petersen NJ, et al: A controlled trial of arthroscopic surgery for osteoarthritis of the knee. *N Engl J Med* 2002;347(2):81-88.

11. Fender D, Harper WM, Thompson JR, Gregg PJ: Mortality and fatal pulmonary embolism after primary total hip replacement: Results from a regional hip register. *J Bone Joint Surg Br* 1997;79(6):896-899.

12. Ubel PA, Silbergleit R: Behavioral equipoise: A way to resolve ethical stalemates in clinical research. *Am J Bioeth* 2011;11(2):1-8.

13. Maloney WJ: National joint replacement registries: Has the time come? *J Bone Joint Surg Am* 2001;83(10):1582-1585.

14. Capozzi JD, Rhodes R: Examining the ethical implications of an orthopaedic joint registry. *J Bone Joint Surg Am* 2010;92(5):1330-1333.

15. Rhodes R: Response to de Melo-Martin: "On a Putative Duty to Participate in Biomedical Research." *APA Newsletter on Philosophy and Medicine* 2008;7(2):12-13.

16. Rhodes R: In defense of the duty to participate in biomedical research. *Am J Bioeth* 2008;8(10):37-38.

17. Rhodes R: Rethinking research ethics. *Am J Bioeth* 2005;5(1):7-28.

18. Rhodes R: Response to commentators on "Rethinking Research Ethics." *Am J Bioeth* 2005;5(1):W15-W18.

19. Veatch HB: *Human Rights: Fact or Fancy?* Baton Rouge, LA, Louisiana State University Press, 1985.

20. Faden RR, Beauchamp TL: Decision-making and informed consent: A study of the impact of disclosed information. *Soc Indic Res* 1980;7(1-4):313-336.

Index

A

AAOS. *See* American Academy of Orthopaedic Surgeons
Abatacept, 24
Abduction torques, knee joint, 269–270
ACCP. *See* American College of Chest Physicians
ACI. *See* Autologous chondrocyte implantation
ACL. *See* Anterior cruciate ligament
ACL-deficient knees, 274f, 275. *See also* Knee joint
ACL transection, 301–302
    animal models, 301–303
Acquired neuromuscular disorders
    cerebral palsy, 383–384
    poliomyelitis, 375–376
    spinal cord injury, 380–383
    stroke, 376–377
    traumatic brain injury, 377–380
Action potentials
    of peripheral nerves, 242–244, 242f
    propagation, 243
    skeletal muscle contraction and, 231–232
Acute disseminated encephalomyelitis, 374
Acute hematogenous osteomyelitis, 414
Adalimumab, rheumatoid arthritis, 109
ADAMTS, 192
Adaptive immunity, 21–22
Adult somatic stem cells, 10, 10f. *See also* Stem cells
Adult stem cells, 92–93
    exogenous, articular cartilage repair and, 318–319, 319f
Age/aging
    articular chondrocytes, 188–189
    bone
        changes and, 288–289, 289t, 290f, 291f
        osteoporosis and, 179
    ECM, 193
    ligament functions and, 223
    OA and, 311
    skeletal maturation, 223
Aggrecan, 190–191
Alkaline phosphatase (ALP), 163
Alloys
    Co-Cr, 76
        rod, 70
    general structure of, 73, 74f
    manufacturing, 73–75, 75f
        postmanufacture treatments and, 75
        techniques for, 74–75
    metal alloy rod, 70
    shape memory, 78
    tantalum, 78
    titanium, 76–78
        rod, 70
ALP. *See* Alkaline phosphatase
α2HS-Glycoprotein, 161

ALS. *See* Amyotrophic lateral sclerosis
Alumina, 82
American Academy of Orthopaedic Surgeons (AAOS)
    guideline development, 471, 471t
    outcomes instruments, 469
    study quality evaluation, 473, 475t
American College of Chest Physicians (ACCP), 122
American Society for Testing and Materials (ASTM), 73, 76
American Spinal Injury Association (ASIA)
    Impairment Scale, 381, 381t
    Motor Score, 381, 381t
Ampicillin, periprosthetic joint infection, 416
Amyotrophic lateral sclerosis (ALS), 373–374
aNAC. *See* Nascent polypeptide-associated complex and
        coactivator α
Anakinra, 24
Anesthesia, thrombogenesis during, 121–122
Angiogenesis, cancer and inducing, 393
Animal models
    of ACLT transection, 301–303
    of intra-articular fracture, 299–300, 301f
    of meniscectomy, 301
    OA, 299t
    of tissue engineering, 99–100
Anisotropy, 71
Anterior cruciate ligament (ACL), 262
    injury, 274–276, 275f, 276f
        meniscal tears and, 303
        short-term complications, 275
        studies of, 302
    tears
        meniscal, 303
        OA and, 295–296
Anticoagulants, newer selective, 125–127
Antimicrobial agents
    bioavailability of, orthopaedic infection and, 412–413
    elution characteristics of, orthopaedic infection and, 413
    orthopaedic infection, 412–413
        principles of, 408
Apixaban, 127
Arginine-glycine-aspartic acid (RGD), 202
Argument from beneficence, subject selection and, 517
Argument from justice, subject selection and, 516–517
Articular cartilage
    articular chondrocytes and, 186–189
    biomechanical function, 185–186
    biomechanics
        friction and, 194–195
        load transfer and, 193–194
        lubrication and, 194–195
        tissue wear and, 195
    brief overview of, 309–311
    chondrocytes in, 310

BSP. *See* Bone sialoprotein
BSUs. *See* Bone structural units

C

$(Ca_3[PO_4]_2)$, *See* β–tricalcium phosphate
$(Ca_{10}[PO_4]_6[OH]_2)$. *See* Hydroxyapatite
Calcitonin
  mineral metabolism and, 358
  osteoclast, 168
  osteoporosis, 360
Calcium, daily dietary intake requirements, 357, 357t
Cancellous bone, 150–151
Cancer
  bone formation and, tumor-induced, 397, 398f
  cell death in, 393, 394f
  cytokines and, 393–394
  epigenetics and, 396–397, 397f
  growth factor and, 393–394
  hallmarks of, 391–393, 392f
    activating invasion and metastasis, 392–393
    evading growth suppressors and, 392
    inducing angiogenesis and, 393
    replicative immortality and, 393
    resisting cell death and, 392
    sustaining proliferating signaling and, 391–392
  inflammation and, 394
  mitosis in, 393
  musculoskeletal tumors, 391–404
  oncogenes and, 395–396, 395t
  osteolysis and, tumor-induced, 397, 398f
  retinoblastoma and, 396
  tumor suppressor genes and, 395–396, 395t
CANCERLIT, 448
Carcinogenesis, orthopaedic implants and, 348–349, 348f
Cartilage. *See also* Articular cartilage
  biologic regulator delivery
    clinical state of the art and, 97
    recombinant protein, 95
  biomechanical stimulation, in vitro, 97–98, 98f
  cell technology, 94
  chondrocytes and, 186–188
  collagens, 189
  degeneration, 310–311
  disorders, 48
  ECM
    biochemical composition of, 189–193
    matrix fragmentation, 192–193
    proteins of, 189, 189t, 190f
  failure, 310–311
  scaffold technology, 90–91, 91f
  skeletal dysplasias, 48
  water, 189
Cartilage oligomeric matrix protein (COMP), 47, 191
Cartilaginous tumors, molecular pathophysiology of, 398–399
Case-control study, 427, 429–430

Case report, 427
Case series, 427, 429
Case studies, 429–430
  types, 429
Cathepsin K (CatK), 166
  inhibitors, 168
  osteoporosis, 361
Cauda equina syndrome, 382
CD44, 192
CEA. *See* Cost-effectiveness analysis
C/EBP, 15. *See also* Transcription factors
Cell-based implants grown in laboratory, articular cartilage repair, 317–318
Cell death
  in cancer, 393, 394f
  resisting, 392
Cell-matrix interactions, 20–21
Cell-mediated immune response, 106
Cell technology
  cell delivery
    local, 93–94, 94f
    systemic, 93
  cell sources, 92
  clinical state of the art, 94, 94f
  differentiated cells, 92
  research directions, 95
  stem cells
    adult, 92–93
    embryonic, 93
    fetal, 93
Cell transfer-based therapies, tendon-to-bone repair and, 337
Cellular biology, 3–38
  basic cellular structures and function, 25–31, 26t, 27t
  cytokines, 7–10
    clinically relevant, 3–4, 4f
  DNA and, 31
  functional matrix biology, 20–21
  immunology, 21–24
  ligament, 221–222
  musculoskeletal cell function and, proteins affecting, 4–7
  musculoskeletal developmental biology and, 13–20
  proteins and, 31
  RNA and, 31
  stem cells, 10–13
  tendon, 213–215
Cellular solid fabrication, 88–89, 89f
Cellular structures and function, basic, 26t, 27t
  cytoskeleton and, 31
  endoplasmic reticulum and, 28
  Golgi apparatus and, 28
  lysosome and, 28–30
  mitochondrion and, 30–31
  nucleus and, 25
  RNAs and, 25, 29t
Cement, bone, 79
  PMMA, 78–79, 79f

gait and, 264–271, 267*f*, 267*t*
  kinematics of, 266–269, 268*f*
  kinetics of, 269–270, 269*f*
ground reaction forces, 270, 270*f*
injuries
  ACL, 274–276, 275*f*, 276*f*
  kinematics of, 272–276
  PCL, 276, 276*f*
kinematics, 264
  patellofemoral joint, 271–272, 272*f*, 273*f*
  step-up, 270–271, 271*f*
kinesiology of, 261–276
kinetic chain, 262–263
motions, anatomic planes and, 262, 266*f*
muscles and structures surrounding, 261, 262*f*, 263*t*
PCL injury, 276, 276*f*
stabilizers, 261–262, 264*t*, 265*f*
structure and motion, 261–264
Knee meniscus
  anatomy, 199–200, 200*f*
  attachments, 199, 201*f*
  biochemical content, 200–202, 202*f*
  cells of, 202
  form and function, 199–208
  functional aspects, 202–203, 203*f*
  healing and repair, 207
    future of, 207–208
  injury, 206–207, 206*f*
    OA and, 205–206
  mechanical behavior, 203, 204*f*
  pathology, 205–206
  properties, biomechanical evaluation of, 203–204
    compressive properties, 205
    shear properties, 205
    tensile properties, 204–205
  regional variations, 200, 201*f*
  tears, 206–207, 206*f*
Kneist syndrome, 45
Kugelberg-Welander syndrome, 371
Kyphosis, 139

L

Lateral collateral ligament (LCL), 262
Leflunomide, rheumatoid arthritis, 109
Levodopa, Parkinson disease, 375
Ligament
  biologic regulator delivery
    clinical state of the art and, 97
    recombinant protein, 95–96
    small molecules, 97
  biomechanical stimulation, in vitro, 98
  blood supply, 222
  cell technology, 94
  classification and anatomy, 221
  form and function, 213–226
  functions

anatomic location and, 223
biologic factors influencing, 223
exercise and, 223
experimental factors influencing, 223–224
immobilization and, 223
mechanical, 222, 222*f*
proprioception, 223
sex and, 223
skeletal maturation and aging, 223
viscoelastic, 222–223
grafting, 224–226
  functional tissue engineering and, 225–226, 225*f*
  normal tissues for, 225
gross morphology, histology, microanatomy, and cell
    biology, 221–222, 222*f*
injuries, clinically relevant, 224
innervation, 222
repair
  clinically relevant variables affecting, 224
  healing processes, principles, and deficiencies, 224
  reconstruction *versus*, 224–225
replacement, 224–226
scaffold technology, 91
Limb, 141
  patterning, 139–141, 140*f*
    signaling, 141
  VATER/VACTERL association, 44
Limb-girdle muscular dystrophy, 368–369
  autosomal dominant, 370*t*
  autosomal recessive, 369*t*
Lineage cells
  lymphoid, 104, 104*t*
  myeloid, 103
Literature
  outcome probabilities of decision analysis and, 497–498
  scientific
    common statistical misperceptions and, 489–490
    confidence intervals *versus* P values, 490–491
    critical analysis of, 489–492, 489*t*, 490*t*, 491*t*
    effect size and, 491–492
    sample size and, 491–492
    subgroup analyses and, 491
    type II error and, 491
  search of, systematic reviews in, 447–448, 448*f*
Lmx1b, 140–141
Load-deformation curve, bone, 175, 176*f*
Load-displacement tests, 176
Load transfer, articular cartilage, 193–194
Long bone, 150
  development, 142, 142*f*
Loose metal-on-polyethylene implants, 343–345, 344*f*, 345*f*
Lordosis, 139
Losartan, 236
Low density lipoprotein receptor related protein-5 (LRP-5), 7
Low-molecular-weight heparin, 124, 125
  chemoprophylaxis, 126